Current Urologic Therapy 3

E. JAMES SEIDMON, M.D.
Associate Professor
Department of Urology
Temple University School of Medicine
Philadelphia, Pennsylvania

PHILIP M. HANNO, M.D.
Professor and Chairman
Department of Urology
Temple University School of Medicine
Philadelphia, Pennsylvania

W.B. SAUNDERS COMPANY
A Division of Harcourt Brace & Company

Philadelphia, London, Toronto, Montreal, Sydney, Tokyo

W. B. SAUNDERS COMPANY
A Division of Harcourt Brace & Company

The Curtis Center
Independence Square West
Philadelphia, PA 19106

Library of Congress Cataloging-in-Publication Data

Current urologic therapy / [edited by] E. James Seidmon, Philip M. Hanno. — 3rd ed.
p. cm.
Includes index.
ISBN 0-7216-5033-3
1. Genitourinary organs—Diseases—Treatment. I. Seidmon, E. James. II. Hanno, Philip M.
[DNLM: 1. Genital Diseases, Male—therapy. 2. Urologic Diseases—therapy. WJ 166 C976 1994]
RC871.C86 1994
616.6′06—dc20
DNLM/DLC 94-6845

CURRENT UROLOGIC THERAPY 3 ISBN 0-7216-5033-3

Printed in the United States of America.

Last digit is the print number: 9 8 7 6 5 4 3 2 1

To our wives, Nancy and Linda, and our children,
Eric, Emily, Adam, David and Rebecca,
for their patience and forbearance

CONTRIBUTORS

G. FORBES ABERCROMBIE, M.B., F.R.C.S.
Consultant Urologist, St. Mary's Hospital, Portsmouth, Hampshire, England
Retroperitoneal Fibrosis

DAVID M. ALBALA, M.D.
Assistant Professor of Urology; Head, Section of Endourology, Loyola University Medical Center, Maywood, Illinois
Vesicoureteral Reflux in Adults

GERALD L. ANDRIOLE, M.D.
Associate Professor of Urologic Surgery, Washington University School of Medicine, St. Louis, Missouri
Tumors of the Scrotum

RODNEY A. APPELL, M.D., F.A.C.S.
Head, Section of Female Urology and Urodynamics, Department of Urology, The Cleveland Clinic Foundation, Cleveland, Ohio
Treatment of the Nonfunctioning Urethra in Females; Endoscopic Injection of Teflon, Fat, and Collagen for Female Urinary Incontinence

ANTHONY ATALA, M.D.
Instructor in Surgery, Harvard Medical School; Assistant in Surgery, Division of Urology, Children's Hospital, Boston, Massachusetts
Congenital Megacalyces; Ureteral Diverticulosis

GOPAL H. BADLANI, M.D., F.A.C.S.
Associate Professor of Urology, Albert Einstein College of Medicine; Associate Chairman, Department of Urology, Long Island Jewish Medical Center, New Hyde Park, New York
Balanitis and Balanoposthitis

DEMETRIUS H. BAGLEY, M.D.
Professor of Radiology, Jefferson Medical College, Thomas Jefferson University, Philadelphia, Pennsylvania
Ureteroscopic Treatment of Distal Ureteral Calculi

THOMAS P. BALL, JR., M.D.
Professor of Urology, University of Texas Health Science Center, San Antonio, Texas
Epididymitis and Orchitis

MARC P. BANNER, M.D.
Professor of Radiology and Urology, University of Pennsylvania School of Medicine; Director of Uroradiology, University of Pennsylvania Medical Center, Philadelphia, Pennsylvania
Renal Pyelocalyceal Diverticula

CHRISTINE P. BASTL, M.D.
Professor of Medicine, Temple University Health Sciences Center; Chief of Nephrology, Temple University Hospital, Philadelphia, Pennsylvania
Acute Renal Failure; Chronic Renal Failure; Hepatorenal Syndrome

STUART B. BAUER, M.D.
Associate Professor of Surgery; Harvard Medical School; Senior Associate in Surgery (Urology), Children's Hospital, Boston, Massachusetts
Sacral Agenesis

JOHN A. BELIS, M.D.
Professor of Urology, The Milton S. Hershey Medical Center, The Pennsylvania State University, Hershey, Pennsylvania
Surgery of the Ureteral Stump

ARIE S. BELLDEGRUN, M.D.
Associate Professor of Surgery/Urology, UCLA School of Medicine, Los Angeles, California
Renal Cell Carcinoma

MITCHELL C. BENSON, M.D.
Associate Professor of Urology, Department of Urology; Director, Oncology Department, Columbia-Presbyterian Medical Center, New York, New York
M-VAC Therapy for Transitional Cell Cancer of the Bladder

RALPH C. BENSON, JR., M.D.
Co-Director, The Center for Urological Treatment and Research, Nashville, Tennessee
Leukoplakia of the Urinary Tract; Photoradiation for Superficial Bladder Tumors and Carcinoma In Situ

WILLIAM BIHRLE, III, M.D.
Senior Consultant, Urology, Lahey Clinic Medical Center, Burlington, Massachusetts
Foreign Bodies in the Urinary Bladder and Urethra

JERRY G. BLAIVAS, M.D.
Clinical Professor of Urology, Cornell University Medical School, New York, New York
Diabetes, Multiple Sclerosis, and Parkinson's Disease

NORMAN L. BLOCK, M.D., F.A.C.S.
L. Austin Weeks Professor of Urologic Research, Professor of Urology, Oncology, Biomedical Engineering, University of Miami, Miami, Florida
Renal Pelvic Tumors

GERALD B. BROCK, M.D., F.R.C.S.C.
Assistant Professor, Department of Urology, McGill University, Montreal, Quebec, Canada
Priapism

STANLEY A. BROSMAN, M.D.
Santa Monica Urologic Medical Group, Santa Monica, California
Adrenal Hemorrhage; Blunt and Penetrating Bladder Trauma

ANTHONY A. CALDAMONE, M.D.
Professor of Surgery (Urology), Brown University School of Medicine, Director of Pediatric Urology, Hasbro Children's Hospital, Rhode Island Hospital, Providence, Rhode Island
Megalourethra

DOUGLAS A. CANNING, M.D.
Assistant Professor of Urology in Surgery, University of Pennsylvania School of Medicine, Philadelphia, Pennsylvania
Renal Cell Carcinoma in Children

JOSEPH C. CERNY, M.D.
Clinical Professor of Urology, University of Michigan Medical School; Chairman, Department of Urology, Henry Ford Hospital, Detroit, Michigan
Urethral Diverticula

MARK J. CHELSKY, M.D.
Instructor in Urology, Temple University School of Medicine, Philadelphia, Pennsylvania
Management of Fournier's Gangrene

MICHAEL COBURN, M.D.
Assistant Professor, Department of Urology, Baylor College of Medicine; Chief of Urology, Ben Taub General Hospital, Houston, Texas
Renal and Perinephric Abscess; Blunt Renal Trauma

ARNOLD H. COLODNY, M.D.
Clinical Professor of Surgery, Harvard Medical School; Senior Surgeon and Associate Director, Division of Urology, Children's Hospital, Boston, Massachusetts
Ectopic Ureteroceles

ROY J. CORREA, JR., M.D.
Clinical Professor of Urology, Virginia Mason Medical Center, University of Washington, Seattle, Washington
Other Conditions of the Adrenal Gland

JOSEPH N. CORRIERE, JR., M.D.
Professor of Surgery, The University of Texas Medical School at Houston, Houston, Texas
Bladder Injuries with Pelvic Fracture

SAKTI DAS, M.D.
Associate Clinical Professor of Urology, University of California School of Medicine, Davis, California; Chief of Urology, Kaiser Permanente Medical Center, Walnut Creek, California
Renal Venous Thrombosis; Male Genital Lymphedema; Fracture of the Penis

DANIEL T. DEMPSEY, M.D.
Associate Professor of Surgery, Temple University Hospital, Philadelphia, Pennsylvania
Retroperitoneal Sarcoma

DAVID A. DIAMOND, M.D.
Associate Professor of Urology and Pediatrics, University of Massachusetts Medical Center, Worcester, Massachusetts
Urologic Intervention for Fetal Hydronephrosis

ANANIAS C. DIOKNO, M.D.
Clinical Professor, Section of Urology, Department of Surgery, University of Michigan, Ann Arbor, Michigan; Chief of Urology, William Beaumont Hospital, Royal Oak, Michigan
Clean Intermittent Catheterization in Children and Adults

JOHN P. DONOHUE, M.D.
Professor and Chairman of Urology, Indiana University Hospital, Indianapolis, Indiana
Cushing Syndrome and Cushing Disease

STEPHEN P. DRETLER, M.D.
Director, M.G.H. Kidney Stone Center, Massachusetts General Hospital, Boston, Massachusetts
Percutaneous Dissolution of Urinary Calculi

JOHN W. DUCKETT, JR., M.D.
Professor of Urology (in Surgery), The University of Pennsylvania, School of Medicine; Director, Division of Urology, Children's Hospital of Philadelphia, Philadelphia, Pennsylvania
Modern Hypospadias

RICHARD M. EHRLICH, M.D., F.A.C.S., F.A.A.P.
Clinical Professor of Surgery-Urology, UCLA Medical School, Los Angeles, California
Current Treatment for Wilms' Tumor

T. ERNESTO FIGUEROA, M.D.
Assistant Professor, Section of Pediatric Urology, Departments of Surgery (Urology) and Pediatrics, University of South Florida School of Medicine, Tampa, Florida
Congenital Adrenal Hyperplasia; Congenital Ureteral Abnormalities; Prune-Belly Syndrome

HUGH A.G. FISHER, M.D.
Associate Professor of Surgery; Head, Urologic Oncology, Albany Medical College, Albany, New York
Malacoplakia of the Ureter and Kidney; Malacoplakia of the Bladder

IRVING J. FISHMAN, M.D., F.R.C.S. (C), F.A.C.S.
Associate Professor of Urology, Scott Department of Urology, Baylor College of Medicine; Associate Chief of Urology, St. Luke's Episcopal Hospital, Houston, Texas
Female Incontinence and the Artificial Urinary Sphincter

STUART M. FLECHNER, M.D., F.A.C.S.
Associate Professor of Surgery/Urology, Department of Surgery, Stanford University School of Medicine, Stanford, California; Department of Urology, Cleveland Clinic Hospital, Cleveland Clinic Foundation, Cleveland, Ohio
Cyclosporine in Renal Transplantation; Renal Allograft Rejection

ISRAEL FRANCO, M.D., F.A.A.P.
Assistant Professor of Urology, New York Medical College; Instructor of Urology, Albert Einstein College of Medicine, Bronx, New York
Myelomeningocele

JOHN A. FREEMAN, M.D.
Urologic Oncology Fellow, Clinical Professor of Urology, University of Southern California, Los Angeles, California
Invasive Bladder Cancer

KEVIN K. GANDHI, M.D.
Fellow, Children's Memorial Hospital, Chicago, Illinois
Congenital Sponge Kidney

KENNETH I. GLASSBERG, M.D.
Director, Division of Pediatric Urology, Professor of Urology, State University of New York at Brooklyn, Brooklyn, New York
Multicystic Kidney

MARC GOLDSTEIN, M.D.
Professor of Urology, Cornell University Medical College; Staff Scientist, Center for Biomedical Research, The Population Council, New York, New York
Microsurgical Vasovasostomy and Vasoepididymostomy

LEONARD G. GOMELLA, M.D.
Assistant Professor, Jefferson Medical College, Thomas Jefferson University, Philadelphia, Pennsylvania
Benign Testicular Masses; Paratesticular Tumors and Masses

EDMOND T. GONZALES, JR., M.D.
Professor of Urology, Scott Department of Urology, Baylor College of Medicine; Head, Department of Surgery and Chief, Urology Service, Texas Children's Hospital, Houston, Texas
Renal Trauma in Children; The Subcoronal Meatus

JAMES GORDON GOW, M.D. Ch.M., F.R.C.S.
Lourdes Private Hospital, Liverpool, England
Genitourinary Tuberculosis

JOHN G. GREGORY, M.D., F.A.C.S.
Metropolitan Urological Services, Inc., St. Louis Institute of Male Medicine, St. Louis, Missouri
Urinary Tract Calcium Oxalate Stone Disease Following Bowel Resection

GABRIEL P. HAAS, M.D.
Assistant Professor and Chief, Section of Urologic Oncology, Wayne State University School of Medicine, Detroit, Michigan
Cytoxan Cystitis; Adenocarcinoma of the Bladder; Sertoli Cell Tumors of the Testis

MONEER K. HANNA, M.D.
Clinical Professor of Urology, New York University, New York; Clinical Professor of Surgery, University of Medicine and Dentistry of New Jersey, Camden, New Jersey
Bladder Exstrophy

PHILIP M. HANNO, M.D.
Professor and Chairman, Department of Urology, Temple University School of Medicine, Philadelphia, Pennsylvania
Interstitial Cystitis; Carcinoma of the Prostate—Stage C

MICHAEL HEIFETS, M.D.
Associate Professor of Medicine, Temple University School of Medicine, Philadelphia, Pennsylvania
Renal Involvement by Diabetes Mellitus; Analgesic Nephropathy; Renal Transplantation and its Failure; Progressive Systemic Sclerosis (Scleroderma)

W. HARDY HENDREN, M.D., F.A.C.S., F.A.C.P., F.R.C.S. (I) HON.

Robert E. Gross Professor of Surgery, Harvard Medical School; Chief of Surgery, Children's Hospital, Boston, Massachusetts

Urethral Valves

TERRY W. HENSLE, M.D.

Professor of Urology, Columbia University College of Physicians and Surgeons; Director, Pediatric Urology, Babies Hospital, Columbia Presbyterian Medical Center, New York, New York

Hyperalimentation in Urology

ERNEST E. HODGE, M.D., F.A.C.S.

Head, Section of Renal Transplantation, Cleveland Clinic Foundation, Cleveland, Ohio

Effect of Deliberate Third-Party Transfusion in Nonidentical Living-Related Donor Renal Allograft Survival

MARK HOROWITZ, M.D.

Fellow, Pediatric Urology, University of Washington; Children's Hospital and Medical Center, Seattle, Washington

Experience with Transurethral Incision of Ureterocele in Children; Urethral Fistula

ROBERT P. HUBEN, M.D.

Chief of Urologic Oncology, Roswell Park Cancer Institute; Associate Professor of Urology, State University of New York at Buffalo, Buffalo, New York

Medical Therapy for Metastatic Renal Cell Carcinoma

MARK V. JAROWENKO, M.D.

Associate Professor of Surgery, Division of Urology, The Pennsylvania State University, The Milton S. Hershey Medical Center, Hershey, Pennsylvania

Acute Pyelonephritis; Lymphocele Following Renal Transplantation

ROBERT D. JEFFS, M.D.

Professor of Pediatric Urology, The Johns Hopkins University, Baltimore, Maryland

Epispadias Repair in Males with Classic Bladder Exstrophy

ALAN D. JENKINS, M.D.

Associate Professor of Urology, University of Virginia School of Medicine, Charlottesville, Virginia

Renal Tubular Acidosis

KATHERINE F. JETER, EdD, ET

Clinical Assistant Professor in Urology, Medical University of South Carolina (Spartanburg); Adjunct Professor of Nursing, Mary Black Schook School of Nursing, University of South Carolina, Spartanburg, South Carolina

Care of Patients Following Urinary Diversion

GEORGE W. KAPLAN, M.D., F.A.A.P., F.A.C.S.

Clinical Professor of Surgery and Pediatrics, University of California at San Diego School of Medicine, San Diego, California

Enuresis

LESTER J. KARAFIN, M.D.

Professor of Surgery, Chief, Division of Urology, Medical College of Pennsylvania, Philadelphia, Pennsylvania

Chyluria

YOUNG C. KAUH, M.D.

Clinical Professor, Vice Chairman and Clinical Director, Department of Dermatology, Thomas Jefferson University Hospital, Philadelphia, Pennsylvania

Skin Lesions of the External Genitalia; Herpes Genitalis

LOUIS R. KAVOUSSI, M.D.

Associate Professor of Urology, The Johns Hopkins School of Medicine; Chief of Urology, Hopkins Bayview Hospital, Baltimore, Maryland

Advances in Ureteral Surgery

MICHAEL A. KEATING, M.D.

Assistant Professor of Urology, Indiana University School of Medicine; Attending Pediatric Urologist, James Whitcomb Riley Hospital for Children and Affiliated Hospitals of the Indiana University Medical Center, Indianapolis, Indiana

Surgical Management of Megaureter

KALISH R. KEDIA, M.D.

Chief, Division of Urology, Lutheran Medical Center, Cleveland, Ohio

Testicular Malignancy After Orchiopexy

ELLIE KELEPOURIS, M.D.

Associate Professor of Medicine, Temple University Medical School, Philadelphia, Pennsylvania

Alport Syndrome; Systemic Lupus Erythematosus Nephritis

A. RICHARD KENDALL, M.D.

Professor of Urology, Temple University Medical School, Philadelphia, Pennsylvania

Papillary Necrosis; Treatment of Benign Prostatic Hyperplasia

WILLIAM A. KENNEDY II, M.D.

National Kidney Foundation Research Fellow, Department of Urology, Columbia University College of Physicians and Surgeons, New York, New York

Wegener's Granulomatosis

ERIC A. KLEIN, M.D.
Head, Section of Urologic Oncology, Department of Urology, Cleveland Clinic Foundation, Cleveland, Ohio
Urethral Carcinoma

MARTIN A. KOYLE, M.D., F.A.A.P., F.A.C.S.
Associate Professor of Surgery/Urology, University of Colorado School of Medicine; Chief, Section of Pediatric Urology, The Childrens Hospital, Denver, Colorado
Feminizing Adrenal Tumors in Children

EVAN BARRY KRISCH, M.D.
Assistant Professor of Surgery, Robert Wood Johnson Medical School at Camden, Camden, New Jersey
Nonspecific Urethritis; Treatment of Gonorrhea and Chylamydia Infections

R. LAWRENCE KROOVAND, M.D.
Professor of Surgery (Pediatric Urology) and Pediatrics; Head, Section of Pediatric, Adolescent, and Reconstructive Surgery, The Bowman Gray School of Medicine of Wake Forest University, Winston-Salem, North Carolina
Imperforate Anus, Persistent Cloaca, and Urogenital Sinus Outlet Obstruction

DONALD L. LAMM, M.D.
Professor and Chairman, Department of Urology, West Virginia Hospital, Morgantown, West Virginia
Bacille Calmette-Guerin Intravesical Therapy for Superficial Bladder Tumors and Carcinoma In Situ

BETTE LAZZARO, M.D.
Assistant Professor of Pathology, Temple University School of Medicine, Philadelphia, Pennsylvania
Sarcomas of the Prostate

JOHN A. LIBERTINO, M.D.
Assistant Clinical Professor of Surgery, Harvard Medical School; Chief of Surgery and Chairman of Urology Department, Lahey Clinic Medical Center, Burlington, Massachusetts
Percutaneous Transluminal Angioplasty and Renovascular Hypertension; Surgery for Renovascular Hypertension; Percutaneous Transluminal Angioplasty for Treatment of Renal Transplant Artery Stenosis

MICHAEL M. LIEBER, M.D.
Professor of Urology, Mayo Medical School, Rochester, Minnesota
Renal Oncocytoma

J. KEITH LIGHT, M.D.
Professor and Chairman, Department of Urology, SUNY Health Science Center, Syracuse, New York
Treatment of Urinary Incontinence in the Male; Salvage of the Infected Inflatable Penile Prosthesis

MARGUERITE C. LIPPERT, M.D.
Associate Professor of Urology, University of Virginia College of Medicine, Charlottesville, Virginia
Autosomal Dominant Polycystic Kidney Disease

TOM F. LUE, M.D.
Professor of Urology, University of California, San Francisco, San Francisco, California
Work-up of the Impotent Male and Selection of Therapy

S. BRUCE MALKOWICZ, M.D.
Assistant Professor of Urology, University of Pennsylvania; Co-Director of Urologic Oncology, Hospital of the University of Pennsylvania, Division of Urology, Philadelphia, Pennsylvania
Interstitial Cell Tumors of the Testis; Leydig Cell Tumors of the Testis

TERRENCE R. MALLOY, M.D.
Professor of Urology, University of Pennsylvania; Chief, Section of Urology, Hospital of the University of Pennsylvania, Philadelphia, Pennsylvania
Penile Prosthesis in the Treatment of Erectile Impotence

JOEL L. MARMAR, M.D.
Professor of Clinical Urology, Robert Wood Johnson Medical School at Camden; Head, Division of Urology, Cooper Hospital/University Medical Center, Camden, New Jersey
Male Subfertility; Techniques of Andrology

FRAY F. MARSHALL, M.D.
Professor of Urology, Director, Division of Adult Urology, The Johns Hopkins University, Baltimore, Maryland
Embolization of the Kidney

JACK W. McANINCH, M.D.
Professor of Urology, University of California, San Francisco; Chief of Urology, San Francisco General Hospital, San Francisco, California
Scrotal Trauma, Including Avulsion and Lacerations

BRETT C. MELLINGER, M.D.
Assistant Professor of Urology, Albert Einstein College of Medicine, Bronx, New York; Attending Surgeon, Department of Urology, Long Island Jewish Medical Center, New Hyde Park, New York
Echinococcal Disease of the Kidney

ROBERT M. MOLDWIN, M.D.
Assistant Professor of Urology, Albert Einstein College of Medicine at Long Island Jewish Medical Center, New Hyde Park, New York
Trichomonal Infections in Men

MICHAEL MORRIS, M.D., F.A.C.S.
Associate Professor of Surgery, Temple University School of Medicine; Director, Section of Transplantation, Albert Einstein Medical Center, Philadelphia, Pennsylvania
Transplantation Techniques and Pitfalls

HARRIS M. NAGLER, M.D., F.A.C.S.
Professor of Urology, Mount Sinai School of Medicine, New York, New York
A Clinical Approach to Testicular Torsion

ANDREW C. NOVICK, M.D.
Chairman, Department of Urology, The Cleveland Clinic Foundation, Cleveland, Ohio
Primary Aldosteronism; Donor-Specific Blood Transfusion in Living-Related Renal Transplantation

DONALD E. NOVICKI, M.D.
Associate Professor of Surgery, University of Texas Health Science Center at San Antonio, San Antonio, Texas; Associate Professor of Surgery, Mayo Medical School, Scottsdale, Arizona
Nephrogenic Adenoma

JOSEPH E. OESTERLING, M.D.
Associate Professor of Urology, Mayo Medical School; Consultant, Department of Urolology, Mayo Clinic and Mayo Foundation, Rochester, Minnesota; Editor-in-Chief, Urology
Adenocarcinoma of the Prostate—Clinical Stages B_0, B_1, and B_2 (T1c, T2a & b and T2c)

CHRISTOPHER K. PAYNE, M.D.
Acting Assistant Professor and Director, Center for Neurosurgery, Stanford University, Stanford, California
Stress Urinary Incontinence in Females

LESTER PERSKY, M.D.
Emeritus Professor of Urology, Case Western Reserve University; Professor of Urology, University of South Florida, Tampa, Florida
Ureteral Injuries

ROBERT O. PETERSEN, M.D., Ph.D.
Professor of Pathology, Department of Pathology and Cell Biology, Thomas Jefferson University College of Medicine, Philadelphia, Pennsylvania
Schistosomiasis of the Urinary Bladder and Ureters

WILLIAM C. PIERCE, M.D., Ph.D.
Fellow, Hematology/Oncology, UCLA School of Medicine, Los Angeles, California
Management of Genitourinary Sarcomas in Adults

MICHEL A. PONTARI, M.D.
Assistant Professor of Urology, Department of Urology, Temple University School of Medicine, Philadelphia, Pennsylvania
Perinephric Abscess; Penetrating Renal Trauma and Its Treatment; Urinary Extravasation; Crohn's Disease and the Urinary Tract; Phimosis and Paraphimosis

J. EDSON PONTES, M.D.
Professor and Chairman, Department of Urology, Wayne State University, Detroit, Michigan
Adjuvant Treatment of Metastatic Renal Cell Carcinoma; Nonseminomatous Testicular Tumors

GLENN M. PREMINGER, M.D.
Professor of Urologic Surgery, Duke University Medical Center, Durham, North Carolina
Shock-wave Lithotripsy for the Treatment of Renal Calculi

HYMAN H. RABINOVITCH, M.D.
Professor of Surgery (Urology), Temple University School of Medicine, Philadelphia, Pennsylvania
Vesicoureteral Reflux in Children; Urethral Meatal Stenosis

PAUL D. RADECKI, M.D.
Department of Radiology, Magnetic Resonance Imaging Section Fellow, Thomas Jefferson University Medical School and Hospital, Philadelphia, Pennsylvania
Emphysematous Pyelonephritis

JACOB RAJFER, M.D.
Professor of Surgery/Urology, UCLA School of Medicine; Chief of Urology, Harbor-UCLA Medical Center; Head, Section of Male Sexual Dysfunction, Center for the Health Sciences, UCLA, Los Angeles, California
Reduction Clitoroplasty; Cryptorchidism

SHLOMO RAZ, M.D.
Professor of Urology, UCLA School of Medicine, Center for Health Sciences, Los Angeles, California
Treatment of Nonradiated Vesicovaginal Fistula

EDWARD F. REDA, M.D., F.A.A.P.
Assistant Professor of Urology, New York Medical College; Associate Director of Pediatric Urology, Westchester County Medical Center, Valhalla, New York
Hematuria in Childhood

JOHN F. REDMAN, M.D.

Professor and Chairman, Department of Urology, University of Arkansas College of Medicine; Chief, Section of Urology, University Hospital, University of Arkansas Medical Sciences Campus; Chief, Section of Pediatric Urology, Arkansas Children's Hospital, Little Rock, Arkansas

Circumcision

MARTIN I. RESNICK, M.D.

Lester Persky Professor of Urology; Chairman, Department of Urology, Case Western Reserve University School of Medicine, Cleveland, Ohio

Cystine Stones

ALAN B. RETIK, M.D.

Professor of Surgery (Urolology), Harvard Medical School; Chief, Division of Urology, Children's Hospital, Boston, Massachusetts

Neuroblastoma; Congenital Mesoblastic Nephroma; Congenital Megaureter in Children; Congenital Bladder Diverticula; Urachal Anomalies

LOUIS J. RILEY, JR., M.D.

Associate Professor of Medicine, Temple University Medical School; Associate Chief, Renal Section, Director, Clinical Nephrology, Temple University Hospital, Philadelphia, Pennsylvania

Hypokalemic Nephropathy; Interstitial Nephritis; Bartter Syndrome

RICHARD C. RINK, M.D.

Associate Professor, Urology, Indiana University School of Medicine; Chief, Pediatric Urology, James Whitcomb Riley Hospital for Children, Indiana University Medical Center, Indianapolis, Indiana

Ureteroceles

GILBERT ROSS, JR., M.D.

Professor and Chief, University of Missouri-Columbia Division of Urology; Chief, Division of Urology, University of Missouri-Columbia Hospital and Clinics, Columbia, Missouri

Ureterovaginal Fistula

ARTHUR I. SAGALOWSKY, M.D.

Professor of Urology, The University of Texas Southwestern Medical Center, Dallas, Texas

Athletic Hematuria

GRANNUM R. SANT, M.D.

Professor and Vice Chairman, Department of Urology, Tufts University School of Medicine; Associate Urologist-in-Chief, New England Medical Center Hospitals, Boston, Massachusetts

Pyelonephritis; Prostatic Calculi

ANTHONY J. SCHAEFFER, M.D.

Professor and Chairman, Department of Urology, Northwestern University Medical School, Chicago, Illinois

Bacteriuria: Prevention and Treatment

PAUL F. SCHELLHAMMER, M.D.

Professor and Chairman, Department of Urology, Eastern Virginia Medical School; Medical Director, The Sentara Cancer Institute, Sentara Norfolk General Hospital, Norfolk, Virginia

Carcinoma of the Penis

STEVEN M. SCHLOSSBERG, M.D.

Associate Professor of Urology and Anatomy, Eastern Virginia Medical School; Director, Fellowship for Adult and Pediatric Urology, Eastern Virginia Graduate School of Medicine; Chief, Department of Urology, Sentara Hospital, Norfolk, Virginia

Injury of the Anterior Urethra; Medical and Surgical Treatment of Peyronie's Disease

SANDRA F. SCHNALL, M.D.

Associate Professor of Medicine, Division of Medical Oncology/Hematology, Temple University School of Medicine, Philadelphia, Pennsylvania

Retroperitoneal Lymphomas

GERRI A. SCHULMAN, M.D.

Associate Professor of Medicine, Temple University School of Medicine; Attending Physician, Internal Medicine and Nephrology, Temple University Hospital, Philadelphia, Pennsylvania

Amyloidosis; Fanconi Syndrome; Polyarteritis Nodosa

MICHAEL J. SCHUTZ, M.D.

Assistant Professor of Urology, Department of Urology, University of Arkansas School of Medicine, Little Rock, Arkansas

Peripelvic Renal Cysts Xanthogranulomatous Pyelonephritis

JOSEPH W. SEGURA, M.D.

Carl Rosen Professor of Urology, Mayo Medical School, Rochester, Minnesota

Renal Colic; Cacium Phosphate Urolithiasis

E. JAMES SEIDMON, M.D.

Associate Professor of Urology, Temple University School of Medicine; Attending Physician, Temple University Hospital, Medical College Hospitals, St. Christopher's for Children; Consultant, Shriner's Hospital for Crippled Children, Philadelphia, Pennsylvania

Idiopathic Renal Hematuria Percutaneous Nephrostolithotomy and the Application of Ultrasonic Lithotripsy and Electrohydraulic Lithotripsy; Percutaneous Cryosurgery of the Prostate Using Transrectal Ultrasound Guidance; Seminoma

LINDA M. DAIRIKI SHORTLIFFE, M.D.

Professor of Urology, Stanford University School of Medicine; Chief of Pediatric Urology; Lucile Salter Packard Children's Hospital at Stanford and Stanford University Medical Center, Stanford California

Inflammatory Renal Processes in Children; Prostatitis

CRAIG L. SILVERMAN, M.D.

Associate Professor of Radiation Oncology, Temple University School of Medicine; Consultant, St. Christopher's Hospital for Children; Attending Physician, Albert Einstein Medical Center, Philadelphia, Pennsylvania

Radiation Nephritis; Definitive Radiotherapy in the Treatment of Invasive Traditional Cell Carcinoma of the Bladder; Radiation Therapy After Radical Prostatectomy

RANDALL P. SINGLETON, M.D., F.A.C.S.

Associate Clinical Professor of Urology, University of Texas, San Antonio, Texas

Simple Renal Cysts

ARTHUR D. SMITH, M.D.

Professor and Chairman, Department of Urology, Long Island Jewish Medical Center, The Long Island Campus for the Albert Einstein College of Medicine; Chairman, Department of Urology, Long Island Jewish Medical Center, New Hyde Park, New York

Surgical Treatment of Hydronephrosis Secondary to Ureteropelvic Junction Obstruction; Clinical Application of Percutaneous Nephrostomy

JOSEPH A. SMITH, JR., M.D.

William L. Bray Professor and Chairman, Department of Urology, Vanderbilt University Medical Center, Nashville, Tennessee

Laser Treatment of Bladder Cancer; Carcinoma of the Prostate—Stage A_1 and A_2

ROBERT B. SMITH, M.D.

Professor of Surgery/Urology, UCLA School of Medicine; Chief of Staff, UCLA Medical Center; Chief of Urology, Wadsworth Veterans Administration Hospital, Los Angeles, California

Bilateral Renal Cell Carcinoma and Renal Cell Carcinoma in the Solitary Kidney

PRAMOD C. SOGANI, M.D.

Associate Professor of Surgery, Cornell University Medical Center; Associate Attending Surgeon, Memorial Sloan-Kettering Cancer Center, New York, New York

Treatment of Superficial Bladder Tumors

R. ERNEST SOSA, M.D.

Associate Professor of Surgery and Urology, The New York Hospital, Cornell Medical Center; Director of Brady Stone Center and Director of Urologic Endoscopy, New York, New York

Ureteral Tumors

J. PATRICK SPIRNAK, M.D., F.A.C.S.

Associate Professor, Department of Urology, Case Western Reserve University; Director of Urology, Metrohealth Medical Center, Cleveland, Ohio

Calcium Oxalate Stones of the Kidney; Uric Acid Calculi

ROBERT E. STECKLER, M.D.

Instructor in Surgery/Pediatric Urology, UMDNJ/Robert Wood Johnson Medical School at Camden, Camden, New Jersey

Treatment of Genitourinary Rhabdomyosarcoma in Children

BARRY S. STEIN, M.D.

Professor and Chairman, Division of Urology, Brown University; Surgeon-in-Chief, Department of Urology, Rhode Island Hospital, Providence, Rhode Island

Carcinoma of the Prostate—Stage D

NELSON N. STONE, M.D.

Associate Professor of Urology, Mount Sinai School of Medicine; Director of Urology Department, Elmhurst Hospital Center, Elmhurst, New York

Bladder Calculi; Varicocele

STEVAN B. STREEM, M.D.

Head, Section of Stone Disease and Endourology, Department of Urology, Cleveland Clinic Foundation, Cleveland, Ohio

Treatment of Urinary Fistulas after Kidney Transplantation

GERALD SUFRIN, M.D.

Professor and Chairman, Department of Urology, School of Medicine and Biomedical Sciences, State University of New York at Buffalo; Director of Urology, Buffalo General Hospital, Erie County Medical Center, Millard Fillmore Hospitals, Buffalo, New York

Endometrial Carcinoma of the Prostate; Transitional Cell Carcinoma of the Prostate

ROBERT M. SWENSON, M.D.

Professor of Medicine and Microbiology, Section of Infectious Diseases, Temple University Health Sciences Center, Philadelphia, Pennsylvania

The Acquired Immunodeficiency Syndrome

RODNEY J. TAYLOR, M.D.
Chairman, Division of Urologic Surgery, University of Nebraska Medical Center, Omaha, Nebraska
Treatment of Renal Angiomyolipoma

KEITH N. VAN ARSDALEN, M.D.
Associate Professor of Urology, University of Pennsylvania School of Medicine; Chief, Urology, Philadelphia Veteran's Administration Medical Center, Philadelphia, Pennsylvania
Infectious Calculi

E. DARRACOTT VAUGHAN, JR., M.D.
James J. Colt Professor of Urology, Cornell University Medical College; Urologist-in-Chief, The New York Hospital, New York, New York
Pheochromocytoma; Primary Reninoma of the Kidney

ZEV WAJSMAN, M.D., F.A.C.S., F.R.C.S. (C)
Professor of Surgery, University of Florida; Chief, Urologic Oncology, Division of Urology, Shands Teaching Hospital, Gainesville, Florida
Squamous Cell Carcinoma of the Urinary Bladder

JOHN W. WEIGEL, M.D.
Professor of Surgery-Urology, University of Kansas Medical Center, Kansas City, Kansas
Management of Trauma of the External Genitalia and Urethra

ALAN J. WEIN, M.D.
Professor and Chairman, Division of Urology, University of Pennsylvania School of Medicine; Chief of Urology, Hospital of the University of Pennsylvania, Philadelphia, Pennsylvania
Diagnostic Evaluation of Neuromuscular Disorders of the Bladder; Drug Therapy for Neurogenic and Non-Neurogenic Bladder Dysfunction

GILBERT J. WISE, M.D.
Clinical Professor, Department of Urology, Health Science Center, State University of New York; Director of Urology, Maimonides Medical Center, Brooklyn, New York
Treatment of Fungal Diseases of the Kidney, Urether, and Bladder

AUGUST ZABBO, M.D.
Assistant Professor, Brown University; Chief, Section of Urology, Providence VA Medical Center, Providence, Rhode Island
Condylomata Acuminata

MARK R. ZAONTZ, M.D., F.A.C.S., F.A.A.P.
Associate Professor of Urology, University of Medicine and Dentistry of New Jersey/Robert Wood Johnson Medical School at Camden; Head, Section of Pediatric Urology, Cooper Hospital/University Medical Center, Camden, New Jersey
Renal Hypoplasia and Dysplasia Congenital Microphallus

STEPHEN A. ZDERIC, M.D.
Assistant Professor of Urology, University of Pennsylvania School of Medicine; Attending Surgeon, Children's Hospital of Philadelphia, Philadelphia, Pennsylvania
Chancroid; Granuloma Inguinale (Donovanosis); Lymphogranuloma Venereum; Hydrocele and Spermatocele

PREFACE

This is the third issue of *Current Urologic Therapy*, a text which first appeared in 1980. Dr. J.J. Kaufman guided the first two issues with great expertise and common sense. We are grateful that he approached us with the honor of updating what has been an extremely valuable resource for the practicing urologist, and all physicians involved in the care of urologic diseases.

It has now been eight years since this text last appeared, and the management of many disorders has changed dramatically. However, the philosophy of the book remains faithful to what Dr. Kaufman wrote in his preface to the first two issues. Authors were selected who had written or spoken of a particular facet of urology and were asked to describe their current ideas with regard to management of the disorder in a "concise, even casual, fashion." Hopefully, it will still be perceived as a "How I do it" or "How I think about it" volume. For this reason we asked each contributor to author his contribution alone so it would more fully represent his individual ideas rather than a consensus. Where overlap of material is present, it is not altogether unintentional, as some topics warrant multiple opinions. References have been added to allow for further reading and pictures, graphic illustrations, and tables appear where they might help illustrate and justify treatment approaches.

We are indebted to our contributors. We also wish to thank Clarissa Graham Crawford for her secretarial and organizational skills. The editorial assistance and encouragement of Richard Zorab and Sandra Valkhoff from W.B. Saunders were invaluable.

The book is dedicated to all those readers who will hopefully find it a useful, readily available treatment reference, and helpful in their daily practice of medicine.

E. James Seidmon, M.D.
Philip M. Hanno, M.D.

CONTENTS

SECTION 1 THE ADRENAL GLAND

SECTION 2 THE KIDNEY

KIDNEY TRANSPLANTATION AND HYPERTENSION

SECTION 3 THE URETER

CONGENITAL DISORDERS

BLADDER TUMORS

SECTION 5 THE PROSTATE AND SEMINAL VESICLES

PROSTATE INFLAMMATION AND INFECTIONS

PROSTATE TUMORS

SECTION 8 THE TESTIS AND EPIDIDYMIS

CONGENITAL DISORDERS

INFLAMMATIONS

TUMORS

SECTION 9 INFERTILITY AND STERILITY

SECTION 10 MISCELLANEOUS

SECTION 1

THE ADRENAL GLAND

ADRENAL HEMORRHAGE

STANLEY A. BROSMAN, M.D.

Los Angeles, California

Adrenal hemorrhage is being detected with increased frequency. Ultrasound screening examinations in the newborn have found adrenal hemorrhage in as many as 30 per cent of infants. Fortunately, this finding is of little clinical consequence in the vast majority. Risk factors include "large-for-date babies," intrauterine or perinatal hypoxia, prolonged labor, forceps or vacuum extractions, and difficult or traumatic delivery.

The right adrenal gland tends to be particularly susceptible. A possible explanation is that a sudden increase in pressure in the inferior vena cava is transmitted to the right adrenal gland through the short right adrenal veins, whereas the longer and larger left renal vein can absorb the pressure. Bilateral adrenal hemorrhage occurs in 10 per cent of infants.

In those patients with a significant hemorrhage, the clinical findings are apparent within the first few days of life. The triad of adrenal insufficiency, hemorrhage, and abdominal mass is not always apparent. The symptoms of acute adrenal insufficiency—tachypnea, pyrexia, petechiae and purpura, metabolic disturbances, abdominal pain, vomiting and diarrhea, convulsions, and cyanosis—more often are associated with bilateral adrenal hemorrhage and are life threatening. Immediate fluid and steroid replacement is essential to correct the metabolic problems.

A large blood loss can occur in a short period of time. The rapid occurrence of pallor, cold extremities, a weak and rapid heart rate, shock, air hunger, abdominal distention, and an abdominal mass is indicative of the degree of hemorrhage that can occur and the need for a rapid replacement of blood and fluids.

Most infants with adrenal hemorrhage will have neither symptoms of adrenal insufficiency nor symptoms of massive blood loss. Instead, an abdominal mass will develop as a result of a slower or shorter episode of adrenal bleeding that is self-limited. The differential diagnosis includes hydronephrosis, multicystic kidney disease, neuroblastoma, cortical renal cyst, adrenal cyst, an obstructed upper pole segment in a duplicated kidney, and mesoblastic nephroma.

Ultrasonography is the primary diagnostic imaging study in these patients. Serial sonography usually is effective in establishing the diagnosis because of the changes that occur over time. This helps to avoid radiographic investigations and laparotomies. Initially the mass tends to be highly echogenic. Irregular, complex and cystic masses commonly are seen. Later studies show a progressive decrease in size of the mass, and a cystic appearance begins to develop because of liquefaction and reabsorption of the hematoma. Calcification may be apparent as early as 7 days. Ultrasonography or a radiograph of the abdomen will show peripheral shell-like calcification, whereas stippled calcification and widening of the paravertebral soft tissues are suggestive of neuroblastoma. Excretory urography, angiography and computerized tomographic (CT) scanning seldom are necessary. Initially, ultrasonography may not distinguish between adrenal hemorrhage and neuroblastoma. Although the serial changes associated with adrenal hemorrhage are diagnostic, determination of serum catecholamine levels and urinary vanillylmandelic acid and homovanillic acid levels are necessary.

The ipsilateral kidney should be evaluated with ultrasonography because of the possibility of concomitant renal vein thrombosis. This is particularly true if there is gross or microscopic hematuria or proteinuria.

Magnetic resonance imaging (MRI) is helpful when morphologic changes, clinical appearance, and follow-up studies do not differentiate between adrenal hemorrhage and neuroblastoma. Using artifact-suppressing sequences, a typical signal behavior has been identified with adrenal hemorrhage. Gadolinium-DTPA scanning is helpful in demonstrating vascular tumors. MRI is valuable in defining the hemorrhagic nature of echogenic and hypoechoic suprarenal masses and in delineating thrombi within the renal veins and inferior vena cava.

Most patients with adrenal hemorrhage can be managed conservatively. The disorder resolves spontaneously with adequate hydration, and with blood and steroid replacement when indicated. Most infants will not require lifelong steroids. Even in severe cases, adrenal function is restored within 3 months. In rare instances surgical intervention may be necessary if the diagnosis is in doubt, uncontrollable hemorrhage is occurring, or an abscess has developed.

There are reports of adrenal hemorrhage occurring in adults in association with trauma and thromboembolic phenomenon. The patients tend to be diagnosed as having septic shock instead of acute adrenal insufficiency. Most of these patients have been diagnosed by sonography or CT scan. Early steroid replacement therapy usually is essential but may be discontinued when the patient's clinical status has stabilized.

Suggested Readings

Bergami G, Malena S, Di Mario M, et al: Echography in the follow-up of neonatal adrenal hemorrhage: The presentation of 14 cases. Radiol Med (Torino) 79:474, 1990

Brill PW, Jagannath A, Winchester P, et al: Adrenal hemorrhage and renal vein thrombosis in the newborn: MR imaging. Radiology 170:95, 1989

Jöjärt G, Nagy G, Päsztor J, et al: Bilateral neonatal adrenal hemorrhage associated with hypoadrenalism. Orv Hetil 133:1179, 1981

Rubecz I, Gasztonyl V, Szauer E, et al: Neonatal adrenal gland hemorrhage. Orv Hetil 130:2519, 1989

CONGENITAL ADRENAL HYPERPLASIA

T. ERNESTO FIGUEROA, M.D.

Tampa, Florida

Congenital adrenal hyperplasia (CAH) represents a number of hereditary syndromes produced by specific enzymatic deficiencies in the steroidogenesis pathway. The most recognized abnormality arising from the breakdown of steroidogenesis is the virilization of the female fetus. The overproduction of the fetal adrenal androgens primarily affects the formation of the external genitalia. CAH is the most common cause of ambiguous genitalia in the newborn. These patients, although phenotypically altered, have normal and corresponding chromosomal and gonadal features.

The production of adrenal corticosteroids follows a well-outlined pathway of enzymatic modifications of cholesterol. The ultimate products of this pathway are cortisol, testosterone, and aldosterone. Cortisol is of foremost importance because it exerts an inhibitory effect on the pituitary production of adrenocorticotropic hormone (ACTH), the primary stimulating hormone of the adrenal cortex. Lack of cortisol, as seen in CAH, leads to an excessive production of ACTH, inducing hyperplasia of the remaining adrenal cortical tissue. Depending on the enzymatic defect, the hyperplastic adrenal tissue produces vast amounts of alternate corticosteroids—for the most part, androgens. Although under normal conditions adrenal androgens do not influence the development of the external genitalia, the elevated amount of androgens in CAH exerts a profound virilizing alteration of the female fetal genitalia.

Figure 1 depicts the pathway of corticosteroid biosynthesis and the enzymatic links necessary for the production of cortisol (glucocorticoid pathway), testosterone (androgen pathway), and aldosterone (mineralocorticoid pathway). Specific enzymatic blocks sway the biosynthetic flow into alternate pathways. The rate of the biosynthesis is controlled by hydrocortisone and its inhibitory feedback on pituitary ACTH. ACTH stimulates the conversion of cholesterol to pregnenolone.

Each enzymatic defect is determined by hereditary factors. CAH, although the most common cause of sexual ambiguity in the newborn, is still a rather infrequent disorder. The most common cause of CAH, 21-hydroxylase deficiency, occurs in 1 of 15,000 births in the United States. Both 21-hydroxylase deficiency and 11-hydroxylase deficiency are transmitted as autosomal recessive disorders, as are the 17-hydroxylase and 3β-hydroxysteroid dehydrogenase deficiencies. Other defects, such as 17,20-desmolase deficiency and 17β-hydroxysteroid dehydrogenase deficiency, may be transmitted as X-linked recessive mutations, although the small number of patients with these deficiencies does not permit accurate determination. It also is known that some of these deficiencies may be partial, according to the degree of penetration of the

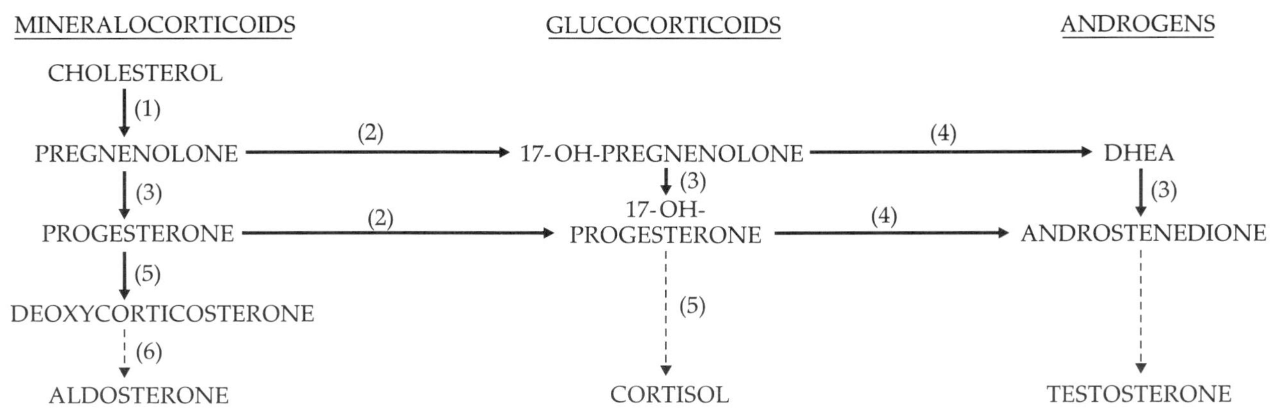

1. Cholesterol desmolase
2. 17α-Hydroxylase
3. 3β-Dehydrogenase
4. 17,20-Desmolase
5. 21-Hydroxylase
6. 11β-Hydroxylase

FIGURE 1. Corticosteroid biosynthesis: specific enzymatic blocks sway the biosynthetic flow into alternate pathways.

given gene. This variability in genetic expression accounts for variability in the phenotype alteration (virilization) seen in these patients.

The overproduction of certain adrenal corticosteroids can be assessed by measuring specific hormones in the blood or urine. This becomes extremely important in two situations. First, an elevated level of a hormone (in blood or urine) assists in the diagnosis of CAH as the cause of ambiguous genitalia in the newborn period. Second, the effect of replacement therapy can be monitored by the urinary levels of biosynthetic by-products. Elevated plasma levels of 17-hydroxyprogesterone and urinary levels of 17-ketosteroids and pregnanetriol indicate androgen overproduction as seen in 21-hydroxylase deficiency. Measurement of other biosynthetic precursors may be necessary when the more exceptional forms of CAH are suspected.

CLINICAL MANIFESTATIONS

CAH produces a number of clinical manifestations determined by level of the enzymatic block and degree of genetic expression producing the block. The most important clinical manifestation of CAH is the virilization of the female external genitalia. This occurs mainly because of 21-hydroxylase deficiency, by far the most common cause of CAH (95 per cent of cases). This enzymatic block results in an overproduction of adrenal androgens. Under this influence in the female fetus, the clitoris is enlarged, the labia majora become scrotalized, and the urogenital sinus persists and elongates. These changes may vary from minimal clitoromegaly with normal-appearing labia majora to a severe phallomegaly with a phallic urethra (sinus) terminating in the glans and complete scrotalization of the labia majora. This sexual ambiguity in the female is referred to as female pseudohermaphroditism.

Of equal clinical importance in 21-hydroxylase deficiency is the lack of mineralocorticoid production. Depending on the degree of genetic expression, this lack of mineralocorticoids may lead to severe, life-threatening salt wasting or to a more subtle subclinical form of mineralocorticoid deficiency. It is estimated that 40 to 60 per cent of patients with 21-hydroxylase deficiency have the salt-wasting variety. This characteristic is of critical importance. This condition may be life threatening if untreated, leading to dehydration, shock, and possibly death. Males affected with 21-hydroxylase deficiency are particularly prone to the metabolic alteration from mineralocorticoid deficiency. Unlike females, the external genitalia are normal in the newborn male, preventing recognition of the syndrome. In the non–salt-wasting variety, males tend to present later on in childhood because of precocious puberty.

The other forms of CAH are extremely rare, but merit mention because of the variability of clinical presentations. Besides the well-recognized form of CAH producing female pseudohermaphroditism, salt wasting, and precocious puberty in the male (21-hydroxylase deficiency), the 11β-hydroxylase deficiency produces virilization of the female and hypertension. Elevated levels of the precursor 11-deoxycorticosterone, a potent mineralocorticoid, account for the fluid retention and hypertension. The 3β-hydroxysteroid dehydrogenase deficiency, a rather proximal block, produces deficiencies in all three metabolic pathways. Its clinical significance stems from the impaired testicular steroidogenesis, producing inadequate virilization of the male, or male pseudohermaphroditism. These patients, as expected, are salt wasters. More distal deficiencies, like 20,22-desmolase deficiency, also impair adrenal and testicular production of androgens, resulting in male pseudohermaphrodites. Mineralocorticoid production is spared in this deficiency. Females are unaffected because of the X-linked origin of this deficiency. It is common to notice increased pigmentation of the labioscrotum in female pseudohermaphrodites secondary to CAH. The elevated levels of ACTH are responsible for this pigmentation.

EVALUATION

The majority of patients with CAH will be diagnosed in the process of evaluating a newborn with ambiguous genitalia. CAH is the most important abnormality to exclude in the child with ambiguous genitalia because of the following reasons. First, CAH is the most common cause of ambiguous genitalia in the newborn. Second, the most common cause of CAH is 21-hydroxylase deficiency, which produces salt wasting in almost two thirds of these patients. As previously mentioned, if untreated, this condition will cause dehydration and shock. Finally, female pseudohermaphrodites are potentially fertile, having coordinate chromosomal and gonadal sex (fertility in the male usually is compromised because of the inability to detect those patients with the non–salt-wasting variety; excess androgens inhibit gonadotropin production).

Protocols for the evaluation of newborns with sexual ambiguity are well described. Initially, any previous family history of intersex, maternal androgen intake, or maternal virilization must be determined. On physical examination, the appearance and length of the phallus, location of the urethral orifice (sinus), and findings on palpation of the labioscrotum are noted. Of critical importance is the presence of gonads in the labioscrotum. Palpable gonads more than likely represent testes, excluding the child as a female pseudohermaphrodite. (Although other causes of CAH may account for impaired virilization in the male, these are extremely rare, and other more common causes of intersex should be entertained.) A rectal examination may reveal a cervix or uterus.

Laboratory evaluation should include chromosomal analysis, serum electrolytes, and levels of plasma 17-hydroxyprogesterone and urinary 17-ketosteroids and pregnanetriol. Serum electrolytes will be normal initially, but progressive hyponatremia becomes evident after five to seven days of life in the salt-wasting varieties.

Radiographic evaluation consists of abdominal and pelvic ultrasound and a retrograde genitogram. This latter study should be performed with an occlusion device (e.g., Christmas tree connector) to delineate clearly the length of the urogenital sinus. This information is of utmost importance in planning the reconstructive surgery. The level of takeoff of the vagina from the sinus determines the type of vaginoplasty to be performed. A voiding cystourethrogram is inadequate in evaluating the urogenital sinus. A cervical impression by genitography suggests the presence of female internal organs. The pelvic ultrasound is confirmatory by demonstrating the ovaries and uterus. Laparotomy and gonadal biopsies are not needed in CAH.

MANAGEMENT

The management of patients with ambiguous genitalia starts at birth by notifying the various medical services of the patient's problems. A well-coordinated multidisciplinary approach encompassing pediatric endocrinologists, geneticists, neonatologists, and pediatric urologists is mandatory to avoid unnecessary delays in diagnosis.

All of these cases elicit a high level of parental anxiety because of the inability to immediately assign a sex of rearing to their newborn. The physician should have a warm, reassuring talk with the parents, informing them that the baby (not "it") has an incomplete development of the genitalia that prevents accurate sex assignment at that point. They should know that the child will undergo a number of tests to determine the sex, and that they should not name the baby until these tests are done. It also is wise to counsel the parents to avoid using certain androgynous names.

Once the diagnosis of CAH is made, the management will depend on: (1) presence or absence of salt wasting, (2) degree of virilization of the external genitalia, and (3) ability of the parents to accept the appearance of the genitalia.

As mentioned previously, the majority of these patients will be of the deficient 21-hydroxylase variety. These patients will exhibit elevated 17-hydroxyprogesterone and urinary levels of 17-ketosteroids. When this diagnosis is entertained, biochemical assays of 21-hydroxylase activity can be performed. All of these patients should be monitored closely in a hospital setting, and replacement cortisone (hydrocortisone and prednisone) and mineralocorticoids (Florinef) started at the slightest indication of salt wasting. Replacement glucocorticoid therapy is essential to reverse or prevent the progression of the excessive virilization. In the clinically stable patient, sequential or serial measurement of 17-hydroxyprogesterone, ACTH, urinary 17-ketosteroids, and plasma renin can be used to assess adequacy of therapy.

The management of the male infant with 21-hydroxylase deficiency merits discussion. These patients present with lethargy and physical evidence of dehydration or shock. Laboratory values will show hyponatremia. These patients should have their urine tested for sodium: an elevated urinary sodium in a patient with hyponatremia suggests adrenal insufficiency. Replacement glucocorticoid therapy along with Florinef should be administered. These patients exhibit a concomitant volume loss along with the hyponatremia. Careful replacement with intravenous isotonic saline is essential.

Most of the controversy surrounding the management of the female pseudohermaphrodite stems from the timing of the reconstructive surgery. Proponents of early reconstruction (neonatal period) claim that the normal appearance of the genitalia leads to greater parental acceptance of and identification with the child. Proponents of delayed repair (9 to 12 months) argue that reconstructive neonatal surgery is an arduous operation in a metabolically impaired patient, potentially endangering the life of the patient. Additionally, a delayed repair permits stabilization of the metabolic deficits, which often results in a diminution in the size of the phallus. Finally, Perlmutter has argued that the older child has more proportionate genitalia as compared to the newborn, allowing for a more symmetrical reconstruction.

Each surgeon has his or her bias regarding early or delayed reconstruction. However, two factors are important in making the decision. The degree of virilization, if extensive, may sway the surgeon to delay surgery. Of most importance, however, is the parental acceptance of the child. Most parents will always do what is best for the child, and they will depend on the surgeon to inform them of the choices.

The reconstruction of the virilized genitalia is referred to as feminizing genitoplasty. This involves a reduction in the size of the phallus, or reduction clitoroplasty and a type of vaginoplasty. The most accepted form of clitoroplasty involves preservation of the glans and neurovascular bundles with resection of either the entire corporal bodies or spongy tissue. The vaginoplasty usually is performed at the time of the clitoroplasty, usually by advancing a wide, posteriorly based skin flap into the spatulated posterior wall of the vagina.

Suggested Readings

Kogan SJ, Smey P, Levitt SB: Subtunical total reduction clitoroplasty: A safe modification of existing techniques. J Urol 130:756, 1983

Perlmutter AD, Reitelman C: Surgical management of intersexuality. *In* Walsh PC, Retik AB, Stamey TA, Vaughn ED (eds): Campbell's Urology, 6th ed. Philadelphia, WB Saunders, 1992, pp. 1951–1966

Snyder HM, Retik AB, Bauer SB, Colodny AH: Feminizing genitoplasty: A synthesis. J Urol 129:1024, 1983

PRIMARY ALDOSTERONISM

ANDREW C. NOVICK, M.D.

Cleveland, Ohio

The clinical syndrome of primary aldosteronism was first described in 1955 by Conn and represents hypersecretion of aldosterone from the zona glomerulosa of the adrenal cortex. The most common underlying disorder is a benign unilateral adenoma; however, some cases, termed idiopathic, are secondary to bilateral adrenal hyperplasia. Adrenal cortical carcinoma is an extremely rare cause of primary aldosteronism.

CLINICAL PRESENTATION AND DIAGNOSIS

Primary aldosteronism is considered to account for approximately 1 per cent of all cases of hypertension. The usual age of patients with this syndrome ranges between 30 and 50 years. Muscle weakness is the most common symptom and hypertension is the most common sign. Primary aldosteronism should be suspected in any patient with hypertension and hypokalemia, recognizing that the latter also may be secondary to chronic diuretic therapy or secondary aldosteronism associated with renovascular hypertension.

The diagnostic hallmarks of primary aldosteronism include elevated urinary and plasma aldosterone levels, unprovoked hypokalemia, and a low peripheral plasma renin level. Although relative hypernatremia and hypervolemia exist, the serum sodium may not be markedly elevated. Some patients have metabolic alkalosis, but this is not invariably present. The two most reliable findings for establishing a biochemical diagnosis of primary aldosteronism are (1) failure to suppress aldosterone output during sodium loading, and (2) a persistently low level of plasma renin activity in the face of sodium deprivation.

EVALUATION AND SELECTION OF MEDICAL VERSUS SURGICAL TREATMENT

The two main causes of primary aldosteronism are an adrenal cortical adenoma and adrenal cortical hyperplasia, which occur in approximately 60 per cent and 40 per cent of cases, respectively. The distinction between these two processes is important, because surgical intervention is much more likely to be effective in the former than in the latter. Adenomas almost always are unilateral, and removal of the affected adrenal gland is curative in most cases. In adrenal hyperplasia, because both glands are involved, unilateral adrenalectomy is much less likely to be curative, although hypertension is relieved in some patients, presumably because of the reduction in adrenal mass. The preferred management of primary aldosteronism secondary to hyperplasia is medical treatment with spironolactone, which inhibits the action of aldosterone on the distal renal tubule. Occasionally, agents that interfere with renal tubular ion transport, such as triamterene or amiloride, also are incorporated into a pharmacologic treatment program. Bilateral adrenalectomy has no place in the management of primary aldosteronism, because complete adrenal insufficiency may be more difficult to treat than hypertension from aldosteronism.

The distinction between an adenoma and hyperplasia can be established prospectively in most cases. An adenoma is more likely to be present when: (1) there is no increase in plasma aldosterone with upright posture, (2) a radiographic imaging study demonstrates a discrete adrenal mass, (3) the blood pressure returns to normal or near normal with spironolactone therapy, and (4) the serum potassium concentration is persistently low during normal dietary sodium intake.

When the biochemical diagnosis of primary aldosteronism is established, radiographic evaluation is indicated to determine the presence and location of an adrenal adenoma. Such adenomas are unilateral and more commonly involve the left adrenal gland. They are small tumors, generally 1 to 2 cm in diameter, and often grow inward toward the center of the gland, making them difficult to localize. Adrenal venous sampling for plasma aldosterone measurement is the most precise technique for identification and localization of an aldosterone-producing adenoma. Computerized tomographic (CT) scanning and adrenal venography also are useful but somewhat less accurate in this regard. The localization efficacy of magnetic resonance imaging (MRI) is equivalent to that of CT scanning in the detection of an aldosterone-producing adrenal adenoma.

In patients with a biochemical diagnosis of primary aldosteronism, a useful approach is first to perform CT, MRI, or both, because they are noninvasive. If these studies do not demonstrate an adrenal mass, adrenal venous sampling should be done. It may be difficult to cannulate one of the adrenal veins, particularly on the right side; in this event, the diagnosis of an adenoma on that side still can be inferred if aldosterone secretion from the contralateral gland is suppressed. Adrenal venography should be considered only when an adenoma is strongly suspected and the above studies are negative or nondiagnostic. This algorithm, combined with postural plasma aldosterone studies if necessary, allows the differentiation of adenoma from hyperplasia with good reliability.

The treatment of choice for an aldosterone-producing adenoma is surgical adrenalectomy, which carries minimal morbidity and provides definitive therapy in most cases. Medical therapy with spironolactone is indicated for patients with hyperplasia or for poor-surgical-risk patients with adenomas. Potential side effects of spironolactone include gynecomastia, impotence, nausea, vomiting, sweating, pigmentation, and weakness. Occasionally, an adrenal gland removed for a suspected adenoma is found to contain one or more hyperplastic nodules. Although the results of adrenalectomy for hyperplasia are less satisfactory, some patients experience cure or improvement of hypertension postoperatively. This therapeutic response is not completely understood and may result from a simple reduction in the amount of adrenal tissue.

SURGICAL TREATMENT

Patients with primary aldosteronism have a significant potassium deficit, which must be corrected preoperatively because hypokalemia increases the risk of cardiac arrhythmias during anesthesia. Supplemental oral potassium alone is not sufficient to overcome the kaliuresis experienced by these patients. Spironolactone also is necessary, and should be administered routinely prior to surgery both to correct hypokalemia and to facilitate blood pressure control. Some patients with a unilateral adenoma develop contralateral mineralocorticoid suppression, which may become manifest postoperatively as clinical hypoaldosteronism. This problem also may be prevented by preoperative spironolactone therapy, because this allows reactivation of the renin-angiotensin-aldosterone system. There is no need for glucocorticoid administration prior to surgery unless the patient recently has received exogenous steroids for another condition.

It is currently possible to determine the location of an aldosterone-producing adenoma prior to surgery in almost all cases. Therefore, bilateral adrenal explorations to discover and remove the causative adenoma are no longer performed. Because aldosterone-producing adenomas invariably are small and benign, unilateral adrenalectomy may be performed through an extraperitoneal approach. I prefer to employ a posterior surgical incision in such cases, although occasionally a flank incision is used.

Following removal of an aldosterone-producing adenoma, there will be a moderate urinary diuresis of sodium and retention of potassium. This requires appropriate volume replacement and close monitoring of serum electrolyte levels for the first week postoperatively. In some cases, hyponatremia and hyperkalemia develop in the immediate postoperative period secondary to suppression of the contralateral zona glomerulosa, with a resulting aldosterone deficiency. This phenomenon will necessitate mineralocorticoid replacement until the remaining adrenal gland recovers. In general, patients experience a rapid and uneventful postoperative recovery from adrenalectomy for hyperaldosteronism. Hypertension may take several weeks to resolve completely; however, ultimately, 80 per cent of patients are cured.

Suggested Readings

Bravo EL, Tarazi RC, Dustan HP, et al: The changing clinical spectrum of primary aldosteronism. Am J Med 74: 641, 1983

Lim RC, Nakayama DK, Biglierri E, et al: Primary aldosteronism: Changing concepts in diagnosis and management. Am J Surg 152:116, 1986

Novick AC: Surgery for primary hyperaldosteronism. Urol Clin North Am 16:535, 1989

Novick AC, Straffon RA, Kaylor W, et al: Posterior transthoracic approach for adrenal surgery. J Urol 141:254, 1989

FEMINIZING ADRENAL TUMORS IN CHILDREN

MARTIN A. KOYLE, M.D.

Denver, Colorado

Feminizing adrenal tumors in childhood are very rare, yet they may be potentially life-threatening disease processes. Approximately 95 per cent of adrenocortical neoplasms (benign and malignant) are hormonally active, compared to only 50 per cent of adrenocortical tumors in adults. Because of the functioning nature of adrenocortical tumors, children with these tumors commonly will present clinically with virilization, feminization, or signs of hypercortisolism. Most commonly, the child presents with virilization or a combination of virilization and hypercortisolism. The least common presentation of a functioning adrenocortical tumor is feminization. The mean age at presentation for an adrenocortical tumor is 4.63 years, with a range of 5 days to 16.5 years. Adrenocortical tumors, in general, affect females twice as often as males; however, feminizing adrenal tumors appear to affect males more frequently than females. There are as few as 22 case reports in the literature describing feminizing benign and malignant adrenal tumors in children.

When girls are affected by a feminizing tumor, they most commonly will present with symptoms of isosexual precocious puberty. Breast enlargement, galactorrhea, accelerated growth, advanced bone age, and even vaginal bleeding can occur. When feminization occurs in a prepubertal female, the differential diagnosis must include other causes of precocious puberty, such as pituitary hyperactivity and ectopic chorionic gonadotropin–producing tumors. Premature thelarche, or early benign breast enlargement, may be distinguished from a feminization syndrome by the fact that there is no associated accelerated growth, advanced bone age, or vaginal bleeding.

The most common presenting sign in boys who harbor a feminizing tumor is gynecomastia (Fig. 1). Advanced bone age and delayed isosexual pubertal development also can be seen. As in girls, galactorrhea may occur, although rarely. Importantly, in boys with evidence of feminization, testicular or extragonadal neoplasms secreting chorionic gonadotropin or estrogens must be excluded. A thorough scrotal examination and testicular ultrasound thus are mandatory. Idiopathic benign prepubertal or pubertal gynecomastia can occur in normal boys, but there is no associated growth spurt, advanced bone age, or any other signs of virilism.

The suspicion of a feminizing adrenocortical tumor requires radiographic and biochemical investigation. Historically, excretory urography and arteriography with adrenal vein sampling were the radiologic diagnostic standards. Currently, computerized tomography (CT) and magnetic resonance imaging (MRI) are the studies of choice to image the adrenal gland. Both of these studies are valuable to determine the extent of local disease and to ascertain the presence of overt abdominal metastases. Recently it has been suggested that MRI is superior in distinguishing malignant from benign adrenal lesions, and it thus has become the study of choice in assessing adrenocortical tumors.

Serum biochemical assessment of a feminizing adrenal tumor usually will reveal an elevated 17-ketosteroid (17-KS) level (a nonspecific indicator of adrenal androgen metabolism) as well as elevated estradiol, estrogen, and testosterone levels. Although testosterone may be elevated, the estradiol/testosterone ratio favors estradiol and thus feminization occurs. A 24-hour urine collection for 17-KS also is valuable in helping to distinguish malignant tumors (wherein the 17-KS usually is markedly elevated) from benign tumors (wherein 17-KS may be only mildly elevated).

The differentiation between benign and malignant adrenocortical neoplasms can be very difficult. The only reliable predictor of biologic behavior other than the presence of metastases has been tumor size. The majority of adenomas are less than 100 gm and most adenocarcinomas are greater than 500 gm; tumors between 100 and 500 gm represent a grey zone and are indeterminate. On gross examination, malignant tumors tend to be lobulated, with a heterogeneous color pattern ranging from tan to reddish brown. Benign tumors are well encapsulated and have a more homogeneous color. Microscopically, even malignant tumors may appear very much like normal adrenal tissue, with rare mitoses, but they also may appear aggressive, with bizarre mitotic figures and pleomorphism. Vascular or capsular invasion, necrosis, and calcification also typically are seen with malignant tumors when compared with adenomas. Many investigators have attempted to develop a microscopic correlation of many characteristics to define malignant disease, but currently tumor size is still the best predictor of biologic activity.

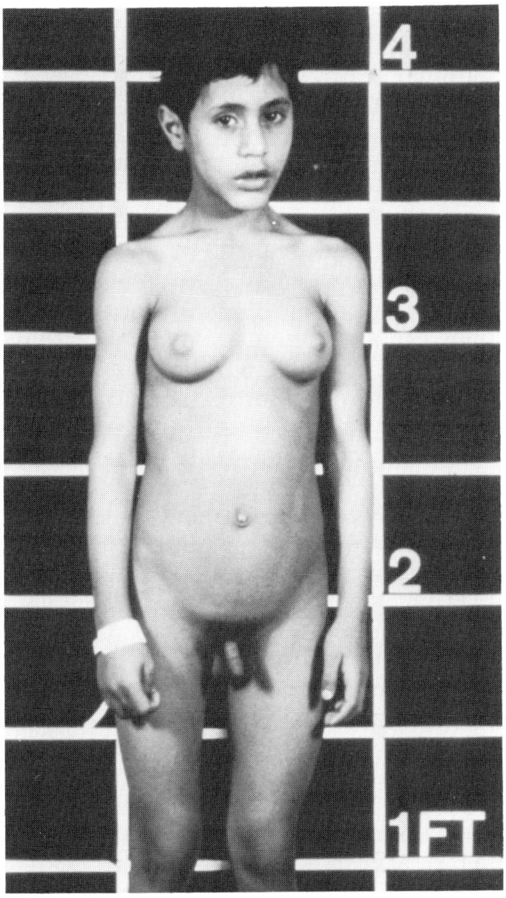

FIGURE 1. Significant gynecomastia with advanced phallic and pubic hair growth. Note height (97th percentile with bone age 11.5 years).

The treatment for feminizing adrenocortical neoplasms is surgery. For tumors that are considered to be malignant, radical aggressive surgical approaches are justified because adjuvant therapy is minimally effective. In boys, gynecomastia may regress incompletely (50 per cent or less) by six months after successful treatment of an adrenocortical tumor. Although complete regression eventually may occur, early reduction mammoplasty is valuable in these boys because it may diminish the potential psychological trauma.

It has been well demonstrated that adrenocortical carcinomas in adults are radioresistant. There is a report of a secondary renal cell carcinoma appearing within the radiation fields of a child successfully treated with surgery and radiation for an adrenocortical carcinoma years before. Mitotane has been used extensively in adults; however, there is little experience with it in children. Although there are anecdotal cases of cure using mitotane for metastatic disease, most studies demonstrate only a short partial response to this therapy. Other chemotherapeutic agents have been used with little proven success.

The prognosis for feminizing adrenal neoplasms depends primarily on whether the tumor is benign or malignant. Unfortunately, even with aggressive multimodal therapy, there is a significant two- and three-year mortality rate for pediatric adrenocortical carcinomas.

Feminizing syndromes in children are a rare entity. They are associated with benign and malignant adrenocortical tumors in rare instances, and therefore evaluation must distinguish such tumors from nonadrenal hormonally active tumors and even normal development. When an adrenocortical tumor is found, aggressive surgical therapy presently remains the cornerstone of therapy.

Suggested Reading

Chudler RM, Kay R: Adrenocarcinoma in children. Urol Clin North Am 16:469, 1989

Kay R, et al: Adrenocortical carcinoma in children. J Urol 130:1130, 1983

Morales L, et al: Adrenocortical tumors in childhood: A report of four cases. J Pediatr Surg 24:276, 1989

Neblett WW, et al: Experience with adrenocortical neoplasms in childhood. Am Surg 53:117, 1987

Wohltmann H, et al: Sexual precocity in a female infant due to feminizing adrenal carcinoma. J Clin Endocrinol Metab 50:186, 1980

CUSHING SYNDROME AND CUSHING DISEASE

JOHN P. DONOHUE, M.D.

Indianapolis, Indiana

Cushing syndrome refers to a constellation of symptoms and signs that derive from excess cortisol. The most common cause is iatrogenic (i.e., cortisol administration). However, unless the physician has an index of suspicion, many of these clinical manifestations can be overlooked and the more important and curable Cushing disease may remain undiagnosed.

The clinical diagnosis of Cushing syndrome is characterized by history and physical findings that must be taken together in order to compile the picture of the syndrome. Historically, the patients often complain of decreased libido, some weakness, and emotional instability that can range from irritability to depression or even manic behavior. One physical sign is polyuria, secondary to cortical suppression of antidiuretic hormone; glucose intolerance is a regular part of this syndrome, but only a quarter of the patients will have frank hypoglycemia. On physical examination, the most classic appearance is facial rounding and upper body obesity supplemented by the so-called buffalo hump (dorsal fat around the lower neck and supraclavicular fullness). Many patients feel a bit weak and jittery. Most also will have mild to moderate hypertension.

Laboratory tests to confirm the diagnosis chemically begin with a routine screening test using 1 mg of dexamethasone in the evening and then collecting serum cortisol the following morning. Normally the serum cortisol level would be 3 μg/dl or less. Anything above this suggests the syndrome is a real manifestation of cortisol excess.

Following the low-dose suppression tests, the most reliable test is a 24-hour urine measurement of free cortisol. This requires a careful collection but, if done, patients with Cushing syndrome exhibit a urine free cortisol well in excess of 100 μg/dl.

Once the syndrome is confirmed, the next step is to determine the source of cortisol excess. It can be the result of adrenal overstimulation by excess adrenocorticotropic hormone (ACTH), usually from the pituitary or less commonly from an ectopic source. ACTH overproduction is the cause of about 90 per cent of Cushing syndrome cases. The other possible cause (i.e., in the remaining 10 per cent) is independent cortisol production from an adrenal source.

The most practical test to help in making this distinction is high-dose dexamethasone suppression. This was classically described as a set of six consecutive 24-hour urine studies for urine steroids. Following two baseline days, two days of 2 mg of dexamethasone per day in four divided doses was followed by 2 days of 8 mg of dexamethasone per day in four divided doses. The criterion for a positive test was suppression of 24-hour urine and plasma steroids to less than 50 per cent of baseline, indicating pituitary Cushing syndrome. Failure to suppress to less than 50 per cent of baseline pointed to an adrenal ACTH–independent source or possibly an ectopic source.

With the recent availability of radioimmunoassay for ACTH, identification of ACTH-dependent forms of Cushing syndrome is much easier. Also, this can be done in the context of dexamethasone suppression testing. ACTH levels usually are suppressed to less than 5 pg/ml in ACTH-independent Cushing syndrome, such as that caused by adrenal tumors. In contrast, patients with pituitary tumors will have an elevated ACTH, usually greater than 10 pg/ml, and those with ectopic ACTH source often have higher levels than that. If the high-dose dexamethasone suppression test is positive and if the plasma ACTH assay shows suppression of ACTH, one can proceed to imaging the adrenal glands with high expectation of success. The most practical imaging exam is a computerized tomographic (CT) scan, which is sensitive to over the 90th percentile in detecting adrenal adenomas. Usually adenomas producing Cushing disease are much larger than those causing aldosteronism and are very easy to confirm by CT scan.

The differentiation of ectopic from pituitary ACTH-secreting tumors often is difficult. As a rule of thumb, ACTH levels are higher in the ectopic cases and pituitary imaging is negative. An ectopic source also is more common in men. Most ectopic ACTH-producing tumors are bronchial carcinoids. Some are not radiographically apparent on routine CT scans of the chest, but occasionally they can be demonstrated by magnetic resonance imaging (MRI) instead.

Also, it was shown recently in a research setting that corticotropin-releasing factor (CRF) can be used in conjunction with venous sampling from both inferior petrosal sinuses, which drain the venous effluent from the anterior pituitary. CRF will stimulate the pituitary to produce ACTH if the source is a pituitary adenoma but not if the source is an ectopic tumor. Although not yet generally available, this procedure shows great promise as a test to make the distinction between pituitary and ectopic sources.

Again as a rule of thumb, most patients with an ectopic ACTH source will have hypokalemia because they have a more severe cortisol excess and very high ACTH levels. Extreme excess cortisol overwhelms the normal enzymatic inactivation mechanisms of cortisol, which then is left free to bind with the mineralocorticoid receptors in the kidney that would otherwise bind aldosterone. The result is potassium wasting and hypokalemia, as seen in aldosteronism.

The most common source, representing about 80 to 90 per cent of Cushing syndrome cases, is pituitary adenoma. Modern microsurgical techniques permit subtotal excision of the pituitary with removal of adenoma but preservation of much of the anterior gland. The only difficulty with this is the recurrence rate, which is in the range of 20 per cent over long-term follow-up. The treatment of an ectopic ACTH-producing tumor is to localize the tumor (usually in the chest), which often is best done by MRI of the lungs, which will reveal a lucent lesion in the hilum or lung itself. These are usually bronchial carcinoids. The treatment of the primary adrenal tumor, representing about 10 per cent of causality in the overall syndrome, is total adrenalectomy. It should be remembered that the patient requires supplementation with steroids in the perioperative period. Injectable cortisone acetate preoperatively and intravenous hydroxycorticoid intraoperatively are useful and are required in this context.

The diagnosis of Cushing syndrome is not difficult if the practitioner has a reasonable index of suspicion. The diagnosis of Cushing disease is more difficult, as noted above, and usually is best done in consultation with the endocrinologist. It is most gratifying, however, to establish the source of the cortisol excess because appropriate surgical treatment is curative.

Suggested Readings

Donohue JP: Adrenal tumors: II. Surgery of the adrenal gland. *In* Crawford ED, Doss S (eds): Current Genito-Urinary Cancer Surgery. Philadelphia, Lea & Febiger, 1990

Findling JW: Cushing syndrome: An etiologic workup. Hosp Practice, October 15, pp 107–122, 1992

Kaye TB, Crapo L: The Cushing syndrome: An update on diagnostic tests. Ann Intern Med 112:434, 1990

Orth DN: Differential diagnosis of Cushing's syndrome. N Engl J Med 325:957, 1991

OTHER CONDITIONS OF THE ADRENAL GLAND

ROY J. CORREA, Jr., M.D.

Seattle, Washington

ADRENOCORTICAL CARCINOMA

Adrenocortical carcinoma is relatively uncommon. Despite its high mortality rate, it has been estimated to account for only 0.2 per cent of all deaths from cancer. Traditionally, the tumor has been classified as functional or nonfunctional, depending on the presence or absence of certain clinically apparent endocrinologic manifestations and/or abnormal laboratory determinations. This classification has little correlation with the primary treatment of this cancer or the prognosis. Its importance in clinical management relates primarily to the converse—that is, when an endocrine abnormality is suspected or proved, one must try to determine the presence or absence of cortical carcinoma. Abnormal endocrine patterns secondary to adrenal cancer, in decreasing order of reported frequency, include Cushing syndrome, virilization, feminization, and hyperaldosteronism.

In earlier literature, a higher percentage of

these tumors were reported as functional, but more recent papers would suggest that about 50 per cent of adrenocortical cancers are in the nonfunctional category. Many of the latter may produce precursor steroids without functional hormonal activity. About 60 per cent of the cases have been reported in females. This sexual discrepancy is not so marked if the cancers seen in the first three decades are recorded separately. In this latter category the female preponderance is striking. There appears to be a bimodal curve in the age incidence. The first peak is during the first two decades, with a second peak in the sixth and seventh decades. The disease seems to be reported more commonly on the left side. Bilateralism has been noted in 10 per cent of cases.

Except for the previously mentioned endocrinologic syndromes, common presenting symptoms and findings are relatively nonspecific. Weight loss, weakness, and fever are recorded frequently. A painful abdominal mass is often noted. Indeed, many of the patients have the diagnosis established only at the time of surgical exploration for abdominal mass or pain.

As the use of abdominal ultrasonography, computerized tomographic scanning, and magnetic resonance imaging has expanded, many asymptomatic adrenal tumors are discovered at an earlier and smaller stage. However, the differentiation of a benign versus a malignant adrenal cortical tumor has not been accurately defined. None of the accepted imaging studies are specific enough to make this differentiation certain. To date, the best determinant of categorizing these so-called incidentalomas is size. All tumors over 4 cm should be considered malignant and warrant surgical exploration and removal; those tumors of lesser diameter can be followed if shown to be nonfunctioning.

Some authors believe that a large tumor size portends a favorable outcome, but others disagree. The pathologic stage of the tumor is the best prognostic indicator, although all tumors classified higher than Stage I (less than 5 cm in size without evidence of invasion, nodal disease, or metastases) have a poor long-term prognosis. The histologic grade of the tumor does not correlate well with either functional characteristics or prognosis.

The primary therapy for adrenal carcinoma is surgical removal. Unfortunately, the rate of cure is quite low. Most tumors are discovered after they have progressed to advanced stages, with invasion into the lymphatics, contiguous organs, and vasculature, and, too often, with distant metastatic spread. A wide operative exposure is necessary for satisfactory removal. This usually can be achieved by a generous transabdominal subcostal incision for right-sided tumors and by a thoracoabdominal or supra–11th rib approach when the tumor is located on the left. Injury to the spleen commonly occurs when operating on left-sided lesions. If invasion of the ipsilateral kidney is discovered or suspected, a nephrectomy should be performed en bloc with the tumor mass. (For this reason, satisfactory renal function on the contralateral side must be ensured before surgery.) All regional nodes should be removed. The contralateral adrenal gland should receive adequate operative assessment because of the 10 per cent incidence of bilaterality. Adequate steroid replacement must be achieved during the immediate preoperative, intraoperative, and postoperative periods.

The response to radiation therapy is generally poor, although some significant palliation can be achieved, especially when irradiating peripheral bony metastases. No satisfactory study has been recorded relating the effects of preoperative radiotherapy.

o,p'-DDD (mitotane), a compound known to destroy specifically adrenal tissue, has been utilized with varying results. Some reduction of the tumor mass occasionally is seen, but this minimal response is usually of short duration. When administered at therapeutic dosage levels, the drug causes significant nausea, vomiting, and headaches. Combining adjunctive chemotherapy with surgery has not proved rewarding.

ADRENAL CYSTS

Adrenal cysts can be both congenital and acquired. Most initially are discovered at the time of intravenous pyelography for other conditions. If benignity can be assured through sophisticated radiologic studies and/or cyst aspiration, surgical exploration is not necessary. However, surgical excision may be required to establish a firm level of confidence in this regard.

ADRENAL ADENOMAS

Small cortical nodularity of the adrenal gland is not uncommon; indeed, it is reported in as many as 20 per cent of all autopsy cases. There is some controversy regarding nomenclature in the vast majority of these situations. Pathologically, most of these are simply hyperplastic nodules and are better categorized as nodular hyperplasia rather than true adenoma. Occasionally, a large, histologically benign tumor is seen arising from the adrenal gland. This mass has a true capsule and can be called an adenoma. As discussed above, nonfunctional adrenal masses over 4 cm in diameter should be removed surgically.

Suggested Readings

Bodie B, Novick AC, Pontes JE, et al: The Cleveland Clinic experience with adrenal cortical carcinoma. J Urol 141:257–260, 1989

Francis IR, Gross MD, Shapiro B, et al: Integrated imaging of adrenal disease. Radiology 184:1–13, 1992

Herrera MF, Grant CS, van Heerden JA, et al: Incidentally discovered adrenal tumors: An institutional perspective. Surgery 110:1014–1021, 1991

PHEOCHROMOCYTOMA

E. DARRACOTT VAUGHAN, Jr., M.D.

New York, New York

Pheochromocytoma is an uncommon entity that is the causative factor of hypertension in less than 1 per cent of the hypertensive population. However, the entity has fascinated both clinicians and investigators. Because of the potential lethal side effects of pheochromocytoma, all hypertensive patients should be evaluated to rule out this entity. Fortunately, we now have accurate measures for identification and localization of these tumors.

The clinical manifestations of pheochromocytoma are all due to the physiologic effects of the amines produced by the lesion. It is interesting that often small lesions that bind catecholamines poorly will lead to high epinephrine and norepinephrine secretion and severe symptoms, whereas larger tumors that have high catecholamine content bind and metabolize the amines and often are characterized by less severe hypertension and higher levels of catecholamine breakdown products in the urine.

SIGNS AND SYMPTOMS

Approximately 85 per cent of adults and 90 to 95 per cent of children will by hypertensive. This finding is the usual reason for initial evaluation. Approximately a third of the patients will have sustained hypertension, about 50 per cent will have paroxysms of hypertension, and the remaining patients will have sustained hypertension with "spells" or "dramatic attacks" of the symptoms usually considered to be associated with pheochromocytoma; those most commonly found are excessive sweating, palpitations, and anxiety. In children, nausea and vomiting, weight loss, and visual complaints are more common, sustained hypertension is more common, and paroxysms are less common. The frequency of paroxysmal attacks varies, but one or more episodes a week occur in 75 per cent of patients. Obviously stressful situations can bring about attacks, and patients are particularly prone to hypertensive crisis during induction of anesthesia for surgical procedures or during pregnancy. Maternal and infant mortality exceeds 40 per cent in patients with undiagnosed pheochromocytoma.

The adrenal medulla is composed of chromaffin cells that are derived from the neural crest and are part of the amine precursor uptake and decarboxylation (APUD) cell system, which explains the association of pheochromocytoma with other entities. The most common association is Sipple syndrome, consisting of pheochromocytoma, medullary thyroid carcinoma, and parathyroid adenomas; this more recently has been termed multiple endocrine neoplasia type II. Pheochromocytoma also may be associated with neuroectodermal dysplasias such as von Recklinghausen disease, Sturge-Weber syndrome, and von Hippel–Lindau disease.

Multiple pheochromocytomas are seen in three situations: in association with the multiple endocrine adenopathy syndromes, in children (15 to 30 per cent of cases), and in familial pheochromocytomas. The vast majority of patients with pheochromocytoma have a solitary lesion. The pheochromocytoma can be located at any site where there are neural crest cells, from the level of the adrenal down to the bladder and the organ of Zuckerkandl.

LABORATORY DIAGNOSIS OF PHEOCHROMOCYTOMA

The clinical diagnosis of pheochromocytoma is suggested by the subjective evaluation of signs and symptoms; however, all hypertensive patients should be evaluated. Fortunately, laboratory confirmation has become extremely accurate. Excellent methods now are available for demonstrating elevated levels of catecholamines in the blood or urine, which occur in 95 per cent of patients with pheochromocytoma. Thus, a patient can have blood drawn for determination of plasma norepinephrine and epinephrine during a hypertensive crisis or can have 24-hour urine sampling of urinary catecholamines, vanillylmandelic acid (VMA), and metanephrine. One caveat is that plasma catecholamines are extremely labile, and false-positive plasma values can be obtained when a patient is stressed. Accordingly, the patient should be at rest prior to measuring blood levels.

Once elevated catecholamines are determined, it is most likely that the patient has the disease and radiographic localizing studies are in order. The current imaging technique of choice is magnetic resonance imaging (MRI). This technique has a number of advantages over computerized tomography. There is a characteristic "bright light bulb" on the T_2-weighted study that is quite characteristic of neural tumors, although it also can be seen in situations of adrenal hemorrhages or some adrenal cysts. Moreover, the sagittal and coronal images can give excellent anatomic information concerning the relationship between the tumor and the surrounding vasculature, as well as the draining venous channels. Finally, MRI can identify the presence of multiple lesions.

One adjunctive test that is sometimes useful is the 131-Iodine–labeled meta-iodo-benzylguanidine (MIBG) scan. MIBG is a precursor of catecholamines and will be localized in an active tumor.

PREOPERATIVE PREPARATION

Catecholamine production leads to hemoconcentration and volume constriction, and it is now the consensus that patients should have preoperative stabilization prior to adrenalectomy. The standard therapy is phenoxybenzamine hydrochloride (dibenzyline), a long-term alpha blocker that generally is begun at 20 to 30 mg orally per day and increased until blood pressure control is obtained. Beta blockade generally is not utilized unless there are concurrent arrhythmias. Short-term alpha-blocking agents have not been as effective. If the catecholamine levels are extremely high, we would add alpha-methylparatyrosine (DEMSA) to decrease the rate of catecholamine synthesis. The combined treatment is particularly important if a patient demonstrates decreased cardiac function as a result of what has been termed "catecholamine cardiomyopathy." Thus, one can not only block the adrenergic receptors but also decrease catecholamine production. Immediately preoperatively the patient is given increased crystalloid to raise intravascular volume to avoid hypotension following removal of the pheochromocytoma. In general, blood transfusions are no longer used.

ANESTHETIC MANAGEMENT

The operative approach to pheochromocytoma takes a coordinated effort between the urologist and the anesthesiologist. In the best-prepared patients alpha blockade will be in place; however, there may be marked fluctuations in blood pressure, particularly during induction of anesthesia or manipulation of the tumor.

The safest anesthetics available appear to be enflurane and isoflurane, agents that decrease myocardial irritability. During the procedure, arterial lines and Swan-Ganz catheters are utilized and systemic hypertension is controlled with the addition of phentolamine (Regitine) or sodium nitroprusside. Both lidocaine and propranolol should be available for the occurrence of arrhythmias.

When the blood supply to the tumor has been divided, there will be a fall in circulating catecholamines and resultant hypotension. Volume replacement is the treatment of choice, with careful cardiovascular monitoring, but at times norepinephrine (Levofed) at low dosage is needed.

SURGICAL THERAPY

Because these tumors can be multiple and extra-adrenal, the traditional approach to pheochromocytoma has been through a chevron or a midline abdominal incision. However, in patients who are not at high risk for multiple lesions, because of the extremely high accuracy of localizing studies we now would utilize a flank approach directed toward the offending lesion. If the lesion is large or suspected to be malignant, a thoracoabdominal approach is utilized; if not, a standard 11th rib approach is adequate. The operative technique should include a "hands off" approach, one in which the goal is to "dissect the patient from the tumor." These tumors are often friable, and obviously any pressure on the tumor will cause blood pressure elevation. An attempt should be made to obtain early ligation of the adrenal vein, and the anesthesiologist should be notified when the adrenal vein is ligated. Following ligation of the vein, dissection should be from lateral to medial and all cephalad attachments should be taken down initially, leaving the adrenal attached to the kidney. The most difficult technical situations are the early ligation of the short, posteriorly placed right adrenal gland and the sometimes difficult dissection of extra-adrenal pheochromocytomas, which often lie near the renal hilum behind the renal vein with intimate relationship to the renal artery, which can even be incorporated into the tumor.

If the lesion is thought to be malignant, an ipsilateral node dissection should be carried out; often nephrectomy is needed. Surgical aids that are most useful include good head lights, right-angle titanium clips, and a forceps electrocautery to coagulate small vessels.

The success rate of removal of known pheochromocytomas without any attendant morbidity or mortality is currently quite high, but is dependent on close coordination between the anesthesiologist and urologist.

MEDICAL TREATMENT

The standard approach to patients with pheochromocytoma is adrenalectomy. One of two exceptions is that of pheochromocytoma identified during pregnancy; in this setting it is thought that the patient should be treated with control of blood pressure and the tumor removed at the time of cesarean section. The other setting for medical management is in cases of the rare entity of malignant pheochromocytoma, which probably occurs less often than the quoted 10 per cent incidence. In this setting patients can be treated with both an alpha blocker to block adrenergic receptors and metyrosine (DEMSA) to decrease catecholamine production.

NEUROBLASTOMA

ALAN B. RETIK, M.D.

Boston, Massachusetts

Neuroblastoma is the most common extracranial malignant solid tumor of infancy and childhood. It is exceeded in frequency only by leukemia, lymphoma, and brain tumors. The tumor usually arises from the sympathetic nervous system or its precursors, or it may originate from parasympathetic ganglia, the dorsal root ganglia of the spinal cord, or the neurilemma of peripheral nerves. Although the most frequent sites of origin are the adrenal medulla and the abdominal sympathetic ganglia, the tumor may occur in sympathochromaffin tissue in the neck, chest, or pelvis.

Spontaneous regression of neuroblastoma is not an infrequent occurrence. The excellent prognosis of infants, even with metastatic disease, is probably due to the high incidence of spontaneous regression in this age group. Spontaneous regression usually occurs as lysis of tumor with a shrinking tumor mass, although there are many reports of maturation to a benign ganglioneuroma.

CLINICAL FEATURES

An adrenal neuroblastoma commonly presents as an abdominal mass that extends under the costal margin, is hard and fixed, and may cross the midline. Pelvic neuroblastoma may cause urinary retention. The initial symptoms of presentation often are caused by metastatic lesions. Unilateral proptosis with periorbital hemorrhage resulting from a retroocular deposit may also be seen. Infrequently, encephalopathy with myoclonus, opsoclonus, and ataxia may be seen as the first evidence of neuroblastoma.

DIAGNOSIS

The mass may be demonstrated by radiography as a soft tissue mass, commonly with stippled calcification. Excretory urography often demonstrates displacement of the kidney downward and laterally. Computerized tomography also may be helpful. Approximately 75 per cent of neuroblastomas secrete the catecholamines dopamine, norepinephrine, and epinephrine. These hormones and their breakdown metabolites, vanillylmandelic acid and homovanillic acid, are excreted in excessive amounts in the urine.

STAGING

The staging of neuroblastoma is important with regard to treatment and ultimate prognosis.

Stage I: The tumor is confined to the organ or structure of origin.

Stage II: The tumor extends in continuity beyond the organ or structure of origin but does not cross the midline. Regional lymph nodes on the homolateral side may be involved.

Stage III: The tumor extends in continuity beyond the midline. Lymph nodes may be involved bilaterally. The tumor may be incompletely resected at surgery.

Stage IV: There are distant metastases.

Stage IV-S: Patients who are less than 1 year of age at diagnosis who would otherwise be Stage I or II, but who have remote disease confined to one or more of the following sites: liver, skin, or bone marrow.

TREATMENT

Stage I: Surgery is performed to remove the entire lesion through a transabdominal incision. Additional therapy is not required.

Stage II: In children under 1 year of age, the tumor is removed surgically and no further treatment is given. In children over 1 year of age, radiation therapy and chemotherapy are used as well. The chemotherapy regimen at our institution is MADDOC, which consists of nitrogen mustard, Adriamycin (doxorubicin), DDT (chlorophenothane), DTIC (dacarbazine), vincristine, and cyclophosphamide.

Stage III: In Stage III disease, the tumor cannot be completely resected and is "debulked." In addition, chemotherapy and radiotherapy are used.

Stage IV: Children with Stage IV disease are treated in a fashion similar to those with Stage III. Neuroblastoma is sensitive to radiation, and bone pain often can be relieved by simple doses of 300 to 500 rad.

Stage IV-S: This group of patients probably have spontaneous regression of their disease. They usually require little, if any, treatment. Surgery is performed to remove the primary, if identifiable. Tumors in the liver or skin frequently require no treatment, although our usual regimen is chemotherapy until there is no evidence of disease.

PROGNOSIS

The prognosis for the child with neuroblastoma depends primarily on the site of the tumor, the degree of differentiation, the age of the patient, and the stage of the disease. The most important are age and stage. Age and stage are independent factors, with survival ranging from 100 per cent for Stage I at any age in a recent series to less than 5 per cent for Stage IV disease in children older than 1 year of age at the time of diagnosis. In Stage I disease in patients under 1 year of age, the survival rate may be as high as 96 per cent; over 2 years of age, it is approximately 90 per cent. With Stage II patients under 1 year of age, the prognosis has been reported to be 91 per cent cure; over age 2, the figure decreases to 48 per cent. With Stage III patients under age 1, the cure rate has been reported to be 77 per cent; over age 2, it is 28 per cent. With Stage IV patients under age 1, the cure rate has been reported to be 27 per cent; over age 2, 3 per cent. With Stage IV-S patients under age 1, the cure rate has been reported to be 95 per cent; over age 2, it decreases markedly to approximately 40 per cent. The prognosis is best when the tumor is highly differentiated, the child is under the age of 1 year, and the stage is I or IV-S. The outlook is best for intrathoracic tumors and worst with adrenal and other abdominal origins. Other factors reported to be associated with an improved prognosis include nonadrenal or extra-abdominal primaries, lymphoid infiltration of tumor, and degree of differentiation toward ganglioneuroma.

Suggested Readings

Brodeur GM, Seeger RC, Barrett A, et al: International criteria for diagnosis, staging and response to treatment in patients with neuroblastoma. J Clin Oncol 6: 1874–1881, 1988

Evans AE, D'Angio GJ, Propert K, et al: Prognostic factors in neuroblastoma. Cancer 59:1853–1859, 1987

Grosfeld JL: Management of solid tumors in infancy and childhood: The Indiana experience. Jpn J Pediatr Surg 19:256, 1983

Silber JH, Evans AE, Fridman M: Models to predict outcome from childhood neuroblastoma: The role of serum ferritin and tumor histology. Cancer Res 51:1426–1433, 1991

Sitarz A, Finklestein J, Grosfeld S, et al: An evaluation of the role of surgery in disseminated neuroblastoma: A report from the Children's Cancer Study Group. J Pediatr Surg 18:147, 1983

SECTION 2

THE KIDNEY

Congenital Disorders

UROLOGIC INTERVENTION FOR FETAL HYDRONEPHROSIS

DAVID A. DIAMOND, M.D.

Worcester, Massachusetts

Over the past decade, maternal ultrasound has become a routine diagnostic procedure for the assessment of fetal/maternal anatomy. As a result, the diagnosis of prenatal hydronephrosis has become increasingly common, occurring in approximately 1 of every 600 routine maternal ultrasound studies.

DETECTION AND INDICATIONS FOR INTERVENTION

The relationship of embryologic development of the urinary tract to the diagnosis of prenatal hydronephrosis is a critically important one. Fetal urine production first can be detected at about 9 weeks of gestation. The earliest reported diagnosis of prenatal hydronephrosis has been at 13 1/2 weeks of gestation. For obstetric purposes, such as amniocentesis, the optimal timing for prenatal ultrasound is at 16 weeks of gestation, when only severe hydronephrosis is detectable. In general, the diagnosis of prenatal hydronephrosis cannot be made with certainty until 18 to 20 weeks of gestation. The question is whether urologic intervention at mid-gestation is more protective of renal function than is postnatal drainage.

Harrison has outlined clearly the indications for considering intervention for prenatal obstructive uropathy, which include bilateral hydronephrosis or unilateral hydronephrosis in a solitary kidney, evidence of a dilated bladder, and oligohydramnios. The reasons for considering intervention are the experimental evidence that suggests potential preservation of renal and pulmonary function following in utero drainage as well as the enhanced ability to deliver the child vaginally. Yet the risks that one accepts with intervention include the induction of premature labor, perforation of fetal bowel and bladder, and hemorrhage and infection in the fetus and mother.

CLINICAL RESULTS OF INTERVENTION

Among those fetuses with a prenatal diagnosis of hydronephrosis, Harrison's criteria are very rarely met. Peters recently presented the Boston experience with 136 cases of prenatal hydronephrosis, among which only 3 (2 per cent) met the criteria for prenatal intervention. All three patients had posterior urethral valves. One underwent in utero vesicostomy and ultimately died; one child was the product of an induction of labor at 32 weeks and is on dialysis; and the third underwent a vesicoamniotic shunt at 21 to 22 weeks and has demonstrated good infant renal and pulmonary function. At birth, this child had bowel protruding through a shunt puncture site, requiring laparotomy. Thus, only one of the three seemed clearly to benefit from prenatal intervention, and not without complication.

The results of prenatal intervention for fetal hydronephrosis between 1982 and 1985 were reported by the International Fetal Surgery Registry. This included 73 children undergoing catheter shunts for obstructive uropathy diagnosed at a mean of 23 weeks' gestation (range 16 to 34 weeks), with intervention at a mean of 24 weeks (range 17 to 36 weeks). The largest group of fetuses so treated (45 per cent) had an indeterminate cause of their prenatal hydronephrosis. Among those fetuses with a clear etiology of their hydronephrosis, posterior urethral valves was the leading cause (29 per cent). The survival rate among valves patients was 76 per cent, second only to the 100 per cent survival among three patients with prune-belly syndrome. Because prune-belly babies often are found to have unobstructed upper and lower tracts, despite their dilated collecting systems, their excellent survival was not surprising. More significant, perhaps, was the survival rate among valves babies—those with true lower tract obstruction. Although 76 per cent survival would seem to represent a commendable result, it may differ little from the natural history of valve patient survival. In 1973, Johnston had shown that, among valves patients presenting within the first month of life, 50 per cent ultimately survived. In a recent series, Nakayama noted 55 per cent survival among valves patients presenting clinically within the first week of life. One would expect Johnston and Nakayama to have seen the most clinically severe cases early on, whereas prenatal ultrasound would detect milder cases in utero. Thus, a 76 per cent survival rate among the prenatal posterior urethral valves babies may not represent a dramatic clinical achievement.

Perhaps as important as the success rates were the causes of fetal deaths described in the Fetal Registry Report. As one might expect, pulmonary hypoplasia accounted for the majority of deaths (63 per cent), and elective termination of pregnancy (26 per cent) comprised the second largest group. Seven per cent of deaths were procedure related. These cases represented a 5 per cent risk of death among those fetuses undergoing prenatal treatment. Two deaths occurred at the time of shunt placement as a result of fetal trauma. One occurred 6 weeks following shunt placement and was associated with central nervous system abnormalities. Premature labor occurred in only one patient (48 hours following shunt placement), but the fetus survived. With such considerable risk associated with fetal intervention, the establishment of significant benefit of the procedure becomes essential.

In order to evaluate more critically the potential benefit of in utero intervention, Elder reviewed the American experience with prenatal intervention through 1985. This included 58 cases, with vesicoamniotic shunts having been placed in 37 per cent. Elder noted a 44 per cent complication rate, which included inadequate shunt drainage or migration (19 per cent), onset of premature labor within 48 hours (12 per cent), urinary ascites (7 per cent), and chorioamnionitis (5 per cent). Of 28 fetuses with associated oligohydramnios, only 6 (21 per cent) survived. In no case could Elder clearly demonstrate an improvement in renal function as a result of prenatal intervention. In two cases, restoration of amniotic fluid dynamics by vesicoamniotic shunting seemed to have allowed normal pulmonary development to have occurred.

Thus, it seems that the fetus with bilateral obstructive uropathy and oligohydramnios is most likely to die from pulmonary hypoplasia. Prenatal drainage of the urinary tract seems unlikely to influence renal function. Perhaps it is more appropriate to concentrate on restoring amniotic fluid dynamics to improve pulmonary development rather than relieving obstructive uropathy in order to maximize fetal survival.

CONCLUSION

Our appreciation for the complexity of the diagnosis of prenatal hydronephrosis has evolved considerably since Harrison's case report of 1982. Although laboratory investigations have suggested the potential physiologic benefit of in utero intervention, unequivocal confirmatory clinical evidence has been lacking. As our ability to select those few fetuses that may benefit from in utero intervention is refined, so, too, should our assessment of this modality develop. Clearly, for the present, the greatest benefit of diagnosing hydronephrosis prenatally is identifying the child who can be treated promptly postnatally to preserve renal function and prevent serious illness.

Suggested Readings

Elder JS, Duckett JW, Snyder HM: Intervention for fetal obstructive uropathy: Has it been effective? Lancet 2: 1007–1010, 1987

Harrison MR, Golbus MS, Filly RA, et al: Fetal surgery for congenital hydronephrosis. N Engl J Med 306:591–593, 1982

Manning FA: Fetal surgery for obstructive uropathy: Rational considerations. Am J Kidney Dis 10:259–267, 1987

Manning FA, Harrison MR, Rodeck C: Catheter shunts for fetal hydronephrosis and hydrocephalus. N Engl J Med 315:336–340, 1986

CONGENITAL MEGACALYCES

ANTHONY ATALA, M.D.

Boston, Massachusetts

Congenital megacalyces, or megacalycosis, was first described by Puigvert in 1963. The renal calyces, although usually ectatic, may be normal in number but often are increased to as many as 36 (instead of the normal 8 to 12). The renal pelvis is not dilated and has a normal wall thickness. The ureteropelvic junction is normal, without any evidence of obstruction. Although the cortex is normal in thickness, the medullary pyramids are underdeveloped. There is generally a malformation of the renal papillae and a defect in tubular concentrating ability. The collecting tubules are not dilated but are shorter than normal, with a transverse rather than a vertical orientation from the cortical medullary junction. Glomerular filtration, tubular isotope uptake, and plasma flow are normal.

The embryologic cause of congenital megacalyces is unknown. Several theories have been proposed, including a faulty metanephric ureteral bud embryogenesis. It is believed that there may be a transient delay in the recanalization of the upper ureter after the branches of the ureteral bud hook up with the metanephric blastema. This delay may produce a limited period of obstruction when the embryonic glomeruli start producing urine. The calyces may dilate and then retain their obstructed appearance despite the lack of postnatal obstruction. The increased number of calyces may be due to an arrest of the coalescence of terminal ureteral buddings and may occur in response to the transient period of obstruction at a critical time in development. Other theories proposed for the etiology of congenital megacalyces include hypoplasia of the juxtamedullary glomeruli, which may account for a lack of renal concentrating ability, as well as maldevelopment of the pelvicalyceal muscle.

Megacalycosis occurs predominantly in males in a ratio of 6:1. Segmental unilateral involvement is seen exclusively in females, whereas bilateral disease has been seen only in males. This distribution suggests that an X-linked, partially recessive gene with reduced penetrance in females is a possible causative factor.

Megacalycosis may lead to urinary stasis, which predisposes children to urinary tract infection and adults to stone formation and hematuria. The diagnosis usually is made with an excretory urogram. Although the ureteropelvic junction does not appear obstructed, there may be segmental dilation of the distal third of the ureter. In addition, megacalycosis has been associated with an ipsilateral megaureter. This combination of anatomic abnormalities may be mistaken for congenital ureteropelvic or ureterovesical junction obstruction, but no obstruction at these locations has been demonstrated. It is important, therefore, to be aware of this condition so as to avoid unnecessary surgery. Once this condition has been diagnosed, an increased fluid intake is recommended in order to reduce the chances for stone formation and other complications that might arise.

Suggested Readings

Kimsche D, Lask D: Megacalycosis. Urology 19:478, 1982

Talner LB, Gittes RF: Megacalyces. Clin Radiol 23:55, 1972

Talner LB, Gittes RF: Megacalyces: Further observations and differentiation from obstructive renal disease. Am J Roentgenol Radium Ther Nucl Med 121:473, 1974

Vargas B, Lebowitz RL: The coexistence of congenital megacalyces and primary megaureter. Am J Roentgenol 147:313, 1986

RENAL PYELOCALYCEAL DIVERTICULA

MARC P. BANNER, M.D.

Philadelphia, Pennsylvania

Pyelocalyceal diverticula are round or oval outpouchings of the collecting system into the renal parenchyma. They contain urine that is derived by passive filling from the adjacent normal collecting system, with which they communicate via a narrow channel. Diverticula are smooth walled, lined by nonsecretory transitional cell epithelium, and usually small (<1 cm in diameter), asymptomatic, and incidentally discovered during excretory urography (frequency of 0.2 to 0.4 per cent). They are most often unilocular but may be multilocular or septated. Most are congenital in origin, resulting from abnormal branching of the ureteral bud, but they may develop from traumatic calyceal laceration or erosion of a renal abscess into the collecting system. The great majority are related to polar calyces (usually the upper pole); a few originate from the renal pelvis or infundibula—hence the proper terminology, pyelocalyceal diverticula. Both kidneys and sexes are affected equally.

Radiologic diagnosis is usually straightforward, although diverticula may be mistaken for acquired hydrocalyces with stenotic infundibula or even communicating renal cysts or abscesses on urography, ultrasonography, or computerized tomography. Demonstration of a normal adjacent calyx differentiates calyceal diverticula from papillary necrosis.

Small diverticula rarely require treatment, but larger ones may be symptomatic either by virtue of their size alone or by associated complications, such as flank pain related to infection, poor drainage, abscess formation, pressure on adjacent calyces or renal parenchyma, or calculi (formed stones or milk-of-calcium). Calculi result from stasis of urine. They have been noted in from 9.5 to 39 per cent of pyelocalyceal diverticula but may not be symptomatic. They rarely pass spontaneously because of the narrow diverticular neck. When a calculus is present, there often is scarring and atrophy of the overlying parenchyma.

Indications for intervention include chronic or recurrent pain, infection, or evidence of progressive local renal damage.

Treatment for symptomatic pyelocalyceal diverticula has changed dramatically. Previously managed by surgical unroofing, nephrotomy with closure of the narrow communication with the collecting system, marsupialization onto the surface of the kidney and fulguration, or partial or even complete nephrectomy, symptomatic pyelocalyceal diverticula currently are managed with endourologic techniques.

Direct percutaneous puncture of a diverticulum, dilation of its neck, and intubation with a large nephrostomy catheter for several weeks usually traumatizes the lining of the diverticulum sufficiently to eventuate in its obliteration by granulation once the nephrostomy is removed. Approaching diverticula indirectly via their infundibula with flexible instruments does not produce as favorable an obliteration rate as the direct approach.

Fulguration of the wall has been used for large-volume diverticula. Percutaneous drainage of a diverticular abscess can be followed by sclerosis with absolute alcohol if the diverticulum no longer communicates with the collecting system.

Nonoperative treatment of stones in calyceal diverticula has generated considerable controversy. Extracorporeal lithotripsy may relieve symptomatology (70 per cent in the short term but only 39 per cent long term) but leaves 80 per cent of patients with residual stone fragments. Although noninvasive, it may not be a cost-effective method of managing diverticular stones. Primary percutaneous nephrostolithotomy can render 87.5 per cent of patients stone free and relieve symptoms in all. Obliteration of the diverticulum (with or without fulguration) is an added advantage of percutaneous management.

Suggested Readings

Ellis JH, Patterson SK, Sonda LP, et al: Stones and infection in renal caliceal diverticula: Treatment with percutaneous procedures. AJR 156:995, 1991

Hulbert JC, Reddy PK, Hunter DW, et al: Percutaneous techniques for the management of caliceal diverticula containing calculi. J Urol 135:225, 1986

Jones JA, Lingeman JE, Steidle CP: The roles of extracorporeal shock wave lithotripsy and percutaneous nephrostolithotomy in the management of pyelocaliceal diverticula. J Urol 146:724, 1991

Psihramis KE, Dretler SP: Extracorporeal shock wave lithotripsy of caliceal diverticula calculi. J Urol 138:707, 1987

Wulfsohn MA: Pyelocaliceal diverticula. J Urol 123:1, 1980

CONGENITAL SPONGE KIDNEY

KEVIN K. GANDHI, M.D.

Chicago, Illinois

Congenital sponge kidney is a well-defined clinical entity characterized by cystic dilation of the collecting tubules in one or more renal papillae. The radiographic features initially were described in 1939 by Lenarduzzi. Ten years later, Cacchi and Ricca coined the term "medullary sponge kidney" (MSK) to describe the radiographic and gross pathologic features that on transection appeared similar to a sponge.

MSK is generally an asymptomatic condition and may go undetected if complications of the disease never become manifest. For this reason, the true incidence remains unknown but is estimated to be 1:5000 to 1:20,000. Initially, men and women were thought to be involved equally, but new data support the conclusion that symptomatic cases are more common among women. MSK does not appear to be inherited and, although considered a congenital disease, it is rarely seen in children as an isolated lesion. More commonly, it is associated with hemihypertrophy, Ehlers-Danlos disease, Caroli's disease, and adult polycystic kidney disease. A wide spectrum of changes are seen in MSK. On occasion, the disease is limited to a single pyramid on one kidney, although in more than 75 per cent of cases both kidneys are involved, with many pyramids in each kidney being affected.

Renal colic, infection, and hematuria are complications that can transform MSK into a serious illness. These symptoms usually occur in the third to fifth decade of life and, if not treated, may result in sepsis and renal failure. Dilation of the collection tubules and stasis may be responsible for the increased susceptibility to infection and stone formation. Characteristically, calcium oxalate and hydroxyapatite stones form, and may result from renal tubular acidosis and hypercalciuria. Hematuria associated with MSK is usually without proteinuria and of little concern. Remarkable proteinuria should alert the clinician to concurrent disease processes.

The diagnosis of MSK is made radiographically with an intravenous pyelogram. Common findings include an enlarged kidney, papillary blush, cystic dilations filled with contrast, and elongated papillary tubes. Also, nephrocalcinosis is found in 50 per cent of patients with MSK. The diagnosis can be difficult because there exist a spectrum of radiolographic findings, some subtle, that define MSK. Other diagnostic tests, such as computerized tomography and ultrasound, have proven inferior to intravenous pyelography.

On pathologic inspection, the kidney is reniform in shape and may be slightly enlarged. The cystic dilatation is between 1–5 mm and may be lined with columnar, cuboidal or transitional epithelium. The cystic tubes are continuous with the collecting system but may be blocked with desquamated cells.

The management of MSK is aimed at aggressively treating infections and stone disease. Urinary tract infections should be treated with antibiotics and manipulation of the genitourinary system should be discouraged. If infection is associated with stone disease, it is an exercise in futility to treat the infection without eradicating the stones. This can be done with extracorporeal shock-wave lithotripsy. If stones are present, it has been shown that thiazide therapy can reduce the number of recurrent stone episodes and calcifications. Surgical intervention should be avoided in children because MSK can be a diffuse bilateral process and resection may remove precious renal tissue. In adults, surgical intervention should be limited and kidney sparing.

Suggested Readings

Gednoyc WMW, Saxton HM: More medullary sponge variants. Clin Radiol 39:423, 1988

Ginalski JM, Schynder P, Portmann L, et al: Medullary sponge kidney on axial computed tomography: Comparison with excretory urography. Eur J Radiol 12:104, 1991

Osther PJ, Hansen AB, Rohl HF: Renal acidification defects in medullary sponge kidney. Br J Urol 61:392, 1988

Parks JH, Coe FL, Straoss AL: Calcium nephrolithiasis and medullary sponge kidney in women. N Engl J Med 18:1088, 1982

Yendt ER: Medullary sponge kidney and nephrolithiasis. N Engl J Med 306:1106, 1982

Yendt ER, Cohanim M: Prevention of calcium stones with thiazides. Kidney Int 13:397, 1978

SIMPLE RENAL CYSTS

RANDALL P. SINGLETON, M.D.

San Antonio, Texas

The diagnostic dilemma of asymptomatic simple renal cysts lies in determining whether the mass lesion is a cyst or a renal carcinoma. Therefore, the treatment of the mass lesion is predicated on the ability to differentiate it from a renal adenocarcinoma. With the advent of many diagnostic procedures, the diagnosis of renal cysts should be in the 98th percentile of accuracy. With the use of nephrotomography, ultrasonography, cyst puncture, computerized tomography (CT), and renal angiography, there is seldom a situation in which the diagnosis of simple renal cysts cannot be ascertained, but, when tumor cannot be excluded, surgical exploration of the renal mass is indicated.

Renal cysts are usually asymptomatic but occasionally present with flank discomfort; therefore, the diagnosis of renal cyst usually is made when one is found on routine intravenous pyelogram. After routine nephrotomography was combined with intravenous pyelogram, more asymptomatic renal cysts have been found. This technique also has been helpful in distinguishing a solid renal mass from a typical radiolucent renal cyst. After the diagnosis of a renal mass has been made, the stepwise progressive work-up of this lesion becomes controversial. Before the advent of the CT scan, the standard work-up usually began with ultrasonography of the lesion. If the lesion was found to be without any internal echoes (sonolucent), one proceeded directly to percutaneous aspiration of the lesion. If the lesion was solid or appeared suspicious for tumor, one went directly to renal angiography. If renal angiography demonstrates tumor staining and puddling or neovascularity, the diagnosis of adenocarcinoma was made. When angiography demonstrates an avascular mass, the clinical decision of whether to proceed with cyst puncture or surgical exploration had to be made.

The dilemma of sticking a needle into a tumor versus an open renal exploration for a benign cyst is then encountered. Even though it is against basic tumor principles to needle a tumor, because of the theoretic possibility of seeding the needle tract with tumor cells, vast clinical experience has shown that this rarely happens. The technique of cyst puncture may vary, but the basic principle advocated by Lange is the one most commonly used. The exact location of the cyst is ascertained by preliminary intravenous pyelogram with fluoroscopy or by the use of ultrasound. The patient then is placed in the prone position, and the skin is anesthetized with a local anesthetic. A 20-gauge, short-beveled spinal needle is introduced through the skin into the lesion with the aid of fluoroscopy or ultrasonography. The patient is instructed to hold his or her breath while the needle is slowly advanced into the lesion to prevent tearing of the cyst wall. Once the lesion has been entered, a flexible plastic tube is attached to the needle, and a measured amount of cyst fluid is removed. Most of the fluid removed is then replaced with contrast material. The needle is withdrawn, and a number of radiographs are taken from different positions to inspect all sides of the cyst wall. If all the sides of the cyst wall appear smooth, this corresponds to the typical appearance of a simple cyst and rules out the presence of a possible tumor in the cyst wall.

The cyst fluid that has been removed is sent for cytologic testing (Papanicolaou smear) and analysis of fat content. The fat content is almost always zero in a typical renal cyst, with an occasional trace amount. In almost all tumors, the fat content is high, but this also may be the case in an inflammatory cyst. The cytology is extremely important because the results are positive in almost 100 per cent of cases if it is a tumor. The appearance of the cyst fluid is also very important, because cyst fluid is usually clear. The presence of bloody fluid in an atraumatic cyst puncture is a definite indication to proceed with further diagnostic tests or surgical exploration. The cyst puncture has another advantage in addition to confirming the diagnosis of renal cysts. It has been reported that approximately 25 to 35 per cent of the cysts will disappear after needle aspiration alone.

With the advent of CT, another important tool has been added to the diagnosis of the mass lesion of the kidney. CT has the advantage of being totally noninvasive but also the disadvantage of being an expensive procedure. The final word on the diagnostic accuracy of the CT scan has not been determined as yet, but it appears to be very high. It has the ability to show clearly the demarcation of the mass from the normal renal parenchyma and the thickness of the wall of the mass, and it can assign attenuation value to the mass itself to determine if it is of water or tissue density. The technique of CT scanning is very simple. The only requirement is that the patient be able to stop breathing for 18 seconds, which is the time required to complete each scan. The scan is done both with and without contrast material to enhance visualization of the collecting systems and to distinguish tissue and water densities. The densitometer values used in CT vary for different types of equipment, but cyst fluid essentially should have a zero reading, as does water, versus 30 to 50 Hounsfield units for normal renal parenchyma. CT has an extremely high accuracy for a noninvasive test, and is in the 90 to 95 per cent range.

Once the diagnosis of renal cyst has been made, there is no indication for surgical treatment unless complications arise. The indications for surgical intervention with renal cysts are: (1) infection; (2) persistent pain that has not been relieved with cyst puncture; (3) obstruction of the ureter or renal calyx causing progressive hydronephrosis and destruction of renal parenchyma; and (4) to rule out a possible carcinoma if all diagnostic tests were indeterminate. Another rare indication for surgery is the presence of polycythemia, because renal cysts have been known to produce erythropoietin.

The flank approach is used for the removal of renal cysts unless there is a high suspicion of carcinoma. If the kidney is explored for a carcinoma, it is best to explore it transabdominally or thoracoabdominally so that the renal vessels can be exposed and clamped before removing the renal lesion. Once the kidney is visualized through the flank approach, the typical blue dome cyst is exposed after Gerota's fascia has been removed. The cyst wall then is opened and the cyst fluid is drained. The cyst wall is excised, and any suspicious areas should be biopsied and sent for frozen section. The base of the cyst that is within the renal parenchyma should be left alone and not excised. If it is excised, it causes excessive bleeding and also damages the renal parenchyma. The remaining cyst wall then is secured with 3-0 chromic suture in a running lock stitch around the edges for hemostasis. The incision is closed, and a small Penrose drain is inserted for a few days. This procedure has a very low morbidity rate and a less than 2 per cent mortality rate.

Suggested Readings

Bosniak MA: Difficulties in classifying cystic lesions of the kidney. Uro-Radiology 13:91–93, 1991

Castillo OA, Boyle ET Jr: Multilocular cysts of kidney—a study of 29 patients and review of literature. Urology 37:156–162, 1991

Dalton D, Neiman H, Grayhack JT: The natural history of simple renal cysts—a preliminary study. J Urol 135: 905–908, 1986

MULTICYSTIC KIDNEY

KENNETH I. GLASSBERG, M.D.

Brooklyn, New York

Schwartz, in 1938, was probably the first to propose the term "multicystic kidney" when he described a kidney that he removed from a 7-month-old child that contained multiple cysts of various sizes without evidence of normal renal tissue. Because they translate to the same meaning, the terms "multicystic" and "polycystic" have been confused all too frequently. However, as stressed by Spence in 1955, when used to describe clinical entities they clearly imply separate conditions.

The typical multicystic kidney has a "bunch of grapes" appearance, without a well-defined hilum or hilar vessels. It is nonrenoform in shape and there is little intervening stroma between the cysts. Those multicystic dysplastic kidneys that are made up predominately of cysts and have little stroma are referred to as the typical multicystic kidney, and those kidneys made up predominantly of stroma, having small cysts and more solid in appearance, sometimes are referred to as solid cystic dysplasia. It has become clear from clinical reports that a large percentage of multicystic kidneys get smaller with time, and may get so small they may not be identifiable by sonography. At this involuted stage, these kidneys represent a form of renal aplasia in which a "nubbin" of nonrenoform tissue is found in the renal fossa.

Multicystic dysplasia may involve one side of a horseshoe kidney or one pole of a duplex kidney.

HISTOLOGY

The cysts range in size from microscopic to grossly palpable. They are lined by epithelial cells and are separated by stroma that contains fibrous tissue and primitive dysplastic tissue. Primitive ducts must be present for the diagnosis. These ducts are lined by cuboidal or tall columnar cells. The ducts are surrounding by concentric rings composed of collagen and smooth muscle cells. Immature glomeruli and cartilage also may be present. The ureter is partly or totally atretic, and a renal pelvis-like structure may be present. Those kidneys with a pelvis-like structure may have connecting structures between the cysts and the pelvis. Multicystic kidneys without a pelvis have been referred to by Griscom et al. as pyeloinfundibular atresia. When a pelvis is present, Felson and Cussen have referred to that variety of multicystic kidney as the "hydronephrotic type." Kidneys that have some primitive glomeruli may on occasion even demonstrate a few percentage points of function on a dimercaptosuccinic acid renal scan.

ETIOLOGY

There is no genetic predisposition, so it is hard to account for why the abnormality develops. Felson and Cussen suggested that it is the outcome of hydronephrosis secondary to atresia of the ureter, pelvis, or infundibuli, findings that usually coexist. The condition appears predominantly on the left side and more often in males, just as do other conditions that are obstructive in nature, such as ureteropelvic junction obstruction and primary obstructive megaureter. If obstruction is the cause, it must happen early because dysplasia can be induced experimentally only in early gestation.

CLINICAL PRESENTATION

Gordon et al. estimated the incidence of unilateral multicystic kidneys to be 1 in 4300 live births. It is one of the two most common genitourinary causes for an abdominal mass in infancy (the other being ureteropelvic junction obstruction). The diagnosis is made more often now antenatally because of the prevalence of ultrasound studies during pregnancy. In many instances, there is either a ureteropelvic junction obstruction or a dilated but not necessarily obstructed renal pelvis on the contralateral side, another finding suggesting multicystic kidney to be secondary to obstruction. The condition may be bilateral. Bilaterality is associated with the findings of classic Potter syndrome and is not compatible with life.

The condition may be present in adulthood as an incidental finding when an abdominal imaging procedure is done for some other reason, or may on occasion be a cause for abdominal pain in an adult. In some of these adults, Ambrose found removal of the kidney to be associated with relief of the abdominal pain.

IMAGING STUDIES

The diagnosis most often is made by renal ultrasound and most often is confused with severe hydronephrosis. The most characteristic sonographic findings of a multicystic kidney are a non–renal-shaped cystic flank mass with visible interfaces between the cysts, a nonmedial or noncentral location of the largest cyst, absence of visible communications between the cysts, and absence of an identifiable renal sinus. If a renal sinus is identifiable, if the most medial cyst is the largest, or if there is communication of the peripheral cyst with a central large cyst, the diagnosis of hydronephrosis is more likely. It is easy to overlook a renal sinus on ultrasound exam, so the absence of one may not be that pertinent. In multicystic dysplasia, the cysts usually are distributed in a haphazard way, whereas in severe ureteropelvic junction obstruction, the cysts (i.e., calyces) are situated on the periphery around a central cyst (i.e., renal pelvis) (Fig. 1).

Radioisotope studies may be helpful. Rarely, is any function seen in multicystic kidneys unless there are a significant number of primitive glomeruli or the hydronephrotic form of multicystic kidney is present. In severe ureteropelvic junction obstruction, almost always there is some function.

Percutaneous contrast studies may or may not demonstrate communication between the cysts. We have demonstrated communications between cysts by contrast injection both percutaneously and ex vivo.

A hemitrigone may be seen on cystoscopy, but more often a ureteric orifice is present and associated with an atretic ureter. Cystoscopy and retrograde ureterography rarely if ever are indicated in the work-up.

Contralateral vesicoureteral reflux is present in a significant number of patients, making it advisable to obtain a voiding cystourethrogram routinely. Heikkinen et al. found 4 of 13 patients with a multicystic kidney to have contralateral reflux. Sixty-five of 441 cases included in the Multicystic Kidney Registry of the American Academy of Pediatrics, Section of Urology, have had a voiding cystourethrogram, and in 43 per cent contralateral reflux was found.

PROGNOSIS AND MANAGEMENT

The decision of whether or not to remove a multicystic kidney should be based on what the expected outcome is for a multicystic kidney. On the basis of preliminary data accumulated by the Multicystic Registry of the American Academy of Pediatrics, Section on Urology, Wacksman and Phipps have concluded that the multicystic kidney does not need to be removed immediately. Of course, exceptions occur, such as when the kidney is so large that it is causing respiratory or feeding problems or when the pediatric urologist is not confident in the diagnosis. If it is decided to remove a multicystic kidney, the surgery is straightforward, with little risk of bleeding because the vessels supplying these kidneys are usually quite small. The kidney is mobilized easily, and, if its size creates difficulty for removal, the cysts can be punctured to make the kidney considerably smaller.

The multicystic kidney is a dynamic condition that changes both in utero and in the years following birth. The same criteria used to diagnose multicystic kidneys in infants and children may be used to diagnose multicystic kidneys in utero.

There are enough reports in the literature to suggest that, when a multicystic kidney is diagnosed early in pregnancy, the kidney and its cysts will continue to grow initially but

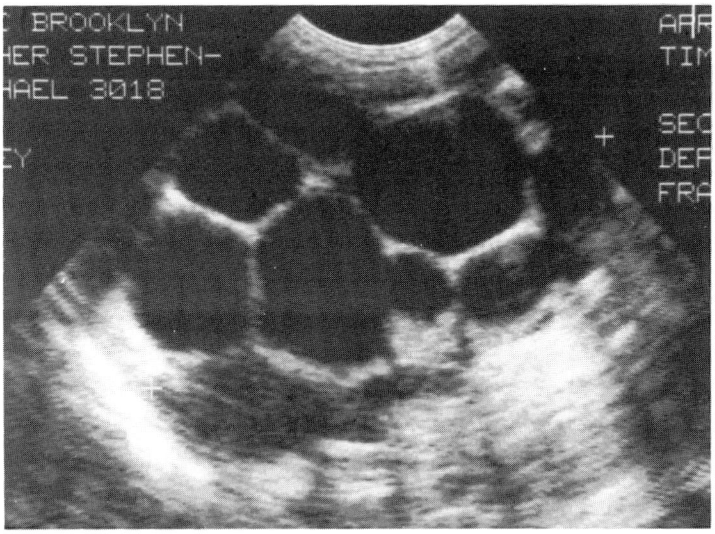

FIGURE 1. Typical sonographic appearance of a multicystic kidney.

that many of these kidneys get smaller prior to birth and still more will continue to get smaller after birth (Table 1). Not only do they get smaller, but a large percentage will involute with time and not be identifiable by ultrasound study. In the Multicystic Kidney Registry 18 per cent disappeared on ultrasound studies in the first year of life, 13 per cent in the next 2 years, and 23 per cent between the third and fifth year of life. On the basis of these statistics, within 5 years, 54 per cent of multicystic kidneys will become nonidentifiable on imaging studies. Hashimoto et al. suggested that a decrease in function may account for the decrease in size in many of these kidneys. The fluid present in some kidneys at first may represent fluid produced by primitive glomeruli or even a few mature glomeruli. With time, some of the nephrons will fibrose, causing the kidneys to shrink as less fluid accumulates within the cysts.

It frequently is recommended to remove these kidneys because of the possibility of hypertension or malignant degeneration. As regards hypertension, Gordon et al. found only nine well-documented cases with hypertension in the literature over the previous 20 years, and in only three did the hypertension disappear after nephrectomy. In the Multicystic Kidney Registry of 441 patients, none presented with hypertension and none have developed hypertension, with some patients having been followed for 5 years.

The likelihood of malignant degeneration seems to be very small. Only seven such patients have been described in the literature, and in none of them was the kidney previously recognized to be a multicystic one. With perhaps as many as 1000 children being born with multicystic kidneys per year, the incidence of malignancy seems to be almost negligible. Two of the seven cases were reported

TABLE 1. Long-Term Follow-up of Neonatal Multicystic Kidneys

	No. of Infants	Follow-up (months)	Decreased in Size*	Increased in Size	No Change in Size
Gordon et al.	11	Greater than 12 (mean 15)	8 (2)	0	3
Avni et al.	9	1–36	7 (3)	0†	2
Rickwood et al.	33	14–73 (mean 36)	19 (10)	0	14
Multicystic Registry (Wacksman and Phipps)	215	12–36	132 (29)	3	80

*Number in parentheses indicates those kidneys that are no longer identifiable by sonography.
†One kidney became more solid and was removed, probably representing solid cystic dysplasia.

as Wilms' tumor, one in a 10-month-old child and the other in a 4-year-old; four cases were reported as renal cell carcinoma in patients 15 to 68 years of age; and one 68-year-old had an embryonal carcinoma. The fact that none of these kidneys were diagnosed as multicystic kidneys prior to presentation makes the diagnosis questionable in some, although in those with an absent or atretic ipsilateral ureter, the diagnosis of multicystic kidney was probably the correct one. To date, in no case in the Wilms' tumor registry (over 260 kidneys) was there an associated multicystic kidney.

Jung et al. have obtained flow cytometric analysis on multicystic kidneys from 30 patients. They found no evidence of tetraploidy or aneuploidy, findings that, if present, would be considered preneoplastic. Some reports have identified nephrogenic rests of nodular renal blastema or Wilms' tumorlets and suggest these findings may support removing multicystic kidneys. However, these findings may be present in a small percentage of normal kidneys and in the vast majority will involute and never be identified.

Wacksman and Phipps suggested that 8000 multicystic kidneys will need to be removed to prevent one tumor, and perhaps 20,000 nephrectomies will need to be performed to prevent one death secondary to the tumor. A greater number of nephrectomies done to prevent one tumor, of course, would be associated with an increasing chance of causing a death secondary to the anesthesia.

It is hoped that the long-term follow-up of multicystic kidney (i.e., beyond 5 years, as the Multicystic Kidney Registry plans to do) will better define the expected outcome. Questions still must be answered. Does the disappearance on an imaging study of a multicystic kidney mean that the patient is no longer at risk? If there is a potential for cancer, should not that potential still exist, because the cells and dysplastic tissue remain and only the fluid has disappeared? It is important to know how long these patients must be followed, because many will become lost to follow-up. What we do know is that the vast majority of multicystic kidneys that are not removed will never cause a clinical problem.

Suggested Readings

Ambrose SS: Unilateral multicystic renal disease in adults. Birth Defects 13:349, 1976

Avni E, Thova Y, Lalmand B, et al: Multicystic dysplastic kidney: Natural history from in utero diagnosis and postnatal followup. J Urol 138:1420, 1987

Felson B, Cussen LJ: The hydronephrotic type of congenital multicystic disease of the kidney. Semin Roentgenol 10:113, 1975

Glassberg KI: Renal dysplasia and cystic disease of the kidney. *In* Walsh PC, Retik AB, Stamey TA, et al. (eds), Campbell's Urology, 6th ed, Philadelphia, WB Saunders, 1992, pp 1443–1495

Gordon AC, Thomas DFM, Arthur RJ, et al: Multicystic dysplastic kidney: Is nephrectomy still appropriate? J Urol 140:1231, 1988

Griscom NT, Vawter FG, Gellers FX: Pelvoinfundibular atresia: The usual form of multicystic kidney: 44 unilateral and two bilateral cases. Semin Roentgenol 10: 125, 1975

Hashimoto B, Filly R, Cullen P: Multicystic dysplastic kidney in utero: Changing appearance of US. Radiology 159:107, 1986

Heikkinen ES, Herva R, Lanning P: Multicystic kidney: A clinical and histologic study of 13 patients. Ann Chir Gynaecol 69:15, 1980

Jung WH, Peters CA, Mandell JA, et al: Flow cytometric evaluation of multicystic dysplastic kidney. J Urol 144: 143, 1990

Rickwood MK, Anderson PAM, Williams MPL: Multicystic renal dysplasia detected by prenatal ultrasonography. Natural history and results of conservative management. Br J Urol 69:538–540, 1992

Wacksman J, Phipps L: Report of the Multicystic Kidney Registry: A long term follow up. J Urol (in press).

AUTOSOMAL DOMINANT POLYCYSTIC KIDNEY DISEASE

MARGUERITE C. LIPPERT, M.D.

Charlottesville, Virginia

Autosomal dominant polycystic kidney disease (ADPKD) is the most common form of cystic renal disease and is one of the most common hereditary diseases that is potentially fatal. It accounts for 6 to 12 per cent of patients on chronic renal dialysis. ADPKD is characterized by bilateral cystic disease in enlarged kidneys, often associated with hepatic cysts, cardiac valve lesions, and intracranial aneurysms.

CLINICAL FEATURES

In the absence of family screening, ADPKD patients can present symptomatically with hematuria, pain (abdominal or flank), headache, or urinary tract infection between the ages of 30 and 40 years. Renal failure requiring dialysis or renal transplantation occurs after age 50, although creatinine can begin to rise between ages 40 and 50 years. Without dialysis or renal transplantation, patients died of uremia (59 per cent), heart failure, or cerebral hemorrhages, with a mean age of death of 50 years. However, with family screening, asymptomatic ADPKD patients are being diagnosed at a much younger age because renal ultrasound typically can reveal asymptomatic renal cysts between the ages of 10 and 30 years. With earlier diagnosis, asymptomatic ADPKD patients are being treated for hypertension early, which may partially account for why currently only 53 per cent of ADPKD patients reach end-stage renal disease (ESRD) by age 73. However, the ability to diagnose asymptomatic ADPKD patients also is allowing us to identify phenotypes who do not develop ESRD or other symptoms until their 70s, regardless of treatment.

Less than 10 per cent of ADPKD patients present in the first decade of life. Children presenting at an early age with symptomatic ADPKD are a distinctly different group than those who are diagnosed by family screening. Those children diagnosed as having ADPKD under 1 year of age may have a deterioration of renal function early in life. Neonates typically are diagnosed because of renomegaly, although severe disease can result in stillbirth or respiratory distress. Ultrasound screening in children at risk for ADPKD has revealed many asymptomatic children with the disease. Simple renal cysts are so rare in children that detection of any renal cyst on ultrasound in a child at risk for ADPKD is probably diagnostic. In children who present with symptoms after 1 year of age, usual symptoms are renomegaly, hypertension, and hematuria. Early and late symptomatic presentations of ADPKD can occur within the same family.

ADPKD patients may develop cysts in the liver, pancreas, ovaries, testes, thyroid, spleen, pineal gland, and subarachnoid space. Liver function remains normal despite the fact that 50 per cent of ADPKD patients have hepatic cysts. With the advent of dialysis of ESRD, more ADPKD patients are surviving with cystic liver changes. Although usually asymptomatic, the liver cysts may cause abdominal pain or swelling.

Cardiovascular abnormalities such as cardiac valve anomalies and possibly aortic aneurysms have been reported with increased incidence in ADPKD patients. Routine echocardiography with Doppler analysis revealed 26 per cent incidence of mitral valve prolapse, 31 per cent incidence of mitral incompetence, 8 per cent incidence of aortic incompetence, and 6 per cent incidence of tricuspid prolapse in ADPKD patients. Other nonrenal manifestations of ADPKD involve increased incidence of inguinal hernias, hiatal hernias, colonic diverticula, and cholangiosarcoma.

ADPKD patients may present with rupture of an intracranial aneurysm. Four to 40 per cent of ADPKD patients have asymptomatic, unruptured cranial aneurysms on both autopsy and prospective angiography studies. However, familial clustering of intracranial aneurysms has been observed. Perhaps the increased rupture of intracerebral aneurysms in ADPKD patients is secondary to the hypertension that is common in ADPKD. Perhaps earlier treatment of hypertension in ADPKD patients will result in fewer deaths from intracranial hemorrhage. In addition, ADPKD patients with family histories suggestive of subarachnoid hemorrhage or intracranial aneurysms could be screened with magnetic resonance imaging (MRI), angiography, or high-resolution computerized tomography (CT).

Mild to moderate hypertension antedates the onset of ESRD in about 60 per cent of ADPKD patients. Prior to ESRD, ADPKD patients with larger renal volume as a result of increased numbers and sizes of cysts had a higher incidence of early hypertension. Enlarging cysts theoretically could compress renal vessels, causing renal ischemia, and thereby activate the renin-angiotensin-aldosterone system. Angiotensin-converting enzyme inhibitor therapy in hypertensive ADPKD patients with massive cystic involvement and chronic renal insufficiency has caused reversible renal deterioration, perhaps because these patients are more likely to rely on angiotensin-mediated efferent arteriolar tone to maintain glomerular filtration rate. The pathogenesis of hypertension may be caused by different mechanisms at different stages of ADPKD. However, this mild to moderate hypertension responds well to drug treatment. Antihypertensive treatment may retard the development of ESRD and decreases the incidence of rupture of intracranial aneurysms.

Pain in the flank or abdomen is a common presenting symptom of ADPKD. Acute pain could be secondary to cyst hemorrhage, obstruction from stone or blood clot, infection, or tumor. Distinguishing among these various etiologies is difficult but important, because early treatment of obstruction or infection can help preserve future renal function. Chronic pain occurs as the renal cysts enlarge and may be secondary to stretching of the renal capsule or pressure on adjacent organs.

Hematuria, gross or microscopic, also is common, occurring in up to 64 per cent of ADPKD patients. Etiologies of hematuria include calculi, rupture of hemorrhagic cyst into the collecting system, tumor, or infection. Hematuria evaluation must exclude all of these diagnoses with history and imaging studies.

PATHOGENESIS

Cysts in ADPKD patients initially develop as diverticuli or outpouchings in any part of the normal renal tubules (including collecting ducts and glomerular capsule). In these early stages, the cyst fluid is from glomerular filtrate, but, as the cyst enlarges, the fluid is secreted from the epithelium because the cysts lose connection from the tubule of origin.

Multiple theories have struggled to explain why ADPKD kidneys form renal cysts. One theory suggests that renal cyst epithelium is hyperplastic. The frequency of micropolyps and hyperplasia in ADPKD kidneys would support the hyperplastic epithelium theory. Biologically active substances in the cyst fluid may be synthesized by the epithelium and modulate the progression of enlargement of ADPKD kidneys. A second theory offers a structurally altered tubular basement membrane with resultant altered compliance of the tubular wall. Such a system-wide hereditable defect in basement membrane could account for other ADPKD defects, such as hepatic cysts, cerebral artery aneurysms, prolapsed mitral valves, and colonic diverticula, and cysts in the pancreas, spleen, lungs, and epididymis. A third theory suggests defective proteins in the extracellular connective tissue matrix, which also would account for the aforementioned abnormalities in other organs. These theories probably are all interrelated but the initiating factor is controversial.

As the cysts enlarge, normal parenchyma is thinly displaced, which may account for the development of renal failure. However, there is an ADPKD phenotype without renal failure.

MORPHOLOGY

ADPKD kidneys are huge because they are filled with hundreds of fluid-filled cysts ranging in size from a few millimeters to a few centimeters. The kidneys retain their reniform shape but are studded with cysts in the cortical and medullary parenchyma.

The cysts are lined by a single layer of flattened cuboidal or columnar epithelium. Cysts involve all elements of the nephron and collecting ducts. Islands of normal renal parenchyma can be found between cysts. When renal failure is imminent or present, arteriosclerosis and interstitial fibrosis are common. As renal function deteriorates, the incidence of hyperplastic polyps in ADPKD kidneys increased despite dialysis.

RADIOLOGIC EVALUATION AND DIAGNOSIS

CT scanning with contrast enhancement is the most sensitive diagnostic procedure for ADPKD. However, renal ultrasonography may be a more pragmatic screening tool because patients avoid radiation exposure. Renal ultrasound should pick up 7.2 per cent of those patients at risk for ADPKD between ages 15 and 25 years (Fig. 1). Both abdominal CT scan and renal sonography are advantageous over intravenous pyelography (IVP) because both allow concomitant examination of the liver for cysts (Fig. 2). IVP may reveal calyceal distortion on the pyelogram phase (mass effect), bilateral renal enlargement, and a Swiss cheese appearance in the nephrogram phase. Renal arteriography reveals stretching of vessels around avascular masses in large kidneys in the arterial phase and a mottled or Swiss cheese appearance in the nephrogram phase.

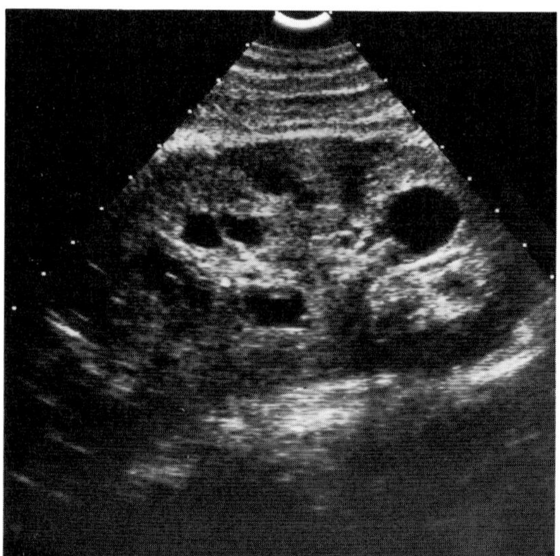

FIGURE 1. Renal ultrasound demonstrates multiple cysts in early ADPKD.

Unfortunately, the distorted anatomy of ADPKD kidneys often reduces the diagnostic accuracy of imaging procedures that are quite reliable in patients with normal kidneys. Therefore, the diagnosis of the etiology of hematuria or flank pain in ADPKD kidneys is difficult despite good imaging modalities. Obtaining a baseline CT scan is helpful in the asymptomatic ADPKD patient. Enhanced and unenhanced CT scanning is the desired technique in ADPKD kidneys for evaluating infection in renal parenchyma, renal cyst, or cyst hemorrhage, and for determining the location of renal calculi to be parenchymal or within the collecting system. Renal cell carcinoma can be diagnosed best by unenhanced and enhanced CT scanning or renal arteriography.

The level of ureteral obstruction by stones or blood clots is best evaluated by retrograde pyelography or IVP. However, retrograde pyelography should be avoided in ADPKD patients because of the high risk of introducing infection. If intravenous contrast is contraindicated in an ADPKD patient, CT scanning without contrast is the most useful test to rule out obstruction (but not to find the level of obstruction) because renal ultrasonography may not distinguish between parenchymal cysts and dilated calyces. Radiogallium and indium-111 leukocyte scanning may help detect and localize infected cysts in some individual patients. Renal MRI does not appear to offer advantages over CT except perhaps to diagnose an acute renal hemorrhage.

GENETICS LEADING TO DIAGNOSIS

The mutant gene in ADPKD is expressed in an autosomally dominant pattern with a 50 per cent chance of inheritance. However, within a given family, there is variable penetrance and variable age of onset. As many as 25 per cent of patients have no history for ADPKD, possibly because (1) affected relatives died of other causes before their disease was diagnosed, (2) affected living relatives may not be aware of their diagnoses, (3) there is nonpaternity, or (4) the case is a spontaneous new mutation.

In 1983, Reeders et al. localized the abnormal gene to the α-globulin locus on the short arm of chromosome 16 using reverse genetics. This locus has been named PKD_1 because about 4 to 10 per cent of ADPKD patients have no linkage with the PKD_1 locus. These nonlinked families have a later onset of renal failure and may not necessarily share the same locus.

Because the ADPKD gene has not been identified, diagnosis using genetic markers in PKD_1 families is dependent on the distance between the marker genes and the ADPKD gene. Closely linked genetic markers flanking

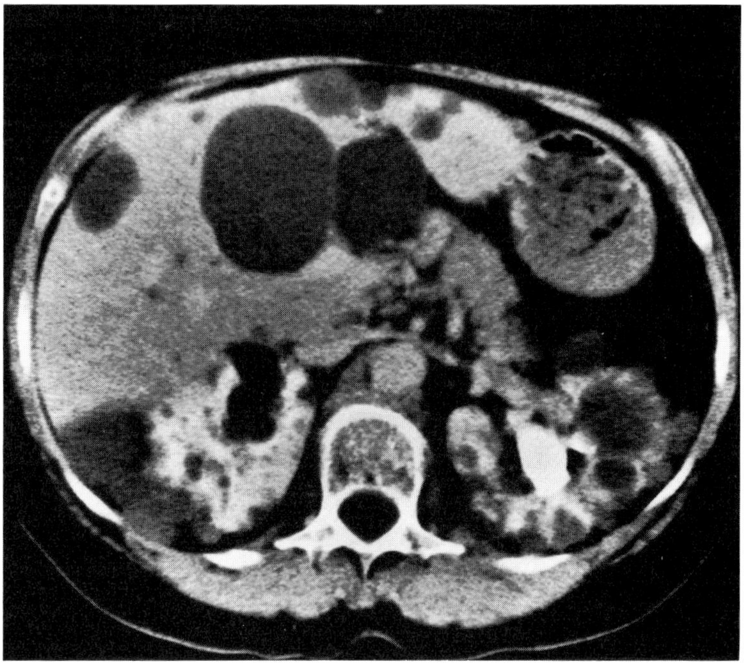

FIGURE 2. Abdominal CT scan reveals multiple liver and renal cysts in an ADPKD patient with a normal serum creatinine level.

both sides of PKD_1 have been characterized and have improved the reliability of diagnosing ADPKD. However, two related clinically affected persons are required as a minimum to diagnosis ADPKD in an asymptomatic PKD_1 family member at risk with an accuracy of 95 per cent. Hence, prenatal and presymptomatic diagnosis of ADPKD is possible, which facilitates genetic counseling and rational decision making about reproduction. Individuals at risk for ADPKD who have fewer than two affected family members or who are in unlinked families are dependent on traditional methods such as ultrasound for diagnosis. Many individuals at risk for ADPKD avoid presymptomatic diagnoses because of difficulty in getting life and medical insurance as well as future employment. Genetic testing also can be offered to potential living related transplant donors.

MANAGEMENT

ESRD can occur at any time in ADPKD and affects about 50 per cent of ADPKD patients. The kidney is unable to concentrate urine maximally before other signs of renal failure occur. Early treatment of hypertension and urinary tract infections may slow progression of renal failure. Eventually, patients will require either hemodialysis or peritoneal dialysis. Kidney transplantation results in cases of ADPKD are good, with both graft and patient survival equivalent to those of other transplant patients. However, ADPKD transplant patients have a higher risk of ruptured cerebral and aortic aneurysms and infected hepatic cysts. Elective pretransplant nephrectomy should be considered in patients with a history of urinary tract infections, kidney tumors, problematic hematuria, and chronic pain.

Urinary tract infections (UTIs) in ADPKD are more common in women than men, and pose a greater risk of complications than in the general population. ADPKD renal infections can be divided into three types: (1) acute bacterial interstitial nephritis (infection of the noncystic parenchyma with an unobstructed collecting system); (2) pyonephrosis (infection of the upper collecting system, which may be obstructed by stone, blood clot, or compressing cyst); and (3) pyocyst (infected cyst). UTIs in ADPKD are thought to be ascending in origin. Urinary tract instrumentation (cystoscopy, retrograde pyelograms, and bladder catheterization) should be avoided if possible in ADPKD patients because of the higher risk, morbidity, and mortality of resultant infections. Although a urine culture should be positive in acute bacterial interstitial nephritis, it may be negative in pyonephrosis and pyocyst because of the confined infection. Hence, the diagnosis of cyst infection can be difficult. Furthermore, flank pain can be secondary to other causes. A poor response to antibiotics should suggest a pyocyst, which is difficult to diagnose and to treat. CT scan, gallium scan, and indium-III–labeled leukocyte scanning may help distinguish between an infected cyst and pyelonephritis.

Lipophilic antibiotics (ciprofloxacin, norfloxacin, ofloxacin, trimethoprim, tetracycline, chloramphenicol, clindamycin, erythromycin, and metronidazole) penetrate renal cysts well, but lipophobic antibiotics (aminoglycosides, cephalosporins, and penicillins) penetrate poorly. If prolonged treatment with cyst-penetrating antibiotics is unsuccessful and if obstruction of the collecting system has been ruled out, percutaneous puncture and drainage or laparoscopic or open surgical drainage of the infected cysts should be aggressively pursued before resorting to a nephrectomy.

Evaluation of flank pain in ADPKD patients must include an evaluation to rule out obstruction from calculi, blood clots, and cyst compression. Imaging studies must distinguish between obstructing calculi in the collecting system, renal parenchymal calcifications, and cyst wall calcifications. CT scanning with and without contrast best achieves these goals, plus it can differentiate cysts from dilated calyces, which may not be possible on ultrasound. CT scanning reveals that 11.6 per cent of ADPKD patients have renal calculi, whereas 44.2 per cent have parenchymal calcifications. Uric acid stones and calcium oxalate stones are most common and both well seen on CT. Metabolic abnormalities include low urine citrate, elevated serum uric acid, and low urine pH in ADPKD patients. Obstructing ureteral and renal calculi have been treated successfully with extracorporeal shock-wave lithotripsy. Retrograde procedures such as ureteroscopy with basket extraction and/or fragmentation with laser or ultrasound have been used successfully but potentially can cause ascending infections. Occasionally, appropriate open stone surgery may be necessary.

Cyst hemorrhage or hematuria in ADPKD patients usually can be diagnosed by CT and treated conservatively with bed rest and observation. More severe hemorrhage can be treated with segmental renal artery embolization or nephrectomy (complete or partial).

Percutaneous cyst decompression can treat urinary tract obstruction or chronic pain in ADPKD patients caused by cyst compression. If the pain or obstruction is relieved initially but returns when the cyst refills, open surgical unroofing of the cysts has a longer beneficial result. Open surgical unroofing of ADPKD cysts does not appear to cause further renal deterioration.

Renal cell carcinoma must be excluded in ADPKD patients with flank or abdominal pain, intrarenal hemorrhage, or hematuria. The risk of unilateral renal cell carcinoma in ADPKD patients is the same as that in the population in general. However, ADPKD patients in renal failure and on dialysis can develop acquired renal cyst disease, which has a higher incidence of renal cell carcinoma.

Suggested Readings

Hossack KF, Leddy CL, Johnson AM, et al: Echocardiographic findings in autosomal dominant polycystic kidney disease. N Engl J Med 319:907, 1988

Reeders ST, Breuning MH, Davies KE, et al: A highly polymorphic DNA marker linked to adult polycystic disease on chromosome 16. Nature 317:542, 1985

Sedman A, Bell P, Manco-Johnson M, et al: Autosomal dominant polycystic kidney disease in childhood: A longitudinal study. Kidney Int 31:1000, 1987

Sklar AH, Caruana RJ, Lammers JE: Renal infections in autosomal dominant polycystic kidney disease. Am J Kidney Dis 10:81, 1987

PERIPELVIC RENAL CYSTS

MICHAEL J. SCHUTZ, M.D.

Little Rock, Arkansas

Peripelvic renal cysts are cysts that develop in the renal sinus. They also are known as parapelvic cysts, peripelvic lymphatic cysts, and peripelvic lymphangiectasia. These cysts may be single or multiple. As the above terms suggest, they are believed to arise from lymphatic ectasia secondary to pelvic lymphatic obstruction. Other possible causes include parenchymal cysts, wolffian duct remnants, renal duplication, and trauma.

Peripelvic cysts usually are found incidentally. A cyst occasionally may cause obstruction with hydronephrosis or pain or compression of the renal vascular structures. Most are identified during imaging of the urinary tract.

An excretory urogram may reveal a diffuse, ill-defined mass effect in the renal sinus, displacement or splaying of a calyx, or elongation of the infundibula. Occasionally obstruction of the infundibula or renal pelvis will be seen.

Ultrasound examination of the kidneys may reveal single or multiple echo-free areas in the renal sinus. These may be confused with hydronephrosis unless one observes communication of the dilated calyces with the renal pelvis. In the case of a suspected mass on excretory urography, ultrasonography frequently is used to confirm the presence of a cyst.

Computerized tomographic scanning usually demonstrates solitary or multiple masses with attenuation values equal to water. Because the cysts are adjacent to the collecting structures, intravenous contrast enhancement is helpful in differentiating the cysts from collecting structures.

Peripelvic renal cysts do not require treatment unless they cause pain or obstruction. With pain or obstruction, the cyst may be drained percutaneously and ablated with 95 per cent ethanol. Rarely, marsupialization of the cyst is required. Exploration may be required if there is a question of a malignant process and a diagnosis cannot be made radiographically.

Suggested Readings

Amis ES: Cyst of the renal sinus. *In* Pollack HM (ed): Clinical Urography. Philadelphia, WB Saunders, 1990, pp 1185–1192

Amis ES, Cronan JJ: The renal sinus: Imaging review and proposed nomenclature for sinus cyst. J Urol 139:1151–1159, 1988

RENAL HYPOPLASIA AND DYSPLASIA

MARK R. ZAONTZ, M.D.

Camden, New Jersey

Renal dysplasia and renal hypoplasia fall under the broader umbrella of renal dysgenesis, which encompasses all developmental abnormalities of the kidney. To avoid confusion over terminology, the Section of Urology of the American Academy of Pediatrics in 1987 rendered the specific definitions described herein.

RENAL DYSPLASIA

Renal dysplasia is an abnormality of the kidney solely defined by its histology and whose etiology is unclear. The presence of primitive ducts on microscopic examination is the hallmark lesion. Cartilage, primitive glomeruli, cysts, and haphazard areas of loose mesenchymal and fibrous tissue are found commonly in cases of dysplasia but are not diagnostic. Primitive ducts must be present for this diagnosis. Kidneys so affected may have segmental, focal, or diffuse areas of dysplasia.

Table 1 lists the various abnormalities seen with renal dysplasia. Various-size cysts may be noted in these kidneys. The term "*cystic dysplasia*" is used if cysts are present in addition to primitive ducts. If a kidney is both diffusely cystic and dysplastic, it is called a *multicystic dysplastic kidney* (MCK). Multicystic kidneys fall into two well-described presentations. The classic type of MCK consists of typical grape-like clusters of varying size noncommunicating cysts, with intervening dysplastic tissue. This differs from the hydronephrotic type of MCK, which also has a variety of cysts that may communicate and that are abutting a hydronephrotic renal pelvis.

Today, because of the predominance of antenatal ultrasound testing, multicystic kidneys are diagnosed frequently in the prenatal period. On renal scan, the classic MCK will show no function on early or delayed films, whereas a minor amount of renal function has been shown in the hydronephrotic variety.

TABLE 1. Abnormalities Associated with Renal Dysplasia

Multicystic kidney
Ureteral orifice ectopia
Ureterocele
Vesicoureteral reflux
Posterior urethral valves
Prune-belly syndrome
Familial renal dysplasia
Renal retinal dysplasia
Beckwith-Wiedemann syndrome (Wilms' tumor)
Meckel-Gruber syndrome (microcephaly, cleft palate, hepatic dysgenesis)
Simopoulos syndrome (hydrocephalus)
Dandy-Walker syndrome (Goldston syndrome)
Mirada syndrome (cerebral dysgenesis)
Jeune syndrome (asphyxiating thoracic dystrophy)
Zellweger syndrome
Trisomy D

Courtesy of Dr. David A. Bloom.

Wacksman, through the National Multicystic Kidney Registry, has shown that the previously common practice of elective nephrectomy for such kidneys probably is not necessary. Potential but rare complications from nonoperative management include tumor, of which there have only been six documented cases, infection, hypertension, and pain. Despite the exceedingly low risk for problems related to these abnormal kidneys, there are still strong proponents in some pediatric centers for elective nephrectomy in the first year of life.

Familial dysplasia, as described by Squiers, is thought to be an unusual autosomal dominant disease involving a hereditary renal dysplasia syndrome. Most cases of multicystic dysplasia, however, are considered random.

The "ureteral bud" theory of Mackie and Stephens postulates that the presence of an ectopic ureter results from an abnormal takeoff of the ureteral bud, and this, in turn, induces metanephric development abnormalities such as dysplasia. Dysplasia can be seen in either single or duplex collecting systems in the presence of ureteral ectopia. *Ureteroceles* may be present in single collecting systems but mostly are associated with the ureter subtending the upper pole of the kidney in duplex systems and frequently are associated with dysplasia at this level. If radiographic imaging, such as nuclear scintigraphy, shows a nonfunctional upper pole moiety, upper pole nephrectomy should be performed to prevent the future possibility of infection or other morbidity. However, if satisfactory function is present, surgery aimed at salvaging the upper pole should be performed utilizing techniques such as ureteral reimplantation or ipsilateral ureteroureterostomy.

It is important to realize that dysplasia is not a cause of urinary tract infection, nor is it a sequela of infection. Pyelonephritis may occur in the presence of dysplasia but generally is due to urinary stasis and/or reflux of infected urine into a patent urinary tract.

Controversy still exists as to whether dysplasia may be a result of obstruction as opposed to being its cause. Stephen's work suggested that the more distal the obstruction, the more severe the dysplasia. An example of this is *posterior urethral valves*. In these patients both kidneys frequently have evidence of dysplasia; the worst cases develop renal failure. A variety of "pop-off" mechanisms do exist that, when present, may preserve function in one or both kidneys.

As demonstrated by Filmer, dysplasia is irreversible. However, often there is present salvageable, nondysplastic renal tissue that may recover or maintain its function after relieving the distal obstruction. Techniques include primary valve ablation, vesicostomy, or upper tract urinary diversion with delayed valve ablation. Patients with posterior ureteral valve and dysplastic nonfunctioning kidneys should undergo nephrectomy because of a significant risk of infection and attendant morbidity. If the situation includes reflux, nephroureterectomy should be considered.

APLASIA, ATROPHY, AGENESIS

Renal *aplasia* represents the most severe form of dysplasia. These kidneys consist of a small nubbin of nonfunctioning dysplastic tissue. *Renal atrophy* refers to secondary shrinkage of the kidney after development already has occurred. Infection and ischemia most commonly are implicated as the causative agents of renal atrophy. *Renal agenesis* refers to congenital absence of the kidney. Unilateral renal agenesis is found in 1:1500 urologic cases, occurs more commonly on the left side, and is more common in males. The solitary kidney is usually normal in appearance and function, except for the finding of compensatory hypertrophy. Endoscopy in these patients may reveal a hemitrigone. The finding of a blind ending or atretic ureter may signal the possibility of renal aplasia. Although there is no treatment for unilateral renal agenesis, the patient with a solitary kidney must be counseled regarding his or her condition and potential problems such as glomerulosclerosis. Also, consideration must be given to other anomalies associated with unilateral agenesis (Table 2). Finally, bilateral renal agenesis, a rare condition, commonly is accompanied by other anomalies and uniformly is fatal.

RENAL HYPOPLASIA AND HYPODYSPLASIA

Whereas dysplastic kidneys are always hypoplastic, the converse may not occur. *Renal hypoplasia* or *oligonephronia* refers to small kidneys that have less than the full complement of calyces and nephrons without being dysplastic. Hypoplasia may occur segmentally, unilaterally, or bilaterally. *Renal hypodysplasia* is the combination of hypoplasia and dysplasia.

The etiology of the small kidney may be acquired diseases or an embryologic malformation. Common causes of acquired hypoplasia include reflux nephropathy, chronic pyelonephritis, glomerulonephritis, and renal ischemia. Radiographically, a screening ultrasound that reveals one or two small kidneys suggests renal hypodysplasia. If hypoplasia is noted unilaterally, the contralateral kidney may show compensatory hypertrophy. Intravenous urography or renal scintigraphy demonstrates small kidney(s) and also may reveal evidence of parenchymal damage (scarring). A voiding cystourethrogram always should be performed in such instances to specifically rule out reflux. Renal biopsy is helpful in differentiating the different types of hypoplasia.

Less common types of hypoplasia include the *Ask-Upmark kidney* (segmental hypoplasia). This is now thought to be a form of reflux nephropathy. The Ask-Upmark kidney is more common in females and generally is found in older children. Because of the association of significant hypertension, nephrectomy or partial nephrectomy is advocated in unilateral cases. When bilateral, however, medical management is the treatment of choice. Correction of reflux, if present, generally does not improve the hypertension but

TABLE 2. Anomalies Associated with Unilateral Renal Agenesis

Sireno-monomelia
Albright syndrome
Arnold-Chiari syndrome
Imperforate anus
Urethral diverticula
VATER syndrome
Myelomeningocele
Spina bifida
Sacral agenesis/hypoplasia
Cardiac septal defects
Tracheoesophageal fistula
Pulmonary anomalies
Poland syndrome
FEMALES
Uterine anomalies
Tube and ligament abnormalities
Ovarian ectopia
Vaginal atresia
Turner syndrome
MALES
Undescended testis
Absent vas, seminal vesicles, and ejaculatory ducts
Hypospadias
Testicular agenesis
Epididymal abnormality

Courtesy of Dr. David A. Bloom.

can promote renal sparing for the unaffected renal segments.

Congenital causes of hypoplasia include the rare *oligomeganephronia*. This is predominantly a nonfamilial condition affecting males three times more frequently than females. This disorder is usually bilateral and frequently diagnosed shortly after birth. The infants present with symptoms of dehydration, vomiting, fever, proteinuria, polyuria, and polydypsia. Renal function generally is impaired from birth, although it can remain stable up to adolescence. When these children reach adolescence, the renal function generally deteriorates quickly and develops into full-fledged end-stage renal failure. At this point, dialysis and/or renal transplantation are indicated. Histologically, oligomeganephronia kidneys show a reduced number of nephrons but with significantly enlarged glomeruli. As these kidneys reach end-stage disease, the histologic findings are consistent with those seen in glomerulonephritis. No dysplasia is present. Despite the renal insufficiency and ultimate end-stage renal failure in these patients, hypertension usually does not occur.

As mentioned previously, management of the patient with a hypoplastic kidney must take into consideration associated factors. Those patients with normotension and significant renal function require long-term observation, whereas those with hypertension should undergo nephrectomy if the contralateral kidney is normal. The presence of reflux should be managed according to the usual clinical guidelines.

Hypodysplasia occasionally may be seen when the ureteral orifice is in the normal position with or without associated obstruction. Conditions such as *ureteropelvic junction obstruction* and *primary obstructive megaureter* with normal ureter orifice positions are not commonly associated with dysplasia. More often, hydronephrosis and thinned-out parenchyma are found. In the unusual instance when dysplasia is present, two possible explanations include early development of the obstructive lesion and a poor response of the metanephric mesenchyme to induction by the normal ureteric bud.

More commonly, hypodysplasia is associated with abnormally situated ureteral orifices, as is seen with ureteroceles, refluxing megaureters, posterior urethral valves, and prune-belly syndrome. Although uncommon, the most severe cases of prune-belly syndrome may have urethral obstruction or atresia. In these patients, the spectrum of renal appearance and function is quite wide and varies from normal kidneys to marked hypodysplasia. In the latter case, the ureters frequently are dilated and tortuous, with laterally displaced ureteral orifices. As with the other forms of hypodysplasia described, treatment generally is directed toward renal salvage where possible.

Suggested Readings

Glassberg KI, Filmer RB: Renal dysplasia, renal hypoplasia, and cystic disease of the kidney. *In* Kelalis PP, King LR, Bellman AB (eds), Clinical Pediatric Urology, 3rd ed. Philadelphia, WB Saunders, 1992, pp 1121–1184

Glassberg KI, Stephens FD, Lebowitz RL, et al: Renal dysgenesis and cystic disease of the kidney: A report of the Committee on Terminology, Nomenclature and Classification, Section of Urology, American Academy of Pediatrics. J Urol 138:1085, 1987

Mackie GG, Stephens FD: Duplex kidneys: A correlation of renal dysplasia with position of ureteral orifice. J Urol 114:274, 1975

Wacksman J: Dilemma of the multicystic kidney. *In* Kramer SA (ed), Problems in Urology (Recent Advances in Pediatric Urology, vol 4, no 4). Philadelphia, JB Lippincott Co, 1990, pp 574–582

SURGICAL TREATMENT OF HYDRONEPHROSIS SECONDARY TO URETEROPELVIC JUNCTION OBSTRUCTION

ARTHUR D. SMITH, M.D.

New Hyde Park, New York

Although reputed to be congenital, ureteropelvic junction (UPJ) obstruction also can be secondary to infection, extrinsic compression, or, more commonly, intrinsic scarring. Congenital causes are likewise either extrinsic or intrinsic. The intrinsic causes are thought to be abnormal muscle fibers at the UPJ or mucosal folds, whereas the extrinsic causes include retroperitoneal bands, kinks, and, occasionally, aberrant vessels. There has been significant controversy about whether the aberrant vessels actually cause the obstruction or are incidentally present. In any event, if open surgery is performed, the anastomosis always should be made anterior to any aberrant vessels.

SYMPTOMS

Patients are commonly asymptomatic most of the time, with episodes of abdominal or flank pain being precipitated by a fluid load or infection. Other manifestations of UPJ obstruction include hematuria, hypertension, and, occasionally, azotemia. Patients with congenital obstruction frequently manifest symptoms in the neonatal period and then again in childhood and adolescence. The condition can present at any age in adults, but it tends to peak in the fourth.

DIAGNOSIS

The classic findings on intravenous urography are delayed excretion of contrast material, dilation of the calices and renal pelvis, and narrowing of the UPJ. On delayed films, there may be a holdup of contrast material in the renal pelvis. If the disease is long standing, parenchymal atrophy may be present.

The differential diagnosis encompasses various other causes of dilation, such as megacalicosis (in which there usually is a normal renal pelvis and UPJ), pyelonephritis, papillary necrosis (in which there is a normal UPJ), and reflux nephropathy. Diagnosis can be aided by a diuretic renal scan, with furosemide being injected at the time of maximal renal concentration of the radioactive material. If the concentration within the renal pelvis decreases rapidly (sharp downward slope on the graph), obstruction is unlikely to be present. In equivocal cases, particularly in patients who have already undergone a pyeloplasty, a pressure-flow study (Whitaker test) can be performed across the UPJ.

Prior to the repair of the UPJ, it is essential to outline the length of the ureter with contrast material. This study is best performed immediately prior to surgery because delay in correcting the stasis afterward may cause severe sepsis.

INDICATIONS FOR AND EXPECTED RESULTS OF SURGERY

Surgery in the patient with UPJ obstruction is performed to prevent further deterioration or relieve severe symptoms. If parenchymal atrophy is already present, no operation can correct it. Therefore, in patients with severe parenchymal atrophy in whom differential renal function testing shows a creatinine clearance rate of less than 15 ml/min on the affected side, nephrectomy should be performed. Surgery of the UPJ is indicated in a symptomatic patient for significant UPJ obstruction and some parenchymal atrophy but not in the patient with mild fullness of the renal pelvis alone. The extremes are easy to discern, but the in-between cases require further evaluation and, if necessary, repeated studies over time.

OPTIONS FOR TREATMENT

In the past, the treatment of choice was undoubtedly a dismembered pyeloplasty. This operation has stood the test of time and has a success rate of greater than 90 per cent. It still is appropriate if the stricture is long (>2 cm). Recently, however, there has been a trend toward correction by means of percutaneous endopyelotomy. The success rate of this procedure is slightly lower, ranging from 75 to 87 per cent, but it is appealing because of the diminished morbidity. Patients have a 1-cm incision, are in the hospital for approximately 3 to 4 days, and can recommence work within 10 to 14 days. They require less analgesics, but blood loss and operative time for the two approaches are similar.

TECHNIQUE OF ENDOPYELOTOMY

There are at present several slight variations in the technique involved in this procedure. The UPJ can be incised by a percutaneous approach or, alternatively, ureteroscopically.

Percutaneous Approach

We begin an endopyelotomy by inserting a ureteral catheter retrograde to instill contrast medium. A percutaneous nephrostomy tract is created and dilated through a central or upper-pole calix that will provide a good working angle with the UPJ. Control of the target area then is gained with a guidewire. An easy way to do this in most cases is to retrieve the ureteral catheter with forceps and pass a guidewire through it.

At this point, any stones are removed from the renal pelvis and the UPJ is enlarged to 12F or 14F with Amplatz dilators. The area is examined systematically with the nephroscope to identify areas of arterial pulsation so these can be avoided when making the incision. In our experience, this measure is sufficient for incision planning, and we do not perform renal arteriography routinely.

Various devices have been used for the incision. I prefer a purpose-built (Karl Storz) endopyelotome, which uses a cold hook-shaped knife that lifts the tissue for the operator's examination before cutting it. Hot knives have not been satisfactory in the experience of most surgeons because of later excessive scar formation. The incision is made posterolaterally, is deep enough to reveal the periureteral fat, and is 1.5 to 2 cm long.

In the 1940s and 1950s, Davis, Oppenheimer, and Hinman showed that an incised ureter will heal with a larger lumen if it has a good vascular supply and is kept open for 6 weeks with a stent. This research was the basis for the intubated ureterotomy, from which endopyelotomy is derived. The stent must be narrower in the lower ureter (8.2F in adults, 5F in children) than in the area of the incision (14F and 10F, respectively), because a nontapered stent that is large enough to hold the UPJ open is likely to cause pressure necrosis distally. We use an internal-external stent designed for endopyelotomy that can be clamped after a nephrostogram confirms the absence of extravasation. There also are double-pigtail endopyelotomy stents with the same tapering design, which have the advantage of being entirely internal. However, if these stents become obstructed, the patient must return to the hospital immediately, whereas with the internal-external design, the patient can unclamp the stent in the flank. We leave the stent in place for 6 weeks.

Ureteroscopic Approach

Endoscopy of the upper third of the ureter, and particularly the UPJ, is often technically difficult, and the initial attempts at ureteroscopic endopyelotomy were thwarted by several mechanical problems. Thomas avoided some of these problems by inserting a double-pigtail stent for 2 weeks prior to the intended procedure. This allowed dilation of the ureter and more ready access to the UPJ.

The retrograde endopyelotomy procedure is essentially the same as in the antegrade approach, the UPJ being incised under direct vision through a ureteroscope either with a straight knife, a special hook knife, or even electrocautery. At the termination of the procedure, a double-pigtail stent is inserted. Essentially, the results have been fairly good, but the procedure is still technically difficult in a muscular male patient and in children. However, there are reports of strictures of the ureter after ureteroscopic endopyelotomy, possibly as a result of pressure damage by the endoscope during the lengthy procedure. As a result of this complication, some urologists have stopped performing retrograde endopyelotomies. Other operators have not seen problems, possibly because of their use of indwelling stents in advance of the procedure to dilate the ureter thoroughly.

Fluoroscopic Approach

Clayman has designed a balloon catheter with a wire that can be activated by the electrocautery. Under fluoroscopic control, he inflates the UPJ with this "Acusize" balloon catheter and activates the electrode. This results in the "waist" of the balloon disappearing and the UPJ opening up extensively. Following this, a double-pigtail stent can be inserted. Orientation for the site of the incision can be achieved by visualizing the position of the wire in relation to the catheter and positioning it so that the incision is posterolateral. Large series of operations with this catheter have not been reported.

OPEN SURGERY

Several methods have been devised to correct UPJ obstruction by open surgery, with various flap operations (Foley, Culp-DeWeerd, Scardino-Prince) and the Anderson-Hynes dismembered pyeloureteroplasty being the most popular. All of these operations aim to create a dependent, funnel-shaped UPJ that permits unimpeded passage of urine from the collecting system.

The Anderson-Hynes operation is particularly appropriate when the renal pelvis is redundant or the upper ureter is tortuous or has a high insertion. The redundant portion of the renal pelvis is excised in a way that permits closure without tension. The ureter is transected below the stricture and spatulated on its lateral margin for approximately 1 cm. A dependent V flap is created with a wide base and fitted into the spatulated ureter with care not to twist the ureter. The anastomosis should be calibrated before the kidney is anchored back in position. A watertight anastomosis is critical to the success of this repair. Some authors use nephrostomy drainage, stenting, or both, but the designers of the operation stressed the value of avoiding both external drainage and stenting.

LAPAROSCOPIC REPAIR OF THE URETEROPELVIC JUNCTION

With the rapid expansion of laparoscopic techniques in urology, application of these methods to the UPJ was inevitable. Recently, Sheussler and Preminger reported a small series of patients in whom they performed laparoscopic pyeloplasty. Laparoscopic cannulas are placed in much the same way as in the access for a nephrectomy. The UPJ initially is intubated, and the renal pelvis then is exposed laparoscopically. The redundant portion of the renal pelvis is excised and a dismembered pyeloplasty performed.

At the present time, this procedure is very tedious and mechanically demanding, so that each operation takes 5 or 6 hours. However, I think that once staples are developed that are not subject to encrustation, this procedure may become more popular.

CAUSES OF FAILURE

One of the most common causes of failure in endopyelotomy is the development of adhesions between the site of the incision and a vessel. A band of scar tissue forms and this results in kinking of the UPJ. At the time of exploration, this adhesion may be found to be to either a normally situated or an aberrant vessel. There are other causes of failure, such as a long stricture or external compression, but, in terms of numbers of cases, these are not as important. In view of the cause, the treatment of choice for a failed endopyelotomy is a dismembered pyeloplasty. Attempts at repeat endopyelotomy yield a success rate of less than 50 per cent, and therefore I do not feel that this is advisable.

In patients who have undergone a dismembered pyeloplasty, the most common cause of failure is a technical error. For example, there may be some ischemia of the tissue, which will result in scarring, or some extravasation at the site of the anastomosis, which results in perianastomatic extravasation and scarring. Another problem is the removal of excessive amounts of the renal pelvis to reduce the redundancy, which may give rise to infundibular narrowing.

SUMMARY

In this era in which patients are demanding less invasive surgery, I think that the treatment of choice for UPJ obstruction should in most cases be endopyelotomy. If that fails, the patient should undergo a dismembered pyeloplasty. We have found that our results in patients initially treated percutaneously have been no less successful than in a "control" group in whom pyeloplasty was performed de novo. The patient therefore loses very little with the conservative approach, and 85 per cent of them will not suffer the morbidity associated with a formal open procedure.

Inflammation and Infection

PYELONEPHRITIS

GRANNUM R. SANT, M.D.

Boston, Massachusetts

Bacterial pyelonephritis typically involves the pyelocalyceal system and renal interstitium but spares the glomeruli. Bacteria reach the kidney as a result of ascending, retrograde spread from the bladder via the ureters. At least 250,000 cases of acute pyelonephritis occur annually in the United States, and the majority are due to the Enterobacteriaceae group of bacteria, particularly *Escherichia coli*. The spectrum of illness associated with acute pyelonephritis is wide, ranging from mild to serious with gram-negative bacteremia and intrarenal or perinephric abscesses.

PATHOPHYSIOLOGY

In patients with anatomically and functionally normal urinary tracts, uropathogenic bacteria with a propensity for adhesion to urothelial cells in the bladder and kidney gain a foothold in the kidney and lead to infection. A number of bacterial virulence factors, including pili (fimbriae), hemolysin, and aerobactin production, enable pathogenic bacteria to colonize and infect the urinary tract. However, in normal urinary tracts, host factors are more important than bacterial pathogenicity in the causation of urinary tract infections. This particularly obtains in males, children with vesicoureteral reflux, and individuals with neurogenic bladder dysfunction, renal calculi, or indwelling catheters.

The risk of pyelonephritis is increased in diabetics, immunocompromised patients, and alcoholics and in patients receiving immunosuppression (e.g., after renal transplantation). The colonized prepuce in noncircumcised boys may predispose to the development of urinary tract infections, as does insertive anal intercourse in sexually active men. Asymptomatic bacteriuria in pregnant women is a significant risk factor for the development of acute pyelonephritis, which more commonly occurs in the right kidney. Diabetics are at increased risk because of glycosuria, papillary necrosis secondary to vascular medullary lesions, and stasis.

CLINICAL FEATURES AND DIAGNOSIS

The clinical onset of acute pyelonephritis is usually sudden and associated with typical signs and symptoms. Patients present with fevers (103° to 104°F), chills, nausea, vomiting, flank pain, malaise, and headaches. Symptoms of lower tract infection, such as frequency, urgency, and dysuria, are variable and gross hematuria is uncommon.

Flank and costovertebral angle tenderness on the affected side usually are present. The clinical manifestations of pyelonephritis in the elderly and in children may be nonspecific and this can lead to misdiagnosis. Pyelonephritis in the elderly can be mistaken for diverticulitis, appendicitis, or cholecystitis. Localized flank pain may not be present in children, who frequently complain of malaise and abdominal pain. In young, sexually active women, acute pyelonephritis can be confused with appendicitis as well as gynecologic diseases such as ruptured ovarian cyst, pelvic inflammatory disease, and ectopic pregnancy.

Urinalysis typically reveals numerous polymorphonuclear leukocytes (>5 to 10 leukocytes per high-power field). Grams stain of an uncentrifuged specimen or urinalysis of a spun specimen establishes the diagnosis of bacteriuria. The presence of at least one bacterium per oil immersion field correlates with a bacterial count of greater than 10^5 bacteria per milliliter of urine culture. Microscopic hematuria usually is present, as are white cell casts. The presence of casts in a freshly voided urine specimen strongly supports the diagnosis of acute pyelonephritis. Midstream urine culture establishes the diagnosis of infection, identifies the causative organism, and serves as a guide to appropriate antibiotic therapy. The bacterial count in pyelonephritis is usually greater than 10^5 bacteria per milliliter of urine, with a single pathogen identified in 80 to 90 per cent of patients with normal urinary tracts.

Gram-negative aerobic bacilli, particularly *E. coli,* are the organisms responsible for the majority of community-acquired cases of acute pyelonephritis. Mixed polymicrobial infections occur in patients with urinary tract abnormalities, a history of recent instrumentation, indwelling catheters, or foreign bodies. In this cohort of patients, infections caused by other gram-negative bacilli (e.g., *Proteus* species, *Klebsiella, Serratia,* and *Pseudomonas*) are common. Gram-positive cocci (e.g., *Staphylococcus saprophytics* and *Enterococcus* [*Streptococcus faecalis*]) account for only 5 to 10 per cent of cases of community-acquired pyelonephritis. Blood cultures should be obtained on all patients with suspected acute pyelonephritis because up to 20 per cent of patients will have associated bacteremia.

TREATMENT

In the past, most patients with acute pyelonephritis were treated on an inpatient basis because of the need for initial intravenous antimicrobial therapy. The introduction of powerful oral antibiotic agents (e.g., the fluoroquinolones), the emphasis on the reduction of health care costs, and the use of emergency room observation units have altered the management philosophy for patients with acute pyelonephritis.

Individuals with signs of systemic sepsis and impending bacteremia require hospital admission. Such signs include hypotension, tachycardia, high fever, shaking chills, and altered mentation. Admission also is recommended for males, children, the elderly, immunocompromised or diabetic patients, and women who are pregnant. Outpatient treatment of acute pyelonephritis in otherwise healthy young women with anatomically normal urinary tracts is possible. Patients so treated should have no nausea or vomiting and lack signs of volume depletion or impending sepsis. The diagnosis of pyelonephritis should be clear cut and the patient reliable. A 10 to 14 day course of trimethoprim-sulfamethoxazole (TMP-SMX), trimethoprim alone, or norfloxacin or ciprofloxacin is recommended for outpatient treatment. Ampicillin should not be used because up to 30 per cent of bacteria isolated from patients with acute pyelonephritis are ampicillin resistant.

Hospitalized patients initially are treated with parenteral antibiotics. Until the results of urine and blood cultures and bacterial sensitivity testing are known, empiric treatment is based on the local sensitivity patterns of the microbial strains causing pyelonephritis. Our usual preference is for combination therapy with an aminoglycoside (gentamicin, 1.5 mg/kg IV q 8 h) plus ampicillin (2 gm IV q 6 h). The spectrum of coverage afforded by this combination is useful against the common gram-negative and gram-positive uropathogens. Single-dose treatment with an aminoglycoside or a third-generation beta-lactam cephalosporin can be substituted for the combination therapy. The drugs used to treat acute pyelonephritis should be bactericidal, achieve high tissue and urinary levels, and be active against the usual infecting organisms.

The pain and fever associated with pyelonephritis usually take 3 to 4 days to subside, and complete sterilization of the kidney takes longer. This is because bacteria in the medullary regions of the kidney are slowly eradicated because of decreased blood flow and the hypertonicity that inhibits antibody killing of bacteria and exudation of leukocytes. Thus, 10- to 14-day courses of treatment are required for effective kidney sterilization. Supportive treatment with bed rest, hydration (oral or intravenous), antipyretics, and analgesics is employed *pari passu* with the systemic antibiotic therapy.

The therapeutic objective in uncomplicated pyelonephritis is the relief of symptoms and eradication of bacteria using antibiotics that are least likely to cause toxic side effects. An early therapeutic paradigm is the utilization of results of culture and sensitivity testing to replace potentially harmful drugs (such as tobramycin or gentamicin) with less toxic oral agents such as the cephalosporins, TMP-SMX, or one of the third-generation fluoroquinolones. The fluoroquinolones offer excellent oral bioavailability and a broad spectrum of antimicrobial activity.

Within 72 hours, 75 to 80 per cent of patients will be clinically improved and afebrile, and therapy then can be switched to the oral route if the patient is not vomiting or nauseated. If afebrile for a further 24 to 36 hours, the patient can be discharged and the antibiotic treatment continued on an outpatient basis. Even in patients with positive blood cultures, a 10- to 14-day course of treatment is adequate. The patient should be seen 4 to 6 weeks after discharge for reexamination, reassessment, and a repeat urine culture to ensure bacteriologic and clinical cure. Patients who are treated as outpatients from the onset should be seen 2 to 3 days after beginning treatment to ensure that clinical improvement has occurred and to check the bacterial sensitivity patterns against the prescribed antibiotics. Outpatient treatment for 10 to 14 days is the norm, and the follow-up is similar to that of hospitalized patients.

RADIOLOGIC IMAGING

In both groups of patients, hospitalized and outpatient, a careful reassessment is needed if there is no clinical response within 2 to 3 days of appropriate therapy, or if there is clinical deterioration. Such patients should be screened carefully to exclude drug-resistant strains of bacteria, anatomic and/or physiologic urinary tract abnormalities, and urinary obstruction. Radiologic imaging is indicated with either intravenous urography or ultrasonography and appropriate urologic or radiologic intervention should be carried out in cases of obstruction, calculi, or the like. An intravenous urogram is an important part of the initial evaluation of patients with acute pyelonephritis whenever an obstruction to the upper urinary tract (kidney, ureters) from stones, strictures, or other causes is suspected. An obstructed kidney is unable to concentrate antimicrobial agents adequately to clear the infection within it. Expeditious relief of obstruction by indwelling stents or percutaneous nephrostomy drainage speeds recovery and reduces the chance of bacteremia or septicemia and their associated morbidity.

Pyelonephritis resolves without renal scarring or impairment of renal function in the majority of patients. Failure to respond to antibiotic therapy may be an early clue to the development of an intrarenal or perinephric abscess. Abscesses may require percutaneous or open surgical drainage.

SPECIAL SITUATIONS

Pyelonephritis in pregnancy requires special attention. It usually develops in patients with asymptomatic bacteriuria and can lead to premature labor with the risk of fetal abnormalities in the offspring. All pregnant patients with pyelonephritis should be hospitalized. There is a limited choice of antibiotics available for this group of patients. The drugs that are regarded as safe in pregnancy include the penicillins (amino-, ureido-, and carboxy-), the cephalosporins, aztreonam, and the aminoglycosides. The fluoroquinolones and TMP-SMX are contraindicated in pregnancy. Most cases of pyelonephritis in pregnancy can be prevented by the identification and prompt treatment of asymptomatic bacteriuria early in pregnancy.

All males and children with pyelonephritis should be evaluated radiologically to exclude anatomic abnormalities. Vesicoureteral reflux and prostatic diseases (prostatitis, benign prostatic hyperplasia) are common associated conditions in these patients. Children should undergo voiding cystourethrography to rule out vesicoureteral reflux. Once the pyelonephritis is treated and the urine sterilized, definitive urologic treatment of anatomic abnormalities should be carried out. Ultrasound is particularly useful in pregnancy because it avoids the risk of radiation to the developing fetus. Computerized tomography is helpful for the diagnosis, localization, and percutaneous drainage of intra- or perirenal abscesses.

Suggested Readings

Lipsky BA: Urinary tract infections in men. Epidemiology, pathophysiology, diagnosis and treatment. Ann Intern Med 110:138, 1989

MacNeeley SG: Treatment of urinary tract infections during pregnancy. Clin Obstet Gynecol 31:480, 1988

Pinson AG, Philbrick JT, Lindbeck GH, et al: Oral antibiotic therapy for acute pyelonephritis: A methodologic review of the literature. J Gen Intern Med 7:546, 1992

Roberts JA: Etiology and pathophysiology of pyelonephritis. Am J Kidney Dis 17:1, 1991

Safrin S, Siegel D, Black D: Pyelonephritis in adult women: Inpatient versus outpatient therapy. Am J Med 85:793, 1988

ACUTE PYELONEPHRITIS

MARK V. JAROWENKO, M.D.

Hershey, Pennsylvania

Acute pyelonephritis arises from bacterial invasion of renal tissue. Its presentation includes fever greater than 38°C, flank pain, costovertebral angle tenderness, and malaise with or without rigors. Dysuria or frequency may be present, as may nausea or vomiting resulting from ileus. In children, findings are less specific (diarrhea or failure to thrive).

Laboratory results helping to confirm the diagnosis of acute pyelonephritis include white cell casts on microscopic examination of the urine. Typical laboratory findings include leukocytosis, bacteriuria, pyuria, hematuria, an erythrocyte sedimentation rate greater than 20 mm/h, C-reactive protein level of 20 mg or greater, or an elevated interleukin-6 level (>20 units/ml). A clean-catch urine culture will yield 10^5 or more colony-forming units (CFU) per milliliter of a single organism in 80 to 90 per cent of patients; however, lower counts of a single pathogen may occur. A count of 10^4 CFU/ml or higher is diagnostic of infection except for coliforms (10^2 CFU/ml). Upper tract infections may be demonstrated by the presence of antibody-coated bacteria (using fluorescein-tagged antihuman globulin).

Fecal flora serve as the reservoir of infection, with *Escherichia coli* accounting for 85 to 90 per cent of acute pyelonephritis cases and *Klebsiella, Proteus, Pseudomonas* species, and *Staphylococcus saprophyticus* occurring less frequently. The primary route of infection is ascending from the gut and perineum, with urethral-bladder-ureteral ascent and renal invasion. Hematogenous infection with *Staphylococcus aureus, Candida albicans,* or less often *Mycobacterium tuberculosis* is uncommon.

RISK FACTORS

Risk factors for pyelonephritis consist of host and bacterial factors. Host factors include compromised immunity; anatomic or functional abnormalities, including bladder outlet obstruction or neurogenic bladder; vesicoureteral reflux (VUR), indwelling foreign body (e.g., Foley catheter, suprapubic tube, ureteral stent or nephrostomy tube); urinary calculi; urinary diversion; recent urinary tract instrumentation; and pregnancy. Alternatively, the Tamm-Horsfall protein, which is produced by the kidney and has bacterial receptors, may be protective against infection.

Bacterial phenotypes associated with acute pyelonephritis (versus asymptomatic bacteriuria), such as certain fimbriae (P-pili), O antigens (lipopolysaccharides), and K antigens (capsular polysaccharides), are markers of increased bacterial virulence. Other markers include aerobactin production, hemolysin synthesis, cytotoxic necrotizing factor production, and resistance to human serum. Serum resistance and hemolysin production do not differentiate between pyelonephritis- and cystitis-causing *E. coli.* Although bacterial virulence factors continue to be defined, it is clear that bacterial adherence is critical to the development of acute pyelonephritis.

Bacteria such as *E. coli* have extensions (protein filaments)—pili or fimbriae—that adhere to human uroepithelium. Fimbriae and adhesions allow bacterial binding to cells in the gut, perineum, urethra, bladder, and like tissues, permitting colonization, proliferation, and efficient endotoxin delivery. These lead to inflammation (e.g., cystitis or paralysis in the ureter [lipid A acting on alpha-adrenergic receptors]), resulting in ureteral dilation and functional obstruction or pyelitis and renal parenchymal invasion by bacteria, leading to further inflammation and possible scarring. Thus, although abnormal voiding or VUR facilitate pyelonephritis, they are not necessary (e.g., only one third of infants with pyelonephritis had VUR in one study). Type I fimbriae agglutinate red blood cells in the presence of mannose, allowing vaginal, buccal, and uroepithelial attachment, and are associated with cystitis. P-pili agglutinate red blood cells in the absence of mannose, the receptor being the P blood group antigen (the disaccharide moiety alpha-galactose-1,4-beta-galactose). P-fimbriated pathogenic *E. coli* adhere with greater avidity to mucosal surfaces than do nonpathogenic *E. coli,* and are associated with pyelonephritis. In animal models, *E. coli* with P-pili ascend the urinary tract and cause pyelonephritis in the absence of any anatomic advantage, such as VUR. In one series, 94 per cent of patients with pyelonephritis had P-positive *E. coli,* compared to 19 per cent with cystitis and 14 per cent with asymptomatic bacteriuria, but other studies are not consistent with this.

Other bacteria are capable of adhesion (*S. saprophyticus*), or may alter the environment. For example, *Proteus* and other urease-producing organisms promote calculus (struvite) production, which increases resistance to antimicrobial sterilization of the urinary tract.

DIAGNOSTIC IMAGING STUDIES

Imaging options include intravenous urography (IVU), ultrasonography, computerized tomography (CT), and renal scintigraphy. Imaging is necessary in diabetics, patients with a history of calculi, pregnancy, males, patients with recurrent infection, immunocompromised patients, septic patients, and all patients not responding to antimicrobial therapy within 48 to 72 hours.

IVU, although normal in 75 per cent of patients, may demonstrate renal obstruction, calculi, and congenital anomalies. It is less diagnostic for renal abscess or parenchymal involvement with infection than is CT scanning. Failure to improve clinically increases IVU findings from 8 to 36 per cent.

CT provides definitive evaluation of parenchymal or perinephric abscesses or scars, while still effectively evaluating for function, obstruction, and calculi. Unlike IVU, CT scans may demonstrate focal parenchymal inflammation or acute lobar nephronia as hypodense areas with decreased Hounsfield units (30 to 80) versus normal parenchyma (120 to 130).

Ultrasonography is a noninvasive, rapid imaging study that can rule out obvious obstruction, perinephric or renal abscess, and large calculi, but it cannot assess nonhydronephrotic obstruction or renal function. In pyelonephritis, typical findings include renal enlargement, focal hyper- or hypoechoic areas, and loss of corticomedullary differentiation.

Renal cortical scintigraphy with technetium-99m–labeled dimercaptosuccinic acid (DMSA) or glucoheptonate provides the most sensitive imaging for pyelonephritis. Lesions typically occur in upper and lower poles, showing an uptake defect without associated loss of volume. Less often, a diffuse decrease in uptake may be seen. Scar development is seen effectively.

SEQUELAE OF ACUTE PYELONEPHRITIS

Acute pyelonephritis may progress to sepsis, shock, or abscess (cortical or perinephric) formation. Sequelae of acute pyelonephritis include renal scarring, hypertension, proteinuria, and renal failure or toxemia of pregnancy. Twenty per cent of end-stage renal disease is a consequence of pyelonephritis, usually with associated VUR. Although VUR may facilitate pyelonephritis and scarring, it is not a requirement. Studies have shown that new scars may be found with equal frequency in patients with and without VUR. Renal parenchymal infection is the key to scar formation. Prevention and prompt therapy are critical. As infection and inflammation progress via bacterial parenchymal invasion, bacterial lipopolysaccharides trigger chemotactic factor release, promoting granulocyte migration, bacterial ingestion, and lysozyme release with oxygen radical generation (as described by Roberts), with bacterial death and tubular cell injury as a result. Edema and vascular occlusion by granulocytes produce focal renal ischemia. CT scan studies by Soulen and Meyrier show greater frequency of scarring from a single episode of pyelonephritis (up to 50 per cent) than previously thought. These studies also suggest scar development is gradual and may require months. Acute renal failure from a single episode of pyelonephritis is rare.

Patients with diabetes, obstruction, or pregnancy may suffer significant sequelae from acute pyelonephritis. Diabetics are at risk of emphysematous pyelonephritis (extensive tissue injury by gas-forming organisms), which carries a 10 to 70 per cent mortality rate and frequently requires nephrectomy. Patients with recurrent infection (*Proteus*), frequently with associated obstruction, may develop xanthogranulomatous pyelonephritis, producing a tumor-like appearance on renal imaging caused by diffuse infiltration of the renal cortex by foam cells, giant cells, and leukocytes. Therapy typically includes partial or total nephrectomy.

Acute pyelonephritis occurs usually in the second or third trimester in 1 to 2 per cent of obstetric patients, commonly starting as asymptomatic bacteriuria (4 to 7 per cent of patients). Complications include shock, adult respiratory distress syndrome, low-birth-weight infants and preterm delivery.

TREATMENT

Inpatient therapy is recommended for infants, the elderly, diabetics, pregnant women, immunocompromised patients, and patients with chronic renal disease or signs of dehydration and/or sepsis. Urine and blood cultures are obtained and hydration and intravenous antibiotics begun. Traditional antibiotic treatment in the severely ill patient (diabetic, immunocompromised) includes ampicillin (1 gm IV q 6 h) and an aminoglycoside (1.5 to 2 mg/kg loading dose followed by 1 mg/kg IV q 8 h), with modification based on serum levels and renal function. Recent studies suggest that trimethoprim-sulfamethoxazole (TMP-SMX; 160 to 800 mg/kg IV q 12 h) should replace ampicillin in this combination. Once culture results are available, therapy is narrowed. Other regimens include ticarcillin and aztreonam, imipenem-cilastatin, or clavulanate potassium, or single-drug therapy using a third-generation cephalosporin, TMP-SMX, or a fluoroquinolone. If the patient does not respond within 48 to 72 hours, imaging (IVU, CT scan, ultrasound, renal scan) and further intervention (i.e., surgical or percutaneous drainage of abscess or obstructed urinary tract) is indicated.

After 48 to 72 hours of IV therapy with the patient having defervesced, conversion to oral therapy based on culture results is appropriate. TMP-SMX or one of the fluoroquinolones is recommended for a minimum of 2 weeks, or longer (6 weeks) if bacterial prostatitis coexists or poor renal function is present. Others suggest TMP-SMX therapy (after the acute infection is treated) to rid the gut flora of P-fimbriated organisms. Treatment in pregnancy should increase to 5 days of IV cephalosporin alone or in combination with an aminoglycoside, followed by full-dose oral therapy and suppression (e.g., nitrofurantoin 100 mg PO q d) until delivery or close follow-up. Up to 60 per cent of patients not placed on prophylaxis will have recurrence.

In minimally ill patients, outpatient therapy with a 14-day course of TMP-SMX or an oral quinolone appears superior to cephalosporin or ampicillin. Urine cultures should be obtained initially and 2 weeks after treatment is begun to detect relapse. Relapse mandates full urologic evaluation, including urinary tract imaging. In the absence of any findings (calculi, abscess, etc.) extended therapy is recommended (6 weeks). Following successful therapy, urines should be followed at regular intervals because recurrence is high (25 per cent in 6 months).

Suggested Readings

Majd M, Rushton HG: Renal cortical scintigraphy in the diagnosis of acute pyelonephritis. Semin Nucl Med 22: 98, 1992

McNeely SG Jr: Treatment of urinary tract infections during pregnancy. Clin Obstet Gynecol 31:480, 1988

Meyrier A, Marie-Claude C, Fernet M, et al: Frequency of development of early cortical scarring in acute primary pyelonephritis. Kidney Int 35:696, 1989

Roberts JA: Is routine circumcision indicated in the newborn? An affirmative view. J Fam Pract 31:185, 1990

Soulen MC, Fishman EK, Goldman SM: Sequelae of acute renal infections: CT evaluation. Genitourin Radiol 2: 423, 1989

Tehner SM, Yadven MW, Kimmel PL: Acute pyelone-

phritis: Preventing complications through prompt diagnosis and proper therapy. Postgrad Med 92:261, 1992
Tullus K, Jacobson SH, Katouli M et al: Relative importance of eight virulence characteristics of pyelonephritis *Escherichia coli* strains assessed by multivariate statistical analysis. J Urol 146:1153, 1991

INFLAMMATORY RENAL PROCESSES IN CHILDREN

LINDA M. DAIRIKI SHORTLIFFE, M.D.
Stanford, California

Renal inflammatory lesions in children include a spectrum of processes from pyonephrosis, pyelonephritis, focal pyelonephritis, and chronic atrophic pyelonephritis to renal and perirenal abscesses and xanthogranulomatous pyelonephritis. These processes are similar to those occurring in adults, but diagnosis may be more difficult because of the vague, nonspecific symptomatology characteristic of many childhood diseases. The organisms causing these renal inflammatory lesions enter the kidney in two ways: by direct hematogenous seeding or retrogradely by access from the ureter and collecting system. Determining the portal of bacterial entry is especially important in a child in order to determine treatment and future management.

PYELONEPHRITIS

Pyelonephritis is defined as inflammation of the kidney and renal pelvis, and is most often a diagnosis made clinically. This is because efforts to differentiate upper versus lower urinary tract infections using either clinical symptoms or simple noninvasive tests have been unsuccessful. It generally is agreed that pyelonephritis results from bacteria that gain access to the urinary collecting system and renal parenchyma retrogradely through the bladder and ureter. Two important factors determine this access: bacterial virulence factors and host factors of bacterial adherence—in children specifically, vesicoureteral reflux. Some bacteria demonstrate greater virulence than others for the urinary tract, as mediated by increased adherence. For instance, it has been found that bacterial P-fimbriae are present more commonly on *Escherichia coli* causing pyelonephritis in children than on *E. coli* that do not cause urinary infections. If children who have vesicoureteral reflux become bacteriuric, they clearly risk pyelonephritis because the infected urine will be washed into the renal pelvis.

When renal inflammation must be confirmed for diagnostic or treatment purposes, the intravenous pyelogram (IVP) is poorly diagnostic. Findings compatible with pyelonephritis are present in only 25 to 30 per cent of cases. Although renal ultrasound may be more helpful in visualizing poorly functioning or nonfunctioning renal segments and urinary tract dilation, it is no more likely than the IVP to detect actual renal involvement of infection. Renal cortical scintigraphy with technetium-99m–labeled dimercaptosuccinic acid (DMSA) detects renal inflammation greater than 80 per cent of the time, and may be useful in differentiating cystitis from pyelonephritis. In addition, when scanned serially, DMSA scans may be used to follow renal growth and scarring.

Another radiologic finding in pyelonephritis may be generalized or focal renal enlargement, probably resulting from renal inflammation and edema. When inflammation involves only a segment of the kidney, focal renal enlargement (focal bacterial nephritis or acute lobar nephronia) may occur. This may appear to be a mass on ultrasound and must be differentiated from a neoplasm or intrarenal abscess.

When pyelonephritis is diagnosed in a neonate or infant, a child with elevated temperature and flank pain, a child unable to take fluids, an immunocompromised child, or child with a highly resistant organism, broad-spectrum parenteral antimicrobial agents should be started and continued until bacterial sensitivity testing allows selection of an antimicrobial agent with a narrower antimicrobial spectrum. Parenteral treatment should be continued for at least 7 to 10 days in the neonate or immunocompromised child. Parenteral treatment in the older child should continue until the child is afebrile and well for 48 hours, and then an oral agent may be given until a total of 10 to 14 days of treatment are completed. Most important, however, after this initial treatment the child should be given a daily prophylactic antimicrobial agent (e.g., low-dose trimethoprim-sulfamethoxazole, nitrofurantoin, and cephalexin), until full radiologic evaluation can be performed to examine the child for associated congenital renal anatomic abnormalities and vesicoureteral reflux.

Children who are diagnosed as having pyelonephritis (or any bacteriuria) must be evaluated for vesicoureteral reflux with a voiding cystourethrogram once the urine is sterile. In addition, renal imaging must be obtained to look for congenital anatomic abnormalities that may cause difficulties in treatment. In situations in which symptoms are particularly severe or do not improve after a few days, renal imaging to evaluate a child for anatomic abnormalities or renal abscess should be performed more urgently.

When young children have had scarring and multiple episodes of acute pyelonephritis, they often are said to have "chronic pyelonephritis" or, synonymously, interstitial nephritis, reflux nephropathy, chronic atrophic pyelonephritis, or focal coarse renal scarring. These kidneys are diagnosed radiologically and pathologically to be scarred and shrunken, with microscopic evidence of inflammation and fibrosis. The importance of these findings should be noted and followed because 10 to 20 per cent of children with focal coarse renal scarring develop early hypertension, and some of these children also develop progressive renal dysfunction.

PYONEPHROSIS

Pyonephrosis must be diagnosed and treated rapidly to avoid renal parenchymal loss and urosepsis. Although the symptoms often are similar to those of acute pyelonephritis, these children usually have obstructive hydronephrosis as well. Children having their first episode of pyelonephritis are particularly suspect because congenitally obstructive ureteropelvic junctions, ureterovesical junctions, ectopic ureters, ureteroceles, and posterior urethral valves all have been reported to be first diagnosed with an episode of pyonephrosis.

Renal ultrasound is the initial radiologic study most useful to diagnose pyonephrosis because it often will diagnose the cause of the hydronephrosis as well as the pyonephrosis. Because the involved renal segment may be poorly functioning or nonfunctioning, IVP is less helpful. In simple hydronephrosis, the dilated pelvis shows good ultrasonic transmission. In pyonephrosis, however, there is usually a dilated pelvis with poor ultrasonic transmission and a fluid-debris level in the renal pelvis that moves as the patient changes position.

Treatment involves placing the child on appropriate parenteral antimicrobial agents and prompt drainage of the obstructed urinary collecting system. Whereas this may be accomplished transurethrally in cases of valves or ureteroceles, in other situations the cause of the obstruction may not be so easily diagnosed or treated. In these cases of young, severely ill children in whom definitive surgery would involve pyeloplasty or ureteral reimplantation, placement of a good-size percutaneous nephrostomy tube to relieve obstruction under ultrasonic or computerized tomographic (CT) guidance is quicker, less morbid, and more likely to drain the kidney than ureteral manipulations or retrograde ureterograms. In an older child, placement of a ureteral catheter may be therapeutic. Once the child is hemodynamically stable and on appropriate antimicrobial drugs, more definitive evaluation and treatment can be performed. If the child needs an operative correction, this can be done when tissues are less inflamed.

XANTHOGRANULOMATOUS PYELONEPHRITIS

Xanthogranulomatous pyelonephritis is an unusual form of renal inflammation characterized by yellow nodules and pericalyceal granulation with lipid-laden histiocytes (xanthoma cells) that has been reported in children as young as a few months. It almost always is associated with both infection and urinary tract obstruction and may involve the kidney diffusely or segmentally (pericalyceal tissue alone).

Most of the children have fever and chills, persistent bacteriuria, vague constitutional symptoms, such as malaise, and often a renal mass. Radiologic evaluation usually reveals a poorly or nonfunctioning kidney associated with a renal mass, pyonephrosis, and often stones.

Although treatment involves surgical removal of areas of xanthogranulomatous pyelonephritis by segmental or total nephrectomy, preoperative diagnosis is uncommon. In most patients the diagnosis is made postoperatively with the renal abnormality misdiagnosed as a renal tumor.

PERINEPHRIC AND RENAL ABSCESSES

Perinephric and renal abscesses differ in their anatomic locations. Renal abscesses are intraparenchymal subcapsular lesions that show displacement of the renal capsular artery away from the kidney. Perinephric abscesses are thought to occur when renal capsular infections rupture into the perirenal space or from direct hematogenous seeding from other sites of infection. The organisms involved reflect the origin of the infection. Before the advent of powerful antimicrobial agents, *Staphylococcus* was the primarily causative bacterium; now, however, in most communities with easy access to antimicrobial agents, the gram-negative bacteria that commonly infect the urinary tract are more usual. This probably reflects modern rapid antimicrobial treatment of staphylococcal skin and wound infections. It may be, however, that in children as opposed to adults, substantial numbers of staphylococcal abscesses still occur. The classic history of a skin or urinary tract infection followed in 1 to 2 weeks by fever and flank pain is uncommon. More commonly, vague complaints of fever, flank or abdominal pain, and abdominal mass may be present. In many cases urinalyses may be normal.

During the last decade ultrasonography and CT have been used to diagnose and guide treatment of perinephric and renal abscesses in adults. Most reported series now include children as well. In most cases abscesses have been diagnosed by renal ultrasound as round or oval hypoechoic lesions. Because these lesions may represent focal bacterial nephritis (lobar nephronia), however, CT or other imaging may need to be performed as well.

If the abscess is small and the patient not severely ill, parenteral antimicrobial treatment alone has been successful. However, if the child is severely ill, the abscess large, or the child has not responded to initial antimicrobial treatment, drainage should be performed while the child is on appropriate antimicrobial agents. The majority of these drainages can be performed percutaneously with ultrasonic or CT guidance. The abscess is aspirated for cultures of routine aerobic, anaerobic, and acid-fast bacilli and cytology, and a catheter or nephrostomy tube is left in place until the cavity is adequately drained and begins to close. In most instances percutaneous drainage has been successful, and only the minority of abscesses with multiple loculations or complications must be drained by further surgical exploration. Once the abscess has been treated, however, unless there was an obvious non–urinary tract source of hematogenous seeding, it is still necessary to evaluate the urinary tract for congenital abnormalities and vesicoureteral reflux.

FASTIDIOUS ORGANISMS CAUSING RENAL INFLAMMATION

Anaerobes, *Mycobacterium tuberculosis*, and other atypical mycobacteria have been described as causing renal inflammatory disease; it is important to remember to culture for these organisms. When anaerobes are involved in renal and perirenal abscesses, diagnosis and treatment are the same as with other causative agents except that an appropriate spectrum of antimicrobial agents must be used. The treatment for renal *M. tuberculosis* is systemic chemotherapy. Further treatment of renal tuberculosis differs depending on the severity of the genitourinary involvement. This organism must be sought whenever sterile pyuria is present.

Suggested Readings

Asin F, Scholtmeijer RJ: Xanthogranulomatous pyelonephritis in childhood—report of two cases and review of the literature. Neth J Surg 38(2):56–60, 1986

Barker AP, Ahmed S: Renal abscess in childhood. Aust N Z J Surg 61:217–221, 1991

Conway JJ: The role of scintigraphy in urinary tract infection. Semin Nucl Med 18:308–319, 1988

Sty JR, Wells RG, Schroeder BA et al: Diagnostic imaging in pediatric renal inflammatory disease. JAMA 256: 895–899, 1986

Wippermann C-F, Schofer O, Beetz R, et al: Renal abscess in childhood: Diagnostic and therapeutic progress. Pediatr Infect Dis J 10:446–450, 1991

RENAL AND PERINEPHRIC ABSCESS

MICHAEL COBURN, M.D.

Houston, Texas

Renal and perinephric abscesses represent part of the spectrum of infectious disease ranging from acute pyelonephritis to frank abscess formation. Acute focal bacterial nephritis ("lobar nephronia"), multifocal bacterial nephritis, renal abscess (cortical, corticomedullary, medullary), perinephric abscess, and xanthogranulomatous pyelonephritis all represent differing stages and forms of such inflammatory disease. Advances in renal and retroperitoneal imaging have improved our understanding of these various entities, allowing improved sensitivity and specificity of detection and more discriminating selection of therapy.

Whereas historically most renal abscesses

resulted from dissemination of cutaneous or other remote infection with staphylococcal organisms, most now represent extensions and complications of ascending primary infections of the urinary tract. Overall, suppurative renal or perinephric infections result in 1 to 10 of every 10,000 hospital admissions.

For discussion purposes, abscesses involving the kidney can be divided anatomically into intrarenal versus perinephric, with intrarenal abscesses being further classified as renal cortical versus corticomedullary. This classification is used in the discussion that follows.

INTRARENAL ABSCESSES

Renal Cortical Abscess

Although much has been written about the classic "renal carbuncle" or renal cortical abscess, this is a relatively uncommon entity, with different anatomic, pathophysiologic, and bacteriologic characteristics than the corticomedullary abscess. Renal cortical abscess results from hematogenous dissemination of bacteria from a remote site—most commonly from cutaneous infections or endovascular origin. Predisposing factors, in addition to cutaneous staphylococcal infection, include diabetes mellitus (particularly if poorly controlled), hemodialysis, and intravenous drug abuse. In about one third of cases, the primary infectious site may not be evident clinically but only suspected by history. Often a delay of several weeks may occur between the initiating primary infection and the subsequent presentation with renal abscess. Renal cortical abscesses result from *Staphylococcus aureus* in 90 per cent of cases. Infection in the kidney presumably results from staphylococcal bacteremia, with the occurrence of multiple microabscesses that coalesce, resulting in a renal parenchymal abscess that is usually solitary and unilateral, with a slight predominance for the right kidney. This type of abscess is significantly more common in the male, with a 3:1 ratio. In immunocompromised patients, such as those with human immunodeficiency virus infection or malignant disease or those on immunosuppressive medical regimens, seen now with increasing frequency, atypical infectious agents should be anticipated.

Typical presenting findings include chills, fever, and flank or abdominal pain, although localizing symptoms may be lacking. Guarding or a mass effect may be noted on examination. The urinalysis is frequently negative, in keeping with the pathophysiology of the disease, which does not arise from the urinary tract per se. Leukocytosis is the rule.

Diagnosis may be delayed if localizing symptoms are absent or adequate renal parenchymal imaging studies are not obtained. Excretory urography may reveal distortion of the collecting system by the cortical mass, or may demonstrate relatively diminished function if the abscess is large and results in diffuse renal inflammation, but often this study is negative or nonspecific. The kidney axis is usually normal, as is the kidney position, unless there is a concomitant perinephric infectious process. Ultrasound examination, although its accuracy is operator dependent, may yield specific useful information. A cystic lesion containing a thickened, irregular wall and debris evidenced by internal echoes is suggestive of an abscess in the appropriate clinical setting. When evaluating a fever of unknown origin, gallium citrate radionuclide scanning may localize inflammation to the kidney and may be useful in distinguishing an inflammatory cystic mass from a noninfectious cyst, although it does not provide sufficient anatomic detail to plan surgical management. In recent years, the most accurate study for suppurative processes of the kidney or perinephric space has been the computerized tomographic (CT) scan. Precise anatomic localization, evaluation of the perinephric space, and imaging of the urinary collecting system are among the advantages of CT scanning. Used in conjunction, ultrasound and CT may provide complementary information in equivocal cases, in which the presence of liquefaction is in question.

Arteriography, once the gold standard for renal abscess diagnosis, now is applied less commonly with the availability of high-quality CT and ultrasound imaging, but still may be useful occasionally in planning the surgical approach when partial nephrectomy is contemplated, or in cases in which the differentiation from renal neoplasm is problematic.

Differential diagnosis includes other complex renal masses such as renal cell carcinoma, angiomyolipoma, oncocytoma, renal medullary or corticomedullary abscess, and xanthogranulomatous pyelonephritis. Distinguishing abscess from renal neoplasm may be challenging at times, although the clinical setting and the results of needle aspiration, which presents minimal if any risk of tumor dissemination, usually clarify this issue.

Treatment consists of antibiotic therapy and

surgical drainage in selected cases. Although recent medical literature supports the contention that many renal cortical abscesses will resolve with medical therapy alone, the decision not to perform aspiration or drainage should be made with caution and selectively. If staphylococcal infection is suspected, either from the clinical setting or from Gram stain or culture of aspirated material, antistaphylococcal therapy should be instituted promptly. Parenteral therapy with a semisynthetic penicillin, cephalosporin, or vancomycin should be initiated and continued until the patient has remained afebrile for at least 48 hours, or for an empiric period of 10 to 14 days, followed by a prolonged course of oral antibiotics, for at least 2 to 4 weeks, to be able to expect an acceptably low recurrence rate.

Some studies would suggest reserving percutaneous or open surgical drainage for patients who do not respond clinically to medical therapy within 48 to 72 hours, although complete aspiration of abscess contents is therapeutic in some cases and is useful to confirm the bacteriologic diagnosis. If an abscess is located in an area amenable to safe percutaneous drainage, placement of a drainage tube into the abscess cavity under ultrasound or CT guidance generally can be performed safely and may speed recovery. Large or multiloculated abscesses are more likely to require drainage than smaller ones. Even multiloculated abscesses often can be drained successfully by a percutaneous route by a skilled operator. Open surgical drainage, performed through an extraperitoneal posterior or flank approach, generally is reserved for abscesses that reaccumulate or are inadequately drained after percutaneous attempts. Nephrectomy seldom is indicated at the time of surgical drainage, being better reserved for a subsequent setting after the control of the infectious process, and after further renal functional evaluation. Follow-up using serial renal ultrasound or CT scanning until normal anatomy returns should be performed. Control of any underlying predisposing disease process is of obvious importance.

Renal Corticomedullary Abscess

This entity describes the more common type of renal abscess, which results most often from ascending infection of the urinary tract. Important predisposing factors include obstructive uropathy, calculous disease, neurogenic bladder dysfunction, vesicoureteral reflux, renal scarring from prior infection, and urinary tract dysfunction related to diabetes mellitus, among others. Renal infection results from ascension via the renal papilla and medulla, with progression to corticomedullary tissue infection and suppuration. As mentioned above, renal corticomedullary abscess is one aspect of the continuum of corticomedullary infection, which includes focal and multifocal bacterial nephritis. Development of an abscess in such infections may result from the combination of relative tissue ischemia with necrosis and liquefaction, as influenced by bacterial virulence factors, and may progress to perinephric abscess, an event made more likely by the presence of urinary tract obstruction with extravasation and perforation at the fornix or capsule.

Renal corticomedullary abscess occurs with roughly equal frequency in the male and female, and most commonly is due to aerobic gram-negative bacilli such as *Escherichia coli, Klebsiella* species, and *Proteus* species. Typical presenting symptoms include fever, chills, and flank pain. A chronic, walled-off abscess can result in a nonspecific picture of insidious, progressive medical deterioration and present a true diagnostic challenge, with constitutional complaints and weight loss being the presenting picture. Leukocytosis most often is present, and the urinalysis usually suggests infection, although it may be normal in one third of the patients, especially after partial treatment of urinary infection.

Diagnostic and imaging considerations are similar to those discussed above for renal cortical abscess. Ultrasound or CT scanning generally will be diagnostic; difficulty may be encountered in infectious states in which significant focal or multifocal renal inflammation with edema is present but has not progressed to frank liquefaction. Serial studies, demonstrating either evolution of the process toward liquefaction or resolution toward normal tissue appearance, usually will clarify the issue. Imaging studies also must demonstrate satisfactorily lack of obstruction of the upper urinary tract; contrast opacification of the system by intravenous or retrograde pyelography may be necessary if doubt exists.

Treatment depends on the anatomy (size and location) of the abscess, the clinical condition of the patient, the stage of the illness at presentation, and the response to initial medical therapy. Antibiotic therapy should be based on the knowledge that most corticomedullary abscesses result from typical urinary organisms, as mentioned above.

Aminoglycosides, second- or third-generation cephalosporins, extended-spectrum penicillin compounds, and fluoroquinolones are useful agents for initiation of therapy while awaiting culture data to choose culture-specific therapy.

A critical issue in the management of these abscesses, because they often occur as a result of intrinsic urinary tract disease, is whether obstruction or some other correctable lesion is present that should be addressed at the time of presentation. Antegrade or retrograde drainage of an obstructed collecting system is an important part of early therapy, with definitive management of the obstruction (e.g., ureteroscopic stone manipulation) better performed at a later date after the inflammatory process has resolved.

Most corticomedullary abscesses should be drained, and most can be managed percutaneously under ultrasound or CT guidance. Medical management alone has been applied less frequently in this setting, although it occasionally may be appropriate for a small abscess in a patient who is responding favorably to antibiotic therapy, and in whom serial studies show progressive spontaneous resolution of the collection. Open surgical drainage most often is selected for cases in which percutaneous drainage is either unsuccessful or presents an undue risk of vascular or contiguous organ injury, when the abscess is so large or multiloculated that percutaneous drainage is thought to be unlikely to succeed, or when débridement of devitalized tissue is necessary. Complicating infectious processes such as emphysematous pyelonephritis may require a combined medical and open surgical approach for optimal results. The selection of percutaneous versus open surgical drainage must be individualized, considering the details of anatomy and the skill and experience of the radiologic personnel available to perform a percutaneous drainage procedure.

Nephrectomy seldom is indicated at presentation but may be appropriate in selected cases, such as in an elderly patient, as a lifesaving measure, or in a patient with diffuse parenchymal disease. An appropriate period of fluid resuscitation, metabolic stabilization, and initiation of antibiotic therapy should precede nephrectomy in such cases, when medically feasible. Initial abscess drainage, followed by renal functional assessment as to the merits of delayed nephrectomy, is the safest approach in most cases.

Antibiotic therapy should be continued for a sustained course of at least 4 to 6 weeks to minimize the likelihood of recurrent pyelonephritis or abscess reformation. Definitive anatomic and functional diagnostic evaluation of the urinary tract should be pursued after the acute phase of infection is resolved, to exclude any treatable etiologic condition.

PERINEPHRIC ABSCESS

Perinephric abscess may be defined as a collection of purulent material in the tissues around the kidney, most often contained within the perinephric fascia of Gerota. Perinephric abscesses are of primary renal origin in 75 per cent of cases, resulting from rupture of renal cortical or corticomedullary abscess into the perinephric space, forniceal extravasation of infected urine from an obstructed collecting system, or complications of urinary tract surgery. Primary non–urinary tract sources include subphrenic and psoas abscesses from nonurologic surgery or trauma; abscesses of bowel, pancreatic, or hepatic origin; and extension of process related to empyema or osteomyelitis. Abscesses arising from the kidney reflect the same underlying disease mechanisms as noted in the above sections on cortical or corticomedullary abscess.

Mortality rates of 5 to 50 per cent have been described for perinephric abscess, higher than those commonly quoted for intrarenal abscess, reflecting differences in the stage of diagnosis, the magnitude of the inflammatory process involving the retroperitoneum, and host characteristics. Mortality often results from delayed diagnosis, which often is due to the marked variability in clinical presentation.

Early diagnosis is the key to successful outcome in this condition. One study described the correct diagnosis being made after a mean of 12 days of hospitalization on a medical service, with an attendant 70 per cent mortality rate, versus 2 days on a surgical service with a 25 per cent mortality rate. This difference probably reflects the admission of patients with nonfocal findings and atypical presentations to medicine services, whereas patients with obvious signs and symptoms of intra-abdominal infection were admitted to surgical services, with earlier imaging and definitive treatment.

Perinephric abscess of renal origin generally is confined to Gerota's fascia. This perinephric space is continuous with the retroperitoneal fat of the pelvis inferiorly and fuses with the diaphragm superiorly and the transversalis fascia laterally, and continues across the midline to the perinephric fascia of the contralateral side, with variable fusion over the great vessels. Abscesses therefore may extend down into the pelvis, superiorly to the subphrenic space, and medially to the tissues around the great vessels and renal hilum, or occasionally may penetrate through the confines of Gerota's fascia to involve the muscles of the posterior abdominal wall or to the peritoneal cavity.

Although most perinephric abscesses are of renal origin and are therefore similar bacteriologically to corticomedullary or renal cortical abscesses, other etiologic origins may introduce different flora, including *Mycobacteria* species, *Candida* species, or anaerobes, most commonly *Bacteroides fragilis.* As for renal corticomedullary abscess, structural or functional abnormalities of the urinary tract, or medical renal diseases such as diabetes mellitus that result in ischemia and decreased resistance to infection, may be important contributing factors. Immunocompromise of any etiology, chronic renal failure, or polycystic kidney disease should raise suspicion of an abscess when febrile urinary infection occurs. Prior blunt or penetrating renal trauma also may precede abscess formation, particularly if devitalized parenchyma and urinary extravasation occur, and especially in the setting of preexisting bacteriuria or with concomitant visceral retroperitoneal injury.

Fever is a common presenting complaint, seen in 50 to 90 per cent of cases, and flank pain is present in 40 to 70 per cent. Flank tenderness or a palpable flank mass is noted in 50 to 60 per cent of cases. Seventy to 80 per cent will have pyuria on presentation, and about 25 per cent will be anemic, which often represents long-standing infection and debilitation. Persistence of fever for more than 4 days after initiation of therapy for febrile urinary infection is an important predictor of a complicating factor such as upper or lower tract obstruction or abscess formation. In some cases, an abscess may be chronic and walled off, presenting with a more insidious onset manifested by nonspecific constitutional complaints and signs of chronic disease without focal complaints and physical findings, making diagnosis difficult and often delaying definitive therapy.

Imaging considerations are similar to those noted in the preceding sections. Plain abdominal radiographs may show psoas margin obliteration or an altered intestinal gas pattern resulting from displacement of bowel by the inflammatory process. Intravenous pyelography may reveal collecting system distortion or decreased function of the involved kidney but is relatively insensitive, as is ultrasound, in its ability to image the perinephric space clearly. CT scanning is superior for imaging the involved area thoroughly, providing qualitative renal functional information while demonstrating the full extent and location of the abscess and the status of contiguous organs in the abdomen and chest. Differential diagnosis between perinephric abscess and hematoma, tumor, and urinoma can be difficult at times, but clinical history and radiographic features usually allow accurate diagnosis.

Treatment for perinephric abscess involves combined medical and surgical management. A recent review described a 75 per cent mortality rate with medical treatment alone, compared with only 10 per cent when combined with surgical drainage. In selecting antibiotic therapy, the potential high mortality rate should be considered and aggressive broad-spectrum therapy instituted pending culture results. Urine cultures are positive in 75 per cent of patients with perinephric abscess, whereas blood cultures are positive in only 40 per cent; importantly, a second or different organism is cultured from the abscess material in anywhere from 10 to 70 per cent of cases. Accordingly, antibiotic therapy that provides broad coverage for gram-positive and gram-negative bacteria—and, in selected cases, anaerobes—is appropriate until culture data from the abscess are available. Gram stains obtained immediately after abscess aspiration are also useful in guiding early selection of antibiotics.

Drainage may be accomplished by a percutaneous route in the majority of cases. Very large or multiloculated abscesses may not be drained effectively percutaneously, although it is often difficult to determine if apparent loculations actually freely communicate until percutaneous aspiration is attempted. Multiple catheters may be placed in large, separate loculations as an alternative to open surgical drainage. If percutaneous drainage is unsuccessful, in cases of infected hematomas or when significant necrotic debris is present, open drainage may be accomplished through a posterior or posterolateral flank approach. The likelihood that nephrectomy eventually may be required is higher with extrarenal than intrarenal abscesses, but nephrectomy generally should be performed at a subsequent time unless required initially as a lifesaving maneuver. In addition to drainage of the perinephric collection, detection and drainage of any upper tract obstruction that exists is essential. Abscess drains should remain in place until the cavity is fully collapsed, purulent drainage has ceased, and the infection has resolved clinically. Serial imaging studies may aid in the decision to remove drains at the appropriate time.

CONCLUSION

Intrarenal and perirenal abscesses constitute potentially life-threatening complications of renal or systemic infection, requiring a high index of suspicion and an aggressive diagnostic approach to decrease the mortality rate through early diagnosis and treatment. Combined medical and surgical approaches generally result in the most favorable outcomes, although carefully selected cases of intrarenal abscess may be managed safely by medical therapy alone. Comprehensive clinical evaluation aimed at identification and correction of underlying etiologic conditions, whether involving acquired or congenital urinary tract disorders or non–urinary tract abnormalities, is essential.

Suggested Readings

Edelstein H, McCabe RE: Perinephric abscess: Modern diagnosis and treatment in 46 cases. Medicine 67:118, 1988

Goldman SM, Fishman EK: Upper urinary tract infection: The current role of CT, ultrasound and MRI. Semin Ultrasound 12:335, 1991

Hutchison FN, Kaysen GA: Perinephric abscess: The missed diagnosis. Med Clin North Am 72:993, 1988

Patterson JE, Andriole VT: Renal and perirenal abscess. Infect Dis Clin North Am 1:907, 1987

XANTHOGRANULOMATOUS PYELONEPHRITIS

MICHAEL J. SCHUTZ, M.D.

Little Rock, Arkansas

Xanthogranulomatous pyelonephritis (XGP) represents an unusual form of severe chronic renal infection. It may be seen in patients of any age, from infants to the elderly, but it usually occurs in the fifth to seventh decades of life. Women are affected three times more frequently than men. The etiology of XGP is unclear. Chronic infection, obstruction, and calculus disease are associated with XGP but are not found in every case.

XGP is difficult to diagnose clinically. The typical presenting symptoms include flank pain, fevers and chills, malaise, and weight loss. These symptoms may be associated with tuberculosis or renal cell carcinoma. One third of the patients may have symptoms of lower urinary tract irritation, including urgency, frequency, dysuria, and hematuria.

Physical examination may reveal a flank mass or tenderness. Weight loss and hypertension also may be seen. The hemogram may show an elevated erythrocyte sedimentation rate, anemia, and leukocytosis. Examination of the urine may reveal bacteriuria, pyuria, hematuria, or foam cells, which represent lipid-laden macrophages. The most common organisms found on urine culture are *Escherichia coli* and *Proteus* species.

Radiographic studies are crucial in making the diagnosis. Excretory urography usually will show a poorly functioning or nonfunctioning kidney associated with a calculus. In children, the disease is usually more focal, with varying amounts of normal-functioning renal parenchyma. Renal masses or calyceal distortion may be seen.

In the past, renal angiography commonly was employed to further evaluate the process, but computerized tomography (CT) is used today. CT characteristics of XGP include the absence of contrast excretion, a large calculus in the collecting system, spherical areas arranged in a hydronephrotic pattern with higher attenuation than urine, no enhancement or rims of enhancement of tissue that correspond to compressed normal parenchyma, large ill-defined lesions that extend beyond the kidney into the perirenal space, and diffuse enlargement of the kidney.

Treatment is usually nephrectomy because the diagnosis is difficult to make preoperatively and XGP can be confused with renal cell carcinoma. Patients with focal disease and otherwise preserved renal function in the affected kidney may be candidates for partial nephrectomy. Selected patients with XGP have been treated with drainage and antibiotics with good results. This may become more common in the future as diagnostic improvements allow for more accurate diagnosis and better evaluation of residual renal function of the affected kidney. If there is any doubt about the diagnosis, surgical exploration should be undertaken.

Patients treated with drainage will require correction of any underlying anatomic defects that may have contributed to the development of XGP. Close follow-up to evaluate for the progression of disease is important. If there is any question of malignancy, exploration is required.

Suggested Readings

Cohen MS: Granulomatus nephritis. Urol Clin North Am 13:653–655, 1986

Kenney PJ, Breatnach FS, Stanley RJ: Chronic inflammation. *In* Pollack HM (ed), Clinical urography. Philadelphia, WB Saunders, 1990, pp 827–835

Malik RS, Elder JS: Xanthogranulomatous pyelonephritis: A critical analysis of 26 cases and other literature. J Urol 119:589–593, 1978

PERINEPHRIC ABSCESS

MICHEL A. PONTARI, M.D.

Philadelphia, Pennsylvania

A perinephric abscess most commonly results from the extension of an intrarenal abscess into the perinephric space. In this setting, *Escherichia coli*, *Proteus*, and *Pseudomonas* are most often the responsible organisms. In the era before widespread use of antibiotics, perinephric abscesses frequently developed from the hematogenous seeding of the perinephric space by a distant infection, usually from a cutaneous site. *Staphylococcus aureus* was overwhelmingly the most frequent cause of infection in these cases. This condition also can result from the spread of extraperitoneal infections into the perinephric space, such as seen with diverticulitis and bowel perforation or, rarely, the spread of an osteomyelitis of the thoracolumbar spine. Patients who develop a perinephric abscess often have had prior urologic surgery, such as percutaneous or open lithotomy, an ileal loop, or ureteral surgery. A history of urinary tract infection, urinary tract stones, diabetes, or IV drug abuse also frequently is found in these patients.

Fever is the dominant symptom, along with pain in the flank and/or abdomen. Pleuritic chest pain can result from involvement of the diaphragm. Spread of the infection to the psoas muscle can produce pain referred to the ipsilateral hip or inguinal area. Voiding symptoms are found in the minority of cases. On examination, one can find costovertebral angle tenderness and a mass palpable in the flank or abdomen. Results of laboratory studies are variable. There is usually a leukocytosis with a left shift. Pyuria and microscopic hematuria are common. Blood and urine cultures may be negative in up to half of all cases.

Findings on kidney-ureter-bladder radiographs and intravenous pyelography include the loss of the renal outline, displacement and rotation of the kidney, renal fixation with breathing, nonvisualization, calyceal stretching, thoracolumbar scoliosis with concavity toward the affected side, absence of the ipsilateral psoas shadow, and extravasation of contrast from the collecting system to the perinephric space. A renal ultrasound can demonstrate a perirenal mass or complex collection, but this may be confused with a urinoma, hematoma, or fat. Perinephric abscess can be seen on gallium- or indium-labeled white blood cell scans. These tests take several days to complete, and are most useful when other tests are equivocal. Because of its high accuracy and precision in delineating the retroperitoneum, computerized tomographic (CT) scanning is the imaging study of choice. On CT, an abscess will appear as an irregular soft tissue mass with a central area of low attenuation. Perinephric gas may be demonstrated. The abscess wall, but not the central area, will enhance after the administration of IV contrast (the rind sign).

Historically, open surgical drainage with or without nephrectomy has been the mainstay of therapy. Now, the first line of therapy is percutaneous catheter drainage guided by CT or ultrasound. This will be curative in up to two thirds of cases, and also can temporize patients who later will need an open procedure for definitive therapy, such as a stone removal or repair of a bowel rupture. After percutaneous drainage, the patient should defervesce in 24 to 48 hours. Failure to do so should prompt a repeat CT scan to look for areas of loculation that were not adequately drained during the initial catheter placement. Open surgical drainage will be needed only in those cases refractory after an adequate percutaneous trial, or for treatment of a specific underlying problem. A nonfunctioning or poorly functioning kidney should be removed.

While waiting for results of cultures of the material obtained at percutaneous drainage, empiric coverage with an aminoglycoside and an antistaphylococcal agent, such as oxacillin or nafcillin, is recommended. Vancomycin can be used in patients allergic to penicillin. Mortality from perinephric abscess is relatively rare in the modern era, but is directly associated with delays in diagnosis and therapy.

Suggested Readings

Deyoe LA, Cronan JJ, Lambiase RE, et al: Percutaneous drainage of renal and perirenal abscesses: Results in 30 patients. AJR 155:81, 1990

Edelstein H, McCabe RE: Perinephric abscess: Modern diagnosis and treatment in 47 cases. Medicine 67:118, 1988

Lang EK: Renal, perirenal, and pararenal abscesses: Percutaneous drainage. Radiology 174:109, 1990

Morgan WR, Nyberg LM: Perinephric and intrarenal abscesses. Urology 26:529, 1985

Sheinfeld J, Erturk E, Spataro RF, et al: Perinephric abscess: Current concepts. J Urol 137:191, 1987

EMPHYSEMATOUS PYELONEPHRITIS

PAUL D. RADECKI, M.D.

Philadelphia, Pennsylvania

Emphysematous pyelonephritis is a potentially life-threatening gas-producing infection of the renal parenchyma that may extend into the perirenal space or collecting system. This condition is a rare complication of acute pyelonephritis, and poorly controlled insulin-dependent diabetics account for 90 per cent of cases. Urinary tract obstruction is present in 20 to 40 per cent of all patients. In cases occurring in nondiabetics, obstruction of the kidney nearly always is present. At least 70 cases have been described, likely underestimating the true occurrence of this entity. A 1.8:1.0 female-to-male ratio presumably is due to the higher frequency of urinary tract infection in women. Average patient age is 54, with a range of 19 to 81 years; pediatric cases have not yet been reported. Up to 7 per cent of cases are bilateral, and this condition has been described in solitary, polycystic, transplanted, and xanthogranulomatous kidneys. Concomitant emphysematous cystitis is very uncommon.

ETIOLOGY

Gas within the kidney can be explained by a variety of causes. Iatrogenic manipulation, including diagnostic and therapeutic procedures, can introduce gas into the collecting system and possibly the renal parenchyma. Gas may enter by fistula formation from the alimentary tube or pulmonary or cutaneous fistulas, whether on an inflammatory basis, such as in Crohn's disease, or from trauma. Fermentation of glucose or other substrates by micro-organisms producing carbon dioxide and other gases is responsible for gas seen in emphysematous pyelonephritis and pyelitis. Causes for renal parenchymal gas other than potentially life-threatening suppurative infection thus should be excluded before a diagnosis of emphysematous pyelonephritis is made.

Emphysematous infection in the kidney, ureter, or bladder usually requires the presence of gas-forming bacteria, a high local tissue glucose level, and impaired tissue perfusion. Impaired immunity also should be considered a contributing factor, and diabetic patients often are compromised hosts and possess an impaired defense mechanism for bacterial infection. Actual gas analysis in emphysematous pyelonephritis demonstrates nitrogen as the major gas component (likely as a result of equilibration with other gases present), with hydrogen, carbon dioxide, and oxygen present in variable amounts. The actual mechanism of gas production is not entirely clear but is likely glucose fermentation via the glycolytic pathway, with carbon dioxide produced from a glucose or protein substrate. Mixed acid fermentation of tissue glucose by gas-forming bacteria will produce hydrogen and carbon dioxide, which initially are removed by the bloodstream. Impaired transportation of the fermentation by-products secondary to diabetic microangiopathy, compounded by defective immune responses, produces gas expansion in infected tissue. With increasing quantities of gas, rupture into adjacent tissue occurs. Nonetheless, emphysematous pyelonephritis is extremely rare even in the diabetic patient, despite the relatively common occurrence of bacterial infections in these patients. Other mechanisms of gas production likely exist to explain gas production in the nondiabetic obstructed kidney and the nonobstructed diabetic kidney.

In most cases reported, aerobic, facultative anaerobic coliform gram-negative rods, predominantly *Escherichia coli*, have been identified as the causative bacterial agent. *E. coli* is recovered in 65 to 75 per cent of cases, with *Klebsiella*, *Aerobacter*, and *Proteus* less common. Multiple organisms are present in 15 per cent of cases. Unusual organisms include *Candida albicans*, *Candida tropicalis*, and *Cryptococcusneoformans*. Anaerobic bacteria have been demonstrated in 1 per cent of cases, and *Clostridium,* despite its propensity for gas production, has not yet been reported as a sole causative agent but has been identified as part of a mixed bacteria population.

DIAGNOSIS

Renal emphysema describes gas within the kidney, whether in the renal parenchyma or restricted to the collecting system. Emphysematous pyelonephritis is characterized by gas within the renal parenchyma, whereas gas from infection restricted to the collecting system is emphysematous pyelitis. Although these conditions may coexist, they should be considered distinct entities with significant differences in prognosis and treatment; even recently gas in the collecting system alone without any parenchymal involvement or perirenal extension has been diagnosed as emphysematous "pyelonephritis" by some authors, which can limit objective assessment of therapeutic modalities.

The diagnosis of renal emphysema, whether pyelitis of pyelonephritis, is definitively made by radiologic imaging. An abdominal radiograph may demonstrate a mottled renal parenchyma with streaks of gas arranged radially (Figs. 1 and 2). Evolution to a more bubbly pattern, perhaps associated with perirenal crescentic gas, may be seen preceding focal or diffuse retroperitoneal gas. Gas outlining the collecting system only (Fig. 3) is seen in ephysematous pyelitis. Nonintravenous contrast nephrotomography preceded by oblique views of the abdomen can be a useful adjunct to anterior-posterior supine radiographs but is inferior to computerized tomography (CT), especially when ileus is present. Excretory intravenous pyelography will allow an assessment of renal function and possible obstruction, but should be regarded as relatively contraindicated in the acutely ill diabetic patient, given commonly associated renal insufficiency. Retrograde pyelography usually is not needed if CT is performed and no signs of obstruction on ultrasound are present. When excretory urography is performed, nonfunction is evident in the affected kidney in 45 per cent of cases. Ultrasound usually will not be useful in identifying perirenal gas and may not be able to distinguish renal calculi from gas with or without calculi. An abnormal ultrasound in the appropriate clinical setting requires further evaluation preferably with CT. A normal renal ultrasound exam by a skilled examiner should exclude emphysematous pyelonephritis. CT provides the most precise localization of gas within the kidney and retroperitoneum, and, although intravenous contrast during CT is useful in evaluating iodine excretion, it is not required.

CLINICAL FEATURES

The clinical presentation of emphysematous pyelonephritis is that of acute bacterial pyelonephritis with chills, fever, flank pain, and pyuria. Lethargy and confusion may be present. Diabetic ketoacidosis is uncommon. Pneumaturia is not present except in the unusual concomitant emphysematous cystitis. An indolent course prior to presentation is not uncommon. Physical findings other than costovertebral tenderness usually are not helpful. Flank crepitus is associated with a poor outcome. Laboratory findings include leukocytosis (>10,000/cu mm) in 80 per cent of patients and pyuria, glycosuria, and hyperglycemia (>200 mg/dl) in 90 per cent. These values are less abnormal in pyelitis. Azotemia is present in 65 per cent of patients.

MANAGEMENT

The mortality rate in patients treated with antibiotics has been greater than 70 to 75 per cent, and, in those patients that survive, function in the affected kidney is usually greatly reduced or virtually absent. Mortality rates of greater than 75 per cent have been reported previously; however, current therapy with a combined medical and surgical approach has improved survival rates to greater than 90 per cent in the last 10 years. The significant decline in mortality likely is due to earlier diagnosis, improved resuscitative and perioperative care, and the realization that medical therapy alone may be fatal.

Aggressive control of diabetes, proper fluid management, and treatment for shock are essential even before the diagnosis is confirmed radiologically. It is important to distinguish emphysematous pyelitis from pyelonephritis as the source of renal gas (easily accomplished with CT), because gas confined to the collecting system usually will respond to antibiotic therapy if any obstruction present is corrected. Adequate urinary drainage is essential in all patients. Antibiotic therapy with broad-spectrum antibiotics should be instituted as soon as the diagnosis is suspected, and modified according to blood or urine cultures. Efficacy of antibiotic therapy may be less than optimal because of impaired tissue perfusion. Persistence of gas on serial radiographs or CT indicates persistent infection, and prompt disappearance of gas may obviate surgery. After initial stabilization with medical management, further intervention with percutaneous catheter placement, incision and drainage or nephrectomy should be performed. The specific procedure should be based on the likelihood of recoverable function in the involved kidney, the presence or absence of a normal contralateral kidney, and the general medical status of the patient. Radionuclide imaging with technitium-99m–labeled dimercaptosuccinic acid (DMSA) to assess the extent of renal cortical function can be combined with the infection-avid agent gallium-67 to determine response to medical therapy. Focal intrarenal gas collections can be treated with percutaneous catheter placement alone, similar to abscesses elsewhere in the abdomen. Catheter placement with aggressive medical management may result in a satisfactory outcome and is a viable alternative to

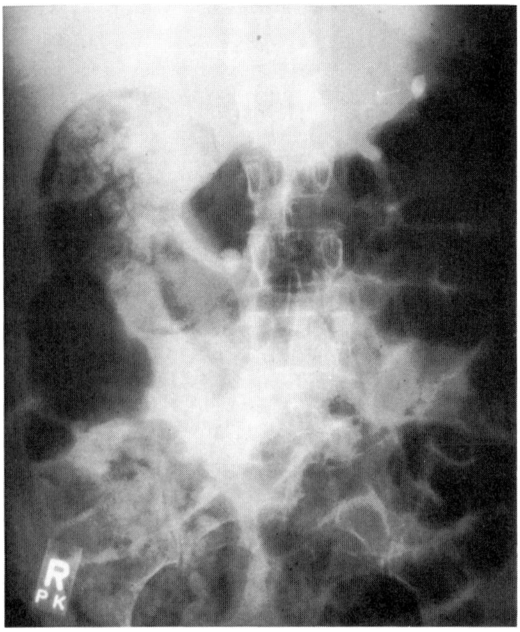

A

FIGURE 1. Emphysematous pyelonephritis. *A*, Abdominal radiograph of a 65-year-old woman with diabetes mellitus demonstrates a mottled gas collection with vague radiating bands replacing the entire right kidney. *B*, Computerized tomographic scan of the right kidney demonstrates virtually complete replacement of the right kidney by gas, with extension into the perirenal space.

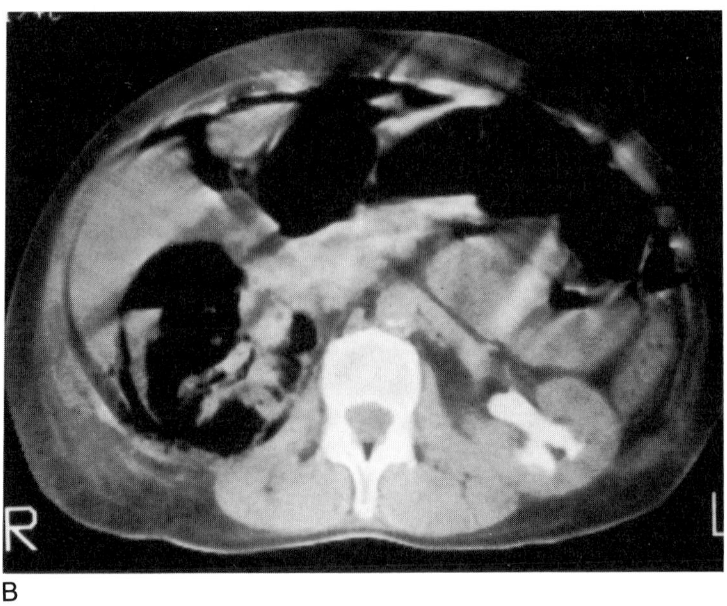

B

FIGURE 2. Emphysematous pyelonephritis. *A*, Coned-down abdominal radiograph demonstrates gas replacing the left kidney in a manner similar to that in Figure 1. *B*, Computerized tomographic (CT) scan with standard soft tissue technique demonstrates gas replacing the left kidney. The renal cortex is not identified. *C*, CT scan at the same level as *B*, but with different CT window level and window width settings, demonstrates an identifiable renal cortical edge. Gas is present in the perirenal space.

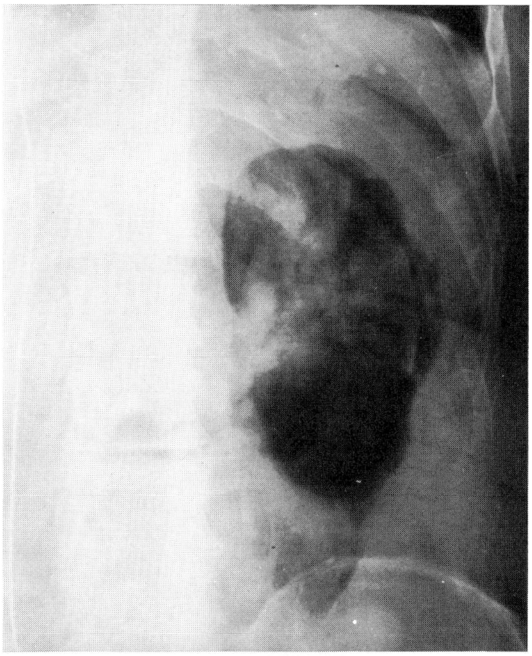

A

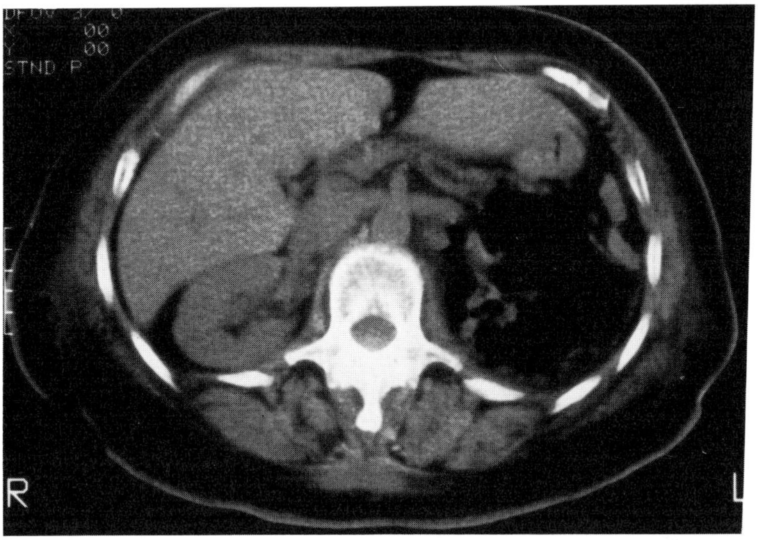

B

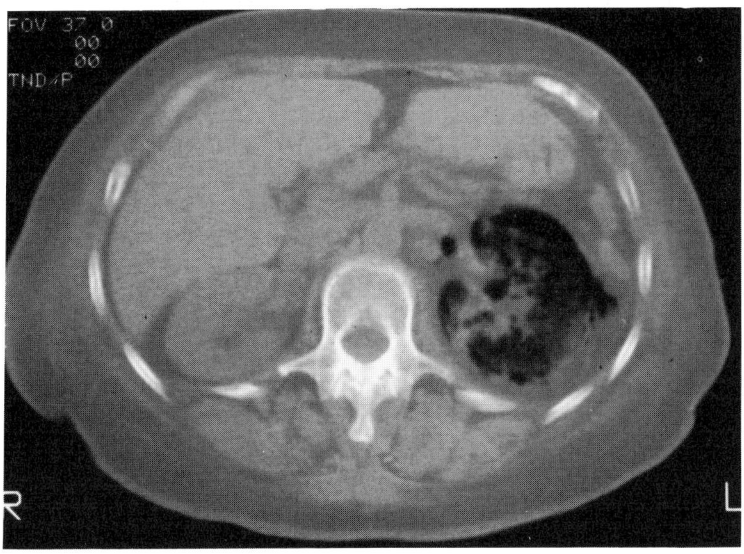

C

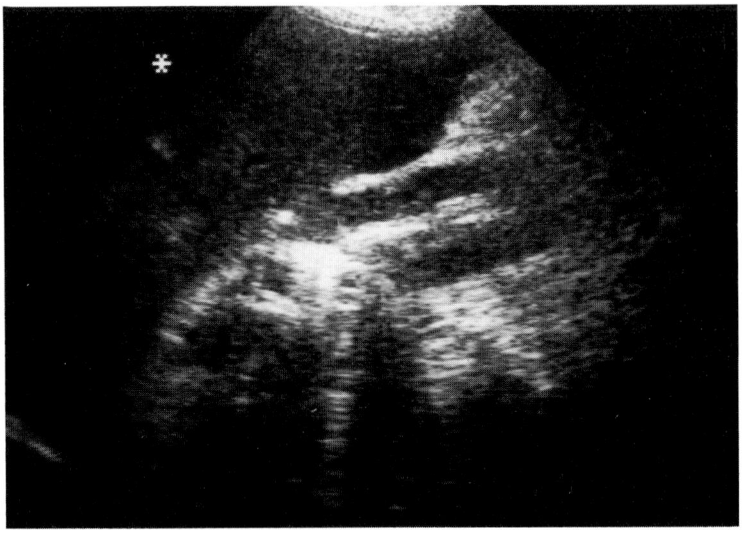

A

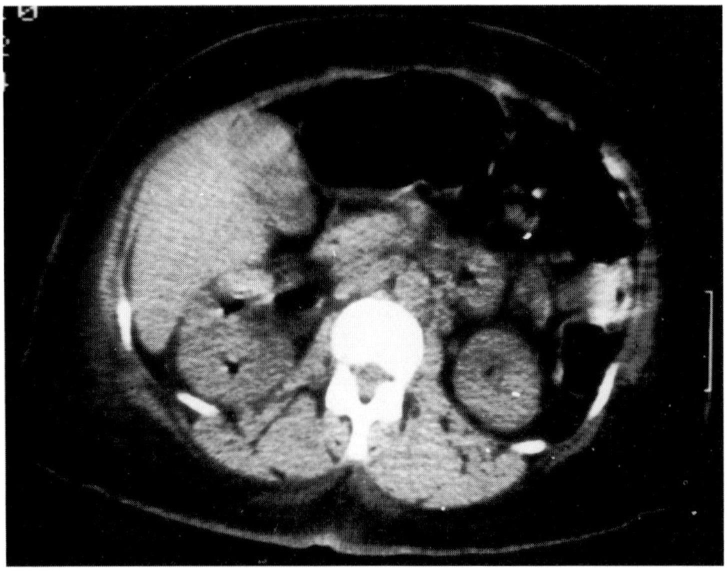

B

FIGURE 3. Emphysematous pyelitis. *A*, Ultrasound of the right kidney demonstrates right echoes in the upper half of the kidney without evidence for posterior acoustic shadowing, as would be expected for renal calculi. *B*, Computerized tomographic scan of the same patient demonstrated gas restricted to the collecting system.

major surgery in severely ill patients, who often have significant impairment of renal function, and those patients with a solitary kidney or bilateral emphysematous pyelonephritis.

Suggested Readings

Ahlering TE, Boyd DS, Hamilton CL, et al: Emphysematous pyelonephritis: A 5 year experience with 13 patients. J Urol 134:1086–1088, 1985

Bohlman ME, Sweren BS, Khazan R, et al: Emphysematous pyelitis and emphysematous pyelonephritis characterized by computerized tomography. South Med J 84:1438–1443, 1991

Evanoff GV, Thompson CS, Foley R, et al: Spectrum of gas within the kidney. Am J Med 83:149–154, 1987

Hall JRW, Choa RG, Wells IP: Percutaneous drainage in emphysematous pyelonephritis—an alternative to major surgery. Clin Radiol 39:622–624, 1988

Hudson MA, Weyman PJ, Van der Vlict AM, et al: Emphysematous pyelonephritis: Successful management by percutaneous drainage. J Urol 136:884–886, 1986

Michaeli J, Megle P, Periberg S, et al: Emphysematous pyelonephritis. J Urol 131:203–208, 1984

Paivansalo M, Hellstrom P, Siniluoto T, et al: Emphysematous pyelonephritis. Acta Radiol 30:311–315, 1989

Shahatto N, Alawadhi NZ, Ghazali S: Emphysematous pyelonephritis: Surgical implications. Br J Urol 66:572–574, 1990

Zagoria RJ, Byer RB, Harrison LH, et al: Percutaneous management of localized emphysematous pyelonephritis. JVIR 2:156–158, 1991

GENITOURINARY TUBERCULOSIS

JAMES GORDON GOW, M.D.
Liverpool, England

During the last two decades, there has been a marked change in the management of genitourinary tuberculosis, a change that has been experienced in many medical disciplines. When it is realized that tuberculosis predates written history, the results of modern treatment are an outstanding achievement. Following the introduction of modern chemotherapy, the incidence of genitourinary tuberculosis has declined in proportion to other manifestations of the disease in the Western World, but the downward trend in the developing countries is hardly noticeable because of a combination of natural immunity, failure of diagnosis, and a lack of compliance in taking medical treatment.

SIGNS AND SYMPTOMS

Males predominate over females at the ratio of 2:1, and 80 per cent of patients are in the 20- to 40-year age group, although, in recent years, more patients are being seen in the 50- to 60-year age group. The most common initial complaint is a painless frequency of micturition, usually at night but later both day and night. The urine is normally sterile and dysuria is present only if there is a coincidental urinary infection. If the urine is sterile, pyuria of 20+ cells per high-power field is present in many cases. Hematuria is noticed in only 10 per cent of cases, and renal pain is uncommon.

Suprapubic pain is experienced if there is a severe bladder infection or when there is marked painful frequency of micturition. Hematospermia is rare but should not be ignored. Ureteral colic occurs when a clot or flake of calcification passes down the ureter. Occasionally, the first symptom is an enlarged painful testis, which must be distinguished from nonspecific epididymo-orchitis. Finally, the disease may be discovered as an incidental finding following a transurethral resection of the prostate.

DIAGNOSIS

A diagnosis depends on the isolation of *Mycobacterium tuberculosis*, an acid- and alcohol-fast organism, in three or preferably five consecutive early morning specimens of urine. The urine is cultured on two types of culture media: (1) one for the isolation of *M. tuberculosis* and (2) one for *Mycobacterium bovis*, an organism that is becoming more important. A direct smear is not sufficient for diagnosis because there are other nonpathogenic mycobacteria, such as *Mycobacterium smegmatis*, that cannot be differentiated from *M. tuberculosis* on a direct smear. Until a culture has isolated the organism, treatment should not be started unless there is overwhelming clinical evidence of the disease. Every positive culture should be tested for sensitivity to all the common chemotherapeutic agents so that the most appropriate regimen of treatment can be started. Intravenous urography is the most important investigation because it outlines the pelvic calyceal system, excludes any calcification in the renal tract, and outlines the ureter and the bladder. Cystoscopy is indicated only if there is clinical evidence of bladder involvement.

MANAGEMENT

Patients in the Western World should be treated as outpatients unless there are specific contraindications, such as social problems or a serious infection. They should be seen weekly, and at each visit liver function tests should be carried out and the urine inspected to ensure that the drugs are being taken. (If the urine is not orange, as a result of the rifampin, it is evident that the drugs have not been taken for at least 48 hours.) In the developing countries, however, the situation is very different because of poor living conditions, primitive transportation, malnutrition, and coincidental diseases such as malaria and worm infections. It is important to admit these patients to give them a sufficient diet and to be certain that all drugs are taken regularly. Compliance is the most important part of chemotherapeutic treatment.

Antituberculous Drugs

Antituberculous drugs are divided into two categories: bacteriocidal and bacteriostatic. Bacteriocidal drugs are rifampin, isoniazid, pyrazinamide, and streptomycin. Bacteriostatic drugs are ethambutol and ethionamide. The modern approach to the disease is aimed at killing the organisms and curing the infection. The days of prolonged drug taking are now over, because clinical research in the pulmonary manifestations of tuberculosis has confirmed the potency of the drugs and reliability of short courses. It is now standard practice for chemotherapy to be given for 6 months for the pulmonary infection and 4 months for genitourinary disease; the latter is possible because there are physiologic conditions in the renal tract that are an advantage and allow drug treatment for this shorter period of time.

The recommended regimen is as follows (Table 1). For the first 2 months, the patient should take a daily combination of pyrazinamide 25 mg/kg body weight (maximum dose 2 gm); isoniazid 300 mg; and rifampin 450 mg. (I have found the best way for the patient to take these drugs is together with milk at bedtime.) Clinical studies have confirmed that, if streptomycin is added to the regimen, no additional advantage is obtained; however, it could be considered if there was a severe bladder infection. For the second 2 months, pyrazinamide is discontinued and the isoniazid and rifampin are taken three times a week, 600 mg isoniazid and 900 mg rifampin. With these doses of isoniazid, it has not been found necessary to give pyridoxine. Urine is examined for *M. tuberculosis* at the end of the 2- and 4-month periods, and thereafter at a further 6 months and then 1 year. In my experience, if the urine is negative for *M. tuberculosis* after 1 year, the patient can be discharged and told to report back if any urinary symptoms recur. Only if there is resistance to any of the bacteriocidal drugs are the two bacteriostatic drugs considered.

In developing countries, because of cost, the three drugs (pyrazinamide, isoniazid, and rifampin) can be given three times a week for 3 months from the start of treatment, because there is good evidence that such a regimen can be very effective.

Toxicity

Antituberculous drugs do not often cause toxicity but, if they do, it usually occurs in the first 2 months of treatment. The two main reactions are hypersensitivity and hepatotoxicity (pyrazinamide). Should either occur, the drugs should be stopped, the offending one isolated, and a desensitizing course started. If ethambutol is being used, careful monitoring is essential because it can cause optic atrophy and blindness.

Surgery

Surgery is an essential part of the modern management of genitourinary tuberculosis. About 80 per cent of patients require some operative procedure. The indications are extensive organ destruction or reconstruction. Nephrectomy is necessary when the organ is extensively destroyed, when the disease is the cause of hypertension, or when there is coexisting renal carcinoma. It is most important when short courses of chemotherapy are being used because surgery removes the potentially dangerous side effects of the disease. Nephroureterectomy is never indicated because, as long as most of the ureter is removed at the time of nephrectomy, the remainder will give no trouble and will often fibrose.

Partial Nephrectomy

This operation is becoming less and less frequent because of the effect of modern chemotherapy. There are only two indications: a polar lesion containing calcified deposits that has not responded to chemotherapy, or a localized area of calcification that is steadily increasing in size, so that it ultimately will destroy the whole kidney.

Cavernostomy

This procedure has no place in the modern management of genitourinary tuberculosis

TABLE 1. Regiments of Chemotherapy

	Western World		Developing Countries
	1st 2 Months	2nd 2 Months	(3-Month Course)
Pyrazinamide (25 mg/kg body weight)	max dose: 2 gm daily	—	max dose: 2 gm 3×/week
Isoniazid	300 mg daily	600 mg 3×/week	600 mg 3×/week
Rifampin	450 mg daily	900 mg 3×/week	900 mg 3×/week

because the abscess can be aspirated under radiographic control and, if required, the cavity can be instilled with a solution of 5% rifampin and 1% isoniazid.

EPIDIDYMECTOMY

Tuberculous epididymitis is a declining method of presentation, but it does occur and must be differentiated from nonspecific epididymo-orchitis. Epididymectomy will be required when there is a caseating abscess that has ulcerated through the scrotal skin and that is not responding to chemotherapy. The testis is involved rarely, and orchidectomy is required in only 5 per cent of cases. All the operations carried out on extensively diseased organs should be covered by an umbrella of chemotherapy. It is a wise precaution to give the patient a full course of treatment for 4 weeks minimum before surgery is undertaken.

Ureteric Strictures

Strictures occur commonly at the ureteropelvic junction, at the ureterovesical junction, and in the middle ureter. The most common site is the ureterovesical area, which is involved in 9 per cent of cases. A ureteropelvic stricture is rare but requires urgent treatment with some form of surgical repair because, if the obstruction is left too long, the combination of obstruction to the outflow of urine and an acute infection can cause irreparable damage to the kidney. Strictures in the middle third of the ureter are very rare and will require treatment by some intubation technique using a double-J stent. Autonephrectomy (complete nonfunction of the kidney) occurs with unrecognized complete ureteral obstruction.

Obstruction at the lower end of the ureter in the acute phase of the disease may be due to edema. The patient should be kept under close supervision because the obstruction may respond to antituberculous chemotherapy. However, if there is no improvement in 3 weeks, corticosteroids 20 mg tid should be added to the normal chemotherapy. This is a high dose because rifampin doubles the excretion of steroids. If at the end of this time the stricture remains unchanged, further measures will be required. Dilation of the ureteric orifice has been tried but is not recommended because there is a high failure rate and the necessity of frequent dilations and anesthetics. Reimplantation of the ureter into the bladder gives excellent results using an antireflux procedure with an intramural tunnel of at least 5 cm. When a stricture is more than 5 or 6 cm in length, either a psoas hitch or a Boari flap technique is necessary, again using an antireflux procedure.

Augmentation Cystoplasty

Intolerable painful frequency of micturition is the definitive indication for bladder augmentation. Either the ileum, colon, or cecum can be used depending on the surgeon's preference, but I have found the cecum most satisfactory because the ureters can be anastomosed into the terminal ileum using an antireflux technique as an added advantage in preserving renal function.

Suggested Readings

Gow JG: Genito-urinary tuberculosis. *In* Walsh PC, Retik AB, Stamey TA, et al (eds): Campbell's Urology, 6th ed. Philadelphia, WB Saunders, 1992, pp 951–981

TREATMENT OF FUNGAL DISEASES OF THE KIDNEY, URETER, AND BLADDER

GILBERT J. WISE, M.D.

Brooklyn, New York

GENERAL OBSERVATIONS

Fungi that can cause genitourinary infection can be classified as primary or opportunistic pathogens. However, in the era of the immunocompromised patient, the distinctions between primary and opportunistic infection may not be clearly delineated.

The primary pathogenic fungi, indigenous to the environment, include *Blastomyces dermatitidis, Coccidioides immitis*, and *Histoplasma capsulatum*. They cause infection in individuals exposed to the fungal germ spores and who may have defective cell-mediated immunity.

Opportunistic fungal infections develop in patients who are immunosuppressed from a variety of causes that include metabolic dysfunction, chronic disease, and steroid or immunosuppressive therapy. Opportunistic fungi may be indigenous to the external environment (e.g., *Aspergilla* and *Cryptococcus*) or exist as saprophytes of the gastrointestinal tract or external genitalia (e.g., *Candida* and *Torulopsis*).

The opportunistic organisms often infect the patient who is immunosuppressed following complicated surgery, therapy with steroids, immunosuppressive agents, or antineoplastic agents. Patients with diabetes mellitus or vascular disease are most vulnerable to candidal infection. The prolonged use of indwelling urethral catheters or IV hyperalimentation lines and excessive administration of broad-spectrum antibiotics increase patients' vulnerability to fungal infections.

Recognition of these predisposing factors not only alerts the urologist to the possible development of mycoses, but also helps in management of fungal colonization. Correction or amelioration of these factors may in itself resolve fungal colonization at an early stage. For example, removal of an indwelling urethral catheter, discontinuance of broad-spectrum antibiotic therapy, and modification or termination of immunosuppressive therapy may permit the patient's natural host factors to rid the body of early fungal infection or colonization. Unfortunately, these steps often are ineffective in the management of fungal infections that have become invasive.

Nonhospital environmental factors also have been incriminated in increasing the patient's vulnerability to fungal infection. As an example, individuals whose occupations expose them to chronic moisture, such as bartenders, bakers, and kitchen workers, have susceptibility to skin infection that may serve as an entry for fungus. Birds, particularly pigeons, are a source of *Aspergillus* and *Cryptococcus* organisms; in one case, a successful kidney transplant has been compromised by secondary aspergillar infection traced to the patient's avocation of raising pigeons. Recognition and avoidance of these environmental sources may prevent secondary fungal infection in vulnerable patients such as renal transplant recipients.

There is a third group of fungi that are so unusual that development of genitourinary infection in a patient may be worthy of a case report. Many fungi in this group can be considered environmental pathogens; they include *Geotrichum, Paecilomyces, Paracoccidioides,* Phycomycetes, *Penicillium, Rhinosporidium,* and *Sporothrix.*

PRIMARY FUNGAL INFECTIONS

Blastomycosis

Blastomyces dermatitidis inhabits soil that is high in water content and animal excreta. Blastomycosis usually occurs after inhalation of the fungus, with the initial onset of pulmonary infection after inhalation. Sexual transmission has been reported infrequently.

In a retrospective analysis of 51 patients with systemic blastomycosis, the prostate was involved in 8 cases (16 per cent) and the epididymis in 10 (20 per cent). The kidney, testis, and prepuce were involved in one case (2 per cent) each. Clinical manifestations of genitourinary *Blastomyces* infection focus on prostatic involvement. These include clinical findings compatible with prostatic abscess, irritative voiding symptoms, and urinary retention. Although relief of obstructive uropathy by transurethral resection may be helpful, systemic therapy with amphotericin B is advised.

Infected organs such as the testis and epididymis should be removed in conjunction with systemic antifungal therapy. Ketoconazole (400 mg daily for >1 month) has been utilized as the first line of treatment for systemic blastomycosis in nonimmunosuppressed patients. In isolated cases of prostatic blastomycosis, ketoconazole has been efficacious; however, prostatic infection may be a manifestation of systemic disease, so IV amphotericin B (up to 3 gm total dose given over 3 months) is indicated.

A newer antifungal agent, itraconazole, has been successful in the treatment of *Blastomyces* infections that have failed ketoconazole therapy. Unlike ketoconazole, itraconazole does not inhibit steroidogenesis. However, the use of itraconazole in genitourinary blastomycosis has not been documented.

Coccidioidomycosis

Coccidioides imitis is indigenous to semiarid regions. Coccidioidomycosis generally develops as a transient pulmonary infection. Risk factors for dissemination include increased skin pigmentation, pregnancy, and immunosuppression. Postmortem studies of patients with systemic coccidioidomycosis have revealed infection of the kidneys in 35 to 60 per cent, the adrenals in 16.8 to 22 per cent, the prostate in 4.6 to 6 per cent, and the scrotal contents in 1 to 5 per cent. Patients with human immunodeficiency virus/acquired immunodeficiency syndrome (AIDS) are at increased risk for development of systemic coccidioidal infection.

Genitourinary coccidioidomycosis generally occurs in association with disseminated infection. Systemic (IV) amphotericin B (>2 gm total dose) is required in these cases. The imidiazole ketoconazole (200 mg daily for 1 year) and the newer triazoles, itraconazole and fluconazole (200 mg daily), have been utilized for chronic therapy to prevent relapse. Insufficient clinical experience with the triazoles has not clearly defined the length of therapy or effectiveness in genitourinary infection.

Histoplasmosis

The fungus *Histoplasma capsulatum* is world wide in distribution, but infections have been most prevalent in the Mississippi and Ohio river valleys. The fungus is found in soil that is contaminated by bird excreta. Outbreaks have occurred among spelunkers exploring bat-infested caves. Infections have developed in urbanites exposed to construction excavations.

Approximately 90 per cent of infections result in mild and clinically insignificant respiratory histoplasmosis. Immunosuppression may enhance the patient's vulnerability to disseminated infection. The patient with AIDS is at increased risk for developing disseminated infection.

Disseminated histoplasmosis can involve the genitourinary system. In a 1959 (pre-AIDS) review of 17 autopsy cases of patients with disseminated histoplasmosis, the adrenal was involved in 14 (82 per cent), the kidney in 3 (18 per cent), the testes in 1 (6 per cent), and the prostate in 1 (6 per cent). Clinical manifestations of disseminated histoplasmosis include fever, weight loss, cough, chest pain, hepatosplenomegaly, and lymphadenopathy. Disseminated histoplasmosis also may involve the penis. Surgical treatment may be indicated, but systemic therapy with IV amphotericin B (>1 gm) is the first line of treatment. Itraconazole (200 mg daily) may have a role in long-term therapy of systemic infection.

OPPORTUNISTIC INFECTIONS

Aspergillosis

Species of *Aspergillus* are second in frequency to *Candida* as sources of opportunistic fungal infections. Underlying malignancy, particularly lymphoma, increases the patient's susceptibility to aspergillar infection. Other predisposing factors include steroid use, diabetes mellitus, and IV drug abuse.

Twelve per cent of patients with systemic aspergillar infection may have kidney involvement. The fungal hyphae may invade blood vessels, causing ischemia with organ infarcts. Renal abscesses and fungal balls may cause obstructive uropathy and destruction of the kidney. Pyelography may reveal filling defects within the collecting system and also necrotic changes in the renal parenchyma. Treatment modalities have included nephrectomy, nephrostomy with removal of fungal ball, irrigation of renal collecting system and ureter with amphotericin B (500 mg/day), and systemic intravenous amphotericin B (> 1-gm). Long-term itraconazole (200 mg/day for 1 year) may be required for disseminated aspergillar infection.

Candidiasis

Candidal species may exist as a saprophyte in the external genitalia or urethra. In a general hospital, 5 per cent of urine cultures may yield *Candida*. Most of these cultures are evanescent (i.e., transient) and occur in one culture only, and thus do not necessarily represent infection. In the immunocompromised patient, *Candida* has emerged as a significant nosocomial infection. In a tumor center study of 135 patients with fungemia, *C. albicans* was the most prevalent species (51 per cent), followed by *C. tropicalis* (25 per cent), *C. parapsilosis* (12 per cent), and other species (3 per cent). *Torulopsis*, often considered a variant or close relative of *candida*, comprised 9 per cent of cases of blood-borne fungal infections.

Factors that predispose the patient to candidal infection include diabetes mellitus, broad-spectrum antibiotics, corticosteroids, obstructive uropathy, and prolonged urinary catheter drainage. Congenital anomalies may predispose the pediatric patient to candidal infection of the urinary tract. Low birth weight and intravascular catheters increase the newborn risk for systemic candidal infection. In the adult, most lower urinary tract infections are caused by retrograde infection from an indwelling catheter or genital or perineal colonization, whereas renal infections often are the result of hematogenous infection.

Microscopic pyuria, yeast, and hyphae are

often nonspecific findings on urine cultures. A urinary colony count of *Candida* may differentiate infection from colonization. Culture of a clean-catch urine specimen (obtained by midstream or single-catheter collection) showing 15,000 colonies per milliliter indicates infection. In the presence of an indwelling catheter, however, a candidal count cannot be utilized to differentiate colonization from infection. The persistence of candiduria and the presence of fever (low grade or spiking), lethargy, or weakness may be indicative of invasive fungal infection.

Other clinical findings, such as multiple positive cultures for *Candida* and retinal lesions, indicate disseminated infection, which requires systemic therapy (1 gm amphotericin B IV). Mild anemia, leukocytosis, and increased serum gamma globulin are laboratory findings often found with chronic candidal infection. Evaluation of serologic markers such as candidal antigen may be helpful in differentiating local (bladder) from invasive (renal) or systemic infection.

The removal of an indwelling urethral catheter or discontinuance of broad-spectrum antibiotic therapy may eradicate colonization of early noninvasive (bladder) candidal infection. If these steps fail, treatment with bladder irrigation with amphotericin B (50 mg/liter of water per day) via three-way urethral catheter or urethral catheter and suprapubic tube is effective. Treatment is required for 5 to 7 days; a repeat course may be necessary. An alternate treatment is the use of miconazole (50 mg/liter of saline per day). Both treatments have had a greater than 90 per cent success rate in the treatment of localized bladder funguria. Ambulatory patients may be treated with a daily instillation of amphotericin B (200 mg) administered on a daily or alternate-day basis for 3 to 5 treatments. Following instillation, the patient should not void for 2 hours. The results of this form of therapy have not been well documented, but anecdotal observations suggest it is efficacious.

Persistence of funguria indicates invasive bladder, upper tract, or systemic infection; hence, other treatment modalities are indicated. The new triazole fluconazole (200 mg/day administered orally for 14 days) has been effective in the treatment of bladder candiduria. However, its role in the management of upper tract candidiasis has not been defined clearly. The availability of both oral and IV fluconazole may provide a useful agent for upper tract infection. Invasive or disseminated infection requires systemic therapy with IV amphotericin B.

Fungal infection by *C. albicans* has developed in two patients with artificial urethral sphincters and in one with a penile prosthesis. Systemic therapy with amphotericin B without removal of the sphincter was effective in those two cases, whereas removal of the penile prosthesis and systemic therapy with amphotericin B (>1 gm) and ketoconazole (400 mg/day for 14 days) was necessary in the other patient. Careful evaluation of skin for possible fungal infection is necessary prior to surgical placement of protheses.

Candidal infection of the upper tracts (i.e., collecting system or ureter) can be caused by direct ascent from the lower urinary system or disseminated infection. Upper tract infection may cause fungal accretions known as fungal balls, which can cause obstructive uropathy. Indwelling urinary catheters, pre-existing obstructive uropathy, diabetes mellitus, or immune suppression often is the predisposing factor. The patients often are clinically ill, with fever and flank pain. They may be oliguric or anuric, with fungal material found in the urine. Imaging studies will demonstrate filling defects within the renal collecting system. Upper tract obstruction caused by fungal balls also has occurred in infants. Predisposing factors have included congenital anomalies, prematurity, antibiotic therapy, and parenteral feeding. In the adult, percutaneous nephrostomy and antifungal irrigation (amphotericin B, 50 mg/day), often in conjunction with systemic antifungal therapy (IV amphotericin B, 1 gm), are necessary to control the infection and alleviate the obstructive uropathy.

Disseminated candidiasis frequently infects the kidney. Autopsy studies of 39 patients with disseminated infection revealed kidney involvement in 32 (82 per cent). Predisposing diseases included leukemia in 18 (46 per cent), major surgery in 12 (31 per cent), and other malignancies or chronic disease in 9 (23 per cent). Pathologic study of renal involvement in patients with disseminated candidiasis has revealed multiple abscesses in the interstitium or glomeruli. Candidal infection of the kidney has demonstrated budding yeast and pseudomycelia in peritubular vessels and collecting tubules. Papillary necrosis has been observed in pathologic specimens and clinical settings. Clinical manifestations of renal candidal infection may include fever, chills, and flank pain. Renal infection may be indicative of parenchymal and/or disseminated disease.

Systemic therapy with IV amphotericin B is indicated. Therapy should continue until the patient is clinically well (i.e., afebrile, normal white count, negative cultures).

Anecdotal and isolated case reports suggest that fluconazole may be effective in the treatment of invasive genitourinary candidal infection. The drug may be used in patients who are not critically ill (i.e., no fever, leucocytosis, or positive blood culture). In critically ill patients, systemic amphotericin B is the treatment of choice.

Cryptococcosis

The initial focus of infection with *Cryptococcus* is usually the respiratory tree, and infection usually occurs following inhalation of the fungal spores. Dissemination may occur with involvement of the central nervous system, bone, skin, and genitourinary system. Cryptococcal infection of the genitourinary system can affect the adrenal, kidneys, prostate, or external genitalia. In 39 patients with disseminated cryptococcal infection, 20 (51 per cent) had renal involvement. Pathologic changes ranged from sparse lymphocytic infiltrate to intense granulomatous reaction. In no case could renal insufficiency be attributed to cryptococcal infection. Of 23 male patients with infection, 6 (26 per cent) had prostate involvement as evidenced by large granulomatous nodules with focal caseation. Cryptococcal pyelonephritis has been known to precede the onset of meningeal infection.

In AIDS patients, the prostate is often a reservoir of cryptococcal infection following treatment of cryptococcal meningitis with systemic IV amphotericin B and oral flucytosine. In these cases, fluconazole (200 mg/day for 6 months) has been efficacious in the treatment of cryptococcal prostatitis.

Penile lesions caused by cryptococcis have been treated by surgical excision, amphotericin B, ketoconazole, and/or flucytosine.

RARE AND UNUSUAL INFECTIONS

Geotrichum candidum has been known to cause a urinary tract infection. Systemic amphotericin B stabilized but did not cure the infection.

Hansenula fabianii caused prostatitis in a 57-year-old patient with chronic lymphocytic leukemia and schizophrenia. Urethral self-manipulation was the putative source of entry. The infection did not respond to ketoconazole and required amphotericin B (2 gm).

Paecilomyces pyelonephritis has occurred in a patient with nephrolithiasis. The infection resolved following removal of the stone.

Paracoccidioidomycosis is common in South America; urologic manifestations are rare. Pulmonary exacerbation has occurred in a patient who required immune suppression for renal transplantation. The infection was controlled with amphotericin B (2 gm) and ketoconazole.

Phycomycosis (mucormycosis, zygomycosis) has been documented in patients on chronic dialysis for end-stage renal disease. Mucormycosis affects primarily the sinuses and respiratory system. In systemic infection, the kidneys may be involved; poor renal function and obstructive uropathy may be caused by fungal hyphae occluding both the vascular and collecting systems. Disseminated infection is usually fatal, whereas isolated renal infection may be successfully treated with systemic amphotericin B and nephrectomy.

Rhinosporidiosis is indigenous to India and Sri Lanka. This fungus can cause chronic granulomatous lesions of the urethra. Surgical excision is adequate treatment.

PHARMACOLOGIC THERAPY

Amphotericin B

Amphotericin B is an antifungal antibiotic derived from the fungus strain *Streptomyces nodosus*. It can be fungistatic or fungicidal depending on dosage and vulnerability of the fungus. The drug induces its effect by binding to sterols in the cell wall membrane, resulting in disruption of cell membrane permeability.

Amphotericin B (Fungizone) is available as a topical cream for cutaneous fungal infections and is available for IV administration as a powder for colloid suspension. Supplied in sterile bottles of 50 mg, the powder is suspended in 10 ml of (nonbacteriostatic) sterile water to yield a 5 mg/ml colloid suspension. This suspension is further diluted in 500 ml of 5% dextrose and water with a resultant 0.1-mg/ml colloid suspension. Amphotericin B can be inactivated by light and heat, and it thus should be prepared on the day of administration. During IV administration, the bottle and IV tubing should be protected with aluminum foil to prevent light inactivation.

Amphotericin B can induce toxic reactions; therefore, the patient initially is given low doses of 0.25 mg/kg per day, with a gradual increase to 1 mg/kg per day. The total dose level should never exceed 1.5 mg/kg per day. The patient may develop chills, fever, gastrointestinal upset, or even hypotension during therapy, which will necessitate temporarily discontinuing the IV amphotericin B. Rising creatinine and/or electrolyte imbalance (hypokalemia) indicates the need for modification or discontinuation of therapy. Adequate saline maintenance may mitigate renal toxicity. Concomitant IV steroids have been used to ameliorate the toxic effects of amphotericin B treatment.

The primary fungal infections (blastomycosis, coccidioidomycosis, and histoplasmosis) require long-term (6 to 8 weeks) therapy with a total dosage of more than 2.0 gm of amphotericin B. In mycotic infection caused by the opportunistic fungi (i.e., *Candida, Cryptococcus*, or *Torulopsis*), amphotericin B may be given in modified doses in conjunction with flucytosine therapy, as discussed later in this section.

In cases in which fungal infection appears to be confined to the kidney or bladder, the localized infection can be treated by amphotericin B irrigation, which does not have the toxic effect of systemic treatment. Irrigation with amphotericin B is described subsequently.

BLADDER IRRIGATION WITH AMPHOTERICIN B

At present, the drug insert found with amphotericin B and its description in the *Physicians' Desk Reference* do not indicate use of amphotericin B for bladder or kidney irrigation. Nevertheless, amphotericin B has been successfully used for many years for treatment of candidal cystitis by means of bladder irrigation without adverse affect. The method used is as follows.

One ampule of IV amphotericin B (50 mg suspended in 1 liter of sterile water) is slowly run through a three-way Foley or urethral catheter and suprapubic tube for period of 12 h/day. This procedure is continued for 5 to 7 days. Following this course of therapy, urine should be recultured for candidal infection. Treatment may have to be repeated for another course of 5 to 7 days. The amphotericin B irrigant should be prepared daily, and both the bottle and irrigation tubing should be covered with aluminum foil to protect it from light and excess heat. Most cases of candidal infection confined to the bladder will be resolved by this treatment alone. If the patient has systemic manifestations (i.e., fever, anemia, or elevated serum antibody titer to candidal antigen), systemic treatment with fluconazole or IV amphotericin B may be necessary.

Flucytosine

Flucytosine (5-FC, fluorocytosine, Ancobon) is an effective drug for the treatment of *Candida, Cryptococcus, Torulopsis*, and some strains of *Aspergillus*. Flucytosine presently is available in 250-mg or 500-mg capsules for oral administration only. The dosage schedule is 150 mg/kg of body weight per day, administered in four divided doses. Treatment generally is required for 3 to 4 weeks. Because the drug is excreted primarily by the kidneys, dosage should be modified in the presence of compromised renal function, with the reduction of dosage commensurate with the level of kidney function. For example, if creatinine clearance is 50 ml/min, halve the dose or increase the dose interval relative to creatinine clearance (i.e., every 12 hours instead of every 6 hours). Flucytosine is a compound with small molecular weight; it is readily dialyzable and can be given to patients by hemodialysis or peritoneal dialysis.

Fungal cultures should be tested for in vitro sensitivity to 5-FC by tube dilution methods. Organisms whose sensitivity is greater than 12.5 μg/ml of flucytosine will not respond to 5-FC treatment. Most hospital strains of *Candida* initially may be sensitive to 5-FC; however, if the dose is too low or inadequate, secondary resistance may develop.

Adverse reactions to flucytosine may include skin rash, gastrointestinal upset (a few cases of enteritis have been reported), and agranulocytosis (which is reversible). One case of aplastic anemia has been reported associated with flucytosine therapy. Transient hepatocellular dysfunction has been known to occur. These adverse reactions are infrequent and, for the most part, reversible. Flucytosine should not be given during pregnancy. However, there have been case reports of successful treatment of candidal infection in pregnancy without adverse effect on the fetus.

In recent years flucytosine has lost favor in the treatment of genitourinary candidiasis because of the development of resistant strains of candida, the potential for bone marrow toxicity, and the availability of the newer drug fluconazole. Nevertheless, flucytosine still has a role in the treatment of cryptococcal infections. In view of its relatively low toxicity and ease of administration (the patient may be treated on an ambulatory basis), flucytosine may still have a role in the treatment of noninvasive urinary candidiasis.

The Imidazoles and Triazoles

In the 1970s a group of antifungal agents, the imidazoles, were introduced for the treatment of fungal infections. These included clotrimazole, miconazole, and ketoconazole.

Clotrimazole's rapid metabolic breakdown and toxic effects limit its use to a topical agent. Miconazole is not rapidly metabolized but it has toxic effects caused by Cremophor EL, a polyethoxalated castor oil required for colloidal stabilization for intravenous use. The low level of renal excretion further limits miconazole's use as a systemic agent in the urologic patient. As indicated above, miconazole can be utilized as a bladder antifungal irrigant. It is supplied in 200-mg ampules that can be diluted into 4 liters of saline to provide a 50-mg/liter solution that can be utilized as an antifungal bladder irrigant. Care must be taken that the solution is mixed in a glass container because some plastics will elute the drug.

Ketoconazole fulfills the criteria desirable for an effective antifungal agent. It is readily absorbed (in nonachlorhydric patients) by the gastrointestinal tract and achieves good tissue distribution. Ketoconazole interacts with the ergosterol of fungal membranes and the cholesterol of mammalian cells. It also interferes with the cytochrome P-450 enzyme systems of several organ systems, including the testis, ovary, adrenal gland, liver, and kidney. Single doses of 200 to 400 mg of ketoconazole may interact with C_{17-20} lyase in the testis and adrenal, causing impairment of steroidogenesis. This effect has been utilized clinically in the treatment of patients with carcinoma of the prostate and Cushing disease.

Ketoconazole's role as an antifungal agent has been in the treatment of nonimmunocompromised patients with non–life-threatening blastomycosis, chronic mucocutaneous candidiasis, histoplasmosis, and paracoccidioidomycosis. However, ketoconazole has the potential for hepatic dysfunction. Most significantly, ketoconazole has not been very effective for urologic patients because low levels of renal excretion result in inadequate therapeutic urine drug levels. Clinical studies of 20 patients with genitourinary fungal infections indicated that ketoconazole was effective in only 50 per cent of patients with candiduria.

Newer antifungal agents known as the triazoles, itraconazole (Sporanox) and fluconazole (Diflucan), have been developed. The mode of action of the triazoles is similar to that of ketoconazole—inhibition of the synthesis of ergosterol, a component of the fungal cell membrane. The step required to convert 14-alpha-methylsterol to ergosterol is dependent on cytochrome P-450 activation, which is inhibited by the imidazole moiety.

Itraconazole has poor water solubility and minimal urine excretion, but may be used in primary fungal infections at a dose of 200 mg/day. Fluconazole has good water solubility, which results in high levels of urinary excretion, which makes it useful in most urinary fungal infections.

Fluconazole has excellent absorption from the gastrointestinal tract (>90 per cent). It is available as both an oral and an IV preparation. Unlike ketoconazole, it is not dependent on gastric acidity. Peak serum concentrations are reached in 2 hours. There is minimal protein binding (12 per cent) and the drug is metabolically stable, with renal excretion accounting for 80 per cent of elimination. The plasma half-life is approximately 30 hours; rifampin decreases the half-life of fluconazole, but to a lesser degree than it does of ketoconazole. There is minimal interaction with warfarin, phenytoin, and cyclosporin. Fluconazole does not inhibit steroidogenesis to the degree that ketoconazole does.

The dosage of fluconazole should be modified in the presence of renal failure. The drug can be administered in patients undergoing hemodialysis.

SUMMARY

In the era of the critically ill immunosuppressed patient, fungal infections will increase. Many of these infections will cause genitourinary disease. The patient who is recovering from major urologic surgery (e.g., cystectomy) or who is immunosuppressed (e.g., renal transplant patient) may be vulnerable to secondary fungal infection. Recognition and treatment of these fungal infections may avoid the final and critical insult to the patient.

Suggested Readings

Hamory BH, Wenzel RP: Hospital associated candiduria: Predisposing factors and review of the literature. J Urol 120:444, 1978

Irby PB, Stoller ML, McAninch JW: Fungal bezoars of the upper urinary tract. J Urol 143:447, 1990

Larsen RA, Bozzette S, McCutchan JA, et al: The Collaborative California Treatment Group: Persistent *Cryptococcus neoformans* infection of the prostate after successful treatment of meningitis. Ann Intern Med 111: 125, 1989

Rippon JW: Characteristics of fungi. *In* Medical Mycology: The Pathogenic Fungi and the Pathogenic Actinomycetes, 3rd ed. Philadelphia, WB Saunders, 1988, pp 121–153

Wise GJ: Amphotericin B in urological practice. J Urol 144:215, 1990

Wise GJ: Fungal infections of the urinary tract. *In* Walsh PC, Retik AB, Stamey TA, et al (eds): Campbell's Urology, 6th ed. Philadelphia, WB Saunders, 1992, pp 928–950

Wise GJ, Silver DA: Fungal infections of the genitourinary system. J. Urol 149:1377, 1993.

WEGENER'S GRANULOMATOSIS

WILLIAM A. KENNEDY II, M.D.

New York, New York

Wegener's granulomatosis is a disease characterized by necrotizing granulomatous angiitis involving the upper and lower respiratory tracts and the kidneys. Pathologically, the necrotizing angiitis causes a segmental focal glomerulonephritis in the kidney. Although renal involvement is common (83 per cent of reported cases) and renal failure is the most common cause of death in Wegener's granulomatosis, other involvement of the genitourinary tract is not as rare as once suspected. Cases of penile necrosis, prostatic involvement, and retroperitoneal fibrosis secondary to Wegener's granulomatosis have now been reported.

In the past, there has been some conflict as to whether Wegener's granulomatosis, limited Wegener's granulomatosis, and midline granuloma were really the same disease or different disease entities. Recent evidence suggests that Wegener's granulomatosis is a disease spectrum in which there is frequently progression of disease from one anatomic site to another. Most frequently, patients with symptoms of Wegener's granulomatosis present with symptoms of upper respiratory involvement, suggesting that the upper airway may be the portal of entry for the agent or agents that cause the disease. It has become clear from this that patients presenting with upper airway and pulmonary lesions secondary to Wegener's granulomatosis should be thoroughly screened for genitourinary involvement.

In most cases, a focal glomerular lesion will not cause an abnormality in the intravenous urogram; however, ureteral involvement will present with varying degrees of obstruction. Virtually all patients with renal involvement secondary to Wegener's granulomatosis will present with microscopic hematuria, and, if the lesion is advanced, there may be some decrease in renal function in terms of blood urea nitrogen, creatinine, and creatinine clearance. We have found renal scanning with technetium-99m–labeled diethylenetriaminepentaacetic acid to be valuable in detecting renal defects not evident by standard intravenous urography or biochemical parameters. The definitive diagnosis of renal involvement, of course, depends on renal biopsy. The renal biopsy shows necrotizing glomerulonephritis in all patients and crescent formation in the majority of patients. Other laboratory findings are highly variable in the patient with genitourinary Wegener's granulomatosis. About half of the patients will have some degree of anemia, and another half will have an elevated erythrocyte sedimentation rate. Rheumatoid factor and C-reactive protein will be positive in only about one third of the patients with genitourinary Wegener's granulomatosis, and elevated immunoglobulin A levels seem to be an unreliable finding in most patients.

The treatment of Wegener's granulomatosis has changed drastically over the last few years. Prior to the introduction of treatment with modern immunosuppressive agents, therapy was based on the use of corticosteroids in moderate to high doses. Corticosteroids alone, despite being relatively effective in controlling upper respiratory and pulmonary involvement, were found to be relatively ineffective in controlling renal involvement with Wegener's granulomatosis. The introduction of other immunosuppressive agents, particularly cyclophosphamide, into the treatment of these patients has changed dramatically the nearly uniform mortality previously seen in the untreated form of the disease. In the past, untreated Wegener's granulomatosis had a mean survival of 5 months, with 82 per cent of the patients dying within the first year and 90 per cent dying within 2 years.

The recommended safe and effective dose range of cyclophosphamide for patients with Wegener's granulomatosis and renal involvement is 2 to 3 mg/kg per day. Prolonged treatment with cyclophosphamide for at least 2 years after clinical remission is associated with improved survival and renal function. The incidence of hemorrhagic cystitis and bone marrow depression is minimal in this dose range. One side effect that has been noted consistently is the cessation of menses in premenopausal women on therapy. Other complications of immunosuppressive therapy include localized herpes zoster, localized and disseminated herpes simplex, and squamous cell carcinoma of the skin. The routine use of immunosuppressive therapy (cyclophosphamide) has become the treatment of choice in patients with Wegener's granulomatosis, particularly those with renal involvement, and such agents have greatly altered the outlook in this once devastating disease process.

Suggested Readings

Andrassy K, Erb A, Koderisch J, et al: Wegener's granulomatosis with renal involvement: Patient survival and correlations between initial renal function, renal histology, therapy and renal outcome. Clin Nephrol 35:139, 1991

Sizeland PCB, Bailey RR, Lynn KL, et al: Wegener's granulomatosis with renal involvement: A 14 year experience. N Z Med J 103:366, 1990

ECHINOCOCCAL DISEASE OF THE KIDNEY

BRETT C. MELLINGER, M.D.

New Hyde Park, New York

Echinococcosis is caused by the larval form of the tapeworm *Echinococcus granulosus*, which resides in the adult form in the intestinal tract of the dog, the definitive host. This disease is rare in the United States but is endemic in South America, South Africa, Australia, New Zealand, central and southern Europe, and parts of the former Soviet Union.

Humans act as intermediate hosts after ingestion of ova. The larva hatch in the duodenum and penetrate the intestinal wall to enter the circulation. The liver is involved most frequently (70 per cent of cases), followed by the lung (10 per cent); renal infection occurs in 2 to 3 per cent of cases. Bilateral renal involvement and infection of other genitourinary organs are rare.

CLINICAL PRESENTATION

Hydatid disease of the kidney evolves slowly, with cysts developing at the rate of about 1 cm/year. Hydatid cysts are usually solitary and located in the renal cortex. Patients frequently present with flank pain, often with a palpable mass and hematuria. The cyst rarely may rupture into the collecting system and the patient may experience colic, with passage of grape skin–like material. Secondary infection of the cyst cavity may lead to development of symptoms and signs indicative of renal abscess. Cysts may rupture into the peritoneum or an adjacent viscus. Cyst fluid is highly antigenic and may lead to a severe anaphylactic reaction.

DIAGNOSIS

Identification of daughter cysts in the urine is pathognomonic. Eosinophilia may be present in 20 to 50 per cent of cases. Complement fixation, hemagglutination, and the Casoni intradermal skin test are positive in 90 per cent of patients when combined. Intravenous urography typically shows a thick-walled cystic mass, which may have a rim of calcification. If the cyst ruptures into the collecting system, daughter cysts may be outlined in the renal pelvis as an irregular mass or multiple solitary lesions. Ultrasound demonstrates a multicystic or multiloculated mass. Shifting hydatid sand may be seen as a falling snowflake pattern after changes in the patient's position. Computerized tomography may demonstrate a cystic mass with discrete daughter cysts and an enhancing membrane, daughter cysts within the mother cyst, or a thick-walled, multiloculated cystic mass.

TREATMENT

Cyst aspiration for diagnosis and treatment should be discouraged because of the risk of dissemination of infection and allergic reaction to the cyst fluid. Marsupialization of cysts also is not recommended for similar reasons. When these two procedures are unavoidable, such as in preservation of renal function in a solitary kidney, the instillation of a scolecidal agent should be used (30% sodium chloride, 2% formalin, 1% iodine, or 0.5% silver nitrate).

Systemic anthelmintic agents, such as mebendazole and albendazole, have been used with limited success. Sterilization of cyst fluid is variable, with significant side effects.

Surgery remains the treatment of choice for renal echinococcosis. The degree of renal involvement will determine the surgical approach. Partial nephrectomy, removal of the intact cyst, or total nephrectomy may be required. Surgical exposure should be generous, with anticipation of a difficult dissection as a result of extensive fibrosis and inflammation. Isolation of the kidney is necessary to prevent spillage of cyst material. If cyst rupture seems imminent, aspiration of cyst fluid and instillation of any of the above sterilizing agents may be performed.

Bench surgery has been used for centrally located cysts when renal preservation is required. The kidney is detached from its pedicle followed by ex vivo aspiration of cyst material, cyst excision, and orthotopic autotransplantation. This method may provide better isolation with less opportunity for spillage of cyst material.

Suggested Readings

Cohen MS: Granulomatous nephritis. Urol Clin North Am 13:647–659, 1986

Schaeffer AJ: Renal infection. *In* Gillenwater JY, Grayhack JT, Howards SS, et al (eds): Adult and Pediatric Urology. Chicago, Year Book Medical Publishers, 1987, pp 648–690

Smith JH, von Lichtenberg F, Lehman JS: Parasitic diseases of the genitourinary system. *In* Walsh PC, Retick AB, Stamey TA, et al (eds): Campbell's Urology, 6th ed. Philadelphia, WB Saunders, 1992, pp 883–927

PAPILLARY NECROSIS

A. RICHARD KENDALL, M.D.

Philadelphia, Pennsylvania

It is quite obvious that papillary necrosis is usually an unsuspected radiologic diagnosis and rarely presents initially as a clinical entity. Thus the vast majority of cases are mild, undiagnosed, and untreated.

Acute papillary necrosis rarely is seen, but when it does occur usually is found in diabetics with acute pyelonephritis with or without obstruction and with or without "gas" formation. This type of fulminating infection was encountered more commonly in the past but now is seen infrequently in clinical practice as a result of improved management of diabetes and urinary tract infections.

Through 25 years of radiologic conferences, Dr. Howard Pollack has taught the use of etiologic mnemonic "POSTCARD." That is, the causes of papillary necrosis include *p*yelonephritis, *o*bstruction, *s*ickle cell disease, *t*uberculosis, *c*irrhosis, *a*nalgesic abuse, *r*enal vein thrombosis, and *d*iabetes. This condition is seen more commonly in adult females and rarely in the pediatric population.

Renal papillary necrosis represents a form of ischemic necrosis occurring usually at the papillary tip or apex of the pyramid, but there may be more extensive involvement of the entire pyramid, often in conjunction with a more diffuse interstitial nephritis. This entity usually involves multiple calyces (papillae) and typically is bilateral, but early on can be limited to lesser involved areas. Vascular ischemia may be the etiologic factor in all cases, with the medullary blood supply being so tenuous. Overall, the most common causes are diabetes and analgesic abuse, with maximal damage in the region of the loop of Henle.

Analgesic abuse with resulting interstitial nephritis and papillary necrosis has been described over the past three decades. Analgesic neuropathy is estimated to be the cause of renal failure in 20 per cent of dialysis patients in Australia but in many fewer such patients in the United States. Phenacetin has been the most often documented drug etiology, but aspirin and nonsteroidal anti-inflammatory agents also can produce renal toxicity, including interstitial nephritis, renal failure, and papillary necrosis.

Although the rare "fulminant" type with sepsis and all the stigmata of acute pyelonephritis may occur, most cases develop insidiously without symptoms of infection. Eventually, either an incidental urogram is obtained, there is evidence of chronic renal insufficiency, or symptoms occur related to passing a sloughed papilla (colic, pyuria, hematuria). In advanced cases, fibrosis of the interstitium and tubular atrophy lead to decreased renal size and end-stage renal disease.

RADIOLOGIC MANIFESTATIONS

Renal size is usually normal in the early stages, and the contour remains smooth. Early in the course of the disease, papillary swelling may be difficult to detect. Later the epithelium will be disrupted, and contrast can be seen extending outside the calyx and eventually revealing the progression to complete papillary slough and cavitary formation. Calcification is not uncommon, especially in analgesic abuse patients. With progression, typical small kidneys result as renal insufficiency becomes a major clinical problem. There have been minimal reports of ultrasound and computerized tomography findings in cases of papillary necrosis. These findings are nonspecific, and this diagnosis is one of the few conditions that still requires an intravenous program.

DIAGNOSIS

The differential diagnosis includes medullary sponge kidney, postinflammatory atrophy, old abscess cavity, and calyceal diverticulum. A sloughed papilla, presenting as colic, must be differentiated from a calculus, tumor, or any other filling defect. The papilla may have some degree of calcification. Retrograde urography is quite valuable in diagnosis while minimizing the invasiveness of the work-up. There is an increased incidence of transitional cell carcinoma in patients with analgesic nephropathy, and these tumors seem to be slow growing, multifocal, and bilateral.

THERAPY

Patients with the acute form of papillary necrosis are treated aggressively, as one would care for acute pyelonephritis. Obstruction, if present, must be relieved. Although not reversible once established, progression can be limited by treatment of the basic problem; therefore, control of infection, relief of obstruction, control of diabetes, and discontinuance of analgesics are the primary steps in the treatment regimen.

Operative intervention is rarely necessary. In the diabetic with emphysematous pyelonephritis who is failing to respond favorably despite intravenous antibiotics and supportive therapy, emergency nephrectomy may be lifesaving.

The sloughed papilla, once properly diagnosed, most often passes spontaneously. If sepsis is present, preferably a temporary percutaneous nephrostomy or a ureteral stent should allow time for antibiotic therapy and decompression to stabilize the patient. The papilla probably will pass, especially after undergoing further necrosis. With persistent obstruction in the stabilized patient, the obstructing papilla can be treated endoscopically as one would any ureteral calculus. Open operation indeed rarely would be necessary.

In general, papillary necrosis either is an incidental finding requiring no aggressive therapy or presents as chronic renal disease requiring medical treatment. Rarely is this a surgical disease requiring operative intervention.

Suggested Reading

Davidson AJ: Chronic parenchymal disease in clinical urography. *In* Pollack HM (ed): Clinical Urology, vol 3. Philadelphia, WB Saunders, 1990, pp 2278–2285

CHYLURIA

LESTER J. KARAFIN, M.D.

Philadelphia, Pennsylvania

Chyluria denotes the presence in the urine of chyle, a combination of lymph and triglycerides, with the fats appearing as milk-like emulsions or mixtures of fatty acids, neutral fats, and soaps. Chyluria is noted by the patient as passage of milky white urine. This represents leakage from a lymphatic–urinary system fistula. Chyluria probably was first mentioned by Hippocrates. In 1670, Moellenbroch described chyluria as the result of a pathologic connection between the lymphatic system and the urinary tract. In 1741, Morgagni associated chyluria with a disturbance in lymphatic circulation. In 1863, Ackerman proposed the obstruction theory.

The lymphatic drainage of the kidney includes an extensive parenchymal plexus that drains the substance of the kidney and converges onto the renal hilus. There is also a subcapsular plexus that drains the tissue beneath the capsule and emerges at the renal hilus. It follows the course of the renal vein to the lateral aortic nodes. Finally, there is a plexus that communicates with the subcapsular plexus and drains independently to the lateral aortic nodes. Filariasis, trauma, tuberculosis, and retroperitoneal tumors are the most frequent causes of obstruction of the renal lymphatics, leading to forniceal rupture and leakage of chyle.

Chyluria can be classified into two groups, parasitic and nonparasitic. The former is associated with filariasis caused by *Wuchereria bancrofti*, a thread-like nematode about 0.5 cm in length that lives in the human lymphatics. Filariasis is endemic in countries bordering the Mediterranean, south China, Japan, and the South Pacific islands (particularly Samoa). Limited infections, as seen in American soldiers during World War II, give an entirely different clinical picture from that seen in the frequent reinfections usually encountered among the native populations. However, diagnosis and treatment are the same. Filariasis leads to protein deposits in the lymphatic system causing obstruction and subsequent chyluria.

Nonparasitic chyluria occurs with mechanical obstruction of the lymphatics proximal to the kidney, with subsequent renal forniceal rupture and leakage into the urinary tract. This can be caused by retroperitoneal tumors, trauma, tuberculosis, or spontaneous rupture. There is one case report of obstruction after percutaneous nephrolithotomy.

RADIOLOGIC DIAGNOSIS

Pedal lymphography is the technique of choice to evaluate the lymphatic channels and nodes. The findings in chyluria may be striking. There may be total obstruction of drainage above the level of the renal pedicle, with lymphaticovisceral backflow into the perirenal lymphatics frequently seen. Lymphorenal reflux is not specific for chyluria and can occur in any obstructing process in the retroperitoneum. Pollack reported that the contrast medium occasionally may find its way into the renal pelvis, ureter, and bladder.

TREATMENT

Conservative treatment consists of a medium-chain fatty acid diet and instillation of sclerosing agents into the renal pelvis. The rationale for the diet therapy is that the fatty acids are transported from the gut directly into the liver by the portal system and not with the chylus, like long-chain fatty acids. The diet is very hard to follow and this treatment may be unsuccessful. The instillation of 1% to 2% silver nitrate is an attempt to sclerose the lymphopelvic fistulas. However, there is associated back pain and a low success rate. Treating the filariasis is usually insufficient because chyluria is a late manifestation of the disease.

Surgical options include lymphovenous anastomosis using the microscope, as suggested by Cockett and Goodwin, with ligation of all remaining lymph vessels leading to the kidney and renal pelvis. Renal autotransplantation is another option, as is nephrectomy. There is one reported case of renal autotransplantation resulting in a cure. The most popular option is stripping of the renal pedicle, with ligation of all lymphatic vessels leading to the kidney and upper ureter. This results in cessation of the chyluria in 66 to 75 per cent of the reported cases.

Suggested Readings

Brunkwall J, Simonsen O, Bergquist D, et al: Chyluria treated with renal autotransplantation: A case report. J Urol 143:793–796, 1990

Pollack H: Radiologic Examination of the Urinary Tract. New York, Harper & Row, 1971

Pool MO, Vanderhem K, Stel HV, et al: Bilateral excision of perinephric fat and fascia in the treatment of intractable chyluria. J Urol 146:1374–1376, 1991

Thrasher JB, Snyder JA: Post-nephrolithotomy chyluria. J Urol 143:578–579, 1990

MALACOPLAKIA OF THE URETER AND KIDNEY

HUGH A. G. FISHER, M.D., F.A.C.S.

Albany, New York

Malacoplakia of the urinary tract is an inflammatory process. Although found primarily in the bladder, malacoplakia of the ureter and renal pelvis with no evidence of bladder involvement is seen in 12 per cent of cases. Renal parenchymal involvement occurs rarely.

The distal ureter is the most common site of upper urinary tract involvement, with other sites, in decreasing frequency, in the proximal ureter, renal pelvis, and renal parenchyma. Malacoplakia of the ureter most often causes narrowing of the ureteral lumen and resultant hydronephrosis. Patients can present with symptomatic hydronephrosis, pyelonephritis, or silent destruction of the ipsilateral kidney. Greater than 90 per cent of patients have infected urine, and the most common organism cultured is *Escherichia coli*. Patients with a solitary kidney or bilateral upper tract involvement may present with azotemia of uremia.

Intravenous urography and retrograde ureteropyelogram reveal rounded filling defects. The papillary lesions may be solitary or multiple and are most commonly several millimeters in size. Circumferential lesions commonly appear as dense narrowing of the ureteral lumen. The differential diagnosis includes ureteritis cystica, tuberculous ureteritis, leukoplakia, blood clot, nonopaque calculi, and papillary transitional cell carcinoma. Renal pelvic malacoplakia can be difficult to distinguish radiographically from ureteral pelvic junction obstruction.

The histologic findings in upper urinary tract malacoplakia are identical to those in the bladder. It is characterized by large histiocytic cells (von Hansemann cells) containing Michaelis-Gutmann inclusions admixed with an infiltrate of lymphocytes, plasma cells, and bundles of fibroblasts and collagen. This must be seen on microscopy to make the diagnosis of malacoplakia with certainty.

Treatment of ureteral and renal pelvic malacoplakia consists of long-term antibiotics and appropriate surgery. Depending on the location of the lesion, distal ureterectomy with ureteroneocystostomy, segmental ureterectomy with end-to-end spatulated uretero-ureterostomy, or a dismembered renal pelvic procedure may be performed. Nephroureterectomy is indicated in cases of diffuse disease.

Renal parenchymal malacoplakia, compared to involvement of the bladder, ureter, and renal pelvis, occurs in older patients (seventh decade), with a greater female predominance (female-to-male ratio of 15:1). Patients present with flank pain and often have a palpable flank mass. Fever is common. When bilateral (60 per cent of cases) or in a solitary kidney, patients may present with azotemia. The majority of patients have urinary infection, most commonly with *E. coli*.

Excretory urography will show an enlarged kidney with multiple filling defects, a solitary large mass, or nonfunction. Arteriography typically reveals a hypovascular mass with peripheral neovascularity. There will be lower urinary tract involvement in 50 per cent of cases.

Renal parenchymal malacoplakia is treated by nephrectomy with hope of cure. Patients with bilateral renal involvement have a poor prognosis and generally survive less than 1 year. When the disease is found to involve a transplant kidney allograft, the kidney is removed and immunosuppression stopped.

Suggested Readings

Deridder PA, Koff SA, Gikas PW, et al: Renal malacoplakia. J Urol 117:428, 1977

Sexton CC, Lowman RM, Nyongo AO, et al: Malacoplakia presenting as complete unilateral ureteral obstruction. J Urol 128:139, 1982

Sunshine B: Malacoplakia of the upper urinary tract. J Urol 112:362, 1974.

IDIOPATHIC RENAL HEMATURIA

E. JAMES SEIDMON, M.D.

Philadelphia, Pennsylvania

Idiopathic renal hematuria can be described as focal glomerulonephritis with recurrent hematuria. This disease affects some of the glomeruli within the kidney and the identification usually is made by light microscopy. However, on further investigation of the kidney biopsy by immunofluorescence and electron microscopy, immunoglobulin (Ig) A nephropathy or IgA-IgG mesangial nephropathy can be demonstrated. There are a wide variety of clinical situations that can lead to focal glomerulonephritis, but this discussion is limited to the benign idiopathic form.

Idiopathic renal hematuria involves children but is more common in young adults, especially males. The cause remains unknown; it is associated with recurrent microscopic, and sometimes macroscopic, hematuria, yet the blood pressure and glomerular filtration rate remains unchanged. There is no family history and no peripheral edema, nor is proteinuria noted. Bleeding occurs most commonly after strenuous exercise or during an upper respiratory infection. The serum creatinine, as well as the creatinine clearance rate, remains unaffected, and a 24-hour urine collection usually accumulates less than 1.0 gm of protein. Recurring episodes of hematuria are known to extend from childhood into adult life, yet rarely is renal failure encountered.

In 1968, Berger's and Hinglais published a paper that delineated this disease, which has since become known as Berger's disease: recurrent hematuria, mesangial IgA deposits diagnosed by means of a renal biopsy, and the lack of a specified disease process, such as

Henoch-Schönlein purpura, systemic lupus erythematous nephritis, or chronic liver disease. Further research into this disease entity has led to the discovery that interleukin-2 (IL-2) plays a central role and may cause the derangement of the cellular immunoregulation pattern in idiopathic IgA nephropathy. Also, thin-basement-membrane nephropathy leads to diffuse thinning of the glomerular basement membrane and has been linked to idiopathic IgA nephropathy.

Over 85 per cent of the cases seen are noted in young male white adults less than 35 years of age. The symptoms are as noted previously and the pathology includes mesangial IgA granular deposits, deposition of C3 and properdin, and no early complement components. Most of the patients will have macroscopic hematuria, and at least 50 per cent of them will develop nephrotic syndrome and unfortunately progress to chronic renal failure requiring dialysis and/or renal transplantation.

If the biopsy does not demonstrate IgA-IgG mesangial deposits, the clinical picture is almost the same except there is no sexual predominance and often there may be associated flank pain. If the protein content of the urine remains low, this is indeed a benign disease; if proteinuria is elevated, further investigation is required to rule out glomerular or vascular dysfunction. Light microscopy of the renal tissue reveals findings that are basically the same as in Berger's disease with a local or segmental effect; however, because of the absence of mesangial IgA deposition, the long-term prognosis is excellent.

The urologist's role is to work with the nephrologist, allowing the latter to make the initial diagnosis via renal biopsy. Only if this does not prove to be diagnostic does the urologist become active in the work-up to rule out a benign or malignant lesion. Routine intravenous urogram, cystoscopy, and possibly rigid or flexible ureteroscopy may become necessary. Additional help may call for interventional radiologic procedures to rule out an arteriovenous fistula. Occasionally, a bleeding site may be observed (papillitis, angioma), and fulguration or instillation of 0.25% to 0.5% silver nitrate (5 to 10 ml qid for several days) via a ureteral catheter may resolve the situation. Regardless of the outcome, it is imperative to follow these patients closely and remain vigilant, because the recurrent bleeding may be the signpost of a small tumor of the endothelium or renal parenchyma.

Suggested Readings

Berger J, Hinglais N: Les dépĉots intercapillaries d'IgA-IgG. J Urol Nephrol (Paris) 74:694, 1968

Parera M, Rivera F, Egido J, et al: The role of interleukin 2 (IL-2) and serum-soluble IL-2 receptor cells in idiopathic IgA nephropathy. Clin Immunol Immunopathol 63:196, 1992

Tiebosch AT, Frederik PM, van Breda Vriesman PJ, et al: Thin-basement-membrane nephropathy in adults with persistent hematuria. N Engl J Med 320:14, 1989

RENAL VENOUS THROMBOSIS

SAKTI DAS, M.D.

Walnut Creek, California

Renal venous thrombosis (RVT) is most common in the neonatal age group, with an autopsy incidence of 0.26 to 0.7 per cent. Occasionally diagnosed in utero, the majority of pediatric RVT cases present during the first 2 weeks of life.

Primary RVT occurs acutely in a previously healthy neonate. Etiologies include primary disease such as membranous or membranoproliferative glomerulonephritis, pyelonephritis, or renal involvement with polyarteritis nodosa, amyloidosis, and sickle cell disease. Nephrotic syndrome, either itself or because of its underlying glomerulonephritis, often is associated with RVT, especially in adults. Other causes include traumatic thrombosis and neoplastic permeation of the renal veins. Secondary RVT, comprising nearly two thirds of the cases, results from preceding illness and ailments like diarrhea, dehydration, and sepsis leading to hypovolemia, decreased renal perfusion, and renal venous stasis.

Clinical presentations depend on the acuteness and completeness of thrombosis. The child is usually very sick, with painful enlarged kidneys and hematuria. Shock and sepsis are often manifestations of the primary disease predisposing to RVT. Laboratory studies reveal anemia, azotemia, thrombocytopenia, and proteinuria in varying degrees.

For definitive imaging diagnosis, contrast radiography has been supplanted by noninvasive abdominal ultrasonography, which depicts renal enlargement with thrombosis in the renal veins and vena cava. Similar findings may be observed with computerized tomography or magnetic resonance imaging, thereby offering no significant advantage over ultrasonography.

The initial management of RVT should be directed at prompt correction of dehydration and electrolyte imbalance. Antibiotic therapy often is necessary as prophylaxis or to control overt infection. Bilateral RVT leading to renal failure occasionally necessitates peritoneal dialysis. In most patients these vigorous medical measures prevent further progression of thrombus, and functional recovery is evident on serial renal scans. The rationale for early nephrectomy is rather tenuous, and this is not recommended except for life-threatening refractory hemorrhage or infection.

Anticoagulant therapy is instituted in patients without prompt response to medical therapy. Heparin is started at a dosage of 100 U/kg q 4 h to maintain clotting time at one to two times normal. Heparin should be continued for at least 2 weeks. As an alternative, combined therapy with heparin and warfarin can be given for 48 hours, followed by continuation of warfarin alone. Thrombolytic therapy with urokinase or streptokinase by systemic intravenous route or administered through a catheter embedded in the venous thrombus has been successful in adults and infants, with acceptable morbidity of rare allergic reactions and hemorrhagic episodes.

Bilateral RVT is a potentially fatal condition with high risk of pulmonary embolism. Most of the reported survivals resulted from surgical thrombectomy. Initial vigorous medical therapy of fluid and electrolyte replacement is mandatory. If ultrasonography demonstrates thrombus in the vena cava propagating into the renal veins, thrombectomy should be carried out. Both kidneys should be left behind even if brisk back-bleeding is not achieved and the kidneys remain grossly congested after extraction of the thrombi. Supportive medical therapy with anticoagulants should be continued with careful monitoring.

As a consequence of RVT, the affected kidney may recover completely or develop varying degrees of scarring and parenchymal damage. There may be diminished function, nonfunction, chronic renal infection, nephrotic syndrome, or renal hypertension. These delayed complications rarely require nephrectomy unless sufficiently severe and refractory to medical therapy.

Suggested Readings

Bromberg WD, Firlit CF: Fibrinolytic therapy for renal vein thrombosis in the child. J Urol 143:86, 1990

Ricci MA, Lloyd DA: Renal venous thrombosis in infants and children. Arch Surg 125:1195, 1990

Kidney Trauma

BLUNT RENAL TRAUMA

MICHAEL COBURN, M.D.

Houston, Texas

Among emergency conditions, renal trauma poses one of the major challenges to the urologist. Renal injury comprises a wide variety of clinical problems: penetrating and blunt trauma, adult and pediatric patients, the otherwise normal and the previously abnormal kidney. Injury may involve the renal parenchyma, vasculature, or collecting system, or be bilateral. Clinical presentations may range from the entirely stable patient with a solitary renal injury to the setting of multiple organ trauma in the unstable patient, when the need for immediate attention to the injured kidney may be overshadowed by the urgency of other injuries.

The approach to diagnosis and management of renal trauma has evolved over the past decade, as a result of changes in imaging technologies and further clinical experience with nonoperative therapies. The basic principles of trauma care continue to apply to these injuries, however, and the surgeon's role in patient care has become, in some respects, more complex and challenging as the therapeutic decisions become more precisely individualized based on detailed staging of injuries.

CLASSIFICATION

Most literature divides renal trauma into some variation of the following designations: minor parenchymal injury, major parenchymal injury, extrarenal collecting system injury, and renal pedicle injury. Minor parenchymal injuries would include renal contusions, subcapsular hematomas, and superficial parenchymal lacerations. Major parenchymal injuries describe lacerations deeper into the kidney, generally involving the deep cortex and/or medulla, often with variable degrees of contrast extravasation on imaging studies indicative of concomitant collecting system injury. Avulsion or devitalization of tissue, significant urinary extravasation, and continued or recurrent bleeding may be important considerations in such injuries, which may range from single deep lacerations to severe crushing with no salvageable renal tissue. Blunt renal pedicle trauma, usually caused by deceleration or acceleration injuries with arterial stretching, intimal tearing, and subsequent thrombosis, is discussed separately below. A formalized classification system (Grades I through V) has been proposed through the Organ Injury Scaling Committee of the American Association for the Surgery of Trauma.

MECHANISM OF INJURY

Blunt trauma comprises about 60 to 90 per cent of renal injuries in most series, although the prevalence of penetrating trauma varies with the patient population, being higher in urban trauma system settings. Vehicular trauma, including auto-pedestrian accidents, as well as falls, industrial accidents, and violent crime, account for most blunt renal injury. Although the normal kidney is somewhat protected by the surrounding abdominal and chest wall, a blow to the flank or abdomen may result in sudden compression of the kidney between the abdominal wall and the spine or rib cage, resulting in crush injury to the renal parenchyma. Similar forces also may result in rupture or avulsion of the extrarenal collecting system. Patterns of multiple organ injury may be recognized that are typical of such blunt abdominal trauma: left renal injury with splenic rupture, right renal injury with liver laceration. Injury to other upper abdominal viscera, especially the duodenum, pancreas, and colon, may accompany renal trauma as well. As previously noted, deceleration trauma may result in pedicle tension with vascular injury. An anatomically abnormal kidney may be particularly prone to injury from seemingly minor trauma; such conditions as ureteropelvic junction obstruction or renal neoplasm may be recognized only after such trauma and the attendant evaluation. Overall, renal injury occurs in 8 to 10 per cent of all cases of abdominal trauma.

PHYSICAL FINDINGS AND LABORATORY EVALUATION

Suspicion of renal injury is based on history, physical findings, or the presence of hematuria. Patients with blunt renal trauma may have overt physical evidence of upper abdominal or flank trauma, or such evidence may be entirely lacking. Flank ecchymoses, costovertebral angle or upper abdominal pain or tenderness, or abdominal mass may be present. The presence of lower rib fractures or vertebral transverse process fractures on plain films also should raise one's suspicion of significant renal trauma.

Hematuria is the classic sign of urinary tract injury, and, although a strong indicator of urinary tract trauma, the degree of hematuria correlates poorly with the severity of injury. Hematuria may be noted grossly and is easily comfirmable by chemical dipstick and microscopic urinary sediment examination.

Recent studies have questioned the need for routine renal imaging in every case of posttraumatic hematuria. Extensive data now exist to support the view that, in the absence of hypotension or gross hematuria, renal imaging is not always essential. In several large reviews, only renal contusion or minor lacerations were found in this population, injuries appropriately managed nonoperatively. Several caveats apply, however, in safely following this formula. First, lack of hypotension refers to any time after the time of injury, including blood pressure determinations obtained by paramedical personnel prior to or during hospital transport. Second, this approach should not be applied routinely in the pediatric population, in which injuries such as ureteropelvic disruption, forniceal avulsion, and renal artery thrombosis are more common than in the adult and often may lack hematuria as presenting signs. Third, in this author's view, a history of trauma of extraordinary magnitude, manifested by the presence of major closed head injury, long bone fracture, physical signs of major abdominal impact, or a history of deceleration injury, should prompt investigation to exclude urinary tract injury regardless of the absence of hypotension or gross hematuria. Furthermore, if the patient's condition changes after initial evaluation to generate an increasing suspicion of major renal injury, full evaluation should commence.

Additional initial laboratory studies for a patient with suspected blunt renal trauma should include a hematocrit, complete urinalysis with microscopic examination, and measurement of serum electrolytes, blood urea nitrogen, and creatinine. Urine culture also should be obtained if the urine sediment or past history suggests infection.

RADIOGRAPHIC IMAGING

When renal imaging is indicated because of a suspicion of injury, several options exist. The traditional approach is to obtain an intravenous pyelogram (IVP) with rapid infusion of contrast (2 ml/kg), and the IVP remains a useful study in many situations. When combined with postcontrast nephrotomograms, the IVP provides adequate information for detection of a significant injury in over 80 per cent of patients, at a substantially reduced cost and generally in less time than that required for a computerized tomographic (CT) scan. The IVP obtained without tomograms, in the emergency center, may not provide the same degree of diagnostic accuracy, and its limitations should be recognized. As a preoperative study in the unstable blunt or penetrating abdominal trauma patient, the "shock room" IVP should demonstrate the presence of two functioning renal units and reveal the presence of significant contrast extravasation or gross renal injury, but less often does it provide sufficiently detailed information for complete staging of the injury.

CT scanning has the advantage of providing thorough imaging of the perinephric space and other abdominal organs, and therefore is used commonly when a single study is desired for abdominal imaging in the blunt trauma setting. It is especially useful in the pediatric patient, and in any patient in whom detailed imaging is required. The renal parenchyma and collecting system are fully demonstrated, and renal pedicle damage also may be identified as lack of renal parenchymal enhancement. Renal ultrasound commonly is used in European trauma centers for both renal imaging after blunt trauma and abdominal imaging in general after injury. Although not as popular in the United States, in the hands of a skilled and experienced operator, good renal imaging can be obtained to exclude the presence of a major laceration, perinephric hematoma/urinoma, and, with the aid of Doppler imaging, presence of renal arterial flow. Arteriography is employed much less commonly now in the era of high-resolution CT scanning, but still may be helpful in selected cases, such as when planning delayed partial nephrectomy or as a prelude to angiographic embolization for hemorrhagic complications.

MANAGEMENT OF BLUNT RENAL INJURY

After complete radiographic staging of the injury, management decisions are based on the specific anatomy of the injured organ and the clinical status of the patient. Choosing between operative and nonoperative management of blunt renal injuries is one of the major areas of controversy in urologic trauma, with strong proponents of each viewpoint. Although there is general agreement that minor injuries are safely manageable nonoperatively and certain major injuries, such as those with complete destruction of the kidney and ongoing hemorrhage, should be managed operatively, managing injuries of intermediate grade is less straightforward. The controversy essentially focuses on the issue of whether operative management should be pursued only in cases of hemodynamic instability, continued bleeding, or postinjury complication, or whether worrisome radiographic findings noted during staging should prompt operation even in a stable patient, because of an anticipated high risk of subsequent complications.

Approximately 70 to 80 per cent of blunt renal injuries are "minor," consisting of contusions or superficial cortical lacerations without significant bleeding and without urinary extravasation. These injuries can be managed nonoperatively with a very low complication rate. After appropriate early observation, strenuous physical activity should be restricted for the early weeks after injury.

Approximately 5 to 10 per cent of blunt renal injuries involve severe damage clearly requiring operative intervention. These include major crush injuries of the kidney with multiple distracted fragments of nonperfused parenchyma and continued bleeding requiring repeated transfusion. Some also would include in this category renal pedicle injuries, the management of which is discussed separately. Patients who have continued significant bleeding from an injured kidney, either into the urinary tract, manifested as gross hematuria, or into the retroperitoneum, may require intervention as a lifesaving measure.

This may involve surgical exploration with renal repair, nephrectomy, or, alternatively, angiographic embolization, either as definitive therapy or, more likely, as a temporizing measure until stabilization allows surgery more safely.

The operative approach in such cases involves exploration through a generous midline incision with early control of or access to the vascular pedicle being obtained prior to exploration of the kidney. Evacuation of hematoma, débridement of devitalized parenchyma, suture control of parenchymal bleeding, and collecting system repair constitute the basic maneuvers of reconstructive renal trauma surgery. Use of absorbable materials for hemostasis or for capsular substitution may be beneficial. Nephrostomy diversion usually is reserved for cases in which collecting system repair is tenuous or incomplete. Nephrectomy is performed if major damage to the renal hilar region makes vascular, parenchymal or collecting system reconstruction impossible or inadvisable considering the patient's condition. A nephrectomy rate of less than 20 per cent for operatively managed blunt trauma can be expected.

Severe renal injuries in the hemodynamically stable patient or injuries of intermediate grade present the most difficult management decisions. This group of injuries confers the highest risk of delayed complications with initial nonoperative management, with 80 per cent of all renal trauma complications occurring in such patients. Careful patient selection, based on knowledge of the radiographic features that predict a high complication rate, is the key to reduction of significant morbidity in such patients. Deep lacerations without devascularized fragments and with limited extravasation have an excellent prognosis and low complication rate. Findings such as major urinary extravasation with distracted, devascularized parenchymal fragments introduce a potentially high complication rate, variably quoted as ranging from 10 to 50 per cent. Patients with extensive extravasation arising medially near the hilum may require further studies, such as retrograde pyelography, to exclude significant extrarenal collecting system injury such as ureteropelvic disruption. The presence of visceral/retroperitoneal injury (pancreas, duodenum, colon) in association with extensive renal damage presents a high risk of postoperative perirenal infection, and may be considered a relative operative indication.

Once nonoperative management of a major renal injury is selected, intensive monitoring and planned reimaging will prevent many adverse outcomes. The patient may be observed best in an intensive care setting with serial hematocrit determinations obtained during the first 24 to 48 hours. The use of antibiotics is encouraged in cases with urinary extravasation managed nonoperatively. High-risk patients should be aggressively reimaged at a specified interval after injury. When complications such as secondary hemorrhage, perinephric abscess, or urinary fistula develop, delayed surgical exploration may be required, leading to a nephrectomy rate of nearly 50 per cent. Some postinjury complications may be managed effectively by percutaneous drainage or embolization, avoiding open surgery.

RENAL PEDICLE INJURY

Blunt injury to the renal vascular pedicle occurs in less than 5 per cent of cases of renal trauma. Nearly 90 per cent occur in the pediatric population or in young adults, more commonly in males. Most occur as a result of blunt trauma and involve the renal artery, more often on the left side. Blunt venous injury and combined arterial and venous trauma is less common, and bilateral pedicle injury occurs rarely. Arterial injury typically results from sudden stretching of the renal pedicle during major acceleration or deceleration trauma, usually from vehicular accidents or falls from a height. The resulting tearing of the arterial intima leads to subintimal dissection and thrombosis. The mortality rate for renovascular injuries remains high, nearly 30 to 40 per cent, largely as a result of extensive associated injuries.

Specific symptoms suggestive of renal pedicle injury are often lacking, although the patient may have typical signs of flank trauma. If the diagnosis is missed initially, fever from renal necrosis may be a late presenting sign. Hematuria may be entirely absent in one third of patients with arterial injuries; one third will have gross hematuria, and one third microscopic hematuria, often reflecting concomitant renal parenchymal contusion or laceration. With bilateral pedicle injury, the patient may be anuric.

The classic suspicious imaging finding of unilateral nonfunction on an IVP after blunt abdominal trauma is, in fact, nonspecific, with congenital renal absence or ectopia, severe contusion, and major parenchymal laceration also potentially producing this finding. If noted, however, renal arterial injury must be considered until disproven. Immediate arteriography, CT scanning, or ultrasound with Doppler all have been suggested as appropriate studies to further evaluate a kidney that appears to be nonfunctioning on IVP. Although arteriography is the gold standard historically for the diagnosis of renovascular injury, recent data suggest that CT scanning also may provide highly specific information. The absence of parenchymal enhancement after intravenous contrast infusion is diagnostic, and in some cases a specific point of cutoff of the renal artery or a thin peripheral rim of cortical enhancement from capsular collaterals may be seen. CT has substantial advantages in being less invasive and often less time consuming and having lower potential morbidity than arteriography, especially in the pediatric population. The major disadvantage of CT is its dependence on parenchymal perfusion as an indicator of arterial integrity, rather than precisely imaging the arterial anatomy itself, as in arteriography. CT therefore may miss intimal disruptions that have not yet progressed to complete thrombosis, which would be detectable by arteriography.

Management of documented renal pedicle injury requires an integrated decision as to the risk of surgical exploration versus the likelihood of a successful outcome from vascular reconstruction. The kidney can tolerate 30 minutes of warm ischemia without significant loss of function; after 2 hours, some degree of irreversible loss of renal function can be expected. It is important to recognize that the time interval from injury to definitive diagnosis does not necessarily represent warm ischemia time, because complete arterial thrombosis may occur at any time after injury and may be delayed, possibly occurring late as subintimal dissection and luminal occlusion progress. In the stable patient who likely could tolerate laparotomy, exploration with attempted revascularization is reasonable within 12 hours after injury, recognizing that the chance of a successful outcome deteriorates with time after injury. Most repairs may be accomplished by excision of the abnormal arterial segment and primary end-to-end anastomosis. Venous interposition grafts and other arterial bypass and substitution techniques also are applicable when primary arterial anastomosis is not feasible. In the pediatric population, interrupted sutures of fine nonabsorbable vascular suture material should be utilized to allow subsequent growth of the vessel. Success rates ranging from 20 to 50 per cent have been described, with the major determining factor apparently being the time from injury to repair. Some degree of diminished renal function is common on long-term follow-up, which may be accurately accomplished using nuclear scanning techniques.

SUMMARY

Modern management of blunt renal trauma is based on a high degree of suspicion to allow early diagnosis, followed by careful injury staging using the currently available armamentarium of imaging techniques, with CT scanning having assumed major importance. Selecting operative versus nonoperative management depends on a thorough knowledge of the injury characteristics that portend a high risk of delayed complications, weighted against a realistic assessment of the practitioner's ability to safely approach an injured kidney operatively with an acceptably low nephrectomy rate. This decision-making process represents a challenge to the urologist, often working as a member of a trauma management team in the care of the multiply injured patient.

Suggested Readings

Bretan PM Jr, McAninch JW, Federle MP, et al.: Computerized tomographic staging of renal trauma. J Urol 136:561, 1986

Carroll PR, McAninch JW: Staging of renal trauma. Urol Clin North Am 16:193, 1989

Cass AS, Luxenberg M: Unilateral nonvisualization on excretory urography after external trauma. J Urol 132: 225, 1984

Turner WW Jr, Snyder WH III, Fry WJ: Mortality and renal salvage after renovascular trauma. Am J Surg 146:848, 1983

PENETRATING RENAL TRAUMA AND ITS TREATMENT

MICHEL A. PONTARI, M.D.

Philadelphia, Pennsylvania

Approximately 15 to 20 per cent of all renal injuries are due to penetrating trauma. Overall, the kidneys are involved in 10 per cent of all abdominal penetrating wounds. An isolated penetrating renal injury is uncommon, and the liver, small intestine, colon, and/or stomach often are involved as well. Renal stab wounds less frequently involve other organs than do gunshot wounds.

Patients with gunshot wounds to the torso and abdomen that involve the kidney often present in hemorrhagic shock from multisystem injury. Careful physical examination often is not possible in the acute setting. Higher velocity bullets will produce more tissue damage because the amount of kinetic energy of the bullet is equal to $\frac{1}{2}mv^2$, where m is the mass of the bullet and v the velocity. Whereas in the past high-velocity (>2000 ft/sec) weapons were limited to military use, now more civilian high-velocity weapon injuries are being seen. For stab wounds, the size of the entrance site has little correlation with the extent of injury and depth of penetration. Patients with stab wounds also can present in hemorrhagic shock. Physical examination should assess for abdominal rigidity, which is indicative of bowel injury.

Hematuria is not a constant sign in penetrating injuries, and the degree of hematuria does not correlate with the severity of injury. Approximately 70 per cent of penetrating injuries will present with gross hematuria. Any patient with a penetrating injury and more than 5 red blood cells per high-power field should undergo an imaging study to assess the kidneys. Patients with no hematuria but in whom there is suspicion of a renal injury based on the path of a bullet or stab wound also should undergo radiologic evaluation.

When a patient presents in hemorrhagic shock, there is no time for a full radiologic work-up prior to open exploration. In these patients, a limited intravenous pyelogram (IVP), either in the trauma area or on the operating room table, should be performed. A dose of 100 to 150 ml of 50% to 60% contrast is recommended. This dose is somewhat larger than the standard IVP dose, but compensates for possible decreased renal perfusion from hypotension and the dilution effect of parenteral fluids. The status of the contralateral kidney may dictate therapy on the involved side. For patients who are stable on admission, the older literature suggests proceeding with an IVP, but currently our study of choice is a computerized tomography (CT) scan with IV and oral contrast. CT is a more sensitive test for evaluating parenchymal lacerations and urinary extravasation than is IVP, and is helpful with determining the presence of nonviable segments of tissue, hematoma size, and the status of associated injuries. For kidneys that are nonfunctioning or hypoperfused, an arteriogram is obtained to rule out a vascular injury. A chest film should be obtained in the emergency room to rule out a hemothorax and/or pneumothorax.

Indications for renal exploration include expanding or uncontained hematoma, pulsatile hematoma, extensive urinary extravasation, large segments of nonviable tissue, and vascular injury. These findings may be encountered at the time of intraoperative consultation in a patient taken to the operating room by the trauma team or on preoperative imaging studies. Small amounts of urinary extravasation most often resolve spontaneously. Even larger amounts of extravasation may subside, but this must be weighed against the risks of urinoma and abscess formation. Most penetrating renal injuries will be explored, but an increasing number of patients with penetrating renal trauma are being managed nonoperatively. For gunshot wounds, this decision must include consideration of the type of weapon if known, because as the muzzle velocity of the weapon used increases, the chance of injury from the blast effect also increases. For stab wounds, there is no such blast effect, and when the entrance site is posterior to the anterior axillary line, the incidence of associated abdominal injury is low. Up to 90 per cent of patients with stab wounds in this area have been successfully managed nonoperatively.

For penetrating renal injuries, the preferred approach is a midline transperitoneal incision. This allows for assessment of other abdominal viscera, as well as quick access to the renal vessels if necessary. Repair of major vascular, liver, spleen, or bowel injuries should precede renal exploration unless the renal bleeding is causing hemodynamic instability. Previous dogma dictated that vascular control should be obtained prior to exploring any renal injury. Some centers now obtain vascular control first only if there is a wound and hematoma overlying the renal vessels suggesting a vascular injury. For an isolated hematoma away from the pedicle, exploration can proceed by entering Gerota's fascia laterally and obtaining rapid manual control of any bleeding that occurs.

When vascular control is necessary, the small bowel is reflected to expose the retroperitoneum. An incision is made over the aorta just above the inferior mesenteric artery. If a large hematoma prevents identification of the aorta, the incision should be made just medial to the inferior mesenteric vein. Once onto the aorta, dissection proceeds up to the level of the left renal vein. At this level, the renal artery and vein on each side can be identified, and vessel loops placed around the vessels ipsilateral to the injury. The vessels are not clamped unless bleeding is excessive. The kidney is then approached by incising the line of Toldt and reflecting the colon to expose Gerota's fascia and the hematoma.

Total renal exposure is carried out. If bleeding necessitates clamping of the vessels for more than 30 minutes, iced slush should be used to cool the kidney. Nonviable tissue is débrided, and as much viable tissue (i.e., any tissue that bleeds when cut) as possible is preserved. For a devitalized polar lesion, a heminephrectomy may be necessary. Bleeding is controlled by suture ligation and figure-of-eight 4-0 chromic sutures. Rents in the collecting system are closed with running 4-0 chromic suture. The integrity of the collecting system can be assessed by injecting indigo carmine via a fine-gauge needle into the collecting system while compressing the ureter distally with the fingers. Renal defects ideally are covered by the renal capsule. If this is not available, omentum can be sutured to the wound margin, or absorbable gelatin sponges can be used to bolster and cover the repair. Absorbable mesh can be placed around the kidney if a larger repair in the mid-portion of the kidney has been performed and the ends of the kidney cannot be approximated without tension. Lacerations of the renal artery or vein are repaired with 5-0 interrupted vascular suture. Extensive injury to a segmental vessel may require ligation. Closed suction drains are placed around the repair, and systemic antibiotics are given.

Postoperatively, the patient ambulates once the urine has cleared of gross blood. The blood pressure is monitored, and at 6 weeks to 3 months a follow-up IVP is obtained to evaluate the reconstruction. After penetrating renal injuries and repair, patients are at risk for developing delayed bleeding, abscess formation, urinary extravasation, fistula formation, and hypertension. Delayed bleeding may represent the formation of an arteriovenous fistula, especially in stab wounds. An arteriogram in this setting can both be diagnostic and allow for therapeutic embolization of the bleeding site. Low-grade fever and continued pain in the area of injury should prompt a CT scan to look for a urinoma or abscess; if present, percutaneous drainage can be carried out. Hypertension may be transient and subside over a few months. If persistent, it usually responds to medical therapy.

Suggested Readings

Bernath AS, Schutte H, Fernandez RRD, et al: Stab wounds of the kidney: Conservative management in flank penetration. J Urol 129:468, 1983

Corriere JN, McAndrew JD, Benson GS: Intraoperative decision-making in renal trauma surgery. J Trauma 31: 1390, 1991

Eastham JA, Wilson TG, Larsen DW, et al: Angiographic embolization of renal stab wounds. J Urol 148:268, 1992

McAninch JW, Carroll PR: Renal exploration after trauma: Indications and reconstructive techniques. Urol Clin North Am 16:203, 1989

Pollack HM, Wein AJ: Imaging of renal trauma. Radiology 172:297, 1989

RENAL TRAUMA IN CHILDREN

EDMOND T. GONZALES, Jr., M.D.

Houston, Texas

Renal injury usually is discussed under two separate headings: blunt renal trauma and penetrating renal trauma. In the pediatric age group, especially in prepubertal children, the incidence of renal injury resulting from blunt trauma is far higher relative to penetrating renal injury than it is in the adult. In the child, injury to the kidney as a result of blunt abdominal trauma occurs proportionately more often than in adults. There are several reasons why this is thought to be the case. First, relative to abdominal volume, the kidney is proportionately larger in a child than it is in an adult and is not as well protected high in the flank tucked under the lower ribs. Second, the kidney is more mobile in the child. Third, the kidney is less well protected by the thick perirenal fatty envelope typical in the adult, and abdominal musculature is less well developed in children. Finally, the kidney in the child retains its fetal lobulations and often seems to split along those anatomic margins—sometimes as a result of what is perceived as relatively minor flank or abdominal trauma. Another unrelated factor is responsible for the increased incidence of injury to the kidney in children: in the presence of congenital anomalies, especially congenital ureteropelvic junction obstruction, the kidney is large and tense and can sustain contusions or lacerations with much less external force than would be needed to injure a normal kidney.

Penetrating renal injury is most often a result of violence in our society—either gunshot or stab wounds. Although prepubertal children are not often involved in this type of violence, they are increasingly becoming victims of family and school violence, and the incidence of this type of renal injury is very definitely increasing in the younger age groups. This article, however, does not discuss penetrating renal injuries specifically.

The significant mobility of the kidney in children also results in two specific renal injuries that are seen more commonly in the pediatric age group and do not involve the renal parenchyma directly. During rapid deceleration and flexion injury, abnormal stresses are put on the region of the ureteropelvic junction as well as on the renal pedicle. In the former, laceration with complete disruption of the ureteropelvic junction can result because of the relative immobility and fixation of the upper ureter as compared to the kidney and renal pelvis. Renal pedicle injuries result because the muscularis and adventitia of the renal artery is more elastic than the intima. With significant stretching of the renal artery, these elastic differences can result in a tear of the intima with subsequent dissection and ultimate occlusion of the renal artery.

DIAGNOSIS

Any child who has sustained a major blunt or penetrating abdominal injury or a significant deceleration injury, such as a fall from a considerable height, or who has blood in the urine, either gross or microscopic, after an abdominal injury of any sort, should be suspect of having a renal injury. However, it remains controversial, as will be discussed later, who in the population of patients with suspected renal injury requires specific renal evaluation as well as the extent of that evaluation. The presence of hematuria is, of course, the most common physical finding suggesting renal injury. The bleeding may be extensive and gross or it may be only microscopic. There are, however, two specific renal injuries that demand prompt evaluation and attention but may not present with hematuria. These include disruption of the ureteropelvic junction and renal artery intimal tears with occlusion of the renal artery. Similarly, hematuria may mean a renal injury but also might be the presenting finding with a bladder or urethral injury. In all patients who sustain significant abdominal trauma, a thorough, organized evaluation should be undertaken as part of the total evaluation of the patient.

Diagnostic studies commonly used to evaluate a patient with suspected renal injury include intravenous urography, renal ultrasonography, abdominal computerized tomography (CT) scanning, radioisotope imaging studies, and renal arteriography. The appropriate diagnostic study depends on the extent of injury, the suspected presence and severity of other visceral injuries, the stability of the patient, and the diagnostic imaging modalities most immediately available to the treating physicians. If only one examination were able to be chosen, an abdominal CT scan with contrast would be the procedure of choice. This imaging evaluation provides a clear delineation of the integrity of the renal parenchyma, is able to identify even minor amounts of urinary extravasation, differentiates between poorly vascularized and normally vascularized parenchyma, and screens the abdomen for other visceral injury. Sooner or later, an abdominal CT scan should be performed in nearly all cases of documented renal injury in order to classify accurately the extent of the injury and allow development of a treatment algorithm. In many situations, however, an intravenous pyelogram is likely to still be the study most immediately available in many hospital emergency rooms and I would choose to proceed with that study if waiting for an abdominal CT scan meant a considerable delay in initial evaluation of the injured patient. If an intravenous pyelogram shows prompt function bilaterally without distortion of the intrarenal architecture and with intact renal margins, it is unlikely that a significant renal injury is present. However, a kidney that has sustained significant injury is likely to function poorly on intravenous urography, and accurate delineation of the extent of injury is often exceedingly difficult.

Renal ultrasonography has a limited role in evaluating a patient with suspected renal injury. The study does not provide any information regarding the presence or absence of function, and thus would not suggest whether a renal arterial injury has occurred. In the presence of a perinephric hematoma, the ultrasound may have difficulty in differentiating the presence or absence of significant parenchymal lacerations. Following a diagnosis of renal injury, the ultrasound can be beneficial in monitoring the extent and expansion of a hematoma or urinoma.

Radioisotope renal scanning has a limited role in the evaluation of renal injury. Perhaps its primary role would be in differentiating whether any function exists in a kidney suspected of having a renal pedicle injury. Isotope scanning also can demonstrate the presence of urinary extravasation, but this also can be defined clearly on CT scanning.

With the introduction of better diagnostic imaging, renal arteriography is not used as commonly today as it was in the past. However, in the presence of suspected main renal artery occlusion, an arteriogram should be obtained to document the suspected diagnosis as well as to outline more clearly the arterial anatomy in preparation for possible vascular reconstruction.

In summary, then, a properly performed CT scan of the abdomen will demonstrate promptly the presence of renal function, will identify segmental injury with segmental nonfunctioning renal segments, and will demonstrate extravasation very clearly. Ultimately, in any renal injury of significance, a CT scan is most likely to provide the information necessary to differentiate those patients who can be followed nonoperatively from those patients who require surgical consideration.

Special consideration must be given to the presence of congenital anomalies in the child who presents with a renal injury. A hydronephrotic nonfunctioning unit can be injured easily and present with hematuria. Initial evaluation with an intravenous pyelogram might suggest a nonfunctioning kidney and one might suspect a renal artery occlusion. In this case, however, a simple ultrasound will differentiate clearly between the two diagnostic possibilities and eliminate the need for more extensive and invasive diagnostic procedures.

A unique situation exists when a urologist is called to evaluate the extent of renal trauma on an unevaluated patient currently undergoing a laparotomy. This most often happens when a patient presents with severe abdominal injury and is rushed to the operating room because of vital sign instability. Most often in these situations, it is best to inject the patient with an intravenous contrast material for an intraoperative intravenous urogram. The purpose of this study is not so much to delineate the extent of injury, but to document the presence of a normal contralateral kidney before initiating active exploration of a stable perirenal hematoma.

Another area of interest and some controversy is how much work-up is indicated in a patient with suspected renal injury. It is tempting to correlate the extent of renal injury with the extent of hematuria. To some extent that relationship is legitimate in that a patient with microscopic hematuria of mild degree without significant abdominal or flank tenderness and with stable vital signs is less likely to have significant renal injury than is someone with gross hematuria, a palpable flank mass, or who is unstable. However, as indicated previously, two major renal injuries can occur and not result in any blood in the urine at all. For this reason, it seems most appropriate to recommend that any patient with a history compatible with a renal injury but with no or only minimal microscopic hematuria should have at least an intravenous pyelogram performed. Further imaging studies might be planned based on the presence or absence of any significant abnormalities on this study.

MANAGEMENT

The management of renal trauma has been a source of controversy for many years. Management schemes generally are based on a classification of renal injury as major or minor. A patient with a minor renal injury would be managed nonoperatively. A patient with a major renal injury might be managed operatively in most cases. Major renal injuries generally would include renal parenchymal lacerations that extend from the capsule to the collecting system or patients with significant renal vascular injury or disruption of the ureteropelvic junction. Lacerations that bridge the entire thickness of renal parenchyma are likely to disrupt major arcuate vessels and result in significant bleeding as well as ischemia of the disrupted parenchyma. Marked hematoma formation and extensive urinary extravasation usually result. Minor degrees of extravasation alone are not considered a major renal injury.

In children, in whom some segmentation of the kidney persists, sometimes parenchymal lacerations will occur between renuculi, and these are not so disruptive of parenchymal blood supply. This is particularly likely to occur when there is a duplication of the renal pelvis, wherein the parenchyma may separate along the anatomic differentiation between upper and lower renal segments.

Statistically, about 85 per cent of renal injuries are classified as minor. Of the 15 per cent of patients said to have major renal injuries, one third will require immediate surgical exploration because of unstable vital signs or because of other severe visceral injury. Therefore, only about 10 per cent of patients who present with renal injury fall into the category that might be considered for surgical exploration. The traditional recommendation for surgery is based on the observation that 90 per cent of the complications associated with renal injury occur in the 15 per cent of patients classified as having a major injury.

Controversy still persists, however, regarding when and whether these 10 per cent of injuries need urgent or even elective exploration. The kidney is contained within a strong fascial envelope, and bleeding usually will tamponade within a relatively short period of time. Sterile urinary extravasation will reabsorb and, in itself, does not appear to be a problem that requires immediate surgical drainage. Ischemic tissue ultimately will undergo atrophy, but if infection does not occur this may not present any long-term problem. Displaced fragments, if they are viable, often will realign as the hematoma and urinoma gradually resorb. A surprisingly normal renal architecture may result after healing despite a frightening appearance of the kidney on initial diagnostic evaluation. There is no doubt, in reviewing the current literature, that the number of primary explorations for renal injury has decreased in incidence with the introduction of more accurate classification of renal injury with CT as well as the ability now to follow the progress of the patient with abdominal CT scans.

In contrast, extensive hematoma and significant amounts of ischemic tissue may be complicated by infection. In other cases, Gerota's fascia may rupture, allowing for life-threatening delayed bleeding. The development of arteriovenous fistulas days after the injury likewise may result in significant hemorrhage several days after the injury. It also seems obvious from the literature that exploration of a kidney because of secondary complications not uncommonly results in nephrectomy. Proponents of elective early exploration suggests a higher rate of renal salvage. Because of the improved diagnostic modalities available, it seems safe today to conclude that fewer kidneys require exploration than was thought in the past based on findings with intravenous pyelography and sometimes angiography. A careful evaluation of the studies and an accurate classification are the only means to judge whether exploration is the appropriate therapeutic modality or not.

In my opinion, the only isolated renal injuries that would justify immediate surgical exploration would be an injury to the renal artery, complete disruption of the ureteropelvic junction, or a significant renal parenchymal injury associated with sustained and significant life-threatening hemorrhage. Other major injuries with major segmental ischemic segments are probably best explored, although this does not have to be done as a surgical emergency in each case. There are times also when one would explore a kidney that is obviously injured (perinephric hematoma) when operating because of other significant visceral injury.

Any time exploration of an injured kidney is considered, in my opinion it is best that this be accomplished transperitoneally and that the major renal vessels be controlled at their origin and insertion before Gerota's fascia is opened and the kidney examined. The approach to the major vessels is well described in numerous surgical texts. With this technique, extensive life-threatening bleeding necessitating urgent nephrectomy is unlikely and elective reconstruction of the kidney can be undertaken.

Surgery for acute renal artery injuries in children do not usually result in salvage of the kidney. By the time the diagnosis is made and surgical exploration accomplished, the warm ischemia time is often too long for renal parenchymal salvage. Successful surgery demands a high index of suspicion and a prompt diagnosis with appropriate vascular surgical management. In addition, in the very young child successful vascular reanastomosis is uncommon because of the small size of the renal vessels.

Total disruption of the ureteropelvic junction is best managed by immediate surgery and primary reanastomosis. Although percutaneous access to the renal collecting system might be considered in some situations, the ultimate fibrosis that will result will make the pyeloureteral anastomosis more difficult. Immediate surgical exploration allows for reanastomosis of healthy tissue that is generally well vascularized. The likelihood of a successful outcome is improved with early versus delayed surgery for this unique injury of childhood.

COMPLICATIONS

The major complication associated with renal injury is the potential for hypertension. All children who sustained major renal injuries should be followed on a regular basis to be sure that blood pressure remains within acceptably normal limits. Occasionally, obstructive changes will occur because of the hematoma and fibrosis that develop after the injury, or urinomas may encyst. However, these are unusual complications. The major concern in dealing with renal injuries is choosing appropriate management to best salvage renal parenchyma and minimize morbidity.

Suggested Readings

Atala A, Miller FB, Richardson JD, et al: Preliminary vascular control for renal trauma. Surg Gynecol Obstet 172:386–390, 1991

Baumann L, Greenfield SP, Aker J, et al: Nonoperative management of major blunt renal trauma in children: In-hospital morbidity and long-term follow-up. J Urol 148:691–693, 1992

Middlebrook PF, Schillinger JF: Hematuria and intravenous pyelography in pediatric blunt renal trauma. Can J Surg 36:59–62, 1993

Smith EM, Elder JS, Spirnak JP: Major blunt renal trauma in the pediatric population: Is a nonoperative approach indicated? J Urol 149:546–548, 1993

Teigen CL, Venbrux AC, Quinlan DM, et al: Late massive hematuria as a complication of conservative management of blunt renal trauma in children. J Urol 147: 1333–1336, 1992

ATHLETIC HEMATURIA

ARTHUR I. SAGALOWSKY, M.D.

Dallas, Texas

Hematuria occurring after athletics may indicate either minor or major genitourinary tract pathology. Alternatively, stress hematuria may occur in a patient with a normal urinary tract and be related to the exercise itself. Physicians should have a broad concept of the differential diagnosis of hematuria (Table 1) and obtain a careful history and perform a thorough physical examination.

Intrinsic coagulation defects often are suggested by a history of easy bruisability or ex-

TABLE 1. Differential Diagnoses of the Cause of Renal Hematuria

1. Trauma
   - A. Acute
   - B. Delayed
2. Tumors
   - A. Kidney
     - a. Malignant cancers
     - b. Angiomyolipoma
   - B. Pelvis
   - C. Ureter
3. Stone disease
   - A. Ureteral
   - B. Pelvic
   - C. Calyceal
4. Obstruction
5. Glomerulonephritis
   - A. Acute
     - a. Postinfectious
     - b. Collagen diseases
   - B. Rapidly progressive
     - a. Goodpasture syndrome
     - b. Wegener's granulomatosis
   - C. Chronic
6. Viral diseases
   - A. Varicella
   - B. Mumps
   - C. Influenza
   - D. ECHO
   - E. Coxsackie
   - F. Measles
7. Congenital hereditary nephritis
8. Focal glomerulonephritis or benign hematuria
9. Subacute bacterial endocarditis
10. Arterial thrombosis and emboli
11. Renal vein thrombosis
12. Pyelonephritis
13. Papillary necrosis or papillitis
14. Tuberculosis
15. Parasitic disease
    - A. Malaria
    - B. Schistosomiasis
    - C. *Echinococcus* or hydatid disease
    - D. Filariasis
16. Polycystic disease
17. Coagulation defects
18. Hemoglobinopathies
19. Vascular malformations
20. Secondary carcinomas
21. Malignant hypertension
22. Endometriosis
23. Exercise-induced hematuria
24. Drug- or chemical-induced hematuria
25. Factitious hematuria

cessive bleeding from minor cuts or surgeries. Prothrombin time, partial thromboplastin time, platelet count, and, occasionally, bleeding time are sufficient coagulation screening tests. A history of drug ingestion may be an important cofactor in the cause of hematuria. Nonsteroidal anti-inflammatory drugs (NSAIDs) are cyclo-oxygenase inhibitors and block the production of cyclic endoperoxides such as thromboxane A_2 and prostacyclin. The net effect of NSAIDs on coagulation is a decrease in platelet aggregation and decreased clotting. NSAIDs have been associated with papillary necrosis, interstitial nephritis, and even acute renal failure in some patients. In one recent retrospective study on causes of hematuria, 54 per cent of patients in the idiopathic group were taking NSAIDs, versus only 1 per cent in the group with an identified cause of the hematuria.

Any degree of hematuria following trauma to the flank or pelvis or physical evidence of such trauma (i.e., ecchymosis, bruises, tenderness, rib or pelvic fractures) necessitates a thorough evaluation. Blunt and penetrating renal trauma are addressed by other authors elsewhere in this section and will not be considered further in this article. Nevertheless, it is worth repeating the maxim that hematuria out of proportion to the trauma suggests preexisting, often congenital, abnormalities such as ureteropelvic junction obstruction and hydronephrosis.

Exercise-induced hematuria per se is the main subject of this article. As early as 1878, proteinuria was reported in soldiers following exercise. In 1907 and 1910, proteinuria was reported in athletes following rowing and long-distance running, respectively. Contrary to earlier reports, there is no difference between the sexes for risk of athletic hematuria with equivalent degrees of exertion. Athletic hematuria may be categorized in the following ways:

Activity—contact versus noncontact
Character—gross versus microscopic
Source—upper tract (kidney) versus lower tract (bladder)

ACTIVITY

The mechanism of hematuria following contact sports most often is simple renal contusion. Urinalyses obtained immediately after the game in football players reveal hematuria in 45 to 65 per cent, gross hematuria in 10 to 15 per cent, and frequent red cell casts. The finding of red cell casts in the urine confirms glomerular injury. Hematuria believed to be due to renal contusion should be managed by rest, fluids, and observation as in any other trauma patient. Most sports-related hematuria clears within 48 hours, and nearly always by 72 hours. In one study of boxers, 73 per cent had hematuria following a bout. Interestingly the degree of hematuria correlated more with the duration of the fight than the number of punches received. This finding suggests that, even in a violent contact sport such as boxing, other nontraumatic consequences of strenuous exercise also may play a role in causing hematuria.

One must review exercise-related changes in renal physiology in order to understand noncontact sports-related hematuria. In the basal state, renal blood flow (RBF) is approximately 1200 ml/min, or 20 per cent of the cardiac output. Renal plasma flow (RPF) is 700 ml/min and glomerular filtration rate (GFR) is approximately 15 per cent of RPF, or 105 ml/min. During exercise, as blood is shifted to muscles to supply oxygen, RBF and RPF decrease. The kidney maintains GFR over wide ranges of RPF by neuronal-mediated vasoconstriction of the efferent arteriole. However, with extreme stress the net effects of markedly decreased RPF and increased efferent arteriolar constriction are decreased GFR and renal injury resulting from hypoxia. Both glomerular and tubular hypoxic injury result in leakage of red blood cells and protein into the tubular lumen, producing hematuria. Thus, strenuous noncontact activities such as calisthenics, swimming, and rowing may produce transient hematuria and proteinuria. Review of the literature reveals that the incidence of hematuria following exercise varies from 15 to 80 per cent. The incidence and severity of hematuria is directly related to the duration and intensity of exercise.

The current popularity of running has provided a wealth of information on sports hematuria. Most microscopic hematuria following jogging is asymptomatic and clears within 48 hours. Further work-up is recommended only in symptomatic patients or those with a history suggestive of genitourinary pathology. Warm-weather marathoners reveal much greater post-race changes in renal function than do their cold-weather counterparts. Hematuria, proteinuria, myoglobinuria, and decreased clearance parameters (inulin, para-aminohippurate, and creatinine) all are more marked in warm-weather runners. Dehydration during exercise adds to the diminished

RPF and increases nephron hypoxic injury. The return to normal urinalysis and normal parameters of renal function is slower in warm-weather runners than in cold-weather runners. Nevertheless, the findings generally are mild and fully reversible except for minimally decreased creatinine clearance in both groups within 1 week after running.

CHARACTER

The urinalysis is the initial test following the history and physical examination in defining the character of hematuria and in narrowing the broad differential diagnosis. The distinction of gross from microscopic hematuria after exercise is important. In one small study, two cases of transitional cell carcinoma and one case each of renal cell carcinoma and renal calculus presented as gross hematuria following jogging. In contrast, the incidence of major urinary tract pathology in athletes with only transient microscopic hematuria is so low that routine evaluation is not recommended. Red urine without red blood cells in the sediment suggests discoloration resulting from hemoglobinuria, myoglobinuria, porphyria, or dye ingestion.

SOURCE

The great majority of athletic hematuria is due to renal leak of red blood cells as described above. Both kidneys should be affected similarly, barring other specific abnormalities. Gross hematuria following exercise should be evaluated with upper tract imaging and cystoscopy. Confirmed recurrent unilateral hematuria may be further evaluated with ureteropyeloscopy or nephroscopy if excretory urography and retrograde pyelography fail to identify the source of bleeding. Numerous recent sports document a high likelihood of identifying benign mucosal vascular abnormalities, which are amenable to curative fulguration, by these improvements in endoscopic instrumentation.

Cystoscopy also may reveal a bladder source of hematuria following exercise, such as a bladder tumor, diverticulum, or stone. Cystoscopy in joggers after a race reveals mucosal erythema and ecchymoses on both the posterior wall and trigone. The bladder is relatively empty during exertion as a result of dehydration and decreased urinary output. During jogging, the posterior wall of the nearly empty bladder may hit against the trigone and anterior wall, producing contusions and hematuria.

SUMMARY

Athletic hematuria is a common finding with several contributing causes. Possible long-term consequences to renal function from repeated episodes of acute, mild renal injury related to exercise remain speculative at this time. Finally, whether or not patients with varying degrees of renal impairment are more susceptible to renal injury from exercise also is uncertain.

Suggested Readings

Abarbanel J, Benet AE, Lask D, et al: Sports hematuria. J Urol 143:887–890, 1990
Boileau M, Fuchs E, Barry JM, et al: Stress hematuria: Athletic pseudonephritis in marathoners. Urology 15: 471, 1980
Kraus SE, Siroky MB, Babayan RK, et al: Hematuria and the use of nonsteroidal anti-inflammatory drugs. J Urol 132:288–290, 1984
Neviackas JA, Bauer JH: Renal function abnormalities induced by marathon running. South Med J 74:1457, 1981
Patterson DE, Segura JW, Benson Jr RC, et al: Endoscopic evaluation and treatment of patients with idiopathic gross hematuria. J Urol 132:1199–1200, 1984
Wendel EF: Urologic aspects of athletic activity. American Urologic Association (AUA) Update Series, Lesson 12, Vol. III, 1984.

URINARY EXTRAVASATION

MICHEL A. PONTARI, M.D.

Philadelphia, Pennsylvania

Extravasation of urine from its normal confines within the urinary tract may occur spontaneously or as the result of trauma. Both the etiology and the specific site of the extravasation dictate therapy. In general, in cases of urinary extravasation, antibiotics are started empirically and continued until the results of a urine culture are obtained.

KIDNEY

In the face of obstruction, extravasation can be a physiologically protective mechanism for the kidney because it decompresses the collecting system and allows for continued glomerular filtration. The spread of the urine around the kidney is limited somewhat by the presence of bridging septa dividing the perirenal space into several compartments, instead of one fat-filled space.

Spontaneous Rupture

Spontaneous rupture of the renal collecting system occurs in response to increased intrapelvic pressure. Extravasation is seen when intrapelvic pressure exceeds a critical level, variously reported as between 20 and 70 mm Hg. Acute ureteral obstruction is the most common cause. The leak of urine is at the weakest site in the renal pelvis, the calyceal fornix. Pre-existing disease can produce other areas of weakness in the collecting system. In general, the extravasation from a fornix is more often from acute distal or mid-ureteral obstruction, whereas frank pelvic rupture is usually from chromic obstruction at a higher level.

Acute processes that can result in renal extravasation include ureteral obstruction from a stone, retrograde pyelography, and external compression applied during an intravenous pyelogram (IVP). Chronic conditions are less likely to lead to extravasation, but retroperitoneal fibrosis, ureteral tumors, congenital ureteropelvic junction obstruction, renal cysts producing compression, and bladder tumors obstructing a ureteral orifice can lead to rupture of the renal pelvis. Spontaneous renal rupture also has been reported during pregnancy, and is thought to occur when the gravid uterus shifts and causes ureteral obstruction, resulting in a rapid increase in intrarenal pressure.

Flank pain, hematuria, and occasional fever are the clinical findings. Flank pain from an underlying obstruction may improve or even resolve as extravasation relieves renal pelvic pressure. In frank rupture, the symptoms usually will be more severe, and the presentation often is one of an acute abdomen. The diagnosis of renal urinary extravasation most often is made on IVP. An IVP also can precipitate extravasation, because the contrast material produces an osmotic diuresis in a patient with already elevated intrapelvic pressure. Plain films can show obliteration of the psoas shadow, blurring of the renal outline, or a calculus. Massive extravasation from frank rupture of the renal pelvis is better seen on delayed films because of the poor function of a chronically diseased kidney, and dilution of the contrast medium by a large volume of peripelvic fluid. In some cases, especially with small amounts of extravasation, the diagnosis is made only by computerized tomography (CT) or ultrasound.

The treatment depends on the amount of extravasation and the presence or absence of infection. Mild amounts of urine leak from the pelvis are usually self-limited. Treatment is aimed at reducing the intrapelvic pressure and restoring normal urinary tract outflow. Urinary stones that produce perirenal extravasation are mostly small, distal ureterovesical junction stones, which have an excellent chance of passing by themselves. In the absence of infection and fever, most of these stones can be observed without a stent. Obstruction that cannot be relieved by a ureteral catheter or recurs after its removal will require further endoscopic or open procedures. For extravasation produced during an IVP or retrograde pyelogram with otherwise normal drainage, the process will stop with termination of the procedure.

Spontaneous frank rupture of the renal pelvis usually results in large amounts of extravasation and requires surgical exploration. If the kidney is relatively normal, as in the case of an obstructing calculus, an attempt at repair is warranted. A ruptured diseased kidney should be removed, as in the case of a malignancy, chronic hydronephrosis, or chronic infection. After nephrectomy, the renal fossa is drained. Recent reports have described treating rupture of the renal collecting system with a stent alone, but more evidence is needed to support this approach.

Trauma

Renal injury and urinary extravasation can be the result of blunt or penetrating trauma. A CT scan can both evaluate the degree of extravasation and assess injuries to surrounding organs. Blunt trauma can produce a range of injuries from mild extravasation to complete avulsion of the ureteropelvic junction. The management depends on the severity of the extravasation, the clinical condition of the patient, and the status of surrounding organs. For mild amounts of renal extravasation in a stable patient with no other injuries, and in whom the ureter is adequately visualized below the injury, observation with serial CT scans is a reasonable option. Some have advocated placing a ureteral stent in this situation. For larger amounts of extravasation, exploration and repair are undertaken if (1) there are associated injuries requiring exploration and/or (2) the patient becomes hemodynamically unstable or requires frequent blood transfusions for ongoing bleeding. In a stable patient with an isolated renal injury, or another injury that does not require exploration, a course of observation with serial CT scans, close hemodynamic monitoring, and prophylactic antibiotics is undertaken. In the setting of large amounts of extravasation and significant parenchymal injury, observation can lead to preservation of the kidney, because in this setting there is a high nephrectomy rate at the time of attempted repair.

There is a growing literature on the nonoperative management of penetrating renal injuries. Stab wounds dorsal to the posterior axillary line have a low incidence of extrarenal injuries and increasingly are being observed, as are selected gunshot wounds. However, most injuries from gunshot wounds will require exploration. If the kidney can be repaired, the area of injury is débrided and the collecting system oversewn. Often for calyceal injuries, a piece of fat can be sewn over the area to act as a bolster. Drains are placed; for a pelvic injury with a large repair, it may be advantageous to drain the repair by a ureteral stent or nephrostomy.

A special case of penetrating trauma is when a ureteral catheter, or even more frequently a guidewire, is placed through the pelvis or calyces. Given a normal kidney with normal ureteral drainage, leaving a ureteral catheter for several days is all that will be required. Iatrogenic perirenal urinary extravasation is also a common sequela of percutaneous nephrostolithotomy, and usually resolves uneventfully provided the kidney is adequately drained and infection controlled.

Complications

Complications of renal extravasation include the formation of a urinoma, which also may obstruct the kidney, and occasionally a perinephric abscess. Both are best treated initially by percutaneous drainage. Extravasated urine also has been found in the pleural space as a urinothorax, presumably moving into the pleural space through lymphatics and moving across the diaphragm. A urinothorax is identified by its characteristic low pH (≤ 7.30) on pleural tap and a serum creatinine level greater than normal.

URETER

Spontaneous Rupture

Most cases of spontaneous rupture of the ureter are associated with erosion of a stone through the ureteral wall. Less common causes are ureteral tumors, infections, or processes of the colon and duodenum that spread to include the ureter. Symptoms and signs similar to those with spontaneous renal extravasation will be found, including flank and lower abdominal pain, microscopic hematuria, and fever. The diagnosis is best made on IVP. Small amounts of extravasation may be treated with a ureteral stent or nephrostomy tube, but larger defects will require open drainage and repair of the ureter. For localized tears of the mid-ureter, a ureteroureterostomy should be performed over a stent. For defects in the lower ureter, a ureteral reimplant with or without a psoas hitch should be tried. Still more length can be obtained by using a Boari flap. Large defects may require an interposition of ileum.

Trauma

Injuries to the ureter by blunt trauma are uncommon. Children can have traumatic disruption of the ureteropelvic junction from hyperextension injuries. The ureter can be injured by gunshot wounds and, less commonly, by stab wounds. Treatment depends on location, as for spontaneous ureteral rupture. Gunshot wounds are best treated by an open surgical approach. The involved segment of ureter must be débrided prior to repair, because the local blast effect can devitalize surrounding tissues and lead to delayed necrosis of the involved areas. The repair should be drained, and antibiotics given. Often a penetrating ureteral injury occurs in the setting of other injuries. If the patient's poor condition precludes a definitive repair at the time of exploration, a nephrostomy or even a cutaneous ureterostomy can be used to establish drainage and temporize.

Most traumatic injuries to the ureter are iatrogenic. A ureteral catheter placed through the wall of the ureter should be removed, and a catheter placed past the injury if possible. If this is unsuccessful, a percutaneous nephrostomy should be placed if the injury is large. Small tears may be observed. An increasingly common cause of ureteral injury and urinary extravasation is misadventure during ureteroscopy, especially when using electrohydraulic lithotripsy (EHL) or pulsed-dye lasers to treat ureteral calculi. If a tear is noted during ureteroscopy, the procedure should be terminated and a ureteral stent placed. If this fails, a percutaneous nephrostomy is placed, and the ureter can be stented from above at a later date. Another source of ureteral extravasation is retrograde pyelography using a bulb-tip catheter. Because of the local injury, edema may develop that can obstruct the ureter temporarily. Small tears can be observed, but, if questionable, a ureteral stent should be placed.

Operative ureteral injuries should be repaired immediately if recognized. If a ureteral injury is suspected at the time of a surgical procedure, one ampule of indigo carmine is given intravenously. If a ureteral injury has occurred, the blue dye will be visible in the periureteral tissues. If diagnosis is delayed, the ureter should be diverted or stented and an elective repair undertaken after waiting several months.

BLADDER

Spontaneous rupture of the bladder in adults resulting in urinary extravasation is uncommon but has been seen in the setting of necrotizing infection, foreign bodies, calculi, inflammatory bowel disease, and bladder ischemia. In the neonatal period, bladder outlet obstruction such as from posterior urethral valves or a neuropathic bladder can produce bladder rupture and urinary ascites. Blunt trauma that causes a pelvic fracture can produce bladder rupture as well. Sudden increases in intra-abdominal pressure can result in rupture of the bladder dome.

Penetrating injuries include gunshots, stabbings, and, more commonly, iatrogenic injuries, either during open procedures or endoscopically. Neonatal bladders can be injured during umbilical artery catheterization.

The signs and symptoms associated with bladder injuries depend somewhat on location. Extraperitoneal bladder defects with extravasation can produce suprapubic pain, fever, and occasionally inability to void. Intraperitoneal rupture will result in peritoneal signs. The diagnosis is best made on cystogram, during which the bladder is filled with 300 to 400 ml of contrast. The bladder cuts on a CT scan are inadequate to evaluate the bladder for extravasation unless the bladder is filled to the same volume of contrast as a cystogram prior to scanning.

Treatment is based on location of the bladder injury producing extravasation. Intraperitoneal injuries require open drainage and bladder repair. A suprapubic catheter is left at the time of repair, as are perivesical drains. Extraperitoneal defects, if limited, can be treated by urethral catheter drainage alone. A cystogram is obtained 7 to 10 days after the injury, and prior to the removal of the catheter. Larger extraperitoneal rents will need open drainage and repair. Intraoperative injuries should be repaired when they are recognized.

URETHRA

Posterior Injuries

Urine that extravasates from the posterior urethra will be cephalad to the urogenital diaphragm. Posterior urethral injuries are almost always traumatic, and those from blunt trauma almost always are associated with pelvic fractures. The prostatomembranous urethral junction can be partially disrupted or completely severed. Intrapelvic hematomas from the pelvic fracture will displace the prostate so on exam it feels to be "high riding" and superior to its usual location. Blood at the urethral meatus also can be seen. Either of these two signs in the setting of a pelvic fracture indicates that a retrograde urethrogram should be performed prior to placement of a urethral catheter.

Whether a posterior urethral disruption is partial or complete, one treatment option is to place a suprapubic tube and come back 4 to 6 months later for definitive repair. In the setting of a partial urethral tear, some would suggest to try to gently place a Foley catheter across the defect, either antegrade or retrograde if the patient is being explored for other injuries. In this approach, if any resistance is met, the effort is abandoned and a suprapubic tube placed because, although potentially beneficial in aiding the healing process and obviating a second procedure, this attempt also could convert a partial tear to a complete one and greatly increase the morbidity of the injury. For a complete posterior urethral disruption, some advocate a primary repair if the patient is stable and will tolerate the procedure. This procedure is made more difficult because of the associated bleeding from the pelvic fracture, and can be technically challenging. In selected cases, this procedure may reduce morbidity.

Penetrating traumatic defects in the posterior urethra occur during transurethral resection of the prostate. Treatment is usually only insertion of a Foley catheter. Occasionally, rather large injuries will require open drainage and closure of the prostatic urethral wall.

Anterior Injuries

Anterior urethral injuries will produce urinary extravasation inferior to the genitourinary diaphragm. Spontaneous anterior urethral extravasation can occur with infection, urethral stricture, and calculi. Symptoms include local tenderness and inflammation, and difficulty voiding from the underlying process. If Buck's fascia is not violated, urine will be confined to the shaft of the penis. If Buck's fascia is not intact, urine will extend into the scrotum. From there, it can proceed on to the anterior abdominal wall, deep to Scarpa's fascia, bounded by Colles' fascia. Urine can extend up to the clavicle, to the level of the insertion of Colles' fascia onto the coracoclavicular fascia. Colles' fascia also inserts posteriorly to the triangular ligament and laterally to the fascia lata of the thigh, so the ischiorectal area and the thighs are protected.

If the extravasated urine is infected, Fournier's gangrene can develop. The necrotizing infection will start in the perineum but can spread quickly to the abdominal wall. This is a surgical emergency and requires wide débridement of all involved tissue and broad-spectrum antibiotics. The patient may need several more trips to the operating room to completely remove all the necrotic tissue. More commonly, the infection is not as severe but still requires placement of a suprapubic tube, antibiotics, and débridement of the involved tissue. Urethral repair is performed at a later date once the infection has been eradicated.

Traumatic injuries of the anterior urethra can be from straddle-type injuries, which result in partial disruption. Retrograde urethrography makes the diagnosis, and treatment is by an indwelling Foley catheter for several weeks. Delay in diagnosis of this injury will require opening the penis to drain the area and placing a Foley. Penetrating injuries can be from gunshot wounds, for which a suprapubic tube is placed, the urethra is débrided, and the edges sewn to the skin as the first stage of a two-stage repair. Primary closure in this setting is contraindicated because the bullet produces a dirty wound. For traumatic amputation, a primary repair of the urethra should be performed.

Suggested Readings

Chapman JP, Gonzalez J, Diokno AC: Significance of urinary extravasation during renal colic. Urology 30:541, 1987

Kaplan LM, Farrer JH, Lupu AN: Spontaneous rupture of the ureter. Urology 29:313, 1987

Khan AU, Malek RS: Spontaneous urinary extravasation. J Urol 116:161, 1976

Rose BS, Ragosi R, LaRosa JL, et al: Pyelosinus extravasation and urinoma associated with malignancy. Urology 31:353, 1988

Webster GD, Mathes GL, Selli C: Prostatomembranous urethral injuries: A review of the literature and a rational approach to their management. J Urol 130:898, 1983

HEMATURIA IN CHILDHOOD

EDWARD F. REDA, M.D.

Valhalla, New York

Hematuria in infancy and childhood is an important symptom and may be a sign of underlying nephrologic as well as urologic disease. The approach to evaluation differs significantly from that in the adult because the spectrum of pathologic causes varies markedly.

INCIDENCE

It is estimated that 3 to 5 per cent of children will demonstrate hematuria at some time during their development. This may take the form of gross hematuria, which is the more dramatic presentation, or, more commonly, it may be discovered incidentally during a routine urinalysis. Age is the other key factor in determining the sequence and nature of clinical and laboratory investigations.

GROSS HEMATURIA

In neonates, gross hematuria generally signifies a potentially life-threatening condition. Renal vein thrombosis must be entertained immediately in the neonate who has associated renal enlargement and thrombocytopenia. A history of maternal diabetes and/or dehydration in the neonate can predispose to this condition. It more frequently affects one kidney, but, if both kidneys are involved, it can result in renal failure. Prompt recognition and attention to fluid replacement and renal failure management is the key to treatment. Anticoagulants have been recommended, but the benefits are questionable, and significant complications may occur from the anticoagulants themselves. Unilateral renal vein thrombosis must be differentiated clinically from hydronephrosis, multicystic kidney disease, and multilocular cystic disease. Infantile polycystic kidney disease, an autosomal recessive inherited entity, is almost always bilateral and is easily differentiated on ultrasonography as well as by the absence of thrombocytopenia. Moreover, this condition generally is associated with microscopic rather than gross hematuria.

Wilms' tumors do occur in infancy but only rarely. Most present between age two to four years. Renal cortical and medullary necrosis are rarer causes of gross hematuria in neonates and generally occur in hypovolemic states. Congenital renal artery stenosis is the other less commonly encountered condition which can present with gross hematuria, hypertension and cardiac decompensation.

Gross hematuria may also be the presenting feature in obstructive uropathy. These conditions include posterior urethral valves as well as hydronephrosis due to ureterovesical and ureteropelvic junction obstructions.

Urinary tract infections in neonates and infants may have accompanying gross hematuria but it is rarely the presenting symptom except when the infection occurs in an obstructed system.

Bloody diapers may result from other than urologic causes and should not be confused with hematuria. The passage of swallowed maternal blood passed per rectum is one such condition. Vaginal bleeding from maternal estrogen withdrawal is another entity that must be entertained in the female neonate. Finally, reddish discoloration of the infant's diaper from urate crystalluria can be confused with hematuria. Dipstick analysis and microscopic evaluation of the urine showing no red blood cells in the presence of urate crystals confirms this entity. Urate crystalluria is a transitory phenomenon resulting from precipitation of urates in acidic urine as it cools to room temperature. It has no clinical significance.

In older children, gross hematuria is most commonly associated with renal or bladder trauma. Self induced gross hematuria from instrumentation is rare, but must be considered. Severe cystitis and urethritis, both bacterial and viral as well as chemical (i.e., chemotherapy related) may have associated gross hematuria as a feature of their presentation.

Circumcised boys with meatal stenosis and meatitis also may present with blood staining in their underwear or have drops of blood at the termination of micturition. Gross hematuria is a not uncommon presentation in boys with "urethrorrhagia." This condition can be transient or can persist over months or years and can result in a urethral stricture.

Gross hematuria also may be a prominent feature in medical renal disease. Immunoglobulin (Ig)A nephropathy or Berger's disease, most commonly encountered in boys, is characterized by IgA and IgG deposits on the mesangial cells of the glomerulus. Intermittent gross hematuria is a prominent feature of this entity, but microscopic hematuria usually is detected between episodes of gross bleeding. The gross hematuria generally follows an upper respiratory tract infection or vigorous exercise. Basement membrane nephropathy, another class of familial disorder of the glomerular basement membrane, is the second most common renal parenchymal condition in children with recurrent gross hematuria. Urologic evaluation, including radiographic and ultrasonographic studies as well as cystoscopy, is normal in these children and therefore is not indicated in these medical conditions.

Sickle cell trait and sickle cell disease may be associated with severe gross hematuria. Sickle cell hemoglobinopathy is said to account for approximately one third of gross hematuria in blacks. Hematuria is a more frequent complication of hemoglobin SS disease than in hemoglobin SA trait. Intravenous urography and cystoscopy are used to localize the side of bleeding, which is generally the left.

MICROSCOPIC HEMATURIA

Microscopic hematuria, defined as two of three urine samples positive for more than five red blood cells per high-power field, is said to occur in 1 to 2 per cent of children between 6 and 12 years of age. Poststreptococcal glomerulonephritis is a common cause and should be considered. It usually occurs in children between 3 and 7 years of age and is rare before 2 years. The classic features include gross, painless hematuria that is tea colored, associated with mild edema and hypertension. Protein also usually is seen on urinalysis. Red blood cell casts define the site of origin to the nephron. Some children demonstrate mild renal functional impairment and an elevated antistreptolysin titer. This merely indicates that a previous streptococcal infection occurred sometime within the past 6 months. The other positive findings on laboratory evaluation include a transiently reduced serum complement (C3) level. The urinary sediment changes often are present for months despite the fact that the other laboratory parameters are usually normal by 6 weeks following the onset of the condition. Poststreptococcal glomerulonephritis rarely progresses to renal failure. Membranoproliferative nephritis with persistent hypocomplementemia, in contrast, is the most common cause of progressive glomerulonephritis. A renal biopsy is mandatory for definitive diagnosis and treatment.

Systemic diseases can produce nephritis as part of their involvement of multiorgan systems. These include collagen diseases such as lupus erythematosus.

DIAGNOSTIC APPROACH

The child's age and the type of hematuria (i.e., gross versus microscopic) allow a selective evaluation. The relative incidence of the various conditions as they present in the child at different ages is the key to the algorithm and directs the sequence of diagnostic tests. A complete and thorough urinalysis for the detection of protein and a search for casts is mandatory. Measurement of the specific gravity is helpful in identifying patients with concentrating defects, which indicate underlying renal parenchymal disease or sickle cell abnormalities. Similarly, significant proteinuria implicates the glomerulus as the cause of the problem. All children with hematuria must undergo imaging of the kidney and bladder to evaluate the anatomy of the urinary tract. Ultrasound is generally the screening test of choice. This examination is used to exclude tumors, cysts of various types, obstructive uropathy, and calculus disease. In some cases, additional imaging studies may be required to define the condition more clearly. The intravenous pyelogram and particularly the computerized tomographic scan with and without contrast material are helpful in this regard. More recently, magnetic resonance imaging has been utilized because it involves no radiation burden. Calcium-to-creatinine ratios determined in a spot specimen of urine will detect cases of hypercalcuria. Protein-to-creatinine ratios determined in random urine specimens will identify children with significant proteinuria. Evaluation of the first morning specimen will exclude orthostatic proteinuria.

Cystoscopic evaluation is reserved for those children with persistent and recurrent hematuria. Most children with gross or microscopic hematuria do not require cystoscopic evaluation because urothelial malignancies are extremely rare. Other malignant conditions, such as rhabdomyosarcoma of the bladder and prostate, are detected by imaging studies. In suspected collagen diseases that involve multiorgan systems, antinuclear antibody testing is essential. However, this is rarely positive unless the hematuria is accompanied by proteinuria and is usually confined to teenage girls. C3 normally is depressed in poststreptococcal glomerulonephritis but also is reduced in membranoproliferative glomerulonephritis as well as in lupus erythematosus. The antistreptolysin-0 titer is less specific in that it may be elevated for up to 6 months following any streptococcal infection. However, it is helpful in completing the battery of tests for acute glomerulonephritis.

Suggested Readings

Baumgardner DT: The infant with a reddish diaper. Postgrad Med 88:199–202, 1990

Diamond DA, Ford C: Neonatal gross hematuria as a presenting sign of posterior urethral valves. Urology 40: 267–269, 1992

Garcia CD, Miller LA, Bruder Stapleton F: Natural history of hematuria associated with hypercalcuria in children. Am J Dis Child 145:1204–1207, 1991

Robson WLM, Leung AKC: Patients with macroscopic hematuria. Caucasian Fam Physician 39:912–913, 1993

Schroeder PL, Francisco LL: Evaluating hematuria in children. Postgrad Med 88:171–176, 1990

Tumors and Related Disorders

CONGENITAL MESOBLASTIC NEPHROMA

ALAN B. RETIK, M.D.

Boston, Massachusetts

It is generally accepted that most primary kidney tumors occurring in the first year of life have a relatively favorable prognosis. Most of these infantile renal tumors had been classified as nephroblastoma (Wilms' tumor), but recently, through retrospective studies, several histologic subtypes have been recognized that dictate that aggressive therapy be tempered in some instances. Bolande and associates introduced the term "congenital mesoblastic nephroma" in 1967 to designate a group of renal neoplasms seen early in life that had a remarkably good prognosis when treated by local excision alone. Since then, the concept of congenital mesoblastic nephroma has expanded, and cases with more cellular histology are now being recognized. This expanded concept has raised some questions regarding optimal therapy and ultimate prognosis.

The usual presenting symptoms of this lesion are related to a nontender abdominal mass that is characterized as being large enough to extend past the midline or below the anterior superior iliac spine.

Ultrasonography and excretory urography usually reveal significant distortion of the pelvicalyceal system by a large intrarenal mass. The differential diagnosis is usually Wilms' tumor versus congenital mesoblastic nephroma. In the neonatal period, the majority of these tumors are congenital mesoblastic nephromas. Grossly, the usual congenital mesoblastic nephroma is firm and resembles a uterine "fibroid" or leiomyoma on cross section. The cellular type of mesoblastic nephroma is generally softer and more variegated, with areas of hemorrhage and necrosis and occasional cystic changes. The conventional congenital mesoblastic nephroma is composed of interlacing fascicles of uniform, spindle-shaped cells having a pale pink fabrillar cytoplasm with indistinct borders. The cellular variant of congenital mesoblastic nephroma has increased cellularity and more mitotic activity.

Surgery for congenital mesoblastic nephroma is performed through a transabdominal incision, and, in general, the tumors are totally resected without difficulty. Local invasion virtually never is seen. Conventional congenital mesoblastic nephroma is an uncommon but distinctive infantile renal tumor having an excellent prognosis when treated by nephrectomy alone. Although local recurrence, presumably from residual tumor, has been reported to date, no metastasis from congenital mesoblastic nephroma has been documented with conventional histology. Chemotherapy and radiation therapy are not indicated.

Infantile renal tumors of the nephroblastomatosis complex and perhaps the cellular variant of congenital mesoblastic nephroma may have a more aggressive biologic potential. The goal of surgery should be complete resection of the tumor as early as possible to eliminate a potentially dangerous focus. It is then that an aggressive approach in terms of chemotherapy and radiation, as well as surgery, would appear to be warranted.

Suggested Readings

Blank E, Neerhout RC, Burry KA: Congenital mesoblastic nephroma and polyhydramnios. JAMA 240:1504, 1978

Bolande RP: Congenital and infantile neoplasia of the kidney. Lancet 2:1497, 1974

Hartman DS, Lesar MSL, Madewell JE, et al: Mesoblastic nephroma: Radiologic-pathologic correlation of 20 cases. Am J Roentgenol 136:69, 1981

Howell CG, Othersen HB, Kiviat NE, et al: Therapy and outcome in 51 children with mesoblastic nephroma: A report of the National Wilms' Tumor Study. J Pediatr Surg 17:826, 1982

Snyder HS, Lack EE, Chetty-Baktavizian A, et al: Congenital mesoblastic nephroma: Relationship to other renal tumors of infancy. J Urol 126:513, 1981

CURRENT TREATMENT FOR WILMS' TUMOR

RICHARD M. EHRLICH, M.D.

Los Angeles, California

In 1969, the National Wilms' Tumor Study (NWTS) Group was formed. This study group proved to be the quintessential example of what can be accomplished through cooperative endeavors among surgeons, pediatricians, oncologists, and radiation therapists. Patients were classified according to age and extent of disease at diagnosis, and comparative treatment regimens were devised accordingly. This landmark chemotherapeutic trial established that double-agent chemotherapy using actinomycin and vincristine gave better relapse-free survival rates than the use of either agent alone. At 2 years, the relapse-free survival rate for patients who were given both drugs was 81 per cent as compared with 55 per cent for those who were given a single drug.

Other pertinent aspects of Wilms' tumor were investigated, and data regarding familial patterns as well as important information were collected, including characteristics of the specimen, unifocal or multifocal disease, and involvement of lymph nodes.

In 1974, NWTS-II was begun. This study was predicated on the results of the first study. As stated, double-agent chemotherapy had been found to be superior to actinomycin or vincristine alone, and this became the baseline for an advanced chemotherapeutic approach. In addition, radiation therapy was found to be expendable as far as the survival or Group 1 children.

Adriamycin (doxorubicin), a known cardiotoxin, was added to the protocol, and the children in Groups 2, 3, and 4 were divided into two subgroups: those who were given actinomycin plus vincristine for 15 months and those who received actinomycin plus vincristine plus Adriamycin for 15 months. All received radiation therapy postoperatively in doses similar to those used in NWTS-I. It was found that the relapse-free survival rate and 2-year survival rate for Group 1 children was well over 90 per cent, despite the length of chemotherapy used. In advanced disease, triple-drug therapy yielded a better 2-year relapse-free survival rate than did double-drug chemotherapy.

The study, however, continued to be mindful of the serious cardiotoxicity and total lifetime dose of Adriamycin that could be given to such children and hoped to change either the duration or dosage of this drug or suggest its elimination if possible.

Patients with "favorable histology" faired well with the treatment regimens described earlier, and those with "unfavorable histology," comprising anaplasia and sarcomatous patterns, faired poorly. In the "favorable" category, only 7 per cent of patients died of Wilms' tumor, as opposed to those in the "unfavorable" category, who had a 57 per cent death rate.

The NWTS-III is now underway and considers the following three categories: (1) additional shortening of the period of chemotherapy for early-stage disease, (2) testing of an intensive regimen to improve survival with the unfavorable histologic type or with metastatic disease at the time of diagnosis, and (3) the development of a more concentrated course of actinomycin and vincristine with the objective of potentially eliminating Adriamycin and its cardiotoxicity from the regimen. Other objectives of this study are to gather information regarding patients and their families, including patterns of cancer within families, in an attempt to identify children and families who are at higher risks for cancer and to study the late consequences of successful treatment given for Wilms' tumor.

NWTS-III is also trying to determine the amount of radiation therapy that is necessary for Group 2 and Group 3 patients, as well as the efficacy of adding a fourth drug for those patients with unfavorable histology. We eagerly await the results of this study, which will probably be the last of this project.

Information is now available on the issue of bilateral Wilms' tumor, and although these data are not prospective, they nevertheless offer interesting insights. Bilateral Wilms' tumors do not behave as aggressively as their unilateral counterpart and have a different natural history. The surgery for bilateral disease should be conservative, with preservation of as much renal parenchyma on one or both sides as possible. The thrust is to remove as little functioning parenchyma as possible with the use of initial biopsy only, followed by a second laparotomy after treatment and even a third laparotomy after further treatment before total nephrectomy is performed.

Even though the exceptional efficacy of chemotherapy and radiation therapy may compensate for a poorly executed nephrectomy, it is incumbent on the surgeon who is dealing with these tumors to be thoroughly familiar with the latest information in diagnosis and treatment. This implies a constant perusal for the pertinent urologic and surgical literature and in-depth familiarity with the guidelines of the NWTS Group.

Suggested Readings

Beckwith JB: Wilms' tumor and other renal tumors in childhood: A selective review from the National Wilms' Tumor Study Pathology Center. Hum Pathol 14:481, 1983

Beckwith JB, Palmer NF: Histopathology and prognosis of Wilms' tumor: Result from the National Wilms' Tumor Study. Cancer 41:1937, 1978

D'Angio GJ, Breslow N, Beckwith JB, et al: Treatment of Wilms' tumor: Results of the Third National Wilms' Tumor Study. Cancer 64:349, 1989b

Farewell VT, D'Angio GJ, Breslow N, et al: Retrospective validation of a new staging system for Wilms' tumor. Cancer Clin Trials 4:167, 1981

Kelalis PP: Bilateral tumor: Surgical treatment: NWTS recommendations. Dialog Ped Urol 8(10):6, 1985

Mesrobian H-GJ: Wilms' tumor: Past, present, future. J Urol 140:231, 1988

RENAL CELL CARCINOMA

ARIE S. BELLDEGRUN, M.D.

Los Angeles, California

Renal cell carcinoma will represent approximately 2 per cent of new cancer cases in the United States in 1993 with approximately 27,200 new cases expected to occur this year. The etiology of the tumor is unclear but recent evidence indicates that deletions on the short arm of chromosome 3 are playing an important role in the development and progression of this tumor.

PRIMARY RENAL CELL CARCINOMA

Radical nephrectomy remains the established therapy for localized renal cell carcinoma, but this treatment is seldom effective if the tumor has spread beyond the confines of Gerota's fascia. The indication for surgery and the surgical approach therefore must be guided by the preoperative staging evaluation. With computerized tomography (CT), considerable information can be obtained preoperatively regarding the extent of local tumor spread. The CT scan also can ascertain reliably the nature of the renal mass, the size of the tumor, invasion of adjacent muscle and organs, renal vein and vena caval involvement, and regional lymph node metastases. However, because complete surgical excision remains the best hope for cure, the urologist must be cautious when denying a patient the potential for surgical cure solely on the basis of CT staging. Evidence of regional extension combined with fine-needle percutaneous biopsy confirmation often is helpful in avoiding unrewarding surgical exploration. Patients with renal masses and nonfunctioning kidneys on intravenous pyelography should be suspected of having renal vein and/or vena caval involvement. In such patients, magnetic resonance imaging or a venocavography should be performed. The two studies have equal sensitivity and are complimentary in evaluating the inferior vena cava.

The most cost-effective method of staging for distant metastases is to obtain a chest radiograph, perform liver function tests, and measure alkaline phosphatase levels. Abnormal serum values, a palpable liver, or skeletal pain should prompt the appropriate radiographs or radioisotope scans. Routine liver and skeletal scans do not seem to be cost-effective, although obtaining this added assurance preoperatively cannot be condemned.

Operative Treatment

The goal of radical nephrectomy in the treatment of localized renal cell carcinoma is the complete removal of Gerota's fascia and its contents and, usually, a regional lymph node dissection. The surgical approach must be designed to accomplish this end and also must allow early ligation of the renal vein to prevent tumor dissemination during surgery.

Many approaches have been championed, and all are effective and satisfactory. Although the choice depends on individual preference, it also should be tailored to the build of the patient and to the size and position of the tumor. For large upper-pole tumors, the thoracoabdominal approach offers excellent exposure, although the subcostal, or chevron, incision is often just as effective, without the need for a thoracotomy. Supracostal 11th- or 12th-rib incisions are excellent for small tumors or tumors in the lower pole and do not require intraperitoneal or intrathoracic dissection. Regardless of the type of incision, the next step in the operation must be the ligation of the renal artery and vein, and the incision must facilitate access to the renal pedicle.

The role of lymph node dissection remains controversial. Most urologists now agree that extensive retroperitoneal lymphadenectomy has proven not to be therapeutic. However, a limited lymph node dissection in the area of the renal hilum and dissection of the ipsilateral para-aortic or paracaval lymph nodes may encompass early lymphatic dissemination and will allow for accurate staging. The staging information obtained from such a dissection currently is becoming important as the new biologic therapies are included in postoperative adjuvant trials.

Because of the low response rates of therapeutic alternatives, the indications for operative treatment of renal carcinoma have been extended. Direct extension into an adjacent organ should not deter surgical treatment, provided the tumor can be completely excised. Although the 5-year survival rate of such patients is poor, an occasional patent will be cured and may achieve significant short-term palliation. Resection of the adjacent structures (e.g., tail of the pancreas, mesocolon, and small bowel)—when technically feasible—should be considered. Because extensive regional lymph node metastasis indicates virtually no chance of a 5-year survival, and because such lymph nodes seldom can be excised totally, nephrectomy is probably not indicated, unless it is based on a planned postoperative protocol therapy or performed for control of severe symptoms.

Improved technical aspects of partial nephrectomy have rekindled interest in nephron-sparing surgery for renal cell carcinoma. A recent review by Novick et al. summarized the results of nephron-sparing surgery in 700 patients reported in the literature since 1980. Mean disease-free survival in these studies was 57 to 100 per cent; the median follow up was approximately 5 years and the local recurrence rate was 0 to 10 per cent. Most of the lesions are well differentiated, and a follow-up of 10 to 15 years may be required to detect the true incidence of low recurrence. Partial nephrectomy with circumferential incision of the parenchyma around the tumor almost always is possible as an alternative to enucleation and much less likely to result in local recurrence. Despite these advances, radical nephrectomy should remain the mainstay in the treatment of localized renal cell carcinoma in patients with two normal kidneys because of the proven cure rate and the published literature demonstrating excellent long-term renal function in living kidney donors. Nephron-sparing surgery is utilized in patients in whom radical nephrectomy would result in the need for permanent dialysis.

Adjuvant Management

The preoperative and postoperative adjuvant management of localized renal carcinoma remains controversial. Routine preoperative percutaneous angioinfarction has been popularized in some centers. The many effective methods that have been devised for occluding the renal artery have prompted this popular adjunct to surgical treatment. In the case of localized renal carcinoma, it is usually carried out immediately before the procedure. Although some kinds of immunologic response have been postulated, no true therapeutic gain has been realized with respect to ultimate survival in these patients. Furthermore, the procedure adds to the cost of therapy and sometimes can be associated with major complications. At most institutions, therefore, it is reserved for the patient with a huge renal tumor, when early access to the renal artery would be difficult. It also may be helpful in the patient with a large vena caval thrombus, which can then be managed before manipulating the renal vein and vena cava while gaining access to the main renal artery.

Preoperative and postoperative adjuvant radiotherapy have proven not to be effective. Preoperative radiotherapy is seldom considered, but postoperative radiotherapy is often attractive in the patient with known localized tumor extension in the renal fossa or in the regional nodes. In the presence of gross residual tumor, radiotherapy may control the regional disease but distant recurrence is almost certain. In the presence of microscopic residual disease, the side effects of therapy outweigh the potential gain. In short, radiotherapy has no proven role in the treatment of localized renal carcinoma.

No effective systematic adjuvant treatment has been proven in patients with locally advanced renal carcinoma. Because interferon-alpha (IFN-α) has demonstrable activity in the treatment of metastatic renal cell carcinoma, studies utilizing IFN-α as adjuvant therapy for locally advanced renal cell carcinoma are in progress. A German study has not demonstrated efficacy for adjuvant IFN-α in patients at high risk for relapse; the results of an Eastern Cooperative Oncology Group (ECOG) study have not been reported. Interleukin-2 (IL-2) has received Food and Drug Administration (FDA) approval in the treatment of metastatic renal cell carcinoma but no adjuvant studies have yet been performed. Hormonal therapy and chemotherapy seem to have little impact on this tumor. Thus, at the present time, no postoperative adjuvant treatment is available or practical, except in the context of a structured clinical trial.

Prognosis

The results of surgical therapy depend on a number of prognostic factors, including the extent of local invasion into the renal capsule and Gerota's fascia, main renal vein and vena caval extension, extension to contiguous organs, involvement of regional lymph nodes, and tumor cell type. The grade of the tumor seems to influence prognosis, and the sarcomatoid, undifferentiated cell type appears to have a worse prognosis than the clear cell variety. The 5-year survival rate of surgically treated patients with tumor within the kidney, surrounded by a normal parenchyma and without lymphatic spread, is approximately 70 per cent. Extension through the renal capsule decreases the 5-year survival rate to approximately 50 per cent. Involvement of the main renal vein or the vena cava usually is associated with a 5-year survival rate of 40 to 50 per cent, and survival of patients with proven regional lymph node metastases is from 0 to 30 per cent. Extension to contiguous organs implies a 5-year survival rate of 0 to 10 per cent.

METASTATIC RENAL CELL CARCINOMA

High-dose IL-2 has received FDA approval in the treatment of metastatic renal cell carcinoma and should be considered the treatment of choice in high-performance patients. The response rate in high-performance patients (ECOG Grades 0 and 1) is 4 per cent complete (disappearance of all measurable tumor) and 11 per cent partial (50 per cent or greater decrease in size of measurable tumor). The median duration of response has been 2 years, and some patients have remained disease free for more than 7 years. Most patients who have received IL-2 have previously undergone nephrectomy.

Because researchers at UCLA and other institutions have noted poor responses of primary tumors to IL-2 therapy, the issue of tumor debulking with nephrectomy prior to IL-2 therapy is currently under investigation. At UCLA, 28 patients who presented with metastatic renal cell carcinoma with the primary tumor in place underwent radical nephrectomy. Tumor-infiltrating lymphocyte (TIL) cells from the nephrectomy specimen were prepared in vitro. Patients were treated with the TIL cells and low-dose IL-2 regimens. Seven patients achieved a complete response, with ongoing responses ranging from 4 to 28 months. These data strongly suggest that metastatic renal cell carcinoma may be a curable disease when treated with optimal immune therapy.

Suggested Readings

Belldegrun A, Figlin R, Danella J, deKernion J: Immunotherapy for renal cell carcinoma. Semin Urol X: 23–27, 1992

Licht MR, Novick AC: Nephron sparing surgery for renal cell carcinoma. J Urol 149:1–7, 1993

Long JP, Choyke PL, Shawker TA, Robertson CR, Pass HI, Walther MM, Linehan MW: Intraoperative ultrasound in the evaluation of tumor involvement of the inferior vena cava. J Urol 150:13–17, 1993

Minasian LM, Motzer RJ, Glusk L, Mazumdar M, Vlamis V, Krown SE: Interferon alfa-2a in advanced renal cell carcinoma: Treatment, results and survival in 159 patients with long-term follow-up. J Clin Oncol 11:1368–1375, 1993

Morgan WR, Zinke H: Management of renal cell carcinoma involving a solitary kidney. AUA Update Series Lesson 21, Vol. X, 1991

Porzsolt F on behalf of Delta-P study group: Adjuvant therapy of renal cell cancer (RCC) with interferon alfa-2-a. ASCO 11:202, 1992

RENAL CELL CARCINOMA IN CHILDREN

DOUGLAS A. CANNING, M.D.

Philadelphia, Pennsylvania

Renal cell carcinoma is rare in children. The overwhelming majority of malignant renal tumors in those under 21 are Wilms' tumors. Summarizing a number of reports, Raney found the incidence of renal cell carcinoma to be 7 per cent in patients under 21 with primary intrarenal tumors. Earlier reports suggest an even lower incidence when compared to Wilms' tumor. Confirming the relative predisposition of this tumor to occur in adults, Castellanos noted that fewer than 0.05 per cent of all renal cell carcinomas occur in children. When one considers the incidence of Wilms' tumor (7.8 in 1 million), and adult renal cell carcinoma (3 per cent of adult malignancies), it is understandable why fewer than 100 cases have been reported.

Unlike renal cell carcinoma in adults, which attacks males twice as frequently as females, girls under 21 develop renal cell carcinoma as frequently as boys. Although renal cell carcinoma has presented in a 3-month-old and a 10-month-old, there is no predisposition toward younger age. Most patients are older than 5 years at presentation. The mean age at diagnosis in Raney's study was 11.8 years, with a range of 14 months to 19 years.

The appearance of renal cell carcinoma in children is sporadic. There is evidence in adults that at least some renal cell carcinomas may be inherited. In one family, it occurred in 10 adult members in what appeared to be an autosomal dominant inheritance pattern.

A characteristic chromosomal translocation was present in each affected member. A higher than expected incidence of renal cell carcinoma exists in adults with von Hippel–Lindau disease and autosomal dominant polycystic kidney disease. These disorders appear most commonly after the second decade and therefore have little bearing on the pediatric patient. No associated hormonal or genetic anomaly exists in children.

PATHOPHYSIOLOGY

The cell of origin for renal cell carcinoma in adults is the proximal renal tubular cell. Immunohistochemical studies, however, have shown expression of a heterogeneous group of cell surface antigens. One such tumor in children expressed the Tamm-Horsfall protein. This protein is found only in the distal tubule or collecting duct. This suggests that at least some tumors in children may originate in the distal tubule or collecting duct. The clear cell tubulopapillary histology pattern predominates in children. However, as in adults, granular cell and mixed tumors also occur. The tumor may invade adjacent organs and has recurred in the tumor bed following nephrectomy. Metastatic spread is most commonly to bone, bone marrow, and lungs, but metastasis to the brain and distant lymph nodes also occurs.

PRESENTATION

Although children with Wilms' tumor generally appear healthy and present with a palpable mass and few other symptoms, children with renal cell carcinoma seem to present with more tumor-related symptoms. At initial evaluation, a palpable abdominal mass is present only about half the time. Children with renal cell carcinoma more frequently present with gross hematuria or abdominal pain than do children with Wilms' tumor. Less specific symptoms such as weight loss, anorexia, nausea, vomiting, and fevers, also unusual in Wilms' tumor, occasionally appear in children with renal cell carcinoma. Hypertension, which occurs one third of the time in adults with renal cell carcinoma, is unusual in children. Abnormal erythrocyte sedimentation rate, elevated liver function test results, anemia, or polycythemia, while reported with some frequency in adults, are rarely present in children.

STAGING AND DIAGNOSTIC IMAGING

Accurate preoperative staging is essential. Because most solid renal tumors in children are Wilms' tumors, the initial work-up should adhere to National Wilms' Tumor Study recommendations. A careful physical examination is essential. Elevated blood pressure, although less common in children, must be identified and controlled prior to surgery. Careful palpation will help characterize the mobility of the mass and its relation to adjacent organs. Lower extremity edema or varicocele may suggest vena caval compression by the primary tumor or associated lymph nodes. Complete blood cell count, urinalysis, and serum electrolyte, creatinine, and liver function tests should be done prior to surgery.

Imaging studies should endeavor to identify local vascular invasion and contiguous organ involvement, and metastasis if present. Ultrasound readily identifies tumors larger than 1 cm. Children are leaner than adults, with less fat within Gerota's fascia. As a result, computerized tomography (CT) scanning less precisely characterizes the renal margins in children. Nevertheless, CT combined with ultrasound will identify and accurately stage most tumors. Although a larger proportion of renal cell tumors than Wilms' tumors appear calcified or hyperdense on enhanced CT, it is impossible to separate Wilms' tumor from renal cell carcinoma prior to surgery. Occasionally the initial diagnostic ultrasound or CT scan does not adequately image the vena cava or renal vein. In these cases a repeat study with the patient well hydrated may help identify the presence of vascular invasion and localize the level of tumor involvement. Magnetic resonance imaging may be helpful to identify flow past a suspected tumor thrombus. Angiography adds little except in patients with bilateral tumors, those suspected of having adjacent organ involvement, or those in whom preoperative tumor embolism is planned. Pulmonary metastasis must be identified if present. Our routine at The Children's Hospital of Philadelphia is to obtain a four-view chest radiograph. No other studies are done routinely before removing the renal tumor.

THERAPY

Despite attempts at salvage with multiple adjuvant chemotherapy regimens, successful surgical eradication of renal cell carcinoma remains the cornerstone of therapy in children as well as in the adult. The goal is en bloc radical nephrectomy with limited retroperitoneal lymph node sampling. Because the preoperative diagnosis is usually Wilms' tumor, surgery should include visualization of the contralateral side. The incision should be large enough to provide adequate exposure of both the tumor and associated vessels. Because the ribs shelter the kidney incompletely in children, a transperitoneal horizontal incision off the tip of the 11th or 12th rib is adequate for all but the largest tumors. The thoracoabdominal approach is less commonly used in children, but may be helpful for a particularly large right-sided tumor.

If vascular invasion exists, particularly if the tumor thrombus extends superior to the hepatic vessels, a midline incision that can be extended into the chest will provide excellent exposure of the cava and atrium. Preoperative embolization may be worthwhile in large tumors with obvious vascular invasion. If tumor extends above the level of the hepatic veins, cardiopulmonary bypass with deep hypothermia may help control blood loss and facilitates a complete excision. Intraoperative sonography helps further characterize the tumor thrombus in these cases. A poor salvage rate with adjuvant chemotherapy justifies even heroic attempts at tumor removal.

PROGNOSIS

Prognosis is much less favorable than for Wilms' tumor. As in adults, survival is about 50 per cent at 10 years. Although Raney's 1983 review suggested a more favorable prognosis for younger patients, clinical stage at presentation appears to be the only consistent predictor of outcome. Patients with tumor confined to the kidney and completely removed appear to do well, with between 80 and 100 per cent long-term survival. Similar success can be anticipated in patients with limited extension to paracaval nodes if resection is complete. Patients with vascular invasion fare poorly, with between 10 and 30 per cent survival. Patients with metastatic disease uniformly die, generally within 3 years.

Attempts to control recurrence or metastasis with high-dose radiation or chemotherapy occasionally have resulted in reduction of tumor volume in adults, but long-term survival does not improve. Actinomycin D and vincristine at Wilms' tumor doses have been used in some patients without clear-cut advantage. Radiation to the tumor bed or to localized metastasis has resulted in dramatic reduction in tumor bulk and probably should be offered, especially in symptomatic patients. Unfortunately, little evidence exists to promote optimism when surgical cure is not possible.

Suggested Readings

Booth CM: Renal parenchymal carcinoma in children. Br J Surg 73:313–317, 1986

Broecker B: Renal cell carcinoma in children. Urology 38: 54, 1991

Castellanos RD, Aron BS, Evans AT: Renal adenocarcinoma in children: Incidence, therapy and prognosis. J Urol 111:534–537, 1974

Hartman DS, Davis CJ Jr, Madewell JE, et al: Primary malignant renal tumors in the second decade of life: Wilms' tumor versus renal cell carcinoma. J Urol 127: 888, 1982

Kabala JE, Shield J, Duncan A: Renal cell carcinoma in childhood. Pediatr Radiol 22:203–205, 1992

Leuschner I, Harms D, Schmidt D: Renal cell carcinoma in children: Histology, immunohistochemistry, and follow-up of 10 cases. Med Paediatr Oncol 19:33–41, 1991

Pochedly C, Surwansirkul S, Penzer P: Renal-cell carcinoma with extrarenal manifestations in a 10 month old child. Am J Dis Child 121:528–530, 1971

Raney RB, Palmer N, Sutow WW, et al: Renal cell carcinoma in children. Med Paediatr Oncol 11:91–98, 1983

Young JL Jr, Miller RW: Incidence of malignant tumors in US children. J Pediatr 86:254, 1975

RENAL ONCOCYTOMA

MICHAEL M. LIEBER, M.D.

Rochester, Minnesota

Renal oncocytoma is a new and common clinicopathologic entity. A recent review of renal tumor registries in various locations has revealed that renal oncocytomas make up 3 to 14 per cent of renal tumors; such tumors previously were classified as renal cell carcinomas. As a best guess, oncocytomas represent 5 to 7 per cent of tumors previously considered to be renal cell carcinomas. Perhaps the most intriguing aspect of renal oncocytoma is that this distinctive and benign-behaving renal neoplasm was nearly totally overlooked by several generations of urologists and pathologists.

HISTOPATHOLOGY

Oncocytes are large neoplastic cells with intensely eosinophilic granular cytoplasms. Histochemical and ultrastructural studies have demonstrated that the eosinophilic granules are seen after staining because the cytoplasm of the oncocyte is packed with mitochondria. By definition, oncocytomas are tumors that are composed solely of oncocytes. Although such tumors have been identified previously in organs other than the kidney, including the salivary, thyroid, parathyroid, and adrenal glands, the cell or tissue origin for oncocytomas is unknown.

Only renal tumors that are made up strictly of well-differentiated eosinophilic granular cells, or *oncocytes*, can be considered oncocytomas. Some renal cell carcinomas are made up of granular cells that are more poorly differentiated and that have an obvious neoplastic nuclear appearance. These tumors behave like malignant neoplasms. Other renal cell carcinomas contain a mixture of clear cells and granular cells. In our experience, these tumors also behave like malignant neoplasms.

The most current immunologic and histochemical studies from Europe suggest that renal oncocytomas in experimental animals and humans arise from the intercalated cells of the collecting tubules of the kidney. This would be in contrast to standard renal cell carcinomas, which are believed to develop from cells of the proximal tubules.

GROSS MORPHOLOGY

Renal oncocytomas often have a typical gross morphology that is distinctive. These tumors are often well encapsulated and rarely, if ever, penetrate the perirenal capsule or invade local structures. The intrarenal collecting system and perinephric fat generally are not invaded. Even when such tumors are quite large, the adjacent kidney parenchyma appears intact. On cut section, renal oncocytomas normally have a homogeneous appearance, with the absence of hemorrhage or necrosis. The cut surface of a tumor usually is tan, brown, or mahogany, which contrasts with the yellowish hemorrhagic and necrotic surface commonly seen with renal cell carcinomas. Large tumors often have a prominent stellate central scar.

CLINICAL PRESENTATION

Renal oncocytomas generally are not symptomatic. Almost all such tumors have been discovered either incidentally during the course of evaluation for some unrelated symptom or at autopsy. For example, among the group of oncocytic renal tumors seen at the Mayo Clinic, 60 per cent were discovered incidentally and were asymptomatic. In other institutions, none of the patients with oncocytomas had any renal-related symptoms. It seems a safe generalization to posit that about 75 per cent of renal oncocytomas will be discovered in an asymptomatic state. Because the techniques for imaging the retroperitoneum and the kidneys, particularly computerized tomographic (CT) scanning, have improved radically since the 1970s, it seems likely that these techniques will be used to help identify even more oncocytomas in the future. In most series that were studied, males have predominated over females at an approximately 2:1 ratio. The age incidence for renal oncocytomas has been close to that commonly seen for "garden-variety" renal adenocarcinomas. Most of the patients have been middle aged, with a median age of approximately 55 years. No anatomic site in the kidney or side (right or left kidney) predilection has been found. Several cases of bilateral renal oncocytoma have been reported. Also, several reports have established that multifocal renal oncocytomas can occur in one or both kidneys. Such cases have been labeled "renal oncocytomatosis."

RADIOLOGIC FINDINGS

Almost all renal oncocytomas have been discovered because excretory urography or CT scanning of the abdomen was performed for some unrelated reason. In some instances, however, renal oncocytomas became so large that a palpable flank mass prompted radiologic investigation. By excretory urography, ultrasound examination, and CT scanning, renal oncocytomas have the typical appearance of a solid renal mass lesion. We have not found these standard imaging techniques useful for differentiating renal cell carcinoma from oncocytoma.

To date, selective renal angiography has been the test that most commonly has suggested the presence of a renal oncocytoma preoperatively. Renal oncocytomas often have a typical angiographic appearance that can suggest (but not prove) their existence. Angiographic signs of renal oncocytoma include the "lucent rim sign" resulting from the thick capsule, a homogeneous capillary nephrogram phase, the absence of clearly wild neoplastic vessels, and the spoke-like appearance of the feeding arteries. At the Mayo Clinic, a typical angiographic appearance suggesting the diagnosis of renal oncocytoma preoperatively was present in about 50 per cent of cases reviewed. Angiographic findings in the other 50 per cent could not be differentiated from renal cell carcinoma.

Thus, at present, no radiologic imaging technique allows the unequivocal preoperative diagnosis of renal oncocytoma. This diagnosis should be considered, however, when an incidental solid renal mass is discovered. Angiography can prove useful in increasing the odds of identifying a renal oncocytoma preoperatively.

SURGICAL TREATMENT

Until recently, nearly all renal oncocytomas were considered to be renal cell carcinomas and generally were treated by radical nephrectomy. It is hard to take serious issue with this approach, because the prognosis for patients with renal oncocytoma treated by radical nephrectomy is excellent and approximates the prognosis for normal age- and sex-matched control groups (see below). Nevertheless, we believe that renal oncocytomas behave benignly. Because the current preoperative imaging techniques, such as CT scanning, are becoming so precise, and because the incidence of multifocal oncocytomas is unusual, we believe that partial renal resection for small and suitably located renal oncocytomas probably will come to be the norm in the future. For example, often a 2- or 3-cm mass lesion of the upper or lower pole of the kidney is detected as an incidental finding during CT examination of the abdomen performed for nonrenal symptoms. Such tumors can be removed totally with an adequate margin of normal parenchyma by relatively uncomplicated guillotine-type partial nephrectomy. We believe that this approach to the surgical treatment of renal lesions (including carcinomas) will be used in the future in young patients who are in good health. There seems to be no justification for thinking that such patients would have a poorer prognosis than patients with similar-stage tumors treated by radical nephrectomy.

Intraoperative frozen-section biopsy may be the most suitable test to evaluate the possibility that a small and easily resectable renal tumor may be an oncocytoma. This attractive approach has not been studied extensively as yet. Although preoperative thin-needle aspiration biopsy of oncocytic renal tumors has been reported in the literature, we do not believe that this method would necessarily give an adequate sampling of the tumor. Rather, we propose that total surgical removal of such tumors will always be the procedure of choice, because oncocytomas can grow quite large, even if they are not locally invasive or metastatic. Except for high-risk patients, we do not believe that the time will come when the preoperative diagnosis and percutaneous biopsy of renal oncocytoma would lead to nonsurgical treatment, such as observation. Because renal carcinomas with malignant behavior can have oncocytic cell components, we believe that the total volume of any renal neoplasm, even one thought to be an oncocytoma, must be thoroughly sampled histologically before the diagnosis of renal oncocytoma can be made confidently.

Because renal oncocytomas have minimal, if any, metastatic potential, there seems to be no appropriate role for regional or retroperitoneal lymphadenectomy for patients with renal oncocytomas. Rather, such tumors should simply be removed totally and safely, sparing the residual normal kidney tissue if this is technically feasible or removing the kidney and tumor totally if it is not. Even for very large renal oncocytomas, the tumor capsule generally is preserved, and, with care, the tumor can be removed safely with minimal blood loss. Such tumors do not have the florid external neovascularity commonly seen with true renal cell carcinomas, and the resultant technical problems of nephrectomy also are not seen commonly. Even for patients with renal oncocytomatosis, enucleation of multiple tumors in the presence of an anatomically or functionally solitary kidney may be possible.

PROGNOSIS

More than 600 cases of renal oncocytoma have been reported in the literature. These reported cases (and many others not reported formally) leave little doubt that the nonaggressive, benign behavior first emphasized for this tumor by Klein and Valensi has been confirmed amply. At the Mayo Clinic, among 62 patients with Grade 1 renal oncocytomas, none developed recurrent or metastatic disease and none died of metastatic cancer. Benign behavior was observed despite a large number of tumors studied and despite the fact that the tumors often reached a large size before they were treated. Indeed, to date, no tumor deaths have been reported in the literature for patients with renal oncocytoma.

In the past, renal oncocytomas were considered to be granular cell renal carcinomas. Because the recent data strongly support the concept that such tumors in fact behave more like adenomas than carcinomas, it now seems reasonable to make oncocytomas of the kidney a separate diagnostic entity. Because oncocytomas have a benign behavior and almost certainly can be treated adequately by localized surgical extirpation, there has been inflation of our survival figures for renal carcinoma over the past years. Because about 5 per cent of renal tumors resected really have been renal oncocytomas, we have been deluding ourselves somewhat about our skills in treating renal cell carcinoma.

CONCLUSION

Review of recent published clinical and pathologic data from many centers around the world leaves no doubt that renal oncocytomas exist and are not so uncommon. Rather, this distinctive clinical and pathologic entity was merely overlooked until recent years. These generally asymptomatic solid renal mass lesions often have a suggestive appearance by renal angiography. The tumors are not locally invasive or metastatic, and total surgical extirpation of the tumor almost seems certainly to control the disease. New imaging methods, such as radionuclide imaging with a labeled compound that could be selectively concentrated by oncocytes or magnetic resonance imaging, seem to be promising techniques for future investigation. Renal oncocytomas do exist as distinctive entities that behave like benign adenomas rather than like carcinomas of the kidney. Adjustment of our urologic practice to take this new knowledge into account seems to be the next logical step.

Suggested Readings

Crotty TB, Lawrence KM, Moertel CA, Bartelt DH Jr, Batts KP, Dewald GW, Farrow GM, Jenkins RB: Cytogenetic analysis of six renal oncocytomas and a chromophobe cell renal carcinoma. Evidence that -Y, -l may be a characteristic anomaly in renal oncocytomas. Cancer Genet Cytogenet 61:61–66, 1992

Klein MJ, Valensi QJ: Proximal tubular adenomas of kidney with so-called oncocytic features: A clinicopathological study of 13 cases of a rarely reported neoplasm. Cancer 38:906–914, 1976

Lieber MM, Tomera KM, Farrow GM: Renal oncocytoma. J Urol 125:481–485, 1981

Lieber MM, Tsukamoto T: Renal oncocytoma. Chapter 20 *In*: Tumors of the Kidney, JB deKernion and M Pavone-Macaluso (eds). Williams and Wilkins, Baltimore, MD, pp 257–273, 1986

Zerban H, Nogueira E, Riedasch G, Bannasch P: Renal oncocytoma: Origin from the collecting duct. Virchows Arch 52:375–387, 1987

ADJUVANT TREATMENT OF METASTATIC RENAL CELL CARCINOMA

J. EDSON PONTES, M.D.

Detroit, Michigan

Approximately 26,000 new cases of renal cell carcinoma are diagnosed annually, with an estimated death rate of about 10,000 patients a year. Between 25 and 50 per cent of patients will have metastatic disease at the time of diagnosis. Furthermore, approximately 50 per cent of the patients seen initially with localized disease will develop metastasis or local recurrence at a later date. Because of this somewhat bleak picture, attempts to develop adjunctive methods of therapy that could improve the survival of these patients have been made over the past few years.

LOCAL OR REGIONAL ADJUNCTIVE TREATMENT

In the absence of local or systemic symptoms, the value of nephrectomy in the presence of disseminated disease is questionable. Although reports of spontaneous regression of metastasis after nephrectomy have been made, their occurrence is rare (0.8 per cent), and the length of response is short. It has been shown that, in the presence of disseminated disease, the survival of patients who are subjected to nephrectomy does not differ from those without nephrectomy. A slight increase in survival has been reported in patients with bone metastasis only, although because of the small number of patients, this may reflect selection. Among patients presenting with extensive vena caval involvement in the absence of distant metastasis, complete excision of the tumor will lead to approximately 50 per cent 5-year survival. Attempts at complete surgical removal should be made in those cases.

Surgical excision of a "solitary" metastasis,

either at the time of nephrectomy or when it appears at a later date, has been shown to benefit patients, and the 5-year survival of such patients has been reported at 34 per cent. Patients who develop a solitary metastasis at the time of diagnosis will do worse than those with asynchronous appearance of metastasis. Recent data have indicated, however, that in large institutional series the results are not as optimistic as has been presented previously.

The use of preoperative or postoperative radiation therapy has been advocated in the past in an attempt to decrease local recurrences. It is evident from analysis of both prospective randomized studies and retrospective studies that neither preoperative nor postoperative radiation has an advantage over radical nephrectomy.

Renal artery embolization before nephrectomy or as a palliative procedure to stop bleeding in patients who are considered poor surgical risks has been popularized since the 1970s. Renal embolization before nephrectomy should be restricted to those patients with very large tumors involving the hilum and to those in whom nephrectomy may present technical problems. There is no place for its routine use otherwise. Embolization is indicated in patients with bleeding who, for medical reasons, are not candidates for surgery, because it often leads to decrease of symptoms. Recent reports of arterial embolization before nephrectomy in patients with metastatic disease have proposed that this procedure may affect the immunologic status of such patients and prolong survival. Although reports suggest an improvement in survival, other factors, such as the concomitant use of hormones, preclude a direct cause-and-effect relationship between embolization and the disappearance of metastasis. These procedures should be viewed as experimental and should be done as part of clinical studies. Recently, we have used embolization of lytic metastatic lesions in the pelvic bones to palliate the pain, with excellent results in six out of seven patients.

SYSTEMIC THERAPY

Because a large percentage of patients with renal cell carcinoma will have widespread metastatic disease, several modalities of treatment have been proposed without significant success.

Hormonal Therapy

Experimental observation that renal cell carcinoma can be induced in golden hamsters by estrogen administration and inhibited by estrogen antagonists has been the basis of hormonal therapy for metastatic renal cell carcinoma. Clinical observations that renal cell carcinoma is more common in men than in women and that the majority of spontaneous regressions are seen in males also are suggestive of the hormonal dependence of this tumor. However, clinical trials using a variety of hormones have been disappointing.

In a recent review of data collected from 463 patients who were treated either by progestational agents or by androgens, the objective response rate was 11 per cent. This percentage probably reflects just the natural history of the disease. However, because no other modalities of therapy are available, and because side effects of hormones are minimal, a trial of hormones in such patients is warranted. The most commonly used agent has been medroxyprogesterone acetate, in a dose of 400 mg intramuscularly twice a week.

Chemotherapy

The objective response of metastatic renal cell carcinoma to a variety of chemotherapeutic agents is weak and unpredictable. Often agents that show responses in initial studies demonstrate disappointing results in larger series. Almost every chemotherapeutic agent has been used in renal cell carcinoma. Woodruff reviewed 270 patients who were treated with a variety of chemotherapeutic agents and found objective response in 5 of 36 patients who were treated with 5-fluorouracil, 2 of 23 who were treated with 6-mercaptopurine, and 1 of 10 who were treated with vinblastine. A similar experience was reported by Bloom, who found only 7.6 per cent objective response in his review of different chemotherapeutic trials. Probably the most commonly used agent has been vinblastine, based on the experience of effectiveness of this antineoplastic in renal cell carcinoma in BALB/C mice. Clinical trials with this agent, however, have been disappointing.

A recent trial using floxuridine (FUDR) chemotherapy delivered by continuous infusion in a circadian cycle has shown some promise, with 43 per cent overall response among 24 patients treated. Further studies using this approach are necessary to confirm these initial observations.

Biologic Response Modifiers

Considerable evidence has been collected suggesting that renal cell carcinoma can be influenced by the host immune system. In the past, most of the trials included the use of nonspecific immunostimulants such as bacille Calmette-Guérin vaccine, immune ribonucleic acid, or transfer factor, with questionable results. Later attempts at specific immunotherapy using autologous tumor cell vaccine, either with radiated tumor cells or with tumor cell membrane, showed occasional responses that, although dramatic in some cases, could not be reproduced. Further attempts at modulation of these trials, with suppression of suppressor cells, demonstrated no further advantage.

In recent years, with the improvement in technology in recombinant DNA, a large number of biologic response modifiers have become available for widespread use.

Interferons

Interferons are glycoproteins produced by mammalian cells in response to viral infection. Three major classes of interferons have been characterized: Interferon-alpha, interferon-beta, and interferon-gamma. Of the three classes, most of the studies done in renal cell carcinoma have been with alpha-interferon. The results of gamma-interferon in metastatic renal cell carcinoma have been disappointing. Among all the compiled trials of alpha-interferon from the literature, it appears that the overall response rate is about 17 per cent. Patients with metastatic lung lesions appear to have a higher response rate. Attempts at combination of alpha-interferon with chemotherapeutic agents have been made, but the results have not been significantly better than those with interferon alone.

Interleukin-2

Interleukin-2 (IL-2) is a potent T cell growth factor, naturally secreted by activated T lymphocytes. IL-2 causes T cell proliferation and differentiation and enhances natural killer cell function. In animal models, IL-2 mediates regression of tumors. IL-2 alone or in combination with lymphokine-activated killer (LAK) cells has shown encouraging results in the initial phase II trials, with an overall response rate of 35 per cent. Other studies demonstrated a significant response rate, although not at the same level as initially reported. In a recent large multi-institutional study, the overall response rate for IL-2 alone was approximately 15 per cent. Toxicity associated with this mode of therapy is significant, especially that related to cardiopulmonary problems. This limits somewhat the widespread use of this lymphokine.

Combination of IL-2 with other cytokines, such as alpha-interferon, tumor necrosis factor, and other interleukins, has been the subject of several small trials; however, the overall results are too premature to evaluate. Based on some animal studies that suggested tumor infiltrating lymphocytes are more specific than LAK cells, attempts to use this approach in renal cell carcinoma have been made, but the results have been disappointing.

Gene Therapy

Progress in molecular techniques has allowed researchers to insert specific genetic material into immunocompetent cells, which could allow for the delivering of high concentrations of cytokines at the tumor site. Initial work in this area for human trials is now in progress in some selected institutions.

BILATERAL RENAL CELL CARCINOMA AND RENAL CELL CARCINOMA IN THE SOLITARY KIDNEY

ROBERT B. SMITH, M.D.

Los Angeles, California

Bilateral renal cell carcinoma or renal cell carcinoma in a solitary kidney represents a challenge to the clinician. In the past, bilateral renal cell carcinoma, especially with a synchronous presentation, indicated a poor prognosis. Recent experience seems to contradict these previously held concepts. Our experience at UCLA confirms that an aggressive treatment is indicated in patients with such carcinomas and that long-term survival is possible.

Previously, it was thought that patients presenting with bilateral renal cell carcinoma had a worse prognosis than patients presenting with renal cell carcinoma in a solitary kidney, when the contralateral kidney had been removed for benign disease. In the UCLA experience of 55 cases of patients with either bilateral renal cell carcinoma or renal cell carcinoma in the solitary kidney, it appears that the fate of the contralateral kidney is not as important as the stage of the lesion at presentation and whether or not the lesion can be totally excised. Even patients with synchronous bilateral renal cell cancer have an excellent chance for survival if all the local lesion can be removed.

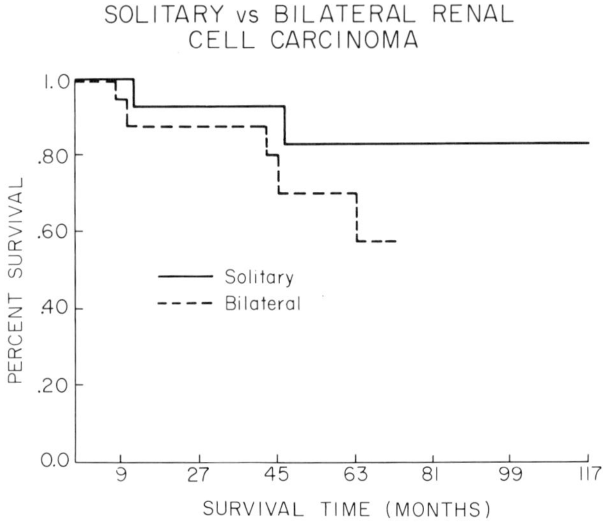

FIGURE 1. Survival rate in months of patients treated for solitary kidney renal cell carcinoma and bilateral renal cell carcinoma in the UCLA series.

PARTIAL NEPHRECTOMY

Most lesions can be managed by in situ partial nephrectomy. In our series of those patients treated with potentially curative resections, only three were not amenable to partial nephrectomy. These three patients required radical nephrectomy to clear the lesion. The surgical principles that are involved in in situ partial nephrectomy include excision of all of Gerota's fascia with perinephric fat, resection of regional lymphatic and lymph nodes if feasible, wound exclusion with a barrier, and wound irrigation with distilled water. The renal pedicle is occluded only when necessary, using intraoperative mannitol infusion and renal cooling if the ischemic time is expected to exceed 30 minutes. Most renal cell carcinomas that are amenable to partial nephrectomy are encapsulated. It is tempting to perform enucleation on such lesions. This should not be done, however, because microinvasion of the tumor capsule is not uncommon. We have had 3 cases of local recurrence out of 52 patients who were treated with partial nephrectomy. All three instances of local recurrence were a direct consequence of such enucleations. Resection of such a lesion should include a margin of normal renal parenchyma.

Ex vivo partial nephrectomy should be reserved for large central complex lesions. Either a large midline transabdominal incision, with the patient in the supine position, or a large flank incision, using a torque flank position, is an acceptable operative approach. A radical nephrectomy with regional lymphadenectomy is performed. The kidney is perfused with an intracellular perfusate (Collins solution), and the tumor excision and reconstruction are performed on a workbench. With the use of intracellular perfusate, the tumor excision and subsequent reconstruction can be performed in a meticulous manner without undue concern about ischemic damage. The ureters should be left intact and occluded with a noncrushing clamp. (Ureteral blood flow may cause some renal warming, increasing the possibility of ischemic damage.) The kidney is then implanted into the iliac fossa, using standard transplantation techniques. Advantages of ex vivo surgery include better visualization and access to the tumor, reduced possibility of tumor spill, more

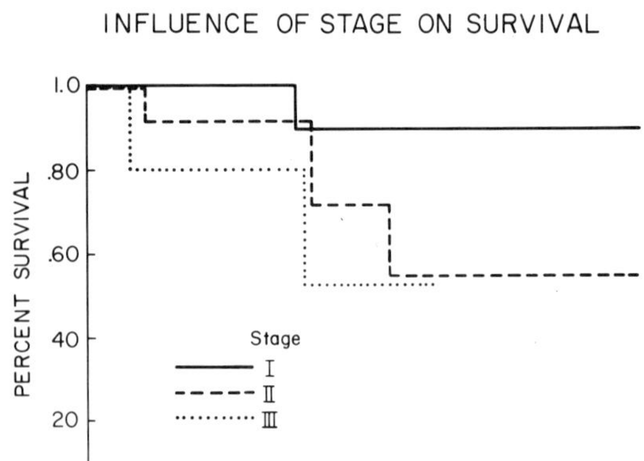

FIGURE 2. Survival time in months of patients with both solitary and bilateral lesions with survival related to stage of presentation. Survival differences related to stage are significant.

complete excision of regional lymph nodes and lymphatics, and lower intraoperative blood loss. Disadvantages include complexity of technique, with the need for arterial and venous anastomoses with attending complications, and increased operating time. Also, there is the increased possibility of ischemic renal damage.

Most lesions are best managed by in situ partial nephrectomy. In only four instances in our series was it necessary to use ex vivo techniques. Jacobs reviewed 51 cases of renal resection, comprising 34 in situ resections and 17 ex vivo resections. The survival rate was the same in those patients having ex vivo resection (82 per cent) as in those having in vivo resection (76 per cent). There was no increased incidence of local recurrence from tumor spill within the renal fossa in patients with in vivo resection.

OPTIONS FOR SIMULTANEOUS BILATERAL LESIONS

Simultaneous renal cell carcinoma, which was once thought to have an ominous prognosis, is not an uncommon occurrence. Half the patients in our series with bilateral renal cell carcinoma presented as synchronous lesions. The approach to simultaneous lesions varies in the literature. Possible treatment options include primary partial nephrectomy operating on the least involved kidney first, while allowing the worse side to remain to lessen the need for postoperative dialysis. Some surgeons believe that the most involved side should be attacked first, making certain that it is resectable, followed later by partial nephrectomy on the contralateral side. This approach allows for some functional compensatory hypertrophy of the contralateral kidney, thus perhaps increasing the likelihood of being able to perform a nephron-salvaging procedure. There is some evidence that a solitary kidney tolerates periods of ischemia better when a contralateral kidney is not present. The simultaneous approach also is possible, with either bilateral partial nephrectomy, combination radical and partial nephrectomy, or bilateral nephrectomy. All approaches are acceptable and have been used in our series. Survival does not seem to depend on which surgical approach is used. It is my feeling that, if a patient is a satisfactory operative risk, simultaneous approach to both kidneys is the best option. If the lesions are complex or the patient is a poor operative risk, the staged approach is best, with a radical nephrectomy on the more involved side first to make sure it is resectable, reserving the partial nephrectomy for later.

Figure 1 shows the survival rate in the UCLA series, comparing the solitary lesions with the bilateral lesions. Figure 2 relates the survival of both groups compared in regard to stage at presentation. Stage for stage, there is no difference in survival between the bilateral group and the solitary group.

SUMMARY

Survival rates of bilateral renal cell carcinoma and renal cell carcinoma in the solitary kidney justify an aggressive surgical approach. Stage for stage, survival rates approximate those for radical nephrectomy for unilateral disease when the contralateral kidney is present. If these results with Stage I lesions treated with partial nephrectomy are similar after a 10-year follow-up, an argument could be made for using partial nephrectomy for Stage I renal cell carcinoma, even when a normal contralateral kidney is present, especially if the lesion is polar. Most lesions are amenable to partial nephrectomy by established in situ techniques. Ex vivo surgery should be reserved for complex central lesions. We caution against enucleation of these lesions, even though a definite capsule may be present, because microinvasion of the tumor in the capsule is common. Current literature, including our experience, challenges the prior concept that the patient's prognosis depends on the fate of the contralateral kidney. The prognosis depends more on adequacy of tumor resection and tumor stage at the time of presentation.

Suggested Readings

Jacobs SC, Berg SI, Lawson RK: Synchronous bilateral renal cell carcinoma: Total surgical excision. Cancer 46: 2341, 1980

Morgan WR, Zincke H: Prognosis and survival after renal conserving surgery for renal cell carcinoma: Experience in 104 patients and extended follow up. J Urol 144:852, 1990

Novick AC, Streem S, Montie JE, et al: Conservative surgery for renal cell carcinoma: A single-center experience with 100 patients. J Urol 141:835, 1989

Smith RB, deKernion JB, Ehrlich RM, et al: Bilateral renal cell carcinoma and renal cell carcinoma in the solitary kidney. J Urol 132:450, 1984

Steinbach F, Stockle M, Muller SC, et al: Conservative

surgery for renal cell tumors in 140 patients: 21 years of experience. J Urol 148:24, 1992

EMBOLIZATION OF THE KIDNEY

FRAY F. MARSHALL, M.D.

Baltimore, Maryland

With the advent of the Seldinger technique of percutaneous angiography, renal masses often could be evaluated more accurately than with intravenous or retrograde pyelography. Initially, angiographic techniques primarily were diagnostic. Then it became apparent that occlusive or therapeutic manipulations also could be performed through the selectively placed catheters. In some cases, chemotherapeutic agents, such as mitomycin, have been instilled directly into the renal artery as a form of selective chemotherapy. In most instances, however, embolization has been occlusive. Agents that have been used for arterial occlusion include autologous clot, oxidized cellulose, absorbable gelatin sponge, wool coils, steel coils, absolute alcohol, vasopressin, tissue glue, and detachable Silastic or silicon balloons.

Embolization of the renal artery and kidney has been performed commonly for renal cell carcinomas. The typical hypervascular patterns with small arteriovenous fistulas create vascular tumors that can produce significant intraoperative blood loss. For this reason, and for the prevention of tumor cell dissemination during surgery, renal arterial embolization has been recommended. We generally have not used this adjuvant technique with most tumors because we have felt that it was unnecessary and that it would have little effect on operative time or blood loss. However, if the tumor is very large or is associated with larger arteriovenous fistulas, embolization may facilitate surgical removal. If there is tumor involvement of the renal vein or in the inferior vena cava, total occlusion of the renal artery may allow dissection and division of the renal vein earlier in the operative procedure. Frequently, however, arterial parasitization can provide significant perfusion of the vascular tumor bed, and early venous occlusion still can result in significant venous hypertension and blood loss if this phenomenon is not recognized. Thus, embolization can be helpful in selected circumstances but is unnecessary in the less complex tumors.

In the past, it has been suggested that embolization of the renal artery may be therapeutic in patients with metastatic renal cell carcinoma. Renal arterial occlusion followed by nephrectomy was thought to stimulate the immune system and affect metastatic disease favorably. Although initial reports were encouraging, and we had one or two patients with dramatic responses, the overall results are not convincing or long lived (South West Cooperative Group Study).

Other benign tumors of the kidney, such as angiomyolipomas, can bleed profusely. With massive hematuria, selective occlusion of such lesions actually may preserve more renal tissue than surgical exploration, which frequently results in nephrectomy. Middle-aged women without stigmata of tuberous sclerosis may present with hemorrhage from angiomyolipomas, and, in such cases, selective embolization and occlusion of these tumors may preserve renal tissue. In patients bleeding from malignant tumors such as renal cell carcinoma or transitional cell carcinoma, embolization may be palliative in the presence of metastatic disease or severe medical problems.

Renal arteriovenous fistulas may occur in carcinoma. Frequently, they occur on a small scale, but occasionally, with tumor necrosis, large arteriovenous connections may cause congestive heart failure or massive hematuria or both.

Intraoperative identification of the precise site of the arteriovenous fistula is often technically impossible. Renal angiography lends itself to the identification and therapeutic management of this clinical problem. A newer angiographic technique using detachable Silastic balloons allows for selective placement before final inflation and detachment of the balloon. This technique has been successful in controlling renal hemorrhage and has resulted in minimal loss of renal tissue. Inadvertent embolization has been uncommon. Embolization in the presence of an arteriovenous fistula can be hazardous, however. These occlusive techniques may be used in hemangiomas or vascular malformations within the kidney. A renal artery aneurysm in a small arterial branch may be occluded without operative intervention. Particulate matter may be used to fill these aneurysms and distal small vessels. The availability of a wide variety of substances with special properties for embolization allows selection of appropriate occlusive techniques in different clinical settings.

In patients with chronic renal failure, renin-mediated hypertension may be a major clinical problem. If the patient is already on dialysis, renal arterial occlusion can provide a "nephrectomy." However, small, capsular, perforating vessels still may allow hypertension to persist. If there is renin-mediated hypertension from a portion of the kidney, selective embolization may allow for occlusion of the segment of the kidney that is responsible for the high renin output.

This technique also lends itself effectively to renal trauma. In patients with massive injuries, angiography will identify injuries to organs such as the liver, the spleen, and the kidney. Occlusive techniques can control bleeding and often preserve more renal tissue than operative explorations. In the majority of such patients, however, other organs are involved with trauma, so that frequently exploration is necessary to identify other injuries.

After renal biopsy, patients also may have hemorrhage. An increasing number of patients are undergoing percutaneous nephrolithotripsy, and a major complication of this technique is hemorrhage. If the bleeding cannot be controlled with compression within the percutaneous tract, selective angiography may be necessary.

The significant risks associated with angiography are injury to the femoral vessels and inadvertent embolization either to the lower extremity or to other organ sites, but the diagnostic and therapeutic advantages of this technique should outweigh these risks. Obviously, the knowledge and use of a wide variety of embolization techniques and agents are required so that appropriate techniques can be selected for the individual patient.

Suggested Readings

Craven WM, Redmond PL, Kumpe DA, et al: Planned-delayed nephrectomy after ethanol embolization of renal carcinoma. J Urol 146:704, 1991

deSouza NM, Reidy JF, Koffman CG: Arteriovenous fistulas complicating biopsy of renal allografts: Treatment of bleeding with super selective embolization. Am J Roentgenol 156:507, 1991

Heyns CF, van Vallenhoven P: Increasing role of angiography and segmental artery embolization in the management of renal stab wounds. J Urol 147:1231, 1991

Marshall FF, White RI Jr, Kaufman SL, et al: Treatment of traumatic renal arteriovenous fistulas by detachable silicone balloon embolization. J Urol 122:237, 1979

Teigen CL, Mitchell SE, Venbrux AC, et al: Segmental renal artery embolization for treatment of pediatric renovascular hypertension. J Vasc Interv Radiol 3:111, 1992

MEDICAL THERAPY FOR METASTATIC RENAL CELL CARCINOMA

ROBERT P. HUBEN, M.D.

Buffalo, New York

Despite unquestionable gains in the treatment of many urologic tumors, metastatic renal cell carcinoma remains a very troublesome and frustrating malignancy for those who treat patients with this disease. About 27,000 new cases of renal cell carcinoma will occur in 1994, and about 11,000 patients will die of this disease. Thirty to 40 per cent of patients have metastases at presentation, and another 30 to 40 per cent eventually will develop metastases. Untreated, metastatic renal cell carcinoma is associated with a 1-year survival rate of about 20 per cent, and a 5-year survival of 0 to 5 per cent. The median survival of patients with metastases is only 8 months.

Presently, some gains are being made in the treatment of this disease, particularly with various forms of immunotherapy, but often at the expense of significant morbidity and occasional treatment-related deaths. Our current challenge is to make further gains in the treatment of metastatic renal cell carcinoma without prohibitive morbidity or treatment complexity and cost. This article reviews the status of various forms of medical management of metastatic renal cell carcinoma.

INTERFERON THERAPY

Interferons (IFNs) are naturally occurring proteins that possess a wide range of immunomodulatory and antiproliferative activity produced by cells in response to antigenic stimulation by viruses, malignant cells, or other inducers. Interferons have antitumor properties that may be mediated through a direct cytotoxic effect on tumor cells, by augmentation of immunogenicity of tumors, by upregulation of histocompatibility and tumor-associated antigens, and/or by activation of macrophages, T lymphocytes, and natural killer cells. There are three major types of IFNs: alpha-IFN, which is produced by leukocytes; beta-IFN, from fibroblasts, lymphoblastoid cells, macrophages, and epithelial cells; and gamma-IFN, produced by activated lymphocytes. There are more than 20 subtypes of alpha-IFN, of which three are commercially available: recombinant IFN alpha-2b, recombinant IFN alpha-2a, and alpha-n3 from human leukocytes. Alpha-IFNs are approved for the treatment of hairy cell leukemia, acquired immunodeficiency syndrome–related Kaposi sarcoma, condyloma acuminata, and chronic viral hepatitis. Recombinant alpha-IFN is the type of IFN most commonly used in the treatment of metastatic renal cell carcinoma. IFN gamma-1b is also commercially available and is approved for the treatment of chronic granulomatous disease.

Single-agent IFN produces overall response rates of about 15 per cent in the treatment of metastatic renal cell carcinoma, including rare but occasionally complete responses. The median duration of response is 6 to 10 months, with few durable responses beyond this period. Intermediate doses of IFN (10 to 20 million units/day) are more effective than low dosages (1 to 2 million units/day) or very high dosages (greater than 30 million units/day). As in the case of other moderately effective treatments for metastatic renal cell carcinoma, favorable responses often correlate with metastases that are predominantly pulmonary, good performance status, previous nephrectomy, and a long interval between resection of the primary tumor and the development of metastases.

The toxicity of IFN is manifested largely by the development of flu-like symptoms, fatigue, and gastrointestinal upset. These side effects are reversible, and often are generally lessened with the use of nonsteroidal anti-inflammatory drugs.

Interferons have been used in combination with various chemotherapeutic agents, but this approach is not proven to be more effective than the use of interferon alone. Interferon also frequently is combined with interleukin-2 in ongoing clinical trials, as is discussed in the next section.

INTERLEUKIN THERAPY

Interleukin-2 (IL-2) first was identified in 1976 by Morgan et al., and initially was described as T cell growth factor. In 1983, large amounts of recombinant IL-2 became available for clinical study through gene cloning, and recombinant IL-2 appears to have equivalent activity to naturally occurring IL-2.

A central feature of an immune response is controlled clonal expansion of the antigen-specific cells to generate sufficient numbers of T cells bearing receptors for a given antigen. For T lymphocytes, this is accomplished by IL-2. Antigen specificity of T cell growth is maintained by secretion of IL-2 and cell surface expression of IL-2 receptors, both of which are dependent on recent antigen activation of the T cell. Only T lymphocytes are able to secrete IL-2, and this requires activation of the T cell. However, the growth-promoting activity of IL-2 is nonspecific; that is, any cell with IL-2 receptors responds to IL-2. Thus, IL-2 appears to have no direct impact on malignant cells, but acts through stimulating host immune reactivity.

IL-2–induced lymphocyte activation causes a cascade of subsequent effects as a result of the interactions of the activated lymphocytes and the cytokines they release with other tissues. Cytokines induced by IL-2 include gamma-IFN, tumor necrosis factor (TNF)-alpha, TNF-beta, IL-1, IL-5, and IL-6.

Interleukin therapy is associated with substantial toxicity, which is characterized by a "vascular leak syndrome" consisting of marked fluid retention, weight gain, hypotension requiring vasopressors, and dyspnea resulting from pulmonary edema. About 5 to 10 per cent of the patients receiving high-dose IL-2 have required intubation and mechanical ventilation. IL-2 toxicity is related to the dose administered, the route of administration, and the treatment schedule. For example, equivalent IL-2 doses given by continuous infusion are more toxic than bolus injections. Several studies have suggested that secondary cytokines, such as TNF and IL-1, may be responsible for the vascular leak syndrome induced by IL-2 treatment.

Interleukin-2 and Lymphokine-Activated Killer Cells

In 1980, Rosenberg's group discovered that incubation of resting murine lymphocytes with IL-2 in vitro led to the generation of populations of cells that could lyse a wide range of fresh autologous and allogeneic cancer cells, but not normal tissues in vitro. These cells were called lymphokine-activated killer (LAK) cells. This discovery led to the development of a form of adoptive immunotherapy in which immune cells that are capable of mediating, either directly or indirectly, antitumor effects are transferred to the tumor-bearing patient. IL-2 is critical for the generation of these immune cells used in adoptive transfer of cellular immunity and is administered along with these cells. Early studies suggested that the combination of LAK cells and IL-2 therapy exerted an antitumor effect that was superior to that of either therapy alone.

Since their initial publication in 1985, Rosenberg and coworkers at the National Cancer Institute (NCI) Surgery Branch have treated more than 300 patients with high-dose IL-2 regimens. About 40 per cent of these patients have had renal cell carcinoma. Treatment regimens with IL-2 and LAK cell transfusions generally have included three phases: a priming phase of IL-2, a second phase of lymphocytaphereses to harvest lymphoid precursor cells used to generate LAK cells in vitro, and a final phase of LAK cell transfusions accompanied by additional IL-2.

In this first clinical trial involving 25 patients, Rosenberg et al. witnessed 11 objective responses, including all 3 patients with renal cell carcinoma. In 1987, a 33 per cent response rate was reported in 36 patients with renal cell carcinoma, with four complete responses and eight partial responses. In 1989, an overall response rate of 35 per cent was reported in 72 patients with renal cell cancer, with 8 (11 per cent) complete responses and 17 (24 per cent) partial responses.

The Interleukin-2/LAK Working Group (ILWG) was sponsored by the NCI to determine whether these results could be duplicated at other centers. Using the same treatment regimen, the ILWG reported a total response rate of 16 per cent in 32 patients receiving at least one LAK cell infusion. It has been suggested that the difference in response rates between the ILWG and the NCI studies (16 versus 35 per cent) may be related to patient selection factors. The ILWG study included fewer patients with pulmonary-only metastases (7 versus 19), and 9 of 35 patients in the ILWG trial had not undergone nephrectomy before receiving treatment. In both studies, soft tissue or pulmonary sites of disease and prior nephrectomy were associated more often with response, whereas a large tumor burden and an intact primary tumor were poor prognostic factors.

In trials of IL-2/LAK for renal cell carcinoma, the ILWG has shown consistent response rates of 15 to 20 per cent. These rates are similar to other NCI studies of IL-2 alone. This suggests that LAK cell coadministration may contribute little to the therapeutic benefit of such therapy, and the ILWG subsequently withdrew the ex vivo production of LAK cells from all future trials. More recent studies again suggest no improvement in survival with combination therapy. In the collective IL-2 studies, an overall survival of 30 per cent was reported at a median follow-up of 15 months, which contributed to Food and Drug Administration approval of IL-2 for the treatment of metastatic renal cell carcinoma in 1992.

Interleukin-2 and Cytokines

In recent studies using combinations of cytokines, subcutaneous IL-2 frequently is used with alpha-IFN. With subcutaneous IL-2, fatigue is a prominent symptom, as is tenderness at the injection site. Hypotension is mild or absent. With this route of administration, patients may develop neutralizing serum antibodies to IL-2. A phase I study of IL-2 and alpha-IFN given by intravenous bolus reported a 38 per cent response rate in patients with metastatic renal cell carcinoma at the highest dose of both agents. Combination therapy appears to be associated with a higher response rate than therapy with either agent alone, although combination therapy is also clearly more toxic at higher doses.

Several studies using IL-2 either alone or in combination with other cytokines have demonstrated responses at extrarenal sites, although objective responses are seen only rarely in the primary tumor. This finding and the fact that patients who have undergone nephrectomy prior to initiation of immunotherapy consistently respond more often than patients with renal tumors in situ suggest that there may be justification to resect the primary tumors in patients with good performance status prior to initiation of immunotherapy. However, in one study, 37 per cent of patients who underwent nephrectomy in preparation for immunotherapy could not be treated because of complications of surgery or progression of disease during the recovery phase. In other studies, patients who have undergone resection of a solitary metastasis after completing immunotherapy have had long-term remissions comparable to those of patients with a complete response to treatment. At present, the role of surgery both prior to and at the completion of immunotherapy is unclear, and this issue would be an appropriate focus of randomized clinical studies.

Interleukin-2 and Tumor-Infiltrating Lymphocytes

The majority of human cancers contain an infiltration of lymphocytes. These tumor-infiltrating lymphocytes (TILs), mainly T cells, proliferate in response to IL-2. TILs can be obtained by culturing tumor fragments with IL-2 for 2 to 4 weeks. This results in a 1000-fold expansion of TILs. However, only certain human tumors, such as melanoma and renal cell carcinoma, are susceptible to IL-2/TIL therapy. In melanoma, TILs are therapeutic against the tumor of origin but not against histologically related but non–cross-reactive tumors, whereas TILs from renal cell cancer may be cytotoxic to both autologous and allogeneic tumor cells. Individually, TILs may be up to 100 times more potent than LAK cells.

In an NCI study of 12 patients receiving IL-2/TIL treatment, two partial responses (17 per cent) were reported, in 1 of 6 patients with melanoma and in 1 of 4 patients with renal cell carcinoma. Toxicity was similar to that of IL-2 alone. However, there are substantial difficulties with the use of TILs. Tumor tissue must be obtained to cultivate the TILs, and a minimum of 4 to 6 weeks is necessary to generate an adequate number of cells. Technical difficulties include high cost, labor intensiveness, and the laboratory expertise required. Also, as in the case of LAK cell therapy, it has been suggested that responses to IL-2/TIL therapy may be due to IL-2 itself. In several studies, radiolabeled TILs did not migrate or distribute in large numbers to metastatic tumor sites.

CHEMOTHERAPY

Historically, vinblastine is the single agent that has been reported to have the highest response rate in the treatment of metastatic renal cell carcinoma. Older studies suggested response rates as high as 24 per cent in patients who were treated with vinblastine at weekly doses in the range of 0.1 to 0.3 mg/kg. However, recent studies have failed to duplicate the results of these earlier reports. Other drugs that have been reported to have some efficacy in the treatment of this disease include nitrosurea compounds, hydroxyurea, cyclophosphamide, 6-mercaptopurine, 5-fluorouracil, nitrogen mustard, chlorambucil, bleomycin, and mitomycin C. However, these agents have exhibited only about a 10 per cent response rate, and most responses were partial. The use of methotrexate with citrovorum rescue has been reported to produce a 20 per cent partial response rate and a stabilization rate of 25 per cent, with prolonged survival of those patients who showed responses.

Generally, combination chemotherapy for metastatic renal cell carcinoma has not been associated with better responses than those reported for single-agent trials. As previously stated, the combination of immunotherapy with conventional cytotoxic agents also has failed to result in responses higher than those to the immunotherapeutic agent alone. In one randomized study comparing alpha-IFN to the combination of alpha-IFN plus intravenous vinblastine, the overall response rate was 13 per cent and that for the INF-alone arm was identical to the response rate to interferon plus vinblastine. The most striking finding in this study was that 7 of 16 patients (44 per cent) with metastases only to the lungs had objective responses. The site of metastasis was the single best predictor of response, time to progression, and survival time. Both performance status and prior nephrectomy were also significant individual predictors of response.

An interesting but controversial approach to the treatment of metastatic renal cell carcinoma is the modulation of drug dosage based on the time of day or the body's circadian rhythm. Circadian timing of treatment has been shown to permit higher chemotherapeutic dose intensities to be given with acceptable toxicity. Several studies by Hrushesky et al. have employed continuous infusion of the S-phase fluoropyrimidine antimetabolite 5-floxuridine (FUDR) for 14 days followed by 14 days with no chemotherapy, during which heparinized saline was administered to keep an implanted Synchromed pump (Medtronic, Inc., Fridley, MN) operational. The starting FUDR dose was 0.15 mg/kg per day for 14 days, after which the dose was escalated monthly by 0.025 mg/kg per day until the dose-limiting toxicity of diarrhea was encountered. The maintenance dose then became the previously tolerated dose. A daily sinusoidal infusion pattern was used in which 68 per cent of the daily dose was administered between 3:00 and 9:00 P.M. It was postulated that normal tissues would be least susceptible to the toxic effect of this drug during this period.

In their most recent report of the clinical results of continuous-infusion FUDR therapy, a total of 68 unselected patients with progressive metastatic renal cell carcinoma received such therapy. Thirty-seven per cent of these patients had previously received and failed systemic therapy. Of 56 evaluable patients, 4 had complete responses (7.1 per cent) and 7 had partial responses (12.5 per cent), for an objective response rate of 19.6 per cent. Objective response duration ranged from 1 to 18 months, with a median of 10.8 months. Gastrointestinal toxicity was dose limiting. Moderate diarrhea occurred in 17 per cent of patients, whereas hemologic, hepatic, renal, neurologic, and skin toxicities were not observed. Tumor site and the history of previous therapy again appeared to influence the likelihood of response, because objective responses were seen in 7 of 21 patients with lung metastases only, whereas only two objective responses were seen in 20 patients who had received prior systemic therapy.

At Roswell Park Cancer Institute, we have treated 25 patients with progressive metastatic renal cell carcinoma with continuous-infusion FUDR chemotherapy. Selection criteria included histologically documented renal cell carcinoma, good performance status with an Eastern Cooperative Oncology Group grade of 0–2, and an estimated life expectancy of greater than 6 months. In our patient group, there were four complete responses (16 per cent) and six partial responses (24 per cent), for a total objective response rate of 40 per cent. The duration of response has been 3 to greater than 60 months. One patient has had durable complete response for more than 60 months, and another patient has had a partial response of the same duration. There were six treatment-related complications in this group, for a complication rate of 24 per cent. There were three surgical complications, including one infected pump site and the development of superior vena caval syndrome in two patients. The three nonsurgical complications consisted of severe diarrhea that required hospitalization for rehydration. Our results indicate that, in carefully selected patients (those with good performance status and limited metastatic burden), continuous-infusion FUDR chemotherapy appears to be highly effective in the treatment of metastatic renal cell carcinoma. A multi-institutional NCI-sponsored study is now underway comparing daily sinusoidal infusion of FUDR to a flat infusion pattern. A preliminary report of the results of this study has confirmed a lower toxicity with sinusoidal infusion, which allows for higher drug delivery.

Despite these encouraging results, a recent review by Yagoda et al. of 72 cytotoxic chemotherapeutic agents used singly or in a limited number of two-drug combinations involving 3502 patients reported objective responses in only 197 patients (5.6 per cent). The authors concluded that, although some data suggest that a few drugs warrant further evaluation, renal cell carcinoma still must be considered a chemotherapeutically resistant cancer. The basis for this resistance has been postulated to be the finding of enhanced expression of the multidrug resistance gene (mdr) with the overproduction of the plasma membrane p-glycoprotein 170 in renal cancer cells. In one report, high mdr1 RNA levels were found in 80 per cent of 50 unpretreated renal tumors. This finding has led to studies that combine cytotoxic agents with those that inhibit mdr action, such as calcium channel blockers or calmodulin inhibitors. To date, the results of these studies have been routinely disappointing. The resistance of renal cell carcinoma to chemotherapeutic agents is undoubtedly multifactorial, and further studies of resistance mechanisms clearly are necessary.

HORMONAL THERAPY

The basis of interest in hormonal therapy for metastatic renal cell carcinoma was the observation that induction of renal cortical tumors in Syrian golden hamsters by estrogen administration could be blocked by progestational agents or testosterone. Reports from the early 1970s suggested an objective response rate of about 16 per cent in patients with metastatic renal cell carcinoma treated with progestines or androgens. However, subsequent reviews of hormonal therapy for metastatic renal cell carcinoma based on a large number of phase II and randomized phase III trials reported a collective response rate of about 5 per cent.

Although estrogen and other hormonal receptors have been demonstrated in both renal proximal tubule cells and renal tumor cells, no correlation has ever been established between receptor levels and response to hormonal therapy. High-dose medroxyprogesterone has been reported to have a partial response of 15 per cent, although these results have not been duplicated in other studies. The antiestrogen tamoxifen, at high doses, has been reported to have a response rate of about 12 per cent in patients with metastatic renal cell carcinoma. This agent also has been combined with vinblastine in past and ongoing clinical trials. The antiandrogen flutamide was reported to have a 4 per cent response rate in 25 evaluable patients and a 27 per cent response rate when combined with alpha-IFN in 52 patients when the latter was given three times a week. It is likely that this response rate is more indicative of the therapeutic effect of alpha-IFN, rather than representing a synergistic effect.

Realistically, the role of hormonal therapy would appear to be limited to use in patients who are not candidates for more aggressive forms of therapy because of extent of disease, poor performance status, or patient preference. Oral droxyprogesterone (Megace) at a dose of 40 mg three to four times daily not infrequently will result in subjective improvement, with very limited toxicity. Such therapy may be offered to patients when the only alternative is no therapy at all.

SUMMARY

As this review of available treatment options for metastatic renal cell carcinoma has suggested, there is no standard therapy for this disease. Immunotherapy, particularly with IL-2, has been the most promising therapy to date, but is also the most toxic. Its use at the present time probably should be restricted to the context of well-controlled clinical trials. Questions of dosage, route of administration, and treatment frequency remain unresolved and must be addressed.

Chemotherapy should not be dismissed as an area of further clinical research in the treatment of this disease. New agents, modification of drug resistance mechanisms, and innovative drug delivery mechanisms are areas of potential breakthrough. Application of various combination therapies awaits further progress in our understanding of renal cell tumor biology at the molecular and cellular level. The outlook for patients with metastatic renal cell carcinoma has improved greatly in the past few years, and further gains are inevitable.

Suggested Readings

Belldegrun A, Figlin R, Danella J, et al: Immunotherapy for renal cell carcinoma. Semin Urol 10:23, 1992

Huben RP: Advances in chemotherapy for renal cell carcinoma. Semin Urol 10:16, 1992

Kradin R: Adoptive immunotherapy with tumor-infiltrating lymphocytes. *In* Atkins MB, Mier JW (eds): Therapeutic Applications of Interleukin-2. New York, Marcel Dekker, 1993, pp. 217–231

Malek TR, Gutgsell NS: IL-2 and its receptor: Structure, function, and regulation of expression. *In* Atkins MB, Mier JW (eds): Therapeutic Applications of Interleukin-2. New York, Marcel Dekker, 1993, pp 3–25

Rao SV, Wadler S: Current use of interferons. Contemp Oncol December:44, 1992

Sunderland MC, Weiss GR: High-dose IL-2 treatment of renal cell carcinoma. *In* Atkins MB, Mier JW (eds): Therapeutic Applications of Interleukin-2. New York, Marcel Dekker, 1993, pp 119–142

Yagoda A, Petrylak D, Thompson S: Cytotoxic chemotherapy for advanced renal cell carcinoma. Urol Clin North Am 20:303, 1993

TREATMENT OF RENAL ANGIOMYOLIPOMA

RODNEY J. TAYLOR, M.D.

Omaha, Nebraska

Angiomyolipoma of the kidney is a rare benign tumor comprised of smooth muscle, thick-walled blood vessels, and mature adipose tissue. In clinical studies, angiomyolipomas may represent up to 3 per cent of all renal lesions diagnosed in nephrectomy specimens. However, in autopsy studies the incidence is much less, with angiomyolipomas accounting for approximately 0.3 per cent of renal lesions found incidentally. Until recently, angiomyolipomas almost always were diagnosed on nephrectomy specimens that had been removed either for clinical symptoms or for suspected renal cell cancer. With improved methods of preoperative diagnosis, specifically computerized tomography (CT) and ultrasonography, these lesions now are diagnosed more frequently nonoperatively and increasingly are being found "incidentally." Current recommendations for treatment stress renal conservation and reserve radical surgery for cases in which the kidney is essentially replaced by the extreme size of the lesion(s), life-threatening hemorrhage has occurred, or there is associated renal cell cancer not amenable to nephron-sparing surgery.

TUBEROUS SCLEROSIS SYNDROME

Angiomyolipomas frequently are associated with the tuberous sclerosis syndrome. However, overall, patients with tuberous sclerosis represent no more than 20 per cent of the patients diagnosed with angiomyolipomas; the others, primarily females, present with "spontaneously" arising angiomyolipomas and no other identifiable stigmata of tuberous sclerosis. Tuberous sclerosis is an autosomal dominant disorder transmitted with variable penetrance. The classic triad includes mental retardation, seizure disorder, and sebaceous adenoma; however, not all patients present with the classic picture. In this condition, angiomyolipomas are present in between 40 and 80 per cent of patients studied and are usually multifocal and bilateral. In addition, renal cysts frequently are found in patients with tuberous sclerosis.

Renal cell cancer has been associated with both spontaneous angiomyolipomas and those associated with tuberous sclerosis. However, the risk of concomitant renal cell cancer appears to be significantly greater in patients with tuberous sclerosis and angiomyolipomas and should be kept in mind when evaluating these patients and deciding on treatment options. If on radiologic evaluation a solid mass is found that does not contain fat on CT scan, or if there also appear to be calcifications within the mass, there should be a high suspicion that this represents a possible renal cell cancer in association with angiomyolipoma. If surgery is indicated, the approach must be carefully planned to avoid unnecessary renal loss.

CLINICAL PRESENTATION

As previously noted, the majority of patients with angiomyolipoma (at least 80 per cent) do not have evidence of tuberous sclerosis. There is an 8:1 female-to-male ratio, and these patients are commonly between the fifth and seventh decade of life at the time of their diagnosis. With increased use of screening ultrasonography and CT scanning for diagnosis of abdominal symptoms, the pattern of presentation is changing and more patients are being diagnosed incidentally.

Presenting symptoms of angiomyolipoma are variable and not specific for the lesion. The most common presenting symptom is flank pain, which is present in between 50 and 80 per cent of the patients with angiomyolipomas. This represents both chronic and acute flank pain. Approximately 50 per cent of patients, at the time of their presentation, will be found to have a flank mass that is palpable on examination. Between 25 and 40 per cent of patients will present with hematuria, either gross or, in most cases, microscopic. Between 10 and 25 per cent of patients will present with either acute retroperitoneal hemorrhage and/or shock.

The likelihood of a patient presenting with symptoms seems to be related directly to the size of the primary lesion. In a study by Oesterling et al., lesions less than 4 cm in size were frequently asymptomatic and discovered incidentally, whereas those greater than 4 cm in size were much more likely to present with symptoms, including spontaneous hemorrhage.

DIAGNOSIS

Currently ultrasound and CT are used as the definitive diagnostic studies of choice for angiomyolipoma. On ultrasound the characteristic appearance is a well-circumscribed, hyperechoic mass. The angiomyolipomas appear to be more echo dense than the remainder of the kidney and more echo dense than other renal tumors. If a lesion meeting these criteria is found on ultrasonography, it is highly likely that it represents an angiomyolipoma, but the diagnostic study of choice remains CT scan. On CT scan, fat has a negative density of between −10 and −80 Hounsfield units, and the finding of fat in a renal lesion complimented with the ultrasound characteristics is diagnostic of angiomyolipoma.

The combined use of ultrasonography and CT scan will permit the noninvasive preoperative diagnosis of angiomyolipoma in up to 75 per cent of cases. However, the diagnosis cannot be made if fat is not present in the lesions or has been obscured by acute hemorrhage. Because of the association of renal cell cancer with angiomyolipoma, if there is a question, the lesion should be considered renal cell cancer until proven otherwise. In patients with known tuberous sclerosis and lesions indistinguishable from renal cell cancer, exploration and excisional biopsies are indicated. In patients with tuberous sclerosis, associated renal cell cancer has been reported in between 10 and 25 per cent of the cases. However, in patients with the more common unilaterally appearing single lesion, the incidence of associated renal cell cancer is less than 10 per cent.

MANAGEMENT

Currently the goals for managing angiomyolipomas are (1) accurate diagnosis and (2) renal conservation. These goals are predicated on the ability to diagnose the lesion accurately and noninvasively. If the CT scan and ultrasound evaluation unequivocally diagnose the renal lesion(s) as angiomyolipoma, for our patients therapy is based primarily on size and whether or not the lesion(s) are symptomatic or asymptomatic (Fig. 1). The literature is not absolute on this point, but it appears that lesions over 4 cm in size are much more likely to be symptomatic at the time of diagnosis and probably more likely to go on to eventual bleeding than lesions less than 3 cm in size. In a review by Oesterling et al., 90 per cent of symptomatic lesions were 4 cm or greater in size at the time of diagnosis.

If an asymptomatic angiomyolipoma less than 4 cm in size is discovered and the patient is not a female of childbearing age, observation using biannual ultrasound or CT scanning may be the only form of therapy needed. The purpose of observation is to detect any increase in size or development of symptoms that might represent progression of the lesion. If an asymptomatic lesion does increase in size and/or becomes symptomatic, therapy is indicated. Experience to date suggests that the majority of these lesions remain unchanged in size and asymptomatic for at least 3 to 5 years of follow-up. With longer follow-up it may be possible to increase the time between observation. If lesions over 4 cm are discovered incidentally, they also may be observed, but we currently recommend that they be followed more closely and checked for any changes every 3 to 4 months or the patient offered angioinfarction. Women of childbearing age must be carefully evaluated before deciding on a course of observation because of the apparent increased likelihood of hemorrhage from angiomyolipomas during pregnancy.

If the lesion is symptomatic regardless of size, the choices of therapy include nephron-sparing surgery, nephrectomy, and/or angioinfarction. Indications for a nephrectomy include patients with lesions so large that they essentially replace the entire kidney, patients with severe life-threatening hemorrhage if control and renal preservation are not possible, and some patients with associated renal cell cancer. Patients who are candidates for renal-sparing surgery include those with multiple lesions or a large symptomatic lesion where excisional biopsy of the lesion(s) is practical. Angioinfarction may be a good option for patients with small, symptomatic lesions or in carefully chosen patients with even larger symptomatic lesions if it appears feasible.

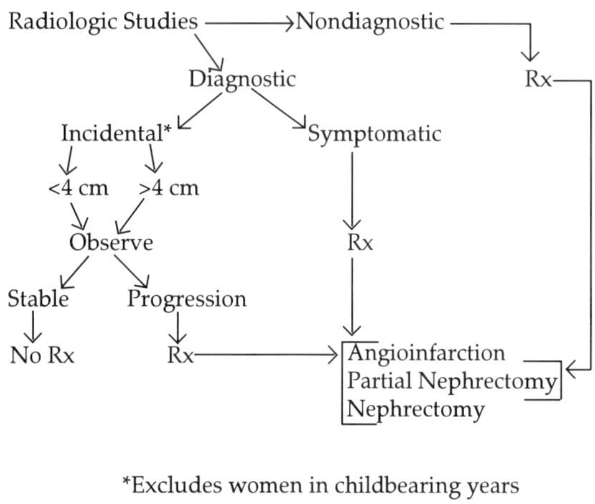

FIGURE 1. Treatment of angiomyolipomas excluding women in childbearing years.

If on initial diagnosis the renal lesion cannot accurately be diagnosed as an angiomyolipoma, additional radiologic studies may be indicated. In these particular cases, renal angiography may be of help for determining the type of lesion and, more importantly, in preparation for possible nephron-sparing surgery. Especially in patients with tuberous sclerosis and bilateral lesions, all attempts should be made to maintain as much kidney mass as possible. Therefore, excisional biopsies and partial nephrectomy are indicated if surgical exploration is undertaken. For the occasional case in which the excisional biopsy and frozen section reveal renal cell cancer, then, depending on the size and location, radical nephrectomy may be the best choice of therapy.

The principles of nephron-sparing surgery are well described in the literature and apply directly in the management of these patients.

CONCLUSION

With current preoperative radiologic imaging, it should be possible to diagnose accurately preoperatively the majority of patients with angiomyolipomas. For those patients with asymptomatic small lesions (<4 cm), conservative observation is our first choice currently. For patients with symptomatic or large lesions, women of childbearing age, or patients with equivocal lesions, surgical or angiographic management is our choice. If surgery is chosen, careful exploration and attempt at nephron sparing is the recommended option.

Suggested Readings

Blute ML, Malek RS, Segura JW: Angiomyolipoma: Clinical metamorphosis and concepts for management. J Urol 139:20, 1988

Drago JR, Nesbitt JA, Leb R: Renal angiomyolipoma. J Surg Oncol 39:64, 1988

Huang J, Ho DM, Wang J, et al: Coincidental angiomyolipoma and renal cell carcinoma—a report of 1 case and review of the literature. J Urol 140:1516, 1988
Oesterling JE, Fishman EK, Goldman SM, et al: The management of renal angiomyolipoma. J Urol 135:1121, 1986
Taylor RS, Joseph DB, Kohaut EC, et al: Renal angiomyolipoma associated with lymph node involvement and renal cell carcinoma in patients with tuberous sclerosis. J Urol 141:930, 1989

RENAL PELVIC TUMORS

NORMAN L. BLOCK, M.D., F.A.C.S.
Miami, Florida

Primary tumors arising in the renal pelvis previously have been thought to be quite uncommon. Recent reports, however, show the incidence to be increasing. Earlier in the century a ratio of 1:18 with renal parenchymal tumors was reported. In recent decades, a ratio of 1:4 seems to have been reached. The reason for this change is unknown, but it may be related, in part, to a rise in carcinogens excreted in the urine from such sources as tobacco smoke and phenacetin. Increasing interest and awareness as well as improving diagnostic capabilities also may play a role.

Renal pelvic tumors (RPTs) now represent 10 to 20 per cent of all renal tumors, the second most common renal tumor. The incidence has been reported as 1:10,000 new patients at the Cleveland Clinic and 0.5 cases per 100,000 in the general population. RPTs accounted for 1600 new cases and 700 deaths in the United States in 1989. The incidence for whites is double that of blacks. Incidence peaks in the sixth and seventh decades of life. Occurrence rates in the two kidneys are equal. Half of patients with RPT will have other urothelial tumors synchronously or metachronously. Mazeman reported a 2 per cent incidence of bilaterality.

PATHOLOGY

RPTs parallel other sites of transitional epithelium with regard to the incidence of development of tumor cell types. The majority are transitional cell carcinomas, with a lesser incidence of squamous cell carcinomas (often associated with calculi) and a still lesser incidence of adenocarcinomas. With relative rarity, the full range of other types of carcinomas and sarcomas have been reported. Occasional benign mucosal lesions, such as inverted papilloma, and benign stromal tumors have been reported.

RPTs may be either papillary or solid. The former account for about 75 per cent of the total and seem to prefer the ureteropelvic junction. Tumors arising in the pelvis itself invade the wall and cause thickening and induration. Tumors arising in the infundibular or calyceal epithelium invade directly into the renal substance. In the solid tumors, this invasion, rather than an exophytic lesion, is the predominant feature and may not be easily distinguishable from areas of chronic inflammatory change, thus complicating diagnosis. This feature is especially common with squamous tumors.

RPTs may spread by invasion of contiguous organs. Local recurrence is seen in 43 per cent of autopsy cases. They involve regional lymph nodes in one third of all post-mortem cases. Hematogenous spread with RPT is less common than with the usual parenchymal adenocarcinoma. In one series, 12 per cent of patients had hematogenous spread; all cases were associated with delayed diagnosis. Invasion of the renal vein is uncommon. Lung and liver metastasis is seen in one third to one half of autopsy cases. Bone metastasis, usually to the spine, is seen in 15 per cent.

SYMPTOMS AND SIGNS

The classic diagnostic triad of renal tumors—hematuria, flank pain, palpable mass—occasionally is seen with pelvic tumors but is uncommon. Hematuria, the most frequent symptom, occurs in 90 per cent of patients. The presence of string-like clots (representing a cast of pelvis or ureter) is pathognomonic. Flank pain and urinary frequency are the next most common symptoms and fever, dysuria, anemia, azotemia, bacteriuria, weight loss, fatigue, and metastatic symptoms frequently are reported. A wide range of humorally mediated symptoms also has been reported. The presence of a bladder tumor may be the first manifestation of RPT.

Although symptoms are generally the reason patients seek medical advice in this disease, they seldom permit the actual diagnosis to be made. One paper suggested that only one third of patients ultimately diagnosed with RPT actually had a correct initial diagnosis.

DIAGNOSTIC EVALUATION

The initial work-up of a patient with hematuria and/or other symptoms and signs suggesting a renal tumor should include intravenous urography and cystoscopy. Pyelography may reveal filling defects, collecting system distortions, or blockage of all or part of the collecting system. All of these may be indicative of tumor, but caution is advised in calling a filling defect a tumor when in fact it is a clot, pyelitis cystica/glandularis, radiolucent calculus, or sloughed papilla. Hydronephrosis or nonfunction may be due to blockage, invasion of the renal vein, or replacement of parenchyma. In one series 8 of 19 patients had nonvisualization; parenchymal invasion caused 6 of 8 cases. In two thirds of patients in whom intravenous urography raised suspicion of RPT, supplementary investigation was useful.

Cystoscopy reveals such suggestive findings as associated tumor in the ureter or bladder, bleeding from a specific orifice, and ureteral obstruction on attempted catheterization. Cystoscopy alone is helpful in about only one third of cases. When cystoscopy is done for hematuria, discovery of a bladder tumor should not act as a decoy against *adequate* upper tract investigation.

Retrograde pyelography during cystoscopy is frequently useful. The tumor diagnosis is established in about one half of cases by this method. Retrograde brushing through the ureteral catheter may be useful. A calculus on the radiograph should not exclude the possibility of concurrent RPT. Antegrade pyelography may be useful when retrograde study is impractical.

Angiography previously was useful in determining the nature of these tumors and their level of involvement of renal parenchyma and other surrounding structures. This method has been mostly superceded by computerized tomographic (CT) scanning. Dynamic CT scanning, in particular, can resolve the issue of parenchymal involvement. Magnetic resonance imaging occasionally is useful for diagnostic delineation of this tumor modality, but a well-defined role has not been established. Ultrasound and isotopic studies are of limited value. Positron emission tomography has not been useful to the best of my knowledge.

Urinary cytology is useful for the diagnosis of RPT and also is useful in the follow-up to monitor for the presence of associated tumors (e.g., bladder, opposite pelvis, and ureter). In one report, 66 per cent of patients with RPT had a positive cytology when three specimens per patient were studied. Specifically, cytology is best reserved for the following situations: (1) detection of an early lesion when other clinical findings are not conclusive, (2) evaluation of a pyelographic filling defect, (3) detection of tumor occurrence in the opposite kidney before radical excision is planned, and (4) follow-up.

In recent years, direct endoscopic evaluation and management of RPT has been described. This may be by ureteropyeloscopy, intraoperative nephroscopy, or percutaneous nephroscopy. The last has the obvious risk of retroperitoneal tumor dissemination (see below).

MANAGEMENT

Because radiation and chemotherapy have limited applicability to the primary treatment of RPT, surgery is the mainstay of the urologist's therapeutic armamentarium.

Kimball and Ferris in 1934 published a classic paper recommending total nephroureterectomy as the optimal management of RPT. Since that time, this has been the "gold standard." This procedure involves removal of the kidney, ureter, and a cuff of bladder at the ureterovesical junction. Gerota's fascia and the fatty layers surrounding the kidney and ureter generally are included. The usefulness of associated lymphadenectomy is debatable.

The rationale for this wide surgical approach lies in Melicow's concept of "field change" in the visually normal mucosa associated with the putative lesion. As the stage and grade of the visible tumor advance, the probability of related carcinoma in situ, dysplasia, or atypia in the surrounding urothelium rises. Evaluation of the patient with RPT therefore should include the entire urothelial surface.

In recent years, as longevity has increased, so has the cumulative risk to renal units from tumor, calculus, infectious problems, and so on. As a result of lost contralateral renal function, or in anticipation of such, attempts at renal-sparing surgery have acquired increasing acceptance. Decisions for conservative treatment should include the consideration that half of tumors so treated will recur. RPT can be treated by partial nephrectomy, simple nephrectomy, open pyelotomy and local excision, or endoscopically (ureteropyeloscopy, operative nephroscopy, percutaneous nephroscopy). All of these present the risk of inadequate tumor control and should be reserved only for the most unusual cases. The endoscopic approaches have this risk plus that of renal intraparenchymal tumor dissemination and tract seeding. Explosion during intrapelvic tumor fulguration has been reported.

In very carefully selected cases, such as multifocal small tumors in a solitary renal unit, intracavitary instillation of various of those topical agents useful for bladder tumors has been successful for RPT. Bacille Calmette-Guérin (BCG) has been used by both Herr and Soloway; due caution against systemic BCG dissemination is advised.

Radiotherapy should be used as primary treatment only for inoperable tumors, poor-risk patients, or localized metastases.

Chemotherapy for metastatic RPT generally has been disappointing, but recently the platinum-based regimens have shown some efficacy.

PROGNOSIS

As expected, survival is directly correlated with grade and stage of tumor. Five-year overall crude survivals are reported at 18 to 55 per cent. In the Sloan-Kettering series (staged by the system of Grabstald et al.), those patients with noninvasive or microfocally invasive tumor had a determinate 5-year survival of 77 per cent; those with invasion into the pelvis or parenchyma but not beyond, 57 per cent; and those extending beyond the kidney, 5 per cent. In the New York Hospital series, 87 per cent of patients with low-grade tumors, 60 per cent of those with intermediate-grade, and only 15 per cent of those with high-grade tumors showed prolonged survival. Mazeman reported, in 737 cases, a 50 per cent late recurrence rate divided equally between local (urothelial), regional, and metastatic disease. The prognosis for squamous and adenocarcinomas of the pelvis is poorer, but the numbers are too small for definitive statistics.

The results of radical versus conservative treatments have been variously compared, but, with patient selection being an usually unstated but important issue, no valid conclusions can be drawn. A comparative series reported by Johansson in 1979 suggested that the more extensive operative procedure resulted in improved survival (intrafascial nephrectomy had a 5-year survival of 51 per cent, whereas perifascial nephrectomy with total ureterectomy and homolateral adrenalectomy had a 5-year survival of 84 per cent). The difference was statistically significant. Simple nephrectomy therefore may be justified only (1) for RPTs so extensive that only palliation is possible; (2) for a squamous tumor, because ureteric recurrence is so rare; and (3) in poor-risk patients. As many as 65 per cent of transitional cell tumors so treated will have recurrence in the ureteral stump.

Those patients with bilateral tumors, renal insufficiency, severe operative risk factors, preoperative evidence of a single, low-grade, superficial tumor, or tumors in solitary kidneys should be the only ones considered for even more conservative surgical treatment. Metachronous bilateral tumors are usually low grade/stage at the second appearance and therefore are reasonably treated conservatively.

Multiple second primary tumors occur in association with RPT. In one series, 75 per cent of autopsy cases had past or current second primaries.

CONCLUSION

RPT shows an increasing incidence. A poorly functional kidney, particularly when associated with bladder tumor, or a bleeding nonfunctional kidney should be suspicious for RPT. Appropriate treatment for renal pelvic cancer is complete nephroureterectomy with bladder cuff. Conservative therapy should be used only in carefully selected cases. Radiologic, cystoscopic, and cytologic follow-up should be similar to that for bladder cancer.

Suggested Readings

Andrews PE, Segura JW: Renal pelvic explosion during conservative management of upper tract urothelial cancer. J Urol 146:407–408, 1991

Grabstald H, Whitmore WF Jr, Melamed M: Renal pelvic tumors. JAMA 218:845–854, 1971

Guinan P, Vogelzang NJ, Randazzo R, et al, and Cancer Incidence and End Results Committee: Renal pelvic cancer: A review of 611 patients treated in Illinois 1975–1985. Urology 40:393–399, 1992

Latham HS, Kay S: Malignant tumors of the renal pelvis. Surg Gynecol Obstet 138:613–622, 1974

Mazeman E: Tumours of the upper urinary tract calyces, renal pelvis and ureter. Eur Urol 2:120–128, 1976

McCredie M, Stewart JH, Day NE: Different roles for phenacetin and paracetamol in cancer of the kidney and renal pelvis. Int J Cancer 53:245–249, 1993

PRIMARY RENINOMA OF THE KIDNEY

E. DARRACOTT VAUGHAN, Jr., M.D.

New York, New York

The term "primary reninoma" applies specifically to a renal cortical juxtaglomerular cell benign tumor first reported independently by both Robertson and Kihara in 1967. The full clinical syndrome, usually found in young people, is characterized by severe hypertension, hypokalemia, hyper-reninemia, and secondary hyperaldosteronism not explainable by renovascular disease or malignant hypertension. The more general term "primary reninism," coined by Conn, includes juxtaglomerular cell tumors and those other neoplasms, such as Wilms' tumor, renal cell carcinoma, and extrarenal tumors, that secrete renin and induce severe hypertension.

Fifteen cases of primary reninoma have been reported by Lam and associates. All but one of the patients were younger than 40 and they had a mean blood pressure of 215/140 mm Hg. All exhibited elevated aldosterone and renin levels, with localization of renin secretion to the affected side in those cases studied by differential renal vein renin sampling. Renal angiography revealed normal renal arterial anatomy in association with an avascular or hypovascular cortical renal mass lesion that was proven to be solid on renal sonography. The mean size was 2.3 cm on pathologic examination, and all tumors were not visualized by angiography. The treatment generally has been nephrectomy, with partial nephrectomies reported.

At present, the diagnosis should be suspected in a patient with severe hypertension, elevated renin and aldosterone levels, the absence of renovascular occlusive disease, and lateralization of renal venous renin secretion. Improved renal anatomic studies, such as renal sonography and computerized tomography, should identify most of the small cortical mass lesions.

The tumors are usually solid (one was cystic), and on light microscopy show spindle-shaped cells containing Bowie-positive granules, vascularity, tubular elements, and mast cell infiltration. Electron microscopy shows electron-dense "renin" granules, and immunofluorescent studies for renin are positive. Renin secretion by the tumor itself can be documented further by demonstrating the presence of renin mRNA or by demonstrating autonomous renin production from cell cultures.

Recently a patient with a renin-secreting tumor underwent a captopril test. The blood pressure dropped but there was not a reactive rise in renin, suggesting different processing and control of renin secretion in these patients. Moreover, long-term captopril treatment was ineffective in controlling either blood pressure or secondary hyperaldosteronism.

Local excision instead of total nephrectomy has been performed occasionally because the tumors have been uniformly solitary and benign. However, the dilemma of differentiating these tumors from small renin-secreting renal cell carcinomas remains. Despite this problem, partial nephrectomy seems reasonable, because limited resection is probably as effective as radical nephrectomy in patients with a small renal cell carcinoma.

Postoperatively, the blood pressure, plasma renin activity, and aldosterone level have fallen to normal in all patients, confirming the etiologic role of the tumor in the hypertension.

Suggested Readings

Corvol P, Pinet F, Galen FX, et al: Primary reninism. *In* Laragh JH, Brenner BM (eds): Hypertension: Pathophysiology, Diagnosis, and Management. New York, Raven Press, 1990, pp 1573–1582

Lam ASC, Bédard YC, Buckspan MB, et al: Surgically curable hypertension associated with reninoma. J Urol 128: 572–575, 1982

RETROPERITONEAL SARCOMA

DANIEL T. DEMPSEY, M.D.

Philadelphia, Pennsylvania

Solid primary retroperitoneal tumors are either mesenchymal (retroperitoneal sarcoma) or lymphoid tissue (lymphoma) until proven otherwise. Rarely, a retroperitoneal mass may represent a large metastatic focus from a heretofore unrecognized primary tumor of the genitourinary or gastrointestinal tract.

Soft tissue sarcomas account for 1 per cent of all solid neoplasms and retroperitoneal sarcomas account for 10 to 15 per cent of all sarcomas. There are only 500 to 1000 new cases of retroperitoneal sarcomas seen annually in the United States, and they represent approximately 50 per cent of all retroperitoneal solid neoplasms. Although these malignancies are relatively rare, primary retroperitoneal sarcoma should be included in the differential diagnosis of any mass in the retroperitoneum.

The majority of sarcomas arise from mesenchymal tissue. The relative frequency of histologic subtypes of retroperitoneal sarcomas differs from that seen in soft tissue sarcomas of the extremity. Malignant fibrous histiocytoma has been recognized as the most common type of extremity soft tissue sarcoma. Contrary to this finding, in most series, liposarcoma remains the most common histologic type found in the retroperitoneum. Leiomyosarcoma and fibrosarcoma follow in relative frequency, with neurosarcomas and undifferentiated sarcomas being unusual.

In most cases of retroperitoneal sarcoma, it is impossible to identify any possible etiologic factors. However, epidemiologic data suggest that previous (>10 years ago) radiation therapy, exposure to certain chemicals (e.g., vinyl chloride, dioxin), and neurofibromatosis are significant risk factors for sarcoma.

CLINICAL FINDINGS

By virtue of their location, retroperitoneal sarcomas often produce very few symptoms until they are quite large. In the Mayo Clinic series, 92 per cent of patients had tumors larger than 5 cm (56 per cent) or tumor fixed to adjacent structures (36 per cent). Although their complaints are vague and nonspecific, most patients are symptomatic at the time of presentation. At the Mayo Clinic, 96 per cent of patients are symptomatic when diagnosed, with a mean duration of symptoms prior to operative treatment of 6.3 months.

Patients most frequently present with a palpable abdominal mass or a history of increasing abdominal girth. They also may report vague abdominal discomfort. Not infrequently, these patients may present with a history of constant low-grade fevers, often accompanied by a mild leukocytosis caused by tumor necrosis. Symptoms of pelvic and lower extremity neurologic involvement can occur secondary to compression. These tumors may become large enough in size to impinge on the lower extremity venous return, thus producing lower extremity edema. Also, numbness, paresthesia, or weakness of the lower extremity may be seen as a result of neural compression.

The most common finding on physical examination is a palpable abdominal mass or increasing abdominal girth on serial examinations. Ascites occasionally can occur as a result of portal venous compression or lower extremity edema caused by vena cava compression. A detailed neurologic examination may reveal sensory or motor deficits in the lower extremity secondary to nerve compression. Serum glucose levels may be found to be abnormally low because of the occasionally produced insulin-like substance.

DIAGNOSTIC TECHNIQUES

One should never exclude the possibility of retroperitoneal tumor being a primary sarcoma. Sarcoma should be included in the differential diagnosis of any retroperitoneal mass. Because of their location, sarcomas of the retroperitoneum usually present as a very large abdominal mass. Almost all retroperitoneal sarcomas are greater than 5 cm in diameter at the time of presentation. Large retroperitoneal masses are more suggestive of sarcoma; however, size alone should not be used to exclude other disease processes. With computerized tomographic (CT) scanning being used more frequently to evaluate nonspecific abdominal complaints, discovery of more sarcomas of smaller size may be expected.

The single most important radiographic study is an abdominal CT scan with oral and IV contrast. This is an excellent modality for defining the character of the mass as well as the extent of retroperitoneal involvement. CT scan can be valuable in differentiating sarcomas from other retroperitoneal malignancies. Diffuse retroperitoneal adenopathy is more suggestive of lymphoma and should prompt a clinical re-evaluation of the lymphatic basins and perhaps a bone marrow biopsy. Retroperitoneal tumors of testicular origin tend to be more homogeneous, and this finding should prompt an evaluation of tumor markers and ultrasound of the scrotum. Abdominal CT scan also may be useful in defining the involvement of other retroperitoneal and intraperitoneal organs that may require resection. The suggestion of aortic or caval involvement on CT is an indication for arteriogram and/or venacavagram prior to operative management. The function of both kidneys and the presence of ureteral obstruction also can be evaluated by CT scan.

Abdominal magnetic resonance imaging (MRI) is a very useful study in the delineation of the tumor extent. Both T_1- and T_2-weighted images can be used to better define the relationship of the tumor to other solid organs and adjacent muscles, respectively. MRI or spiral CT eventually may abrogate the need for angiography because of its excellent delineation of vascular structures. However, we prefer preoperative arteriography in most cases prior to curative resection.

An essential element in the staging work-up of retroperitoneal or extremity sarcoma is the performance of a chest CT scan. Frequently, routine chest radiographs are inadequate in detecting small metastatic lesions; thus a CT chest tomogram is imperative. Another frequent site of metastatic spread from retroperitoneal sarcoma is the liver. Diffuse liver involvement should be ruled out prior to undertaking curative resection.

CT scan can aid in percutaneous biopsy of the retroperitoneal mass. However, it has been our practice not to perform percutaneous needle biopsy in patients in whom the primary differential diagnosis is between retroperitoneal sarcoma and lymphoma. Usually, the specimen obtained by this technique is inadequate to make a definitive diagnosis as to the particular cell type in these cases, and there is significant concern with retroperitoneal sarcoma that contamination of the needle tract with tumor may increase the possibility of local recurrence following a curative resection. Laparoscopic biopsy of obviously incurable lesions might be useful in the future.

Often, open biopsy is performed for potentially curable lesions. Resection of these large tumors without a definitive diagnosis is unwise. Although it is unusual to be able to obtain a definitive histologic diagnosis on frozen section, the differentiation between a lymphoma or a germ cell tumor and a sarcoma should be obvious, even on frozen section, which should also confirm the adequacy of biopsy. It is imperative when performing an open biopsy technique that the abdominal cavity or wound edges not be contaminated with tumor cells, because this might compromise cure. Hemostasis should be meticulous and drains should not be used. Large areas of liquification should be decompressed carefully to avoid inadvertent rupture and massive contamination of the operative site with tumor.

TREATMENT

Surgery

Surgery remains the major method of treating retroperitoneal sarcomas. Optimal treatment is wide local excision with removal of all gross and microscopic disease. The transabdominal approach is favored over the flank approach because of the limitations in exposure via the flank incision. These tumors are often of large size, with contiguous organ involvement. Thus, the latter approach may compromise the extent of resection. Furthermore, the control of large feeding vessels and the evaluation of the aorta, vena cava, and major visceral vessels is best accomplished early in the case with a transabdominal approach. Initial laparoscopic evaluation may detect foci of disseminated disease heretofore unsuspected and obviate the need for a laparotomy for cure.

The retroperitoneum is not compartmentalized as is the extremity; thus, no fascial boundaries exist to contain the neoplasm. This creates a situation in which almost any retroperitoneal or intraperitoneal organ may be involved. Once transabdominal exploration is initiated, the first maneuver is to determine the resectability of the lesion. This can be done by evaluating the relationship of the mass to the aorta, SMA, SMV, and vena cava. If these vessels are free of contiguous spread, the sarcoma usually can be resected for cure in the absence of distant metastases or peritoneal spread. In the Memorial series, 65 per cent of patients with primary sarcoma had complete resection, compared to 51 per cent operated for recurrent disease. Curative resection was not attempted because of vascular involvement (43 per cent), peritoneal studding (28 per cent), distant metastases (17 per cent), or involvement of the root of the mesentery (16 per cent). Retroperitoneal sarcomas rarely invade vessels or nerves, but they may become densely adherent to them. Infrequently, resection of the sarcoma for curative intent involves the resection of a segment of aorta or vena cava. This is the exception rather than the rule and is rarely performed.

Resection for cure should be carried out through normal tissue. Sarcomas often have a pseudocapsule, and "enucleation" is to be condemned because gross tumor will be left behind in the margins. Attached viscera should be considered potentially invaded and should not be separated from the tumor. Instead, en bloc resection should be performed, including the attached organ(s). In decreasing order of occurrence, the kidney, spleen, small bowel, colon, stomach, pancreas, ureter, uterus, or diaphragm may be involved. Again, complete excision of all disease will yield the optimal results. Special care should be given to tumors that have large cystic areas, because inadvertent incision into these areas during an open biopsy, or rupture of these areas during manipulation required for resection, may result in gross contamination of the operative field with tumor. Preoperative evaluation of both kidneys as well as a good bowel preparation should be done.

Overall, about 50 per cent of patients explored for retroperitoneal sarcomas undergo curative resection, and the 5-year survival in this group is about 50 per cent. In the Memorial series, the 5-year actuarial survival for completely resected patients was 74 per cent, compared to 35 per cent after partial resection or cytoreduction and 15 per cent for unresectable disease. This is comparable to other surgical series that report an 8 to 33 per cent 5-year survival with partially resected disease and a 3 to 10 per cent 5-year survival with unresectable retroperitoneal sarcoma. Symptomatic patients with large but incurable tumors probably should have their tumors debulked if this can be done safely, because it may relieve symptoms, give some marginal survival advantage, and increase the efficacy of other treatment modalities (i.e., radiotherapy and chemotherapy). Nevertheless, completeness of resection strongly predicts outcome, as does tumor grade but not type. Because of the greater importance of grade over size in the prognosis of patients with retroperitoneal sarcoma, the current sarcoma staging system relates stage to histopathologic grade (Table 1).

Even after successful excision, retroperitoneal sarcomas have a high rate of local recurrence. More than 90 per cent of patients will develop recurrent disease if follow-up for 10 years after curative resection is performed, and local recurrence is usually the cause of death. The grade of the tumor is significant in predicting the recurrence rate. High-grade tumors tend to recur earlier than low-grade tumors. For the first 5 years, patients should be followed clinically every 3 months, with CT scan done every 6 months to detect recurrent disease, which will be local in 75 per cent of cases. Patients with a completely resected recurrence have a median survival of 48 months compared to 15 months in those with unresectable recurrence.

Radiation Therapy

Radiation therapy as the primary means of eradicating primary retroperitoneal sarcoma is clearly of very little utility. Although complete surgical excision is unequivocally the major method of treating this disease, the high rate of tumor recurrence along with the frequently encountered unresectable disease suggests that other modalities must be defined to enhance local control of retroperitoneal sarcoma. Although the theoretical benefit of adjuvant radiation therapy is recognized from the salutary effects in extremity sarcoma, the doses of external beam radiation must be lower when treating retroperitoneal sarcoma. In the extremity, up to 6000 cGy can be used; however, the small bowel can tolerate only 4500 to 5000 cGy. The liver and kidneys have an even lower radiation tolerance.

To date, no study has shown a distinct survival advantage for external radiation in this disease. To avoid the toxicity of external beam radiation, it has been suggested that intraoperative radiation therapy (IORT) or brachytherapy may be used with greater efficacy and fewer complications. Studies currently are being done to test this hypothesis, but thus far there is no prospective, randomized study showing improved results of IORT over external beam radiation in retroperitoneal sarcoma.

Radiation therapy can be useful in palliating patients with unresectable disease. Results of external beam radiation therapy for retroperitoneal sarcoma may be enhanced substantially by the use of radiosensitizing chemo-

TABLE 1. Sarcoma Staging†

Tumor Designation	Tumor Histopathology	Tumor Grade	Patient Stage‡
G1	Well differentiated	Low	I
G1	Moderately well differentiated	Intermediate	II
G3	Poorly differentiated; undifferentiated	High	III

From Storm FK, Mahvi DM: Diagnosis and management of retroperitoneal soft-tissue sarcoma. Ann Surg 1991; 214(1) 2–10, with permission.

†A tumor less than 5 cm = T1 tumor (substage A); a tumor of 5 cm or greater = T2 tumor (substage B). Bone, nerve, and/or vessel invasion = T3 tumor (substage IVA in past schemas).

‡Currently stage IVA designates patients with nodal metastases; IVB denotes distant disease.

therapy. The high rates of local control seen with radiation and iododeoxyuridine (IUDR) in patients with unresectable disease has prompted a neoadjuvant protocol at the University of Michigan. Resectability rates are high and toxicity low, but data on local recurrence and survival are not yet available.

Chemotherapy

Several trials have investigated the use of postoperative adjuvant chemotherapy. Preoperative, neoadjuvant therapy also has been evaluated, with some suggestion that doxorubicin (Adriamycin) may be of benefit. There are currently no studies to support a survival benefit with the use of adjuvant chemotherapy. More detailed evaluation is needed to define the role of chemotherapy in the management of retroperitoneal sarcoma.

SUMMARY

Retroperitoneal sarcomas represent 15 per cent of soft tissue sarcomas, which are rare malignancies representing 1 per cent of all solid neoplasms. Signs and symptoms of retroperitoneal sarcomas are vague and nonspecific. The most common complaint is increasing abdominal girth or the presence of an abdominal mass. Abdominal pain and fevers also may occur. Abdominal CT scan is essential in defining the extent and character of the mass. MRI is helpful in evaluating vascular involvement and occasionally can provide improved resolution of retroperitoneal tissue planes and structures. Complete surgical excision of the sarcoma provides the best results, but local recurrence is common. The benefit of adjuvant radiation (either external or IORT) and chemotherapy is currently undergoing evaluation, but the obvious benefits seen in patients with extremity lesions are lacking.

Suggested Readings

Bevilacqua RG, Rogatko A, Brennan MF, et al: Prognostic factors in primary retroperitoneal soft-tissue sarcomas. Arch Surg 126:328–334, 1991

Dalton RR, Donohue JH, Macha P, et al: Management of retroperitoneal sarcomas. Surgery 106:725–732, 1989

Jaques DP, Coit DG, Hadju SI, et al: Management of primary and recurrent soft-tissue sarcoma of the retroperitoneum. Ann Surg 212:51–59, 1990

Sondak VK: Sarcomas of bone and soft tissue. *In* Greenfield (ed): Surgery: Scientific Principles and Practice. Philadelphia, JB Lippincott, 1993 pp 2035–2052

Storm FK, Mahvi DM: Diagnosis and management of retroperitoneal soft-tissue sarcoma. Ann Surg 214:2–10, 1991

Willett CG, Suit HD, Tepper JE, et al: Intraoperative electron beam radiation therapy for retroperitoneal soft-tissue sarcoma. Cancer 68:278–283, 1991

RETROPERITONEAL LYMPHOMAS

SANDRA F. SCHNALL, M.D.

Philadelphia, Pennsylvania

The retroperitoneum is the area between the peritoneal cavity and the posterior body wall. Its contents include the abdominal aorta and inferior vena cava and their tributaries, the kidneys and ureters, the adrenal glands, the pancreas, part of the duodenum, lymph nodes, and neural structures. One of the more common retroperitoneal tumors is lymphoma, accounting for approximately 15 per cent of cases. Both Hodgkin's disease (HD) and non-Hodgkin's lymphoma (NHL) may involve the retroperitoneal lymph nodes.

In evaluating a patient for a retroperitoneal mass, an initial step must be establishing a diagnosis. If lymphoma is suspected, a biopsy most often is required to help determine specific histologic patterns (see later in this article) that usually cannot be determined from a fine-needle aspirate. Special handling of the specimen should be undertaken so that immunophenotyping (see later in this article) as well as routine pathologic evaluation can be processed.

Once the diagnosis of lymphoma is confirmed, complete surgical excision is not necessarily warranted as primary therapy. Radiopaque clips placed around the remaining tumor may be helpful to demarcate potential radiation portals.

CLASSIFICATION

Several classification schemas for NHL have been developed over the last several years, some according to histology (Rappaport's), some functional anatomy (Mann's), and some immunomorphology (Lukes and coworkers). In 1982, the National Cancer Institute (NCI) established the Working Formulation to serve as a common basis for comparison. It incorporates many features of the previously established classifications. The Working Formulation is shown in Table 1.

HD classification has been simplified to include four different types based on histopathologic parameters: (1) nodular sclerosis, (2) lymphocyte predominate, (3) lymphocyte depleted, and (4) mixed cellularity.

IMMUNOPHENOTYPING

Once the basic pathology has been established, evaluation of antigen expression by neoplastic cells has become an integral part of the work-up of lymphomas (Table 2). It may be performed by immunofluorescence or immunoenzymatic analysis of cell suspensions and/or fresh frozen sections. Only a limited phenotypic evaluation can be obtained by using paraffin sections, because most antigens do not resist the process of routine tissue embedding. Therefore, it is important that, when considering the diagnosis of lymphoma, the surgeon alert the pathologist so that the appropriate tissue processing may be performed. This special typing is also helpful in determining prognosis and treatment options. It is currently commonly performed in NHL but also may be useful in HD.

More recently, flow cytometry also has been used to study parameters of cell proliferation such as DNA content (ploidy status), DNA synthesis, and S-phase fraction. Genomic and cytogenetic analysis of lymphomas provide further information as to the cell of origin, possible etiology, prognosis, and treatment.

TABLE 1. Working Formulation of Non-Hodgkin's Lymphomas

LOW GRADE
Malignant lymphoma, small lymphocytic
Malignant lymphoma follicular, predominantly small cleaved cell
Malignant lymphoma, follicular, mixed small cleaved and large cell
INTERMEDIATE GRADE
Malignant lymphoma, follicular, predominantly large cell
Malignant lymphoma, diffuse, small cleaved cell
Malignant lymphoma, diffuse, mixed small and large cell
Malignant lymphoma, diffuse, large cell
Cleaved cell
Noncleaved cell
HIGH GRADE
Malignant lymphoma, large cell, immunoblastic
Malignant lymphoma, lymphoblastic
Malignant lymphoma, small noncleaved cell (Burkitt's)

Chromosome Analysis

In addition to the monoclonal antibody evaluation of lymphomas, chromosome analysis provides vital prognostic information for the oncologist. Again, this must be performed on fresh nonfixed tissue.

In low-grade lymphomas, tumors may contain the t(14;18)(q32;q21) chromosome abnormality. This results in an altered expression of the bcl-2 oncogene located at band q21 of chromosome 18. Other chromosome alterations in low-grade lymphomas include partial deletion of 16q, trisomy 7, and trisomy 12.

Many cytogenetic abnormalities are seen in the intermediate-grade lymphomas, including t(14;18)(q32;q21), deletion of 6q, trisomy 12, trisomy 21, and point breaks in 2q and 9q.

The chromosome findings in Burkitt's lymphoma are quite unique. They are similar in both the sporadic and endemic varieties and manifest three potential translocations. Eighty-eight per cent of the patients have the t(8;14)(q24;q32) abnormality. Others less commonly demonstrate the t(8;22)(q24;q11) or t(2;8)(p11–p13;q24). These chromosome translocations juxtapose one of the immunoglobulin gene loci on chromosome 2, 14, or 22 to the c-myc oncogene on chromosome 8.

In T cell lymphomas, there are several reported chromosome abnormalities, including deletion or translation of chromosomes 9, 10, and 11 and inversions of chromosome 14.

Chromosome abnormalities in HD are less common than in NHL. Some more noted common break points include those at 11q23, 14q32, 6q11–21, and 8q22–24.

STAGING AND DIAGNOSTIC STUDIES

One of the most important concepts in managing patients with malignant diseases is

TABLE 2. Monoclonal Antibodies in Lymphomas

LYMPHOMA	TUMOR CELL IMMUNOPHENOTYPE
Hodgkin's disease	CD30+, LCA−, CD15+, T40%, B20%, N50%
Large cell lymphoma	CD30+, LCA+, CD15−, T75%, B15%, N10%
Post-thymic or T cell lymphoma	CD30−, LCA+, CD15±, B−, T+
Mediastinal large B cell lymphoma	CD30−, LCA+, CD15−, B+, T−

determining an accurate tumor stage. Because lymphomas are often curable tumors, staging is an important initial step. The most common staging system for NHL and HD is the Ann Arbor system. Stage I disease is that confined to one nodal site. Stage II disease is that confined to lymphatic tissue of more than one site but on one side of the diaphragm. Stage III disease is that confined to lymphatic organs (including the spleen) on both sides of the diaphragm. Stage IV includes widespread lymphoma with or without extranodal involvement (i.e., bone marrow, liver, skin, etc.).

Once the diagnosis is established, further studies needed to establish the exact clinical stage include a careful physical examination, routine laboratory data, radiographic imaging (i.e., computerized tomographic scan of the chest, abdomen, and pelvis), and bilateral bone marrow biopsies. Further studies may be warranted depending on clinical presentation.

Often, depending on clinical staging of HD, an exploratory laparotomy may be performed to confirm the pathologic state (i.e., occult disease below the diaphragm). If, on surgical exploration, a previously undiagnosed retroperitoneal mass is confirmed as a lymphoma, one may consider a wedge biopsy of the liver, random biopsies of suspicious nodes, and possibly even splenectomy. However, an oncologic evaluation in the operating room may be helpful in determining the direction and necessity of these procedures.

CLINICAL CHARACTERISTICS

Clinical presentations of lymphomas vary depending on cellular classification as well as stage. Patients may present noting a "palpable nodule" or simply complain of constitutional symptoms such as an unexplained weight loss, night sweats, or malaise. Laboratory data, including an elevated lactic dehyrogenase (LDH) level, elevated liver function test results, or some degree of pancytopenia, may be helpful in making a diagnosis. In some low-grade lymphomas, there may even be circulating abnormal lymphocytes in the peripheral blood smear.

Low-Grade Lymphomas

The low-grade histologies consist of the small lymphocytic, follicular small cleaved cell, and follicular mixed categories. Because of their natural history and response to therapy, they often are referred to as "favorable"-prognosis lymphomas. Approximately 25 to 40 per cent of lymphomas are of these histologies. Although they most commonly occur in middle-aged patients, the median age is 50 to 60 years. Approximately 75 per cent of patients, however, are Stage III or IV at diagnosis, with extranodal (liver or spleen) or bone marrow involvement. Most histologies are of B cell "subtype."

Although the median survival is 7 to 8 years, the indolent lymphomas are malignant and can be lethal. With time, these lymphomas may transform into a more aggressive pattern.

Intermediate-Grade Lymphomas

The intermediate histologies consist of the follicular large cell, diffuse small cleaved, diffuse mixed, and diffuse large cell categories. Approximately 50 per cent of all lymphomas present with this intermediate grade. Overall, they tend to occur in a younger age population than the indolent lymphomas. Approximately 60 per cent of patients present with Stage III or IV diseases.

Follicular large cell lymphomas account for only 4 per cent of all lymphomas. Like most follicular (nodular) lymphomas, they present with disseminated disease (Stage III or IV) and are most often of B cell origin. The median survival is approximately 3 years.

Diffuse small cleaved cell lymphoma and diffuse mixed lymphoma account for only 15 per cent of all presentations. Most commonly they are B cell malignancies; however, occasionally they also may be of T cell origin. Most patients are asymptomatic at presentation. The median survival is 2.5 to 3.5 years.

Diffuse large cell lymphomas account for approximately 20 per cent or more of all lymphomas. The tumor presents at an early stage (i.e., Stage I or II) in almost 50 per cent of cases. Disseminated disease is less common in this subtype than in other lymphomas. In the United States, diffuse large cell lymphomas are of B cell origin; however, 10 to 20 per cent will be of T cell immunophenotype. The median survival is approximately 1.5 years; however, many of these patients can be cured with newer treatment regimens (see later in this article).

High-Grade Lymphomas

High-grade histologies consist of the large cell immunoblastic, lymphoblastic, and small noncleaved cell (Burkitt) categories. These tumors behave in an aggressive fashion. Overall, they represent 15 per cent of all cases of NHL. More commonly, they present in a younger age group, with over half the patients diagnosed with lymphoblastic and Burkitt's lymphoma being children or teenagers.

Most of the immunoblastic and Burkitt-type lymphomas are of B cell origin. Lymphoblastic lymphomas are often of T cell origin and may show a male predominance. Many of these patients present with a mediastinal mass and require urgent medical attention for symptoms such as upper airway obstruction, superior vena cava syndrome, and even tumor lysis syndrome. Although only 30 per cent of patients will present with disseminated disease at diagnosis, over 80 per cent eventually will develop bone marrow involvement.

Burkitt's lymphoma is unique in that it has both an endemic and a sporadic variety. The endemic variety occurs in Africa and New Guinea. These are often associated with large nodal masses, commonly in the bone of the jaw and/or abdominal viscera. The retroperitoneal tumor may present with vascular or ureteral compromise, spinal cord compression, or bony destruction. There is an association of this type with elevated titers of the Epstein-Barr virus antigen in 80 per cent of cases. The sporadic type of Burkitt's lymphoma, however, is not as commonly associated with Epstein-Barr virus infections, and less commonly involves the jaw. Interestingly, however, both types are identified with a specific chromosome translocation (see earlier discussion of immunophenotyping).

Hodgkin's Disease

Patients with HD often present with supradiaphragmatic lymph node involvement. Regional disease below the diaphragm accounts for less than 10 per cent of cases. The nodal disease involvement above the diaphragm usually involves the anterior mediastinum, supraclavicular, or cervical regions. These nodes classically are described as feeling rubbery and firm and are often bulky. Patients may complain of a dry cough, decreased exercise tolerance, or shortness of breath. Clinically, one may detect extension into the sternum or chest wall with a large palpable mass.

Bulky intra-abdominal (retroperitoneal) HD is less common than retroperitoneal NHL. Ureteral obstruction, lower extremity edema, and deep venous thrombosis are rare complications. Lymph node involvement of the mesentery or isolated retroperitoneal nodes are rare.

Patients may have symptoms such as unexplained fevers greater than 101° F, drenching night sweats, and weight loss. These "B" symptoms often reflect later-stage disease or bulky disease. Other symptoms may include generalized puritis and painful lymph nodes after alcohol ingestion. Laboratory data may reflect an elevated LDH or uric acid level, mild pancytopenia, or an elevated erythrocyte sedimentation rate.

TREATMENT

Low-Grade Lymphomas

Treatment of low-grade, indolent NHL is depended on stage and symptoms. However, much controversy exists as to when to initiate therapy, if at all, and what type. Although most lymphomas in this classification are responsive to both radiation and chemotherapy, survival often is not altered by early therapy. The patients often have a pattern of remissions and relapses. In view of this, physicians often defer treatment and use the "watch and wait" approach until symptoms develop.

Once therapy is warranted, treatment may include radiation therapy to sites of bulky disease to relieve pain or obstruction. Chemotherapy is not likely to be curative for many of these lymphomas and, therefore, the goal of treatment may be to obtain a partial remission. Options include single-agent oral alkylating therapy (i.e., Cytoxan, chlorambucil) with or without steroids. More intense therapy may include intravenous agents in a combined approach with Cytoxan, vincristine, and prednisone. Recently, therapy with recombinant alpha-interferon has shown considerable promise in the treatment of the indolent NHL.

For the patients with localized, early stage (I or II) lymphoma, attempts at "cure" may include radiation therapy to the involved field followed by two to three cycles of chemotherapy. However, at some centers, an aggressive chemotherapy approach similar to that for intermediate-grade lymphomas (see next section) is sometimes undertaken in Stage I/II disease in patients less than 60 years of age with good performance status.

The goal here is a more durable remission. More recently, bone marrow transplantation has been entertained in this population.

Intermediate-Grade Lymphomas

Diffuse lymphomas are a type of neoplasm that can be cured with combination chemotherapy. Despite stage (i.e., localized Stage I/II or disseminated Stage III/IV), most patients with intermediate-grade lymphomas are recommended for systemic chemotherapy. Occasionally a patient with Stage I tumor can be cured with radiation therapy alone. However, this is dependent on the thoroughness of the pretreatment staging.

In disseminated intermediate-grade lymphomas, the best regimen to use remains uncertain. It is known, however, that combination chemotherapy is superior to single-agent treatment. Seventy to 80 per cent of patients will achieve a complete remission, and 50 per cent will obtain a prolonged disease-free survival.

Certain basic principles must be employed in determining an appropriate regimen. The treatment must be intensive and administered at full doses, and a complete response obtained as quickly as possible. It probably is not necessary to administer more than a few cycles after documentation of a complete remission, because this will likely only increase toxicity and not improve survival.

A summary of the more common treatment regimens are listed in Table 3. The "first-generation" regimen of CHOP is probably still considered the gold standard to which other regimens are compared. A multicenter trial has been completed recently comparing many of these regimens. Bone marrow suppression and dose intensity now will be modulated with the use of growth factors (i.e., G-CSF and GM-CSF).

TABLE 3. Chemotherapy Regimens for NHL

REGIMEN†	CR RATE*	RFS RATE*
CHOP	53%	60%
COP-BLAM^{a}	73%	55%
M^{b}ACOP-B	86%	70%
M^{b}-BACOD	72%	—
ProMACE/Cyta-BOM^{b}	80%	—

*CR = complete remission; RFS = relapse-free survival.
†A = Adriamycin; B = bleomycin; C = Cytoxan; Cyta = cytarbine; D = dexamethasone; E = etoposide; H = Adriamycin; M^{a} = procarbazine; M^{b} = methotrexate; O = vincristine; P = prednisone.

The role of bone marrow transplantation in NHL is still evolving. Whether it is recommended to offer a transplant in first remission or defer it until a second remission is obtained is dependent on many features, including age, initial stage, histology, and rate of remission (i.e., number of cycles required to obtain a remission). However, it should be explored in any patient who has relapsed after initial therapy.

Other novel approaches include alpha-interferon, monoclonal antibodies, and biologic response modifiers.

High-Grade Lymphomas

The treatment of immunoblastic lymphoma is similar to that of intermediate-grade lymphomas. Patients with lymphoblastic lymphoma require a more aggressive and intensive regimen. High response rates have been demonstrated using a regimen similar to that used in acute leukemias. Central nervous systems (CNS) prophylaxis usually is employed.

In addition, patients with Burkitt's lymphoma require intensive treatment with combined therapy and CNS prophylaxis. The 5-year survival rate varies from 20 to 20 per cent depending on prognostic features such as stage, bone marrow involvement, level of LDH, and CNS involvement.

Bone marrow transplantation also may play a role in the treatment of high-grade lymphomas and often are recommended in first remission.

Hodgkin's Disease

Treatment of HD is more dependent on stage than is treatment of NHL. Optimal treatment has yet to be determined. However, there is general agreement that patients with Stage I or IIA HD may be treated with high-dose wide-field radiation therapy. Relapse-free survival and overall survival are commonly greater than 90 per cent.

Patients with Stage IIIB and Stage IV HD require multidrug chemotherapy. Currently this most commonly includes the MOPP-ABVD alternating regimen, or the MOPP/ABV hybrid regimen (M = nitrogen mustard; O = vincristine; P = procarbazine; P = prednisone; A = Adriamycin; B = bleomycin; V = velban; D = dacarbazine). There are other available regimens, however.

Treatment of Stages IIB and IIIA remains controversial. Laparotomy-staged patients with Stage IIB, those with minimal splenic involvement and Stage IIIA HD can be treated with radiation therapy alone. However, treatment of patients with Stage IIIA disease with chemotherapy or combined modality therapy also can be effective.

Special attention must be given to the patient with early-stage disease with a large mediastinal mass encompassing greater than one third of the chest diameter. Chemotherapy often is recommended as an initial approach and, once maximal response is obtained, limited-field radiation therapy is employed. By offering radiation after the chemotherapy, the radiation port is decreased, likely minimizing toxicity. With this approach, disease-free survival at 5 years is greater than 85 per cent.

Patients who relapse after radiation therapy may be offered salvage chemotherapy. They may obtain complete remission with rates and long-term survival greater than 50 to 80 per cent. Those who relapse after chemotherapy may be offered further salvage chemotherapy regimens with or without radiation, or bone marrow transplantation.

ACQUIRED IMMUNODEFICIENCY SYNDROME LYMPHOMA

Patients with acquired immunodeficiency syndrome (AIDS) have been noted to be at an increased risk for developing neoplasms. Currently 5 to 10 per cent of patients with AIDS will develop NHL. HD has also been noted to be an AIDS-related illness. The majority of patients develop lymphomas with intermediate- or high-grade histologies. They may present with large retroperitoneal masses but also may present with tumors in extranodal sites, such as the CNS. Staging and treatment are similar to that for non-AIDS associated lymphomas; however, prognosis is poorer.

Suggested Readings

Cannellos GP (ed): Clinical update: Non-Hodkin's lymphoma. Adv Oncol 7(2):9–29, 1991

Foon KA: Laboratory and clinical applications of monoclonal antibodies for leukemias and non-Hodgkin's lymphomas. Curr Probl Cancer 13:2, 1989

Klein EA, Streem SB, Novick AC: Intraoperative consultation for the retroperitoneum and adrenal glands. Urol Clin North Am 12:411–422, 1985

Urba WJ, Longo DL: Hodgkin's disease. N Engl J Med 326:678–683, 1992

MANAGEMENT OF GENITOURINARY SARCOMAS IN ADULTS

WILLIAM C. PIERCE, Ph.D., M.D.

Los Angeles, California

Adult genitourinary sarcomas are rare, histologically diverse tumors with a generally poor long-term prognosis. Complete surgical extirpation with the achievement of adequate negative margins offers the best hope for long-term disease-free remission or cure. This article reviews the current status of the management of these uncommon tumors.

STAGING AND PROGNOSIS

In an important review, Russo and investigators at the Memorial Sloan-Kettering Cancer Center have reported the outcome of 43 adults with genitourinary sarcomas treated with surgery alone (42 per cent) or surgery plus either doxorubicin-based chemotherapy and/or radiation therapy (58 per cent). Stage I and II patients (n=19), primarily defined by tumors less than 5 cm and low histologic grade, had an 89 per cent 3-year relapse-free survival; the analogous survival for combined Stage III and IV patients was 26 per cent.

KIDNEY

Sarcomas constitute 2 to 3 per cent of malignant tumors of the kidney. Patients usually present with flank mass, pain, or hematuria. The diagnosis usually is not suspected preoperatively. Leiomyosarcomas are the most common, followed in incidence by liposarcomas, hemangiopericytomas, and rhabdomyosarcomas.

Most patients have been treated with radical nephrectomy, but the majority succumb to this disease within 2 years. Russo noted that the 3-year survival rate was 0 per cent for seven patients with renal sarcoma treated at the MSKCC despite achievement of complete resection with negative margins in four patients.

There is little experience with preoperative or postoperative chemotherapy or radiation therapy, but these methods of treatment appear to be effective in a number of case reports. Doxorubicin is probably the drug of choice.

BLADDER

Sarcomas of the urinary bladder account for 0.5 per cent of all malignant bladder tumors. Forty per cent of these are embryonal rhabdomyosarcomas in children. The remaining 60 per cent occur in the fifth to sixth decades and are composed of leiomyosarcomas, mixed mesodermal tumors, and rhabdomyosarcomas. Such tumors are more common in men than in women and present with hematuria or bladder dysfunction. The correct diagnosis usually can be made by transurethral biopsy; open biopsy should not be performed.

Leiomyosarcomas are generally broadly based and extend from the trigone. They tend to remain localized but may metastasize to lymph nodes, lungs, and liver. Most authors recommend radical cystectomy, although some have achieved good results with partial cystectomy for small lesions (<5 cm) that were well differentiated and low stage. In a recent review of UCLA cases, 87 per cent (six of seven patients) achieved disease-free survival lasting from 9 months to 21 years when treated with a protocol that uses intra-arterial doxorubicin (30 mg/day continuous infusions for 1½ days in each hypogastric artery), followed by preoperative radiation therapy (3500 rad) and radical cystectomy. We currently recommend this protocol.

Mixed mesodermal tumors (carcinosarcomas) are neoplasms that are composed of malignant epithelium and malignant stromal components. The prognosis for this tumor has been poor partly because of the high stage of presentation. The median survival is about 17 months. At UCLA, all patients (five) with carcinosarcoma of the bladder died of their disease regardless of stage, grade, or aggressiveness of treatment. Aggressive multimodal therapy is still warranted for localized tumors.

PROSTATE

Sarcomas of the prostate represent only 0.1 per cent of all prostate neoplasms. The majority are embryonal rhabdomyosarcomas in children. Among adults, leiomyosarcomas are the most common, followed in incidence by carcinosarcomas and rhabdomyosarcomas (alveolar and pleomorphic). The clinical picture is that of sudden urinary obstruction with a large and regular gland on examination. The diagnosis usually can be made by needle biopsy.

Leiomyosarcomas occur in the fourth to seventh decades and tend to remain localized and grow slowly. Most authors recommend aggressive multimodality therapy. Intraarterial doxorubicin combined with radiation therapy causes considerable (and at times complete) tumor necrosis noted at subsequent cystoprostatectomy. This protocol currently is recommended for the management of such tumors.

Carcinosarcomas are uncommon, and patients normally present with lung and bone metastases. The carcinomatous element is usually adenocarcinoma of the prostate, and, interestingly, this element appears to be of greater clinical significance. Thus, a number of patients have lived for years with orchiectomy or estrogen therapy.

Alveolar rhabdomyosarcomas tend to occur in young adults, whereas pleomorphic rhabdomyosarcomas tend to occur in older men. Only a handful of these histologic subtypes have been reported and all patients have fared poorly.

PARATESTICULAR STRUCTURES

Paratesticular tumors arise in the spermatic cord, epididymis, or testicular tunica. Ninety per cent of the malignant tumors are sarcomas, but they are still rare. The histologic types include leiomyosarcomas, fibrosarcomas, liposarcomas, and fibrous histiocytomas (in order of relative incidence).

Such tumors present as painless, enlarging masses and tend to invade locally and disseminate hematogenously. The prognosis for paratesticular tumors is considerably poorer than that for testicular tumors. Radical orchiectomy with high ligation of the spermatic cord is the treatment of choice. Local extension into adjacent soft tissue necessitates an adequate wide excision and postoperative irradiation of the field. The role of retroperitoneal lymph node dissection has not been defined, and its use generally has been individualized and guided by computerized tomographic findings. The role of chemotherapy is not known, and this treatment generally has been reserved for recurrences.

URETHRA

Only a few urethral sarcomas have been reported, and they include fibrosarcomas and rhabdomyosarcomas. Determination of the origin of the tumor, whether in the penis or the prostate, may be difficult. Such tumors have been treated with penectomy and, at times, with the inclusion of a prostatectomy, with some survivals.

PENIS

Penile sarcomas are rare and have included a few reported leiomyosarcomas, fibrosarcomas, malignant schwannomas, malignant hemangioendotheliomas, and Kaposi sarcomas. They occur most often in the penile shaft (40 per cent) and glans (37 per cent). Many lesions that are treated with wide local excision will recur. Thus, most authorities recommend partial penectomy for distal lesions and radical penectomy for proximal or deep corporal lesions. The roles of lymphadenectomy, chemotherapy, and radiation therapy have not been defined. The outcome after adequate surgery alone generally is favorable.

HUMAN IMMUNODEFICIENCY VIRUS INFECTION

Although the etiology of sarcomas remains unknown, immunosuppressive therapy, including radiation and the administration of alkylating agents in the treatment of neoplasia and autoimmune diseases has been implicated in the etiology of soft tissue sarcomas. Infection with human immunodeficiency virus-1 leads to a profoundly immunosuppressed state, and Adjiman et al. have described a rapidly fatal renal angiosarcoma and Angulo et al. penile Kaposi sarcomas in these patients. Localized penile Kaposi sarcoma may respond to the initiation of effective antiretroviral therapy. Additional effective therapeutic options include the administration of intralesional vinblastine or systemic agents, including vinblastine, bleomycin, doxorubicin, and interferon-alpha, or the administration of radiation therapy.

Suggested Readings

Adjiman S, Zerbib M, Flam T, et al: Genitourinary tumors and HIV_1 infection. Eur Urol 18:61, 1990

Angulo JC, Lopez JI, Unda-Urzaiz M, et al: Kaposi's sarcoma of the penis as an initial urological manifestation of AIDS. Urol Int 46:235, 1991

Russo P: Urologic sarcoma in adults. Urol Clin North Am 18:581, 1991

RETROPERITONEAL FIBROSIS

G. FORBES ABERCROMBIE, M.B., F.R.C.S.

Portsmouth, England

Retroperitoneal fibrosis is a rare disorder in which fibrous tissue is laid down in the retroperitoneum. It is urologically important because the ureters may be encased in the fibrosis and become obstructed.

The condition affects both sexes and may present in a variety of ways. There is often malaise and backache, not particularly typical of ureteric obstruction, sometimes with symptoms of hypertension, such as headache. Many cases present with renal failure resulting from bilateral obstruction. Occasionally lower limb edema, resulting from venous compression, may be present.

CLINICAL FINDINGS AND DIAGNOSTIC TECHNIQUES

Except for physical signs arising secondarily, such as raised blood pressure, there are no specific abnormalities to be found on examination. The plaque of fibrosis is not usually palpable per abdomen, although in cases in which the pelvic retroperitoneum is involved there may be a mass on pelvic examination. Apart from nonspecific anemia and changes caused by renal failure, the only consistent hematologic abnormality is a raised erythrocyte sedimentation rate (ESR). The ESR reflects the activity of the disorder and, in actively progressive cases in which the fibrous tissue is immature, may be very high indeed.

Urography, ultrasound, and retrograde ureterography ordinarily demonstrate a degree of hydronephrosis bilaterally. The ureters characteristically are deviated towards the midline, and the most common site of this deviation is around the L4–L5 level. At the same level, the ureter is obstructed, typically with a long, smooth narrowing. The pelvic ureter is normal in caliber distal to the obstructed segment. The plaque of fibrosis is usually discernible on computerized tomographic (CT) scanning, but probably is visualized even better by magnetic resonance imaging.

PATHOLOGY

Pathologically the lesion is a grayish white sheet of tissue extending across the central retroperitoneum and investing its structures. The thickness of this sheet may vary from 0.5 to 2 or 3 cm. The plaque is usually more or less symmetrical and most often is centered in the lower abdomen at about the L4–L5 level. It may extend down to invest the bladder, encasing the lower ureter as it does so, or caudally to involve the mediastinum. In this case the region of the pelviureteric junction may be affected.

The cells are essentially fibrocytes, and their maturity reflects the current activity of the process. Treatment with steroids may alter the histologic picture from that of a population dominated by immature fibroblasts to one in which the tissue is composed of mature fibrocytes.

ETIOLOGY

Some drugs, notably methysergide, have been associated with retroperitoneal fibrosis, and other etiologies identified include abdominal aneurysm. There are a number of reports in which trauma, hemorrhage, surgery, and urinary leakage have been considered to be associated with the disease. Most cases are truly idiopathic. Suggestions have been made from time to time that there is an autoimmune element possibly resulting from leakage from arterial vessels.

Malignant disease can, of course, produce ureteric obstruction in the retroperitoneum, either primarily, as in lymphomatous disorders, or secondarily, as in metastatic disease. In the latter case this is usually due to lymphatic spread or the compression of the ureters by tissue masses. This ought not to be difficult to distinguish by CT scanning, and there is usually a lack of symmetry in the urographic findings, which is a good pointer. However, the presence of metastatic malignant cells scattered through the retroperitoneum sometimes may give rise to the same reaction and production of fibrosis as in other identified causes of retroperitoneal fibrosis. In these cases, the histologic picture is one of fibrous tissue with occasional metastatic cells within it. Primary sites for this form of disease include the pancreas, prostate, and breast.

MANAGEMENT

Retroperitoneal fibrosis is rarely encountered in ordinary urologic practice, so the greatest difficulty in making the diagnosis lies in conceiving the possibility of it. Once that has been done, the combination of bilateral, reasonably symmetrical ureteric obstruction with medial deviation of the visualized ureters and a raised ESR makes up a recognizable syndrome. Management then is determined by the degree of renal failure.

Ureteric drainage can be reestablished by the insertion of indwelling ureteric stents, which work well in this disease, although they are often disappointing when the ureter is tightly gripped in a malignant process. This should allow renal recovery to take place before definitive treatment is instituted. It is not wise to visualize the pelvicalyceal systems by retrograde catheterization and then remove the ureteric catheter and do nothing to drain the kidneys. This procedure may upset the remaining ureteric function and lead to more severe obstruction, even immediate anuria, sometimes complicated by the introduction of infection into one or the other kidney. Retrograde urography should be done only if there are plans to proceed to some form of renal drainage at the same time.

Conservative Treatment

The choice of management lies between conservative treatment using steroids and ureterolysis. If conservative management is chosen, it is wise to obtain a tissue diagnosis with particular reference to the exclusion of malignant disease. This is possible with CT-guided needle biopsy. There are good reasons for choosing such a course. Not only is the patient spared from a procedure that necessarily has some disadvantages, but it is encouraging that the natural history of the untreated disease demonstrates a periodicity, with periods of spontaneous improvement as well as exacerbation.

The dose of steroids need not be high, and good response may be seen with 10 mg prednisolone thrice daily. The initial phase may need to be covered by ureteric stenting and the progress of the patient monitored by intermittent visualization of the upper tracts after the stents have been removed, as well as measurement of renal function. It is particularly useful to follow the ESR because it may fall dramatically as soon as steroids are exhibited. It is beneficial to reduce the dose of steroids as quickly as possible. Eventually the condition may settle sufficiently to allow the discontinuation of treatment without the reappearance of problems, but it is, of course, necessary to follow the patients up for life because relapse will remain a possibility.

Ureterolysis

Many urologists prefer surgical management of retroperitoneal fibrosis. Because the condition is bilateral, a transperitoneal approach through a midline incision often is recommended, but there are disadvantages. I prefer to use bilateral flank incisions and approach the ureter extraperitoneally, which is the natural route for open ureteric surgery.

The ureter must be identified and raised from its bed in the fibrosis. This is best done by finding the ureter either above or below the affected portion and freeing it by blunt dissection. Biopsy of the investing tissue is mandatory. Once the ureter is dissected away from the abnormal tissue below, it is necessary to dissect from it the layers of fibrosis that have been raised with it. This is difficult and hazardous because it is important to avoid ureteric perforation. The maneuver is made a little easier if ureteric stents are placed preoperatively.

It is necessary to mobilize the whole ureter from pelviureteric junction to bladder to make certain that continuation of the disease process does not affect the ureter where it has been left undisturbed. The blood supply is perfectly adequate for such a dissection but will not sustain the situation should the ureter be inadvertently divided. The ureter cannot be entirely freed because the pelviureteric junction and the bladder are fixed points that do not allow mobilization, and to that extent the operation is always incomplete.

Once the ureters have been adequately lysed, it is necessary to protect them from further involvement, and a variety of techniques for this have been described. The most common solutions are either to wrap them in mobilized greater omentum or to lateralize them by sewing down the peritoneum to the posterior abdominal wall inside the new line of the ureters. If the operation is done transperitoneally, there are potential kinks where the ureters enter and leave the peritoneal cavity and it is important to ensure that they follow a smooth course.

Postoperatively, remembering that the ureters remain at risk at their upper and lower ends, it is sensible to treat the patient with steroids at least until the ESR drops and remains down.

Suggested Readings

Baker LR, Mallinson WJ, Gregory MC, et al: Idiopathic retroperitoneal fibrosis: A retrospective analysis of 60 cases. Br J Urol 60:497, 1988

Bullock N: Idiopathic retroperitoneal fibrosis. BMJ 23:297, 1988

Mitchinson MJ: Retroperitoneal fibrosis revisited. Arch Pathol Lab Med 100:784, 1986

Yuh WT, Barloon WT, Sickels WJ, et al: Magnetic resonance imaging in the diagnosis and follow-up of idiopathic retroperitoneal fibrosis. J Urol 141:602, 1989

Metabolic Disorders

ACUTE RENAL FAILURE

CHRISTINE P. BASTL, M.D.

Philadelphia, Pennsylvania

Acute renal failure is defined as an abrupt decline in renal function to levels insufficient to maintain body homeostasis. The term does not define the pathophysiology, which is divided into prerenal, renal, and postrenal causes. Prerenal acute renal failure means the renal parenchyma remains intact but renal blood flow is so diminished that glomerular filtration cannot be maintained. This can occur with any type of extracellular volume depletion or inadequate cardiac output. Postrenal acute renal failure means the systemic circulation and the kidney are intact but the urinary drainage system is disrupted. Both kidneys must be involved because measurable renal function is not markedly affected by obstruction of one kidney. Intrinsic acute renal failure can be caused by any type of renal vascular, glomerular, tubular, or interstitial process, with similar biochemical consequences. This article concentrates specifically on the process otherwise called acute tubular necrosis (ATN).

Acute renal failure (ATN) can be divided into two etiologic groups, ischemic and nephrotoxic acute renal failure. Ischemic acute renal failure can occur with any insult that impairs blood flow sufficiently to cause epithelial cell death. The list of nephrotoxins grows yearly with our increasing therapeutic armamentarium. Most cases of ATN occur in the hospital. Thus, in unhospitalized individuals presenting with new-onset azotemia, other etiologies than ATN should be considered strongly. In hospitalized patients, the risk of ATN increases with the number of insults to which the patient is exposed, so the etiology is multifactorial in most patients. For instance, sepsis with volume depletion combined with gentamicin administration will result in ATN more frequently than any of these factors alone.

ATN is identified pathologically by the evidence of tubular cell disruption and death and sloughing off basement membranes in the absence of glomerular or interstitial pathology. The pathology does not correlate with the severity of the disease process. Recent evidence suggests this is because particular segments, the proximal tubule pars recta and the thick ascending limb of the loop of Henle, are the segments at greatest risk. Disruption of only these segments will result in acute renal failure.

In ATN the measured glomerular filtration rate approaches zero. There are four factors that contribute to this drastic decline: (1) decreased renal blood flow resulting from afferent arteriolar constriction, (2) tubular obstruction leading to increased tubular hydrostatic pressure, (3) passive backleak of glomerular filtrate across injured tubular epithelial barriers, and (4) decreased glomerular surface area caused by mesangial contraction.

Previously, ATN usually was diagnosed by the abrupt onset of oliguria (<500 ml of urine/day) or anuria. Recent studies indicate that half the cases of ATN are now nonoliguric. The following reasons are believed to contribute to this change: (1) More widespread determinations of blood chemistries lead to identification of nonoliguric ATN, (2) More cases of nephrotoxic ATN are occurring, and these are more often nonoliguric than is ischemic ATN, (3) Patients are being prepared for procedures with high risk of ATN by increased administration of intravenous fluids to prevent decreases in intravascular volume and decreased tubular flow rate. For instance, most cases of ATN occurring after cardiac surgery now tend to be nonoliguric.

DIAGNOSIS

Diagnosis of ATN requires differentiation of this entity from other etiologies of acute azotemia. Urinary tract obstruction always should be considered in the differential diagnosis. Bladder catheterization with the finding of a large residual urine volume can be both diagnostic and curative. A renal ultrasound should diagnose upper tract obstruction with rare exception.

Prerenal azotemia always should be considered and usually can be differentiated from ATN by several criteria. Vital signs and physical examination should suggest evidence of volume depletion in the former. Urine volume should be decreased in the former unless an osmotic diuresis or diuretics prevent the appropriate response to volume depletion. In ATN, urine volume can vary from anuria to polyuria. In prerenal azotemia the urine should not contain protein or blood. Microscopic examination may reveal only a slight increase in granular and hyaline casts. However, with ATN the microscopic examination should reveal increased numbers of casts, tubular cells, and even tubular cell casts.

Urine chemistries aid in the diagnosis. An intact kidney should respond to decreased renal blood flow by maximally conserving salt and water. Urine osmolality should be greater than 500 mOsm/liter, urine-to-plasma creatinine ratio greater than 40:1, urine Na^+ less than 20 mEq/liter, and fractional excretion of Na^+ less than 1 per cent. The injured kidney cannot maximally conserve salt and water, so urine osmolality is less than 350 mOsm/liter, urine-to-plasma creatinine ratio less than 20:1, urine Na^+ greater than 40 mEq/liter, and fractional excretion of Na^+ greater than 2 per cent.

After the onset of acute renal failure, the blood urea nitrogen (BUN) and creatinine levels will rise progressively. Because the glomerular filtration rate is extremely low, the rate of rise in BUN and creatinine reflects only the rate of production, with creatinine rising 1 to 2 mg/dl per day unless the patient has a reduced muscle mass. BUN rises 10 to 20 mg/dl per day but can rise more rapidly if the patient is hypercatabolic or has gastrointestinal bleeding. During this period, the kidney contributes little or nothing to fluid, electrolyte, or acid-base homeostasis. Without careful control of intake, severe derangements will result.

MANAGEMENT

Frequent monitoring of electrolytes and volume status, including weight, is essential. Sodium loss in urine depends on urine volume and can be negligible to large. Extrarenal losses in the postoperative or trauma patient can be large. In the undialyzed oliguric patient, sodium restriction must be severe to prevent volume overload, whereas in the nonoliguric patient Na^+ intake must match the losses to prevent volume depletion. Water intake also must be controlled. In the oligoanuric patient, water intake may need to be restricted to less than 1 liter/day (replacing only insensible losses) to prevent hyponatremia. Intravenous replacement fluids should be isotonic for extrarenal losses and half-normal for renal losses. Fever or hyperventilation will increase insensible losses, which are pure water losses.

Potassium intake must be limited to less than 60 mEq/day in the uncomplicated oligoanuric patient. However, if there is increased tissue breakdown even this restriction may not be sufficient to prevent hyperkalemia. Administration of the potassium exchange resin Kayexalate may be required.

Metabolic acidosis will occur because of failure to excrete the daily endogenously produced acid load. Under normal circumstances this averages 1 mEq/kg per day, but in the hypercatabolic patient the acid load can markedly increase. Sodium bicarbonate or sodium citrate should be administered to keep the serum bicarbonate above 15 mEq/liter. However, administration of both Kayexalate and alkali also results in sodium administration, with the potential of volume overload.

Severe metabolic alkalosis also can occur in the patient with copious vomiting or nasogastric suction, especially if nonabsorbable antacids are given. Administration of histamine-2 blockers should be used to prevent further loss of gastric acid. Hyperphosphatemia should be controlled by restricting phosphate intake and administration of calcium acetate with meals. However, if the serum phosphate is extremely high, aluminum-containing antacids should be used as the phosphate binder to prevent potential precipitation of calcium-phosphate salts in soft tissue. Magnesium-containing compounds should be avoided to prevent hypermagnesemia.

Moderate protein restriction must be employed to prevent rapid increases in uremic toxins. In addition, virtually all food proteins are high in potassium. However, patients with acute renal failure are catabolic. Thus, these restrictions are bound to result in negative nitrogen balance in these seriously ill patients.

Anemia will develop rapidly in these patients, and transfusions may be required. Packed cells should be given to avoid transfusion of plasma, which may have a very high potassium concentration.

All medications should be reviewed. Any medication that is in part or totally excreted by the kidney will require dose adjustment unless the potential toxicity at high levels is low. Because the creatinine is not stable and rising, the adjustment should be calculated on a glomerular filtration rate of less than 10 ml/min.

DIALYSIS TREATMENT

From the above discussion, it should be apparent that conservation management should be restricted to patients with mild, short-lived courses of acute renal failure. There is no definite level of BUN or creatinine at which dialysis should be started. Dialysis definitely should be started before the onset of uremic symptoms. Early and frequent dialysis is recommended, especially in surgical or trauma patients, in whom sometimes even daily dialysis is necessary to maintain the BUN below 100 mg/dl. Early dialysis is often necessary to control fluid and electrolyte imbalance. Institution of dialysis also allows increased nutritional intake. Dialysis allows administration of parenteral nutrition to decrease or reverse negative nitrogen balance. This may improve morbidity and mortality in selected groups of patients.

The ability to place indwelling subclavian catheters decreases the complexity and risk of hemodialysis. Low-dose heparin or no-heparin dialysis frequently are required to minimize the risk of bleeding. Bicarbonate dialysate should be used to maximize cardiovascular stability and reduce the risk of hypotension in unstable patients. Peritoneal dialysis can be used and may be preferred over hemodialysis in patients with cardiovascular instability and active bleeding. However, adequate clearances may not be obtainable in severely catabolic patients.

Continuous arteriovenous hemofiltration dialysis is a relatively new procedure that allows slow continuous fluid removal and dialysis using the patient's arterial pressure for ultrafiltration. This method allows dialysis and volume removal even in hypotensive patients, thus allowing continued administration of parenteral nutrition. However, it does require an indwelling arterial catheter and continuous heparinization of the dialyzer. No study has yet shown improvement in mortality, so the role of this modality is not yet clearly defined.

No matter which mode of dialytic therapy is employed, care should be taken to avoid hypotension and volume depletion because of emerging data that dialysis might prolong renal ischemia and recovery from ATN.

RECOVERY FROM ACUTE RENAL FAILURE

The onset of recovery usually is heralded by increasing urine volume, called the diuretic phase, followed by a plateauing and finally a decreasing BUN and creatinine. The urine volume can be quite large in the diuretic phase. Although some of this can be attributed to retained fluid, diuresis of retained osmols and tubular dysfunction play a large role. Electrolyte imbalance, including hypokalemia and volume depletion, are potential life-threatening complications. A generally accepted therapy is to replace urine volume and electrolytes completely until the serum creatinine plateaus and then slowly diminish fluid administration while monitoring weight, blood pressure, and serum creatinine. Even after urine volume has decreased, it should be remembered that total restoration of tubular function requires weeks to months. Thus, subtle defects in salt and water reabsorption still place the patient at risk of volume depletion when sodium and water intake are restricted.

Suggested Readings

Honda N, Hishida A: Pathophysiology of experimental nonoliguric acute renal failure. Kidney Int 43:513–521, 1993

Kaufman J, Dhakal M, Patel B, et al: Community acquired acute renal failure. Am J Kidney Dis 17:191–198, 1991

Pattison ME, Lee SM, Ogden DA: Continuous arteriovenous hemodiafiltration: An aggressive approach to the management of acute renal failure. Am J Kidney Dis 11:43–47, 1988

Rudnick MR, Bastl CP, Elfenbein IB, et al: The differential diagnosis of acute renal failure. *In* Brenner BM, Lazarus JM (eds): Acute Renal Failure, 2nd ed. New York, Churchill Livingstone, 1988, pp 177–232

CHRONIC RENAL FAILURE

CHRISTINE P. BASTL, M.D.

Philadelphia, Pennsylvania

Chronic renal insufficiency is a common medical problem. The estimated population of patients on hemodialysis is approximately 170,000. The number of patients with significant renal insufficiency is much larger. Chronic renal failure can result from any significant renal insult. It appears that, once a sufficient level of injury occurs, there will be a relentless progression to end-stage renal disease even if the original disease process is controlled or cured. The rate of progression will vary with the disease entity and the individual patient. The reason or reasons for progression is an intensely investigated question, with several factors implicated. The most popular theory at present is that glomerular hypertension and hyperperfusion of surviving glomeruli leads eventually to glomerular demise.

The kidney is remarkably able to adapt to decreasing renal mass. Single-nephron glomerular filtration rate (GRF) increases markedly, so that GFR is higher than expected for the reduction in renal tissue. Serum creatinine and blood urea nitrogen (BUN) usually remain within the normal range until the GFR is decreased by half. Sodium balance is maintained by a precise mechanism that increases excretion per nephron. Similar adaptive mechanisms exist for water, potassium, and phosphate excretion. Renal ammonia production increases to maintain acid-base homeostasis. Thus, abnormalities in serum electrolytes and acid-base balance usually are not apparent with mild to moderate loss of renal function. With some exceptions, sodium and potassium balance is maintained until the GFR falls below 10 per cent of normal when urine volume begins to decrease. Metabolic acidosis does not appear until the GFR is 20 to 30 per cent of normal unless the disease is one that preferentially results in renal tubular acidosis. The ability to maximally acidify urine and excrete titratable acid usually remains intact even with severe renal insufficiency. Hyperphosphatemia is only seen when the GFR decreases below 30 ml/min, and hypocalcemia is seen in only 40 per cent of end-stage patients. Renal concentrating ability is decreased with only moderate decrease in the GFR, but renal diluting ability remains intact until the GFR is less than 20 per cent of normal.

This remarkable ability to adapt to maintain normal balance in the basal condition belies the loss of ability to respond to pathophysiologic perturbations. Because the kidney already is vasodilated to maximize GFR, small decrements in intravascular volume or blood pressure can significantly acutely decrease renal blood flow and GFR in the compromised kidney, resulting in a rapid rise in BUN and creatinine. The kidney can no longer adapt rapidly to acute sodium restriction, so individuals with significant renal insufficiency are more prone to develop volume depletion as a result of renal salt wasting. Conversely, the excretion of an acute sodium load will require a longer time with the compromised kidney. Because maximal concentrating ability is diminished early, increased urine volume is obligated to excrete the daily solute load (10 mOsm/kg). Thus, a minimum urine volume of 1200 ml would be required to excrete 600 mOsm/day if the maximum urine osmolality is reduced to 500 mOsm/liter. Water restriction will rapidly produce hypernatremia. Excess potassium will be excreted but excretion is more prolonged, so that an acute potassium load will result in acute hyperkalemia.

In addition, a significant minority of patients with moderate renal insufficiency will have "hyporeninemic hypoaldosteronism." Under normal circumstances, despite low aldosterone levels these patients do not develop hyperkalemia, but, when they become volume depleted (usually during hospitalization), the other mechanisms that control potassium excretion become compromised and hyperkalemia develops. A supervening increase in acid production or bicarbonate loss, such as occurs in diarrhea, will result in significant acidosis because ammonium production cannot be further increased to meet the increased requirement. Normalization of serum bicarbonate after the insult also is delayed markedly.

MANAGEMENT OF SPECIFIC PROBLEMS RELATED TO CHRONIC RENAL INSUFFICIENCY

Hypertension

Renal disease is the most common cause of secondary hypertension. Furthermore, at least in some specific entities, hypertension hastens and control of hypertension will slow the progression of renal insufficiency. Control of hypertension is also essential to prevent cardiac and cerebrovascular disease. Any drug that normalizes blood pressure appears to protect renal function. Some classes, such as angiotensin-converting enzyme (ACE) inhibitors and calcium channel blockers, may both decrease proteinuria and specifically retard progression of glomerular disease. However, the ACE inhibitors can decrease GFR and cause hyperkalemia and worsening anemia in patients with advanced renal insufficiency, so they must be used with caution. Patients with glomerulonephritis are more prone to retain sodium and thus may have a volume-responsive component to their hypertension. Diuretics should be given to the edematous patient, but care should be taken not to overdiurese and superimpose prerenal azotemia.

Anemia

Anemia becomes a consistent feature as renal insufficiency advances. The etiology is decreased renal production of erythropoietin, bone marrow suppression by uremic toxins, and decreased red blood cell survival. The anemia can be aggravated further by any infection and gastrointestinal blood loss. With decreased production, blood drawing becomes a significant contributing factor. Iron stores should be evaluated by measurement of serum ferritin because serum iron, and total iron-binding capacity become unreliable indices. Usually the anemia is not severe enough to require transfusions. Selected patients with renal insufficiency not yet requiring dialysis are being treated with erythropoietin. This is probably preferable to transfusion.

Renal Osteodystrophy

It is clear that the bone disease of renal failure begins long before the patient reaches the point where dialysis is necessary. Parathyroid hormone becomes elevated early in renal insufficiency. 1,25-vitamin D also decreases early in renal disease. This combination decreases intestinal calcium absorption and increases bone resorption. Early treatment should involve restricting dietary phosphorus and supplementing dietary calcium. Calcium acetate given with each meal will bind dietary phosphate to keep serum phosphate in the normal range and simultaneously provide calcium. 1,25-vitamin D should be supplemented as renal insufficiency progresses. Long-term use of aluminum hydroxide to bind phosphate should be avoided to prevent aluminum toxicity. However, if serum phosphate is very high, it should be used initially to lower serum phosphate and then the patient should be switched to calcium acetate.

Platelet Dysfunction

There is a bleeding diathesis associated with renal insufficiency as a result of a qualitative platelet defect. This is manifested by a prolonged bleeding time, which may be present with only moderate elevation in creatinine. Bleeding time should be measured in any patient with renal insufficiency who has active bleeding or who needs to undergo a procedure with a high risk of bleeding. Bleeding time can be temporarily normalized with administration of desamino-D-arginine vasopressin (DDAVP) or normalized for longer periods with estrogen therapy.

DIETARY MANAGEMENT

As noted above, diet must be carefully modified to avoid precipitating imbalances. The usual error is that of employing restrictions that are necessary for the oliguric end-stage patient to the nonoliguric patient. Sodium should be restricted only in the volume-overloaded patient or patients with concurrent congestive heart failure. Water should not be restricted unless the serum sodium is less than 130 mEq/liter. Potassium restriction is usually unnecessary on a normal sodium diet. Protein restriction will decrease production of uremic toxins, but this is only necessary with advanced renal insufficiency. Protein restriction also may decrease the rate of decline of renal function in early renal insufficiency, but significant protein restriction can produce protein-calorie malnutrition with increased morbidity. The role and level of long-term protein restriction is not yet defined. Moderate phosphate restriction is advisable even early in the course of renal insufficiency to prevent renal osteodystrophy (see earlier in this article).

MEDICATIONS

Drugs are eliminated either by hepatic metabolism or renal excretion of intact drug or metabolite. Water-soluble drugs tend to be cleared by renal excretion. Protein binding of drugs is altered in renal insufficiency, thus changing bioavailability. The dose of any drug that is cleared by the kidney will need to be adjusted to the degree of renal insufficiency. This is especially true for drugs with a low therapeutic-to-toxic index, such as the aminoglycosides. However, even presumed innocuous substances may be contraindicated. Two examples of the latter are magnesium-containing laxatives or antacids, which can cause hypermagnesemia, and sodium phosphate enemas, which can cause severe hyperphosphatemia.

END-STAGE RENAL DISEASE

As a general rule, patients will not develop uremia until the GFR is less than 10 per cent of normal, a level at which urine volume begins to decrease. However, symptomatic uremia is associated with a high morbidity and mortality even if dialysis is instituted. The mortality rate in the first 90 days of dialysis varies from 10 to 25 per cent according to age and comorbid conditions. Because renal insufficiency usually progresses at an orderly rate, it is important to plan for dialysis or transplant before uremia supervenes. This allows establishment of vascular access in preparation for hemodialysis or peritoneal dialysis catheter placement and avoids the risk of emergency insertion of temporary accesses.

Dialysis should be instituted with the earliest signs of uremia: increasing fatigue, decreased appetite, or weight loss. Even with the universal availability of dialysis, this frequently does not occur, and dialysis must be instituted on an urgent basis for uremia. Life-threatening uremic conditions include pulmonary edema in the oliguric, diuretic unresponsive patient, uremic pericarditis, and uremic encephalopathy. The patient should be evaluated for pulmonary edema, the presence of a pericardial function rub, or the presence of asterexis. Any of these require urgent dialysis. Intercurrent conditions causing severe hyponatremia, severe metabolic acidosis, or severe or sustained hyperkalemia also require urgent dialysis for correction once urine volume has decreased.

Suggested Readings

Bucker NS: Sodium homeostasis in chronic renal disease. Kidney Int 21:886–897, 1982

Delmez JA, Slatapolsky E: Hyperphosphatemia: Its consequences and treatment in patients with chronic renal failure. Am J Kidney Dis 19:303–317, 1992

Lohr JW, Schwab SJ: Minimizing hemorrhagic complications in dialysis patients. J Am Soc Nephrol 2:961–975, 1991

Martinez-Maldonado M, Benabe JE, Cordova HR: Chronic clinical intrinsic renal failure. *In* Seldin DW, Giebish G (eds): The Kidney: Physiology and Pathophysiology, 2nd ed. New York, Raven Press, 1992, pp 3227–3288

ter Wee PM, Donker AJM: Clinical strategies for arresting progression of renal disease. Kidney Int 42:S-114–S-120, 1992

RENAL INVOLVEMENT BY DIABETES MELLITUS

MICHAEL HEIFETS, M.D.

Philadelphia, Pennsylvania

Approximately one quarter of all patients with diabetes are expected to develop renal involvement at some point during their lifetime. More than one third of all patients starting dialysis today have lost their kidney function as a result of diabetic renal disease. Using conservative estimates, this number will exceed 100,000 patients in the mid-1990s, with a price tag counted in billions of dollars! The care of these patients is complicated by the multisystem nature of diabetic end-organ involvement. Retinopathy, neuropathy, and coronary artery disease accompany diabetic nephropathy. Not surprisingly, the life expectancy of a diabetic patient on dialysis is under 4 years.

Renal involvement is more common in patients with type I (insulin-dependent) than type II (non–insulin-dependent) diabetes. However, the higher prevalence of the latter in the general population results in comparable numbers of patients with renal involvement resulting from either type of diabetes.

PATTERNS OF RENAL INVOLVEMENT AND DIAGNOSIS

Diabetic Glomerulopathy

This is the most common form of diabetic renal disease and the most common cause of diabetic end-stage renal disease. Diabetic glomerulopathy was first described in 1936 by Kimmelstiel and Wilson as nodular glomerulosclerosis. Glomeruli develop mesangial thickening, later forming nodules, and eventually there is complete glomerular obsolescence. Arteriolar hyalinosis is seen throughout the kidney and is similar to microvascular involvement elsewhere. Although nodular glomerulosclerosis can be nonspecific, the finding of hyalinosis and narrowing of glomerular *efferent* arterioles along with Bowman capsular drop formation is pathognomonic for diabetic glomerulopathy.

Clinically the disease follows three stages: (1) incipient (silent), (2) microalbuminuria, and (3) gross nephrotic syndrome with progressive azotemia. In the incipient stage, which may last up to 8 to 15 years, no signs of renal disease are detected. Glomerular filtration rate (GFR) usually is increased and could be as high as 180 ml/min. Prolonged hyperfiltration and hypertrophy, as well as exposure to hyperglycemic milieu, are postulated to lead to glomerular hypertension and set off the pathologic changes in the mesangium. When microalbuminuria (24-hour urinary albumin excretion in excess of 40 mg) develops, it may be the only sign of impending renal catastrophe for 2 to 3 years. Development of gross nephrotic-range proteinuria with hypoalbuminemia, hyperlipidemia, and anasarca is associated with a rapid decline of GFR. The magnitude of proteinuria in diabetic glomerulopathy rarely exceeds 12 to 15 gm in 24 hours. If proteinuria far in excess of this range is seen, an alternative glomerular disease must be sought.

Diagnosis of diabetic glomerulopathy usually does not require biopsy in a typical patient with diabetes for over 10 years, associated retinopathy, and urinalysis usually showing protein and hyalin casts. Although hematuria and red blood cell casts occasionally are seen in pure diabetic nephropathy, such a finding must involve the search for other causes of hematuric glomerulopathies. The time from the first detection of the nephrotic syndrome, when serum creatinine is still "normal," to the need for dialysis could be as short as 1 to 2 years. Serum creatinine is an inadequate estimate of GFR in progressive diabetic glomerulopathy and may not become elevated until GFR is well under 50 ml/min. Therefore, plans for dialysis and/or transplantation must be made whenever the patient develops frank nephrotic syndrome, because the disease usually follows a rapid and inexorable progression from that point.

Hyporeninemic Hypoaldosteronism

Decreased renin production by the juxtaglomerular apparatus may stem from arteriolar hyalinosis and leads to depressed aldosterone levels. Patients present with hyperkalemia and hyperchloremic acidosis disproportionate to the reduction in GFR. Factors impairing excretion of potassium, such as volume depletion, use of nonsteroidal anti-inflammatory drugs, potassium-containing salt substitutes, potassium-sparing diuretics, beta blockers, and angiotensin-converting enzyme (ACE) inhibitors, may result in life-threatening hyperkalemia. Diagnosis is made by finding a typical combination of hyperkalemia and hyperchloremic acidosis with normal an-ion gap, with only mild to moderate reduction of GFR and absence of urinary tract obstruction. Measurements of renin and aldosterone are unnecessary in a typical presentation.

Atheromatous Renal Disease

Atherosclerosis is accelerated in patients with diabetes and renal insufficiency. Atherosclerotic disease of the main renal arteries presents as renal artery stenosis and occlusion. Bilateral disease may be a cause of end-stage renal failure. The possibility of renal artery stenosis should be entertained in any patient with sudden development or progressive worsening of hypertension, requiring escalating doses of medications, and rapidly worsening renal function. Development of unilateral abdominal bruit makes the diagnosis nearly certain. Diagnostic procedures include captopril renal nuclear scan, renal vein renin sampling, and renal arteriogram. Nuclear scan may show unilateral decrease in isotope excretion after administration of captopril, indicating a hemodynamically significant renal vascular lesion. Nuclear scanning may not detect bilateral disease as well. Renal arteriogram remains the diagnostic gold standard. It must be noted, however, that diabetic patients are at increased risk for radiocontrast-induced acute renal failure, and adequate volume expansion must accompany the procedure.

Atheroembolic Renal Disease

This is observed in patients with marked atherosclerosis of the aorta after cardiac catheterization, aortic surgery, and similar procedures.

Urinary Tract Involvement

Autonomic neuropathy of the urinary bladder is likely to result in increased postvoid residual and *chronic urinary retention,* leading to obstructive uropathy. Increased susceptibility to infection and impaired voiding results in higher incidences of pyelonephritis and *papillary necrosis.* Pyelonephritis may present as or lead to *emphysematous pyelonephritis* and *perinephric abscess.* Recurrent infection may develop into *xanthogranulomatous pyelonephritis.*

Acute Renal Failure

Patients with diabetes and developing renal insufficiency may be more susceptible than other patients to acute renal insults, such as exposure to radiographic contrast dye. Awareness of the risks and vigilant volume repletion may contribute to a reduced incidence of acute renal failure. Prerenal azotemia resulting from severe hyperglycemia and severe volume depletion is easily reversed with insulin and fluid replacement. Ketone bodies by themselves may interfere with some chemical assays and produce false elevation of creatinine, resulting in unnecessary work-up for a nonexisting problem.

MANAGEMENT

The overall goal of managing the diabetic patient is early detection, intervention, and prevention of end-organ failure, be it heart, kidney, or eye, while avoiding side effects that are specific for a diabetic patient.

Although aggressive insulin therapy has not been shown convincingly to retard the progression of diabetic renal disease, dietary protein restriction down to 0.8 gm/kg per day long has been advocated as an effective means of retarding deterioration of renal function in any progressive renal disease. Its usefulness is limited by lack of compliance, because it requires drastic reduction to approximately half of the average North American daily protein intake. Dietary phosphate and potassium restriction are instituted depending on the degree of renal failure and hyperkalemia.

Hypertension is now recognized as an important risk factor contributing to the development of diabetic glomerulopathy and accelerating progression to renal failure. Several studies in diabetic patients with microalbuminuria indicate that normalization of elevated blood pressures to below 140/90 mm Hg actually may lead to the sustained reduction of albuminuria and delay the progression to overt nephrotic syndrome, thus slowing the progression to end-stage renal disease. Once the disease has reached its final phase of overt proteinuria and progressive decline of GFR, any impact of such intervention would be minimal. It appears that two classes of antihypertensive agents—ACE inhibitors and calcium channel blockers—may confer additional renoprotection and antiproteinuric effects beyond their excellent antihypertensive activity. The use of antihypertensive drugs is complicated by side effects of some classes of agents that become intolerable in diabetics. These include acute renal failure in patients with pre-existing renal disease (ACE inhibitors), worsening hyperkalemia (ACE inhibitors, beta blockers, potassium-sparing diuretics), orthostatic hypotension (all vasodilators), and worsening blood sugar control (beta blockers and thiazide diuretics). Thus, a low-dose diuretic with the possible addition of either a calcium channel blocker, an ACE inhibitor, or both should provide the best combination of effective antihypertensive regimen, safety, patient tolerability, and compliance.

Treatment of hyporeninemic hypoaldosteronism and associated hyperkalemia and acidosis is accomplished by strict potassium restriction and alkali administration (sodium bicitra). Sodium polystyrene resin (Kayexalate) may be useful for short-term therapy, but its long-term use should be avoided. Fludrocortisone (100 to 400 μg/day) may be required for patients with refractory hyperkalemia.

ORGAN TRANSPLANTATION AND DIALYSIS

The dismal life expectancy of a diabetic patient starting dialysis can be improved only by a successful kidney transplant from a relative fully matched for human lymphocyte antigen (HLA). Cadaveric kidney or pancreas transplantation does not significantly extend life expectancy when adjusted for all risk factors. Pancreas transplantation alone may benefit a few patients with exceptionally brittle diabetes, but has not yet been demonstrated to either prolong survival or prevent renal disease. Combined kidney-pancreas transplantation has prevented development of diabetic glomerulopathy in the transplanted kidney in only a few cases and has not improved graft and patient survival to the extent seen with kidney transplant from an HLA-identical relative.

Both chronic hemodialysis (in-center and home) and chronic ambulatory peritoneal dialysis (CAPD) are widely used in diabetics. A few observations indicate a possible increase in the rate of amputations in diabetic patients on CAPD. The major deciding factors remain patient preference, compliance, and access availability.

Suggested Readings

Kasinath BS: Non-diabetic renal disease in patients with diabetes mellitus. Am J Med 75:613, 1983

Makita Z, Radoff S, et al: Advanced glycosylation end products in patients with diabetic nephropathy. N Engl J Med 325:836, 1991

Mogensen CE, Christensen CK: Predicting diabetic nephropathy in insulin-dependent patients. N Engl J Med 311:89, 1984

Parving HH, Hommel E, Smidt UM: Effect of antihypertensive treatment on kidney function in diabetic nephropathy. BMJ 294:1443, 1987

RENAL TUBULAR ACIDOSIS

ALAN D. JENKINS, M.D.

Charlottesville, Virginia

Renal tubular acidosis (RTA) is a syndrome of disordered renal acidification that causes a metabolic acidosis, usually with a concurrently low serum chloride concentration and additional electrolyte abnormalities. The ability to excrete normal amounts of acid into the urine is thought to be responsible for the entire syndrome, because the administration of sodium bicarbonate corrects the hyperchloremic acidosis and the excessive urinary losses of potassium, calcium, and phosphorus.

The fundamental defect in RTA is a failure to acidify the urine, but the mechanisms differ from the two major types of RTA: distal RTA (classical or type I) and proximal RTA (type II). The normal process of urinary acidification involves two sequential steps along the nephron. Virtually all of the filtered bicarbonate is reabsorbed in the proximal tubule, while the secretion of hydrogen ion (H^+) against a large electrochemical gradient produces titratable acid in the distal tubule. A defect in the first step is responsible for proximal RTA, whereas the failure to maintain a steep H^+ gradient in the distal tubule is responsible for distal RTA. The reabsorption of bicarbonate in the proximal tubule is a high-capacity system that is unable to maintain a large H^+ gradient, whereas the distal tubular mechanism is a low-capacity system that achieves a high H^+ gradient.

Under normal circumstances the urinary pH can be reduced to less than 5.5. The ability of the proximal tubule to reabsorb filtered bicarbonate is reduced in proximal RTA. If the plasma bicarbonate concentration is low (15 mmol/liter), the distal tubule still has the capacity to reabsorb the small amount of bicarbonate that is delivered to it by the proximal tubule, and the urine pH can be reduced to 5.5. However, if the serum bicarbonate concentration is normal (25 mmol/liter), the distal nephron is unable to compensate for the deficient reabsorption of filtered bicarbonate in the proximal tubule. This results in a high urine pH (>7.5). As much as 25 per cent of the filtered load of bicarbonate may be excreted in the final urine, compared with a normal excretion fraction of less than 0.1 per cent.

The distal tubule is unable to provide for the net excretion of H^+ in distal RTA. The precise defect is unknown. The H^+ pump in the tubular membrane may be defective, or back-diffusion of secreted H^+ may lead to dissipation of the gradient and inefficient H^+ excretion. Regardless of the precise mechanism, net H^+ secretion is reduced, and the urine pH cannot be reduced below about 6.0 no matter how severe the systemic acidosis.

The different mechanisms responsible for proximal and distal RTA also provide an explanation for why large amounts of sodium bicarbonate are needed to treat proximal RTA but much smaller amounts are needed to treat distal RTA. The correction of the acidosis in a patient with distal RTA leads to little increase in the urinary excretion of bicarbonate. Only enough bicarbonate is needed to balance the daily production of fixed acid. When proximal RTA is treated, the increase in the plasma bicarbonate concentration leads to a dramatic increase in the urinary excretion of bicarbonate. This "wastage" of bicarbonate demands that large amounts of bicarbonate be administered to correct the system acidosis. From 5 to 10 times as much bicarbonate will be needed to treat a patient with proximal RTA as to treat a patient with distal RTA.

DISTAL (TYPE I OR CLASSICAL) RTA

Distal RTA may exist in either a primary or a secondary form. The primary form may be subdivided into an infantile type or an adult type. Adult, or persistent primary, RTA occurs predominantly in females. Most of the cases are sporadic, but the disease may be inherited. The reclamation of filtered bicarbonate is intact in the proximal tubule, but the distal tubule is unable to generate or maintain a steep lumen-peritubular H^+ gradient. Ammonia production is normal.

The electrolyte abnormalities are responsible for the symptoms. Chronic acidosis may contribute to the impaired growth of children with distal RTA. (Tiny Tim in Charles Dickens' *A Christmas Carol* probably was afflicted with distal RTA.) Although urinary wasting of calcium and phosphorus may lead to osteomalacia, the hyperchloremic acidosis is so readily detected that patients rarely are left untreated long enough to develop this complication. Nephrocalcinosis or nephrolithiasis occurs in 75 per cent of patients. Urinary potassium wasting may result in severe hypokalemia and a flaccid paralysis.

The diagnosis is made when a systemic acidosis (serum bicarbonate <20 mmol/liter) is present and the urine pH is not below 5.5. An ammonium chloride (NH_4Cl) load often is used as a stress test to confirm the diagnosis. Liquid NH_4Cl (100 mg/kg, as a 5% solution) is given in the evening. The patient voids at 6:00 A.M., drinks three glasses of water, and voids again at 7:30 A.M.. The pH of this latter urine specimen is measured with a pH meter. This pH will be 5.0 to 5.5 in a healthy individual. If the pH is greater than 5.5 and the serum bicarbonate is greater than 20 mmol/liter, the NH_4Cl load is repeated and the urine pH is rechecked in 4 hours.

Treatment consists of fluid and electrolyte replacement, including sodium, potassium, and bicarbonate. Adults require 90 to 150 mEq of base every 24 hours. Citrate solution (Polycitra, 30 mEq base/15 ml) or sodium bicarbonate may be used: the citrate solution will not produce abdominal bloating or belching. The systemic acidosis should be corrected gradually so that the hypokalemia is not exacerbated.

Infantile (Transient) Primary RTA

This disorder usually begins within the first year of life and is accompanied by renal bicarbonate wasting and the acidification defect of distal RTA (a syndrome once labeled type III RTA). The fraction of filtered bicarbonate excreted in the urine is 6 to 14 per cent in this disorder, compared with 1 to 3 per cent in adult distal RTA. Although nephrocalcinosis is uncommon, patients with this condition have anorexia, vomiting, failure to thrive, and polyuria. Recovery is complete with adequate treatment.

Incomplete Distal RTA

Some patients with recurrent calcium oxalate nephrolithiasis may have a subtle acid-base disorder. Although these individuals do not have a systemic acidosis, they are unable to lower their urine pH sufficiently after an NH_4Cl load. Even though a systemic acidosis is not present, the urinary citrate level is low, as it is in patients with the complete form. This probably is due to an intracellular acidosis. Treatment is the same as that for the complete form.

Secondary RTA

Distal RTA may be a manifestation of an identifiable systemic disease, usually a dysproteinemic state such as hypergammaglobulinemia, macroglobulinemia, or cryoglobulinemia. It is not clear how these disorders produce the acidification defect.

PROXIMAL (TYPE II) RTA

The distal tubular acidification mechanism is intact in this disorder, but the reabsorption of filtered bicarbonate by the proximal tubule is reduced. If the plasma bicarbonate is normal, there is massive bicarbonaturia and a high urine pH. The urine pH will be low in the presence of a systemic acidosis.

Most cases are associated with an underlying disorder of proximal tubular function, such as Fanconi syndrome, hereditary fructose intolerance, Wilson's disease, or multiple myeloma. Vitamin D deficiency may lead to proximal RTA in children. The most common cause of proximal RTA in adults is intestinal malabsorption that leads to vitamin D deficiency, hypocalcemia, secondary hyperparathyroidism, and hypophosphatemia. Nephrolithiasis does not occur in proximal RTA.

Treatment is aimed at the underlying disorder. In patients with vitamin D deficiency, vitamin D therapy usually will correct the acidification defect, and long-term administration of base may not be necessary. The metabolic abnormalities are treated if no causative disorder can be identified. The acidosis is corrected with alkali, and the hypokalemia with potassium (as the alkaline salt: potassium bicarbonate or potassium citrate). Calcium supplementation may be needed for persistent hypocalcemia.

TYPE IV RTA

An acidification defect may accompany a reduction in the renal clearance of potassium. The disorder is thought to involve the cation-exchange segment of the distal nephron, in which aldosterone stimulates H^+ secretion. Type IV RTA occurs most frequently in the syndrome of hyporeninemic hypoaldosteronism, a disorder found in elderly patients with diabetes. Hyperkalemic RTA also has been found in patients with obstructive uropathy.

If hypoaldosteronism is present, the acidosis and hyperkalemia may be corrected by fludrocortisone (0.01 mg/day). Restriction of dietary potassium can be useful, and alkali may be necessary to correct the acidosis. Treatment of the acidosis also will reduce the hyperkalemia.

CARBONIC ANHYDRASE INHIBITION

Urolithiasis is a complication of long-term treatment with carbonic anhydrase inhibitors. Carbonic anhydrase, which catalyzes the hydration of carbon dioxide, is present in both the proximal and the distal nephron. Because carbonic anhydrase aids the proximal reabsorption of filtered bicarbonate and the distal secretion of H^+, the administration of an inhibitor of this enzyme, such as acetazolamide, causes a proximal and distal RTA. Treatment with acetazolamide produces alterations in the ionic composition of urine, such as a low citrate concentration, that closely resemble those found in untreated distal RTA. All of the changes can be reversed by stopping administration of the carbonic anhydrase inhibitor.

Suggested Readings

Batlle DC, Arruda JAL, Kuntzman NA: Hyperkalemic distal renal tubular acidosis associated with obstructive uropathy. N Engl J Med 304:373–380, 1981

Caldas A, Broyer M, Dechaux M, et al: Primary distal tubular acidosis in childhood: Clinical study and long term follow-up of 28 patients. J Pediatr 121:233–241, 1992

Caruana RJ, Buckalew VM Jr: The syndrome of distal (type I) renal tubular acidosis. Medicine 67:84–99, 1988

Kinkead TM, Tan FSJ, Menon M: The varied forms of RTA and how to treat them. Contemp Urol 3:33–54, 1991

Morris RC Jr: Renal tubular acidosis. N Engl J Med 304: 418–419, 1981

Valtin H: Renal Dysfunction: Mechanisms Involved in Fluid and Solute Imbalance. Boston, Little, Brown, 1979, pp 354–370

HYPOKALEMIC NEPHROPATHY

LOUIS J. RILEY, Jr., M.D.
Philadelphia, Pennsylvania

Hypokalemic nephropathy results from chronic potassium depletion and manifests clinically as a vasopressin-resistant polyuria or nephrogenic diabetes insipidus. A number of current hypotheses propose a role for increased prostaglandin synthesis, a common finding in hypokalemic disorders, as partially responsible for the polyuria. This is consistent with the experimental observation that prostaglandin E does antagonize the hydroosmotic effect of arginine vasopressin (AVP). However, the data supporting this hypothesis are not without inconsistencies. Potassium depletion is also proposed to impair the adenylate cyclase response to AVP on the inner medullary collecting duct. Finally, hypokalemia has been associated with failure to maintain a medullary hypertonic interstitium, which would, of course, result in a nephrogenic diabetes insipidus.

Although the pathogenetic mechanism remains to be elucidated, there is a consistent pathologic picture of hypokalemic nephropathy that is characterized by tubular vacuolization. Recently, chronic hypokalemia has been found to be associated with enhanced renal cystogenesis that may lead to interstitial scarring and renal insufficiency.

Hypokalemia of any etiology may result in hypokalemic nephropathy. Therefore, conditions known to be associated with chronic hypokalemia must be identified and treated prophylactically to avoid the complication of nephropathy. Clearly, if the underlying conditions can be treated, this is preferable. In the event one is dealing with a condition for which there is no cure, prudent oral potassium supplementation along with potassium-sparing diuretics such as amiloride, spironolactone, or triamterene are appropriate therapeutic measures. Converting enzyme inhibitors also would decrease kaliuresis and help restore the serum potassium to within normal range. Of note, functional recovery of renal concentrating ability may be prolonged over a period of 1 to 3 months after correction of the potassium deficits.

Therapy of hypokalemic nephropathy beyond potassium repletion is essentially therapy of nephrogenic diabetes insipidus. Thiazide diuretics administered to patients on a restricted salt intake produce volume depletion, reduce the glomerular filtration rate, and enhance proximal tubular avidity for filtrate. In this process, delivery of filtrate to the distal diluting segments is reduced, thereby decreasing polyuria. Caution must be exercised to ensure that hypokalemia is not exacerbated by thiazide use in this setting.

Suggested Readings

Dusing R, Attalah AA, Prezyna AP, et al: Renal biosynthesis of prostaglandin E_2 and F_2: Dependence on extracellular potassium. J Lab Clin Med 92:699, 1978

Earley LE, Ortloff J: The mechanism of antidiuresis associated with the administration of hydrochlorothiazide to patients with vasopressin resistant diabetes insipidus. J Clin Invest 41:1988, 1962

Mannitius A, Levitin H, Beck D, et al: On the mechanism of impairment of renal concentrating ability in potassium deficiency. J Clin Invest 39:684, 1960

Relman AS, Schwartz WB: The kidney in potassium depletion. Am J Med 24:764, 1958

Torres VE, Young WF, Offord KP, et al: Association of hypokalemia, aldosteronism and renal cysts. N Engl J Med 323:129, 1990

AMYLOIDOSIS

GERRI A. SCHULMAN, M.D.

Philadelphia, Pennsylvania

Amyloidosis results when tissues are infiltrated with an insoluble protein that ultimately leads to tissue dysfunction. These proteins form a beta-pleated sheet that is responsible for their resistance to proteolytic digestion and their diagnostic appearance, when stained with Congo red, of reddish pink deposits that show green birefringence when exposed to polarized light. The identity of the amyloidogenic protein is the basis of current classifications.

Primary amyloidosis, now known as AL amyloidosis, results from overproduction of NH_2-terminal fragments of immunoglobulin light chains. Approximately 20 per cent of AL amyloidosis is associated with multiple myeloma. Secondary amyloidosis results from chronic infections or inflammatory diseases and is due to overproduction and perhaps abnormal processing of protein AA, an acute-phase reactant synthesized by hepatocytes. Amyloid AA also is found in familial Mediterranean fever. Other types of amyloidosis usually are associated with more limited tissue distribution. Autosomal dominant familial amyloidosis most often is due to mutations in the gene for transthyretin (prealbumin) and is designed amyloid AF. Amyloidosis seen in patients on chronic hemodialysis is due to accumulations of beta-2–microglobulin ($A\beta_2M$). Localized cerebral amyloid (CAA) and senile cardiac amyloidosis (SSA) also have been identified.

Clinically, patients with AL or AA amyloidosis often present with nonspecific complaints of fatigue and weight loss or with symptoms related to infiltration of the kidney, heart, or nerves. Renal involvement most commonly is due to amyloid deposition in the glomerulus and results in proteinuria, which often is in the nephrotic range. Once nephrotic syndrome develops, rapid progression to end-stage renal disease is likely. Patients who develop renal insufficiency without nephrotic-range proteinuria have prominent interstitial or vascular depositions of amyloid instead of extensive glomerular involvement. Cardiac infiltration results in heart failure initially caused by diastolic dysfunction and later caused by systolic failure. Cardiac amyloidosis less often manifests as arrhythmias caused by infiltration of the conduction system or ischemia from infiltration of small arteries. Nerve involvement can present as paresthesias or autonomic neuropathy leading to orthostatic hypotension, impotence, and diarrhea. Other common manifestations of amyloidosis are carpal tunnel syndrome, hepatomegaly, macroglossia, and upper body purpura. Clinical manifestations of AA amyloidosis are similar to those in AL amyloidosis except that renal involvement and goiter may be more common and cardiac and neurologic disease less common.

The diagnosis of amyloidosis requires demonstration of tissue amyloid deposits. Rectal and abdominal fat pad biopsies are positive in approximately 80 per cent of patients. The presence of monoclonal light chains in serum or urine is necessary to diagnose AL amyloidosis. Serum and urine immunoelectrophoresis is more sensitive than protein electrophoresis. Bone marrow biopsy is required to exclude multiple myeloma.

The prognosis of systemic amyloidosis is poor, especially if cardiac failure has developed. Patients with myeloma who respond to chemotherapy have improved overall survival and may have stabilization of or improvement in renal function. Prospective trials of melphalan and prednisone in patients with AL amyloidosis in the absence of myeloma have shown regression of proteinuria but have not demonstrated improved survival. The only established therapy for secondary amyloidosis is reversal of the underlying chronic inflammation. Steroids are of no benefit, and the efficacy of immunosuppressives has not been evaluated prospectively. Colchicine benefits patients with familial Mediterranean fever when given prior to the onset of renal insufficiency and nephrotic syndrome, but has not been shown to improve the prognosis in patients with other causes of amyloidosis.

Suggested Readings

Gertz MA, Kyle RA: Primary systemic amyloidosis—a diagnostic primer. Mayo Clin Proc 64:1505, 1989

Gertz MA, Kyle RA: Secondary systemic amyloidosis: Response and survival in 64 patients. Medicine 70:246, 1991

ALPORT SYNDROME

ELLIE KELEPOURIS, M.D.

Philadelphia, Pennsylvania

Alport syndrome is an autosomal dominant, hematuric hereditary glomerulonephritis that is characterized by progressive loss of renal function. Eventual end-stage renal disease (ESRD) of nearly all affected male patients is a central feature. Although it may be accompanied by nonrenal features, including hearing loss and ocular defects, their presence is not essential to the diagnosis. Clinically, pathologically, and ultrastructurally identical hereditary nephritis has been found both in kindreds with hearing loss and kindreds with normal hearing, and the latter accounts for 50 per cent of all adult cases of Alport syndrome. There is both a juvenile and an adult-type nephritis, with ESRD occurring before 31 years of age in the former and after 31 years of age in the latter. Hearing loss is a universal accompaniment of the juvenile type.

The diagnosis of Alport syndrome is based on a combination of genetic, pathologic, and clinical criteria. The prime criterion for the diagnosis in kindreds is the demonstration of a family history of chronic glomerulonephritis in multiple closely related persons. Chronic hematuria is the cardinal sign of Alport syndrome, present and persistent from birth in 100 per cent of males and in 80 to 90 per cent of females who have a nephritis gene. Infants present with gross hematuria that also may follow sore throats or other infections, whereas macroscopic hematuria is not common in adults. Proteinuria is variable and mild early in the course of the disease, with heavy or increasing proteinuria implying a worse prognosis and an approach to ESRD. In adult-type Alport syndrome, renal function is normal for years and then progresses to end stage within 6 years from diagnosis. Hypertension usually is present at this stage and worsens as renal function deteriorates. Although renal failure is inevitable for affected males, few females become uremic. In fact, clinically normal gene carriers are preponderantly female and should be identified for genetic counseling and selection of kidney donors.

Although the diagnosis of Alport syndrome is suspected in patients with microscopic hematuria, proteinuria, and a positive family history for nephritis, it is confirmed by renal biopsy. Although there are glomerular lesions and the appearance of foam cells in the interstitium on light microscopy, these are by no means pathognomonic. The diagnosis rests on the presence of glomerular ultrastructural changes such as widespread lamellation of the glomerular basement membrane and a splitting of the lamina densa, resulting in a "basket weave" appearance. The immunofluorescence is characteristically negative and there is no complement deposition.

Recently it has been demonstrated that the nephritis in some Alport families is caused by mutation of an X-linked gene, the COL4A5 collagen gene, which physically maps to the Xq22 chromosomal region. This gene codes for a specific basement collagen monomer chain that is abnormal in some kindreds with Alport syndrome.

No specific treatment is known to affect the underlying process or alter the course of the disease. Control of hypertension is paramount and, when patients progress to ESRD, dialysis and transplantation are offered. Alport syndrome has not recurred after transplantation. In selecting a living related donor, meticulous and repeated urinalyses for hematuria should be done.

Suggested Readings

Atkin CL, Gregory MC: Alport syndrome. *In* Schrier RW, Gottschalk CW (eds): Diseases of the Kidney, 5th ed. Boston, Little, Brown, 1993, pp 617–635

Barker DF, Hostikka SL, Zhou J, et al: Identification of mutations in the COL4A5 collagen gene in Alport syndrome. Science 248:1224, 1990

Milliner DS, Pierides AM, Holley KE: Renal transplantation in Alport's syndrome: Antiglomerular basement membrane glomerulonephritis in allograft. Mayo Clin Proc 57:35, 1992

INTERSTITIAL NEPHRITIS

LOUIS J. RILEY, Jr., M.D.

Philadelphia, Pennsylvania

Interstitial nephritis, or tubulointerstitial nephritis, is an inflammation of the kidney characterized by infiltration of the interstitium with polymorphonuclear cells, mononuclear cells, lymphocytes, eosinophils, and/or plasma cells. Depending on the clinical presentation, interstitial nephritis is classified either as acute or chronic.

ACUTE INTERSTITIAL NEPHRITIS

Acute interstitial nephritis is characterized by a reduction in glomerular filtration rate (increase in the serum creatinine over days to weeks [and in some cases over months]) associated with proteinuria of generally less than 2 gm/24 hours. Microscopic examination of the urinary sediment is likely to reveal white blood cells, white blood cell casts (fairly pathognomonic for interstitial renal inflammation), and red blood cells. Eosinophiluria, more easily detectable in the urine with Wright stain or Hansel stain, helps to confirm the diagnosis. However, the absence of eosinophils in the urine by no means excludes the diagnosis. Peripheral eosinophilia also may accompany interstitial nephritis.

The course of acute interstitial nephritis can vary from mild renal insufficiency bespeaking minimal glomerular involvement to a fulminant course with glomerular involvement, oliguria, and hypertension requiring temporary dialytic support. Usually, however, acute interstitial nephritis becomes clinically manifest because of tubular dysfunction, which may present as a general tubulopathy or with features of either proximal tubule dysfunction (glycosuria, phosphaturia, uricosuria, aminoaciduria, and/or bicarbonaturia) or distal tubule dysfunction (salt wasting, defective acidification and concentration, and defective potassium excretion).

The three broad etiologic categories of acute interstitial nephritis are drug related, infection related, and idiopathic. The list of drugs associated with interstitial nephritis continues to increase, with semisynthetic penicillins, sulfa drugs, nonsteroidal anti-inflammatory drugs, and histamine-2 receptor blockers prominently listed. Infection-related interstitial nephritis has been described in association with viral agents (cytomegalovirus, Epstein-Barr virus, Hantaan virus, influenza, and others), bacteria (e.g., leptospirosis, brucellosis, diphtheria, streptococcosis), and protozoa (toxoplasmosis). Idiopathic acute interstitial nephritis is typified by the uveitis-nephritis syndrome.

The predictable therapy for acute interstitial nephritis is withdrawal of the offending agent or inciting antigen. Clearly, this is more easily done with drug etiologies than with infectious etiologies, and is impossible with idiopathic acute interstitial nephritis. The beneficial effect of steroids in shortening the course of acute interstitial nephritis is controversial.

CHRONIC INTERSTITIAL NEPHRITIS

Chronic interstitial nephritis is a chronic inflammatory process that results in progressive renal dysfunction through renal insufficiency to renal failure and eventually end-stage renal disease. The most widely recognized cause of chronic interstitial nephritis secondary to drugs is analgesic nephropathy, which results from chronic ingestion of cumulatively large amounts of phenacetin-containing analgesics. Presumably, metabolism to cytotoxic reactive metabolites in the renal papillae is responsible for the injury. Diabetes mellitus, although recognized as principally a glomerular disease, is a major cause (if not the leading cause) of chronic tubulointerstitial nephritis; it presents clinically as type IV renal tubular acidosis. Reflux nephropathy with recurrent urinary tract infections may result in chronic tubulointerstitial nephritis as well as a progressive glomerulopathy. Lead nephropathy, typically the consequence of indiscreet ingestion of "moonshine" (alcohol distilled in leaded radiators), is a chronic tubulointerstitial nephritis associated with hypertension and gouty attacks. Unfortunately, once initiated, there is no therapy for chronic interstitial nephritis.

Suggested Readings

Burnier M, Jaeger P, Campiche M, et al: Idiopathic acute interstitial nephritis and uveitis in the adult: Report of 1 case and review of the literature. Am J Nephrol 6: 312, 1986

Linton AL, Clark WF, Driedger AA, et al: Acute interstitial nephritis due to drugs. Ann Intern Med 93:735, 1980

Murray T, Goldberg M: Chronic interstitial nephritis: Etiologic factors. Ann Intern Med 82:453, 1975

Ten RM, Torres VE, Milliner DS, et al: Acute interstitial nephritis: Immunologic and clinical aspects. Mayo Clin Proc 63:921, 1988

FANCONI SYNDROME

GERRI A. SCHULMAN, M.D.

Philadelphia, Pennsylvania

The proximal tubule of the kidney reabsorbs 80 to 85 per cent of filtered bicarbonate and most filtered glucose, phosphate, urate, and amino acids. Abnormalities in proximal tubule bicarbonate reabsorption result in bicarbonate wasting, producing a proximal or type II renal tubular acidosis (RTA). The coexistence of a type II RTA and glycosuria, phosphaturia, uricosuria, and/or aminoaciduria is known as Fanconi syndrome. Thus, Fanconi syndrome results from failure of multiple proximal tubular reabsorptive pathways. The common denominator in all these pathways is that reabsorption occurs by Na^+-dependent, secondary active transport. The low intracellular Na^+ concentration created by the Na^+/K^+-adenosine triphosphatase (ATPase) on the basolateral membrane creates a favorable electrochemical gradient for Na^+ entry from the tubular lumen into the cell. Glucose, phosphate, and amino acid uptake is coupled to Na^+ uptake by luminal membrane cotransporters. Bicarbonate reabsorption is indirectly mediated by the luminal membrane Na^+/H^+ antiport. Because in Fanconi syndrome multiple transport processes are abnormal, it is unlikely that a primary defect in each cotransporter is responsible. Instead, it has been postulated that Fanconi syndrome is caused by a decreased lumen-to-cell Na^+ gradient secondary to abnormalities in Na^+/K^+-ATPase, decreased cell ATP supply or increased membrane Na^+ permeability. Alternatively, rather than decreased solute entry into cells, Fanconi syndrome could be due to increased solute efflux. The exact pathogenesis remains unknown.

The causes of the Fanconi syndrome are divided into inherited and acquired forms. The inherited types can be an isolated abnormality or part of a systemic disorder such as cystinosis, hereditary fructose intolerance, Wilson's disease, and other rare disorders. Although usually presenting in childhood, some inherited cases have not been diagnosed until adulthood. The acquired forms of proximal tubule dysfunction can be due to toxic effects of urinary immunoglobulins seen in multiple myeloma or benign monoclonal gammopathy, or secondary to toxic effects of heavy metals, outdated tetracycline, gentamicin, or streptozotocin. Fanconi syndrome also has been reported in association with Sjögren syndrome, amyloidosis, and nephrotic syndrome and in transplanted kidneys. Vitamin D deficiency or resistance also can cause Fanconi syndrome.

Clinical manifestations are variable and often are related to the underlying disease process rather than to Fanconi syndrome itself. Children with Fanconi syndrome often develop bone disease, especially rickets. This primarily is due to phosphaturia and resultant hypophosphatemia. Adults may have osteopenia or osteomalacia but are often asymptomatic. Muscle weakness and cramps secondary to hypokalemia also occur in a minority of patients before treatment.

The severity of the underlying proximal tubule defect is variable and, in addition, patients may demonstrate abnormalities in some but not all proximal reabsorptive pathways. In full-blown cases, laboratory evaluation reveals a hyperchloremic metabolic acidosis, hypophosphatemia, hypouricosemia, and hypokalemia. Urinary findings include glycosuria, aminoaciduria, and slightly increased protein excretion. Hypercalciuria is common but hypocalcemia, nephrolithiasis, and nephrocalcinosis are unusual. Evaluation of the etiology of Fanconi syndrome in children requires screening for the associated hereditary causes. In adults, all patients should be evaluated for dysproteinemia with serum and urine protein electrophoresis and, if the history is suggestive, for heavy metal poisoning.

Treatment of Fanconi syndrome is directed at correcting the electrolyte disorders. In patients with acidosis, the bicarbonate dose required varies from 2 to 3 mEq/kg per day up to 20 to 30 mEq/kg per day. Bicarbonate therapy will correct acidosis but also increases or induces bicarbonaturia. The resultant bicarbonaturia will increase K^+ excretion. It is crucial, therefore, even if the patient is normokalemic prior to bicarbonate therapy, that increased K^+ losses after bicarbonate administration are anticipated and corrected. Phosphate repletion also may be required in phosphaturic patients to prevent metabolic bone disease.

RADIATION NEPHRITIS

CRAIG L. SILVERMAN, M.D.
Philadelphia, Pennsylvania

There are presently numerous indications for curative and palliative upper abdominal irradiation in both adults and children. These include seminoma, abdominal lymphomas, and ovarian cancer as well as pediatric tumors such as Burkitt's lymphoma and high-stage neuroblastoma and Wilms' tumor, to name but a few. Whenever abdominal irradiation is indicated, the major organ of concern is the kidney because of its high sensitivity to irradiation. Most of the treatment planning effort is directed toward minimizing the renal dose in order to prevent potentially serious or fatal radiation nephritis.

CLINICAL SYNDROMES

There are several well-described clinical syndromes that have been noted following fractionated radiation to the kidney.

Acute Radiation Nephritis

This is an extremely poor term because the changes are neither acute nor truly a nephritis but more correctly a progressive nephrosclerosis. It usually occurs 6 to 12 months following radiotherapy. Patients may complain of lower extremity edema, shortness of breath, headache, and hypertension. The abnormal laboratory studies include albuminuria, epithelial and hyaline casts, a chronic normocytic anemia, and impaired renal function tests, including an elevated blood urea nitrogen level. The kidney itself is normal in size. Treatment involves decreasing the physiologic kidney load and renal blood flow with bed rest, a low-protein diet, restriction of fluid and salt, and correction of the anemia. Steroids probably have no role. The prognosis, however, can be grim. Of the original 27 cases described by Luxton, 7 progressed within 6 months and eventually died of renal insufficiency, chronic congestive heart failure, hypertension, and uremia.

Chronic Nephritis

This usually occurs 18 to 24 months after radiotherapy and has many physical and urine abnormalities similar to those seen in the acute phase. The evaluation of the kidney itself, however, shows significant contraction and shrinkage. Such patients must be approached much as other patients with chronic renal failure, with low-protein and low-salt diets, correction of the anemia, and management of the hypertension. Most of these patients will slowly progress and die of chronic renal failure and uremia. The changes are often progressive and never reversible.

Hypertension

Both benign and malignant hypertension have been described in irradiated patients. This may occur as late as 3 to 7 years after treatment. Radiographically, there is always significant renal contracture and shrinkage. Malignant hypertension is an especially serious but fortunately uncommon finding after unilateral and bilateral renal irradiation. It may appear years after the initial onset of chronic radiation nephritis or even benign hypertension. Its course may be extremely rapid and even fatal and it must be aggressively medically managed. If there was unilateral renal irradiation only, there may be a role for nephrectomy, which has been demonstrated to reverse and cure the hypertension in some patients.

PATHOLOGIC FINDINGS

Histologically, there are numerous changes that occur with time. These are well described by Rubin and Cassaret. The major change is a progressive arterial nephrosclerosis mainly in small vessels, including basement membrane thickening, endothelial swelling, and proliferation. Focal tubular epithelial damage also is seen. It is believed that the progressive vascular changes secondarily can cause tubular epithelial changes, including atrophy and denudation, as well as a reduction in cortical mass.

RADIATION FACTORS

There are well-defined guidelines that must be followed based on empirical observations. The $TD_{5/5}$ (the dose required to produce a 5 per cent incidence of chronic renal damage within 5 years) is 2000 to 2500 cGy. The volume of the kidney irradiated is also of extreme importance, and irradiation of over 50 per cent of the kidney may cause irreversible damage at even lower dose ranges. Predisposing factors such as hypertension also may increase the risk of chronic renal damage as a result of pre-existing vascular damage. There are also recent reports of chronic radiation nephritis appearing in bone marrow transplant patients receiving only 1200 to 1300 cGy. This probably is due to the addition of such chemotherapy drugs as cyclophosphamide, bleomycin, Adriamycin, and actinomycin—all known radiation sensitizers. As bone marrow transplant becomes a more widespread procedure, there may be more such cases encountered at doses not previously believed to cause late renal damage.

The unique structure of the basic functional unit of the kidney is believed responsible for its high radiation sensitivity. Damage to any portion of the functional unit from the glomerulus and proximal tubules to the distal cortical tubules may cause loss of the entire functional unit, thereby increasing the chance of irreversible damage from even moderate doses of irradiation.

CONCLUSION

Radiation nephritis is a serious, irreversible, often progressive complication that has profound long-term consequences. Without hope of reversing the effects and with only minimally effective treatment available, the only reasonable course is to minimize the potential for damage to the kidney by minimizing the dose and volume of kidney irradiated. Obtaining precise knowledge of kidney location in the actual radiation treatment position using computerized tomography scans or magnetic resonance imaging provides the best chance for protection of most of the renal parenchyma. Ultrasonography has been used in the past but may give misinformation and should be discouraged. During the radiation simulation process, IV contrast dye should be used to provide additional information as to the precise anatomic relationship of the kidney to the proposed treatment volume so as to allow maximal shielding of the kidney. Extensive computer treatment planning, including three-dimensional imaging, will also help in minimizing kidney dose. Experimental radiation protectors may in the future provide some degree of protection, but no proof as yet exists that they are effective. Therefore, the best method of protecting the kidney remains avoiding it.

Suggested Readings

Krochak RJ, Baker DG: Radiation nephritis. Urology 27: 389–393, 1986

Luxton RW, Kunkler PB: Radiation nephritis. Acta Radiol 2:169–178, 1964

Moulder JE, Fish BL: Influence of nephrotoxic drugs on the late renal toxicity associated with bone marrow transplant conditioning regimens. Int J Radiat Oncol Biol Physics 20:333–337, 1991

Rubin P, Casaret GW: Urinary tract—the kidney. In Rubin P, Casaret GW (eds): Clinical Radiation Pathology, Vol 1. Philadelphia, WB Saunders, 1968, pp 293–333

ANALGESIC NEPHROPATHY

MICHAEL HEIFETS, M.D.

Philadelphia, Pennsylvania

Analgesic nephropathy emerged as a cause of end-stage renal failure in the mid-1950s, stemming from the popularity of phenacetin-containing analgesics. Typical presentation involved a patient who has consumed 2 to 3 kg of phenacetin over several years. Although the incidence of analgesic nephropathy has declined since phenacetin was banned in several countries, it has not disappeared. Recent observations suggest that any analgesic mixtures containing aspirin, other nonsteroidal anti-inflammatory drugs, and/or acetaminophen may result in progressive renal failure. There is significant worldwide geographic variability in the incidence of analgesic nephropathy. The frequency of terminal renal failure is higher in Australia, parts of Europe (Belgium, Switzerland) and the southeastern United States. Analgesic nephropathy is several times more frequent in women.

The kidneys in analgesic nephropathy are shrunken, with frequent papillary necrosis and interstitial fibrosis. The pathogenesis or renal injury stems from direct depletion of glutathione by phenacetin/acetaminophen and from inhibition of glutathione synthesis through hexose monophosphate shunt by aspirin. Vasoconstriction and medullary ischemia secondary to prostaglandin inhibition by aspirin and other nonsteroidal anti-inflammatory drugs contributes to medullary injury and papillary necrosis. Because these drugs or their metabolites are renally excreted, medullary concentration may increase several-fold in volume depletion, potentiating toxicity. This effect of hypovolemia was proposed to explain the higher incidence of analgesic nephropathy in hot climates, such as Australia and the southeastern United States.

Patients are generally asymptomatic until advanced stages, and the only demonstrable abnormality is progressive loss of urine concentrating ability, which may manifest itself clinically only if patients are subjected to water deprivation or loss (e.g., during a summer heat wave). Sometimes nocturia is the only presenting symptom. Such patients exhibit marked loss of normal nocturnal increase of urinary concentration (hypoisosthenuria). Impaired concentrating ability is documented by reduced urine osmolality (<600 to 800 mOsm/liter, depending on the age) after a standard 14-hour water deprivation test. Papillary necrosis may present with hematuria, renal colic, and obstruction if a necrotic papilla detaches and lodges in the ureter.

Diagnosis is made by eliciting a typical history of cumulative analgesic intake of 1 to 2 kg or more, finding of impaired urinary concentration, and shrunken kidneys with or without papillary necrosis on radiographic examination. Biopsy is unnecessary in such a presentation and would reveal only advanced fibrosis. Urinalysis may show proteinuria, microscopic hematuria, and sterile pyuria. Although proteinuria of less than 2 gm in 24 hours is common, frank nephrotic syndrome (24-hour urine protein >3.5 gm) warrants a search for other nephropathies. There is increased frequency of transitional cell carcinoma of the collecting system. Extrarenal manifestations include hypertension, which worsens when patients become volume depleted. Analgesic abuse frequently is associated with diuretic, laxative, and illicit substance abuse. These patients may have an underlying psychiatric disturbance, complicating the diagnosis of resulting complex fluid-electrolyte disturbance.

Management of patients with analgesic nephropathy must include appropriate counseling and discontinuation of analgesic abuse, with a goal of slowing or arresting the deterioration of renal function. Patients must avoid extremes of heat and humidity and maintain adequate salt and water intake.

Suggested Readings

Dubach UC, Rosner B, Pfister E: An epidemiologic study of abuse of analgesic drugs: Effects of phenacetin and salicylate on mortality and cardiovascular morbidity. N Engl J Med 324:155, 1991

McCredie M, Stewart JH, Carter JJ, et al: Phenacetin and papillary necrosis: Independent risk factors for renal pelvic cancer. Kidney Int 30:81, 1986

Sandler DP, Smith JC, Weinberg CR, et al: Analgesic use and chronic renal disease. N Engl J Med 320:1238, 1989

Wright L, DuVal W: Renal injury associated with laxative abuse. South Med J 80:1304, 1987

BARTTER SYNDROME

LOUIS J. RILEY, Jr., M.D.

Philadelphia, Pennsylvania

Bartter syndrome is characterized by the constellation of hypokalemic metabolic alkalosis, hyperreninemia, normal or elevated plasma and urinary aldosterone levels, normotension, and resistance to the pressor effect of angiotensin II and norepinephrine. The current popular hypothesis regarding generation of the syndrome has increased production of vasodilator prostaglandins playing a role. In fact, hyperplasia of the juxtaglomerular apparatus, a histopathologic trademark of the disorder, is corroborative in that this is also the site of prostaglandin production (as well as renin production). However, not all patients respond to therapy with prostaglandin inhibition, and all patients have not been uniformly found to have elevated levels of prostaglandins, so how important a role is played by prostaglandin in the pathogenesis of Bartter syndrome is as yet not known. Functionally, Bartter syndrome results from defects in both tubular transport of potassium, resulting in kaliuresis, and tubular transport of sodium chloride. There is a familial tendency for the disorder, which is more commonly seen in children.

Clinically, the principal concerns are the consequences of hypokalemia and the metabolic alkalosis. Severe hypokalemia is cardiotoxic and a medical emergency because of its potential for cardiotoxicity and skeletal muscle paralysis; prompt correction is required. In contrast, chronic, mild to moderate hypokalemia may be associated with weakness and result in a nephrogenic diabetes insipidus characterized clinically by polyuria and polydipsia.

The differential diagnosis of Bartter syndrome is the differential diagnosis of hypokalemic metabolic alkalosis without hypertension. Accordingly, surreptitious vomiting, diuretic use and abuse, and magnesium deficiency must be excluded as etiologic before diagnosing Bartter syndrome. Given the rarity of Bartter syndrome, the other entities deserve exclusion as a matter of first course. Urinary chloride measurement and assay of the urine for diuretics will be helpful in establishing these diagnoses.

Therapy of Bartter syndrome is directed at correction of the hypokalemia and metabolic alkalosis. Therapy with prostaglandin synthetase inhibitors (e.g., indomethacin) is successful in correcting the metabolic alkalosis. Potassium chloride supplementation in combination with spironactolone or converting enzyme inhibitors may correct both abnormalities.

Suggested Readings

Bartter FC, Pronove P, Gill JR, et al: Hyperplasia of the juxtaglomerular complex with hyperaldosteronism and hypokalemic alkalosis: A new syndrome. Am J Med 33:81, 1962

Clementsen P, Hoegholm A, Hansen LL, et al: Bartter's syndrome—treatment with potassium, spironolactone and ACE-inhibitor. J Intern Med 225:107, 1989

Fujita T, Ando K, Sato Y, et al: Independent roles of prostaglandins and the renin-angiotensin system in abnormal vascular reactivity in Bartter's syndrome. Am J Med 73:71, 1982

Jest P, Pedersen KE, Klitgaard NA, et al: Angiotensin-converting enzyme inhibitor as a therapeutic principle in Bartter's syndrome. Eur J Clin Pharmacol 41:303, 1991

Stein JH: The pathogenetic spectrum of Bartter's syndrome. Nephrology Forum. Kidney Int 28:85, 1985

POLYARTERITIS NODOSA

GERRI A. SCHULMAN, M.D.

Philadelphia, Pennsylvania

Polyarteritis nodosa (PAN) is a systemic necrotizing vasculitis of small and medium-sized arteries. Two forms have been described. Classic PAN affects medium-sized muscular arteries, especially at branch points, leading to focal aneurysm formation and ischemia of involved tissues. In contrast, microscopic PAN results from vasculitis of small arteries and arterioles. The most common form of PAN is actually an overlap syndrome with features of both classic and microscopic PAN. Classic PAN is the least common type of PAN. The typical pathologic finding is infiltration of affected vessels with granulocytes and fibrinoid necrosis of the vessel wall.

The etiology of PAN is unknown. In approximately 10 per cent of cases serologic evidence of chronic infection with hepatitis B or hepatitis C is present and immune complexes are observed in involved vessels. This suggests that PAN may result from formation and deposition of viral-related immune complexes. PAN also has been reported in association with collagen vascular diseases, drug reactions, and tumors. These cases usually also demonstrate immune complex deposition. However, the majority of cases of PAN are not associated with any of these conditions and therefore are idiopathic. Immune deposits are absent in most cases of idiopathic PAN, arguing against an immune complex—mediated mechanism.

Recently antineutrophil cytoplasmic antibodies (ANCAs) have been reported in many patients with idiopathic PAN, especially the microscopic or overlap forms. These antibodies are not specific for PAN but appear to be a marker for pauci-immune vasculitides such as Wegener's granulomatosis and idiopathic crescentic glomerulonephritis. Two patterns of ANCAs are observed by immunofluorescence, cytoplasmic staining (C-ANCAs) and perinuclear staining (P-ANCAs). PAN has been reported in association with both C-ANCAs and P-ANCAs. Most C-ANCAs react with proteinase 3, a serine proteinase, whereas P-ANCAs react with myeloperoxidase. In vitro studies suggest that both of these antibodies actually may have a pathogenic role in causing vasculitis.

The clinical manifestations of PAN are variable depending on which organs are involved. The peak incidence is in the fifth and sixth decades, and males are affected twice as often as females. Nonspecific constitutional symptoms of fever, weight loss, anorexia, and malaise are present in over 80 per cent of cases. Gastrointestinal involvement occurs in 30 to 50 per cent of patients and presents as nausea, vomiting, abdominal pain, or bleeding. Most often, abdominal complaints are secondary to ischemic intestinal infarctions or intestinal perforation. Less frequently, PAN causes pancreatitis or cholecystitis. Neurologic symptoms of paresthesias, numbness, or weakness are common and are due to mononeuritis multiplex and/or peripheral distal sensorimotor neuropathy. Central nervous system vasculitis occurs in a minority of patients and presents as seizures or strokes. Musculoskeletal involvement is observed in 50 to 75 per cent of patients and leads to myalgias and arthralgias. Cardiac vasculitis may result in ischemia and congestive heart failure. Testicular vasculitis often results in pain and tenderness. The kidneys are affected by PAN in 70 to 100 per cent of cases, although patients usually do not complain of symptoms related to the kidney at presentation.

In classic PAN, vasculitis of the medium-sized renal vessels results in renal ischemia and cortical infarction. In microscopic PAN and overlap PAN, vasculitis of the renal arterioles causes necrotizing glomerulonephritis with crescent formation. Hypertension is more common with vasculitis of the medium-sized renal arteries and is mediated by elevated renin and angiotensin. Rarely, rupture of an aneurysm results in a retroperitoneal hematoma. The ureters and bladder also may be involved. Vasculitis of ureteral arteries resulting in ureteral fibrosis, stricture, and renal obstruction has been reported. Bladder neuropathy also has been observed.

The diagnosis of PAN is based on the typical clinical findings and the demonstration of vasculitis in histologic specimens from involved tissue or angiographic demonstration of typical aneurysms. The American Rheumatologic Association has developed 10 criteria for the diagnosis of PAN. Kidney biopsy changes usually are not diagnostic because both ischemic changes and necrotizing glomerulonephritis are observed in many other conditions. Other diseases associated with PAN, such as hepatitis B and C, collagen vascular diseases, and cryoglobulinemia, must be excluded by appropriate serologic tests. The importance of a positive ANCA test is not known, but a recent reclassification of the systemic vasculitides subdivided PAN into P-ANCA–positive, C-ANCA–positive, and ANCA-negative forms.

Further studies are necessary to determine if treatment and prognosis differ in ANCA-positive and ANCA-negative PAN. Untreated, patients with PAN have a dismal prognosis, with less than 10 per cent 5-year survival. Some patients respond to glucocorticoids alone, but most studies suggest that addition of cytotoxic therapy further improves the prognosis. The safety and efficacy of oral versus intravenous cyclophosphamide as therapy for PAN currently are being investigated.

Suggested Readings

Falk RJ, Hogan S, Carey TS, et al: Clinical course of antineutrophil cytoplasmic autoantibody-associated glomerulonephritis and systemic vasculitis. Ann Intern Med 113:656, 1990

Jennette JC: Antineutrophil cytoplasmic autoantibody-associated diseases: A pathologists perspective. Am J Kidney Dis 18:164, 1991

Jennette JC, Falk RJ: Diagnostic classification of antineutrophil cytoplasmic autoantibody-associated vasculitides. Am J Kidney Dis 18:184, 1991

Lightfoot RW, Michel BA, Bloch DA, et al: The American College of Rheumatology 1990 criteria for the classification of polyarteritis nodosa. Arthritis Rheum 33:1088, 1990

RENAL TRANSPLANTATION AND ITS FAILURE

MICHAEL HEIFETS, M.D.

Philadelphia, Pennsylvania

Kidney transplantation has become a reality for an increasing number of dialysis patients since the introduction of cyclosporine. One-year graft survival rates now frequently exceed 85 per cent for cadaveric transplants and approach 99 per cent for living related transplants fully matched for human lymphocyte antigen. After the first year, however, there is a continuous attrition of functioning grafts. The mean graft half-life of a first cadaveric transplant is 7.5 years, and for living related grafts it is over 22 years. Although there has been a major reduction in acute rejection as the cause of transplant loss in the first year, chronic rejection, cyclosporine toxicity, recurrent disease, noncompliance, and patient mortality from nonrenal problems remain relatively constant as impediments to long-term success.

EARLY POST-TRANSPLANT GRAFT FAILURE (WITHIN 1 YEAR)

Primary Nonfunction

Primary nonfunction implies no urine production and either severe reduction or absence of blood flow to the transplant. The most common cause is irreversible ischemic injury to the kidney during procurement and/or technical problems with vascular anastomosis. Primary nonfunction should be differentiated from hyperacute rejection, reversible ischemic injury, and acute cyclosporine nephrotoxicity.

Hyperacute (Vascular, Humoral) Rejection

Preformed cytotoxic antibodies bind to the graft endothelium and activate complement and coagulation cascades, resulting in thrombosis and loss of transplant within minutes after opening of the arterial clamp. This type of rejection can be prevented by careful screening for cytotoxic antibodies while the patient is on the waiting list. In addition, final cytotoxic cross-matching to detect antibodies not picked up by screening must be performed immediately before transplant. This is a critical requirement for patients with a history of elevated titers of cytotoxic antibodies and those receiving a second transplant.

Cellular Rejection

Accelerated cellular rejection is seen within 2 to 7 days after transplantation and is manifested by massive infiltration of the kidney with activated lymphocytes. This is due to the existence of cytotoxic lymphocytes presensitized to the antigens of the recipient. These lymphocytes may be detected before transplantation using some of the more sophisticated screening methods.

Acute cellular rejection is usually seen 7 to 10 days after transplant and is due to the appearance of a *newly formed* cytotoxic lymphocyte pool sensitized against the new graft. The prevention of cytotoxic lymphocyte proliferation is achieved by using high doses of glucocorticoids (which are directly lymphocytotic) and antilymphocyte preparations (monoclonal or polyclonal) for 7 to 10 days after transplant, followed by varied combinations of prednisone, cyclosporine (an interleukin-2 antagonist), and azathioprine (an antiproliferative agent), with gradual reduction of doses to the lifelong maintenance levels. An alternative approach is to use cyclosporine immediately after transplant to avoid excessive immunosuppression from the antilymphocyte preparations. The limiting factor remains renal intolerance of high doses of cyclosporine. Acute rejections occur in 40 to 60 per cent of all patients, representing a balance between the doses of immunosuppressive medications and the risk of infection. With treatment, only 10 to 15 per cent eventually result in transplant failure within the first year.

DIAGNOSIS OF REJECTION

If elevation of serum creatinine more than 20 per cent above the recent baseline is seen and the cyclosporine level is at the low end of the therapeutic range, urine culture must be done, the patient's fluid volume expanded, and creatinine levels rechecked in 24 to 48 hours. Renal ultrasound and a Doppler or nuclear scan should be done to look for obstruction and adequate blood flow to the kidney. Development of anuria requires immediate renal nuclear scan to exclude complete vascular occlusion. The patient should be off all medications known to interfere with creatinine measurements. If a patient presents with severe elevation of creatinine and has signs of acute illness, such as fever, anuria, or significant peripheral edema, scans should be done immediately. If creatinine remains elevated, a transplant biopsy should be done in an inpatient setting, preferably using ultrasound localization. Because postbiopsy bleeding may result in graft loss, the patient must have a bleeding time under 10 minutes and prothrombin and partial thromboplastin times within normal limits, blood must be available for transfusion, and the patient must have reliable intravenous access. A urine culture must be negative, and blood pressure must be less than 160/100 mm Hg. Biopsy samples should be sent for light microscopy, electron microscopy, and immunofluorescence study. Eighty to 90 per cent of all biopsies of transplant patients with *acute* elevation of creatinine in the first several weeks after transplant will show some lymphocytic infiltrate, consistent with acute cellular rejection.

TREATMENT OF REJECTION

The patient usually receives 1000 mg of methylprednisolone intravenously daily for 3 days, followed by tapering doses of prednisone. The patient is considered to have failed steroid treatment if creatinine remains significantly elevated and/or continues to rise by the fifth to seventh day after the initiation of steroids. The patient should be treated with *OKT3 (monoclonal muromonab CD3)* or another anti–T cell preparation, and must be hospitalized in the intensive care unit for the first two or three doses of OKT3 administration. The patient must be documented to be euvolemic or within 3 per cent of estimated dry weight. A chest radiograph must be without significant congestive heart failure. If the patient is anuric, dialysis must be performed before OKT3 administration to remove excess fluid. The patient must not have any signs of volume depletion or evidence of infection, and a pregnancy test must be negative.

OKT3 (5 mg) is given intravenously as a push over *30 seconds* to avoid localized binding and loss of systemic effect. The patient is pretreated with methylprednisolone intravenously before the first dose, along with antihistamines and antipyretics. These precautions are necessary to minimize the systemic effects of rapid release of cytokines (interleukin-1, tumor necrosis factor-alpha, etc.): disintegration of activated lymphocytes, high fever and capillary leak throughout the body, and resulting pulmonary edema, vascular collapse, and diarrhea. Painstaking attention to maintenance of euvolemia is a must. A physician and a resuscitation cart must be at the bedside for 15 minutes after the first dose. The activated lymphocyte pool usually is depleted after the second dose, and no reactions are observed thereafter. Imuran is discontinued while the patient is on OKT3, and the cyclosporine dose is reduced. Both drugs are brought up to pretreatment doses 2 to 3 days before planned discontinuation of OKT3. Total duration of OKT3 treatment is usually 10 to 12 days. If antibodies to OKT3 are present, the patient should receive a course of *ATGAM* (polyclonal anti T–cell horse immunoglobulin G) instead. ATGAM must be given through a central venous line and requires skin testing before administration.

Some patients may have subsequent rejection(s), and, if biopsies show significant amounts of chronic scarring and the potential for the kidney salvage is significantly reduced, no further antirejection treatment should be considered because of significantly enhanced risk for severe infections.

Acute Tubular Necrosis

Acute tubular necrosis (ATN) may present as either anuria or oliguria immediately after transplant, or it could develop within hours after anastomosis. This represents acute reperfusion injury to the kidney that has suffered prolonged ischemia. The incidence of ATN is directly proportionate to the length of cold ischemia, and many centers will not accept a kidney over 36 hours from the time of harvest. The severity of ATN also may impact on the long-term graft survival and certainly adds to immediate postoperative morbidity, extends hospital stay, and adds to the cost. ATN also may occur as a result of postoperative hypotension from any cause—sepsis, nephrotoxic drugs, and the like.

The course of ATN is highly variable. It may manifest as a nonoliguric azotemia with only several days' delay in the normalization of good renal function or a prolonged anuric state requiring dialysis for as long as several weeks. The diagnosis of ATN is made by a typical finding of impaired tubular function and preserved renal flow on nuclear scan and on Doppler ultrasound. Biopsy shows a variable degree of tubular epithelial injury and lack of lymphocytic infiltrate, although some infiltration with polymorphonuclear leukocytes can be seen. Prognosis for recovery is usually very good as long as there is preservation of blood flow. Management should concentrate on avoidance of additional insults, such as hypotension, severe hypertension, and nephrotoxic drugs.

Acute Cyclosporine Toxicity

Cyclosporine may cause severe renal vasoconstriction, resulting in protracted oligoanuria and azotemia. The effect is dose dependent and is seen mostly with intravenous cyclosporine. Differentiation from ATN in the immediate post-transplant period is difficult and is based on the clinical course and presence of high levels of cyclosporine. Transplant biopsy may differentiate it from rejection, but not from ATN. The management consists of dose reduction or discontinuation and change to antilymphocyte preparations in the immediate post-transplant period. Several studies indicate that calcium channel blockers may protect the kidney against the toxic effect of cyclosporine.

Rarely, cyclosporine produces microangiopathic hemolytic uremic syndrome, occasionally resulting in graft loss. The majority of patients improve after temporary dose reduction.

Acute Pyelonephritis

Acute pyelonephritis may be indistinguishable clinically from acute rejection. It presents with graft tenderness, fever, oliguria, and fluid retention. Urine culture is usually positive for the offending organism, and biopsy shows polymorphonuclear, rather than lymphocytic, infiltrate. As opposed to acute rejection, acute pyelonephritis may be seen several years after the transplant. Usually there is a quick response to the conventional antibiotic therapy, with rapid normalization of renal function.

Ureteral Leak and Obstruction

Ureterovesicular anastomosis detachment or ureteral obstruction may present a complicated management problem but rarely results in graft loss if detected early. For that purpose, an ultrasound examination should be done immediately after the transplant and 1 to 2 days after removal of the indwelling bladder catheter. The treatment of obstruction caused by stenosis is usually percutaneous nephrostomy and subsequent balloon dilation. Ureteral leak management depends on the extent of the leak. Minor leaks usually heal with prolonged bladder decompression with indwelling bladder catheters, and major leaks require either reanastomosis or anastomosis of the transplant pelvis to the native ureter.

DELAYED GRAFT FAILURE

All of the problems encountered in the early post-transplant period may lead to the failure of a transplanted kidney several years after surgery. The frequency of these complications declines with time. *Noncompliance with medications occurs in as many as 50 per cent of all patients with long-term function of the graft.* Abrupt discontinuation of immunosuppressive agents as late as 5 years after transplant will lead to acute rejection, which may be resistant to therapy. Intermittent or partial noncompliance will lead to episodes of "smoldering" acute rejection, which may be missed.

Unless there is a correctable anatomic problem, the therapy of chronic progressive transplant failure is usually unsatisfactory. Efforts should be directed toward dietary adjustments, blood pressure control, and preparation for dialysis and retransplant.

Chronic Rejection

This should be considered in any patient with gradual progressive rise of creatinine more than 25 per cent over baseline without apparent cause (obstruction, vascular occlusion, or nephrotoxins). Biopsy demonstrates diffuse intestitial fibrosis, tubular atrophy, and glomerular dropout. Patients with proteinuria in excess of 1 gm should undergo biopsy to differentiate chronic rejection and cyclosporine toxicity versus primary disease recurrence.

Chronic Cyclosporine Toxicity

This presents as progressive interstitial fibrosis or as glomerulopathy. The interstitial form is practically indistinguishable from chronic rejection both clinically and pathologically. The presumptive diagnosis is made in a patient with elevated levels of cyclosporine over a long time and nonrenal signs of toxicity, and by virtue of *sustained* improvement in renal function after dose and level reduction. Cyclosporine glomerulopathy can be differentiated from other glomerular disease by electron microscopy.

Recurrent Glomerulopathy

Several forms of glomerulonephritides are more likely to recur in a transplanted kidney and lead to its failure. Focal sclerosing glomerulonephritis, immunoglobulin A nephropathy, and membranous nephropathy head the list. Diabetic nephropathy, in contrast, rarely causes transplant failure. Focal sclerosis recurs more often in patients who had rapid progression to renal failure initially and then received a kidney from closely matched donor. Patients usually present with progressive proteinuria, followed by progressive rise of creatinine. Diagnosis is made by biopsy.

Transplant Glomerulopathy

Clinically this is indistinguishable from focal sclerosis. The diagnosis is made by electron microscopy of glomerular basement membrane showing specific changes.

Transplant Renal Artery Stenosis

These patients often present with *progressive* uncontrollable hypertension and rising creatinine and may have an audible bruit over the transplant. The diagnosis is made by captopril-enhanced renal nuclear scan and arteriogram. The preferred therapy is angioplasty. Surgical revascularization is hampered by extensive scar tissue surrounding the anastomosis area.

Suggested Readings

Banfi G, Colturi C, Montagnino G, et al: The recurrence of focal segmental glomerulosclerosis in kidney transplant patients treated with cyclosporine. Transplantation 50:594, 1990

Bohman S, Wilczek HE, Reinholt, FP, et al: Immunopathological patterns in long-term renal allografts. Transplantation 51:610, 1991

Kashi SH, Lodge JPA, Giles GR, et al: Ultrasonography of renal allografts: Collecting system dilatation and clinical significance. Nephrol Dial Transplant 6:358, 1991

Zhang L, van Bree S, van Rood JJ, et al: The effect of individual HLA-A and -B mismatches on the generation of cytotoxic T lymphocyte precursors. Transplantation 50:1008, 1990

PROGRESSIVE SYSTEMIC SCLEROSIS (SCLERODERMA)

MICHAEL HEIFETS, M.D.

Philadelphia, Pennsylvania

Scleroderma is a rare collagen vascular autoimmune disorder, most frequently affecting women over 40 years of age. It is conventionally divided into limited forms (types 1 and 2), affecting only the skin of the digits and/or extremities, and a generalized form (type 3, or progressive systemic sclerosis), affecting the skin and viscera throughout the body. The term "scleroderma" properly describes only skin involvement (literally: hardened skin). The term "progressive systemic sclerosis" should be used to describe the generalized form. The combination of cutaneous calcinosis, Raynaud's phenomenon, esophageal motility disorder, sclerodactyly, and telangiectasia is referred to as CREST syndrome. Morbidity and mortality of patients with systemic sclerosis is proportionate to the extent of visceral involvement. Renal involvement portends the highest morbidity and mortality.

The pathogenesis involves vasospastic hyperreactivity and structural narrowing of arterioles throughout the body. The anatomic changes stem from excessive collagen synthesis and growth of smooth vascular cells. Recent findings suggest that there is a genetic defect in patients with scleroderma that is responsible for uncontrolled production of collagen. The collagen produced in patients with scleroderma is structurally different. Because the vessel lumen is already reduced by collagen production, even slight vasospasm leads to major reduction in blood flow and tissue ischemia. The latter also stimulates collagen synthesis, thus sustaining a vicious cycle. The serum of patients with scleroderma is toxic to endothelial cells in culture. Injury and denudation of endothelial cells exposes the underlying lamina interna and causes platelet activation, adherence, and local inflammatory response. Activated platelets release several growth factors, stimulating proliferation of fibroblasts and vascular smooth muscular cells.

Although fibrotic changes of scleroderma can affect any organ, renal involvement leads to secondary systemic changes, such as malignant hypertension and end-stage renal failure. Pathologic changes in the kidneys arise from vascular injury. Gross examination of kidneys of patients with systemic sclerosis who died of renal failure may show multiple infarcts and glomerular and tubular dropout in the distribution of involved vessels. Involvement of intermediate renal arteries shows typical proliferation of intima and accumulation of collagen leading to concentric obliteration of the vessel lumen, accompanied by periadventitial fibrosis, resulting in an "onionskin" appearance on cross section. Fibrinoid necrosis of small arterioles may extend into the glomeruli and is frequently associated with malignant hypertensive crisis of scleroderma.

These histologic changes resemble those seen in patients with malignant hypertension of other causes, but they occur *before the onset of hypertension or renal failure.* These early histologic changes explain the reduced renal blood flow in early renal involvement by systemic sclerosis, while glomerular filtration rate is not yet affected. Plasma renin activity in patients with systemic scleroderma is elevated prior to the development of hypertension as well and is postulated to be pathogenetic in the development of exaggerated vasospastic response. The hyper-reninemic state has a histologic correlate in the increased size of the juxtaglomerular apparatus. Vascular smooth muscles themselves may serve as an important extrarenal source of renin, thus contributing to the generalized arterial vasoconstriction.

Clinical presentation depends on the organ(s) involved. Renal involvement usually is suspected when a patient with systemic sclerosis (type 3) develops proteinuria, progressive renal failure, and/or uncontrollable hypertension. In rare patients, development of uncontrollable hypertension may be the only clinical sign of systemic sclerosis. "Scleroderma crisis" develops as a result of marked renal vasoconstriction, leading to escalation of arterial hypertension as a result of a sharp increase in renin production. These patients typically develop progressive azotemia and anuria, which may be irreversible. Pathologic findings of near-normal renal histology (outside of scattered infarctions) in anuric patients dying from scleroderma crisis underscore the fact that vasoconstriction, and not intrinsic renal disease, is responsible for renal shutdown. The life expectancy of patients with systemic sclerosis, malignant hypertension, and anuria is under 1 year.

The clinical diagnosis is based on typical symptoms of visceral involvement (e.g., esophageal) and findings of cutaneous scleroderma. Early renal involvement is manifested by the appearance of proteinuria, which rarely exceeds 3 to 4 gm/24 hours. Full-blown nephrotic syndrome is uncommon. Urinalysis may show hyaline casts but is otherwise quite unrevealing. Scleroderma crisis can be recognized readily in a patient with scleroderma who develops malignant hypertension, requiring intensive care management, and exhibits progressive deterioration in urine output and renal function. Although Raynaud's phenomenon is the most common first presenting feature of scleroderma and systemic sclerosis, it is not diagnostic by itself. An antinuclear antibody (ANA) titer greater than 1:80 and significant capillary dropout in the nail bed imply that the Raynaud's phenomenon in such a case is not benign but is likely to be a manifestation of scleroderma. The degree of dropout is predictive of visceral involvement. The fluorescent ANA pattern in scleroderma is typically nucleolar or speckled. Anti-DNA topoisomerase I and anti Scl-70 antibodies correlate better with systemic involvement, whereas anticentromere antibodies are seen more often with local forms.

Successful management of a patient with systemic sclerosis depends on rigorous control of elevated blood pressures as a key to forestalling renal failure and scleroderma crisis. Angiotensin-converting enzyme inhibitors should be used as first-line agents, especially in scleroderma crisis. Captopril, an angiotensin inhibitor drug, also was shown to aid in regression of some skin fibrotic changes, probably because of the presence of a sulfhydryl moiety. Angiotensin-converting enzyme inhibitors should be used with caution in patients with hyperkalemia and rising creatinine in the presence of volume depletion.

Calcium channel blockers are also effective antihypertensive agents and are useful in treating the Raynaud's phenomenon. Other antihypertensive agents should be added as needed. Diuretics generally are not effective, unless used to control secondary volume retention. Beta blockers should be avoided because they can worsen peripheral and renal vasoconstriction.

D-Penicillamine is promising in reducing fibrotic changes because of its collagen cross-linking properties. Most other therapeutic approaches (plasmapheresis, corticosteroids, chlorambucil, and antiplatelet drugs) have not been found effective.

Patients should be advised to avoid any cold exposure because this may trigger vasospasm and ischemia not only in the hands but in internal organs as well.

Suggested Readings

Barnett AJ, Miller M, Littlejohn GO: The diagnosis and classification of scleroderma. Postgrad Med J 64:121, 1988

Beckett VL, Donadio JV, Brennan LA, et al: Use of captopril as early therapy for renal scleroderma: A prospective study. Mayo Clin Proc 60:763, 1985

Lally EV, Jimenez SA, Kaplan SR: Progressive systemic sclerosis: Mode of presentation, rapidly progressive disease course and mortality based on an analysis of 91 patients. Semin Arthritis Rheum 18:1, 1988

Pandolfi A, Florita M, Altomare G, et al: Increased plasma levels of platelet derived growth factor activity in systemic sclerosis. Proc Soc Exp Biol Med 191:1, 1989

SYSTEMIC LUPUS ERYTHEMATOSUS NEPHRITIS

ELLIE KELEPOURIS, M.D.

Philadelphia, Pennsylvania

The incidence of clinically detectable renal disease varies from 15 to 75 per cent in patients with systemic lupus erythematosus (SLE). Histologic evidence of renal involvement in SLE is found in the vast majority of renal biopsies when studied by light microscopy (LM), immunofluorescence (IF), and electron microscopy (EM), even in the absence of clinical renal disease. Analysis of renal biopsies has helped define and classify subgroups of patients with differing therapeutic responses and natural histories, and it is now apparent that renal biopsy in SLE nephritis is mandatory in evaluating patients with this disease and is of considerable value both in the therapeutic choice and in predicting prognosis.

CLASSIFICATION

The World Health Organization (WHO) classification of lupus nephritis has attempted to combine all morphologic modalities of renal biopsy interpretation and assess severity of involvement, and is now widely accepted by both clinical nephrologists and renal pathologists. The WHO classification is superior to previous ones in that it has the advantages of using LM, IF, and EM to classify each biopsy, rather than only one form of microscopy, and of separating the milder pure mesangial patterns from those with focal or diffuse proliferative involvement with a more severe clinical course. In addition, the WHO classes correlate well with the clinical presentation at biopsy.

It is possible that the WHO classes may not be distinct clinical entities and may represent different aspects in a continuum of disease. This is likely because transformation from one lesion to another can occur both spontaneously and as a result of treatment. Transformation from class III to class IV is common and transformation from a diffuse proliferative to a membranous or mesangial lesion can occur during therapy. The mechanism of this transformation is unknown.

WHO Class I (Normal)

This class is rare and is seen only in patients without clinical renal findings early in the course of the systemic disease. Because renal tissue as examined by LM, IF, and EM is usually normal, without morphologic evidence of glomerular damage, this class may not represent a form of renal involvement.

WHO Class II (Mesangial Lesions)

On tissue examination, there is glomerular mesangial hypercellularity by LM and evidence of immune deposits confined purely to the mesangium and dense deposits seen on EM. Clinically, the majority of these patients have mild renal involvement, are never found to have nephrotic-range proteinuria, and have an excellent long-term prognosis. These patients do not require specific treatment directed at their renal lesions.

WHO Class III (Focal Proliferation Nephritis)

On LM, these patients have a focal and segmental glomerulonephritis. The changes may be proliferative, sclerosing, and/or necrotizing, and, if the latter are present, this suggests a higher degree of clinical activity and severity. There are focal interstitial and tubular changes present. Clinically, patients have active lupus serologies, and an "active" urinary sediment with red blood cells, red blood cell casts, and variable amounts of proteinuria.

Approximately 25 per cent of patients with a class III lesion have nephrotic-range proteinuria.

The similarity of the IF and EM findings of class III with those of class IV suggest that the two may represent a continuum of morphologic changes. In fact, patients can evolve or transform from a class III to a class IV pattern. These patients have an aggressive clinical course with a natural history similar to that of class IV patients.

WHO Class IV (Diffuse Proliferative Glomerulonephritis)

All glomeruli are involved, with diffuse hypercellularity and focal areas of necrosis. Some areas of the peripheral capillary loops in the glomerulus are dramatically thickened to form "wire loop" lesions. This class of lesion is characterized by large and abundant subendothelial electron-dense deposits on EM that are pathognomonic for the disease. Patients with class IV lesions have severe renal involvement, nephrotic-range proteinuria, and an active urinary sediment. They frequently have hypertension and often can present with a decrease in renal function and a rising creatinine level. Without therapy, these patients have the worst prognosis because a high percentage of them progress to renal failure.

WHO Class V (Membranous Glomerulonephritis)

Patients with this renal lesion tend to be older on presentation and usually have inactive urine sediment, inactive lupus serologies, and proteinuria in the nephrotic range. In fact, some patients present with the nephrotic syndrome before fulfilling the other accepted systemic criteria for SLE. Although this lesion is characterized by a relatively indolent course with a good short-term prognosis, patients can progress to renal failure over many years. Renal vein thrombosis commonly is seen in association with membranous lupus nephritis.

CLINICOPATHOLOGIC CORRELATIONS

The pattern of renal injury determines the long-term prognosis of renal disease in SLE nephritis and the subsequent clinical course. Recent reports have emphasized the presence and location of electron-dense deposits as important indices of the clinical course. Subendothelial deposits correlate with a higher incidence of heavy proteinuria and renal insufficiency. Furthermore, 60 per cent of patients with subendothelial deposits who were treated with prednisone and azathioprine demonstrated complete disappearance of these deposits on repeat biopsy and had normal renal function with very little proteinuria at the end of a 40-month follow-up period.

In patients with persistence of subendothelial deposits, renal function subsequently deteriorated and proteinuria increased. Additionally, the presence of glomerular sclerosis and interstitial fibrosis are significant predictors of both renal and patient death. The aim of therapy, therefore, is the prevention of necrosis, because tissue fibrosis is the only consequence of inflammation and tissue destruction.

THERAPY

In general, because patients with Class IV lesions on renal biopsy have the worst prognosis, they should be treated aggressively. Patients with Class III lesions with necrotizing foci and large subendothelial deposits also should be vigorously and similarly treated. Aggressive therapy for SLE nephritis includes high-dose oral and/or IV pulse steroids, oral azathioprine or cyclophosphamide, IV cyclophosphamide, and cyclosporine. Plasmapheresis no longer has an active role in the treatment of SLE nephritis because it was recently proven unsuccessful in a major clinical controlled trial.

Glucocorticoids

Glucocorticoids remain the mainstay of treatment for the systemic features of SLE and to curtail the renal inflammatory reaction. High-dose prednisone at 60 mg/day for 3 months, followed by a taper to 20 mg/day for 6 months, has been shown to result in an increase in creatinine clearance and a decrease in proteinuria. In patients with a recent decrease in glomerular filtration rate, diffuse proliferative class IV lesions, and high serologic activity, IV pulse methylprednisone is thought to be more effective in some, but not all, cases. It is administered as a bolus 1-gm dose daily for 3 to 5 days, followed by high-dose oral prednisone as described previously. An improvement in renal function was seen in 30 to 50 per cent of patients on this regimen, and functional improvement was maintained for greater than 1 year. In general, the steroids are continued until clinical evidence of remission appears and discontinued after 3 months if the clinical condition has stabilized. However, recent studies at the National Institutes of Health (NIH) have shown that IV methylprednisone is less effective than IV cyclophosphamide in preventing end-stage renal disease in patients with severe renal lesions.

Immunosuppressive Agents

Cytotoxic drugs are important in the current management of patients with SLE nephritis characterized by diffuse proliferative (class IV) and/or necrotizing lesions and large subendothelial deposits. Oral cyclophosphamide has been effective in many patients with SLE nephritis. Cyclophosphamide administration (1 to 2 mg/kg per day) has been suggested to improve long-term renal survival because it led to a decrease in the number of clinical renal lupus flares when compared to prednisone alone. Recent results of an NIH clinical trial in which patients were randomized to cytotoxic agents with and without prednisone demonstrated that patients treated with cytotoxic agents (either azathioprine or cyclophosphamide) fared better than those with steroid treatment alone. One limb of this trial was IV cyclophosphamide administration, which appeared to be a very effective treatment modality in preventing progressive renal deterioration and also was associated with fewer side effects than oral administration.

Currently, class IV lesions are being treated with a once-monthly intravenous cyclophosphamide administration at a dose of 0.5 to 1.0 gm/sq m body surface area. This monthly regimen, in combination with a rapid steroid taper, is very popular and showing promising short-term results, with stabilization of the serum creatinine, decrease in proteinuria, remission of the nephrotic syndrome, and resolution of the serologic abnormalities and clinical signs of disease activity. As with all forms of treatment, not all patients respond to this regimen, which is complicated by a high infection rate.

Cyclosporine

Recent trials with the use of cyclosporine have been promising in selected patients. Patients unresponsive to conventional treatment have responded to cyclosporine administration with a decrease in serum creatinine and proteinuria. Cyclosporine is particularly promising in membranous lupus nephritis, resulting in a remission of the nephrotic syndrome. Any conclusions about this form of treatment remain speculative.

Summary

In general, although the treatment protocols remain controversial, patients with SLE nephritis are treated with steroids as the first-line drug, with a rapid taper regimen. After 3 months of steroids, the dose should be tapered to the lowest possible dose and administered on an alternate-day regimen. Immunosuppressive agents are next in line for refractory cases and should be given judiciously.

Suggested Readings

Appel GB, Cohen DJ, Pirani CL, et al: Long term follow-up of LN: A study based on the WHO classification. Am J Med 83:1987

Appel GB, Silva FG, Pirani CL, et al: Renal involvement in SLE: A study of 56 patients emphasizing histologic classification. Medicine 57:371–410, 1978

Balow JE, Boumpas DT, Vaughan EM, et al: LN: Controlled trial of pulse methylprednisolone (MP) versus pulse cyclophosphamide (CY). J Am Soc Nephrol 2:263, 1991

Donadio JV, Holley KE, Iulstrup MS: Cytotoxic drug treatment of LN. Am J Kidney Dis 2:178–181, 1982

Kimberly RD, Lockshin MD, Sherman RL, et al: High-dose intravenous methylprednisolone pulse therapy in SLE. Am J Med 70:817–824, 1981

Lemoine R, Favre H, Miescher P, et al: Morphologic evolution of membranous LN on combined treatment of cyclosporine and steroids. Kidney Int 37A:442, 1990

McCune WJ, Golbus J, Zeldes W, et al: Clinical and immunologic effects of monthly administration of cyclophosphamide in SLE. N Engl J Med 318:1423–1431, 1988

Pernis A, D'Agati V, Estes D, et al: IV pulse cytoxan for severe LN. Kidney Int 35:211, 1989

HEPATORENAL SYNDROME

CHRISTINE P. BASTL, M.D.

Philadelphia, Pennsylvania

The hepatorenal syndrome is a unique clinical entity associated with severe liver disease, usually decompensated cirrhosis, in which there is progressive renal failure without apparent cause other than the liver failure. This entity is the most extreme example of what is termed "functional renal failure." Urinalysis does not reveal evidence of glomerular or tubular injury and tubular function remains intact. In fact, functional parameters suggest a very severe prerenal state, with marked oliguria and a urine almost devoid of sodium. In virtually all patients, renal failure relentlessly progresses. Death is the invariable result without liver transplant. It is generally believed that patients die of hepatic failure with renal failure rather than because of renal failure.

It used to be thought that renal insufficiency was of rapid onset in the patient with severe hepatic failure, but recent studies suggest that decreasing renal function occurs more gradually in the patient with decompensated cirrhosis and ascites. The decline in renal function can be masked because hyperbilirubinemia can interfere with the automated assay of serum creatinine, giving falsely low values. Even more important, the serum blood urea nitrogen (BUN) and creatinine levels are inadequate markers of renal disease in the patient with severe liver disease. Because of decreased protein intake and decreased urea production by the liver, the BUN is low in cirrhosis. Marked muscle wasting decreases creatinine production so that, in cirrhotics with normal renal function, a lower than normal creatinine should be seen. A serum creatinine of 1 to 1.5 mg/dl can be seen with a creatinine clearance of 50 ml/min or less. However, because of tubular secretion of creatinine, the creatinine clearance also overrepresents the true glomerular filtration rate (GFR), which can be as low as 25 to 35 ml/min despite a normal creatinine level. It is probably this group with occult decreased GFR that is most at risk for development of hepatorenal syndrome.

The etiology of renal dysfunction in cirrhosis has been partly but not totally defined. There is marked peripheral and splanchnic vasodilation associated with intense renal vasoconstriction, alterations resembling gram-negative sepsis. Peripheral vascular resistance and blood pressure are low, accompanied by an increased cardiac output. Portal hypertension leads to splanchnic arterial dilation. Several hormones and vasoactive substances have been implicated as systemic vasodilators in liver failure. Rapid transudation of fluid into ascites and increased hepatic and abdominal pressure impede cardiac return, leading to venous pooling and decreased effective arterial volume. This decreases renal blood flow and activates renal vasoconstrictor hormones. Increased hepatic sinusoidal pressure also increases renal sympathetic nerve activity. Hepatic failure also leads to increases in other renal vasoconstrictors, even in the absence of decreased arterial volume. The net effect is a dilated systemic circulation that is resistant to vasoconstrictors and a vasoconstricted renal circulation that is resistant to vasodilators.

The potential for precipitation of severe electrolyte abnormalities and renal failure should be kept in mind in caring for the decompensated cirrhotic with ascites. Intense sodium retention makes increasing ascites and edema a constant problem. The less severely affected patient may be controlled with sodium restriction to 1 to 2 gm and bed rest and probably can be safely diuresed with spironolactone. Measurement of creatinine clearance and urine sodium concentration can help identify patients at risk of renal failure. A decreased GFR and very low urine Na^+ suggest that intense renal vasoconstriction is already present. In these patients attempts at volume removal should be done only for clear medical indications such as relief of respiratory distress, and done with extreme care. Paracentesis with intravenous albumin administration appears to be a safer and more effective method to reduce ascites than potent diuretics. Attempted diuresis has been associated with a very high complication rate and increased mortality. Decreases in effective arterial volume have been implicated as a major precipitating cause of hepatorenal syndrome. It is also important to remember that these patients are prone to losses that can rapidly decrease vascular volume, such as gastrointestinal bleeding or development of diarrhea. Lactulose, which is used to decrease gut ammonia production, is an osmotic agent that will increase gastrointestinal losses.

If the creatinine level is elevated, a urinalysis should be done to rule out renal pathology and urine sodium should be measured. If the urine sodium is low, the intravascular volume should be expanded with crystalloid or, preferentially, with colloid or blood to achieve a high-normal pulmonary capillary wedge pressure. If the elevation in creatinine is due to effective intravascular volume depletion, the azotemia should reverse. However, volume expansion will be ineffective in established hepatorenal syndrome, and further attempts at volume expansion should cease if no improvement is found with an initial trial.

The patient with ascites is prone to develop hyponatremia because of increased proximal tubule sodium absorption and high circulating levels of antidiuretic hormone. Therefore, if the serum sodium decreases to less than 130 mEq/liter, water restriction should be instituted. The restriction required is severe, usually less than 1 liter/day. Protein restriction may be required but should be instituted only if there is evidence of impending hepatic encephalopathy because of the negative effect on nutritional status. Acid-base derangements are common; the most common is respiratory alkalosis. However, both hyperchloremia and lactic acidoses are seen, and metabolic alkalosis occurs with vomiting or diuretic use. Urine and gastrointestinal losses of potassium may be high. Potassium should be replaced because hypokalemia increases renal ammonia production.

It is important to remember that the patient with hepatic disease is more prone to complications of drug therapy. The liver is a major route for drug metabolism, so the half-lives of multiple drugs are prolonged. Protein binding and distribution also may be altered. Decreased renal clearance occurs with diminished renal perfusion. Thus, drug toxicity is a common problem. Aminoglycoside toxicity occurs frequently. Nonsteroidal anti-inflammatories markedly decrease renal function. Vasodilators can cause marked hypotension and vasoconstrictors will further compromise renal function.

Dialysis has been attempted in patients with hepatorenal syndrome, but probably only delays death. Dialysis can be used to support a patient awaiting liver transplant or patients with severe acute hepatic failure in whom recovery is expected. Peritoneal-venous shunts have improved renal function in some patients but have a high complication rate. Despite this, the shunt is probably more successful than dialysis in long-term maintenance.

Suggested Readings

Gines P, Arroyo V, Quintero E, et al: Comparison of paracentesis and diuretics in the treatment of cirrhotics with tense ascites. Gastroenterology 93:234–241, 1987

Levy M: Hepatorenal syndrome. Kidney Int 43:737–753, 1993

Papadakis MA, Arieff AI: Unpredictability of clinical evaluation of renal function in cirrhosis, prospective study. Am J Med 82:945–952, 1987

Rocco VK, Ware AJ: Cirrhotic ascites: Pathophysiology, diagnosis and management. Ann Intern Med 105:573–585, 1986

Schelling JR, Linas SL: Hepatorenal syndrome. Semin Nephrol 10:565–570, 1990

Vaamonde CA: Selected renal and electrolyte abnormalities in liver disease. Am Kidney Fund Nephrol Lett 9: 13–28, 1992

Calculus Disorders

RENAL COLIC

JOSEPH W. SEGURA, M.D.

Rochester, Minnesota

Severe pain arising in the flank and radiating anteriorly and caudally toward the groin is called renal colic, even though the stone causing this pain is usually in the ureter. As the stone moves down the ureter, the pain is more likely to be felt in the abdomen in one of the lower quadrants, and, as the stone enters the distal ureter, the pain often is referred to the testis. The pain may be episodic or intermittent, but while present is unremitting and unaffected by changes in body position. Most patients will have tenderness over the affected flank, with guarding, but there are no peritoneal signs, although some patients may have a reflex ileus.

A plain film of the abdomen should be performed as the initial diagnostic step. Although the quality of such a film often leaves much to be desired because of intestinal gas and bowel contents, the diagnosis of ureteral stone is confirmed by finding a stone in the course of the ureter on the affected side. A negative film should be regarded with caution because a small stone easily may be missed and radiolucent stones (usually, uric acid) will not be seen. An intravenous pyelogram (IVP) may be necessary to settle doubtful cases and is desirable if the anatomy of the patient's collecting system is not known from previous such episodes. In "routine" situations, an emergency IVP is usually not necessary. Almost all patients have microhematuria, unless complete ureteral obstruction is present. A Gram stain of the urine should be obtained, as well as a urine culture and sensitivity.

The character and location of colic are such that a stone usually heads the differential diagnosis. Right-sided colic secondary to a lower ureteral stone may be confused for appendicitis. Less commonly, renal vein thrombosis will present symptoms indistinguishable from those of a renal or ureteral stone.

Sometimes, drug addicts or those suffering from Munchausen syndrome are practiced enough to exactly mimic symptoms of colic. Musculoskeletal pain, nerve root pain, and pain originating in the gallbladder all should be considered as diagnostic possibilities. Colic often is accompanied by nausea and vomiting, often requiring intravenous fluids.

Relief of pain should be effected as soon as the diagnosis is suggested. The pain is generally severe enough that morphine is required in doses of 2.0 to 6.0 mg IV, depending on the particular patient. It may be more practical to manage the patient with IM morphine in doses from 8.0 to 16 mg. Meperdine also can be used, but relatively large doses may be required to achieve the same effect. Pain control is the usual reason for hospital admission. Often, after 8 to 12 hours, the pain will have subsided, making discharge from the hospital possible. Home remedies for pain containing aspirin should be avoided because their antiplatelet activity may compromise stone removal if it becomes necessary.

Most patients either are afebrile or have a low-grade temperature. Fever is an ominous sign and may signal pyelonephritis or pyonephrosis. A positive Gram stain confirms the diagnosis of infection in the urinary tract, but the Gram stain still may be negative if the ureter is completely obstructed. Such situations require that the obstruction be bypassed by either a ureteral catheter or a percutaneous nephrostomy. Usually, this should be done as an emergency procedure. If the patient is febrile, or if the urine Gram stain is positive, antibiotics should be administered, and our preference is for intravenous antibiotics. Routine use of antibiotics in renal colic generally is not indicated.

Management of the particular stone event depends on a variety of factors, the most important of which is the size of the stone. As a rule of thumb, stones 4.0 mm or smaller have an 85 per cent chance of passing spontaneously. A 5.0-mm stone will pass about 50 per cent of the time, and, if the stone is greater than 5.0 mm in size, the chances of spontaneous passage drop to 10 to 15 per cent. Those patients with a history of successfully passing large stones may do so again, but those who have previously failed to pass even small stones may be again unsuccessful. The decision to intervene to remove the stone will reflect not only the chance of the stone passing, but a desire to avoid more trips to the emergency room or the need to remove the stone before an upcoming vacation, for example.

Emergency stone removal almost never is indicated. Even if a stent is being placed to relieve infection, the risks associated with the additional manipulation in the face of infection preclude this step. Today, most stones in the upper two thirds of the ureter are first treated with shock-wave lithotripsy (SWL), the goal of which is to further reduce the stone to fragments small enough to pass with minimal pain. Stones in the lower ureter also can be managed with SWL but often are removed using ureteroscopy. Open surgery rarely should be necessary.

Suggested Readings

Lingeman J: Urinary Calculi: ESWL, Endourology, and Medical Therapy. Philadelphia, Lea & Febiger, 1989

McCullough D: Problems in Urology: Calculous Disease, Vol 1, No 4. Philadelphia, JP Lippincott, 1987

Rous S: Stone Disease Diagnosis and Management. New York, Grune & Stratton, 1987

CALCIUM OXALATE STONES OF THE KIDNEY

J. PATRICK SPIRNAK, M.D., F.A.C.S.

Cleveland, Ohio

Stones consisting of calcium oxalate either in the pure form or in combination with calcium phosphate are the most common stones found in North America, and account for about 80 per cent of all calculi. The typical calcium oxalate stone former is usually a white, middle- to upper-class male who lives in the southeastern United States and is employed in a white-collar job with a sedentary life-style. He typically experiences his first stone event in the third decade of life and usually during the hot summer months. The typical first-time stone former usually will pass his stone spontaneously with the aid of fluids and analgesics. The first-time calcium stone former has about a 60 per cent chance of forming a second stone, usually over a 7-year period. Selective medical management based on any detectable metabolic abnormality can reduce the recurrence rate effectively in 90 per cent of calcium stone formers.

All patients who form a single stone should undergo screening laboratory studies consisting of complete blood count, urinalysis with urine culture if bacteria are detected, serum chemistry survey, an excretory urogram (intravenous pyelogram), and 24-hour urine collection for volume and measurement of calcium, phosphorus, uric acid, creatinine, citrate, and oxalate. A more thorough metabolic evaluation is performed only if abnormalities are detected. The most common abnormality identified is a low urine volume, frequently less than 1 liter/day.

Patients with no detectable metabolic abnormalities are encouraged to increase their fluid intake to achieve a minimal urine output of 2 to 3 liters/day. Water is the best fluid because colas, fruit juices, and tea are high in oxalate and should be consumed in moderation. Fluids are effective in controlling stone formation by decreasing the urinary concentration of stone-forming constituents. Repeat 24-hour urine collections are obtained to ensure compliance with this regimen. Patients also are instructed to consume in moderation high-calcium-containing foods such as ice cream and cheese. Foods rich in oxalate, such as tea, rhubarb, spinach, berries, chocolate, and nuts, also should be consumed in moderation.

Patients who continue to form stones in spite of adopting these basic dietary changes undergo more intensive metabolic evaluation consisting of repeated 24-hour urine collection before and after instituting a low-calcium and sodium-restricted diet for 1 week. The urine is studied for calcium, phosphorus, uric acid, magnesium, and creatinine. Blood is obtained for calcium, phosphorus, uric acid, and creatinine measurement both while the patient is on the regular diet and while on the restricted diet. If the serum calcium is elevated, a blood sample is sent to measure the parathyroid hormone level. In addition, the urine pH of all voided specimens is measured. Also, each patient has urine collected while fasting and after receiving a calcium load. By calculating the calcium-to-creatinine ratio in both the fasting and calcium-loaded states, one can differentiate between absorptive and renal hypercalciuria. If the urine pH in the fasting state is consistently above 5.3, renal tubular acidosis must be excluded. Hypercalciuria (300 mg/day on an unrestricted diet) is the most commonly detected abnormality and can be divided into absorptive and renal types.

ABSORPTIVE HYPERCALCIURIA

Absorptive hypercalciuria, present in 50 to 60 per cent of patients with recurrent calcium oxalate stones, is the most commonly detected metabolic abnormality. Individuals with this abnormality have altered intestinal response to vitamin D that causes increased absorption of calcium, elevated serum calcium levels, and depression of parathyroid function, which results in an increased amount of calcium being delivered to the kidney and excreted in the urine. Hypercalciuria present when the diet is unrestricted returns to normal when the dietary calcium is restricted to 150 mg/day. With fasting, the urinary calcium level is normal; after calcium loading, the urinary calcium level again becomes abnormally high, often to two to three times the fasting level.

Patients with absorptive hypercalciuria are encouraged to increase their daily urine output to at least 3 liters/day. Dietary consultation is obtained to instruct the patient in a limited-calcium diet (800 mg/day). In addition, it is known that a diet low in sodium reduces the intestinal absorption of calcium; therefore, sodium is restricted to 100 mEq/day.

Patients with absorptive hypercalciuria who fail to respond to a high fluid intake and a calcium-restricted diet are placed on sodium cellulose phosphate. This nonabsorbable ion-exchange resin corrects hypercalciuria by binding calcium in the intestinal tract and thus inhibiting calcium absorption. In addition to effectively lowering the urine concentration of calcium, cellulose phosphate causes an increase in the urinary phosphate level, a decrease in the serum magnesium level, and an increase in the urinary excretion of oxalate. This drug is not indicated to treat other forms of hypercalciuria because it can overstimulate parathyroid function. It is useful in patients with severe absorptive hypercalciuria or those patients who have failed, or do not tolerate, thiazide therapy. Sodium cellulose phosphate (2.5 to 5 gm) is taken with meals. Oral magnesium supplementation (magnesium gluconate, 1 gm twice per day) is provided while dietary oxalate is restricted.

Orthophosphates have been shown to decrease the incidence of stone formation in patients with absorptive hypercalciuria and in patients with idiopathic recurrent calcium stone disease. Orthophosphates act by decreasing urinary excretion of calcium and increasing excretion of two urinary inhibitors, pyrophosphate and citrate. Treatment with orthophosphates (administered to provide 1.5 to 2.5 gm of elemental phosphorus per 24 hours in three to four divided doses) is considered in patients with absorptive hypercalciuria who have failed changes in dietary and fluid management. Orthophosphates are contraindicated in patients with urinary tract infections and should be used with caution in patients with hypercalciuria or compromised renal function. Gastrointestinal side effects such as diarrhea and bloating may occur during treatment.

RENAL HYPERCALCIURIA

Renal hypercalciuria is found in about 10 per cent of all calcium stone–forming patients. The cause of the kidneys' inability to conserve calcium is unknown; however, it has been suggested that an abnormality in tubular function may be responsible. The urinary calcium level does not typically decrease following fasting, and it may increase following a calcium load. The increased excretion of calcium by the kidney results in a low serum calcium level, which stimulates parathyroid hormone secretion (secondary hyperparathyroidism), increased synthesis of vitamin D_3, and increased absorption of calcium from the gastrointestinal tract.

Thiazide is the treatment of choice for patients with renal hypercalciuria. The thiazides exert their hypocalciuric effect by increasing calcium reabsorption in the distal tuble. Additional reabsorption of calcium occurs in the proximal tubule in response to extracellular volume depletion. The hypocalciuric effect usually begins 2 to 3 days after instituting thiazide therapy, becomes maximal in 6 days, and nearly always is sustained. Thiazides have no effect on oxalate excretion; however, they do increase the urinary concentration of zinc and magnesium, which may further enhance their effectiveness.

Hydrochlorothiazide (50 mg twice a day), chlorthalidone (Hygroton, 50 mg/day), or trichlormethiazide (Naqua, 4 mg/day) are the agents most frequently used. Hypokalemia typically occurs regardless of the drug used and may be responsible for the side effects of weakness and fatigue commonly associated with thiazide therapy. Additionally, hypokalemia also may lower the renal excretion of citrate and thus reduce its effectiveness in inhibiting stone formation. Potassium citrate (10 to 20 mEq twice a day) is given to replace the potassium; the added citrate further opposes new stone formation by reducing the urinary saturation of calcium salts while directly inhibiting the crystallization of calcium. Potassium citrate is contraindicated in renal failure, hyperkalemia, peptic ulcer disease, and active urinary tract infections. Thiazides also increase urinary uric acid excretion, which may promote hyperuricosuric calcium oxalate stones. Urinary uric acid excretion levels should be checked periodically.

NORMOCALCIURIA

Normocalciuric patients who continue to form oxalate stones in spite of adequate hydration and dietary modifications are placed empirically on neutral phosphates to achieve urinary phosphorus levels above 800 mg/day. Thiazides also may be used in these patients.

HYPOCITRATURIA

Patients with idiopathic hypocitraturia (320 mg/day) and recurrent calcium oxalate stone disease are placed on potassium citrate. The slow-release tablet preparation is well tolerated and has been shown to increase citrate levels to normal.

Hypocitraturia, either alone or in combination with another metabolic abnormality, is a known contributor to calcium oxalate stone disease. Citrate inhibits crystallization of calcium oxalate by binding calcium and reducing the saturation of calcium oxalate. It also may inhibit directly the crystallization of calcium salts.

HYPEROXALURIA

Primary hyperoxaluria is a rare autosomal recessive disorder that causes recurrent calcium oxalate stones, nephrocalcinosis, and renal failure, usually before age 40. Medical treatment consists of pyridoxine with phosphate and magnesium supplementation.

Secondary hyperoxaluria may occur in patients with inflammatory bowel disease, and in those who have undergone intestinal bypass surgery for morbid obesity. In the normal intestinal tract, most of the oxalate binds to calcium and exists as the insoluble and nonabsorbable calcium salt. Patients with malabsorption syndromes have excessive amounts of unabsorbed fatty acids that bind to calcium; as a result, less calcium is available to bind oxalate, and thus enteric oxalate absorption is increased. Treatment consists of hydration, limiting oxalate intake, and oral calcium supplementation to bind oxalate and inhibit absorption.

SURGICAL TREATMENT

Surgical intervention is indicated in patients who present with obstruction and persistent pain. Small renal stones (2 to 3 cm) are treated by extracorporeal shock-wave lithotripsy, whereas larger stones are managed with either a percutaneous or an open surgical technique.

Suggested Readings

Coe FL: Treatment of hypercalciuria. N Engl J Med 311: 116, 1984

Drach GW: Urinary lithiasis: Etiology, diagnosis, and medical management. *In* Walsh PC, Retik AB, Stamey TA, et al (eds): Campbell's Urology, 6th ed. Philadelphia, WB Saunders, 1992, pp 2085–2156

Menon M, Mahle CJ: Urinary citrate excretion in patients with renal calculi. J Urol 129:1158, 1983

Pak CYC: Medical management of nephrolithiasis: Update, 1987. J Urol 140:461, 1988

Pak CYC, Britton F, Peterson R, et al: Ambulatory evaluation of nephrolithiasis: Classification, clinical presentation, and diagnostic criteria. Am J Med 69:19, 1980

Spirnak JP, Resnick MI: Urinary stones. *In* Tanagho ED, McAninch JW (eds): Smith's General Urology, 13th ed. Norwalk, CT, Appleton and Lange, 1992, pp 271–298

URIC ACID CALCULI

J. PATRICK SPIRNAK, M.D., F.A.C.S.

Cleveland, Ohio

Uric acid stones account for approximately 5 to 10 per cent of all urinary calculi found in the United States. The occurrence is higher in certain Mideastern countries, where ethnic origin and hot, dry climates probably play a role. Humans and the Dalmation coach hound are the only mammals prone to the development of uric acid stones. Uric acid, which is very insoluble in water, is the major end-product of purine metabolism. All mammals other than humans possess the hepatic enzyme uricase, which converts uric acid to allantoin, a highly water-soluble substance. The Dalmation coach hound possesses uricase, but its proximal renal tubules do not reabsorb all filtered uric acid. Thus, uric acid may be excreted in the urine in abnormally high concentrations.

All uric acid in the serum is filtered by the glomeruli and readily absorbed by the proximal renal tubule. In humans, the reabsorbed uric acid is secreted by the distal renal tubule. In other mammals, it is recirculated to the liver and transformed there into allantoin, which is excreted by the kidneys. The average human excretes about 400 mg of uric acid daily, approximately 10 times more than other mammals.

Uric acid is insoluble in water, which accounts for the formation of uric acid calculi. Once uric acid is secreted into the urine, it exists in two forms: insoluble uric acid and the urate salt, which is 20 times more soluble than the free acid form. Uric acid is a weak acid, with a pK_a of approximately 5.5 (i.e., in a solution with a pH of 5.5, half of the uric acid exists in the insoluble un-ionized form and half in the ionized form). As the urine becomes more acidic, more of the uric acid exists in the insoluble, un-ionized form. Humans secrete predominately an acidic urine with an average pH of 6.2. Individuals who are prone to forming uric acid stones will secrete a predominately acidic urine with a pH of less than 5.5. Therefore, most of the uric acid in susceptible individuals will exist in the insoluble or un-ionized form.

At a pH of 5.0 and at 37° C, urinary saturation occurs with only 60 mg of uric acid per liter of urine. As the pH of the urine is increased to 6, the urine does not become saturated until it contains 220 mg of uric acid per liter, and at a pH of 6.5 nearly all of the uric acid exists in the ionized or readily soluble form. In such a metabolic environment, precipitation of uric acid crystals is unlikely to occur. However, the ionized urate will react with available sodium or potassium to form urate salts. Potassium urate is much more soluble than sodium urate; therefore, increasing the sodium concentration in the urine makes dissolution less likely, whereas increasing the potassium concentration favors the formation of the more soluble potassium urate and favors dissolution.

Most individuals are protected from uric acid stone formation by the temporary elevation in urinary pH that typically follows a meal. Stone formers typically maintain a constant urinary pH in the acidic range (5 to 5.5) and fail to demonstrate the normal postprandial alkaline tide.

A low urine volume also can lead to oversaturation with uric acid and an increased incidence of uric acid stone formation. Patients with inflammatory bowel disease, such as ulcerative colitis, and those with an ileostomy lack the normal colonic reabsorption of water and bicarbonate and typically excrete highly concentrated acidic urine, and are thus more likely to form uric acid stones.

CLASSIFICATION

It is helpful to classify uric acid calculus disease into four categories.

Idiopathic Uric Acid Lithiasis

These patients do not demonstrate elevated serum levels of uric acid or increased urinary excretion of uric acid. They typically excrete a persistently acidic urine (pH 5 to 5.5) without the normal variations in urinary pH. The mechanism to explain this fixed urinary pH is currently unknown.

Calculi Associated with Hyperuricemia

Individuals with a metabolic abnormality such as primary gout or the Lesch-Nyhan syndrome form uric acid calculi. The upper limit of normal for serum uric acid concentration generally is accepted to be 7 mg/dl in men and 5.5 mg/dl in women. About 25 per cent patients with symptomatic gout will form uric acid stones, and about 25 per cent of patients who have formed uric acid stones will prove to have gout. Patients with myeloproliferative disorders such as lymphoma also may exhibit hyperuricemia and hyperuricosuria, presumably as a result of increased cell turnover. Patients receiving chemotherapy for treatment of neoplastic disease also may have increased serum levels of uric acid and hyperuricosuria.

Calculi Associated with Dehydration

Patients with chronic diarrhea or those with ileostomies are more prone to formation of uric acid stones. These patients typically excrete a highly acidic and concentrated urine, which is believed to be due to excessive loss of fluid and bicarbonate. The excretion rate of uric acid is typically normal in these individuals. Strenuous physical activity also may precipitate uric acid stones by reducing the urine output (as a result of fluid loss from perspiration) and lowering the urinary pH (as a result of lactic acidosis).

Calculi Associated with Hyperuricosuria without Hyperuricemia

Hyperuricosuria is defined in men as the presence of more than 800 mg of uric acid in a 24-hour urine specimen, and in women as the presence of more than 750 mg of uric acid per 24-hour urine collection. Drugs such as thiazide diuretics and salicylates can cause hyperuricosuria and lead to uric acid stone formation.

DIAGNOSIS

The typical patient with a uric acid stone will present with acute pain or colic associated with stone passage and urinary obstruction. Pure uric acid stones are typically radiolucent and therefore will not be seen on plain abdominal films. One exception to this is the presence of a large or dense stone, which may be faintly visualized on radiographic examination. An excretory urogram frequently demonstrates a filling defect in the renal pelvis or collecting system. The differential diagnosis of a radiolucent filling defect includes uric acid stone, blood clot, tumor, or sloughed renal tissue. The presence of an acid urine, a negative cytology, and typical findings on either ultrasound or computerized tomographic evaluation of the kidney differentiates a radiolucent uric acid stone from other common urologic abnormalities. Ureteroscopy may prove useful when other less invasive studies have failed to confirm the diagnosis. Once the diagnosis of uric acid stone has been established, a 24-hour urine is obtained to measure the urinary volume, the pH, and the uric acid content.

TREATMENT

Pure uric acid stones are unique in that they initially are treated by attempted dissolution. Surgical intervention is reserved for those that fail medical management. Treatment is based on urinary alkalinization and hydration. Patients are encouraged to drink at least eight 8-oz glasses of water per day in an attempt to increase the daily urine volume to a minimum of 3 liters/day.

A number of treatment options are available to alkalinize the urine. Sodium bicarbonate, in a daily dose of 0.5 to 1.5 mEq/kg, is the least expensive of the available alkalinizing agents. The typical 10-grain sodium bicarbonate tablet contains the equivalent of 7.2 mEq of bicarbonate. The calculated daily dose is usually divided and administered four times daily. The urinary Ph must be checked regularly with a narrow-range pH paper to maintain a urine pH of 6.5 to 7.0. Overalkalinization to a pH greater than 7.0 is to be avoided because additional dissolution does not occur and calcium phosphate may precipitate as a shell around the uric acid stone, thus inhibiting further attempts at dissolution.

Another oral preparation that is being used with increasing frequency is potassium citrate. This potassium preparation is preferred in patients with normal renal function and normal serum potassium levels to sodium-containing preparations because monopotassium urate is more soluble than sodium urate. The average dose of potassium citrate is 15 mEq taken three to four times per day. The citrate is readily metabolized to bicarbonate and sustained levels of alkalinization are readily achieved.

Polycitra (a commercially available mixture of sodium citrate and potassium citrate) is particularly useful in patients with inflammatory bowel disease, who are likely to have chronic diarrhea or malabsorption problems. These patients typically have rapid intestinal transit times, thus inhibiting the absorption of medications taken in tablet form. A typical dose is 30 ml taken three to four times per day.

A trial of intravenous alkalinization is started in patients who require hospitalization for either pain control or persistent nausea and vomiting. Rapid systemic alkalinization is possible with 1/6th-molar lactate administered at a rate of 50 to 75 ml/hr. The urine pH typically reaches 7 within several hours, and the IV rate then is adjusted to maintain an alkaline urine. This method has been shown to be safe and just as effective as direct irrigation with an alkaline solution, and avoids the potential complications associated with nephrostomy tube placement. One disadvantage is the increased sodium load that is administered, which requires careful monitoring for fluid overload and the development of congestive heart failure.

Patients in whom a rapid response to alkalinization is desired and who it has been determined could not tolerate an excessive sodium load may achieve rapid dissolution of their stone by direct irrigation with a sodium bicarbonate solution via either a transureteral or percutaneous catheter approach.

Patients with hyperuricosuria are instructed to consume a diet low in purine-rich foods, such as red meat, beef, chicken, and other high-protein foods such as peanuts. Dietary consultation is obtained to help limit the protein intake to about 90 gm/day.

Hyperuricemic patients or those with hyperuricosuria (greater than 800 mg of uric acid per day) frequently may benefit from the administration of the xanthine oxidase inhibitor allopurinol in doses of 200 to 600 mg/day. Allopurinol inhibits the formation of uric acid and lowers the concentration of uric acid in the serum as well as in the urine. Side effects are uncommon, but may include skin rash, drug fever, diarrhea, and abdominal cramps.

Patients who fail an aggressive attempt at stone dissolution typically have mixed stones of calcium and uric acid. These patients are treated by either extracorporeal shock-wave lithotripsy or ureteroscopic stone extraction depending on the size and location of the offending calculus. New stones are prevented by maintaining adequate hydration and urinary alkalinization.

Suggested Readings

Gutman AB, Yu TF: Uric acid nephrolithiasis. Am J Med 45:756, 1968

Kursh ED, Resnick MI: Dissolution of uric acid calculi with systemic alkalinization. J Urol 132:286, 1984

Lewis RW, Roth JK, Pocanco EJ, et al: Molar lactate in the management of uric acid renal obstruction. J Urol 125:87, 1981

Pal CYC, Sakhaee K, Fuller C: Successful management of uric acid nephrolithiasis with potassium citrate. Kidney Int 30:422, 1986

Rodman JS: Prophylaxis of uric acid stones with alternate day doses of alkaline potassium salts. J Urol 145:97, 1991

CALCIUM PHOSPHATE UROLITHIASIS

JOSEPH W. SEGURA, M.D.

Rochester, Minnesota

Most patients presenting for a metabolic stone work-up either will have passed a stone just recently or will have a stone identified on a radiograph. Because subsequent calculi are usually the same type as previous ones, analysis of any previous stones is important. If the previous stone was a large stone treated with shock-wave lithotripsy or percutaneous ultrasonic lithotripsy, there may be only fragments, and, although analysis of these fragments may reveal calcium phosphate, one should be aware of the possibility that, because of a sampling error, other crystal types may have been present but not analyzed.

The patient should not have had an infection, and magnesium ammonium phosphate, or struvite, should not have been identified in any previous stone analyses. Evaluation of the patient at this point consists of (1) radiographic evaluation with excretory urography and tomograms, and (2) serum creatinine, electrolytes, and serum calcium measurement.

Because of the propensity of these stones to be associated with primary hyperparathyroidism, serum calcium determinations in the high normal range should be repeated. Parathyroid determinations probably are not indicated, at least routinely. Twenty-four–hour urine collections for calcium, phosphorus, oxalate, creatinine, citrate, and uric acid should be performed, as well as a spot test for cystine. Serum pH should be determined, and early morning urinary pH should be determined as a screening test for renal tubular acidosis.

The diagnosis of a specific metabolic abnormality often is possible. If such an abnormality is identified and appropriately treated, there is approximately a 95 per cent chance of eliminating further stone formation.

Primary hyperparathyroidism is described elsewhere in this volume, and is responsible for some 3 to 5 per cent of urinary calculi. Routine measurement of the serum calcium level as part of an automated blood analysis has made the diagnosis of this entity more common than in the past. An elevated serum calcium level confirmed by elevated parathyroid hormone determinations will establish the diagnosis. The surgical removal of a parathyroid adenoma, or of most functioning parathyroid tissue in the case of hyperplasia, usually will reduce serum calcium levels to normal, and patients with previously very active urinary stone formation will cease forming new stones.

The same is true with other metabolic diseases that might be identified, such as renal tubular acidosis, sarcoidosis, vitamin D intoxication, and stone disease associated with immobilization. Radiographic follow-up of any such patients is essential to determine whether or not metabolic activity indeed is present. For example, some patients with residual renal stones who achieve successful metabolic control by removal of a parathyroid adenoma may continue to pass these residual stones on an occasional basis for months and sometimes years to come.

The identification of calcium phosphate stones from previous stone passage or the suspicion of them on radiographs has a bearing on surgical treatment. Smooth, dense stones often are made of calcium phosphate or brushite, and such stones are very hard and may not break up readily with shock-wave lithotripsy. Although stones 2.0 cm or less in size, irrespective of their stone type, usually are treated with shock-wave lithotripsy, and only the failures subjected to percutaneous lithotripsy, it is probably true that borderline cases—those somewhat larger stones composed of calcium phosphate—should undergo percutaneous lithotripsy primarily because of the high risk of extracorporeal shock-wave lithotripsy failure.

Calcium phosphate stones often are associated with magnesium ammonium phosphate, or struvite, stones. These stones occur in the presence of urea-splitting bacteria, and a full discussion is given elsewhere in this volume.

Suggested Readings

Lingeman J: Urinary Calculi: ESWL, Endourology, and Medical Therapy. Philadelphia, Lea & Febiger, 1989

McCullough D: Problems in Urology: Calculous Disease, Vol 1, No 4. Philadelphia, JP Lippincott, 1987

Rous S: Stone Disease Diagnosis and Management. New York, Grune & Stratton, 1987

CYSTINE STONES

MARTIN I. RESNICK, M.D.

Cleveland, Ohio

Cystinuria accounts for approximately 1 to 2 per cent of all urinary stones and is the result of an inherited homozygous recessive disorder of dibasic amino acid transport across epithelial membranes. This defect manifests itself in the gastrointestinal tract of affected individuals, as impaired absorption of amino acids, and in the renal tubule, resulting in excessive excretion of the dibasic amino acids cystine, ornithine, arginine, and lysine. Because of its poor solubility in urine, cystine is the only amino acid involved that causes significant morbidity in affected individuals. Patients who are heterozygous for the inherited disorder usually excrete less than 250 mg of cystine per gram of urinary creatinine and do not reach the supersaturated levels of urinary cystine necessary for stone formation. Interestingly, these individuals are at increased risk for calcium oxalate stone formation. Although there are no known inhibitors of cystine stone formation, urinary electrolyte and macromolecule composition does have an impact on cystine solubility. Patients afflicted with this disorder can develop symptoms at any age from infancy onward, but the peak incidence is during the first two decades of life.

DIAGNOSIS

In the cystinuric patient, microscopic examination of a freshly spun first-voided morning urine often will reveal typical hexagonal cystine crystals. The specimen can be further examined by the cyanide-nitroprusside test, which, in the absence of homocystinuria and ketonuria, will identify correctly urinary cystine excretion in excess of 75 mg/liter. The "paper strip" test is another method by which urinary cystine content can be estimated. Abdominal radiographs in the patient with renal colic will reveal the radiopaque cystine stones provided they are at least 3 to 4 mm in size. In this setting, a 24-hour urine collection for cystine, oxalate, calcium, creatinine, uric acid, and citrate measurement is indicated because cystinuria can be associated with hypocitraturia, hypercalciuria, or hyperuricosuria. Cystine can be quantitated by amino acid analysis or Dionex ion chromatography.

MANAGEMENT OPTIONS

The primary goal in the management of a patient with cystinuria is to prevent urinary cystine concentrations from exceeding the solubility limit, thereby preventing precipitation of calculus. Once a patient fails the observation period or develops a large stone with a low likelihood of spontaneously passing the stone, the treatment options include urinary alkylinization, extracorporeal shock-wave lithotripsy, endoscopic stone retrieval, endoscopic electrohydraulic lithotripsy or laser ablation, percutaneous nephrolithotomy, or combination therapy with percutaneous nephrolithotomy and chemolysis.

Alkylinization

Alkylinization of the urine enhances cystine solubility; if urine pH can be maintained above 7.8, cystine solubility will be increased two- to threefold. This is difficult to accomplish on a consistent basis, but can be achieved with oral alkylinization in the form of 12.6 gm or more of sodium bicarbonate every 24 hours in divided doses, or 60 to 80 ml of a balanced citrate solution per day in divided doses. The citrate preparations are preferred because they enhance calcium solubility and provide for a more constant elevation in urinary pH.

Dietary Changes

Increased oral fluid intake to provide for a daily urine output of not less than 2 liters is another means by which urinary cystine concentrations can be decreased. In a patient with moderate cystinuria (250 to 500 mg/day), this volume of daily urine output often will maintain urinary cystine concentrations below the solubility limit and thereby prevent calculus formation, and will assist in dissolution. All fluids are acceptable with the exception of tea, which is high in oxalate (a known risk factor of calcium stone formation), and milk, which is high in methionine (an essential amino acid in cystine formation). Accordingly, dietary restriction of methionine is reasonable but provides for a very bland, unpalatable diet with which most patients will not comply. However, patients must be counciled on avoiding overconsumption of foods containing high levels of methionine.

Chelation

Chelating agents include D-penicillamine (beta-beta-dimethylcysteine) and alpha-mercaptopropionylglycine (Thiola), which contains a free sulfhydryl group and undergoes thio-disulfide exchange, which disrupts the cys-S-S-cys disulfide bond, acting to generate a more soluble cysteine-S-Thiola compound. Both agents are Food and Drug Administration–approved treatment modalities, and can be administered orally; provided there is an appreciable decrease in excreted cystine, dissolution of an existing stone could occur. Cystine stone dissolution is a very slow process, and these agents tend to be more efficacious when used in a preventive rather than therapeutic setting.

The dose of D-penicillamine is based on the known excreted amount of cystine in the urine. Every 250-mg increment in D-penicillamine can be expected to lower the excreted load of urinary cystine by 75 to 100 mg/day. D-penicillamine does have significant potential side effects associated with its use, including gastrointestinal manifestations (nausea, vomiting, diarrhea, anorexia, generalized crampy abdominal pain, bloating, and flatus) and impairment of taste and smell. Additionally, dermatologic manifestations in the form of pharyngitis, oral ulcers, rash ecchymosis, pruritis, urticaria, pemphigus, elastosis perforans, and skin wrinkling have been reported. Hypersensitivity reactions, including laryngeal edema, dyspnea, respiratory distress, fever, chills, arthralgia, malaise, and adenopathy, also have been recorded. Hematologic abnormalities such as leukopenia, agranulocystosis, thrombocytopenia, anemia, and eosinophilia, as well as hepatic dysfunction and renal complications, including proteinuria, nephrotic syndrome, and glomerulonephritis, also can occur.

Cessation of D-penicillamine may be required in a significant percentage of patients because of its side effects, which tend to reverse spontaneously on discontinuation of the medication. However, the drug can be reinstituted in certain individuals at a later date when the patient will have developed desensitization and can better tolerate the medication. Finally, patients who remain on this medication for extended periods of time or who are receiving doses greater than 1 gm/day should receive supplemental vitamin B_6 because of the excessive binding of pyridoxine that occurs in the gastrointestinal tract.

Alpha-mercaptopropionylglycine (Thiola) is a less toxic oral chelating agent that may serve as an alternative to D-penicillamine in the patient who manifests side effects of the latter medication. Thiola provides for equivalent urinary cystine reduction with considerably less side effects. However, Thiola is probably more effective in the preventive setting than for treatment of existing stones.

Shock-Wave Therapy

Cystine stones tend to be quite hard and somewhat resistant to shock-wave therapy. Larger stones often require higher energy lithotripsy and a greater number of shocks to fragment. Also, the stone-free rate following extracorporeal shock-wave lithotripsy of cystine stones is comparatively much lower than with stones of different composition (i.e., calcium oxalate, magnesium ammonium phosphate, and uric acid).

Surgical Treatment

Depending on the location of the stone, endoscopic stone extraction is an effective means of managing a cystine stone. This procedure is most successful when stones are located in the distal ureter, and can be safely performed in the outpatient setting. After using a ureteral balloon dilator, the stone basket can be advanced to the level of the stone under fluoroscopic or ureteroscopic guidance and the stone then can be extracted atraumatically. The patient then can be sent home with or without an indwelling ureteral stent. Likewise, endoscopic electrohydraulic lithotripsy or laser ablation of a cystine stone can be carried out under direct visualization utilizing a ureteroscope. These patients usually require a ureteral stent after these procedures and often can be sent home the day after the surgery.

Percutaneous nephrolithotomy often is required for upper tract stones that are not amenable to extraction or ablation from below. After achieving percutaneous access, the stone can be approached through the flexible or rigid nephroscope and treated appropriately. Because of the hard consistency of the cystine stone, stone-free status may not be achieved in one treatment session, and debulking may be advantageous. In this setting the nephrostomy tube is left in place and the patient can be re-treated at a later date or can undergo irrigation therapy at the bedside. Fragmentation of the stone provides for a larger surface area to irrigate and chemolysis is more effective. The most efficacious solution to use in the cystinuric patient is 0.3-molar acetylcystine in Tham E. The pH of this solution is approximately 10, and chemolysis of residual fragments can be achieved in a relatively short period of time with low morbidity provided renal pelvic pressures are maintained below 25 cm of water.

LONG-TERM CONSIDERATIONS

Long-term management of the cystinuric patient with frequent episodes of calculus formation should include continued high-fluid intake and chronic treatment with a cystine chelating agent as well as a urinary alkalinizing agent. Periodic evaluation with imaging studies (ultrasound or radiography) to assess the renal stone burden in a patient undergoing chemolysis, which may take months to years to complete, is certainly indicated, as are quantitative urinalyses to determine the effectiveness of the conservative treatment regimens.

First-degree relatives of cystinurics should be evaluated for the disorder by means of a quantitative urine assessment for cystine. However, children of cystinurics who have a very low incidence of cystinuria despite being a carrier for the defective gene warrant evaluation only if the other parent has a familial history or is also a cystinuric.

Suggested Readings

Crawhill JC, Watts RWE: Cystinuria. Am J Med 45:736, 1968

Drach GW: Urinary lithiasis: Etiology, diagnosis, and medical management. *In* Walsh PC, Retik AB, Stamey TA, et al: (eds): Campbell's Urology, 6th ed. Philadelphia, WB Saunders, 1992, p 2117

Pak CYC: Cystine lithiasis. *In* Resnick MI, Pak CYC (eds): Urolithiasis: A Medical and Surgical Reference. Philadelphia, WB Saunders, 1990, pp 133–143

Smith LH: Errors in membrane transport: Cystinuria, renal glycosuria and renal tubular acidosis. *In* Wintrobe MM, Thorn GW, Adams RD, et al (eds): Principles of Internal Medicine, 7th ed. New York, McGraw-Hill, 1974, p 600

INFECTIOUS CALCULI

KEITH N. VAN ARSDALEN, M.D.

Philadelphia, Pennsylvania

Infectious calculi account for 15 to 20 per cent of upper urinary tract calculi. Although a calculus of any composition may become secondarily infected, the terms "infectious" or "infection induced" usually refer to those calculi that are composed of crystals of magnesium ammonium phosphate (struvite) or a combination of magnesium ammonium phosphate and calcium phosphate (triple phosphate) that result from chronic infections with urease-producing bacteria. Infectious calculi are more common in women, consistent with their higher prevalence of urinary tract infections. Patients with neurogenic voiding disorders, with indwelling catheters, and with supravesical urinary diversions also are more susceptible to these infections and stone formation.

PATHOGENESIS

Supersaturation of the urine with OH^-, NH_4^+, and CO_3^- and an alkaline pH are necessary for struvite crystallization to occur. These specific physicochemical conditions are produced in vivo only in the presence of urease-producing bacteria. This enzyme, which was first isolated in 1926, hydrolyzes urea into NH_3 and CO_2. This enzyme is not normally found in humans but may be produced by certain types of bacteria that invade the urinary tract. The most common urea-splitting organisms are the *Proteus* species as well as certain subtypes of *Klebsiella, Serratia, Pseudomonas,* and *Staphylococcus. Escherichia coli* rarely produces urease.

CLINICAL PRESENTATION AND EVALUATION

Patients may present with typical ureteral colic caused by passage of a struvite stone or with symptoms resulting from cystitis or pyelonephritis. Occasionally they may present with fulminant urosepsis resulting from the development of obstruction, pyonephrosis, or parenchymal or perinephric abscess formation. The hallmark of struvite deposition, however, is the staghorn calculus, which may become quite massive without any associated symptoms. These stones may be identified incidentally on other radiographs or may be detected during the evaluation of persistent chronic urinary tract infections.

Plain abdominal radiographs and intravenous urography are the most useful radiologic studies for evaluation of the urinary tract in association with struvite calculi. The radiodensity of these calculi is dependent on the amount of carbonate apatite that is either mixed with the struvite or deposited in layers, giving a laminated appearance of the stone, because pure struvite has a relatively low density. By contrast, increasing amounts of noncrystalline matrix may make these calculi even less apparent on plain radiographs. Other studies, such as retrograde pyelography, radionuclide renography, and computerized tomographic scanning, may be useful to define the extent of the stone, the function of the kidney, and the involvement of the parenchyma in order to plan appropriate therapy. Finally, urinary tract cultures and sensitivities are essential to determine appropriate antibiotic therapy.

THERAPEUTIC OPTIONS

The primary goal of therapy is the elimination of infection, which can be accomplished only by complete removal of all of the stone. It is well documented that bacteria are harbored throughout the entire calculus, which cannot be sterilized even ex vivo with stringent antiseptic techniques. Hence, surgical therapy remains the treatment of choice; however, medical measures may be useful as an adjunct to surgery or occasionally may be indicated as an alternative to surgery when the latter is contraindicated.

Although it is impossible to sterilize the urinary tract in the presence of a struvite calculus or residual fragments following treatment, the chronic use of suppressive antibiotics may slow stone growth and ameliorate symptoms. Penicillin and its derivatives achieve adequate levels in the urine to suppress the growth of most strains of *Proteus*, the most common organism identified by culture. Even in the absence of residual stone fragments, a prolonged course of culture-specific antibiotics is an important adjunctive measure following surgical removal of struvite calculi in order to sterilize the collecting system and parenchyma in cases of long-standing infection.

Griffith has extensively studied the use of acetohydroxamic acid (AHA) as an inhibitor of bacterial urease. AHA proved useful in decreasing stone growth and in reducing urinary ammonia levels compared to placebo; however, neurosensory, hematologic, and dermatologic side effects were not uncommon. Other nonsurgical measures include maintaining a high urine output and urinary acidification, although the latter may be difficult to achieve.

The surgical treatment of infectious calculi involves extracorporeal shock-wave lithotripsy, endourologic techniques, or combinations thereof. Small struvite renal calculi, partial staghorn calculi, and even delicate but complete staghorn calculi may be managed primarily by shock-wave lithotripsy. Adjunctive use of a retrograde catheter or a stent usually is required to ensure that there is no obstruction, and one must be certain that the degree of fragmentation is adequate. Bulky struvite calculi and complete staghorn calculi are treated most frequently with a combination of initial percutaneous debulking followed by shock-wave lithotripsy of residual portions of the calculus that are inaccessible to the percutaneous ultrasonic lithotrite. A combination of these treatment modalities has proved to be more efficacious and less morbid than either modality alone when dealing with stones of increasing size and complexity. This combination also may allow for irrigation of the collecting system with agents such as hemiacidrin or Suby Solution G to eliminate small residual particles that may remain within the collecting system. Ureteral calculi may be managed with stenting and shock-wave lithotripsy or ureteroscopic techniques. The postoperative use of culture-specific antibiotics and other measures has been mentioned.

Open surgical procedures, including anatrophic nephrolithotomy, largely have been replaced by these less invasive modalities. It should be noted, however, that this procedure, other open techniques, or nephrectomy in the case of a poorly functioning, infected kidney may in fact be appropriate in certain circumstances.

Suggested Readings

Drach GW: Urinary lithiasis: Etiology, diagnosis, and medical management. *In* Walsh PC, Retik AB, Stamey TA, et al (eds): Campbell's Urology, 6th ed. Philadelphia, WB Saunders, 1992, pp 2085–2156

Lingeman JE: Staghorn calculus: Percutaneous versus ESWL treatment. *In* Carson CC III (ed): Problems in Urology: Endourology. Philadelphia, JB Lippincott, 1987, pp 346–354

Meacham RA, Griffith DP: Management of the chronic struvite stone former with chronic urinary tract infection. *In* McCullough DL (ed): Problems in Urology: Calculus Disease, Vol 1, No 4. Philadelphia, JB Lippincott, 1987, pp 660–667

Van Arsdalen KN: Pathogenesis of renal calculi. Urol Radiol 6:65, 1984

Van Arsdalen KN, Banner MP, Pollack HM: Radiographic imaging and urologic decision making in the management of renal and ureteral calculi. Urol Clin North Am 17:171, 1990

URINARY TRACT CALCIUM OXALATE STONE DISEASE FOLLOWING BOWEL RESECTION

JOHN G. GREGORY, M.D.

St. Louis, Missouri

The occurrence of urinary calculi following bowel resection was first reported in studies dealing with the surgical treatment of regional enteritis, but it was not until the publication of series made up of large numbers of patients who had undergone massive bowel defunctionalization by small bowel bypass procedures that this subject attracted attention. It was first suggested that the calculi were uric acid, induced, as in ileostomy patients, by conditions of dehydration, protein catabolism, and acidosis. Examination of the calculi showed those formed secondary to bowel resection or defunctionalization consisted of calcium oxalate.

MECHANISM OF HYPEROXALURIA

The mechanism of stone formation following intestinal resection is only partially understood. It does appear certain that, following the removal of segments of small intestine, hyperoxaluria does occur, and that its extent depends on the amount of intestine removed. The occurrence of this hyperoxaluria is also dependent on an intact colon. Those few patients having both small intestinal resections and an ileostomy do not become hyperoxaluric.

Various metabolic pathways have been explored in an attempt to pinpoint the source of the hyperoxaluria. It is now well established that the oxaluria is not predominantly endogenous, but rather is derived from an exogenous source. It appears that, following small bowel resection, dietary oxalate is absorbed in greater quantities, presumably by the colon, than in an intact individual.

Following a small bowel bypass procedure in which all intestine 12 inches distal to the ligament of Treitz and 6 inches proximal to the ileocecal junction is bypassed and in which the bypassed bowel is secondarily drained into the transverse colon, the gut will absorb up to 300 times more of a given oxalate load than was absorbed prior to surgery.

The mechanism explaining this enteric hyperabsorption is not fully understood. It has been suggested that, following bypass, steatorrhea occurs, and the unabsorbed fat combines with calcium in the gut lumen, making a soap and reducing the amount of ionized calcium present in the lumen. It is presumed that, in the normal individual this luminal calcium combines with oxalate, forming an insoluble salt. With insufficient calcium, highly soluble oxalic acid passively diffuses through all gut surfaces. Alternatively, it has been proposed that bile salts and small-chain fatty acids placed in the colon can stimulate an increased active absorption of gut oxalate via the active chloride/bicarbonate system. Once this oxalate is absorbed, patients with enteric hyperoxaluria display an elevated plasma oxalate and a renal excretion in excess of creatinine, indicating active tubular secretion of this acid.

It is possible, by totally avoiding dietary oxalate, to prevent this hyperoxaluria. Small bowel bypass patients placed on a synthetic diet, such as Vivonex, drop their urinary oxalate values to low-normal levels. Unfortunately, such diets are unpalatable for long periods. Also, oxalate is a ubiquitous substance present in many food products, thus making it difficult to design a low-oxalate diet.

It also should be recognized that oxalate measurements are not well standardized, and some knowledge of the particular clinical method used must be obtained before results can be evaluated correctly. The currently available methods suffer primarily from incomplete and inconsistent oxalate recovery. Isotope dilution techniques greatly reduce this source of error, and inclusion of such a step should be looked for in any proposed method of oxalate measurement.

Oxalate levels in food likewise are determined with difficulty. Of even greater importance than the actual total level of oxalate present in a particular foodstuff is the extent of bioavailability of the oxalate present. This information has been worked out only partially for a few foods, with variances from individual to individual of such a magnitude that possible differences between stone formers and non–stone formers are obscured at present.

STONE FORMATION

The recorded incidence of stone formation following intestinal resection varies with the extent of resection. In most small bowel bypass series, the incidence varies from 10 to 25 per cent. In a group of 600 patients followed at our institution for 2 to 6 years, the incidence has been 16 per cent. Fifty-four per cent of these patients have formed only one calculus, but only 1 per cent have had such frequent calculogenesis as to warrant consideration of bypass reversal.

It is interesting that 60 per cent of these calculi have been noted within 1 year of bypass. Two possible explanations for this are urinary calcium concentration and urinary volume.

Following bypass, there is an immediate increase in urinary oxalate excretion, but a more gradual and progressive decrease in urinary calcium excretion also occurs. This decrease in calcium may be due in part to the fecal fat mechanism thought to be responsible for the observed hyperoxaluria. Whatever the mechanism, urinary calcium decreases with time after bypass. Insofar as calcium oxalate calculogenesis is determined by the urinary calcium oxalate ion product, it is at those times when this product is highest that the bypass patient is at greatest risk of stone formation. This period of risk appears to be most marked during the first year following bypass, when the urinary oxalate is high and before the urinary calcium levels have fallen. It is also during this postbypass period that patients are most apt to restrict their fluid intake, hoping to reduce the marked diarrhea that is a hallmark of the small bowel bypass procedure.

TREATMENT

The treatment of enteric calculi is based on several approaches and includes methods designed to (1) prevention of endogenous oxalate production, (2) prevent the absorption of exogenous oxalate, and (3) prevent urinary calcium oxalate saturation (Table 1).

Prevention of Endogenous Oxalate Production

The prevention of endogenous oxalate production is theoretically attractive but difficult to achieve and of limited significance. Agents such as pyridoxine and folic acid direct the oxalate metabolic pathway toward products other than oxalate. Alternatively, the avoidance of products that can be converted to oxalate, such as vitamin C, will not reduce oxaluria sufficiently to prevent stone formation.

Prevention of Exogenous Oxalate Absorption

Oxalate absorption can be prevented entirely by a diet free of oxalate. This is possible to achieve but difficult to maintain. The avoidance of foods known to be high in oxalate, such as tea, spinach, and okra, is sensible but has not been successful in reducing stone formation among our group of frequent small bowel bypass stone formers.

Cholestyramine, an anionic binding agent, was first used to block bile salt reabsorption and, in this fashion, was thought to be a method of preventing endogenous oxalate production. Further work has shown this mechanism to be incorrect. Nevertheless, cholestyramine may reduce oxaluria slightly by binding oxalate and preventing gut absorption, and by complexing with bile salts and decreasing colonic solubility of oxalate. Unfortunately, in the doses necessary for the prevention of oxalate absorption, cholestyramine is an unpalatable product that increases steatorrhea.

Most of the recent therapeutic regimens designed to alter enteric stone formation employ calcium salts. Calcium is given to reverse the loss of calcium, presumably by the steatorrheic mechanism described previously, and to increase the possibility of insoluble calcium oxalate complexes forming in the gut. Calcium will, in fact, reduce oxaluria in small bowel bypass patients by as much as 10 mg/24 hr, but at the expense of increasing the level of urinary calcium. Most clinical investigators who employ calcium therapy report a high incidence of success. Nevertheless, it is important to bear in mind that over one half of the small bowel bypass stone formers pass only one calculus. In our laboratory, we have recorded the incidence and extent of calcium oxalate crystalluria as a means of assessing the likelihood of an individual forming calculi. We are at this time certain that small

TABLE 1. Therapy for Enteric Hyperoxaluria

Prevent Endogenous Oxalate Production	Prevent Absorption of Dietary Oxalate	Prevent Calcium Oxalate Crystallization
Vitamin B Pyridoxine Diet (avoid vitamin C)	Calcium, lanthanum, magnesium, *organic marine hydrocolloids (Ox-Absorb) Cholestyramine *Diet (avoid oxalate-rich foods)	*Hydration Prevent heterogenous nucleation (allopurinol) *Alkalinization (potassium citrate 500 mg tid) *Crystal inhibitor (magnesium glycerophosphate 1 gm bid)

*Most useful.

bowel bypass stone formers pass more urinary crystals than do bypass non–stone formers. We also have observed repeatedly that, following the institution of calcium therapy, the frequency and extent of crystalluria increases. In one patient who has passed at least one calculus per week following the small bowel bypass procedure, we have noted no decrease in the production of calculi following the institution of calcium therapy.

The increase in crystalluria observed following calcium therapy is due to an increase in the calcium oxalate ion product. In this instance, a small decrease in urinary oxalate is many more times offset by the equally small increase in urinary calcium.

Other divalent ions, such as magnesium and lanthanum, have been used as alternatives for calcium as gut-binding agents. Magnesium oxalate or lanthanum oxalate stones do not form because of the higher solubility of these salts. These agents seem theoretically preferable to calcium. With our own patients, magnesium oxide has been ineffective in altering the frequency of calculus formation.

Most recently, organic marine hydrocolloid (OMHs) charged with calcium have been produced (Ox-Absorb) that, when ingested, bind oxalate to the calcium component of the molecule. Because the calcium in this compound is bound to the colloid, it will not be absorbed and will not be a cause of calciuria. In addition to reducing oxaluria, it has been reported that OMHs cause or act to create a urine that is inhibitory to crystal formation. Preliminary reports do show that OMH therapy reduces stone formation in patients suffering enteric hyperoxaluria.

Prevention of Crystallization

Hydration

As is the case in all instances of stone formation, urinary dilution is a major form of therapy. With sufficient hydration it is possible to prevent crystal components from reaching the point at which spontaneous nucleation will occur. Immediately after massive bowel resection or small bowel bypass procedures, it is difficult for patients to achieve the necessary degree of hydration because of the associated diarrhea that is a universal postoperative problem. Nevertheless, it is important to counsel patients that the severe dehydration they often impose upon themselves and occasionally is imposed by their surgeons may result in stone formation. One year after bypass, hydration is possible for most patients, using codeine or Lomotil as needed to prevent excessive loss of ingested fluid by the lower gastrointestinal tract. We try to have all bypass patients void 24-hour urine volumes in excess of 2000 ml.

Allopurinol

Heterogeneous nucleation presently is considered a probable etiology for calcium oxalate calculogenesis, and, in the state of aciduria seen after bypass, uric acid is the most likely initial nidus. Prevention of nidus formation is achieved by the use of allopurinol, 100 mg orally three times a day.

Alkalinization

While developing a method for the quantitative precipitation of calcium oxalate, we observed that crystal formation occurred quickly and completely at an acid pH, but, at an alkaline pH, precipitation occurred only when extremely high concentrations of calcium and oxalate were attained. On the basis of this observation, we have shown that, at an alkaline pH, the urinary level of saturation of calcium oxalate is increased, as is the crystal formation point. We have used this observation experimentally in animals and clinically with small bowel bypass patients and have been able to suppress crystallization by adequate systemic alkalinization.

Bypass patients are difficult to alkalinize, and we have had to use up to 1 gm of sodium bicarbonate four times a day. Under controlled conditions we have been able to prevent the formation of urinary calcium oxalate crystals with this regimen. In our repeat small bowel bypass stone formers, this regimen seems to prevent stone formation. Unfortunately, many small bowel bypass patients find this alkalinization regimen with its associated flatulence intolerable. We have used a combination of Diamox and bicarbonate in these patients, but with only limited success. Various citrate combinations are available in liquid form (Polycitra) and now in tablet form (Citrolith). These alkalinizing agents are more palatable and have been shown to act as in vivo inhibitors of crystal formation.

Treatment

All patients suffering hyperoxaluria secondary to bowel resection should be treated to decrease the oxaluria. This is best accomplished by dietary restriction of fat and oxalate as well as by the use of oxalate binding agents (OMHs). Hydration and the use of inhibitors to crystallization (potassium citrate and potassium glycerophosphate) also are advised. It is important to remember that extensive stone formation occurs in only 1 per cent of enteric hyperoxaluric patients. These patients should consider bypass reversal or, if this is impossible, should receive careful management to prevent obstruction, with the use of lithotripsy or even autotransplantation of the kidneys and the creation of pyelovesicostomies.

CONCLUSION

Although the treatment of patients with enteric oxaluria is challenging, it is of interest that stone formation occurs in only a minority of patients so affected. Stone formation occurred in only 16 per cent of all our bypass patients, but stone formation occurred in 95 per cent of patients who had had a stone prior to bypass surgery. It would appear that oxaluria is a condition that can enhance stone formation but is not a primary cause.

Suggested Readings

Harper J, Mansell MA: Treatment of enteric hyperoxaluria. Postgrad Med J 67:219–222, 1991

Lindsjo M, Fellstrom S, Wikstrom B, et al: Treatment of enteric hyperoxaluria with calcium containing organic marine hydrocolloid. Lancet 2:701–704, 1989

Morgan SH, Watts RWE, Purkiss P, et al: Jejunoileal bypass hyperoxaluria and systemic oxalosis. Clin Sci 15(suppl), 1986

Rose GA, et al: Oxalate Metabolism in Relation to Urinary Stone. Berlin, Springer-Verlag, 1988

CLINICAL APPLICATION OF PERCUTANEOUS NEPHROSTOMY

ARTHUR D. SMITH, M.D.

New Hyde Park, New York

"Endourology" is the term applied to controlled manipulations within a closed urinary tract under fluoroscopic, ultrasonic, or endoscopic guidance. Endourologic procedures often can be performed using a local or regional anesthetic, have fewer complications than do traditional techniques, and thus offer more rapid recovery.

Percutaneous nephrostomy, a means of direct access to the upper urinary tract from outside the body, is the primary procedure in endourology. Since its introduction by Goodwin and colleagues in 1955, percutaneous nephrostomy has proved to be rapid, efficient, and safe as a method of drainage. In addition, the indications have been extended to include stone extraction or destruction, nephroscopy with rigid and flexible instruments, administration of drugs, dilation of strictures, surgery such as ureteral meatotomy, and even management of certain upper tract urothelial carcinomas. Percutaneous nephrostomy, also can be used for tests of renal function and other diagnostic studies and to facilitate such traditional procedures as ureteral stent insertion. The procedure is not absolutely contraindicated in any group, although, if possible, bleeding disorders should be corrected beforehand. In any case, crossmatched blood should be available because serious bleeding sometimes occurs even if the patient's coagulation profile is normal. Broad-spectrum antibiotic coverage is used.

A good understanding of renal anatomy is critical to the creation of a percutaneous nephrostomy. The review of Kaye and Goldberg is recommended.

NEPHROSTOMY TECHNIQUE

Percutaneous nephrostomy can be performed by any of three basic methods: as a blind procedure, under ultrasonic guidance, or under fluoroscopy with or without determination of the renal pelvic depth by ultrasound. The blind method requires insertion of the needle at the junction of the lower border of the 12th rib and the lateral margin of the erector spinae muscle. The center of the left renal pelvis is usually 4.5 to 5 cm below the tip of the spinous process of L1; the center of the right renal pelvis is 1 to 2 cm deeper. The blind method is recommended for infants and children with markedly dilated collecting systems but otherwise is appropriate only for experienced operators, because there may be marked perirenal extravasation if one punctures the kidney without gaining access to the collecting system.

Ultrasound is an excellent means of determining the distance from the skin to the renal pelvis. It is sometimes used in conjunction with fluoroscopy, but punctures done entirely under ultrasonic guidance are common. When the definitive puncture to create the nephrostomy tract is performed with ultrasound, a special transducer is needed.

I prefer to perform percutaneous nephrostomy under fluoroscopic control. The three steps of this approach are opacification of the collecting system, the definitive puncture, and dilatation of the nephrostomy tract and insertion of a drainage tube. Although opacification may sometimes be accomplished with intravenous contrast medium, in an obstructed kidney, it often is necessary to instill the contrast medium either retrogradely through a ureteral catheter inserted cystoscopically or through a 22-gauge Chiba ("skinny") needle passed percutaneously and blindly into the collecting system. If the latter method is used, the Chiba needle should be left in place until the procedure is completed, both to permit instillation of more contrast medium and to prevent extravasation, which can obscure the kidney on the fluoroscope screen. The renal pelvis must not be overdistended, because this may result in pyelovenous backflow and septicemia or in extravasation.

The definitive puncture usually is made by way of a posterolateral route into a middle or lower calix. This facilitates intubation of the ureter, helps stabilize the drainage tube because of the length of the path through the parenchyma, and places the drainage tube somewhat out of the patient's way, so that he or she can lie back more comfortably. We use 1% lidocaine or 0.5% bupivacaine for local anesthesia and supplement it with an intravenous analgesic (fentanyl citrate with droperidol [Innovar]) and sedation (diazepam).

After the trocar needle has been passed, the trocar is removed and a guidewire is passed into the collecting systems and, preferably, down into the ureter. The cannula is removed, and the tract is enlarged with the dilators in the nephrostomy kit. Various dilating methods, including the inflation in the tract of transluminal angioplasty balloons, are available for enlarging the tract further.

Unless the operation is to continue immediately with another endourologic procedure, a nephrostomy drainage tube must be inserted. Each of the available catheters has its pros and cons. Simple pigtail catheters, which are held in the kidney by a loop created by pulling a thread, usually stay in place but can be hard to insert in a small renal pelvis because of the length of the tubing needed to create the loop; they may also be hard to remove. The Stamey-Malecot catheter drains well but is not truly self-retaining and is uncomfortable. The advantages, however, often outweigh the disadvantages, and I use this catheter extensively. The Castanada nephrostomy tube, which is a variant of the Stamey tube, is softer and thus more comfortable, but the retention device is a considerable distance from the catheter tip and is not always effective in stabilizing the tube. The Foley catheter seldom slips out, but the balloon may occlude one or more infundibula, creating intrarenal obstruction. The Councill catheter necessitates dilation of the nephrostomy tract at least 4F larger than the tube unless the catheter is made stiffer by freezing. If long-term drainage is planned, a circle (U-loop) tube should be inserted to ensure catheter stability; this can be done endourologically.

CLINICAL APPLICATIONS

Diagnostic Studies

Despite the increasing sophistication of radioisotopic renal scans, the most reliable means of evaluating an obstructed kidney remains the Whitaker test, in which the suspected obstruction is bypassed by way of percutaneous nephrostomy and the intrarenal pressure is measured during forced flow. Such studies can be done repeatedly to monitor the effects of treatments, including surgery.

Antegrade pyelography by way of a percutaneous nephrostomy is particularly valuable in children and is the most accurate means of differentiating congenital hydronephrosis from multicystic kidney. The method also is useful in delineating the anatomy in patients with hydronephrosis and ectopic ureter and in pinpointing the site of obstruction.

Ureteral Stenting

Essentially, there are two types of stents: those that provide internal drainage only and those that also communicate with the outside. Most of the former types can be inserted with the aid of endourologic techniques. Indeed, in cases of ureteral obstruction, endourologic methods often are preferable to strictly transcytoscopic ones, because it usually is easier to bypass a ureteral obstruction from above. Externally communicating stents obviously require a percutaneous nephrostomy.

A popular ureteral stent is the double pigtail, which is available in polyurethane and in

C-Flex, a new copolymer. This stent has the largest internal diameter in relation to its external diameter and therefore drains well. However, the need for precise measurement of ureteral length can be a drawback, and trigonal irritation is common. The stent can be slipped down the ureter by way of a percutaneous nephrostomy over a Glidewire or Teflon-coated wire, which have a lower coefficient of friction than traditional wires and thus make stent passage easier.

The universal (Smith) stent is a 90-cm, 8.5F tube of silicone rubber that is cut to the proper length. (Because there is no retention device in the bladder, the length is less critical than in the case of the double-pigtail stent). One virtue of this stent is that it can be flushed or reamed at the nephrostomy site if it becomes occluded. Insertion of the stent has been simplified by the marketing of an inserter consisting of a 9F Teflon dilator and an 11F peel-away sleeve. This device is passed over a guidewire down the ureter, and the 9F dilator is withdrawn. The sized, well-lubricated universal stent is advanced down over the guidewire, and the sleeve is pulled out.

New stent designs continue to appear, both to exploit new materials and to attempt to solve problems such as ease of stent loss, patient discomfort, and encrustation (when stents remain in situ for long periods). The multitude of options is clear evidence of the absence of an ideal stent.

Endourologic Dilations and Surgery

Increasingly, the initial approach to postoperative ureteral strictures is through a percutaneous nephrostomy. Strictures can be dilated by the type of tapered or graded dilators with which urologists are familiar or by balloon dilators. The response depends on the type of stricture: recent postoperative strictures usually respond well, whereas late strictures that are caused by extensive extraluminal fibrosis or ischemia usually recur rapidly. Ureterovesical or ureteroileal strictures have been opened by electrocautery with a catheter with an exposed length of wire that is placed in the stricture. Traction on the steel stylet is used to buckle the catheter (much like a Davis loop), so that the wire can be placed against the tissue. The ureter is stented for 4 to 6 weeks afterward.

A superior option is the new Acucise catheter that consists of a balloon to enlarge a stricture and a cutting wire to lay open the scar tissue.

Stone Removal

Percutaneous stone removal (nephrostolithotomy) has received much attention in the literature, including elsewhere in this book, although the indications have declined as extracorporeal shock-wave lithotripsy becomes more widely available. For smaller stones, direct extraction may be possible; larger ones usually must be destroyed by lithotripsy. We continue to believe that percutaneous debulking or removal is the best approach to branched and staghorn stones, because large calculi do not have room to fragment well when exposed to extracorporeal shock-wave lithotripsy. Removal of these masses often necessitates the creation of multiple or Y tracts, but, with patience and skill, patients can be freed of all stone material and thereby of urinary infection. We also find occasion to retrieve large stones from the upper third of the ureter that are not responsive to extracorporeal lithotripsy (embedded; calcium oxalate monohydrate composition).

A technique that is not fully appreciated is chemolysis, which can be used as the primary method or as an adjunct to lithotripsy. The solution should be aimed directly at visible stone pieces, and the intrapelvic pressure must be kept below 25 cm H_2O (we use a central venous pressure manometer). If pain or fever ensues, irrigation should be terminated immediately. The solution used depends on the chemical composition of the stone; a colleague and I have reviewed this elsewhere.

Ablation of Caliceal Diverticulum

A percutaneous approach to a symptomatic caliceal diverticulum has become common. Usually, the diverticulum is punctured directly, and a guidewire is negotiated into the main collecting system or coiled in the lesion. After any stone has been removed with a grasper with or without adjunctive lithotripsy, the infundibular neck is dilated to prevent stasis that can lead to stone recurrence. We also fulgurate the lining of the diverticulum, although not all surgeons agree that this is necessary.

Drug Administration

Fungicidal drugs that have serious adverse effects when given systemically can be instilled through a percutaneous nephrostomy, providing effective treatment for renal infection with few or no side effects. In patients with a universal stent in place, a fungus-infected urinary tract can be made sterile without removal of the stent.

Nephroscopy

Flexible and rigid nephroscopes can be passed percutaneously into the renal pelvis through an Amplatz sheath for examination of the calices and upper ureter and performance of many therapeutic procedures. Proper visibility necessitates wise placement of the tract and, especially with the flexible nephroscope, facility in manipulating the instrument. Practice in cadaver or large-animal kidneys is advised before one attempts nephroscopy clinically.

The nephroscope is used less often in the removal of stones today than in the past. However, it has found a new application in the biopsy and treatment of low-grade, low-stage transitional-cell carcinoma in properly selected patients. Increasingly, the instrument is used to relieve primary and secondary strictures of the ureteropelvic junction, as discussed in another chapter in this volume. Nephroscopy also may be useful for the extraction of foreign bodies.

Conclusion

Since we began doing endourologic procedures in 1977 with instruments that were designed for other uses, many new devices and techniques have been introduced. As a result, many open operations are far less popular than they used to be. These changes certainly will continue, as new technology is introduced. The recent marriage of laparoscopy and urology already has generated minimally invasive evaluation of intersex disorders, orchiopexy, and pelvic and retroperitoneal lymphadenectomy, and reports are beginning to appear of even more elaborate procedures such as laparoscopic nephrectomy. Perhaps urologic uses will be discovered for new instruments being introduced in other specialties. All of these developments make heavy demands on us as urologists, but they will enable us to serve our patients better.

Suggested Readings

Smith A, Castebada, Zuniga, Bronson. Endourology-Principles and Practice. New York, Thieme, 1986
Smith A: Endourology update. Urol Clin North Am 15:3, 1988
Carson C III: Endourology. Prob Urol 6:2, 1992
Carson CC, Dunnick NR: Endourology. New York, Churchill Livingstone, 1985

PERCUTANEOUS NEPHROSTOLITHOTOMY AND THE APPLICATION OF ULTRASONIC LITHOTRIPSY AND ELECTROHYDRAULIC LITHOTRIPSY

E. JAMES SEIDMON, M.D.
Philadelphia, Pennsylvania

Percutaneous nephrostolithotomy (PCNL) was developed primarily for the treatment of upper tract renal calculi. It is also the primary treatment for those patients with upper tract renal calculi that cannot be treated with extracorporeal shock-wave lithotripsy (ESWL) such as those with a pacemaker, pregnancy, gross obesity, scoliosis, and/or decreased flexibility due to chronic disease. Other factors that preclude the use of ESWL should include calcified renal artery or a calcified abdominal aortic aneurysm. Additional problems that may hinder the use of ESWL are a horseshoe kidney, ureteropelvic junction obstruction, a narrow infundibulum with a calculus in a calyceal diverticulum, or a full staghorn calculus. Some urologists now are advocating percutaneous extraction and endopyelotomy for ureteropelvic junction obstruction with an associated calculus rather than open pyeloplasty and stone extraction. PCNL also is useful following incomplete calculus destruction with ESWL. This may be the result of too large a calculus, multiple calculi, stone composition (cystine, mucoid or matrix calculi, dense calcium), or failure of the particles to pass spontaneously. In addition, in those situations in which a calculus becomes lodged or impacted in the proximal, mid-, or distal ureter with significant hydroureteronephrosis, percutaneous access with antegrade flexible ureteroscopy and calculus destruction with an electrohydraulic lithotripsy (EHL) probe has proven to be safe and efficacious.

NEPHROSTOLITHOTOMY TECHNIQUE

As with many other procedures, there are many variables that must be considered for a percutaneous procedure; however, the primary factor remains patient safety. Generally, this procedure is performed either with general anesthesia or with local infiltration of the tract site and intravenous sedation. The choice of a one-stage (tract placement and immediate stone removal) or a two-stage (tract placement followed by next-day dilation and stone removal) procedure is based on the urologist's expertise. Regardless, the initial placement of the tract is obtained following cystoscopy and insertion of a ureteral catheter or an occlusion balloon.

With the patient prone, the kidney is opacified and, under fluoroscopic control, a thin needle is passed into the appropriate calyx. A thin wire then is passed through the needle and then a larger catheter is inserted either down the ureter or into the kidney. At this point, an additional wire is inserted followed by either balloon dilation of the tract or sequential passage of dilators until an appropriate-sized Amplatz sheath is positioned. In most situations a 30F Amplatz sheath is used, but, when treating a large bulky calculus burden (staghorn), dilation up to 36F Amplatz sheath should be considered to reduce the operative time. The working wire is now removed and the safety wire remains present. The procedure now may commence with the correct instrument (a rigid or flexible nephroscope). Irrigation for the procedure is 0.9% saline and not only allows for the visualization of the interior of the kidney and the direct removal or disintegration of the calculus but also does not interfere with the use of EHL or ultrasound lithotripsy if required.

At the end of the procedure a large or small French-size catheter is left and an intraoperative nephrostogram performed to ascertain its location and detect extravasation. My personal experience in over 300 percutaneous procedures has led to the use of the Seidmon antegrade catheter, a 6F, 50-cm single pigtail stent with a retentive coil and side ports. The proximal renal portion of this catheter has a radiopaque painted band 28 cm from the beginning of the intravesical coil that serves as a guide under fluoroscopic control for appropriate positioning of the stent for prevention of extrarenal extravasation of urine. The antegrade ureteral stent is designed to accept a 0.038-inch diameter, 145-cm Teflon-coated guidewire.

Postoperative management is usually unremarkable. Within 1 to several days a repeat kidney-ureter-bladder radiograph to look for retained stone fragments and a nephrostogram are performed and, if normal, the catheter then is removed. The nephrostomy site is covered with an ostomy bag to keep the patient dry and generally closes and seals within 24 hours.

ULTRASOUND LITHOTRIPSY

The ultrasound lithotripter has a transducer at one end that generates a sound wave at a frequency ranging from 23,000 to 27,000 cps. This sound is transferred longitudinally down a hollow metal tube approximately 12F in diameter. Low-level wall suction with a stone fragment collector is attached to the transducer end and, when the activated tip of the probe is placed in direct contact with the calculus, fragmentation of the calculus occurs and the chips (1 to 2 mm in size) then are extracted through the lumen of the probe. During the ultrasonic destruction of the calculus, metal fragments from the tip of the probe often can be seen, but these inert foreign bodies have never led to stone formation and generally wash away at the end of the procedure or pass down the urinary tract.

ELECTROHYDRAULIC LITHOTRIPSY

Electrohydraulic lithotripsy causes fragmentation of a calculus by means of a high-energy discharge that leads to stone disintegration. The release of an electrical discharge by a high-voltage spark across two copper wires in an aqueous medium (0.9% saline) results in vaporization of the solution and the creation of a rapidly expanding plasma (shock wave) that quickly fragments the foreign body (calculus) into pieces. The fragments then can be grasped with a forceps through the working channel of the percutaneous nephroscope and removed through the sheath. The EHL probe should always be in direct view of the operator and be far enough away from the lens to prevent instrument damage; at the same time it must be close enough to the calculus (approximately 1 mm) to allow for its fragmentation. Because of the EHL probe's rigidity, the tip is sharp enough to cause renal or ureteral perforation. Also, heat from the probe can cause tissue damage and/or perforation.

COMPLICATIONS

Complications of the PCNL procedure can be broken down into four specific types: problems with access, equipment-related complications, medicolegal complications, and surgical sequelae. Poor access may be due to poor opacification, the inability to establish contact with the kidney or loss of contact, the use of an improper tract size, and inappropriate placement of the nephrostomy site, precluding the procedure. The equipment must be understood to prevent malfunction. Failure related to the equipment often may occur because the physician does not understand the equipment or does not have the necessary instruments at the time, which leads to a failed procedure. Medicolegal complications may result from unrealistic expectations by both the patient and the physician, failure to obtain proper informed consent, and failure to prepare the patient to expect multiple procedures, which may increase the hospital length of stay.

Minor sequelae in the immediate postoperative recovery period involve nausea, ileus, tract discomfort and/or pain, tube dislodgement, renal damage, retained stone fragments, irritation from the choice of nephrostomy tube used for drainage, and bleeding. More significant complications include infection (perirenal or urinary tract, including sepsis), renal hemorrhage necessitating transfusion, arteriovenous fistula, blood clot retention in the renal pelvis or ureter, urinary tract injury with pelvic or ureteral tear followed by subsequent stricture formation, injury to adjacent bowel or pneumo/hemothorax, and myocardial infarction.

Suggested Readings

Denstedt JD, Clayman RV: Electrohydraulic lithotripsy of renal and ureteral calculi. J Urol 143:13, 1990

Segura JW, et al: Percutaneous removal of kidney stones: Review of 1,000 cases. J Urol 134:1077, 1985

Seidmon EJ: Endourology, introduction of a new antegrade ureteral stent. Urology 34:162, 1989

PERCUTANEOUS DISSOLUTION OF URINARY CALCULI

STEPHEN P. DRETLER, M.D.

Boston, Massachusetts

Percutaneous nephrostomy catheter placement and chemolysis of urinary calculi composed of magnesium-ammonium phosphate, cystine, or uric acid is an alternative in the expanding group of therapies available for patients with renal or ureteral calculi.

GENERAL CONSIDERATIONS

Percutaneous nephrostomy (PCN) and primary dissolution therapy is appropriate only in patients who are not candidates for other modes of intervention. The stone type should be known from prior stone analysis: however, there are exceptions to this rule. Patients with a positive urine cystine (nitroprusside) test may be considered to have cystine calculi without prior stone analysis. Similarly, patients with lucent calculi without infection may be treated as uric acid stone formers, and patients who develop a urea-splitting infection and a calculus after urinary diversion may be treated as struvite ($Mg\text{-}NH_4\text{-}PO_4$) stone formers with a high likelihood of accuracy without prior analysis.

For a stone to be considered for PCN and dissolution therapy, it cannot be sequestered distal to an obstructed infundibulum and must be in a position to allow surface contact with large volumes of infused solution. Patients with calculi that fill the collecting system are poor candidates for dissolution. This is because there is little space in which to place the catheter(s), and the collecting system cannot accommodate a solution flow of high volume, making chemolysis a difficult and lengthy procedure.

Resistant urinary infection, serum creatinine level greater than 3 mg/dl, lack of accurate stone analysis, and the need for other interventions all have been causes for a patient's exclusion from consideration for primary dissolution therapy. Furthermore, increased facilities with percutaneous techniques, the improvement of flexible instruments, and the effectiveness of extracorporeal shock-wave lithotripsy (ESWL) have decreased the usefulness of dissolution therapy. Solitary kidney or urinary conduit is not a reason for exclusion from dissolution techniques.

TECHNIQUE FOR PERCUTANEOUS NEPHROSTOMY IRRIGATION

An 8F to 12F percutaneous nephrostomy tube is placed by the commonly practiced guidance methods. The catheter is placed so as to maximize contact of irrigating fluid and calculus. The preferred site of entry is the upper pole of the kidney, which then allows dependent perfusion and drainage. After catheter placement, the puncture site is given 12 hours to seal. Then initial infusion of saline is done to determine the maximal flow rate that can be tolerated without significant pain or increase in intrapelvic pressure greater than 30 cm H_2O. Intrapelvic pressure is measured by three-way stopcock, similar to the technique for measuring venous pressure. If intrapelvic pressure exceeds 30 cm H_2O with flow rates at less than 80 to 100 ml/hour, a second percutaneous nephrostomy catheter is placed (in dependent position), so that flow rates may reach the 120-ml/hour level. If it is clear from the outset that the calculus is totally, partially, or intermittently obstructing, or that flow is inadequate, placement of a second percutaneous catheter is done at the time of the initial PCN procedure.

If a ureteral calculus is present, the most efficient arrangement is to have the inflow catheter placed in the ureter just above the stone and the outflow catheter placed in the renal pelvis.

During dissolution therapy, the outflow catheter occasionally will obstruct with debris or kink. Increase in intrapelvic pressure suggests this occurrence. Hand irrigation may be necessary to clear the outflow catheter. If this fails, fluoroscopic studies will be needed to determine the cause for poor outflow. Manipulation, adjustment, or repositioning of the outflow catheter may be necessary for proper drainage. Shrinking of calculi during dissolution may result in an intrarenal shift of calculus position and obstruction to outflow and be another cause for repositioning inflow or drainage catheters. To ascertain effectiveness of treatment, kidney-ureter-bladder radiography is done every 3 days and nephrostography is done weekly.

PRECAUTIONS

Two essential precautions must be taken during all intrarenal perfusions. First, the urine must be clear of infection. This usually is ensured by pretreatment with appropriate antibiotics. However, for patients with resistant infections, placement of a PCN catheter and irrigation with saline has hastened conversion to negative cultures. Patients are treated with broad-spectrum or organism-specific antibiotics during irrigation and for 7 to 10 days after removal of the PCN tube. The second essential precaution is the careful observation of intrarenal pressure. Any increase over 30 cm H_2O must be the occasion for slowing perfusion rate, irrigating obstructed outflow catheters, or fluoroscopically altering position of the PCN tube(s).

In addition to daily urine cultures and hourly measurement of intrarenal pressure, other parameters monitored during irrigation are body temperatures, daily complete blood count (CBC), and serum creatinine, phosphate, and magnesium (with hemiacidrin therapy only).

Irrigation is halted temporarily if body temperature is greater than 101.5° F. This may occur during irrigation without a positive urine culture and is most common during the patient's third to fourth day of renal perfusion. Return of temperature to less than 99° F is an indication to restart perfusion. Elevation of serum creatinine greater than 1 mg/dl above pretreatment levels is another indication for temporary cessation. If creatinine returns to pretreatment levels in 48 hours, irrigation is restarted. Any prolonged alteration in serum creatinine or a progressive increase would be an indication for permanent discontinuation of irrigation.

Pain that necessitates the use of analgesics is common for the first 3 to 4 days of irrigation as the renal collecting system accommodates to chronic distention. It has not been a problem significant enough to warrant discontinuation of therapy.

Because of the lengthy time periods that have been required for some irrigation procedures, emotional support of the patient by physician and nurses is of paramount importance. Often leaves of absence are granted, and the patient is allowed to go home for a few days with the PCN tubes on drainage.

TYPES OF CALCULI APPROPRIATE FOR DISSOLUTION THERAPY

Struvite

Magnesium-ammonium phosphate (struvite) calculi are predominantly formed in the presence of urea-splitting alkaline infection and are dissolvable in the acid solvent hemiacidrin (Renacidin).

Renacidin is a multielectrolyte solution with a pH of 4.7. The solution has a high concentration of magnesium and phosphate. When using this solution for intrarenal irrigation, daily plasma measurement of these two ions should be done. An elevation of one and a half times normal PO_4 level or of serum magnesium to 3.4 mg/dl is an indication to halt therapy temporarily. If the patient has an ileal conduit and magnesium elevations occur, the conduit may require catheterization during irrigation.

A single septic episode (temperature greater than 103° F) is an indication to discontinue Renacidin irrigation. Also, failure of any discernible dissolution after 7 days of treatment, or minimal evidence of decrease in stone size after 14 days, would be cause for cessation of irrigation attempts.

The first sign that dissolution is occurring in struvite stone patients is the appearance of brown, muddy sludge in the effluent. If no sludge occurs in the first few days of Renacidin irrigation, it is likely that one is dealing with a stone that is coated with oxalate, that the stone is not a struvite calculus, or that the solution is not coming in contact with the stone.

If the stone is struvite and the irrigation is properly administered, it can be expected that 70 per cent of patients will have total dissolution of their calculus in 5 to 40 days, depending on calculus size. Staghorn calculi have been dissolved successfully by this method. Another 15 per cent will have almost total dissolution but will have 2- to 6-mm–sized fragments remaining. This may represent the portion of the calculus that is not struvite. Overall, 85 per cent of patients with struvite calculi who fit the criteria for dissolution therapy will have treatment successful enough to avoid surgical intervention. Recurrence rates do not differ from conventional methods of treatment.

One of the most difficult aspects of struvite dissolution is the determination of the end point. Renal pelvic or ureteral edema occurs in approximately one third of patients. The edematous mucosal blebs may be indistinguishable from lucent stone fragments. It may be necessary, before removing the PCN tubes, to send the patient on a leave of absence for 7 to 10 days to allow the edema to subside, to be certain no fragments remain. This time period has been adequate to make the distinction between fragments and blebs.

Using the precautions noted, no complications resulting in significant morbidity or mortality have occurred in 8 years of Renacidin use for dissolution of more than 30 renal and ureteral struvite calculi.

The main use for Renacidin is for the occasional patient with multiple small struvite fragments that remain following other endourologic therapeutic efforts.

Cystine

Nonobstructing, asymptomatic cystine calculi may be treated with fluids, alkali, and penicillamine with the expectation that, within 1 year of treatment, 40 per cent of the calculi will dissolve and 20 per cent will decrease in size by one third. The remainder, however, will show either no change or stone growth and must be treated by percutaneous nephrosto-lithotomy, ureteroscopy, or ESWL. The most common clinical circumstance that necessitates the dissolution therapy for cystine calculi is when multiple cystine stones line the ureter ("string of pearls") after inadvertent ESWL of a renal calculus not previously recognized as cystine. In that situation, a small percutaneous nephrostomy tube is placed, and a second one is placed if obstruction of antegrade flow is a problem.

The irrigation is carried out with either *N*-acetylcystine in a bicarbonate solution or tromethamine (THAM), a buffer with a pH of 8.6. (It is cheaper but slower to use two ampules of bicarbonate and a liter of saline [= pH 8].) THAM is available as a commercial preparation from Abbott Laboratories, comes as a powder, and is reconstituted in the hospital pharmacy. Once in solution, it has a shelf life of only 72 hours; therefore, because it is very expensive, attention must be given to planning irrigation volumes, especially over weekends. THAM-E is no longer available but may be reconstructed by the local pharmacy by adding 30 mEq of sodium, 5 mEq of potassium, and 35 mEq of chloride per liter to THAM. This adjusts the pH to 10.2. Because cystine has a sharp rise in solubility over pH 7.5, the pH of 10.2 is very useful for increasing the efficacy of cystine dissolution therapy.

When a patient with a proven cystine calculus (or a positive nitroprusside test) is selected for dissolution therapy, baseline studies including creatinine level, CBC, and urine cultures are carried out. After a PCN catheter(s) is placed and 12 hours are allowed for the puncture site(s) to seal, perfusion of saline is carried out with the same parameters of flow rate and intrarenal pressure guidance methods as described for Renacidin infusion. When the flow is satisfactory and intrarenal pressure is able to be maintained at less than 30 cm H_2O, the alkaline infusion is begun.

Infusions should be halted for pain that cannot be managed with mild analgesics, fever greater than 101.5° F, white blood cell count greater than 12,000/mm^3, a rise in serum creatinine greater than 1 mg/dl, or if a daily urine culture is positive. When these parameters return to pretreatment levels and urine culture shows no growth, infusion may be restarted.

A plain abdominal radiograph is taken every 3 days and a dilute contrast medium nephrostogram done weekly to assess progress. If inflow or outflow appears inadequate, assessment should be made sooner. All patients receive broad-spectrum antibiotics during treatment and for 10 days after removal of the PCN tube. THAM irrigation has produced no local irritation or complication and has not been associated with fever, sepsis, or elevation in serum creatinine.

When attempting to dissolve a cystine stone, it must be kept in mind that other stone elements, such as calcium oxalate, may coat the calculus, making dissolution impossible. Furthermore, in 20 per cent of patients, other stone elements, such as calcium oxalate, $CaPO_4$, or struvite, may be mixed with the cystine, complicating dissolution.

If irrigation is carried out for 7 to 10 days and no decrease in size of a calculus is seen and deopacification of the calculus has not occurred, it is likely that either the stone is not cystine or it is coated with another element.

Experience with cystine dissolution has shown that, for the first 3 to 7 days of irrigation, stone alteration does not necessarily take the form of an overall decrease in stone size, but rather may manifest itself as progressive deopacification, with the stone taking a mottled radiographic appearance. Then, 1 to 3 days after deopacification, continued irrigation will result in stone disintegration. The process appears to be loss of supporting structure and then collapse, rather than progressive erosion. A 2 × 2-cm calculus may be expected to dissolve with approximately 6 to 12 days of irrigation. Larger stones will take longer.

The complications of irrigation are few, dysuria, hematuria, and flank pain being common but manageable problems. Ureteral edema may occur, and the blebs may be indistinguishable from deopacified fragments. These blebs may make the end point of dissolution unclear. Ultrasound or CT scanning may be used to make the distinction.

If the cystine calculus is pure and accessible and the proper irrigation methods and safeguards are used, it can be expected that dissolution of cystine calculi can be successful.

Other Calculi

Uric acid calculi usually are dissolved by oral alkalinization. If a uric acid calculus is obstructing or symptomatic, or if the patient's urine cannot be alkalized properly, percutaneous dissolution may be carried out with either bicarbonate solutions or THAM with almost uniform success. The technique and precautions are the same as those used for cystine calculi.

Calcium oxalate calculi are not dissolvable by clinically approved solutions. The sodium EDTA chelating agent is locally irritating and has systemic complications that make it inappropriate for clinical use.

SUMMARY

Percutaneous dissolution methods have a success rate of 85 per cent in selected struvite stone formers and even higher for appropriate cystine and uric acid stone patients. The method may necessitate lengthy hospitalization and, because it requires attention to many details and precautions, may try the patience of the patient, physician, and supporting hospital staff. However, in the occasional situations where other endourologic methods fail, dissolution therapy may be the only choice.

Suggested Readings

Dretler SP, Pfister RC: Primary dissolution therapy of struvite calculi. J Urol 131:861, 1984

Dretler SP, Pfister RC, Newhouse JH: Renal stone dissolution via percutaneous nephrostomy. N Engl J Med 300:341, 1979

Schmeller HT, Kerting H, Schuller J, et al: Combination of chemolysis and shock wave lithotripsy in the treatment of cystine calculi. J Urol 131:434, 1984

SHOCK-WAVE LITHOTRIPSY FOR THE TREATMENT OF RENAL CALCULI

GLENN M. PREMINGER, M.D.

Dallas, Texas

The removal of renal calculi should be as rapid, safe, and economical as possible. With these criteria in mind, recent developments in endourologic equipment and shock-wave lithotripsy have revolutionized the surgical treatment of renal stone disease. These innovative techniques have greatly facilitated the stone removal procedure while substantially reducing associated morbidity. Current lithotripsy technology is advancing at a rapid pace, making it extremely difficult for the physician to stay on top of these exciting changes. This article briefly describes the basic principles of shock-wave lithotripsy, presents the new developments in lithotripsy technology, and discusses the early results with the use of these new machines.

BASIC PRINCIPLES OF SHOCK-WAVE LITHOTRIPSY

Shock-Wave Physics

Shock waves are high-energy amplitudes of pressure generated in air or water by an abrupt release of energy in a small space. They propagate according to the physical laws of acoustics and are transmitted through media with low attenuation. However, when a shock wave encounters a boundary between substances of differing acoustic impedance (density), compressive stresses are generated that may overcome the tensile strength of that object. Shock waves travel through water and the soft tissues of the body with low attenuation because these materials have similar densities. However, when kidney stones of any composition are contacted by a shock wave of sufficient energy, a compression wave is induced along the front face of the stone. As a result, the anterior surface begins to crumble. As a shock wave crosses the posterior surface of the stone, part of the energy is reflected, creating tensile stress and fragmentation along the posterior surface. Repeated shock waves eventually reduce the stone to small fragments, ideally 2 mm or less in diameter, which may be passed spontaneously.

Lithotripsy Design

All lithotripters have four main features: an energy source, a focusing device, a coupling medium, and a stone localization system. The "standard" Dornier HM-3 design utilizes a spark plug with an elliptical reflector to generate and focus the shock wave, a water bath to transmit the shock waves to the patient, and biplanar fluoroscopy to localize the calculus within the urinary tract. Although this design works quite satisfactorily, there are 10 second-generation lithotripters being developed that are either in clinical use or undergoing animal trials. Table 1 reviews the principal differences between the second-generation machines in their means of shock-wave generation, focusing, patient coupling, and stone localization.

INDICATIONS FOR SHOCK-WAVE LITHOTRIPSY

The majority of symptomatic renal and ureteral calculi can be removed by minimally invasive means that include either some type of endourologic technique or shock-wave lithotripsy. The current indications for shock-wave lithotripsy have not changed with the new technology. The stones should be either symptomatic, obstructing, the cause of significant bleeding, or the source of infection. Currently, most believe that asymptomatic renal calculi should not be treated by shock-wave lithotripsy except in unique circumstances such as airline pilots.

TABLE 1. Comparison of Second-Generation Lithotripters

MANUFACTURER	SHOCK-WAVE GENERATION	FOCUSING	PATIENT COUPLING	LOCALIZATION
Dornier HM-4	Electrohydraulic	Ellipsoid	Membrane	Biplane fluoroscopy
Diasonics	Piezoelectric	Spherical	Membrane	Fluoroscopy/ultrasound
Direx	Electrohydraulic	Ellipsoid	Membrane	Fluoroscopy/ultrasound*
EDAP	Piezoelectric	Spherical	Membrane	Ultrasound
Medstone	Electrohydraulic	Ellipsoid	Membrane	Plain radiograph
Northgate	Electrohydraulic	Ellipsoid	Membrane	Ultrasound
Siemens	Electromagnetic	Acoustic lens	Membrane	2 fluoroscopy tubes
Technomed	Electrohydraulic	Ellipsoid	Pool	Ultrasound
Wolf	Piezoelectric	Spherical	Pool	Ultrasound

*This unit does not come with its own localization system, so the operator must use his or her own ultrasound or fluoroscopy equipment.

Shock-wave lithotripsy is best employed for the treatment of stones less than 2 cm in diameter. One might expect a 75 to 90 per cent stone-free rate at 3 months for these size calculi. However, as the size of the stone increases, the chance that multiple treatments will be necessary to achieve complete elimination increases and the stone-free rate drops. Moreover, the risk of ureteral obstruction from the stone burden increases. Shock-wave lithotripsy is considered the treatment of choice for the majority of stones in the mid and upper ureter if they can be visualized on the lithotripter. The stone-free rate increases if the stone can be manipulated back into the renal collecting system. Lower ureteral stones also can be treated by shock-wave lithotripsy, yet the success rates are not as high as with direct ureteroscopic stone removal.

Current contraindications to shock-wave lithotripsy include an uncorrected bleeding diathesis; obstructive uropathy, such that the stone fragments will not pass; and pregnancy.

RESULTS

A limited compilation of results either published or presented at various meetings is presented in Table 2. None of the current machines offers superiority in overall stone-free rates (efficacy). It should be noted that, although some of the newer devices claim to offer "anesthesia-free" lithotripsy, most require some form of parenteral, oral, or local anesthesia/analgesia/sedation. Only the piezoelectric machines require absolutely no form of anesthesia.

In general, these "less painful" machines are also less powerful, requiring more shocks (with treatments taking more time) and more secondary treatments. Thus, advances made in patient comfort significantly affect the efficiency of these "pain-free" machines, if comparable efficacy rates are to be expected.

Efficiency Quotient

The determination of lithotripter efficiency with regard to adequate stone destruction requires a delicate balance between the completeness of stone fragmentation and the ability to perform lithotripsy procedures without the need for anesthesia or analgesia. Indeed, as the shock wave intensity is diminished to allow for anesthesia-free lithotripsy, the ability to fragment stones adequately also is reduced, thereby decreasing lithotripter efficiency. Diminished efficiency can be represented by an increase in the number of treatments needed to render a patient stone free, as well as the increased need for auxiliary procedures following lithotripsy, again to attain a stone-free status. Such auxiliary procedures include placement of a percutaneous nephrostomy tube, formal percutaneous nephrostolithotomy, ureterorenoscopy, and placement of a ureteral stent to aid in fragment passage. One can therefore calculate an "efficiency quotient" by determining the stone-free rate obtained by various lithotripters in relation to the need for repeat lithotripsy, as well as the number of auxiliary procedures performed to render patients stone free:

$$\text{Efficiency Quotient} = \frac{\%\ \text{of patients stone free}}{\begin{matrix}100\%\ \text{initial} \\ \text{treatments}\end{matrix} + \begin{matrix}\%\ \text{repeat} \\ \text{treatments}\end{matrix} + \begin{matrix}\%\ \text{auxiliary} \\ \text{procedures}\end{matrix}}$$

Using this efficiency quotient, one can make more valid comparisons between the different types of first and second-generation lithotripters.

It appears that it is not possible to have true anesthesia-free capabilities with a lithotripsy device that rates high on the efficiency quotient scale. In order to achieve anesthesia-free status, one has to expect the number of secondary treatments to increase and therefore the efficiency quotient of that lithotripter to be diminished. One would expect this trend to continue as the manufacturers of the ma-

TABLE 2. Results Achieved with Second-Generation Lithotripters

Manufacturer	Secondary Treatment Rate	Stone-Free Rate	Anesthesia Requirement
Dornier HM-3	10–16%	64–84%	General/sedation
Dornier HM-4	18–22%	68–80%	Sedation/general
EDAP	20–40%	68–74%	Sedation
Siemens	10–22%	65–72%	Sedation/local
Technomed	10–13%	46–59%	Sedation/general
Wolf	10–33%	75–84%	None

jority of available electrohydraulic lithotripters modify their shock-wave generators to make them anesthesia free.

COMPLICATIONS

Complications of shock-wave lithotripsy include insufficient stone disintegration and incomplete stone fragment passage, both usually requiring further procedures. Obstructive symptoms such as nausea, vomiting, pain, and even obstructive pyelonephritis may occur during passage of fragments. It has been reported that anywhere from 10 to 25 per cent of patients will require auxiliary procedures to aid in passage of their stone fragments. Perirenal or renal hematoma formation, infection with or without pyelonephritis, or other infrequent acute complications may occur following shock-wave lithotripsy.

In addition to the acute stone-related complications, studies have demonstrated acute morphologic changes in the renal parenchyma and surrounding tissues following shock-wave lithotripsy. Nevertheless, studies have demonstrated that these acute changes will resolve without evidence of long-term sequelae.

Although there have been reports that suggested shock-wave lithotripsy may induce hypertension, recent studies have demonstrated no significant increase in the incidence of hypertension following shock-wave lithotripsy. It is anticipated that carefully conducted multicenter prospective clinical trials will be needed to further investigate the important question of shock-wave lithotripsy–induced hypertension.

THIRD-GENERATION LITHOTRIPTERS

Currently, there are a number of third-generation lithotripters in which the manufacturers have tried to incorporate many of the aforementioned characteristics of the ideal lithotripter. The basic design of the third-generation machines includes dual imaging capabilities as well as variable shock-wave power. Currently, there are a number of third-generation lithotripters undergoing clinical trials both in the United States and in Europe. These include the Dornier MFL 5000 (HM-5), EDAP LT-02, Siemens Lithostar Plus, Storz Modulith SL 20, and Wolf Piezolith 2500 (Table 3).

Dual Imaging

Dual imaging capabilities entail having both fluoroscopic and sonographic localization systems available in the same machine. Such a design has the advantage of utilizing fluoroscopy for imaging stones within the kidney as well as the ureter, while having the option to use sonography for the identification of radiolucent or biliary tract calculi. Another advantage of having sonography capabilities is that this allows one initially to target a stone using fluoroscopy and then switch over to sonography to avoid an excessive amount of ionizing radiation. Moreover, having fluoroscopy capabilities also may lessen the "learning curve" for many urologists who are unfamiliar with sonographic stone localization procedures.

Interestingly, although the Dornier, Siemens, and Storz machines all have added ultrasound capabilities to provide dual imaging, none of these systems provides "in-line" imaging for both the fluoroscopic and sonographic localization devices. For example, with the Dornier and Siemens devices, one can utilize sonography to target a radiolucent calculus, yet the patient must be moved "blindly" to the fluoroscopy unit, which is in-line with the shock-wave generator. Alternatively, one can utilize the fluoroscopic localization system with the Storz machine, yet

TABLE 3. Characteristics of the Third-Generation Lithotripters

Manufacturer	Shock-Wave Generation	Focusing	Patient Coupling	In-Line Localization*
Dornier HM-5	Spark gap	Ellipsoid	Membrane	Fluoroscopy
EDAP LT-02	Piezoelectric	Spherical	Membrane	Ultrasound & fluoroscopy
Siemens Lithostar Plus	Electromagnetic	Acoustic lens	Membrane	2 fluoroscopy tubes
Storz Modulith SL 20	Electromagnetic	Parabolic reflector	Membrane	Ultrasound
Wolf Piezolith 2500	Piezoelectric	Spherical	Membrane	Ultrasound & fluoroscopy

*Indicates which of the localization systems is "in-line" with the shock-wave generator.

only the ultrasound is in-line with the shock-wave generator.

The EDAP LT-02 and Wolf Piezolith 2500 are the only third-generation devices, at this time, that provide both fluoroscopy and sonography in-line with the piezoelectric shock-wave generator. This design permits rapidly changing from fluoroscopic to sonographic stone localization, without moving the patient off of the treatment dish.

Variable Power

All four of the aforementioned third-generation devices have variable-power shock-wave generators that will allow the operator to apply the appropriate amount of shock-wave energy for a particular stone. One can turn down the generator power to provide significantly reduced anesthesia/analgesia requirements with the Dornier, Siemens, and Storz machines, as well as to provide totally anesthesia/analgesia-free lithotripsy with the EDAP and Wolf devices. Moreover, the shock-wave intensity can be increased with all five machines to allow adequate fragmentation of extremely hard or large calculi. However, it is understood that, when using these lithotripters in the "high power mode," various forms of anesthesia/analgesia will be necessary.

So, in fact, we still have not developed the "ultimate shock wave" that allows totally anesthesia-free lithotripsy with maximum efficiency. Yet, by varying the shock wave energy, one can administer a highly efficient shock wave with the need for anesthesia/analgesia when high shock-wave pressures are indicated. In contrast, with a small or soft stone, the shock-wave energy can be decreased significantly to provide minimal-anesthesia or anesthesia-free lithotripsy.

Interestingly, although much of the industry has pushed for anesthesia-free capabilities over the past few years, many physicians have perhaps not been sufficiently aware of and/or ignored the potential deleterious effect that may result from excessive administration of the higher powered electrohydraulic shock waves. Now, with the availability of variable-powered lithotripters that utilize electrohydraulic and electromagnetic as well as piezoelectric energy sources, one must continue to closely monitor the total amount of energy delivered to a particular kidney to limit the incidence of significant renal injury.

Suggested Readings

Bierkens AF, Hendrikx AJ, de Kort VJ, et al: Efficacy of second generation lithotriptors: A multicenter comparative study of 2,206 extracorporeal shock wave lithotripsy treatments with the Siemens Lithostar, Dornier HM4, Wolf Piezolith 2300, Direx Tripter X-1 and Breakstone lithotriptors. J Urol 148:1052–1057, 1992

Fegan J, Camp LA, Wilson WT, et al: Treatment philosophy and re-treatment rates following piezoelectric lithotripsy. J Urol 149:12–14, 1993

Lam HS, Lingeman JE, Mosbaugh PG, et al: Evolution of the technique of combination therapy for staghorn calculi: A decreasing role for extracorporeal shock wave lithotripsy. J Urol 148:1058–1062, 1992

Rassweiler J, Henkel TO, Kohrmann KU, et al: Lithotripter technology: Present and future. J Endourol 6:1–13, 1992

URETEROSCOPIC TREATMENT OF DISTAL URETERAL CALCULI

DEMETRIUS H. BAGLEY, M.D., F.A.C.S.

Philadelphia, Pennsylvania

The advent of ureteroscopy has permanently altered the approach to distal ureteral calculi. Prior to the development of this endoscopic technique, the only choices for the interventional treatment of distal ureteral calculi that had failed to pass were cystoscopic manipulation or ureterolithotomy. The demonstrated success and safety of ureteroscopic stone removal resulted in its rapid acceptance and wide application. Although shock-wave lithotripsy has been employed with considerable success in treating some selected distal ureteral stones, ureteroscopic removal remains the most successful technique for the treatment of essentially any stone in the distal one third of the ureter. The development of smaller endoscopes and more effective endoscopic lithotriptors has improved the success of the procedure while decreasing the morbidity.

URETEROSCOPIC INSTRUMENTATION

The evolution of ureteroscopic instrumentation has resulted in several endoscopes specifically designed for the treatment of calculi within the distal ureter. In the earliest reports on ureteroscopy, pediatric endoscopes were employed for distal ureteroscopy in the female. Adaptation of juvenile endoscopes extended these techniques to the distal ureter in the male and more proximal locations in the female. Specifically designed ureteroscopes based on this standard endoscopic design became available in longer versions to reach the renal pelvis and shorter models designed specifically for the distal ureter. The sizes generally ranged from 9.5F to 12.5F. The larger of these ureteroscopes required dilation of the ureterovesical junction for introduction of the endoscope. Endoscopes with an offset eyepiece and a straight working channel could accept an ultrasound probe for stone fragmentation. Endoscopes with either a straight or angled channel could accept an electrohydraulic lithotriptor probe and flexible working instruments. Clinical series reported through the late 1980s generally reflect the results obtained with these larger rigid endoscopes.

Parallel to these changes in the endoscope, a wider range of lithotriptors have become available. The earliest devices were hollow ultrasound probes that could be passed only through an endoscope with a straight channel. Probes of 1.5 to 1.8 mm were small enough for use in the ureter. A more powerful unit with a solid wire also was used in the ureter with considerable success. Downsizing of electrohydraulic lithotriptor probes made them available for use through endoscopes with smaller channels. The probes decreased from 5F to 3F to the presently available 1.9F and 1.6F.

The pulsed-dye laser represents another major step in urologic instrumentation. The major advantages of this technique are the safety and the small size (250 to 320 μ) of the laser fiber as well as its efficacy in stone fragmentation. Other lasers, including the alexandrite and the holmium, are presently being studied for applications in endoscopic lithotripsy.

Another major advance in allowing convenient, safe endoscopic access to the distal ureter has been the development of fine-caliber endoscopes that utilize the minimal-size channel available and include a fiberoptic bundle for visual optics. Because of the small size of these instruments, they routinely can be passed into the ureteral lumen without prior dilation. The small working channels are adequate for laser fibers and small-diameter working instruments along with adequate irrigation with a pressurized system.

As the size of ureteroscopes used for the distal ureter has decreased from 12.5F to approximately 7F, the need for dilation has changed from routine to rare. For example, use of the 7.2F Candela ureteroscope required dilation in 31 per cent of patients in one reported series, and our experience with the Circon 6.9F endoscope has required ureteral dilation in only 2 per cent of patients. Thus, the problems associated with dilation, including the technical difficulties, the expense of the dilating instruments, and any complications associated with their use, can be eliminated.

SUCCESS RATE OF URETEROSCOPY

Distal ureteral stones can be removed ureteroscopically by intact retrieval if they are small or if the ureteral lumen and orifice are of adequate diameter. Larger stones must be fragmented for removal. The many lithotriptor devices now available can fragment stones with an extremely high success rate. In evaluating the success of ureteroscopic stone removal, the devices employed must be considered because the effectiveness and the associated complications are closely linked to the instruments employed.

The hollow ultrasound probes could fragment well over 80 per cent of stones encountered ureteroscopically. The solid-wire probe increased that success rate to more than 90 per cent. However, to reap the benefits of the small-diameter ureteroscopes, smaller lithotriptor devices are used. The 3F electrohydraulic lithotriptor probe has been successful in fragmenting over 90 per cent of calculi encountered.

The effectiveness of the pulsed-dye laser is related to the energy and the particular fiber employed. When the device was limited to 60 mJ with a 250-μ fiber, it routinely failed to fragment calcium oxalate monohydrate stones. When a laser capable of a higher energy coupled with a larger (320- or 400-μ) fiber became available, in one clinical series all stones encountered were fragmented. This impressive success rate was confirmed as another manufacturer's device was employed at the higher energy settings and increased other investigators' success with calcium oxalate monohydrate stones from approximately 80 to over 90 per cent. Cystine stones remain resistant. Therefore, the endoscopist who has these devices available can expect to fragment essentially any stone encountered with a rigid ureteroscope.

The very high success rate of ureteroscopy in removing distal ureteral calculi has been documented in numerous series. It should be stressed that success in these reports generally has been defined as total removal of the calculus. The authors have considered the procedure a failure if a second procedure is necessary. In addition, there is no delay period waiting for the fragments to pass, as seen in the series with shock-wave lithotripsy. Often, the success of ureteroscopic stone removal gives an average for stones located throughout the ureter. However, every series utilizing rigid endoscopes has documented a high success rate for distal stones and a much lower success rate for proximally located ureteral calculi. Therefore, based on numerous studies documenting treatment in hundreds of patients, it is expected that distal ureteral calculi can be removed ureteroscopically with a success rate of well over 90 per cent, approaching 100 per cent.

COMPLICATIONS OF URETEROSCOPY

Balanced against the high success rate for the procedure must be the negative aspects, including complications and morbidity related to the procedure. Again, multiple series have documented the low complication rate of ureteroscopy. In addition, several have demonstrated that rigid ureteroscopic procedures in the lower ureter are much less prone to complication than those attempted in the mid- and proximal ureter. For example, Stoller et al. demonstrated that, in the treatment of ureteral calculi with rigid ureteroscopy, the rate of ureteral perforation was 31 per cent for proximal stones but only 8 per cent for distal stones ($p<0.01$). Overall, complications have ranged from 5 to 20 per cent. Among the series that related complications to the location of the stone, distal ureteroscopy resulted in an 8 to 10 per cent complication rate.

In comparing ureteroscopic removal to other modalities, it is also important to compare the overall morbidity of the procedure. Stoller documented that, after ureteroscopic stone removal, 32 per cent of his patients returned to work or felt normal within 3 days and 51 per cent within 1 week. Twelve per cent of patients complained about the epidural anesthetic employed in that series.

Watson has reviewed his series of ureteroscopies over several years and related the success and complications to the instruments employed. As he has begun to use smaller instruments with a pulsed-dye laser lithotriptor, he has noted a sharp decrease in complications while the success rate has gradually increased. He has related this to the lack of ureteral dilation and the greater effectiveness of laser lithotripsy.

FLEXIBLE URETEROSCOPES

When considering the endoscopes available for ureteroscopy, flexible ureteroscopes are not suitable for the treatment of distal ureteral calculi. Because of the need to stabilize the flexible ureteroscope for insertion through the bladder into the ureteral orifice, it is very difficult to maintain it in position to manipulate within the distal ureter. The tip often falls back into the bladder and makes re-insertion necessary. In our series, reviewing the treatment of all ureteral calculi with flexible endoscopy, the success in the distal ureter was less than 50 per cent utilizing the flexible ureteroscope alone. All of the failures were immediately treated successfully with rigid ureteroscopy.

SUMMARY

Ureteroscopy has proven to be a safe and extremely effective technique for the treatment of distal ureteral calculi. Stones in the distal ureter that were previously considered major problems for ureteroscopic treatment can now be approached much more successfully. These include the large impacted calculi and multiple calculi. Often these stones cannot be bypassed with a wire and dilation is either difficult or impossible. Modifications in endoscopes and the development of new endoscopic lithotriptors has improved both the success and the safety of the ureteroscopic procedure. A small-diameter ureteroscope usually can be placed into the ureteral orifice without dilation and can visualize the stone directly. Fragmentation then can be accomplished with either a pulsed-dye laser fiber or a small electrohydraulic lithotriptor probe. After the initial fragmentation, a guidewire can be placed. Ureteroscopy remains the most effective technique for treating distal ureteral calculi.

Suggested Readings

Bagley DH: Removal of upper urinary calculi with flexible ureteropyeloscopy. Urology 35:412, 1990

Bagley DH, Grasso M, Shalaby M, et al: Ureteral laser lithotripsy using the Pulsolith. J Endourol 3:91, 1989
Dretler SP, Cho G: Semirigid ureteroscopes: A new genre. J Urol 141:1314, 1989
Stoller ML, Wolf JS, Hofmann R, et al: Ureteroscopy without routine balloon dilation: An outcome assessment. J Urol 147:1238, 1992
Watson GM, Murray S, Dretler SP, et al: The pulsed dye laser for fragmenting urinary calculi. J Urol 138:195, 1987

Kidney Transplantation and Hypertension

TRANSPLANTATION TECHNIQUES AND PITFALLS

MICHAEL MORRIS, M.D., F.A.C.S.

Philadelphia, Pennsylvania

The technical and clinical applicability of renal transplantation was first demonstrated in the now-famous identical twin series reported by Murray et al. in 1954. This series, by eliminating the immunologic barrier to transplantation, demonstrated not only the soundness of the surgical technique but also the significant positive impact such a procedure can have on a recipient's life. The procedure as performed today is very similar to that performed by Murray's group nearly 40 years ago. The major changes that have occurred have involved the increasing adaptability of the procedure to a multitude of clinical circumstances and its greater availability to patients.

Today, patients being considered for renal transplant represent a broad segment of the dialysis population. Traditional barriers such as coronary artery disease, hypertension, and diabetes mellitus are no longer considered absolute contraindications. Associated diseases often can be controlled and/or better managed, allowing the patient to become an acceptable transplant candidate.

The transplant procedure has several general variations. These are cadaveric donor transplantation, living donor transplantation, combined renal-extrarenal transplantation, and retransplantation. Living donor and cadaveric donor transplantations generally are performed in the extraperitoneal iliac fossa. Multiple retransplants and kidney/pancreas transplants are placed intraperitoneally. Historically, much has been said regarding the positioning of the right or left kidney in the right or left iliac fossa. The reasoning behind such argument has been based on subsequent access to the renal pelvis and the anatomic positioning of the renal vessels in relation to the iliac vessels. We have not found these issues to be significant and will place a kidney on whichever side the patient's particular circumstances require.

GENERAL TRANSPLANT TECHNIQUE

The renal transplant process begins with the identification of a potential recipient. This is determined by crossmatching and human lymphocyte antigen typing. The appropriately identified patient is brought into the hospital for final crossmatching and is prepared for surgery. During this interval, the patient is carefully examined and laboratory studies are checked. It may be necessary to dialyze the patient. Special consultations may be required. When called to surgery, the patient will receive the immunosuppressant medications prednisone, cyclosporine, and azathioprine as well as an antibiotic, frequently a second-generation cephalosporin.

Once in the operating room, a central venous catheter is placed to monitor volume states in the perioperative period. A Foley catheter is placed and 200 ml of a dilute gentamycin-saline irrigant is instilled. We find distention of the bladder helps make intraoperative localization easier and dissection simpler. The gentamycin will sterilize the bladder contents. We prefer general anesthesia, although some centers use epidural anesthesia.

The skin incision is made in the appropriate lower quadrant, extending along the lateral edge of the rectus fascia a distance of 15 to 20 cm to the pubic tubercle. The anterior muscular fascia is divided and the peritoneum is carefully dissected and retracted medially. The inferior epigastric vessels are divided. The spermatic cord in the male is retracted medially; in the female, the round ligament is divided. The iliac vessels are identified easily through this extraperitoneal exposure. A self-retaining retractor is quite useful. Care must be taken, however, in placing these retractors so as not to stretch the lateral femoral cutaneous nerve or obstruct arterial inflow.

Dissection of the external iliac vessels involves the ligation of multiple crossing lymphatics. Failure to accomplish this adequately could result in a postoperative peritoneal lymphatic collection. Such collections can serve as a source of ureteral obstruction and perinephric infection. Successful management of the lymphocele frequently requires surgery to establish intraperitoneal drainage. Full mobilization of the external iliac vessels frequently can be accomplished without ligating deep branches; however, if such ligation is necessary, care should be taken to ensure adequate mobilization prior to their ligation to avoid potentially difficult bleeding.

The kidney is prepared for implantation on the back table. There, it is maintained in a saline iced slush solution to keep it cold while it is being prepared. Back table work consists primarily of the débridement of extraneous tissue and fascia and the mobilization and dissection of the renal vasculature and ureter. To avoid injury to the tenuous blood supply to the ureter, care is taken not to skeletonize this structure, particularly near the kidney.

The arterial blood supply to the kidney may be single or multiple. In the dissection of the renal artery, care must be taken in preserving any polar vessels. These branches may occur anywhere along the course of the renal artery, and not infrequently may rise as an independent aortic branch. To accommodate multiple vessels and to simplify anastomosis, a Carrel patch of aorta is used. This patch also may be used as an anchor for vessels inadvertently divided during procurement.

The renal vein also may be single or multiple. Small independent branches may be ligated. The left renal vein is almost always of sufficient length to allow easy anastomosis and little back table work is required. The right renal vein, however, is very short and can be lengthened by using a vena caval patch. This is accomplished by trimming adequate anterior and posterior segments of vena cava and suturing the opposing walls together using fine Prolene sutures. Such a maneuver can effectively extend the length of the vein some 2 to 2.5 cm.

Once the back table work has been completed, the recipient's iliac vessels are prepared for anastomosis. Venous anastomosis is completed first. This will be an end renal vein–to–side external iliac vein anastomosis using a 5-0 Prolene suture. The iliac vein is clamped proximally and distally. Using a Satinsky scissors, a small patch matching the diameter of the renal vein is excised from the anterior lateral aspect of the vein. The sutures are placed in the respective corners. Stay sutures also are placed to distract opposing venous walls. The anastomosis is then routine. With the completion of the venous anastomosis, attention is directed to the arterial anastomosis. This anastomosis is performed on the anterior lateral aspect of the external iliac artery using 6-0 Prolene suture. Positioning of the artery should be done to avoid interference with venous outflow. Redundant artery or vein is of little consequence and should not be of concern.

It is important to note that we do not heparinize either systemically or locally prior to clamping the iliac vessels. We have had no case of thrombosis or distal embolization. Prior to releasing the vascular clamps, we administer 50 gm of mannitol and 100 mg of furosemide intravenously. We believe the mannitol serves as a free radical scavenger and the furosemide will help induce diuresis. Venous clamps are released first. Following the release of the arterial clamps, the kidney should regain normal tone and color rapidly. Its failure to do so should prompt a careful check of all anastomoses and vessels with correction of any identified problems. Hemostasis is established meticulously, with care taken to preserve vascular integrity. We routinely perform a postperfusion wedged renal biopsy. This biopsy serves as a baseline for comparison of future biopsies and has proven itself useful in evaluation of early renal dysfunction.

LIVING DONOR VERSUS CADAVERIC TRANSPLANTS

Living donor transplantation differs from cadaveric renal transplantation in several important areas. Because of the ease of arterial dissection and the extra length of vein, living donor kidneys frequently are left kidneys. We prefer to avoid multiple renal arteries, and we will use a right kidney if it has a single and the left multiple arteries. Multiple-arteried kidneys can be used with back table reconstruction. Such reconstruction will involve the joining of vessels to establish a single inflow orifice in either a fish-mouth side-to-side or an end-to-side fashion. The living donation prohibits the use of a Carrel aortic patch; however, a patch can be fashioned using a segment of the recipient's hypogastric artery.

In living donor transplantation, the venous anastomosis is performed in a fashion identical to that of cadaveric transplantation. Traditionally, the arterial anastomosis is done end to end, renal artery to hypogastric artery. Anastomosis is completed with 6-0 Prolene sutures. Growth factor, as described by Starzl et al., is utilized to avoid anastomotic narrowing. End-to-side renal artery–external iliac artery anastomosis is performed in those circumstances in which a Carrel patch has been fashioned or atherosclerotic disease of the hypogastric artery discourages the use of this vessel.

SIMULTANEOUS ORGAN TRANSPLANTS

Renal transplantation also frequently is performed simultaneously with other solid organ transplants. Most frequently these include pancreas/kidney, heart/kidney, and liver/kidney. Combined kidney/pancreas transplantation is performed in uremic juvenile diabetics. The renal transplant is performed as described above following the implantation of the pancreas. This procedure is most commonly performed intraperitoneally; generally the pancreas is placed in the right iliac fossa and the kidney in the left. We stent the ureteral anastomosis in intraperitoneal transplants. Patients being evaluated for cardiac and liver transplantation increasingly have renal impairment. Many of these patients are considered candidates for combined transplant. The transplant is performed in the usual extraperitoneal position following the completion of the extrarenal transplant.

URINARY TRACT RECONSTRUCTION

The reconstruction of the urinary tract is accomplished via an extravesicular ureteral neocystostomy. The ureter is trimmed to the appropriate length so that there is not too much redundancy. The muscularis of the anterior lateral surface of the bladder is incised, exposing the bulging bladder mucosa for a distance of 2 to 3 cm. In males, the ureter is brought under the spermatic cord. The end of the ureter is spatulated and, following the opening of the bladder mucosa, is anastomosed to the bladder using a 5-0 absorbable suture. The muscular layer is then reapproximated over the anastomosis, creating a submucosal tunnel. This tunnel is thought to help reduce the incidence of reflux. Reflux in adult renal transplantation is of questionable clinical significance.

Certain clinical situations may require other approaches to the ureteral anastomosis. These include end-to-end pyeloureterostomy, bladder extensions, and ileal loop conduits. Occasionally, a double ureter is encountered. This is associated with two independent collecting systems. A double ureter requires separate ureteral neocystostomies or a joined anastomosis.

RETRANSPLANTATION

Current immunosuppression regiments result in 1-year renal graft survivals of 80 to 90 per cent and 5-year graft survivals of approximately 60 per cent. Following a failed graft, many patients are candidates for retransplantation and some may undergo multiple retransplants. The first retransplant is performed in the iliac fossa opposite that of the original transplant. This transplant can be performed in a fashion identical to that of the first. Third or fourth retransplants require reexploration of the iliac vessels. Transplant nephrectomy may or may not have been performed previously. We find a midline intraperitoneal incision to be the most direct approach to multiple retransplantation. This allows clear access to the iliac vessels, simplifies dissection and avoids the potential problem of lymphocele in the reoperative area. We stent all intraperitoneal ureteral anastomoses.

CONCLUSION

Attention to detail and thorough preoperative evaluation makes the operative side of renal transplantation safe for the patient and easy for the surgeon. Advances in immunosuppression have made renal transplantation the therapy of choice for uremia.

Suggested Readings

Bootsma M, Koohe AMM, Van Bockel HJ, et al: The clinical significance of vescico-ureteral reflux into transplanted kidney. Clin Transplant 1:311–315, 1987

Murray JE, Merrill JP, Harrison JH: Kidney transplantation between seven pairs of identical twins. Ann Surg 148:343, 1958

Starzl TE, Iwatsuki S, Shaw BW Sr: A growth factor in fine vascular anastomoses. Surg Gynecol Obstet 159: 164–165, 1984

DONOR-SPECIFIC BLOOD TRANSFUSIONS IN LIVING-RELATED RENAL TRANSPLANTATION

ANDREW C. NOVICK, M.D.

Cleveland, Ohio

In the early years of renal transplantation, acceptable histocompatibility matching criteria for living-related transplants comprised donor-recipient pairs sharing at least two (one haplotype) of the four serologically identifiable A- and B-locus antigens. During the mid 1970s, several transplant centers reported a significant difference in allograft survival in one-haplotype-matched living-related donor transplants, depending on the preoperative results of mixed lymphocyte culture (MLC) testing. Donor-recipient pairs with a high two-way MLC stimulation index were noted to have 1-year graft survival rates of only 40 to 50 per cent. This was in contrast to 80 to 90 per cent 1-year graft success rates in donor-recipient pairs with a nonstimulatory MLC. Based on these data, criteria for living-related renal transplantation became more restrictive and the use of one-haplotype-matched, high-MLC donor-recipient pairs was abandoned.

In 1980, Salvatierra demonstrated that pretransplant administration of donor-specific blood transfusions (DSTs) significantly improved the outcome of living-related renal transplantation in one-haplotype-matched, high-MLC donor-recipient pairs. The original DST protocol involved the administration of approximately 200 ml of fresh whole blood or packed cell equivalent on three separate occasions at 2-week intervals to the potential recipient. During and immediately after DST, the potential recipient's sensitization against blood-donor lymphocytes was monitored by donor-specific cross-match testing of recipient sera. Transplantation was undertaken only when negative T-warm and B-warm donor-specific crossmatches were maintained. Using this DST protocol, many centers reported 90 per cent or better 1-year allograft survival rates in recipients of one-haplotype-matched living-related renal transplants. These rates were comparable to those obtained in human lymphocyte antigen–identical living-related transplants.

A major disadvantage of the above DST protocol was the occurrence of donor-specific sensitization in approximately 30 per cent of potential recipients, which then precluded transplantation with an organ from the blood donor. Several modifications of this protocol subsequently were introduced in an attempt to lower the rate of sensitization. These modifications included the use of stored whole blood, a single transfusion 2 weeks before transplantation, and concurrent administration of azathioprine during the pretransplantation transfusion interval. Using such modified protocols, the rate of donor-specific sensitization was reduced to 9 to 14 per cent. Although many of these sensitized patients subsequently were able to undergo successful transplantation from a cadaver donor, this created a significant reduction in the available donor pool.

The commercial availability of cyclosporine in the mid 1980s led to controversy over the use of DST in living-related renal transplant recipients. With maintenance cyclosporine immunosuppression, the beneficial effect of DST on graft survival was reduced to approximately 5 per cent and donor exclusion resulting from sensitization was avoided. Pretransplant administration of deliberate third-party blood transfusions provided another strategy for obtaining excellent graft success in one-haplotype-matched living-related transplants while minimizing the risk of donor-specific sensitization.

At the present time, DST protocols continue to be employed in some transplant centers for immunologically high-risk live donor transplants such as one-haplotype-matched pairs and living-unrelated transplants. The potential for DST to induce donor-specific hyporesponsiveness with a consequent reduced need for maintenance immunosuppression is attractive. Reed and associates recently showed that three DSTs significantly reduced the incidence of rejection and improved the ability to withdraw steroids when compared with random donor transfusions. Salvatierra and associates recently described excellent results with pretransplant DST followed by antilymphoblast globulin and cyclosporine therapy; this regimen also enabled significant reduction in maintenance prednisone dosages.

Another potential use of DST is based on animal studies that have repeatedly demonstrated that cyclosporine and donor antigen in the form of DST can prolong allograft survival synergistically. Based on this principle, Davies and associates recently reported 90 per cent 1-year graft survival in haploidentical living-related kidney recipients treated with a single DST and cyclosporine 24 to 48 hours prior to transplantation. This single-DST protocol with cyclosporine coverage avoided donor-specific sensitization while maintaining the excellent immunologic efficacy observed in previous multiple-DST–cyclosporine protocols. At this time, the long-term advantage of combined DST and cyclosporine therapy is not established and requires further study.

Suggested Readings

Davies CB, Alexander JW, Cofer BR, et al: Efficacy of a single pretransplant donor-specific transfusion and cyclosporine A administered 24 to 48 hours before one-haplotype-mismatched living related donor kidney transplant. Ann Surg 215:618, 1992

Hodge E, Banowsky L, Novick A, et al: Alternative immunosuppressive strategies in the management of recipients of living-related renal transplants. Transplant Proc 21:1609, 1989

Reed A, Pirsch J, Armbrust MJ, et al: Multivariate analysis of donor-specific versus random transfusion protocols in haploidentical living-related transplants. Transplantation 51:382, 1991

Salvatierra O, McVicar J, Melzer J, et al: Improved results with combined donor-specific transfusion (DST) and sequential therapy protocol. Transplant Proc 23:1024, 1991

EFFECT OF DELIBERATE THIRD-PARTY TRANSFUSION IN NONIDENTICAL LIVING-RELATED DONOR RENAL ALLOGRAFT SURVIVAL

ERNEST E. HODGE, M.D.

Cleveland, Ohio

Significant enthusiasm for the use of pretransplant transfusions was generated by the observation of Salvatierra et al. that pretransplant donor-specific transfusions (DSTs) in recipients of nonidentical living-related renal allografts, including those with stimulatory mixed lymphocyte cultures, could produce 1-year allograft survival of 94 per cent. Although both DST and third-party transfusion (TPT) have been utilized, the overwhelming majority of reports described the use of DST. Numerous concerns have developed with DST, including logistical considerations of having the donor and recipient in close geographic proximity for the time of the transfusions (usually given as single transfusions 2 to 3 weeks apart, with the transplant occurring 4 to 8 weeks after the final transfusion) and a 10 to 30 per cent sensitization rate, which precludes the use of that particular donor. There also have been reports of sensitization to red blood cell antigens. The rate of sensitization to human lymphocyte antigens (HLAs) was markedly reduced by the administration of immunosuppressive medications, initially azathioprine and subsequently cyclosporine, during the time of transfusions. Many patients receiving nonidentical living-related allografts after undergoing DST protocols with or without the administration of immunosuppressive medications experienced early rejection episodes, although these were relatively mild and many were easily reversed. Several reports subsequently emerged describing results similar to those of Salvatierra but with the use of TPT. Advantages of TPT included a reduction in the logistic problems encountered as well as a decrease in the sensitization rate. Most TPTs were administered according to a deliberate schedule but were random with respect to HLA antigen composition. A potential disadvantage of TPT is that, despite improved screening technology, there continues to be significant concern regarding possible viral transmission via transfusions.

Although numerous studies, primarily single center, have emerged describing either DST or TPT protocols, comparative studies of the two strategies have been sparse. Recently, several issues have arisen that have diminished the enthusiasm for pretransplant transfusions in nonidentical living-related renal recipients. Flechner et al. reported that results for nonidentical living-related renal recipients treated with cyclosporine-based immunosuppressive therapy are similar to those for such patients treated with DST or TPT. This has been confirmed by additional centers. In addition, the development of synthetic erythropoietin has markedly diminished the "medical" need for transfusions in patients with end-stage renal disease. There are, however, a few studies that have compared DST to TPT and either DST or TPT to cyclosporine-based therapy.

Initial studies of pretransplant transfusion protocols compared results to patients who had received either no or small numbers of TPTs. Opelz, reporting for the Collaborative Transplant Study, analyzed a large number of recipients of nonidentical living-related renal allografts. The results in patients who had undergone DST protocols similar to that described by Salvatierra were virtually identical to results in patients who had received at least three TPTs. Patients who had received less than three TPTs had significantly worse allograft survival. Interestingly, there was not a linear relation between improvement and numbers of transfusions, because patients receiving more than four transfusions did not demonstrate additional improvement. In a review of the South-Eastern Organ Procurement Foundation data, Sanfilippo et al. found 1-, 2-, and 3-year allograft survival rates of 95, 89, and 84 per cent, respectively, in patients receiving DSTs and 92, 88, and 83 per cent, respectively, in patients receiving TPTs, with no patient in these groups receiving cyclosporine. In patients receiving cyclosporine, 1-, 2-, and 3-year allograft survival rates for DST-treated patients were 91, 87, and 82 per cent, respectively, and were 92, 88, and 83 per cent, respectively, in patients given TPTs.

Reed et al. recently reported a retrospective analysis of 127 recipients of haploidentical living-related renal allografts in which 74 patients received DSTs plus azathioprine and 53 patients received TPTs under no immunosuppressive umbrella. In the DST group, recipients received three transfusions of stored blood at 2-week intervals and azathioprine at 1 to 2 mg/kg per day, whereas the TPTs were administered randomly at nonspecific intervals. A past history of at least three TPTs satisfied criteria for the TPT group, and transplants occurred in both groups a minimum of 3 weeks following the last transfusion. In the DST group, 50 per cent of patients received a median of three transfusions prior to entering the DST protocol. Rejection episodes were treated with a prednisone bolus, and OKT3 monoclonal antilymphocyte therapy was utilized for refractory rejections. There was a sensitization rate of 9.6 per cent ($n = 7$) in the DST group and 1.9 per cent ($n = 1$) in the TPT group. Two-year graft survival was 95 and 91 per cent for the DST and TPT groups, respectively. More frequent and earlier rejection episodes were seen in the TPT group, with 50 per cent of the DST patients experiencing at least one rejection episode by the end of 1 year compared to 75 per cent in the TPT group. DST and pregnancy were found to have protective benefits against rejection. As indicated by the 2-year allograft survival rates mentioned, the difference in frequency and timing of rejection between the groups has not had a significant impact on survival thus far.

In an attempt to address the question of whether to continue to pretreat nonidentical living-related allograft recipients with transfusions prior to transplantation, a prospective study was conducted at the Cleveland Clinic Foundation and Humana Hospital, San Antonio. From September 1984 to September 1986, 59 haploidentical recipients were prospectively assigned to either of two treatment groups. The assignment was based on the transfusion history of the patient at the time of initial presentation for evaluation for transplantation. Patients who had received two or fewer TPTs were given no additional transfusions and were treated with prednisone and cyclosporine following transplantation. Patients having received three or four TPTs at the time of initial evaluation were given additional units for a minimum of five TPTs and received prednisone and azathioprine following transplantation, whereas those who had already received a minimum of five TPTs were given no additional transfusions and also treated with prednisone and azathioprine. Patients requiring transfusions for purposes of the protocol received leukocyte-poor units (250 to 400 ml) given as single units 2 weeks apart, with transplantation occurring at least 3 to 4 weeks following the last transfusion. The timing of the transfusions was deliberate, although donor selection was random because there was no attempt to avoid or match for HLA antigens. Forty-one per cent of patients in the TPT group required deliberate transfusions prior to transplantation. No recipient became sensitized to the potential donor as a result of deliberate TPT. No difference was seen between the cyclosporine and TPT groups with respect to per cent reactive antibodies nor the number of patients with reactive antibodies greater than 60 per cent. One-year patient survival was 95 and 94 per cent, respectively, for the cyclosporine and TPT groups, with 1-year allograft survival of 81 and 91 per cent, respectively. Significantly more rejection was observed in the TPT group, with a mean of 1.4 rejection episodes per patient compared to 0.7 episodes per patient in the cyclosporine group ($p = .003$). Fifty-one per cent of the cyclosporine group remained rejection free compared to only 14 per cent of the TPT group. The mean serum creatinine 1 year after transplantation was 1.7 mg/dl in the cyclosporine group compared to 1.9 mg/dl for the TPT group. In summary, despite more frequent rejection in the TPT group, overall patient and allograft survivals were similar between the two groups.

Unfortunately, data currently available are insufficient to answer the question of whether DST or TPT is superior or whether cyclosporine has completely obviated the need for pretransplant transfusions in nonidentical living-related renal allograft recipients. Several reports have described additional improvement with a combination of cyclosporine and either DST or TPT in nonidentical living-related renal allograft recipients, although this has not been universally true nor has it been true for HLA-identical recipients. This variation in results probably has been related to the inability, to date, to identify the specific mechanism (selecting out high-risk patients, induction of suppressor or anti-idiotypic antibodies) by which transfusions impact on transplant outcome. Clearly, the transfusion mechanism and effect could be different in different donor-recipient pair combinations. The principal concern of sensitization with DST remains problematic. Although azathioprine and cyclosporine have decreased sensitization rates, it is unknown whether there is a tradeoff in terms of inhibiting suppressor or anti-idiotypic antibody formation, thus counteracting the transfusion benefit. As screening technology continues to improve, the primary concern of disease transmission with TPT should become extremely remote. Currently, there appears to be a trend toward fewer transfusions prior to transplantation and new immunosuppressive agents such as FK506, RS 61443, rapamycin, and brequinar sodium may well signal the end of pretransplant transfusions altogether. Certainly, additional follow-up of existing studies will be important to assess the continued need for and long-term benefit of pretransplant transfusions.

Suggested Readings

Brynger H, Frisk B, Larsson O, et al: Planned third-party transfusions prior to first transplantations from living related donors. Scand J Urol Nephrol Suppl 64:152–156, 1981

Flechner SM, Kerman RH, Van Buren CT, et al: The use of cyclosporine in living-related renal transplantation. Donor-specific hyporesponsiveness and steroid withdrawal. Transplantation 38:685, 1984

Hodge EE, Banowsky LH, Novick AC, et al: Conventional immunosuppression after deliberate third party transfusions versus cyclosporine in living related renal transplant recipients. J Urol, 141:495–498, 1989

Opelz G, for the Collaborative Transplant Study: Comparison of random transfusions with donor-specific transfusions for pre-treatment of HLA one-haplotype-matched related donor kidney transplant recipients. Transplant Proc 17:2357, 1985

Pfaff WW, Fennell RS, Howard RJ, et al: Planned random donor blood transfusion in preparation for transplantation. Sensitization and graft survival. Transplantation 38:701, 1984

Raftery MJ, Lang CJ, O'Shea JM, et al: Controlled trial of azathioprine and cyclosporin to prevent anti-HLA antibodies due to third-party transfusion. Nephrol Dial Transplant 3:671–675, 1988

Reed A, Pirsch J, Armbrust M, et al: Multivariate analysis of donor-specific versus random transfusion protocols in haploidentical living-related transplants. Transplantation 51:382–384, 1991

Salvatierra O, Vincenti F, Amend W, et al: Deliberate donor-specific blood transfusions prior to living related renal transplantation. A new approach. Ann Surg 192: 543, 1980

Sanfilippo F, Vaughn WK, for the South Eastern Organ Procurement Foundation: Results in live-donor renal transplantation: the SEOPF Multicenter Study. Transplant Proc 19:1489, 1987

CYCLOSPORINE IN RENAL TRANSPLANTATION

STUART M. FLECHNER, M.D., F.A.C.S.

Stanford, California

The practice of clinical transplantation has been the result of incremental advances built on previous experiences. The goal continues to be the provision of allografts to patients with end-stage organ failure for the longest period of time with the least morbidity. Many of these incremental advances, such as proper recipient selection, judicious use of antirejection therapy, and the early and definitive management of technical problems, were based on the avoidance of complications. The goal of tolerance, or specific unresponsiveness to the organ allograft, remains elusive and is the focus of most scientific investigation in transplantation biology. Although not a panacea, the most significant recent advance in clinical transplantation has been the widespread introduction of cyclosporine A (CsA) during the last decade. The use of CsA not only has produced the most dramatic incremental advance in kidney and heart graft survival, but has reawakened the dormant fields of liver, pancreas, pulmonary, and small bowel transplantation. The methods employed during the clinical and laboratory evaluations of this agent are now the yardsticks by which newer agents are measured.

CHEMICAL STRUCTURE

Cyclosporine is a fungal fermentation product, first isolated from soil samples in 1972 during a screening program for new antibiotics. Its novel chemical structure, a neutral, cyclic polypeptide with a molecular weight of

1203, contains 11 amino acids, 7 of which are *N*-methylated. The 9-carbon amino acid at position 1 had not been previously observed in nature. The molecule is extremely hydrophobic, only soluble in organic solvents and lipids. Although the molecule can be synthesized de novo in the laboratory, numerous substitution maneuvers and analogues have not been shown to provide greater immunosuppressive efficacy or diminished toxicity than the parent compound.

CLINICAL PHARMACOLOGY

For clinical use, the drug can be given by either the intravenous (IV) or the oral route. The parenteral preparation is stabilized in a cremaphor base, and is best given by a slow continuous infusion to minimize toxicity. Two oral preparations currently are available. The liquid form, with CsA dissolved in olive oil at 100 mg/ml, is perhaps easiest to titrate. However, most patients prefer the drug delivered in soft gelatin capsules. The two oral formulations are bioequivalent, and the IV preparation has a bioequivalence with the oral forms of about 1:3. Allergic reactions to the oral formulations have not been reported, whereas about 1 per cent of patients experience hypersensitivity to the IV drug, presumably as a result of the cremaphor vehicle. The IV route is preferred during periods of gastrointestinal dysfunction.

Oral CsA is absorbed primarily in the small intestine through a process enhanced by bile salts. The bioavailability of CsA fluctuates from 10 to 40 per cent (mean 30 per cent), but tends to increase with time after transplantation. Interestingly, the administration of CsA with food seems to enhance absorption, whereas rapid gut motility, reduced gastric emptying (diabetics), cholestasis, pancreatic insufficiency, and cholestyramine impair absorption. Although absorption may vary among individuals, most reach peak plasma concentration 3 to 4 hours after an oral dose. Circulating CsA is bound almost exclusively to lipoproteins. A small unbound "free" fraction can be measured but does not correlate with clinical events or total plasma concentrations. The drug appears to accumulate in the liver, pancreas, fat, blood, gut, heart, lung, and muscle, in descending order. The volume of distribution in the body is large, but the drug does not seem to preferentially accumulate in the non–lean body mass. Accurate dosing therefore is calculated better according to the ideal body weight.

The liver is the principle site of CsA metabolism and elimination. The cytochrome P-450 oxidase system, through a series of hydroxylation and/or demethylation reactions, renders the parent compound more hydrophilic as it is excreted through the gut. Although some enterohepatic recycling of metabolites may occur, the metabolites uniformly display less immunosuppressive potency when compared to the parent compound. Less than 6 per cent of an oral dose appears in the urine, so renal failure has little impact on CsA metabolism. Those agents that are known to interact with cytochrome P-450 also directly alter CsA circulating blood levels, and can cause changes in clinical events. For example, agents such as rifampin, phenobarbital, dilantin, and carbamazepine, which induce hepatic cytochrome P-450, lower CsA blood levels. Drugs that inhibit cytochrome P-450, such as erythromycin, oral contraceptives, androgens, ketoconazole, and corticosteroids, increase CsA levels. The coadministration of these agents with CsA necessitates careful monitoring of blood levels to avoid either enhanced drug toxicity or underimmunosuppression. The median elimination half-life of CsA is 6 to 8 hours in most patients, which permits once-daily oral dosing. Some adult patients and most children experience shorter elimination half-lives and require more frequent dosing intervals. Intercurrent illnesses, especially hepatobiliary and gastrointestinal disease, may require an altered dosing schedule or route of administration.

MECHANISM OF ACTION

In early experiments, both in vivo and in vitro, it was observed that CsA caused profound immunosuppression, predominantly against cell-mediated responses. Uniquely, CsA-induced immunosuppression not only was reversible but appeared to be selective for lymphocyte function, especially that of the T cell. The sparing of granulocyte, platelet, and macrophage function translates into a greater degree of safety in clinical use. Early experiments also confirmed that CsA acted early during T cell activation, because drug-induced suppression of a mixed lymphocyte reaction (MLR) could be prevented if CsA was added to the culture several hours after incubation. Therefore, once activated, the T cell activation cascade cannot be overridden by CsA. This occurs because CsA appears to inhibit primarily the activation of several lymphokine genes.

The key target of CsA action is the CD4-positive T helper cell. Initially, CsA appears to prevent macrophage-derived interleukin-1 (IL-1) from performing its role in the activation of resting T helper cells. This action is coupled with a profound inhibition of IL-2 biosynthesis, release, and receptor expression by T helper cells. Because IL-2 is a necessary second signal for the clonal expansion of antigen-activated T helper cells as well as cytolytic T cells, the drug acts at an essential step in the amplification of the immune response. More recent studies have demonstrated that CsA acts at the transcriptional level, preventing the release of IL-2, IL-3, and gamma-interferon mRNA. It would also appear that CsA action is not mediated by cell surface events. The drug seems to be passively taken up by lymphocytes and bound to an intracellular carrier termed "cyclophillin." The degree of binding to cyclophillin has been reported to be proportional to the degree of immunosuppression as measured in the MLR. Although not completely understood, it would appear that CsA-cyclophillin, possibly in a calcium-dependent fashion, inhibits the action of one or more transcriptional factors that lead to lymphokine production in alloactivated lymphocytes.

DRUG-RELATED TOXICITY

The side effects associated with clinical CsA use include those related to immunosuppression in general and those related to specific organs and tissues. Compared to a control population, any patient given chemical immunosuppression displays a greater incidence of infections and malignancies, presumably as a result of impaired immune surveillance. Comparative reports have demonstrated that CsA-treated transplant recipients experience fewer bacterial infections and about the same number of viral infections as those treated with other agents or combinations. This may be the result of the limited action of CsA on granulocytes, macrophages, and T cell–independent B cell functions. In addition, CsA-treated patients seem to respond to bacterial infections with the same rate of recovery as nonimmunosuppressed patients given antimicrobials. The herpes viruses, *Cytomegalovirus*, and Epstein-Barr virus, which are controlled by T cell responses, continue to be found in at least 20 per cent of patients. Fungal and parasitic infections are infrequent in the CsA-treated population, and likely are related to the total amount of immunosuppression administered.

Lymphoreticular malignancies and those from rapidly dividing epithelial elements of skin, uterine cervix, and gut long have been associated with immunosuppression. Clusters of these cancers have been reported at certain transplant centers, and they have been universally associated with high doses of multiagent therapy. Currently, there is no evidence that CsA use resulting in trough blood levels under 250 ng/ml causes a higher incidence of these tumors. Individual factors such as age, sex, genetic predisposition, and immune status may impact on the development of post-transplant malignancies, but as yet are difficult to measure.

After 10 years of widespread use, CsA has been found to cause relatively little chronic toxicity. This is perhaps the product of an empirical pattern of drug administration that begins with induction doses of 10 to 14 mg/kg (higher in selected patients and children), and ends in stable maintenance doses of 3 to 5 mg/kg by 1 year and beyond. Thus, the drug-related side effects are most evident the first few months after transplantation and diminish as the dose is lowered. Occasionally a side effect may be so severe in a particular patient that switching to another agent becomes necessary. The side effects include neurologic manifestations such as tremors, headache, burning paresthesias, depression, somnolence, and seizures; hypertrichosis of the face, arms, and back; and gingival hyperplasia, most pronounced in those recipients with poor dental hygiene. Anorexia, bloating, nausea, and vomiting, when reported, may be alleviated by using the gelatin capsule formulation. Hepatotoxicity, manifested by elevation of transaminases and bilirubin, usually is self-limited. However, jaundice has been reported, as well as a possibly increased incidence of cholelithiases.

NEPHROTOXICITY OF CsA

The Achilles heel of CsA has been its toxic effect on renal function, observed among the first group of renal transplant recipients given the drug in 1978. More than any other clinical finding, this has led to much consternation and tinkering with dosage regimens. CsA nephrotoxicity is most severe when CsA doses are highest, renal function is impaired, and a coexistent ischemic renal injury occurs. In clinical practice, this happens in recipients of cadaveric cold-preserved kidneys, heart transplant recipients undergoing cardiopulmonary bypass, and liver recipients with severe fluid overload and decreased renal perfusion. CsA nephrotoxicity is characterized by decreased glomerular blood flow and filtration rate causing serum creatinine elevations, hypertension, fluid retention, and hyperuricemia. These changes are thought to be functional and reversible, and directly due to afferent arteriolar vasoconstriction, even in the denervated transplant kidney. The most widely held hypothesis is that CsA inhibits the prostacyclin synthetase system, resulting in a diminished concentration of the local vascular dilator prostacyclin and an increased concentration of the vasoconstrictor thromboxane A_2. Additional theories relating to altered vascular endothelial calcium and other ionic fluxes also have been proffered.

A histologic pattern for CsA nephrotoxicity has been described but remains controversial. The end results of chronic ischemia and chronic allograft rejection also display many of the same features. Nevertheless, a pattern of tubular atrophy, interstitial edema, tubular vacuolization, microcalcification, giant mitochondria, and moderate to severe interstitial fibrosis has been reported. A macroscopic pattern of so-called striped fibrosis is associated with long-term use. Unfortunately, the varied histologic features described do not necessarily correlate to the level of renal function in a particular kidney. The once-held theory that long-term CsA use led to an inexorable permanent loss of renal function has not been observed in clinical practice. However, early excessive doses, such as 20 mg/kg or more, given during coexistent renal ischemia may impart permanent renal injury.

RENAL TRANSPLANT RESULTS

CsA is now considered the immunosuppressive agent of choice for recipients of renal allografts. Most centers achieve 1-year patient survival of about 95 per cent and graft survival of about 80 per cent for recipients of first cadaver transplants, and about 70 per cent for retransplants. Recipients who receive kidneys from living-related donors generally achieve over 90 per cent graft survival at 1 year for haplotype-matched kidneys, whereas recipients of HLA identical kidneys experience very little immunologic graft loss. These results have been obtained with the combination of daily CsA and prednisone as maintenance therapy. Most subsequent immunosuppressive strategies have been developed to combat the nephrotoxicity caused by CsA. Unfortunately, these excellent early results do decay over time, and chronic rejection may be more of a problem than originally thought. Graft loss of 2 to 5 per cent per year highlights the need for strategies to induce true immunologic tolerance.

MANAGEMENT STRATEGIES

Fortunately, the progressive increase in bioavailability of CsA permits significant dose reduction, by one half to one third, during the first year. Even so, 10 to 15 per cent of recipients may experience a reduction in glomerular filtration rate such that the dose may have to be lowered below a suitable immunosuppressive threshold. This has led to the introduction of azathioprine (AZA) as a substitute agent. Although renal function may improve temporarily after switching from CsA to AZA, the inferior efficacy of AZA results in acute rejection in 30 per cent of these patients, and graft loss at a rate that exceeds that of patients who remain on CsA. Therefore, the concept of triple therapy—lower doses of CsA (2.5 to 4 mg/kg), AZA (1 to 1.5 mg/kg), and prednisone (Pred)—has evolved as maintenance therapy. To combat early CsA toxicity that may exacerbate recovery from post-transplant acute tubular necrosis, some have recommended withholding CsA and adding an antilymphocyte globulin (ALG) the first post-transplant week. CsA is introduced after recovery from acute tubular necrosis, when it is better tolerated. This so-called quadruple therapy (ALG-CsA-AZA-Pred) is popular at centers that experience long cadaveric preservation times. Although such multidrug regimens may help to diminish the toxicity of an individual agent, they may sacrifice the important lymphocyte specificity that has been attributed to CsA. In fact, some reports have questioned whether multidrug regimens produce a greater incidence of infectious complications and/or neoplastic transformation.

Another approach designed to limit the negative aspects of CsA therapy has been the monitoring of blood levels. Because in vitro assays revealed that maximum immunosuppression is attained with concentrations of 100 to 200 ng/ml, it was satisfying to observe that a similar blood level would provide ample rejection prophylaxis with minimal toxicity in the clinical setting. Extensive pharmacokinetic studies subsequently showed that this concentration could be obtained in most patients. However, the variable absorption, metabolism, and elimination of CsA results in less than uniform dosing regimens for all patients. In addition, the ideal tool for measuring CsA parent compound in the blood, high-performance liquid chromatography often is too cumbersome for widespread clinical use. Currently, most centers achieve these target blood levels using commercially available assay kits that include some metabolites in the determinations. Usually, a polyclonal antiserum or a nonspecific murine monoclonal antibody are used for binding in a radioimmunoassay or the fluorescent polarization technique. Such monitoring also may be useful to determine which patients are undertreated and require a divided daily schedule. This can be very helpful in differentiating drug toxicity from other similar events.

FUTURE STRATEGIES

After a decade of widespread use, CsA has become the prototype of a new generation of agents with lymphocyte-specific action. Because CsA does not induce true immunologic tolerance, the quest for selective organ acceptance without the unwanted side effects of nonspecific immunosuppression continues to drive experimental efforts. However, the lessons learned from the introduction of CsA provide a yardstick to measure future agents, as well as those with possible synergy to CsA. Drugs such as FK-506, rapamycin, RS-61443, Brequinar, and 12-deoxyspergualin are on the horizon, and are awaiting trials in the clinical laboratory.

Suggested Readings

Flechner SM, Kolbeinsson ME, Tam J, et al: The impact of body weight on cyclosporine pharmacokinetics in renal transplant recipients. Transplantation 48:806, 1989

Harding MW, Handschumacher RE: Cyclophilin, a primary molecular target for cyclosporine. Transplantation 46:295, 1988

Kahan BD, Flechner SM, Lorber MI, et al: Complications of cyclosporine immunosuppression in 402 renal allograft recipients at a single center for 1–5 years. Transplantation 43:197, 1987

Lorber MI, Flechner SM, Van Buren CT, et al: Cyclosporine toxicity: The effect of combined therapy using cyclosporine, azathioprine, and prednisone. Am J Kidney Dis 9:476, 1988

Mihatch MJ, Thiel G, Ryffel B: Histopathology of cyclosporine nephrotoxicity. Transplant Proc 20:759, 1988

RENAL ALLOGRAFT REJECTION

STUART M. FLECHNER, M.D., FACS

Stanford, California

The major roadblock to universally successful human renal allotransplantation has been, and remains, rejection. The precise reason why some patients reject kidney transplants promptly and repeatedly, whereas others retain grafts of similar immunologic disparity for longer than 20 years, continues to be a mystery. At the present time, graft survival is based on the administration of nonspecific immunosuppression, with the hope that treatment will be adequate to delay the rejection process without exposing the host to significant immunologic morbidity.

THE REJECTION RESPONSE

The rejection response to transplanted tissue can be divided into three phases: (1) the afferent limb, which involves recognition of and sensitization to the graft; (2) the central limb, which involves processing and the development of immunity; and (3) the efferent or effector limb, which involves the response to foreign tissue, leading to graft destruction. The effector limb incorporates both humoral (antibody) and cellular mechanisms, which act in concert.

Specific sensitization of the recipient to the graft begins as cell surface and soluble factors are processed by the immunocompetent cells of the recipient, including macrophages and antigen-presenting cells. These factors are glycoproteins, such as foreign human lymphocyte antigens (HLAs), and are found most prominently on the vascular endothelium of the graft and on so-called passenger leukocytes. Once processed, they are re-expressed on the surface of antigen-presenting cells, and, in conjunction with self-major histocompatibility complex (MHC) class I and class II antigens, begin to trigger resting T lymphocytes. The soluble lymphokine interleukin-1 (IL-1), produced by macrophages, is a necessary second signal in this process. In one schema, expressed foreign antigen plus self-MHC class I antigen is required to trigger the T cell receptor of resting CD8-positive cytolytic cells, whereas antigen plus self-MHC class II antigen is required to trigger the T cell receptor of resting CD4-positive helper cells.

Activated T helper cells rapidly proliferate and produce a wide array of lymphokines, most notably IL-2, which is required for the clonal expansion of specifically sensitized cytolytic T cells and antibody-producing B cells. The sensitized populations then will generate both cell-mediated and humoral responses against the foreign antigens on the graft. Activated cytolytic lymphocytes and complement-dependent and -independent antibody formation cause direct injury and vascular occlusion, eventuating in tissue necrosis. This process requires the interaction of immunocompetent cells acting both locally and at distant sites (lymph nodes, spleen, marrow, etc.). It also confers memory to the immune system, which permits specific recall to the same foreign antigens.

Clinically, the rejection response is manifested by a constellation of both local and systemic signs and symptoms that reflect a severe inflammatory reaction. A recipient may exhibit fever, chills, sweating, lassitude, hypertension, weight gain, peripheral edema, and diminished urine output. The graft may be enlarged, tender to palpation, and associated with edema of overlying tissues or ascites (intraperitoneal kidneys). Laboratory values reflect renal dysfunction, with a decrease in glomerular filtration, increased serum creatinine and blood urea nitrogen, electrolyte abnormalities (hyperkalemia, acidosis), and leukocytosis. Proteinuria frequently is present (>1.5 gm/24 hr) and often is of high molecular weight (>55,000) when significant glomerular basement membrane injury has occurred. Decreased renal arterial perfusion occurs, which can be detected on radiographic studies and nuclear scans. However, many of the criteria cited are present to varying degrees during rejection, and also can be found in other nonimmunologic conditions. Therefore, other conditions, such as sepsis, transplant pyelonephritis, urinary fistulas or obstruction, renal arterial or venous thrombosis, lymphocele, hyperglycemia, nephrotoxic drugs, or recurrent renal parenchymal disease, should be ruled out before administering antirejection therapy. A renal biopsy frequently is required to differentiate these confounding conditions.

CLINICAL REJECTION

In an unmodified host—for example, a recipient not receiving any immunosuppressive agents—the rejection response will begin after about 7 days and progressively destroy the graft. In order to control or limit the response, patients must take daily immunosuppressive drugs to nonspecifically depress the immune system. Even though every recipient must take maintenance therapy, about 50 per cent of cadaveric recipients will suffer at least one breakthrough acute rejection episode during the first year. Currently, the most frequently employed maintenance regimens are cyclosporine based. These usually are combined with either daily oral corticosteroids (double therapy) or steroids plus azathioprine (triple therapy). Rejection episodes usually are treated by adding additional high doses of immunosuppressive agents for a short period of time.

TREATMENT

The following agents are currently in use to treat renal allograft rejection. They often are used in combination.

Corticosteroids. Steroid preparations given in high doses are the most frequently used therapy to treat acute rejection. They can be administered intravenously as methylprednisolone, usually 15 to 20 mg/kg. When given over 1 to 3 days, the term "steroid pulse" is used. Some centers prefer to treat with oral prednisone in tapering doses over a few weeks, beginning with 2 to 3 mg/kg. This is termed a "cycle." Prednisone most often is given as maintenance therapy of 0.1 mg/kg per day.

Azathioprine. Azathioprine is a purine analogue that acts by disrupting nucleic acid synthesis and therefore lymphoid differentiation and expansion. It is given orally as a daily maintenance drug at a dose of 1 to 2 mg/kg. It is not useful to treat acute rejection episodes. The major side effect is myelosuppression, which can limit the total daily dose that can be administered.

Cyclosporine. Cyclosporine is a fungal peptide with selective antilymphocytic activity, used primarily as a daily maintenance drug. It has limited activity to treat acute rejection, and the major side effect is nephrotoxicity.

Antilymphocyte Globulin. The purified serum globulin fraction derived from heterologous species (equine, rabbit) immunized with human lymphocytes is a potent immunosuppressive agent. Antilymphocyte globulin can be given prophylactically as an induction agent (20 to 30 mg/kg) the first 2 weeks after transplant, and has gained favor as a replacement agent in order to withhold cyclosporine while kidneys recover from acute tubular necrosis (ATN). It also can be used to treat acute rejection episodes as a 7- to 10-day course of 15 to 20 mg/kg, especially in cases of steroid-resistant rejection.

Monoclonal Antibodies. Antibody preparations with specificity for human T cell antigenic determinants have been developed using murine hybridoma technology. The most widely used is the antibody to the CD3 molecule (OKT3, Ortho Co.). This preparation has been used both to treat acute rejection episodes and as induction therapy the first week. Reuse can be limited because human antimouse antibody is generated against the murine sequences. Agents that bind to the T cell receptor, the interleukin-2 receptor, and CD4 are in their early phases of study.

X-Irradiation. Ionizing radiation given locally to the graft (150 rads for 3 days) can be cytotoxic to invading lymphocytes and may be helpful in tender, swollen grafts. It is rarely necessary. Higher doses of radiation (3500 rads), given in fractions to the lymph-bearing tissues in a field similar to the treatment area of Hodgkin's disease, result in profound immunosuppression. This is termed "total lymphoid irradiation" and is used in experimental protocols in a few centers.

Plasmapheresis. Plasma exchange to remove donor-directed antibody and antigen-antibody complexes from recipient serum has been used to treat the humoral component of the rejection response. This technique may have a role in the treatment of resistant rejection episodes or those caused by unintentional ABO incompatibility.

Newer Agents. There are a number of new agents currently in various stages of investigation that have immunosuppressive promise. Some appear to be lymphocyte specific (FK506, rapamycin), some are antiproliferative (Mizorbine, RS-61443, Brequinar), and others (deoxyspergualin) have unique actions.

TYPES OF REJECTION EPISODES

From a clinical perspective, there are four types of rejection episodes, each with a different time of occurrence, etiology, response to therapy, and natural history.

Hyperacute Rejection

Hyperacute rejection can occur immediately after renal revascularization and during the first 24 hours after transplant. When it occurs in the operating room, the kidney remains pale and flaccid; hours later it is dark and necrotic. Hyperacute rejection is caused by circulating preformed cytotoxic antibodies that immediately bind to the vascular endothelium of the graft, with subsequent fixation of complement. Microvascular clotting, fibrin deposition, and occlusion follow, which result in tissue necrosis and dense granulocyte infiltration. The only therapy for this catastrophic event is immediate graft nephrectomy. A severe toxic syndrome and possibly cardiovascular collapse can occur if the graft is not removed. Hyperacute rejection implies presensitization of HLA (and other) antigens on the donor kidney, but usually can be prevented by careful pretransplant crossmatching. Recipient serum must be screened before transplantation for any complement-dependent cytotoxic antibody that will lyse donor lymphocytes in vitro.

Accelerated Rejection

This term describes an often severe rejection episode occurring during the first posttransplant week. Such events usually are associated with many of the overt clinical features of rejection. The term "primary nonfunction" is used to describe kidneys that never work. Many of these represent cases in which a kidney with slowly resolving posttransplant ATN is hit with an accelerated rejection and becomes nonviable. Because accelerated rejection occurs before the time necessary to generate a primary immune response, some form of donor-specific presensitization is present. The mechanism is thought to be on a cellular basis because it occurs even when the direct lymphocyte crossmatch is negative. Because it occurs during the first week, other nonimmunologic causes of renal dysfunction must be ruled out.

The treatment of accelerated rejection is usually with a steroid pulse. Antilymphocyte preparations may be necessary if the response is incomplete. Local X-irradiation can be used for the painful and swollen graft. Although it may take several days to see a response to therapy, many grafts are left with permanent injury. Grafts that do not respond to therapy should be removed because of the tissue necrosis that usually is present after a severe immune response.

Acute Rejection

This is the most common form of renal transplant rejection and can occur at any time after transplant. Most acute rejection episodes occur during the first year, with the majority occurring during the first 3 months. An acute rejection also can recur immediately after therapy for a previous episode is completed. The presentation is variable; acute rejection can be insidious, occurring over a few weeks, or sudden, occurring over 24 hours. If many of the clinical criteria for rejection are not present, a renal biopsy is most helpful to make the diagnosis. Histologic examination of kidneys undergoing acute rejection reveals marked and diffuse interstitial edema and mononuclear cell infiltration of the graft. Early in the course, infiltrates are perivascular and periglomerular, but eventually they become diffuse throughout the cortex and medulla.

The therapy for acute rejection is usually a steroid pulse. Some centers have begun using polyclonal or monoclonal antilymphocyte preparations as first-line therapy for rejection, whereas others withhold these agents for those cases in which there is no response to steroids. In general, it is not prudent to persist with antirejection therapy after two or three rejection episodes, especially in high-risk patients (e.g., diabetics, age >60). The major cause of renal transplant recipient morbidity and mortality is overzealous antirejection therapy, with resultant opportunistic infection.

Chronic Rejection

Chronic rejection can occur at any time after about 3 months after transplant, and is associated with gradual progressive renal deterioration. Chronic rejection can be accompanied by hypertension and proteinuria, which can precede the biochemical serum abnormalities. Proteinuria, if severe, can result in the nephrotic syndrome, with edema, ascites, and weight gain. Kidneys are usually small and fibrotic, without tenderness and edema. Radiographic studies demonstrate a marked decrease in renal perfusion. The histologic features of chronic rejection include a dense interstitial fibrosis with sclerosed tubules and hyperplasia, causing the arterioles to have an onionskin appearance.

Chronic rejection is thought to be mediated primarily through humoral mechanisms, but some cellular component is present. There is no reliable therapy for chronic rejection because much of the process (fibrosis) is irreversible. Acute rejection episodes may occur in a graft with background changes of chronic rejection. However, the longer the time that has elapsed since transplant, the less likely that antirejection therapy will be effective. Smoldering chronic rejection may exist for many years and supply life-sustaining renal function to the recipient, as long as hypertension and proteinuria are not severe. Chronically rejected grafts usually can be left in place if the patient returns to dialysis and all immunosuppression is discontinued. However, they should be removed if infected, or if they cause pain, fever, hematuria, or severe proteinuria or hypertension.

Suggested Readings

Dallman MJ, Morris PJ: The immunology of rejection. In Morris PJ (ed): Kidney Transplantation, 3rd ed. Philadelphia, WB Saunders, 1988, pp 15–37

Milford EL, Carpenter CB: Immunopathogenetic mechanisms of allograft rejection. In Tisher CC, Brenner BM (eds): Renal Pathology with Clinical and Functional Correlations. Philadelphia, JB Lippincott, 1989, pp 1506–1518

Modena FM, Hostetter TH, Salhudeen AK, et al: Progression of kidney disease in chronic renal transplant rejection. Transplantation 52:239, 1991

Salmela KT, Von Willebrand EO, Kyllonen LE, et al: Acute vascular rejection in renal transplantation—diagnosis and outcome. Transplantation 54:858, 1992

TREATMENT OF URINARY FISTULAS AFTER KIDNEY TRANSPLANTATION

STEVAN B. STREEM, M.D.

Cleveland, Ohio

The incidence of urologic complications of renal transplantation has decreased markedly in the last decade as a result of refinement in surgical techniques and advances in immunologic therapy. Furthermore, when urologic complications do occur, the historically high rates of morbidity and mortality associated with them also are decreased, in part as a result of earlier diagnosis and treatment. In most contemporary series, urinary extravasation occurs in less than 3 per cent of patients and only rarely results in graft loss or mortality.

URINARY EXTRAVASATION

Urinary extravasation is generally an early complication of transplantation. The clinical presentation can include pain, tenderness or a palpable mass over the graft, ipsilateral leg edema, declining graft function, or leakage of fluid from the incision. If the fluid can be collected from the incision, or aspirated percutaneously, electrolyte, urea, and creatinine determinations will help differentiate urine from lymph or serum. Radiographic studies are invaluable in diagnosing urinary extravasation. These include nuclear renography, cystography, ultrasonography, and computerized tomography (CT) scanning. When renal function is adequate, intravenous contrast can be given during the CT scan to help differentiate urine from other types of fluid. A plain film obtained immediately after CT scanning with intravenous contrast then may provide anatomic information equivalent to that obtained with intravenous pyelography.

In many cases, the level of renal function at the time urinary extravasation is diagnosed is not adequate to allow administration of intravenous contrast. Therefore, alternative diagnostic modalities must be utilized to define further the level of extravasation. In our practice, retrograde pyelography is only rarely utilized for imaging of the collecting system in transplant recipients because retrograde cannulation of the ureteral orifice is often difficult in this setting. An excellent alternative to retrograde pyelography for further delineation of urinary extravasation is placement of a percutaneous nephrostomy tube, which then allows initial proximal diversion and access for subsequent antegrade radiographic studies that will delineate definitively the site of extravasation. Appropriate therapy then is instituted depending on the overall clinical stability of the patient and the site of extravasation.

TREATMENT OF URINARY FISTULAS

Ureteral Fistulas

The incidence of ureteral fistula has decreased, in part as a result of recognition of the importance of preserving periureteral blood supply and, more recently, as a result of the routine use of an extravesical ureteroneocystostomy. However, when ureteral fistulas do occur, the etiology is almost always a compromise of ureteral vascularity, which results in ureteral necrosis and sloughing. A local technical factor associated with the ureteroneocystostomy itself can occur, but is a less frequent cause of a distal ureteral leak.

Classically, the management of a ureteral fistula has been immediate open operative intervention. When the fistula is limited to the most distal ureter, a repeat ureteroneocystostomy is a viable option. In such cases, a soft, self-retaining internal stent should be placed intraoperatively and left indwelling for 4 to 6 weeks. For more extensive ureteral involvement, an almost universally applicable reconstructive procedure is utilization of the native ureter for a ureteroureterostomy to the proximal transplant ureter, or ureteropyelostomy to the transplant renal pelvis. When using the native ureter, the native kidney is usually left in place and the proximal ureter simply ligated. In the face of infection, however, native nephrectomy should be considered. An alternative to native nephrectomy is anastomosis of the native ureter in a side-to-side manner to the transplant renal pelvis, thus precluding the possibility of complications associated with simple ligation of the native ureter. For all patients undergoing either ureteroureterostomy or ureteropyelostomy, an internal stent again should be left indwelling during the initial postoperative period and removed 4 to 6 weeks later. In cases in which a percutaneous nephrostomy tube had been placed prior to definitive open operative repair, it is our preference to leave this nephrostomy tube indwelling during the initial postoperative period to provide temporary urinary diversion as well as access for postoperative radiographic studies.

Rarely, the native ureter is either not available or otherwise inappropriate for use in operative reconstruction. In such cases, several "salvage" reconstructive procedures may be utilized, including an ileal interposition or vesicopyelostomy, with or without a Boari flap. In rare instances in which the transplant pelvis cannot be accessed, reconstruction with a native ureterocalycostomy or vesicocalycostomy can be accomplished. For complicated reconstructive procedures like these, or in the face of associated infection, externalized drains should be placed near the anastomosis and nephrostomy drainage instituted for postoperative diversion if a percutaneous nephrostomy tube had not been placed preoperatively.

More recently, percutaneous nephrostomy drainage has gained a role in the definitive management of transplant ureteral fistulas. The best candidates for definitive percutaneous management are those in whom antegrade studies suggest the extravasation is limited to the distal ureter and in whom contrast enters the bladder during antegrade pyelography. The presence of more proximal extravasation suggests extensive ureteral necrosis and sloughing, and therefore management by percutaneous techniques alone are unlikely to be successful. Similarly, failure of any contrast to enter the bladder on antegrade pyelography suggests complete disruption of the anastomosis, and, again, percutaneous treatment will not obviate the need for eventual open operative reconstruction.

For those patients in whom percutaneous management seems appropriate by these criteria, an attempt should be made to pass a floppy-tipped guidewire, and subsequently a stent, across the site of extravasation. Eventually, the patient should be left with either an internal/external stent placed to external drainage, or a nephrostomy tube and an internal stent. Once internal and external drainage is established and the patient is stabilized, serial radiographic studies are performed and percutaneous management is continued as long as the patient remains clinically stable and the fistula is resolving radiographically. If a urinoma is present, it is drained separately with a percutaneous catheter if it is infected, particularly large, or in any way symptomatic. Once the extravasation itself has resolved radiographically, external drainage with the nephrostomy tube or internal/external stent may be discontinued. However, we prefer to leave an internal stent indwelling for approximately 1 month following radiographic resolution. In some cases, apparently successful management of the ureteral fistula with percutaneous techniques results in ureteral stenosis as a late complication. Therefore, long-term monitoring of the anatomic and functional result is mandatory.

Calyceal Fistulas

Calyceal fistula of a renal allograft is a rare complication that almost always results from segmental renal infarction. Contemporary vascular techniques with "bench" repair of multiple vessels fortunately has relegated this problem to an extremely rare cause of urinary fistulas.

Historically, standard operative intervention consisted of open exploration with débridement and drainage, along with primary closure of the involved portion of the collecting system. However, such management was associated with high rates of graft loss and mortality. Eventually, improved results were obtained with operative placement of nephrostomy tubes and institution of external drainage. More recently, calyceal fistulas have been shown to resolve with externalized drainage alone. Currently, management of this rare complication should consist of placement of a percutaneous catheter at the site of extravasation. If there is any evidence of urinary obstruction, percutaneous nephrostomy drainage with or without internal stenting also should be instituted. With adequate drainage, most calyceal fistulas should resolve without the need for operative intervention.

Bladder Fistulas

Bladder fistulas most commonly arise from the anterior bladder suture line when transvesical ureteroneocystostomy is performed. In such cases, the diagnosis is made with a cystogram that reveals extravasation of contrast. If a catheter had not been indwelling at the time the complication became evident, a cautious trial of bladder catheter drainage alone can be instituted. Failure of catheter drainage to result in clinical and radiographic resolution should prompt open exploration with débridement and repair.

The recent widespread acceptance of an extravesical ureteroneocystostomy to restore urinary continuity has had the additional advantage of decreasing the incidence of bladder fistulas. In these patients, demonstration of contrast extravasation at the time of a cystogram is generally diagnostic of leakage at the ureteroneocystostomy. In such case, catheter drainage alone rarely will be successful. However, when the extravasation is limited to the distal ureter as defined by intravenous or antegrade pyelography, a trial of percutaneous management may be instituted following the guidelines outlined earlier regarding ureteral fistulas.

Suggested Readings

Bennett LN, Voegeli DR, Crummy AB, et al: Urologic complications following renal transplantation: Role of interventional radiologic procedures. Radiology 160: 531, 1986

Bretan PN Jr, Hodge E, Streem SB, et al: Diagnosis of renal transplant urinary fistulas. Transplant Proc 21: 1962, 1989

Campbell SC, Streem SB, Zelch M, et al: Percutaneous management of transplant ureteral fistulas: Patient selection and long-term results. J Urol 150:1115, 1993.

Leibermann RP, Glass NR, Crummy AB, et al: Nonoperative percutaneous management of urinary fistulas and strictures in renal transplantation. Surg Gynecol Obstet 155:667, 1982

Salvatierra O Jr, Olcott C IV, Amend WJ Jr, et al: Urological complications of renal transplantation can be prevented or controlled. J Urol 117:421, 1977

Schiff M Jr, McGuire EJ, Weiss RM, et al: Management of urinary fistulas after renal transplantation. J Urol 115: 251, 1976

Streem SB, Novick AC, Steinmuller DR, et al: Percutaneous techniques for the management of urologic renal transplant complications. J Urol 135:456, 1986

LYMPHOCELE FOLLOWING RENAL TRANSPLANTATION

MARK V. JAROWENKO, M.D.

Hershey, Pennsylvania

A lymphocele, or collection of lymphatic fluid, has been reported with variable frequency (1 to 50 per cent) following renal transplantation. These collections are frequently loculated and variable in size and location. The time of presentation may be the initial postoperative period or many years after transplantation.

Lymphocele formation is a consequence of severed, unligated lymphatics investing the recipient's iliac vessels or the hilum of the allograft. Investigators using lymphangiography and technetium-labeled sulfur colloid have demonstrated external iliac lymphatic communication with lymphoceles. Adequate lymphatic ligation is preferred to electrocautery, and extensive dissection of the allograft hilum should be avoided. Other suggested contributing etiologic factors include retransplantation, acute rejection (which has been shown experimentally to increase allograft lymph flow), anticoagulation, steroid administration, diuretic use, and allograft placement on the side of a lower extremity arteriovenous shunt.

Clinically, the lymphocele may be an asymptomatic collection identified by routine post-transplant ultrasonography or may present with a variety of signs and symptoms. Hydronephrosis, oliguria, a rising serum creatinine level, lower extremity edema (unilateral or bilateral), fever, abdominal discomfort, abdominal mass, cutaneous fistula, voiding symptoms, deep venous thrombosis, and venous compression (including inferior vena cava and portal vein compression with pulmonary embolus) have been reported. Most lymphoceles are asymptomatic and found incidentally.

The diagnosis of a clinically significant post-transplant lymphocele is made by ultrasound-guided needle aspiration. This does not require a specific level of renal function and allows exclusion of other collections such as abscess, seroma, hematoma, and urinoma.

The management of a post-transplant lymphocele depends on its symptoms and complications. Small, incidentally discovered lymphoceles require no treatment. Infected lymphoceles require external drainage either by percutaneous or open surgical techniques with drain placement. Lymphocutaneous fistulas generally may be expected to close spontaneously after several weeks of sterile dressing changes.

A number of therapeutic options exist for the large uninfected symptomatic lymphocele. Needle aspiration alone is associated with an unacceptable recurrence rate (up to 100 per cent). Aspiration combined with sclerosant instillation (ampicillin, tetracycline, povidone-iodine) has been used with variable success, and it is more likely to work for smaller collections. External drainage catheters may introduce infection or induce hemorrhage and the lymphocele may persistently drain. Until recently the therapy of choice was transabdominal exploration with internal transperitoneal drainage of the lymphocele via marsupialization of the lymphocele into the peritoneum, preferably with placement of an omental pedicle or tongue to prevent closure of the opening into the peritoneal cavity. This allows lymph flow from the lymphocele into the peritoneum, where it is absorbed. This method is effective but requires 3 to 5 days of hospitalization and the morbidity and discomfort of an open surgical procedure.

Laparoscopic lymphocele marsupialization can be accomplished, achieving internal lymphocele drainage with minimal morbidity and hospitalization. Omental fixation also has been performed laparoscopically. This approach avoids a large incision and prolonged hospitalization and is applicable to most lymphoceles.

Suggested Readings

Bry J, Hull D, Bartus SA, et al: Treatment of recurrent lymphoceles following renal transplantation: Remarsupialization with omentoplasty. Transplantation 49: 477, 1990

Khauli RB, Rosenthal AC, Caushalt PF: Treatment of lymphocele and lymphatic fistula following renal transplantation by laparoscopic peritoneal window. J Urol 147:1353, 1992

McCullough CS, Soper NJ: Laparoscopic drainage of a post-transplant lymphocele. Transplantation 51:725, 1991

Pollak R, Veremis SA, Maddux MS, et al: The natural history of and therapy for perirenal fluid collections following renal transplantation. J Urol 140:716, 1988

PERCUTANEOUS TRANSLUMINAL ANGIOPLASTY AND RENOVASCULAR HYPERTENSION

JOHN A. LIBERTINO, M.D.

Boston, Massachusetts

Since Dotter and Jedkins introduced the procedure of percutaneous transluminal angioplasty in 1964 and the subsequent development by Grüntzig of a modified technique enabling renal angioplasty in 1978, there has been considerable interest in the application of this procedure in patients with renal artery disease. Percutaneous transluminal angioplasty now has been used widely to treat patients with renovascular hypertension.

The technique used for percutaneous transluminal angioplasty of the renal artery was reported by Tegtmeyer and Sos. The preferred route is through the femoral artery. The balloon diameter chosen is equal to the original diameter of the vessel. The vessel is seen on the preliminary aortogram without correcting for magnification. Therefore, stenotic lesions generally are overdilated by 20 to 30 per cent.

Percutaneous transluminal angioplasty has been shown to cause cracking of the intima, atherosclerotic placques, and tunica media in the renal artery. Fragmentation of the internal elastic membrane and of the elastic lamella and the media occurs. Dotter and Jedkins' original description of the dysplacement and redistribution of atheromatous material into cracks of the renal artery wall has been disputed by most investigators.

In the patients with atherosclerotic renal artery stenosis who underwent transluminal renal angioplasty, the technical success rate ranges from 67 to 100 per cent depending on the investigator and the selection criteria used. The mean duration of follow-up after angioplasty ranged from 11 to 26 months. Of 360 patients, hypertension was cured by angioplasty in only 68 (19 per cent). These patients did not require any medication to maintain the diastolic pressure below 90 mm Hg. The blood pressure was improved in 51 per cent. One third of all patients did not receive any benefit from transluminal angioplasty.

Several factors influence the success of transluminal angioplasty. The technical success rate is markedly diminished in patients with atheromatous disease who present with an occluded renal artery or stenosis of the ostium of the renal artery at the aortic wall. In these patients, the reported technical success rate is only 25 per cent, compared with 75 per cent in patients with a nonostial and nonoccluded atheromatous lesions.

It also has been demonstrated that patients with unilateral disease had better long-term results than those with bilateral involvement. In patients with renovascular hypertension and azotemia, a clinical and technical success was reported in only 47 per cent. The influence of the age of the patient on the degree of technical success is indicated by the fact that, in patients over the age 60 with severe generalized disease, the technical success rate was only 67 per cent in comparison to 100 per cent in patients who were younger than 60 years of age.

In patients with fibromuscular disease, the technical and success rates average between 90 and 100 per cent. In terms of clinical success, 46 per cent of patients are cured and 45 per cent improved, a markedly higher success rate than in patients with atheromatous disease who undergo angioplasty. This degree of success in patients with mural dysplasia is comparable to the results achieved in patients who undergo surgical revascularization. Percutaneous transluminal angioplasty in patients with focally stenotic true fibromuscular hyperplasia appears to be only slightly less successful both technically and clinically (85 per cent) than in patients with the more common medial fibroplasia.

In a literature review encompassing 691 renal angioplasty procedures, complications were reported in 63 (9.1 per cent). There were three fatalities resulting from cholesterol embolism, bowel infarction, and cerebral hemorrhage. The most frequently reported complications were renal artery dissection (2 per cent), renal artery thrombosis or occlusion (1.5 per cent), segmental renal infarction (1 per cent), and hematoma formation (1 per cent). Additional complications included cerebrovascular accident and myocardial infarction.

Suggested Readings

Archambault GR, Beckmann CF, Libertino JA: Focal renal artery stenosis caused by fibromuscular dysplasia: Treatment by percutaneous transluminal angioplasty. Am J Radiol 151:593, 1988

Brawn LA, Ramsay LE: Is improvement "real" with percutaneous transluminal angioplasty in the management of renovascular hypertension? Lancet 2:1313, 1987

Dotter CT, Jedkins MP: Transluminal treatment of atherosclerotic obstruction: Description of a new technique and a preliminary report of its applications. Circulation 30:654, 1964

Gruntzig A, Kuhlmann U, Vetteor W, et al: Treatment of renovascular hypertension with percutaneous transluminal dilatation of a renal artery stenosis. Lancet 1:801, 1978

Tegtmeyer CJ, Sos TA: Techniques of renal angioplasty. Radiology 161:577, 1986

SURGERY FOR RENOVASCULAR HYPERTENSION

JOHN A. LIBERTINO, M.D.

Boston, Massachusetts

The diagnosis and treatment of patients with renovascular hypertension have changed dramatically in the last decade. Some of the newer diagnostic modalities available include digital subtraction angiography and isotopic scans of the kidney after administration of captopril. These tests provide greater sensitivity and specificity than older screening studies and are less invasive. Balloon angioplasty, alternative bypass procedures, and other newer surgical modalities have changed many of the management concepts that once were held in the treatment of patients with renovascular hypertension. The newer diagnostic and therapeutic modalities have altered the nature of the patient population referred for renal artery reconstruction. Balloon angioplasty successfully treats many of the younger, healthier patients with mural dysplasia, leaving many of the older patients with diffuse atherosclerotic disease, azotemia, uncontrollable hypertension, and coronary artery and cerebrovascular disease for surgical reconstruction.

DIAGNOSIS

The presence of renal artery stenosis in a patient with hypertension does not establish the diagnosis of renovascular hypertension. Functional tests—that is, divided renal vein renin assays and captopril isotopic scans—must be performed to determine whether the stenosis is the cause of the patient's hypertension. Frequently, these studies follow digital subtraction angiography, which is the primary screening test performed to unmask renal artery stenosis. The indication to proceed with formal standard renal angiography is the need to assess the segmental blood supply in patients who have mural disease, because the distal renal circulation is not well visualized with intravenous digital subtraction angiography.

The true prevalence of renovascular hypertension in unselected patients with hypertension is unknown. This aspect of renovascular disease is covered in another section of this textbook. In the Lahey Clinic experience, renovascular hypertension, on the basis of renal artery stenosis, is not a rare entity and should be searched for in patients with the appropriate clinical presentation.

In the Lahey Clinic experience with more than 500 patients who have undergone surgical procedures for renovascular hypertension, we believe any patient, particularly a young one who has severe or acute hypertension of short duration or who has sudden acceleration of a chronically elevated blood pressure, should be evaluated for renovascular hypertension. This entity also should be suspected in patients in whom hypertension develops after the onset of acute flank pain, in patients who have progressive symptomatic hypertension in the absence of primary renal disease, and in patients who have no familial history of hypertension. Other subsets of patients who should be studied for renovascular hypertension are patients in whom hypertension is not adequately controlled with antihypertensive drugs and patients in whom azotemia develops after administration of angiotensin-converting enzyme inhibitors.

From an etiologic point of view, atherosclerosis accounts for two thirds of the intrinsic lesions of the renal artery and mural dysplasia accounts for the other one third. Extrinsic causes, such as dissecting aortic aneurysm, traumatic injury to the renal pedicle, and tumor that compresses the renal artery, are uncommon. Atherosclerosis affects the left main stem renal artery more commonly than the right artery, although these lesions may be bilateral in 30 to 40 per cent of patients. Atherosclerosis is more common in men than in women, and the mean age of patients at presentation is 55 years. In contrast, mural dysplasia is more common in women, and, when the disease is unilateral, the right renal artery is affected more often than the left artery. The mean age of patients at presentation with mural dysplasia is 35 years.

In digital subtraction angiography, a noninvasive procedure, contrast material is injected through a peripheral vein as it is for excretory urography. Complementary arteriography and excretory urography can be carried out with the same injection. This method has become Lahey Clinic's screening procedure of choice. Intra-arterial digital subtraction angiography also can be performed when looking at the segmental arterial blood supply of the kidney. At the time of angiography, oblique views are obtained in addition to the anterior and posterior views to evaluate the aorta and alternate sources of arterial inflow, such as the hypogastric, splenic, and hepatic arteries. Angiography permits precise localization of the lesion, accurate determination of the nature and degree of stenosis, and assessment of the extent of cortical atrophy and renal scarring.

TREATMENT OPTIONS

After the diagnosis of renovascular hypertension secondary to a functionally significant renal artery stenosis is made, several treatment options are available. Therapeutic modalities range from antihypertensive drugs to percutaneous transluminal renal angioplasty and surgical reconstruction. In 70 per cent of the patients who are referred for surgical reconstruction, hypertension is refractory to antihypertensive medication despite multiple drug therapy. Uncontrollable hypertension despite aggressive appropriate antihypertensive medication is an indication for either balloon angioplasty or surgical treatment.

We have had favorable results with balloon angioplasty in treating patients with mural dysplasia. We now use balloon angioplasty as the procedure of choice in the treatment of patients with renovascular hypertension secondary to mural dysplasia. In patients in whom recurrent disease develops or in whom the lesion is not capable of dilation, renal artery reconstruction is necessary. Our interventional radiologists believe that the complications attending redilation indicate the need for renovascular surgery, and we concur. Conversely, the poor results that are associated with balloon dilation in the atherosclerotic lesions have led us to abandon this procedure as a viable treatment option in patients with atherosclerotic disease. However, occasional instances of a short isolated middle main renal artery atherosclerotic lesion may respond to balloon angioplasty.

Patients with a functionally significant renovascular lesion are candidates for surgical intervention under the following circumstances: poor control of hypertension after aggressive appropriate drug therapy, poor patient compliance, total renal artery occlusion or dissection, deterioration of renal function as manifested by an elevation of either the blood urea nitrogen or creatinine level, excretory urographic evidence of renal parenchymal loss, angiographic evidence of progressive renal artery disease, severely symptomatic or accelerated hypertension, anuria from arterial occlusion in a solitary kidney, or any combination of these factors.

From a surgical point of view, the aortorenal bypass procedure was the universally preferred operation. With the change in the nature of the patient population, however, alternative bypass procedures have emerged as the preferred procedure in patients with diffuse atherosclerotic disease. For a difficult or heavily atherosclerotic aorta, splenorenal bypass or hepatic-to-renal artery bypass is preferable. These alternative bypass procedures have reduced dramatically the number of complications associated with clamping a diseased aorta. With left-sided lesions and a difficult aorta, we prefer to carry out splenorenal bypass, usually through a supracostal 11th rib flank approach. With right-sided lesions and a troublesome aorta, we prefer to use the hepatic-to-renal saphenous vein bypass graft.

Renal autotransplantation has become a popular procedure for renal revascularization. Under unusual circumstances, workbench surgery and autotransplantation are indicated, especially in patients who have mural dysplasia extending into the segmental vessels or associated with aneurysms. However, I must emphasize that the indications for autotransplantation should not be overzealously extended or abused when acceptable forms of in situ surgery can be accomplished with less hazard and with equally good or better results.

PROGNOSIS

Over the past two decades, we have treated more than 500 patients who required surgical procedures for renovascular hypertension. Of the patients with mural dysplasia, 85 per cent are satisfactorily cured or improved after percutaneous balloon angioplasty. In high-risk patients with atherosclerosis, 50 per cent are cured by operation, 45 per cent are improved, and 5 per cent fail to show any beneficial blood pressure response after reconstructive surgery. In more than 100 patients who underwent bypass surgery because of deteriorating renal function, 85 per cent had stabilization of or improvement in renal function after renal revascularization. The preoperative serum creatinine level was not a predictor of whether the patient would achieve improvement or stabilization of renal function.

Suggested Readings

Libertino JA: Renovascular surgery. *In* Walsh PC, Retik AB, Stamey TA, et al (eds): Campbell's Urology, 6th ed. Philadelphia, WB Saunders, 1992, pp 2521–2551

Libertino JA, Selman FJ: Alternatives to aortorenal revascularization. J Cardiovasc Surg 23:318, 1982

Libertino JA, Zinman L: Surgery for renovascular hypertension. *In* Libertino JA (ed): Pediatric and Adult Reconstructive Urologic Surgery, 2nd ed. Baltimore, Williams & Wilkins, 1987, pp 119–161

Libertino JA, Zinman L, Breslin DJ, et al: Hepatorenal artery bypass in the management of renovascular hypertension. J Urol 115:369, 1976

Libertino JA, Zinman L, Breslin DJ, et al: Renal artery revascularization: Restoration of renal function. JAMA 244:1340, 1980

PERCUTANEOUS TRANSLUMINAL ANGIOPLASTY FOR TREATMENT OF RENAL TRANSPLANT ARTERY STENOSIS

JOHN A. LIBERTINO, M.D.

Boston, Massachusetts

Nearly 10 per cent of renal allograft recipients may develop renal artery stenosis. This frequently causes hypertension that is unresponsive to medical therapy and also may decrease renal function. Renal transplant artery stenosis (RTAS) either involves the anastomosis itself or consists of a tubular narrowing at a site distinctly distal to the anastomosis. In most previous reports, surgical treatment of RTAS has been successful in about 60 per cent of patients; however, the operation has been associated with a 15 per cent graft loss rate, a 13 per cent reoperation rate, and a 5 per cent mortality rate.

A simpler method of treating RTAS, percutaneous transluminal angioplasty, was greeted enthusiastically by surgeons and radiologists alike. The angiographic catheter is advanced across the stenosis and a dilating balloon catheter then is substituted by passing it over a rigid guidewire. Polyethylene balloons of 5 to 6 mm proved to be the most satisfactory. To evaluate the immediate results, postdilation angiograms are obtained.

Lohr et al. reviewed the literature on percutaneous transluminal angioplasty in transplant renal artery stenosis. Of 90 patients, 76 (84 per cent) were successfully treated by transluminal angioplasty; there were only two patients with recurring stenosis and only one with graft loss. When these results were compared with those of vascular surgical repair, they found a successful outcome in 130 of 180 postsurgical patients (72 per cent). Graft loss occurred in 20 patients (11 per cent) and recurrent stenosis in 11 patients (6 per cent). It can be concluded that transluminal angioplasty should be the initial treatment of choice in patients with RTAS. The beneficial effects of percutaneous transluminal angioplasty on blood pressure appear to be maintained during follow-up, with corresponding improvements in serum creatinine values.

Suggested Reading

Lohr JW, MacDougall ML, Chonko AM, et al: Percutaneous transluminal angioplasty in transplant renal artery stenosis: Experience and review of the literature. Am J Kidney Dis 7:363, 1986

SECTION 3

THE URETER

Congenital Disorders

CONGENITAL URETERAL ABNORMALITIES

T. ERNESTO FIGUEROA, M.D.
Tampa, Florida

Developmental abnormalities of the ureter encompass a wide range of disorders that may vary from totally asymptomatic conditions of radiographic interest only to severe conditions that compromise renal function. Consequently, clinically relevant disorders present with either obstructive lesions or lesions associated with urinary tract infection. Other conditions—for example, ureteral duplications—are considered variations of normal when not affected by either obstruction or urinary tract infections. Furthermore, congenital ureteral disorders may be subdivided into categories according to the location of the abnormality. Bauer et al. have outlined a comprehensive classification of all possible abnormalities of the ureter, according to number, structure, termination, and position. For the sake of brevity, only the more common abnormalities are reviewed in this chapter.

EMBRYOLOGY

A clear understanding of the embryology is essential to appreciate the different disorders related to the ureter. The ureteral bud, the early precursor of the ureter, can be identified as an evagination of the mesonephric duct by the 28th day of gestation. This bud elongates and reaches the metanephric blastema cranially, stimulating the formation of the kidney. Caudally, the mesonephric duct is incorporated into the cloaca, allowing the ureteral bud to form part of the developing trigone. The ureter is initially tortuous, and, according to sophisticated histologic analyses, sections of the fetal ureter vary between solid and patent. These findings have been used to explain the origin of ureteral strictures and valves.

Duplications of the ureters have a well-outlined developmental process. In cases of complete duplications, two separate ureteral buds are incorporated into the bladder. The more distal bud, corresponding to the lower pole of the kidney, enters the bladder first and moves cranially and laterally. The more proximal bud, draining the renal upper pole, migrates caudally and medially in the bladder. This sequence of events, known as the Weigert-Meyer law, is highly predictable, with few exceptions having been documented. This pattern explains why lower pole ureters are associated with reflux (lateral and cranial), whereas upper pole ureters usually are obstructed and ectopic (distal and medial).

The location of origin of the ureteral bud on the mesonephric duct also affects the development of the ureter. Early entrance of the bud into the fetal bladder produces a more lateral ureteral orifice, predisposing this unit to reflux. This is seen when the bud arises in the most caudad portion of the mesonephric duct. Similarly, a cranial origin may produce an ectopic ureter. Furthermore, Stephens has theorized that there is an optimal location for the ureteral bud, resulting in normal induction of the renal blastema. Abnormal locations of the bud lead to suboptimal blastemal induction and, possibly, to renal developmental abnormalities.

COMMON ABNORMALITIES

Vesicoureteral Reflux

Vesicoureteral reflux (VUR) is a common disorder, estimated to occur in approximately 1 per cent of all healthy children. When urinary tract infections are the reason for investigation, up to 50 per cent of these children will be found to have refluxing ureters. VUR is divided into primary, or congenital, reflux, and secondary, or acquired, reflux. Common causes of secondary reflux include posterior urethral valves and neurogenic bladder.

Primary VUR results from an inadequate submucosal tunnel. This shortened length prevents an efficient flap-valve mechanism. As mentioned previously, a caudad ureteral bud arising from the mesonephric duct and entering the bladder "early" accounts for this abnormality.

Primary VUR is classified according to severity; grading of the reflux is based on the radiographic appearance during the cystogram. The International Classification divides reflux into five grades, Grade I being minimal reflux and Grade V being the most severe. This classification is also helpful as a prognostic indicator, because approximately 80 per cent of cases of Grades I through III will resolve with time, whereas only 40 to 50 per cent of cases of Grades IV and V will eventually disappear. The more severe grades of reflux typically exhibit a shortened ureteral submucosal tunnel and lateral implantation into the bladder wall.

The most important aspect of VUR is its association with urinary tract infections. The exact reason for this association is not clear, although urinary stasis and turbulent flow within the ureter are believed to predispose a refluxing system to infections. The combination of reflux and infections is potentially problematic because of the injurious effects on the kidney. The growing kidney is particularly susceptible to these infections, or pyelonephritis, leading to the formation of renal scars or parenchymal damage. Progressive damage can lead to loss of renal function and renal failure.

The management of VUR is one of the most controversial in urology. The goal of all forms of treatment is to protect the kidney from infections. The medical approach is offered initially to all patients. This consists of antibiotic suppression, or the administration of an antibiotic that has high urinary levels at a fraction of the usual therapeutic dose. The most common agents are trimethoprim-sulfamethoxazole and nitrofurantoin, because of their minimal effects on the gastrointestinal bacterial flora. The patient is maintained on this suppressive protocol until the disappearance of reflux has been demonstrated by cystography, a process that may take 4 to 8 years in some cases. Repeated urine cultures are necessary to detect possible asymptomatic bacteriuria.

Surgical therapy is considered only when the medical approach has failed. Breakthrough urinary tract infections are the strongest indications to proceed with ureteral reimplantation. Additionally, poor family compliance with the medical protocol, or unwillingness to carry out long-term antimicrobial suppression, also encourages surgical repair. Finally, high-grade reflux in a solitary kidney may be managed best surgically.

The goal of ureteral reimplantation is recreation of a submucosal tunnel of adequate length. This length has been shown to be four to five times the diameter of the ureter (4:1 ratio). The most common techniques are those of intravesical advancement (Cohen, Glenn-Anderson), creation of a new hiatus (Politano-Leadbetter), or extravesical reimplantation (Lich-Gregoire, Zaonts). Most reimplantations are highly successful, with rates of 95 to 99 per cent being common. However, these operations are highly technical, and the grade of reflux and ureteral dilation, plus the surgeon's experience, affect the outcome. Delicate handling and mobilization of the ureters are mandatory to avoid possible complications. Known complications include persistent reflux, ureteral obstruction, and ureteral fistula.

Megaureters

Megaureters are broadly classified into primary and secondary based on either intrinsic or extrinsic causes for their appearance. As in VUR, common causes of secondary megaureters include bladder neck obstruction, neurogenic bladder, or previous surgery. Their management is directed at the correction of the abnormal lower urinary tract.

Primary megaureters are subdivided into four categories: obstructed, refluxing, nonobstructed-nonrefluxing, and obstructed-refluxing. Obstructed lesions, as determined by intravenous pyelography and nuclear renography, always are corrected surgically by various techniques of ureteral reimplantation. Similarly, refluxing megaureters present minimal likelihood of resolution, for which reimplantation usually is needed. Nonrefluxing-nonobstructed megaureters are mostly of radiographic interest, although some of these eventually may become obstructed and require surgical intervention.

The timing of surgical reconstruction is controversial. Although some have argued that neonatal relief of the obstructed megaureter is necessary, a ureteral reimplantation in a neonate is a procedure of great magnitude and demanding of solid surgical skills. Alternative temporizing approaches to the neonate with an obstructed megaureter and documented compromise of renal function include a terminal or end-ureterostomy or a percutaneous nephrostomy tube. In neonates with bilateral refluxing megaureters, a cutaneous vesicostomy may be used as a temporizing maneuver.

Once the decision to reimplant the ureter is made, the need for ureteral tailoring is determined based on the diameter of the ureter. Minimal degrees of dilation usually do not require tailoring as long as a satisfactory tunnel (4:1 ratio) can be created. Ureteral tailoring may be excisional or nonexcisional. Proponents of the excisional method claim that the narrower ureter can be reimplanted more easily than the bulkier plicated or imbricated megaureter. Concerns of vasculature compromise and ureteral fistulization are voiced by those who oppose excisional tapering. Parrott and Woodard have demonstrated similar results utilizing both techniques.

Ureteroceles

Ureterocele is a cystic dilation of the terminal or infradetrusor portion of the ureter. The exact etiology of ureteroceles is not known, although an obstruction of the ureteral meatus appears as an attractive explanation. Ureteroceles are classified as either orthotopic or ectopic, depending on the location of the ureteral meatus. Ectopic ureteroceles are associated with ureteral duplications, and, more specifically, with the upper pole moiety.

In the past, most ureteroceles were discovered during the evaluation of a child with urinary tract infections. With the advent of fetal sonography, more cases are being detected in utero, typically recognized by the presence of a dilated ureter and the intravesical "cyst." Once a ureterocele is detected, or its presence suspected, the function of the affected kidney, particularly the upper pole, must be determined. Nuclear renography is the best tool to image the upper urinary tract in cases of ureteroceles. A voiding cystourethrogram should be performed utilizing diluted contrast so that the ureterocele is not masked by the density of the contrast. Finally, in dubious cases, an intravenous pyelogram often demonstrates a large filling defect in the bladder, confirming the presence of a ureterocele.

The management of ureteroceles is dictated by four factors: (1) presence of urinary infections, (2) single versus duplicated systems, (3) function of the affected renal segment, and (4) presence of ipsilateral or contralateral reflux. Patients with infections in an obstructed system should be stabilized rapidly and surgical decompression should be done either by transurethral unroofing of the ureterocele or placement of a percutaneous nephrostomy tube. In the nonemergent case, the management of the ureterocele is subject to much debate. Alternative surgical procedures include extravesical approaches (nephrectomy, upper pole nephrectomy, ipsilateral ureteroureterostomy) and intravesical maneuvers (transurethral incision, ureterocele excision, and ureteral reimplantation). The selection of any of these approaches is dictated, again, by the factors previously outlined. Extravesical approaches avoid the immediate dissection of the ureterocele, which often may be extremely challenging. Ureteroceles may produce a significant deformity of the bladder and bladder neck by displacement of the normal detrusor. Reconstruction of the bladder, and possibly bladder neck, may be necessary at the time of reimplantation. Extravesical procedures, however, ultimately require a subsequent intravesical procedure in 25 to 30 per cent of cases. Proponents of surgical incision cite the ease of this procedure in decompressing the ureterocele. However, vesicoureteral reflux may arise in 40 to 100 per cent of these incised ureteroceles, necessitating a subsequent ureteral reimplantation.

RARE DISORDERS

Ureteral Ectopia

Ectopic ureters occur when the ureteral bud arises cranially on the mesonephric duct. Because of the embryologic path, the ureters may terminate at the bladder neck, prostate, seminal vesicle, or vas in the male, and bladder neck, urethra, vestibule, vagina, or uterus in the female. This difference in location of the ectopic ureter is critical in understanding the symptoms that may occur. Males may present with ureteral obstruction, whereas females may present with constant urinary incontinence. Treatment depends on the function of the involved upper pole. If adequate function is demonstrated, an ipsilateral ureteroureterostomy should be performed. When no function is present, an upper pole nephroureterectomy is curative.

Retrocaval Ureter

A retrocaval ureter is an abnormality of the venous system, produced by a persistence of the cardinal veins of the fetus. The presentation is usually secondary to pain, with hydronephrosis and medial displacement of the lumbar ureter. A retrograde pyelogram is useful in confirming this abnormality. When indicated, treatment consists of ureteroureterostomy.

Ureteral Valves

These are extremely rare causes of hydronephrosis. Persistent folds or lack of canalization of the fetal ureter may produce ureteral valves. Valves often mimic ureteropelvic junction (UPJ) obstructions. Oftentimes, at exploration, the UPJ is found to be dilated secondary to a more distal ureteral valve. Treatment consists of resection of the affected portion of the ureter and ureteroureterostomy.

Ureteral Strictures

Intrinsic ureteral strictures are most common at the UPJ and at the ureterovesical junction. These strictures produce the common UPJ obstruction and the obstructed megaureter. Other ureteral strictures are exceedingly rare.

Suggested Readings

Bauer SB, Ketik AB, Perlmutter AD: Anomalies of the upper urinary tract. *In* Walsh PC, Retik AB, Stamey TA, et al (eds): Campbell's Urology, 6th ed. Philadelphia, WB Saunders, 1992, pp 1357–1442

Decter RM, Roth DR, Gonzalez ET: Individualized treatment of ureteroceles. J Urol 142:535, 1989

Gonzalez ET: Reconstruction of anomalies of the distal ureter and ureterovesical junction. *In* Wesbster G, Kirby R, King R, et al (eds): Reconstructive Urology. Boston, Blackwell Scientific Publications, 1993, pp 361–388

Kass EJ: Megaureter. *In* Kelalis PP, King L, Belmon AB (eds): Clinical Pediatric Urology, 3rd ed. Philadelphia, WB Saunders, 1992, pp 781–820

ADVANCES IN URETERAL SURGERY

LOUIS R. KAVOUSSI, M.D.

Baltimore, Maryland

Ureteral pathology traditionally has been approached through open surgical intervention. With recent advances in endoscopic techniques, many disease entities once managed by incisional surgery now can be treated successfully with less morbidity. Moreover, the advent of operative laparoscopic techniques has provided surgeons with an even wider array of minimally invasive approaches to ureteral pathology.

ENDOPYELOTOMY

Open surgical treatment of ureteropelvic junction obstruction has been very successful. Traditional pyeloplasty, however, has several drawbacks, including significant postoperative pain, prolonged convalescence, and a prominent skin incision. In an effort to decrease postoperative morbidity, several authors have advocated endopyelotomy as an alternative to open pyeloplasty for both primary and secondary obstruction. Endoscopic incision is usually accomplished by an antegrade approach via a percutaneous nephrostomy through a middle pole calix. Alternatively, a retrograde incision can be attempted using a ureteroscope. The advantage of the ureteroscopic incision is that the patient avoids the discomforts and risks of a percutaneous nephrostomy. However, visualization and manipulation of the cutting element to incise the ureteropelvic junction is much more difficult compared with an antegrade approach. There is no difference in success rate between an antegrade and a retrograde approach.

Karlin and associates compared the postoperative course of patients treated by open pyeloplasty or endopyelotomy. Adult patients undergoing dismembered pyeloplasty required an average postoperative stay of 10 days, compared to 6.2 days for those undergoing endopyelotomy. Moreover, complete convalescence took 41 days following open pyeloplasty, compared to 19 days with endopyelotomy. Finally, there was a 30 per cent decrease in pain medication requirement in the endopyelotomy group.

Unfortunately, there are several shortcomings associated with endopyelotomy. The success rates reported with endopyelotomy (72 to 89 per cent) are lower when compared with open pyeloplasty. Stenting can be required for up to 6 weeks, and some patients may find the stent uncomfortable. Finally, endopyelotomy commits patients to a secondary procedure for stent removal.

CUTTING BALLOON CATHETER

More recently, investigators have been studying the use of a dilating balloon/cutting catheter for treating ureteropelvic junction obstruction and ureteral strictures. The Acucise catheter (Applied Urology, Inc., Laguna Hills, Ca.) is a dilating balloon that has a surgical wire electrode running longitudinally along the outside of the balloon. Under intravenous sedation, a guidewire is passed up into the renal pelvis. The cutting balloon catheter is passed over the guidewire and positioned such that the balloon straddles the area of obstruction. The cutting wire is positioned by rotating the catheter until the wire is located in the posterior position. The balloon is slowly inflated and, as the stricture waste is noted, electrocautery is applied to the cutting electrode to incise the area of obstruction. Once the waste is completely gone from the balloon, adequacy of incision is assessed by injecting contrast and noting extravasation. Following this, an indwelling ureteral stent is advanced over the guidewire.

The initial reports with the Acucise balloon catheter demonstrate success rates similar to those seen with visual endopyelotomy. The advantage with this procedure is that it can be done under intravenous sedation on an outpatient basis, with the average operative time being less than 45 minutes.

ENDOSCOPY FOR URETERAL STRICTURES

Ureteral strictures as long as 5 cm have been treated successfully with endoscopic incision. A cold knife incision with a rigid ureteroscope can be performed for distal ureteral strictures. With these strictures, the goal is to marsupialize the stricture into the bladder. Mid-ureteral strictures are the most difficult type of stricture to approach. The rigid ureteroscope is utilized if the stricture is below the level of the iliac vessels; the flexible ureteroscope is preferred when strictures are above this level. When utilizing a flexible endoscope, an electrocautery or laser fiber can be used to incise the stricture. For proximal ureteral strictures, the goal is to marsupialize the ureter into the renal pelvis. A posterior and lateral incision therefore is made routinely. When approaching completely obstructing strictures or upper ureteral strictures, combining an antegrade and a retrograde approach may be necessary.

The Acucise cutting balloon catheter also can be used to treat ureteral strictures. Care must be taken when incising strictures over the iliac vessel. Cases have been reported of the incision extending into the iliac vessels, leading to significant hemorrhage.

For total ureteral occlusion, a "cut to light" procedure may be necessary. A flexible antegrade nephroureteroscope is passed down to the level of the stricture while performing simultaneous ureteroscopy. The light from the antegrade endoscope then is disconnected and the light from the ureteroscope is sought. The end of a stiff guidewire can be used to perforate the stricture toward the light. Alternatively, a direct cold knife or electrocautery incision can be made. An exchange wire then is passed to establish through-and-through access. An incision is made finally leaving a 7/14F stent in place with the 14F portion traversing the site of stricture.

The results of endoscopic incision of ureteral strictures are promising, with success rates of 57 to 82 per cent noted. The success of the procedure is dependent on stricture length, density, etiology, and prior surgery. Success rates are much lower with long or completely obstructing strictures. Likewise, patients with a prior history of radical surgery, radiation, or ischemic injury are less likely to respond to endoscopic incision.

The flexible actively deflectable ureteronephroscope also has been used via a percutaneous tract to incise ureteroenteric anastomotic strictures. Meretyk and associates reported on 19 strictures in 15 patients and had an overall patency rate of 64 per cent with follow-up of 9 to 54 months. It was necessary to leave a permanent external stent in five strictures because of metastatic disease. Only one patient in the study required subsequent open surgical correction.

EXPANDABLE METAL STENTS

In an effort to avoid an open operative procedure in patients who have failed primary endoscopic management, some centers have begun utilizing expandable metal prostatic stents. Lugmayr and associates used stents in two patients with obstruction resulting from malignancy. In both patients, continued tumor growth and encrustation resulted in recurrent obstruction at 6 months. Locke and associates reported on placing stents in five patients with ureteroileal anastomotic strictures. At mean follow-up of 12 months, all stents were patent; however, patients developed recurrent episodes of symptomatic bacteriuria. Gonzales and associates treated four patients with ureteroenteric strictures, with mean follow-up of 5 months. All patients have maintained normal kidney function and continued ureteral patency.

BLADDER UROTHELIAL GRAFT

Clayman and Denstedt reported on four patients with distal ureteral strictures greater than 5 cm in whom a free graft of bladder urothelium was placed in the bed of the incised stricture. With follow-up of greater than 1 year, all ureters are patent. Unfortunately, data are lacking to demonstrate that the graft tissue actually was incorporated into the ureter.

LAPAROSCOPIC TECHNIQUES

Modern endourologic techniques have obviated the need for open surgical removal of ureteral calculi in the vast majority of cases. However, there are instances in which ureteroscopy or lithotripsy are not successful in treating ureteral stones, and open ureterolithotomy may be necessary. Recently, there have been reports out of several centers on laparoscopic ureterolithotomy. Utilizing three to four trocar sites, the hydronephrotic ureter usually can be identified and followed down to the level of the calculus. A longitudinal incision is made under direct vision and the stone removed. The ureteral wall then can be approximated loosely. With limited follow-up, these patients have had markedly decreased morbidity when compared with those treated with open techniques.

In an effort to obtain both the advantages of a high success of an open dismembered pyeloplasty and the decreased morbidity of endoscopic techniques, investigators have reported on laparoscopic pyeloplasty. Using three or four laparoscopic ports, the colon can be reflected and the ureteropelvic junction identified. Both blunt and sharp dissection are used to free the ureter and then the scarred segment can be excised. The ureter can then be spatulated and reapproximated to the pelvis with interrupted 4-0 or 5-0 Vicryl sutures. The initial results with these have been promising; however, long-term data will be necessary to assess the true efficacy.

Laparoscopy also has been used to treat retroperitoneal fibrosis. We have had experience in four patients who presented with unilateral ureteral obstruction. After reflecting the colon medially, the ureter can be identified where it is not involved by the fibrotic process. The magnification afforded by laparoscopy allows one to dissect the ureter carefully from the surrounding tissue. Once the ureter is completely free, it can be placed in an intraperitoneal position by using a hernia stapler to tack the colon behind the ureter. In three out of four patients with a mean follow-up of 1½ years, there has been no evidence of obstruction; one patient developed recurrent obstruction as a result of an occult carcinoma. It is very important to obtain multiple biopsies during laparoscopic ureterolysis to be sure that the presence of malignancy is excluded.

Nezhat and associates have reported on successive primarily endoscopic repair of ureteral transection during laparoscopy. Endoscopically, a catheter can be passed to bridge the area of injury, which is then reapproximated with sutures.

ENDOSCOPIC TUMOR TREATMENT

Endosurgical approaches to upper tract transitional cell carcinomas have been utilized. Small ureteral tumors may be biopsied or fulgurated with a ureteroscope. Some models of rigid endoscopes allow a small elecrocautery loop to be utilized to resect tumors and obtain muscle for staging. Through a flexible ureteroscope, a 2F electrode or 400-μ laser fiber may be used to ablate tumors. It should be noted that it may be difficult to obliterate the proximal end of a tumor with the ureteroscope.

In selected cases, an antegrade percutaneous method for resecting low-grade ureteral tumors may be utilized. Independent reports by Guiness and Meretyk have shown that thiotepa can be injected via a retrograde catheter just prior to creation of a nephrostomy tract to minimize the risk of tract seeding.

The initial experience in approaching ureteral tumors is favorable. The recurrence rate at 2 years for ureteral tumors treated endoscopically is 15 per cent, with progression to open ablative surgery 13 per cent. Advocating this technique to treat ureteral tumors in patients with two normally functioning kidneys without preexisting renal compromise remains controversial.

CONCLUSION

Many of the aforementioned techniques have been developed only recently, and therefore long-term efficacy and morbidity data are lacking. However, almost every surgical disease affecting the ureter has been treated endoscopically with less morbidity than by traditional open means. As the techniques improve and urologists become more comfortable with endoscopic approaches, the need for open operative ureteral surgery likely will be limited.

Suggested Readings

Blute ML, Segura JW, Patterson DE, et al: Impact of endourology on diagnosis and management of upper urinary tact urothelial cancer. J Urol 141:1298, 1989

Clayman RV, Denstedt JD: New technique: Ureterorenoscopic urothelial endoureteroplasty: Case report. J Endourol 3:425, 1989

Ghoneim MA, Nabeeh A, El-Kappany H: Endourologic treatment of ureteral strictures. J Endourol 20:263, 1988

Karlin GS, Badlini GH, Smith AD: Endopyelotomy versus open pyeloplasty: Comparison in 88 patients. J Urol 140:476, 1988

Kavoussi LR, Clayman RV, Brunt LM, et al: Laparoscopic ureterolysis. J Urol 147:426, 1992

Meretyk S, Albala D, Kavoussi LR, et al: Endosurgery: Noncalculus applications in the upper urinary tract. Monogr Urol 12:67, 1991

Nezhat C, Nezhat F, Green B, et al: Laparoscopic ureteroureterostomy. J Endourol 6:143, 1992

PRUNE-BELLY SYNDROME

T. ERNESTO FIGUEROA, M.D.

Tampa, Florida

The term "prune-belly syndrome" (PBS) characterizes the most apparent abnormality of this syndrome, the hypoplasia of the abdominal musculature. This syndrome, also known as Eagle-Barrett or triad syndrome, involves three specific abnormalities: (1) muscular deficiency of the abdominal wall; (2) ureteral tortuosity and a large, hypotonic bladder; and (3) bilateral cryptorchidism. The complexity of these abnormalities poses a persistent challenge to the reconstructive urologist trying to "normalize" these patients.

A rare syndrome, PBS is estimated to occur in 1:50,000 live births. The full-blown syndrome, by definition, applies only to boys, although scattered reports exist of females with abdominal musculature deficiencies and ureteral tortuosity. The preponderance of males in PBS suggests an X-linked, recessive gene transmission, although most evidence points to sporadic selection without a genetic component.

PBS is a serious syndrome with high morbidity and mortality. Most patients with PBS have some degree of renal compromise. Twenty per cent of those affected perish in the neonatal period. Approximately 30 per cent of PBS patients die during the first 2 years of life from urinary sepsis or renal failure. Surviving patients are prone to upper respiratory infections and chronic constipation. Lack of abdominal musculature prevents these patients from performing many childhood activities. Those patients surviving the first 2 to 3 years of life face an uncertain future, determined primarily by the degree of renal functional impairment. There is ardent debate among those who propose complete reconstruction of the urinary tract to improve or conserve renal function, and those who propose a "hands off" attitude toward the urinary tract, arguing that the ultimate fate of the kidneys cannot be altered by reconstructive surgery.

ETIOLOGY

The cause of PBS remains uncertain. Two main theories have been proposed.

1. Urinary obstruction of the level of the prostate produces marked vesical distention and ureteral tortuosity. The vesical distention impairs the development of the abdominal wall musculature and testicular descent.
2. An intrinsic mesenchymal defect leads to the abnormalities in abdominal wall and urinary tract.

DEVELOPMENT ABNORMALITIES

Abdominal Wall

The wrinkled appearance of the abdomen stems from deficient musculature. The deficiency is quite variable, and different groups of muscles are affected with more or less frequency. The rectus muscle is affected most commonly and the internus least. The muscular fibers are often hypoplastic, although sections of musculature also may be absent. The severity of the muscular deficiency does not have prognostic significance.

Urinary Tract

The appearance of the ureters is characteristic of PBS. Ureteral dilation and serpentigenous tortuosity, more pronounced distally, with or without vesicoureteral reflux, typically is present in these patients. The configuration of the ureters, plus a distended, hypotonic, anteriorly displaced bladder and a wide bladder neck, are specific findings of PBS. On histologic sectioning, the ureters demonstrate fibrosis and scarce musculature. These changes are more pronounced in the distal ureters, leading to impaired peristalsis. The histologic appearance of the bladder is similar to that seen in the ureters: sparsity of detrusor muscular bundles, with interposed sections of fibrosis. These bladders are thickened, although trabeculation is infrequent. The urachus may be patent in some patients; in others, the bladder extends to the umbilicus. Voiding pressures are commonly within normal range, but voiding may be inefficient because of the large capacity of the bladder and lack of continuous detrusor muscle, resulting in elevated urinary residual volumes.

The prostatic urethra is usually wide and conical, with its apex at the urogenital diaphragm. It has been postulated that this conical or triangular appearance occurs secondary to obstruction of the prostate, perhaps producing the other abnormalities of PBS. Obstruction, however, is seldom demonstrable at this level in surviving infants. It is possible that obstruction at this level may be present during intrauterine life. Duckett has expanded on this concept by suggesting that a delay in the canalization of the urethra is the reason for fetal obstruction of the urinary tract.

Of more prognostic importance for these patients is the appearance and morphology of the kidneys. Chronic pyelonephritic changes and the presence of renal dysplasia significantly worsen the function of these kidneys. The histology of the kidneys, however, cannot be predicted based on the appearance of the rest of the urinary tract.

Testes

Bilateral cryptorchidism is characteristic of PBS. The testes are located intra-abdominally, at the level where the ureters cross the iliac arteries. Obstruction of the prostatic urethra with resultant massive dilation of the bladder has been proposed as the cause of the testicular maldescent. More recently, elegant histochemical analyses of infant testes by Kogan and associates have demonstrated atypical germ cells, suggesting a developmental arrest of these testes. PBS patients experience azoospermia and infertility, and often have elevated levels of follicle-stimulating hormone and luteinizing hormone, indicating a seminiferous tubular dysfunction. Secondary sexual characteristic, erections, and libido usually are present in these patients.

Other Abnormalities

A number of other abnormalities also may be present in patients with PBS. Urethral diverticula (scaphoid and fusiform varieties) have been described in some patients. Nonurologic manifestations include cardiovascular, musculoskeletal, and pulmonary abnormalities. Compression injuries result from oligohydramnios or distention of the urinary tract. As with other known causes of fetal urinary tract obstruction, pulmonary hypoplasia is related to the degree of renal dysplasia and oligohydramnios. Pulmonary hypoplasia critically affects these infants and accounts for the high percentage of perinatal deaths.

EVALUATION

The widespread use of fetal ultrasonography has allowed the detection of patients with obstructive uropathy in utero. The findings of fetal bilateral hydronephrosis, a large bladder, and oligohydramnios should suggest PBS as one of the possibilities. These findings, however, are not specific for PBS. In the mid-1980s, much enthusiasm was given to prenatal intervention for presumed obstructive uropathy. Recently, these efforts have been tempered by the recognition that fetal renal damage may occur early in development, perhaps prior to the time when hydronephrosis is detected in utero. The finding of severe oligohydramnios is a very poor prognostic indicator, and aggressive intrauterine attempts to correct this abnormality may not alter the ultimate outcome of these patients.

In the newborn period, patients with PBS should be evaluated carefully for pulmonary hypoplasia and possible pneumothoraces. An initial chest radiograph is mandatory. Physical examination will indicate the laxity of the abdominal wall, bladder distention, and undescended testes. Cardiac murmurs should be evaluated by echocardiography. Suspected orthopedic problems should be confirmed radiographically. The anus should be assessed for patency. Serum electrolytes and creatinine levels are obtained routinely.

Urographic evaluation of the newborn patient with PBS should be thorough and well planned. Ultrasonography of the kidneys, ureters, and bladder provides valuable information about the degree of hydronephrosis and preservation of renal parenchyma. Loss of corticomedullary differentiation and hyperechoic kidneys suggest renal dysplasia. Prior to obtaining a voiding cystourethrogram (VCUG), a urine culture is obtained and the patient started on antibiotic prophylaxis. Amoxicillin at 20 mg/kg per dose is the usual agent for prophylaxis. If the child is stable and voiding well, the VCUG may be delayed until the child is about 1 month of age.

It is often beneficial to schedule a diuretic renogram with a urethral catheter in place to assess upper tract drainage. At the completion of the study, the catheter is left in place and the child transported to a fluoroscopy table, where the VCUG can be performed. This sequence minimizes the need for repeated catheterization of these infants. In the patient with a nonobstructed urinary tract, a renal sonogram and diuretic renal scan are obtained alternatively every 6 months.

MANAGEMENT

Although controversy exists regarding the extent and timing of surgical reconstruction of the dilated urinary tract, the critical factors in preserving renal function are assuring adequate urinary drainage and prevention of urinary tract infection. If obstruction is suspected, a cutaneous vesicostomy usually provides adequate drainage. Upper ureteral diversion should be avoided because it may compromise the section of the ureters most likely to be normal in these patients. Consequently, if upper tract diversion is needed, cutaneous pyelostomies are preferred to cutaneous ureterostomies. Proponents of total urinary tract reconstruction recommend excision of the dilated distal half of the ureters and reimplantation of the plicated, more normal upper ureters into the bladder. A reduction cystoplasty also is done at the time by excising the dome of the bladder and urachus.

Bilateral orchiopexies usually are done utilizing the Fowler-Stevens technique. Some authors advocate early orchiopexy, at 6 months of age, citing the ability to perform a transabdominal orchiopexy at this age without the need for ligation of the spermatic vessels. The surgeon also may consider a staged approach by combining the orchiopexies with a simultaneous operation on the urinary tract.

The abdominal wall defect may be managed in a number of ways. Nonsurgical approaches include observation and use of abdominal corsets. Surgical approaches include the transverse "vest over pants" abdominoplasty; the longitudinal "double-breasted" abdominoplasty, as popularized by Ehrlich; and the plication technique described by Monfort.

Suggested Readings

Ehrlich RM, Lesavoy MA, Fine RN: Total abdominal wall reconstruction in the prune belly syndrome. J Urol 136: 282, 1986

Greskovich EJ, Nymberg LM: The prune belly syndrome: A review of its etiology, defects, treatment, and prognosis. J Urol 140:707, 1988

Reinberg Y, Manivel JC, Fryd D, et al: The outcome of renal transplantation in children with the prune belly syndrome. J Urol 142:1541, 1989

Rich MA, Duckett JW: The prune belly syndrome. A.U.A. Update Series XI(17), 1992

CONGENITAL MEGAURETER IN CHILDREN

ALAN B. RETIK, M.D.

Boston, Massachusetts

Management of the dilated ureter in children has been a controversial topic in pediatric urology during the past 50 years. A variety of therapeutic measures and procedures have been used to treat this disorder. These have included observation alone, multiple micturition, antibiotics, cystoscopic dilation of the ureter, ureteral meatotomy, presacral neurectomy, ureterostomy, the ileal sleeve procedure, and urinary diversion. During the last 25 years, ureteral tailoring and reimplantation have been used with varying degrees of success. It has become apparent that there are a number of different causes of wide ureters in children and that treatment, to a great extent, depends on their etiology.

A number of different classifications of megaureter have evolved. In 1975, a "Working Party to Establish International Nomenclature of the Large Ureter" met in Philadelphia and established a complete classification of wide ureters. The primary categories were refluxing megaureter, obstructed megaureter, and nonrefluxing-nonobstructed megaureter. These all had primary and secondary categories.

Whatever classification is used, it is extremely important to ascertain which wide ureters should not be operated on. For example, severe urinary infection in the neonate may cause ureteral dilation mimicking obstructed megaureter. In the presence of a normal voiding cystogram and prompt response of the infection to antibiotics, these babies should be maintained on antibiotics, and repeat radiologic studies should be obtained in 4 to 6 weeks. If the upper urinary tract dilation regresses, one is dealing with the effects of infection, and surgery is not indicated. (We have seen very severe hydronephrosis and hydroureter improve dramatically in a month and revert to normal over a 6- to 12-month period in a number of infants.) If there is no change in the degree of ureteral dilation, the diagnosis of congenital obstructed megaureter is made and surgery is indicated. Similarly, the hydronephrosis and hydroureter associated with urethral obstruction most often secondary to posterior urethral valves usually will subside gradually after the obstruction is relieved by valve fulguration. Therefore, most of these wide ureters will not require surgical correction (see below). In addition, the mild variety of congenital obstructed megaureter in which the dilation is not severe and is confined to the lower ureter usually is not progressive and also does not require surgical correction.

CLINICAL FEATURES

The typical congenital obstructed megaureter shows severe dilation proximal to a relatively normal-caliber segment of intravesical ureter and, on occasion, extravesical ureter as well. The affected ureteral orifice calibrates to a normal size. The musculature of the undilated segment may be disorganized, abnormal, or absent, and its orientation is often predominantly circular. There is usually an increase in collagen between muscle bundles and cells. There is progressive improvement in muscle cell morphology extending more proximally by the dilated portion of the megaureter. In the absence of an anatomic stenosis, the obstruction is a functional one, caused by failure of peristalsis transmission through the distal ureteral segment. Peristalsis proximal to the undilated segment is abnormal, primarily because of the failure of the dilated ureter to coapt. This leads to stasis and infection. Obstructed megaureter also may be secondary to anatomic obstruction of the distal ureter and ureteral orifice, as seen with ureteroceles and bladder diverticula.

Megaureters sometimes are associated with very severe (Grade 5) vesicoureteral reflux. Children with these have megatrigones with laterally placed golf-hole ureteral orifices.

SURGICAL TREATMENT

Surgical treatment of dilated ureters may be necessary in a small percentage of children for persistent, significant reflux or ureterovesical obstruction after removal of the urethral obstruction (e.g., fulguration of posterior urethral valves). Ureteral dilation may be due to an impaired ability of the ureters to empty or impaired bladder emptying, not necessarily to ureterovesical obstruction. It is very important to make this differentiation. Whitaker's direct measurements of ureteral pressures have shown that only wide ureters with obstructive pressures should be reimplanted. In addition, it is not advisable to perform surgery on megaureters that drain into bladders that do not empty properly. If there is a suspicion of abnormal bladder function, preoperative urodynamic evaluation may be most helpful.

Surgical Technique

Through a Pfannenstiel incision, the bladder is opened and a Denis-Browne retractor is placed within the bladder. A 4-0 chromic catgut traction stitch is placed beneath the involved ureteral orifice. A circumferential incision is made around the orifice with cautery, and the ureter is dissected out sharply with tenotomy scissors from its intravesical and extravesical attachments. The ureter then is dissected extravesically to the level of the ileac vessels. Special care is taken not to disturb the blood supply of the adventitia of the ureter. The normal-caliber intravesical ureter is excised, and the dilated ureter is tailored over a 10F red rubber catheter in infants and a 12F red rubber catheter in older children by resecting the lateral portion of the ureter. The ureteral repair is done using a one-layer continuous 5-0 chromic catgut stitch, with interrupted 5-0 chromic catgut stitches for the most inferior segment of the repair. A new hiatus is made on the posterior wall of the bladder, and a tunnel is made inferiorly into the trigone. The redundant portion of the ureter is excised, with care taken to avoid ureteral angulation. A fine feeding tube should pass without any difficulty and is left indwelling for approximately 7 to 10 days.

Results of Surgery

Review of our patients has led to several conclusions. Forty-eight of 49 obstructed or refluxing megaureters showed postoperative improvement. Lower ureteral tailoring and reimplantation into a normal bladder is therefore a highly successful method of dramatically improving even the most tortuous ureters and the most severe hydronephrosis—with or without reflux. The results are not quite as satisfactory in children with abnormal bladders that do not empty properly. There are several reasons for failure in these patients. They generally have thickened, scarred, inflamed bladders. A large residual urine, whether the result of obstruction, myogenic failure, or neurologic dysfunction, may well lead to a poor result. Therefore, it is extremely important to evaluate bladder function and emptying, as well as ureterodynamics, prior to surgically correcting megaureters in children who have had multiple bladder operations or severe urethral obstruction.

Another observation in our series was that none of the children required upper ureteral tapering. We believe that a dilated ureter, when relieved of obstruction, reflux, and infection and allowed to drain into a normal bladder, will return to a relatively normal functional state. Often, a dramatic improvement in the degree of dilation of the upper ureter and kidney is observed within a few months postoperatively. However, in some instances, radiologic improvement is gradual and may not be maximal until 18 to 24 months after surgery on the lower ureter. Therefore, in the child who is doing well clinically, it is certainly worthwhile to wait for a considerable period of time prior to performing reconstructive surgery on the upper urinary tract. In a few children, however, when obvious ureteropelvic obstruction was present, pyeloplasty was performed prior to lower ureteral surgery. More accurate urodynamic evaluation of the bladder and ureteral function in the future should decrease the number of unsatisfactory results in the treatment of the secondary megaureter.

Suggested Readings

Belman AB: Megaureter classification, etiology, and management. Urol Clin North Am 1:497, 1974

Keating MA, Retik AB: Management of the dilated obstructed ureter. Urol Clin North Am 17:291–306, 1990

Peters CA, Mandell J, Lebowitz RL, et al: Congenital obstructed megaureters in early infancy: Diagnosis and treatment. J Urol 142:641–645, 1989

Pfister RC, Hendren WH: Primary megaureter in children and adults: Clinical and pathophysiologic features of 150 ureters. Urology 12:160, 1978

Retik AB, McEvoy JP, Bauer SB: Megaureters in children. Urology 11:281, 1978

SURGICAL MANAGEMENT OF MEGAURETER

MICHAEL A. KEATING, M.D.

Indianapolis, Indiana

The spectrum of anomalies known as megaureter continue to challenge today's urologist just as they have since their original description more than 90 years ago. The surgical solutions for the dilated ureter have improved, but the decision as to when to address certain variants fuels one of the livelier debates in our field.

The dilated ureter or megaureter can be classified into one of four groups, each having a basis in the dilatation's underlying cause: (1) refluxing, (2) obstructed, (3) both refluxing and obstructed, and (4) nonrefluxing-nonobstructed. Further subdivisions into primary or secondary causes assume additional importance for obvious reasons. Therapeutic recommendations depend on proper categorization, and a thorough evaluation of the entire urinary tract is necessary in every case.

EVALUATION

Ultrasonography should be the initial diagnostic study in any child suspected of having a urologic abnormality. Noninvasive and relatively inexpensive, ultrasound provides useful anatomic detail of the renal parenchyma, collecting system and bladder. It also offers an invaluable standard of the degree of hydroureteronephrosis for follow-up studies. Once ureteral dilatation is detected, a voiding cystourethrogram is obtained to rule out reflux as its cause and to assess the quality of the bladder and urethra, where neurogenic dysfunction or outlet obstruction are common causes of secondarily refluxing or obstructed megaureters. A study also is obtained to judge renal function and the degree of obstruction, if any. In this regard, excretory urography's anatomic detail is sometimes helpful, but functional data must be inferred from the study. Instead, radionuclide scans (DTPA or MAG3) are preferred because, although not without flaws, they offer objective, reproducible parameters of function and obstruction. Cystoscopy and retrograde imaging rarely are included in the initial evaluation. Whitaker's perfusion test and flouroscopy provide little additional data with regard to obstruction but are helpful when concerns about ureteral motility exist.

RECOMMENDATIONS

Historically, ureteral dilatations typically were discovered with evaluations of a palpable abdominal mass, urinary tract infection, or an episode of hematuria. The need for surgery was almost universal. In contrast, during the past decade an increasing number of megaureters have been serendipitously discovered with the advent of antenatal ultrasonography. Most are not associated with reflux. The natural history of these asymptomatic dilatations, which in the past might have been categorized as primarily obstructed, is being defined only now. What is becoming apparent, however, is that many will either resolve entirely or persist merely as nonobstructive congenital distortions if left alone. Discerning these benign variants from others that actually endanger the renal parenchyma and patient presents a difficult therapeutic dilemma, especially because the diagnostic parameters of obstruction are so ill defined.

Deciding between surgery or expectant medical management often becomes a function of one's clinical impressions and experience. Any haste in correcting newborn megaureters must be tempered by the realization that their repair presents a formidable technical challenge in smaller infants. In addition, affected kidneys appear to be somewhat buffered from the deleterious pressures of partial congenital obstruction by their compliant ureters. As long as renal function is unaffected and the infant remains infection free, medical management with antibiotic suppression and close radiologic surveillance are appropriate. If the degree of hydroureteronephrosis is severe and shows no signs of improvement or the clinical status worsens, correction is undertaken when technically feasible, usually between the ages of 1 and 2. For the occasional newborn who presents with massive ureteral dilatation, distal ureterostomy provides an effective panacea for poor drainage until the child's growth allows for ureteral reconstruction.

The classic management of primary refluxing megaureters, which until now have been corrected routinely, also is receiving scrutiny because of altered detection. Historically, the likelihood of seeing spontaneous resolution with the high grades (4 and 5) of reflux found with megaureters was virtually nil. Recently, however, preliminary studies have shown higher rates of resolution with perinatally diagnosed refluxing megaureters than those described in historic projections based on symptomatic presentations in older children. Medical management is appropriate during infancy and is continued if a trend to resolution is noted. Otherwise, surgery remains the recommendation for persistent high-grade reflux in older children and adults. In the rare infant who fails medical management but is considered too small to definitively reconstruct, unilateral ureterostomy or vesicostomy for bilateral disease should be considered as a temporizing solution.

Finally, the management of secondary megaureters is directed at their etiology. For example, impressive degrees of reflux and dilatation often improve with the ablation of urethral valves or management of a neurogenic bladder. Other cases having secondary etiologies, including the prune-belly syndrome, diabetes insipidus, or infection, where bacterial endotoxins sometimes cause transient ureteral paralysis, require no more than observation alone. Chronic congenital distention, regardless of its source, imprints permanent dilatation on many collecting systems. As a result, some degree of nonobstructed hydroureteronephrosis can be expected to persist in most systems, even after primary or secondary causes have been addressed.

SURGICAL TECHNIQUES

The principles held for successful reimplantation of ureters having normal caliber also apply here. Effective ureteroneocystostomies are created by implanting ureters beneath submucosal tunnels having adequate muscular backing and a length approximately five times the ureteral diameter. Achieving this ratio depends on the size of the recipient bladder as well as that of the affected megaureter(s), and adaptability in technique selection is crucial to success.

A Pfannenstiel incision and Denis-Browne retractor afford excellent exposure. A 5F feeding tube placed in the ureter and sutured to its meatus provides traction and helps minimize trauma during mobilization. After making a circumferential incision around the orifice, the ureter is detached from intra- and extravesical tethers that are defined with sharp dissection and cauterized selectively. Many megaureters can be mobilized adequately by staying within the bladder, but there should be no hesitation in moving extravesically, especially with larger ureters. In any case, care is taken to preserve the blood supply of the ureteral adventitia. This is classically taught as emanating from the medial aspect of the lower ureter, but in actuality the vascularity of megaureters is quite variable.

After completion of mobilization, and excision of the adynamic distal segment with cases of obstruction, ureteral calibration is done using a soft red rubber catheter. When the ureter is larger than an 8F catheter in infants or a 10F catheter in children and adults, it should be tailored to these sizes to help achieve the diameter-length ratio desired for reimplantation. Two techniques, nonexcisional plications and excisional tapering, are equally effective in decreasing ureteral size. Plications are simply performed, avoid suture lines that risk leakage, and may be more effective in preserving vascularity. Their removal and repositioning also offer a greater margin for error than tapering, which is less forgiving when avoiding vascularity or adjusting size. One detriment of plications is the bulk that accompanies the refashioned ureter. This makes the reimplantation of larger ureters, especially into smaller bladders, difficult.

Tapering is reserved for larger ureters where plications' bulk would be excessive or luminal reduction (estimated at only 50 to 60 per cent at best) using plications might not be sufficient. Megaureter clamps are helpful in isolating the segment of megaureter that can be sacrificed without compromising the vasculature to the ureter that will remain. After its excision, the ureter is repaired using a running locking 6-0 polydiaxanone suture that incorporates mucosa and muscularis. This is followed by a similar stitch reapproximating adventitia. Regardless of the technique, reduction is planned to include reimplanted ureter as well as a short segment remaining outside the bladder. Total ureteral tailoring is rarely, if ever, indicated, and complete mobilization and unkinking of more proximal ureter is unnecessary.

Reimplantation is completed using either the cross-trigonal advancement technique or ipsilateral Leadbetter-type tunnels, with care taken to avoid ureteral kinking. Intermittent passage of a fine feeding tube is a good test of the patency of any repair. The technically simpler cross-trigonal technique is especially applicable to trabeculated, neurogenic-type bladders and smaller bladders. Ipsilateral tunnels are created with unilateral reimplants or when extravesical ureteral mobilization becomes necessary. Here the somewhat "blind" nature of the Leadbetter technique is eliminated and a new obstacle-free hiatus for the ureter into the bladder is easily defined. Occasionally the feasibility of creating two adequately long tunnels is limited by the size of the bladder regardless of the method used to narrow or reimplant the ureter. When this is the case, transureteroureterostomy and psoas hitch of the recipient megaureter provides an effective option in reconstruction. The psoas hitch also can provide additional tunnel length for unilateral megaureter repairs without altering bladder dynamics.

Stents are not used routinely with plications but are left across tapered megaureters and remain for 5 days to allow for perioperative edema to subside. Postoperative stentograms are no longer obtained. Leaks rarely occur, and past studies typically demonstrated no more than the absence of flow around the tube that served to obstruct the edematous intramural tunnel. Instead, if the patient is doing well clinically, radiographic follow-up consists of a renal scan 6 weeks after surgery and a voiding studying and ultrasound 9 months later. When the repair has been successful, ultrasound alone can be used for subsequent follow-up.

Using the techniques discussed herein, success rates of better than 95 per cent can be cited to patients and their families. When suboptimal results are obtained, they often are related to altered dynamics of the bladder or ureter, where peristalsis and the ability to coapt are sometimes impaired by chronic infection or myogenic failure. The latter perhaps accounts for the higher rates of failure associated with the reimplantation of refluxing megaureters when compared to their obstructed counterparts. Thorough preoperative evaluations and a high index of suspicion are instrumental to minimizing these types of occurrences. Otherwise, strict attention to surgical detail and adherence to the principles that define successful ureteral reimplantation serve to maximize the chances of obtaining a satisfactory result.

Suggested Readings

Brock JW III: Congenital obstructive megaureter: Etiology, diagnosis and treatment. Dial Pediatr Urol 16:2, 1993

Hendren WH: Operative repair of megaureter in children. J Urol 101:491, 1969

Keating MA, Escala J, Snyder HM, et al: Changing concepts in management of primary obstructive megaureter. J Urol 142:636, 1989

King LR: Megaloureter: Definition, diagnosis and management. J Urol 123:222, 1980

URETEROCELES

RICHARD C. RINK, M.D.

Indianapolis, Indiana

One of the more challenging anomalies facing the urologist from both the diagnostic as well as the therapeutic standpoint is the ureterocele. It presents a spectrum of anatomic abnormalities that may cause changes in the entire urinary tract from kidney to urethra. This results in varying clinical presentations with a wide variety of treatment options.

A ureterocele is a cystic dilation of the terminal intravesical ureter. Although ureteroceles have been classified in many ways, it seems easiest to place them into one of two groups depending on the renal unit they subtend—single system versus duplex system. Either may be orthotopic or ectopic.

Embryologic development of the ureterocele has been debated over the years, with no single mechanism being proved. Proposed mechanisms range from ureterovesical obstruction to widening of the ureteral bud as it is incorporated into the urogenital sinus to poor muscular development of the distal ureter. Some even believe there is an acquired form.

DIAGNOSIS

In most instances, particularly in children, the initial diagnostic study is an ultrasound. Ultrasonography allows visualization of a cystic bladder mass. A dilated ureter behind the bladder generally can be seen to extend to the kidney level. A duplex system often is defined easily, with the upper pole being hydronephrotic. Significant reflux or obstruction also may result in hydronephrosis of the lower pole. At times, hydronephrosis may be absent, with only an echogenic cap of a dysplastic upper pole seen at the kidney level and a ureterocele noted in the bladder (ureterocele disproportion).

A voiding cystourethrogram should be done in suspected ureterocele cases. This not only defines the size and extent of the ureterocele but also notes the presence of vesicoureteral reflux, the degree of detrusor backing of the ureterocele, and the extent of bladder outlet obstruction.

Nuclear renal scans will provide an estimate of function and salvageability of the affected renal segment. Intravenous pyelography is often diagnostic in adults with single system ureteroceles. It is used infrequently in children.

SINGLE-SYSTEM URETEROCELES

Ureteroceles associated with a single ureter are found more commonly in adults than children. They most often are intravesical and orthotopic and when so have been designated simple ureteroceles. Simple ureteroceles usually have a pinpoint meatus, but the degree of upper tract change is less than in those seen with duplex systems. In adults, the amount of obstruction is usually not significant and treatment, if necessary at all, has been done endoscopically. The ureteroceles in children usually are detected following a urinary infection or by antenatal ultrasound. Adults tend to present with urinary tract infection, stones within the ureteroceles, or irritative voiding symptoms. The classic "cobra-head" defect of the distal ureter seen within the bladder on intravenous pyelography is usually diagnostic. Vesicoureteral reflux is rare.

Treatment of the more significant single-system orthotopic ureteroceles in children generally has been by excision of the ureterocele and reimplantation of the ureter. Historically, endoscopic unroofing has resulted in reflux and therefore has met with disfavor. More recently, a resurgence in endoscopic management has occurred. A transurethral small transverse incision on the medial aspect of the ureterocele is now the initial procedure of choice. This allows the obstructed dilated ureter to decrease in caliber, with relief of obstruction, and allows assessment of recoverable renal function. Frequently there is no reflux following this incision, but, if present, lower tract reconstruction can still be done, often without the need for ureteral tapering.

The rare ectopic single-system ureterocele generally subtends a nonfunctioning kidney and is treated by nephroureterectomy and ureterocele decompression. Only rarely will this ureterocele require excision.

URETEROCELES IN A DUPLEX SYSTEM

As opposed to single-system ureteroceles, those associated with the upper pole of a duplex system are much more commonly seen in children than adults and have approximately a 4:1 female-to-male incidence. Contralateral duplication is seen in up to 45 per cent of cases. Ureteroceles in duplex systems generally are found during evaluation of a urinary tract infection, and frank sepsis may be noted. Although antenatal ultrasound is an increasingly common means of detection, children still present with a palpable abdominal mass, failure to thrive, or prolapse of a ureterocele through the urethra. Older children occasionally are seen with irritative voiding symptoms.

These ureteroceles can be orthotopic, but an ectopic location is the norm. Ectopic ureteroceles generally are associated with a dysplastic upper pole having severe functional impairment. Less than 10 per cent of these upper poles visualize on pyelography. Some degree of contralateral ureteral obstruction has been noted in 25 per cent.

Vesicoureteral reflux into the ipsilateral lower pole is present in one half of these patients and occurs most commonly with easily compressible ureteroceles. The tensely distended ureterocele is more likely to cause lower pole obstruction. Reflux into the ureterocele and its upper pole ureter is uncommon but may occur following spontaneous or iatrogenic ureterocele rupture. Decompression of a tense ureterocele occasionally may result in reflux to the lower pole that was not initially noted.

Treatment is dependent on the degree of renal function, size and location of the ureterocele, presence of massive reflux, and age of the child. There is no unanimous support for any given form of therapy. Endoscopic incision of the ectopic ureterocele in a duplex system is used primarily to drain the obstructed infected system in a severely ill child.

Therapy at the renal level is better agreed on than that for the bladder level. For the nonfunctioning upper pole segment, upper pole heminephrectomy should be done. In those unusual times when there is salvageable renal function, two forms of therapy have been recommended. If the ureterocele is small, ureterocele excision and common sheath reimplantation of the duplicated ureters could be considered. If the upper pole ureter is quite dilated, some recommend ureteropyelostomy or ureteroureterostomy with ureterocele decompression. Generally these functioning upper pole segments are somewhat dysplastic, adding only minimally to overall renal function, and are best excised. If only the renal level is addressed, at least 50 per cent later will require bladder surgery for persistent reflux, a distended ureterocele, or poor detrusor backing resulting in bladder diverticulum formation. For this reason, some authors have recommended total reconstruction (upper pole heminephroureterectomy, ureterocele excision, and lower pole reimplantation) in one setting. In the best of hands this is an extremely difficult and time-consuming procedure in the neonate, and we therefore recommend upper pole heminephrectomy and partial ureterectomy with ureterocele decompression in this age group as the initial procedure. Any necessary bladder surgery can be done at a later date. Potentially one half of the patients are spared lower tract surgery. In older children in whom lower tract surgery is likely (i.e., those with prolapse, massive reflux, or diverticulum formation), total reconstruction should be considered.

When the ureterocele itself is addressed surgically, we believe it should be excised completely, reconstructing the detrusor defect and trigone. However, some authors believe that marsupialization of the ureterocele alone is all that should be done, to avoid potential injury to the continence mechanism of the bladder neck and urethra. It is clear in either form of therapy that an obstructing distal mucosal lip must be avoided.

For the rare situation of no function of the upper or lower segment, total nephrectomy and ureterocele excision are appropriate.

CONCLUSION

Diagnosis and treatment of ureteroceles can be challenging. The care should be individualized, with every effort made to preserve renal function, and eliminate urinary stasis.

Suggested Readings

Caldamone AA, Snyder H McC III, Duckett JW: Ureteroceles in children: Follow-up management with upper tract approach. J Urol 131:1130, 1984
Decter RM, Roth DR, Gonzales ET: Individualized treatment of ureteroceles. J Urol 142:535, 1989
Gonzales ET Jr: Ureteroceles. *In* Kelalis PP, King LR, Belman AB (eds): Clinical Pediatric Urology, 3rd ed. Philadelphia, WB Saunders, 1992, pp 554–576
Mandell J, Colodny AH, Lebowitz R, et al: Ureteroceles in infants and children. J Urol 123:921, 1980
Rich MA, Keating MA, Snyder HM, Duckett, JW: Low transurethral incision of single system intravesical uteroceles in children. J Urol 144:120, 1990.
Rink RC, Adams MC, Mitchell ME: Ureteral abnormalities. *In* Ashcraft KW (eds): Pediatric Urology. Philadelphia, WB Saunders, 1990, p 125
Scherz HC, Kaplan GW, Packer MG, et al: Ectopic ureteroceles: Surgical management with preservation of continence—review of 60 cases. J Urol 142:538, 1989

EXPERIENCE WITH TRANSURETHRAL INCISION OF URETEROCELE IN CHILDREN

MARK HOROWITZ, M.D.

Seattle, Washington

The diagnosis of ureterocele is being made with increasing frequency prior to birth. In addition to those children discovered by antenatal ultrasonography, some are found during the evaluation of a urinary tract infection. The traditional classification has depended on the location of the orifice, however small, of the ureterocele. Hence terms such as "orthotopic," "ectopic," and "cecoureterocele" have been used. Perhaps a better way to think of ureteroceles is by the size of the detrussor defect. A small defect in the detrussor muscle may allow protrusion of a huge intravesical ureterocele, which is actually easy to deal with. Conversely, the large muscular hiatus will tend to involve the other ureters and be more problematic. All ureteroceles, however, tend to be obstructive and infection prone. For this reason we recommend prophylactic antibiotics as soon as the diagnosis is made prior to completion of the evaluation. In addition to ultrasonography and voiding cystourethrography, a functional study such as Lasix renogram or intravenous pyelogram is helpful prior to surgical decision making.

Treatment options include upper pole heminephrectomy for ureteroceles associated with duplication and poor upper pole function, with or without resection of the distal ureter and ureterocele, with repair of the bladder floor and ureteral reimplantation. Another treatment option includes simple endoscopic incision of the ureterocele. This is especially attractive in the newborn period, when the anesthetic risk is increased and the anatomic structures are tiny and fragile. Although ureterocele incision often is viewed as a temporizing procedure to decompress an obstructed ureter (with subsequent decreased infection risk), we have found that it is often the only procedure required. This is especially true in those ureteroceles that have a small detrussor muscle defect.

Our technique involves the use of a small cold knife urethratome (8.5F sheath) with a variety of cold knife tips, including a small blade and a sharpened hook. Under general anesthesia, the instrument is placed under direct vision and the contralateral ureteral orifice and ipsilateral lower pole ureteral orifice are located. We suggest a vertical incision in the distalmost aspect of the ureterocele. The extent of the ureterocele sometimes can be appreciated by directing the water from the cystoscope at it and noting the fluttering of the mucosa. The vertical slit tends to avoid the formation of flaps that can be obstructive. Bleeding is usually minimal. Prophylactic antibiotics are continued until a postoperative cystogram can be performed, which may or may not demonstrate reflux following incision.

Whereas the ureterocele with a small muscular defect may not require further intervention, we expect that those with a large muscle defect will require definitive open reconstruction.

ECTOPIC URETEROCELES

ARNOLD H. COLODNY, M.D.

Boston, Massachusetts

Ectopic ureteroceles are a major cause of renal damage, usually in association with duplex systems. Early diagnosis (frequently prenatal) and appropriate treatment may avoid urosepsis and further compromise of renal function in many cases.

CLASSIFICATION

Common usage in the past implied that a "simple" ureterocele was associated with a single system and usually was small and completely within the bladder and not causing severe obstruction. Acceptable synonyms for a simple ureterocele were orthotopic or adult. The term "ectopic ureterocele" usually was used to characterize a ureterocele associated with the upper pole ureter of a completely duplicated collecting system. Because some simple ureteroceles may be large and obstructing, and some ectopic ureteroceles may be small or associated with single systems, a new classification was devised. This classification was based on the position of the orifice of the ureterocele (whether it is in the bladder or at the bladder neck or distal to it). Because a simple ureterocele occasionally may be associated with a duplex system, and it is not uncommon to be unable to identify with certainty just where the orifice of a ureterocele is, the above classification has led to some uncertainty about exactly what each author was reporting.

In 1984 the Committee on Terminology, Nomenclature and Classification of the Section on Urology of the American Academy of Pediatrics proposed a new classification. They suggested two terms, one being *intravesical* and one being *ectopic*:

Intravesical ureterocele: "A type of ureterocele that is located entirely within the bladder. An intravesical ureterocele may be associated with a single system but also may be associated with the upper pole ureter of a completely duplicated system; only rarely is it associated with a lower pole ureter."

Ectopic ureterocele: "A type of ureterocele in which some *portion* of the ureterocele is situated permanently at the bladder neck in the urethra. The *orifice* may be situated in the bladder, at the bladder neck, or in the urethra. Ureteroceles can be characterized further as stenotic, sphincteric, sphinctero-stenotic, cecoureteroceles, blind and non-obstructive."

Some authors have adopted the newer terminology, but several still are using the earlier classification described above. This article is limited to a discussion of ureteroceles associated with the upper pole ureter of a completely duplicated system.

ANATOMIC DESCRIPTION

***Stenotic Ureterocele* (*40 Per Cent*):** The orifice of the ureterocele is so small that it produces obstruction. It may be located anywhere on the ureterocele.

***Sphincteric Ureterocele* (*40 Per Cent*):** A portion of the ureterocele is within the grasp of the bladder neck and/or the urinary sphincter. The orifice may be normal or larger than normal, but obstruction usually ensues because the sphincter is closed except when voiding occurs. Reflux to the upper pole may occur only during voiding and may require cyclic voiding to be demonstrated.

***Sphincterostenotic* (*5 Per Cent*):** The stenotic orifice of the ureterocele is obstructive and is located on the floor of the urethra or beyond.

***Cecoureterocele* (*Rare*):** The orifice of the ureterocele is located within the bladder but the ureterocele itself extends submucosally down the urethra. The actual orifice usually is large and incompetent.

***Blind Ureterocele* (*Rare*):** A ureterocele with no detectable orifice.

***Nonobstructive Ureterocele* (*Rare*):** A ureterocele with a large orifice in the bladder.

***Ureterocele Disproportion*:** A ureterocele with a striking dissimilarity in size between the large ureterocele and its diminutive or atretic ureter and calyces. In the past some of these were thought to be trigonal cysts.

PATHOPHYSIOLOGY

The main consequence of the presence of a ureterocele is the obstruction it produces and the associated vesicoureteral reflux that often is present. Obstruction to the developing fetal kidney may be the cause of the dysplasia and the poorly functioning or nonfunctioning renal moiety that usually is associated with the ureterocele. Obstruction of the opposite kidney or bladder neck or the lower pole of the duplicated system also may lead to further problems. The associated reflux into the lower pole may be considered as a form of obstruction to the fetal kidney and often leads to some dysplasia and/or diminished renal function in the involved renal segment.

CLINICAL PRESENTATION

Prior to the almost universal use of maternal and fetal ultrasonography, the most common mode of presentation of a patient with a ureterocele was with a urinary tract infection (80 per cent). In infants this often developed into true urosepsis with septicemia and in some cases a positive spinal tap. The largest group of these children presented in the first 6 months of life. There often was a significant delay from the onset of symptoms to a definitive diagnosis. Other modes of presentation were urinary retention (10 per cent), prolapse of the ureterocele out through the urethra in girls (6 per cent), or the presence of a palpable abdominal mass (5 per cent). Other less common symptoms often seen in association with urinary infections in the older child were failure to thrive, hematuria, and abdominal or back pain. Associated anatomic anomalies are uncommon but do occur.

With the advent of prenatal ultrasonography, many patients (16 per cent) can be started on prophylactic antibiotics at birth and can have a definitive diagnosis made early enough usually to prevent urosepsis and further renal damage. Approximately 15 per cent of ureteroceles associated with duplex systems will be bilateral. They are more common in girls than boys (7:2). Two thirds of unilateral ureteroceles are on the left side. Over half of these patients have ipsilateral hydronephrosis of the lower pole; usually this is due to reflux but sometimes it is secondary to obstruction by the ureterocele or to obstruction of the lower pole ureter by the crossing megaureter of the upper pole.

DIAGNOSIS

Intravenous Urogram

In 70 per cent of the patients with ureteroceles associated with a duplex system, there was nonvisualization of the upper pole at the time of an intravenous urogram (IVU). If the upper pole is hydronephrotic, with an associated hydroureter, one usually will see the functioning lower pole displaced downward and outward, with a concentric indentation on the upper aspect of the lower pole pelvis (Fig 1). There often is dilation of the lower pole and its ureter, as noted above. The lower pole ureter may have a scalloped appearance caused by its intimate association with the dilated tortuous upper pole ureter. The ureterocele itself usually is clearly outlined on the early bladder views of the IVU. It is nonopaque, usually off center, and frequently quite large, almost filling the bladder. It may extend into the urethra. If the upper pole is functioning, the ureterocele may be filled with contrast and delineated by a halo around it.

Voiding Cystourethrography

Voiding cystourethrography (VCUG) must be done with care and a high index of suspicion of the presence of a ureterocele based on the pre- or postnatal ultrasound and/or the clinical presentation. To prevent obliteration and/or effacement of the ureterocele, diluted contrast material should be used and early films should be taken. The VCUG also will be helpful in detecting and grading lower pole and/or contralateral reflux, whether the ureterocele everts or intussuscepts into its ureter, and whether there is a deficient detrusor backing of the ureterocele. Prolapse of the ureterocele through the bladder neck and into the urethra with voiding may be apparent.

Ultrasound

Because maternal (and fetal) ultrasounds currently are done in the vast majority of pregnancies, congenital anomalies of the urinary tract of the fetus are one of the most common abnormalities detected. The fetal urinary tract is easily visualized once the fetal kidneys start to make urine because of the interface between the fluid (urine) and the solid (parenchyma). The diagnosis of a ureterocele (or an ectopic ureter) would be suggested by the presence of a duplex system with hydroureteronephrosis of the upper pole, with or without hydronephrosis of the lower pole. The ureterocele itself may be visualized within the bladder. This finding may be dependent on a number of factors, and lack of visualization of the ureterocele does not eliminate it as a possibility.

In patients who have had a prenatal diagnosis of a urinary tract abnormality or in those patients who first present with a urinary infection, an ultrasound exam is usually the first diagnostic evaluation performed. A careful exam of the kidneys, ureters, and bladder by an experienced observer usually allows the correct diagnosis to be made. However, there are some pitfalls. The ureterocele may be so large that it may be thought to represent the urinary bladder. If the bladder is overfilled, the ureterocele may be effaced and not visible or it may be everted and give the impression it is a diverticulum. If the upper pole is severely dysplastic and tiny, and ureterocele disproportion is present, a duplex system may not be recognizable; a diagnosis of primary megaureter may be considered in those cases in which the ureterocele is not visualized.

Nuclear Scanning

The type of therapy elected may depend on the functional status of the upper pole moiety.

Nonvisualization on an IVU does not equate to nonfunction. Although it is true that most of the upper poles are dysplastic and do not make any significant contribution to overall renal function, some (15 per cent) may have enough function to warrant preservation. A more exact evaluation of the function may be obtained by isotopic scanning with technetium-99m–labeled dimercaptosuccinic acid (DMSA), even though a precise outlining of the upper versus lower pole function may be problematic.

Endoscopic Evaluation

Cystoscopy usually is done at the time of the initial operative procedure. It usually is not too helpful. It may confirm the imaging studies or identify a smaller, previously overlooked contralateral ureterocele. It also may be helpful in delineating the urethral extension of the ureterocele. Cystoscopic findings may be difficult to evaluate. If the ureterocele is large, visualization may be less than optimal. Cystoscopy should be initiated after emptying the bladder, and filling should be done slowly, or the ureterocele may be effaced or everted and missed or misinterpreted as a diverticulum. Direct injection of contrast material into the ureterocele may outline the status of the ureter and the upper tract if they had not been delineated previously.

THERAPEUTIC OPTIONS

Currently there are five acceptable therapeutic options (Fig. 2). The choice among these is based on the age of the patient, the presence or absence of pyelonephritis, the grade of reflux if present, the amount of function remaining, whether or not the ureterocele everts (indicating poor detrusor backing), the degree of ureteral dilation, and whether or not the ureterocele has prolapsed or extends into the urethra.

Transurethral Incision

This was tried years ago but was largely abandoned because, although it relieved the associated obstruction, it created reflux in most of the patients. This probably was related to the technique utilized at that time. Recently the technique of transurethral incision has been modified and has been utilized

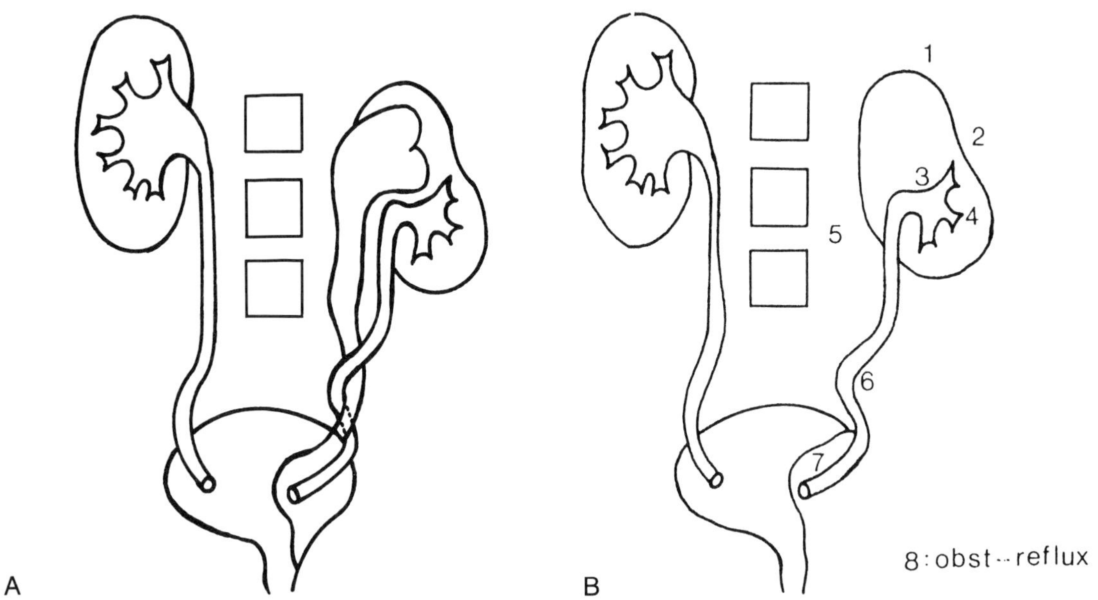

FIGURE 1. *A*, The anatomic situation in a patient with a ureterocele obstructing the upper pole. This would be defined by an ultrasound exam. *B*, Since the upper pole usually does not visualize when contrast is injected, its presence has to be inferred when an intravenous urogram is obtained. (1—no upper calyces will be seen; 2—there may be an indentation in the renal outline where the upper pole joins the lower pole; 3—a concavity in the lower pole pelvis may be apparent. 4—The lower pole calyces will be displaced downward and out; 5—The lower pole pelvis and ureter will be displaced laterally from the spine; 6—The lower pole ureter may be sinuous; 7—There will be a filling defect in the bladder; 8—There may be obstruction of or reflux into the lower pole.)

with increasing frequency and improved results. Although the results are not perfect, in selected cases it is highly effective. It certainly is a procedure of choice in an infant with significant urosepsis. It also may be necessary to incise an incarcerated ureterocele that has prolapsed out the urethra and is causing urinary retention, and is otherwise irreducible. If the ureterocele has not prolapsed and does not extend into the urethra, endoscopic incision has resulted in quite satisfactory results, with secondary operative procedures required in only about 8 per cent of cases. Several authors advocate this technique because it may preserve function of the upper pole. However, in almost all these reports the actual function is not documented or quantitated. In 75 per cent of the usual cases the contribution of this segment is probably inconsequential. The main advantage of the endoscopic technique is that it is simple and, when successful, relieves the obstruction of the upper pole segment and its ureter and any other obstruction (ipsilateral, lower pole, opposite renal unit, and/or bladder outlet) and, it is hoped, obviates the need for open surgery. In addition, if further surgery at the bladder level (such as ureteral reimplantation) becomes necessary, it will be easier to do after the ureterocele has been decompressed for a period of time. If the ureterocele is prolapsed or extended into the urethra, endoscopic incision is less satisfactory. Secondary open surgical procedures will be required in a minimum of 50 per cent of the patients.

Other Procedures

Upper Pole Heminephrectomy, Partial Ureterectomy, and Ureterocele Decompression. Before the resurrection of transurethral incision, this was the procedure of choice in the majority of cases with no significant function of the upper pole and with no or minor grades of reflux. It also was utilized as the first stage of a planned two-stage procedure where ureteral reimplantation was anticipated after the ureterocele had been decompressed. In those patients who had this procedure as a planned one-stage procedure, 21 per cent required a second operative procedure.

Excision of Ureterocele, Reimplantation of Lower Pole Ureter, and Upper Pole Heminephrectomy. Some authors advocated a complete one-stage reconstructive procedure in those patients with no useful function of

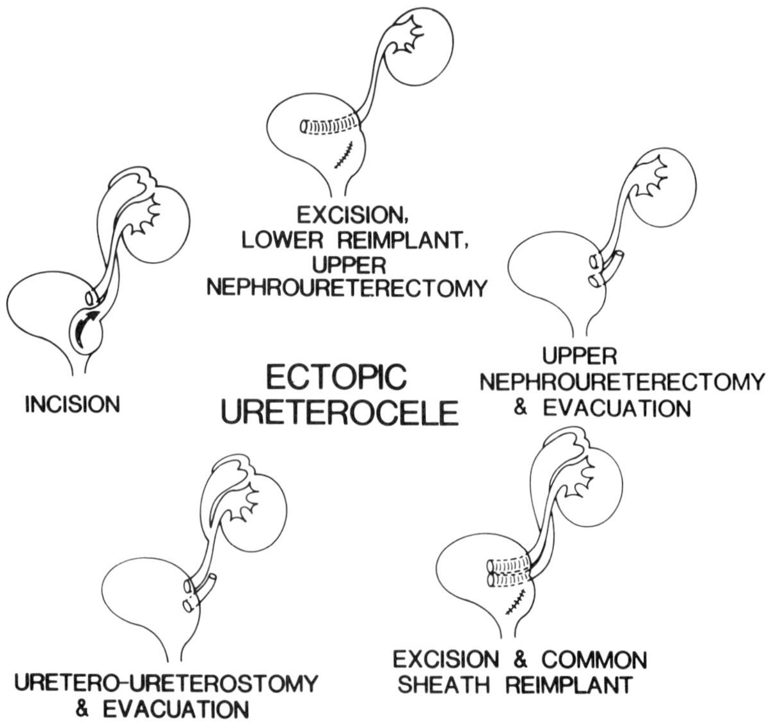

FIGURE 2. The various surgical options available to treat a patient with a ureterocele. The choice will depend on the anatomy and the pathophysiology present (see discussion in text).

the upper pole segment and severe reflux into the lower pole with poor detrusor backing. This is an extensive upper and lower reconstructive procedure in the presence of a large ureterocele and is not utilized very often today.

Ureteroureterostomy and Ureterocele Decompression. When there is significant function remaining in the upper pole segment and either no reflux or only mild to moderate reflux that stands a good chance of disappearing spontaneously, a ureteroureterostomy or ureteropyelostomy with partial upper pole ureterectomy and decompression of the ureterocele from above is a viable option.

Excision of Ureterocele and Common Sheath Reimplant. When there is significant reflux into the lower pole and some function of the upper pole, excision of the ureterocele and common sheath reimplantation may be done. Even if one or both ureters require tailoring, this can be done successfully. This also is a delicate procedure and will require extensive reconstruction of the trigone. This procedure is more suitable when there is ureterocele disproportion and the upper pole ureter is not dilated.

Total Nephroureterectomy (Rare). If the upper pole does not function secondary to obstruction and dysplasia and the lower pole does not have significant function secondary to reflux or obstruction, nephroureterectomy should be done.

CONCLUSIONS

Ureteroceles represent a wide spectrum. The choice of therapeutic options must be individualized. Transurethral incision of the ureterocele is becoming a more attractive option in selected patients.

Suggested Readings

Blyth B, Passerini-Glasel G, Camuffo C, et al: Endoscopic incision of ureteroceles: Intravesical versus ectopic. J Urol 149:556–560, 1993

Decter RM, Roth DR, Gonzales ET: Individualized treatment of ureteroceles. J Urol 142(pt 2):535–537, 1989

Scherz HC, Kaplan GW, Packer MG, et al: Ectopic ureteroceles: Surgical management with preservation of continence—review of 60 cases. J Urol 142(pt 2):538–541, 1989

Share JC, Lebowitz RL: Ectopic ureterocele without ureteral and calyceal dilatation (ureterocele disproportion): Findings on urography and sonography. AJR 152: 567, 1989

Stephens FD: Caecoureterocele and concepts on the embroyology and aetiology of ureteroceles. Aust N Z J Surg 40:239–248, 1971

Weinstein AJ, Bauer SB, Retik AB, et al: The surgical management of megaureters in duplex systems: The efficacy of ureteral tapering and common sheath reimplantation. J Urol 138:328–331, 1988

URETERAL DIVERTICULOSIS

ANTHONY ATALA, M.D.

Boston, Massachusetts

Ureteral diverticulosis refers to multiple ureteral diverticuli. This condition is extremely rare, more so than a single ureteral diverticulum. Less than 30 cases of ureteral diverticulosis have been reported in the literature. The diverticuli are usually small in size (under 5 mm).

This condition usually is diagnosed with excretory urography, particularly with the use of high-dose, high-concentration contrast agents. A few cases in the literature have been diagnosed with retrograde pyelography and none when high-dose urography, even with compression, was used. Such lesions, shown only by unphysiologic pressures, may be congenital variants with weaknesses of the ureteral wall rather than acquired conditions. Others believe that ureteral diverticulosis is a result of chronic infection alone. Currently there is no evidence to support either hypothesis.

Ureteral diverticulosis is usually asymptomatic. If symptoms do occur, they are usually the same as those associated with a single ureteral diverticulum (ureteral obstruction, hematuria, infection, and stone formation). The surgical approach depends on the location of the diverticuli and the state of the associated kidney(s). Simple diverticulectomy with a watertight reanastomosis of the ureteral wall is usually all that is necessary in the rare instances in which surgical therapy is indicated.

Suggested Readings

Hansen EI, Frost B: Multiple diverticuli of the ureter. J Urol Nephrol 12:93, 1978

Navani S, Hipona FA, Shapiro JH: Ureteral diverticulosis. Am J Roentgenol Radium Ther Nucl Med 104:364, 1968

Shoborg TW, Florence TJ: Ureteral diverticulosis. J Urol 116:107, 1976

VESICOURETERAL REFLUX IN CHILDREN

HYMAN H. RABINOVITCH, M.D.

Philadelphia, Pennsylvania

Vesicoureteral reflux (VUR) refers to the regurgitation of urine from the bladder back up to the kidney(s) and is always considered abnormal. The association of VUR, urinary tract infection (UTI), and renal scarring was first described by Hodson and Edwards in 1960. Bailey in 1973 used the term "reflux nephropathy" to describe the renal scarring associated with VUR, replacing the previously used term "chronic pyelonephritis." As seen on the intravenous urogram (IVU), reflux nephropathy can vary from mild changes of calyceal blunting or clubbing on the one hand to end-stage renal atrophy on the other. Between these two extremes, one may see focal to generalized renal scarring with loss of associated parenchyma. These changes seen on the IVU of a child are due to VUR unless proven otherwise. Failure to identify VUR on voiding cystourethrogram (VCUG) does not negate the possibility of previously present reflux that has since resolved spontaneously.

The distal ureter traverses the detrusor (intramural ureter) at the immobile base or floor of the bladder (Fig. 1). It then passes submucosally (submucosal ureter) for a distance equal to approximately five times the diameter of the ureter before it opens into the bladder as a ureteral orifice. The intravesical (intramural and submucosal) ureter is 5 mm in length at birth and elongates to reach a maximum length of 13 mm at puberty.

VUR is prevented normally by compression of the submucosal ureter against the detrusor muscle beneath it by intravesical pressure. Reflux results if the integrity of this anatomic arrangement is altered.

The classification of VUR (International Reflux Study Group) is as follows:

- Grade 1: Reflux up the ureter only
- Grade 2: Reflux to the pelvicalyceal system of the kidney without dilation
- Grade 3: Reflux to the pelvicalyceal system of the kidney with mild dilation
- Grade 4: Reflux to the pelvicalyceal system of the kidney with moderate dilation
- Grade 5: Reflux to the pelvicalyceal system of the kidney with severe dilation

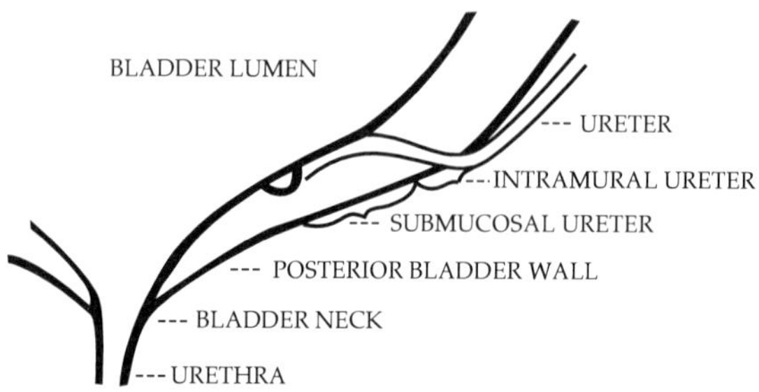

FIGURE 1. Normal ureterovesical junction.

ETIOLOGY

Primary VUR is due to congenital shortening of the submucosal ureter. The pattern of genetic transmission is unknown but it would appear to be multifactorial. It has been reported to occur in up to 45 per cent of siblings of children with reflux and is rare in black children.

The incidence of primary VUR in girls far exceeds that in boys. This may be entirely related to the fact that it usually is diagnosed on investigation following UTI, to which girls are far more susceptible. Sterile reflux is asymptomatic and, therefore, its true incidence in both boys and girls is unknown.

Secondary VUR may be a consequence of any of the following conditions:

1. Outlet obstruction
   a. Urethral valves (posterior or anterior)
   b. Urethral stricture
   c. Vesical-external sphincter dyssynergia
2. Cystitis
3. Neurogenic bladder dysfunction
4. Complete ureteral duplication
5. Ectopic ureterocele
6. Ureteral ectopia
7. Hutch diverticulum
8. Bladder exstrophy
9. Prune-belly syndrome
10. Iatrogenic (incision of ureteral orifice)

Except for two conditions that merit special comment, it is beyond the scope of this presentation to discuss the causes and management of secondary reflux.

Vesical-external sphincter dyssynergia is a common condition in children that must be recognized as a frequent cause of secondary VUR in girls and managed accordingly. It is characterized by inappropriate external sphincter contraction at the time of voiding and is, therefore, a cause for outlet obstruction. It occurs far more commonly in girls than in boys (8:1) at any time beyond the potty-training period (2½ years), with a peak incidence at age 8 years. Untreated, there is a tendency for spontaneous resolution by puberty. The diagnosis is suspected by the characteristic findings of bizarre voiding habits (frequency, urgency, diurnal incontinence, squatting and the like to hold back urination), negative physical (including neurologic) exam, and negative urinalysis. Treatment consisting of instruction in proper voiding habits and a short course of anticholinergics (Ditropan, bid) will eliminate the outlet obstruction and lead to resolution of the secondary VUR.

Cystitis, by causing edema of the bladder mucosa and thereby altering the normal ureterovesical junction (UVJ), may result in reflux in a previously marginally competent junction or, alternatively, may increase the degree of reflux of a previously incompetent UVJ. To distinguish primary VUR from that secondary to cystitis, it is important to delay the VCUG for 4 weeks following the acute UTI to allow for complete resolution of the bladder edema. This distinction is crucial because one of the indications for surgical correction of primary VUR is high-grade (4 or 5) reflux. Thus, Grade 4 or 5 VUR demonstrated during or shortly after a UTI (secondary reflux) may be downgraded to Grade 3 when studied after a 4-week infection-free period (primary VUR). Mistaking secondary for primary reflux may, in this instance, lead to unwarranted surgery.

INVESTIGATION

A voiding cystourethrogram is essential to detect VUR. The initial study should be a radiologic VCUG performed when the child has been infection free for at least 4 weeks. It will allow for accurate grading of the reflux and also rule out possible causes of secondary reflux (Hutch diverticulum, posterior urethral valves, etc.).

Follow-up studies to monitor the progress of the previously documented reflux can be by radionuclide cystogram, which delivers significantly less radiation exposure to the gonads.

Urinalysis and urine culture with sensitivities are necessary for initial diagnosis of UTI and follow-up monitoring. *Blood urea nitrogen and creatinine* levels are usually normal unless over 66 per cent of renal function has been lost.

Hypertension may be a late development of reflux nephropathy and, therefore, follow-up is essential long after the reflux has ceased, whether spontaneously or surgically. The incidence of hypertension is directly related to the extent of the renal scarring—11 per cent when the scarring is unilateral and up to 18 per cent when the scarring is bilateral.

Ultrasound of the kidneys and bladder is noninvasive and provides invaluable information about the urinary tract when performed shortly after a UTI. There is a tendency at an adult facility to obtain an ultrasound of the kidneys only for urinary tract study. This is erroneous in the case of a child, in whom both kidneys and bladder must be studied. Although a normal ultrasound does not rule out VUR, it does rule out obstructive uropathy, calculi, and the like as a cause of the UTI. A small hyperechoic kidney or distal ureteral dilation at the level of the bladder may provide a clue about the presence of VUR.

Isotope renography has replaced the IVU as a functional study of the kidneys in patients with VUR. Its advantages include:

1. No interference with visualization of the kidneys by bowel gas or content.
2. No concern for allergic reaction.
3. Provision of differential renal function.
4. More sensitive in cases of impaired renal function.
5. More sensitive in neonates beyond 4 to 6 weeks of age.

Technetium-99m diethylenetriaminepenta-acetic acid (DTPA) renal scan is used to assess differential (glomerular filtration rate) renal function. The study usually is obtained when the diagnosis of VUR is made, to establish a baseline. It should be repeated following cessation of VUR and at intervals thereafter if necessary to document the long-term effect of reflux nephropathy. Technetium-99m dimercaptosuccinic acid (DMSA) renal scan is used to evaluate the presence and degree of renal cortical scarring.

Cystoscopy is not necessary in the evaluation of a child with reflux because the endoscopic findings do not enter into management decisions. Once the decision to proceed with reimplantation has been made, however, cystoscopic examination just prior to surgery is helpful. The finding of edema and hyperemia of the bladder mucosa caused by UTI or severe trabeculation resulting from voiding dysfunction may alter the decision to proceed with surgery.

TREATMENT

Medical

Sterile reflux in the absence of outlet obstruction does not appear to lead to new or progressive renal scarring. The exception is the young child under age 4 years with a high grade (4 or 5) of reflux, who may present with renal damage even in the absence of previous documented UTI.

Medical management consists of the prevention of UTI by the use of continuous low-dose antibacterials. The antibiotics of choice for prophylaxis are either trimethoprim-sulfamethoxazole (Septra or Bactrim) or nitrofurantoin macrocrystals (Macrodantin) given as a single nightly dose. Periodic (every 4 to 6 weeks) urine checks to rule out UTI are recommended. A follow-up radionuclide cystogram is obtained on a yearly basis.

Any suggestion of voiding dysfunction must be dealt with to eliminate it as a cause of secondary reflux. Voiding five times a day (on wakening, at noon, at midday, at supper time and at bedtime) in an unhurried manner without straining is encouraged. The parent of the same sex is made responsible for "teaching" the child proper voiding technique by example. Constipation is avoided or treated if present and, in the case of girls, wiping front to back is mandatory.

In a review of 98 patients with primary VUR by the author, 41 per cent were found to have low-grade reflux (Grades 1 and 2), 19 per cent had high-grade reflux (Grades 4 and 5), and the remaining 40 per cent had intermediate reflux (Grade 3). The vast majority of those with low-grade reflux ceased spontaneously on medical management. All those with Grade 5 and most with Grade 4 reflux required surgical intervention.

Of the patients with Grade 3 reflux, 50 per cent required operation, only 12 per cent ceased spontaneously, and the remainder continued medical management at the end of the study period. The average duration to cessation of reflux in the Grade 3 group was 3 years. McLorie et al. suggested that moderate grades of VUR (Grades 3 and 4) almost always resolve within a 4-year period but are unlikely to resolve after that period.

Surgical

Surgical management by ureteroneocystostomy (ureteral reimplantation) is indicated for primary VUR if there is:

1. Failure of medical management with recurrent UTI despite antibiotic prophylaxis.
2. Noncompliance.
3. High-grade VUR—Grade 5 and possibly Grade 4.
4. Puberty, beyond which spontaneous resolution of reflux is unlikely.
5. No significant improvement in the degree of Grade 3 VUR after 3 years of medical management.

The success rate of reimplanting ureters of normal caliber in otherwise normal bladders is high (95+ per cent). Antibiotics are continued 4 to 6 weeks postoperatively, with follow-up studies (ultrasound of the abdomen and radionuclide cystogram) at 3 months postoperatively to verify the success of the surgery. A renal scan at 1 year after surgery will indicate the degree, if any, of renal damage. Follow-up renal scans at 3 and 5 years postoperatively may be considered if there is concern about progressive renal scarring. Completion of the scarring process can take up to 2 years following the acute renal insult, so the 3.8 per cent incidence of postreimplant scarring may have been due to preoperative pyelonephritis.

Although primary reflux is a frequent cause of morbidity, it is an infrequent cause of end-stage renal failure.

Suggested Readings

Bailey RR: The relationship of vesico-ureteral reflux to urinary tract infection and chronic pyelonephritis—reflux nephropathy. Clin Nephrol 1:132, 1973

Beetz R, Schulte-Wisserman H, Troger J, et al: Long term follow-up of children with surgically treated vesicoureteral reflux: Postoperative incidence of urinary tract infections, renal scars and arterial hypertension. Eur Urol 16:366, 1989

Hodson CJ, Edwards D: Chronic pyelonephritis and vesicoureteral reflux. Clin Radio.l 11:219, 1960

Hutch JA: Theory of maturation of the intravesical ureter. J Urol 86:534, 1961

International Workshop on Reflux and Pyelonephritis. J Urol 148 (5 pt II), 1992.

Kramer SA: Vesicoureteral reflux. *In* Kelalis PP, King LR, Belman AB (eds): Clinical Pediatric Urology, 3rd ed, vol 1. Philadelphia, WB Saunders, 1992, pp 441–499

McLorie GA, McKenna PH, Jumper BM, et al: High grade vesicoureteral reflux: Analysis of observational therapy. J Urol 144:537, 1990

Van den Abbeele AD, Treves ST, Lebowitz RL, et al: Vesicoureteral reflux in asymptomatic siblings of patients with known reflux: Radionuclide cystography. Pediatrics 79:147, 1987

Wallace DMA, Rothwell DL, Williams DI: The long term follow-up of surgically treated vesicoureteric reflux. Br J Urol 50:479, 1978

VESICOURETERAL REFLUX IN ADULTS

DAVID M. ALBALA, M.D.

Maywood, Illinois

Vesicoureteral reflux is a complex phenomenon involving the biomechanics of the bladder and pelvic muscles, ureteral peristalsis, urinary output, and the anatomy of the vesicoureteral junction. Much attention has been directed to vesicoureteral reflux and nephropathy in children; however, relatively few series of the disease in adults have been published. Spontaneous resolution of reflux in adults seldom can be expected, and, if the urine is infected, reflux is undoubtedly harmful. In patients with intravesical obstruction or upper motor neuron lesions, reflux acts like a water hammer, transmitting the high intervesical pressure to the kidney, which can potentially lead to corticoatrophy.

One feature of this disease in adults is the marked predominance in women. This predominance may be explained by the fact that patients with the most severe cases present with manifestations of renal failure. Milder cases of reflux are largely clinically inapparent in men, but apparent in women because of their predisposition to urinary tract infections. Symptomatic infections are more common in women. Pregnancy may be another cause of this discrepancy, because women are naturally under close medical supervision. During pregnancy, urinary tract infections, hypertension, proteinuria, and impaired renal function are likely to worsen in patients with the disease.

Although congenital factors and recurrent urinary infections have been the most commonly cited reasons for this condition, the exact cause of reflux nephropathy is unknown. Most renal scarring occurs early in childhood, and is associated with vesicoureteral reflux and infection. Although the degree of reflux nephropathy depends on the severity of vesicoureteral reflux early in life, nephropathy does not appear to depend on the frequency or pattern of late urinary tract infections or on the persistence of vesicoureteral reflux into adulthood.

Vesicoureteral reflux may be classified in several ways: according to the degree (partial or complete), according to timing (during filling or voiding, low- or high-pressure reflux), or according to the degree of associated ureterectasis. These classifications are useful primarily to define and compare the disease, because any type of reflux may be associated with gross renal changes. In adults, vesicoureteral reflux also may be categorized as either primary (congenital) or secondary (acquired). Patients with primary reflux usually have some degree of renal failure, and hypertension is common in these patients. Secondary reflux may result from previous surgery with chronic bladder contracture and infection, from interstitial cystitis or tuberculosis, or from radiation injury. This form of reflux is not usually associated with pyelonephritis or any other damage to the upper urinary tract.

The diagnosis of reflux is deceptive because the condition may be sporadic, depending on the changes in urinary output. A high urinary output can abolish reflux; the larger volume of urine transported toward the bladder by each ureteral contraction counteracts regurgitation. Derangements in muscle fibers along the transmural portion of the ureter and wide-open ureteral orifices are factors known to coexist with reflux. Little is known about the possible mechanisms involved in the development of progressive renal insufficiency in later life when scarring has occurred at an early age. Heavy proteinuria has been seen in a number of patients with vesicoureteral reflux nephropathy, and an associated vascular and glomerular lesion might play a major role in the progression to renal failure.

A history compatible with acute pyelonephritis implies the presence of vesicoureteral reflux. Persistence of recurrent cystitis in a patient should suggest the possibility of reflux. In its later stages, vesicoureteral reflux may lead to significant hypertension.

Studies performed at the Mayo Clinic suggest that unilateral vesicoureteral reflux is a relatively benign disease in adults. In adults with unilateral vesicoureteral reflux, the goal of all therapy is to maintain renal function—that is, to prevent progressive renal scarring, hypertension, and nephrolithiasis—and to avoid the morbidity associated with recurrent infections of the upper urinary tract. In patients with low-grade or infrequent urinary tract infections without any evidence of damage to the upper urinary tract, simple treatment with the antibacterial medicine is best. The strongest indication for surgical correction of unilateral vesicoureteral reflux in adults is either febrile upper urinary tract infections in either sex that cannot be controlled satisfactorily with antibiotics or unilateral vesicoureteral reflux in women of childbearing age, even if they have no trouble and are not taking medication, in whom pyelonephritis would pose a major risk to the fetus and mother.

Surgical correction of vesicoureteral reflux in patients with severely damaged kidneys does not seem to halt the progress of renal damage. However, those individuals with damaged but only slightly abnormal renal function benefit significantly from surgical correction of the reflux. An antireflux operation may decrease the occurrence of urinary tract infections from 75 to 10 per cent. When recurrent urinary tract infections persist postoperatively, however, prophylactic antibiotic therapy should be instituted. The possible surgical complication of contralateral vesicoureteral reflux also should be considered and discussed with these patients before surgery. Twenty-five per cent of patients are likely to have this complication and only about 10 per cent require an antireflux operation for the contralateral side. Therefore, the apparently nonrefluxing orifice should be evaluated carefully preoperatively. If there is a history of bilateral vesicoureteral reflux or the orifice on the nonrefluxing side appears to be marginally competent and the kidney is scarred, a bilateral antireflux operation may be considered. Surgical reimplantation may be accomplished through a number of techniques in which the surgeon develops a submucosal tunnel. The many procedures applicable to children also may be used in adults.

The presence or absence of proteinuria seems to be an excellent indicator of overall renal function associated with vesicoureteral reflux. Proteinuria greater than 1.5 gm/24 hours, especially in association with renal scarring and decreased renal function, is indicative of progressive reflux nephropathy. Under these circumstances, antireflux surgery is rarely justified or beneficial unless recurrent symptomatic pyelonephritis becomes uncontrollable.

In summary, vesicoureteral reflux should be suspected not only in patients with clinical pyelonephritis, but also in those with recurrent cystitis, asymptomatic bacterial infections, or urinary tract infections during pregnancy. Radiologically evident nephropathy cannot be reversed, but progressive renal damage and urinary tract infection may be arrested through effective treatment.

Suggested Readings

Guthman DA, Malek RS, Neves RJ, et al: Vesicoureteral reflux in the adult. V. Unilateral disease. J Urol 146:21, 1991

Malek RS, Svensson J, Neves RJ, et al: Vesicoureteral reflux in the adult. III. Surgical correction: Risk and benefits. J Urol 130:882, 1983

Malek RS, Svensson JP, Torres VE: Vesicoureteral reflux in the adult. I. Nephropathy hypertension and stones. J Urol 130:37, 1983

Neves RJ, Torres VE, Malek RS, et al: Vesicoureteral reflux in the adult. IV. Medical versus surgical management. J Urol 132:882, 1984

Torres VE, Malek RS, Svensson JP: Vesicoureteral reflux in the adult. II. Nephropathy hypertension and stones. J Urol 130:41, 1983

URETERAL INJURIES

LESTER PERSKY, M.D.

Tampa, Florida

Ureteral injuries often are considered to be an uncommon entity. However, with increasing violence in the cities and with experience garnered from recent armed conflicts, including the Vietnam War, it is obvious that the ureter is injured more frequently by external violence than previously suspected. Such injuries often are overlooked at the time of surgery, elective or emergency. The attending surgeon usually must pay attention to a host of other problems: bleeding, ruptured viscera, and a field contaminated by feces and external matter brought into the abdomen by missiles. It is easy, therefore, to miss a thin tubular structure that lies behind the peritoneal cavity and that ordinarily is protected by overlying sheltering viscera, by its diminutive nature, and by its elasticity.

In the Vietnam War, a review of all the fatalities associated with a variety of organ disruptions revealed that injuries to the ureter were associated with the highest mortality. This seemed to stem from the fact that the ureter is so readily forgotten, often neglected, and not searched for. The injuries usually are not discovered until sepsis, fever, or urinary drainage has occurred. In civilian life, the patient who is having a pelvic laparotomy is prey to disruption of the ureter by a variety of surgical misadventures—for example, ligatures, tranfixions of a portion of the ureter, division, angulation, and excision of all or part of it. All of these things can occur, and, if neglected or discovered late, ultimate loss of the kidney may ensue. If bilateral ureteral injuries occur, anuria is apparent. The presence of anuria, of course, leads to immediate attention on the part of the surgeon and attending physicians, so that repair is attempted and usually accomplished immediately. Ordinarily, great success attends those efforts that are carried out at the time of surgery. If one can discover the ureteral injury before extravasation, reaction, and infection develop, it is possible to accomplish immediate restoration of continuity of the urinary tract in various ways.

DIAGNOSIS

The symptoms attending an overlooked ureteral injury are the same for both military and civilian injuries as well as for those stemming from external trauma or of iatrogenic origin. The trauma can be penetrating or blunt. Although the latter is infrequent, the ureter can be disrupted without what appears to be significant external force to the patient. When such injuries are overlooked, the patient most often will have a degree of ileus out of proportion to the extent of the previous surgery. Such a patient will have fever and flank pain, which often is disregarded because of the recent surgical procedure with attendant pain in the area of the incision. The patient may well have extravasation of urine with abdominal swelling and with an abdomen silent to auscultation. With further prolongation of the overlooked injury, actual seepage of urine will occur and give a clue as to the existing train of events.

Diagnosis rests now on recognizing the site of extravasation of urine. This is often best and most readily diagnosed by the use of excretory urography in the postoperative period when injury is suspected. Excretory urography may reveal the actual extravasation, may show poor visualization, or may simply show some dilation with hydronephrosis and a poorly visualized ureter. Ultrasound will reveal a distended pelvis and ureter and a fluid collection. Computerized tomography also may reveal a collection of urine and obstruction.

PREVENTIVE MEASURES

The frequently repeated admonition about an ounce of prevention is worth a pound of cure is especially applicable to ureteral injuries. In the course of an anticipated difficult surgical procedure in the true pelvis, whether it be gynecologic, surgical, or even urologic, it is wise to have indwelling ureteral catheters placed and left in situ during the procedure so that the surgeon, during the course of exploring a complex surgical situation, can readily palpate the ureter with its identifying stent. It is difficult to palpate a ureter without such an indwelling tube.

There is discussion about contractility and the suggestive rigidity of the ureter and its tubular nature when palpated by experienced hands. This is a difficult thing to do and not recommended for the individual surgeon unless he or she has had a great deal of experience with such maneuvers and is familiar with the course and location of the ureters.

SURGICAL REPAIR

As stated earlier, best results in the correction of a ureteral injury, whether it be a partial tear, crushing, laceration, disruption, or excision of an actual segment of the ureter, occur with immediate intraoperative repair. Sometimes the discovery of a possible ureteral tear is facilitated by the use of indigo carmine dye intraoperatively. The dye can be given intravenously and the field of surgery observed for possible extravasation as evidenced by the appearance of the typical blue urine. At times, the surgeon, if worried about the possible crushing of the ureter by a hemostatic clamp or concerned about actually ligating the ureter, may have to expose the ureter and trace it down to the operative field to make sure of its continuity. When the ureter has been crushed by a hemostat, it is possible to remove the offending instrument and inspect the area. The surgeon may then elect to stent the area of injury. This can be done currently with the use of intraoperative J-tubes, which can be plucked out later at cystoscopy. Such modern stenting devices have helped a great deal and provide security to the occasional surgeon. Leakage may be obviated by the use of an indwelling stent, which certainly should be placed if there is any doubt in the surgeon's mind as to the integrity of the restoration of ureteral continuity.

In the course of all these repairs, whether with or without stenting, one's judgment as to the state of the traumatized ureteral ends is important. If one thinks that any tension exists with the repair, steps should be taken to eliminate this possibility. The ends can be approximated with interrupted, fine atraumatic chromic catgut sutures, which should be placed through the full thickness of the ureteral wall and achieve a watertight closure. The ureter may be spatulated; it can be vented in order to widen the area of anastomosis. We believe that tension should be avoided at all costs so that the repair is done atraumatically. Again, in this primary repair of transected ureters, the use of a stent can be of great help. We believe that, if possible, such a foreign body should be avoided; however, if one has any qualms about the capability to repair this, or if worried about the state of the anastomosis, a stent is advisable. All areas of possible extravasation should be drained extraperitoneally with a soft rubber drain so that no intraperitoneal or extraperitoneal accumulation develops to threaten and jeopardize the integrity of the ureter. To avoid tension, the kidney may be mobilized downward or the bladder up by a psoas hitch.

If one thinks that the lower segment of a divided ureter is of questionable length or viability, the ureter should be reimplanted. A variety of techniques are available. Usually a modified Politano-Leadbetter anastomosis can be accomplished without difficulty. At times, if there has been a substantial loss of length of the lower end of the ureter, some form of Boari flap can be used in order to gain several additional centimeters to help bridge the gap. When mobilizing the ureter, the location of the blood supply is of great importance. In the upper portion of the ureter the vessels to the ureter enter medially; in the lower third access is made laterally. Antireflux anastomoses are the most desirable; however, when the patient's condition does not warrant it, and it is imperative to complete the reanastomosis quickly, a simple fishmouth anastomosis can be done with or without a stenting catheter. A quick repair directly into the dome or side of the bladder can be accomplished with a great deal of success. Occasionally, it may be necessary to do a psoas hitch to give added length. A psoas hitch in conjunction with a Boari flap can achieve a surprising length and will avoid any tension at the reimplantation site.

MEDICAL MANAGEMENT

For many years it was believed that ureteral injuries should be repaired only after there has been an opportunity to decompress the kidney. Certainly, if the patient is sick, febrile, and has an infected hydronephrosis, the better part of valor is to drain the kidney proximal to the obstruction. This now can be done without need for a formal surgical nephrostomy. Percutaneous efforts have been successful in draining obstructed, septic, distended kidneys. Such procedures can be accomplished with great facility in the hands of experienced radiologists or urologists using ultrasound and fluoroscopy. If this effort fails, it may be necessary to do an open nephrostomy. In many situations, if a ligature has been placed around the ureter, immediate re-exploration will relieve the obstruction secondary to the surgical tie and obviate the need for proximal decompression or formal reanastomosis. Also, in some instances, what appears to be an impassable obstruction or angulation can be bypassed at cystoscopy with passage of a ureteral catheter from below. All these steps are part of the management of patients with ureteral injuries. The use of appropriate antibacterials, the proper administration of fluids, and the overall maintenance of good homeostasis for the patient are imperative.

TRAUMATIC INJURY

When the ureter has been damaged by high-velocity missiles, it is important to determine the extent of the impaired devascularized tissue that will have to be sacrificed. This may be difficult to determine on the operating table. In such situations, we think that the kidney should be drained proximally with a nephrostomy tube and that a stent should be used to help maintain the continuity of the ureter. Often what appears to be a dismal situation may be salvaged. It is important, however, to realize that, when ureteral injuries are extensive and great lengths of ureter have been lost, the urologic surgeon does have several options.

A segment of ileum can be used to bridge the gap between the proximal ureter and the bladder. This is a successful operation and should be familiar to all urologists. Autotransplantation is another alternative that permits a kidney to be saved, bringing it to the true bony pelvis and reconstructing a complete renal unit even though a great length of ureter has been lost. Third, it is important to remember that a defect in the ureter that appears to be impossible to correct can be handled by a transureteroureterostomy, thus salvaging an otherwise irretrievably lost kidney. These techniques should be used only when a length of ureter has been lost and if the patient's condition warrants it. Occasionally, these can be done immediately; otherwise, proximal decompression with later resolution of the problem can be done in any of the aforementioned ways when the situation has been stabilized and the patient's condition is optimal.

CONCLUSION

Ureteral injuries are a challenge, mostly because they are easily overlooked. Efforts to use foreign materials or anatomic structures other than the ileum to replace the ureter generally have been unsuccessful. However, with perseverance and care, most situations can be rectified, an intact genitourinary tract achieved, and litigious actions avoided.

Suggested Readings

Spirnak P, Hempel N, Resnick M: Ureteral injuries complicating vascular surgery—is repair indicated? J Urol 141:13, 1989

Spirnak P, Resnick M, Persky L: Management of civilian gunshot wounds: Review of 8 cases. J Urol 134:733, 1985

URETERAL TUMORS

R. ERNEST SOSA, M.D.

New York, New York

The optimal management for transitional cell carcinoma (TCC) of the upper urinary tract is considered to be nephroureterectomy with excision of a bladder cuff. However, retrospective studies of patients treated by nephroureterectomy have revealed that the grade and stage of a urothelial tumor decide the malignancy's biologic potential. Similar results can be obtained in the treatment of low-grade malignancies with conservative or radical surgery. The aggressive natural history of high-grade TCC does not have a more favorable outcome with radical surgery. At present, several therapeutic options are available for the management of ureteral TCC. This article reviews the rationale for selecting conservative versus radical surgery for the treatment of ureteral tumors.

Primary TCC of the ureter often represents a diagnostic and therapeutic challenge. Clinical confirmation of a ureteral malignancy in patients with unilateral hematuria, flank pain, or a lucent ureteral filling defect was difficult in the preureteroscopy era. Current evaluation for ureteral TCC includes the history, physical examination, voided cytologies, and one or more of the following imaging modalities: excretory urography, retrograde pyelography, computerized tomography, ultrasonography, and possibly magnetic resonance imaging. The definitive diagnosis is made by direct inspection of the lesion and pathologic evaluation of selective cytologies and/or a sample of the tumor. Ureteroscopy facilitates inspection and biopsy of a lesion for stage and grade. Adjacent and remote urothelium also may be biopsied for mapping studies.

A rigid ureteroresectoscope, which is similar to a standard resectoscope, is used to biopsy the ureteral urothelium. Alternatively, a small stone basket can extract a tumor on a thin pedicle, or a cold-cup biopsy forceps can be used to sample a tumor. The latter device may be more useful for learning the grade of a ureteral TCC than its stage. It is advisable to have the pathologist in the operating room to view the gross appearance of the primary tumor and to process the small tissue samples.

The lower ureter is more stable than the upper ureter for ureteroscopic manipulation. It is enclosed in Waldeyer's sheath, and it is backed by the detrusor muscle in the submucosal portion. Biopsies adequate to establish the grade and stage of the tumor usually may be obtained. The base of the lesion and immediate surrounding urothelium should be fulgurated by electrocautery or laser. In contrast, ureteroscopic access of the upper ureter is more difficult to attain. The ureter is not as well supported for biopsy. A flexible ureteroscope is often necessary for inspection of an upper ureteral TCC. A cold-cup biopsy forceps or a brush can be used under visual guidance to sample a lesion.

Primary TCC of the ureter is not common. Tumors of the upper urinary tract represent 5 per cent of all urothelial tumors. Ureteral tumors account for no more than 25 per cent of upper tract TCCs. Patients with a primary upper tract TCC have a 40 to 80 per cent risk of subsequent formation of a similar neoplasm in the bladder, and a 2 to 4 per cent risk of developing a tumor in the contralateral collecting system. High-grade tumors are more likely to display multicentricity than low-grade tumors (23 per cent for Grade 1 tumors vs. 37 per cent for Grade 2 tumors). Moreover, an increased incidence of abnormalities has been documented in the adjacent and remote urothelium as the stage and grade of a primary tumor increase. Tumors of higher anatomic origin also are associated with a greater likelihood of multicentricity. Thus, recurrence rates are likely to increase when high-grade tumors or tumors in higher locations are managed with conservative surgery.

Survival and recurrence rates are similar for low-grade distal ureteral lesions managed by segmental resection of the ureter with a neovesical reimplant or by nephroureterectomy. Lesions of the lower ureter are well suited for endoscopic resection. First, they are readily accessible for diagnosis, treatment, and periodic surveillance; second, the distal ureter is thick walled and stable, permitting adequate biopsy and resection; third, multicentricity is less frequent; fourth, recurrence rates with segmental resection are on the order of 15 per cent; and fifth, if surveillance fails, surgical excision can be performed. In fact, in several series, endoscopic resection of distal ureteral lesions has been reported to be associated with recurrence rates of 15 per cent.

Tumors in the upper ureter should be treated by nephroureterectomy. These malignancies are difficult to reach ureteroscopically. Multicentricity is more probable and recurrence rates are higher than for lesions of the lower ureter. A solitary low-grade tumor could be considered for treatment by segmental excision or possibly by ureteroscopic means if mapping studies prove the adjacent and remote urothelium to be free of disease and if periodic surveillance is possible. Patients managed by renal-sparing techniques are at risk for local and distal urothelial recurrences. Therefore, close follow-up should include cystoscopy with bladder and ureteral washings every 3 months and a periodic pyelogram.

The ureteroscope is a useful tool for surveillance of the ureter following removal of a TCC by segmental or ureteroscopic resection. Ureteroscopy of the upper ureter is reserved for further evaluation of suspicious cytology studies and ureteral filling defects. The lower ureter can be inspected with a miniaturized ureteroscope at the time of follow-up cystoscopy. Recurrent lesions must be biopsied and not just fulgurated. Evidence of progression of the grade and stage of a tumor, or formation of a ureteral stricture that prevents periodic surveillance, or unsatisfactory patient compliance are indications to abandon conservative management and perform a nephroureterectomy.

Ureteroscopic surveillance of the distal ureter also may be indicated in patients with multifocal superficial tumors of the bladder. Retrospective studies at Memorial Sloan Kettering Cancer Center strongly suggest that this subgroup of patients is at an increased risk for developing distal ureteral tumors. Thirty-five per cent of 109 cystectomy specimens with diffuse bladder disease had evidence of carcinoma in situ (CIS) in the excised distal ureters. Moreover, 15 of 66 patients with CIS who responded to intravesical BCG developed CIS in the distal ureter in 13 to 30 months. In patients who were "cured" of multifocal bladder tumors with BCG, 4 out of 24 developed distal ureteral tumors.

In conclusion, rigid and flexible ureteroscopy facilitates the diagnosis and surveillance of primary ureteral TCC. Carefully selected patients with ureteral tumors may derive benefit from ureteroscopic resection. The ideal patient for renal-sparing management of ureteral TCC has a distal ureteral lesion that is monocentric, of low grade and stage, and with normal adjacent and remote urothelium and negative urine cytologies. However, conservative therapy for ureteral TCC may be appropriate in other clinical settings, when local control of the disease can be ascertained. Periodic surveillance of the upper urinary tract must be technically possible and scheduled to take place at regular intervals. If surveillance is not possible or if the lesion progresses in stage or grade, nephroureterectomy must be performed.

Suggested Readings

Blute ML, Segura JW, Patterson DE, et al: Impact of endourology on diagnosis and management of upper urinary tract urothelial cancer. J Urol 141:1298–1301, 1989

Huffman JL: Ureteroscopic management of transitional cell carcinoma of the upper urinary tract. Urol Clin North Am 15:419–424, 1988

Huffman JL, Bagley DH, Lyon ES, et al: Endoscopic diagnosis and treatment of upper-tract urothelial tumors. Cancer 55:1422–1428, 1985

Klotz L: Management of ureothelial carcinoma of the upper tracts. A.U.A. Update Series, Vol 7, Lesson 4, 1988

Mazeman E: Tumors of the upper urinary tract calyces, renal pelvis and ureter. Eur Urol 2:120, 1976

McCarron JP, Mills C, Vaughan ED Jr: Tumors of the renal pelvis and ureter: Current concepts and management. Semin Urol 1:79–81, 1983

SURGERY OF THE URETERAL STUMP

JOHN A. BELIS, M.D.
Hershey, Pennsylvania

EPIDEMIOLOGY

A ureteral stump is usually left after a radical nephrectomy for renal carcinoma or nephrectomy for benign conditions. Because of the known incidence of recurrent transitional cell carcinoma in the lower ureter following nephrectomy for transitional cell carcinoma of the kidney, the entire ureter is removed with the kidney. After nephroureterectomy for transitional cell carcinoma of the kidney, a tumor recurrence may occur if a bladder cuff is not taken and the intramural ureter is not removed. The incidence of recurrence of transitional cell carcinoma in the ureteral stump has been reported to range from 30 to 50 per cent and appears to increase with the length of ureter left behind. If it is elected to leave the ureteral stump in these patients, they should be followed with retrograde ureterograms at the time of bladder tumor checks with cystoscopy.

When nephrectomy is performed for indications other than transitional cell carcinoma, a complete ureterectomy usually is not performed because of the low incidence of complications from the retained distal ureter and the necessity of an extended incision or a second incision to remove the distal ureter. Although the distal ureteral stump seldom causes a problem, approximately 1 per cent of patients will develop complications in the ureteral stump after simple nephrectomy for conditions such as pyonephrosis or loss of kidney function secondary to obstruction, calculi, or tuberculosis. Because of the potential for recurrent infection when a calculus in the ureter or ureteral stricture is the reason for nephrectomy, the ureter above the obstruction should be removed at the time of nephrectomy. When a ureteral stump remains, pathologic conditions may develop many years after the initial nephrectomy.

NATURAL HISTORY

The natural history of pathologic conditions of the ureteral stump may take many forms:

1. The ureteral stump can act as a vesical diverticulum.
2. Reflux of urine into the ureteral stump accompanied by poor drainage may lead to ureteritis and urosepsis.
3. The ureteral stump with reflux may develop a wound sinus or cutaneous fistula.
4. Inflammation and pyoureter may develop secondary to retained distal ureteral calculi or strictures. Secondary stone formation may develop in a poorly drained ureteral stump. Poorly opacified lower ureteral calculi may be overlooked at the time of nephrectomy. When calculus disease is the reason for nephrectomy, the entire ureter should be evaluated by retrograde or antegrade pyelography to rule out this possibility.
5. Primary tumors may arise in the ureteral stump, with an increased incidence of squamous carcinoma as well as transitional carcinoma. There appears to be an increased incidence of transitional cell carcinoma in ureteral stumps of patients with known recurrent superficial bladder transitional carcinoma. A complete ureterectomy should be considered at the time of nephrectomy for benign conditions in this group of patients.

CLINICAL PRESENTATION

The signs and symptoms of pathologic conditions of the ureteral stump may be confusing and nondiagnostic. They include obscure abdominal or suprapubic pain, sepsis, and recurrent fever. These signs and symptoms may mimic gastrointestinal or gynecologic conditions. The differential diagnosis initially includes diverticulitis, appendicitis, pelvic inflammatory disease, ovarian cysts, and biliary disease. The most common presentation for pathologic conditions of the ureteral stump is urosepsis. This may be associated with retained or new calculi in the stump, ureteral stricture, and subsequent empyema. Other conditions include massive reflux into the stump, recurrent urinary tract infections with voiding symptoms, ureteritis cystica, strictured ectopic ureter with vaginal discharge, and tuberculous ureteritis. Primary tumors of the ureteral stump may present with gross hematuria. Urinalysis will reveal pyuria or microhematuria in most patients, and urine cultures frequently will be positive in nonmalignant conditions. The ureteral stump may be difficult to catheterize at cystoscopy. Retrograde ureterography may reveal stricture, calculi, or tumors. Urinary tract infection or sepsis may preclude the performance of retrograde ureterography. A voiding cystourethrogram may demonstrate vesicoureteral reflux.

SURGICAL PROCEDURES

Three surgical techniques may be considered: laparoscopy, ablation in situ, and open surgery. Removal of a ureteral stump may be difficult because of periureteral inflammation and fibrosis. If carcinoma is present in the ureteral stump, open surgical excision should be performed.

Laparoscopic ureterectomy may be attempted after nephrectomy for benign conditions, including distal ureteral calculi, strictures, and reflux. The laparoscopic approach also may be used for ureterectomy after radical nephrectomy for renal parenchymal masses that have the radiographic characteristics of renal cell carcinoma but subsequently are found to be transitional cell carcinoma on pathologic examination. Depending on the length of ureter to be excised, a laparoscopic camera port and four additional ports are placed in the abdomen on the side of the involved ureter. The patient is placed in the modified flank position to permit intra-abdominal contents to fall away from the involved ureter. The colon on the involved side is reflected. Instrumentation into the ureter via cystoscopy using catheters or ureteroscopes is often necessary to aid in the identification of the ureter. The ureter is excised as closely as possible to the bladder and divided between surgical clips. The specimen is removed through a 10-mm port.

Endoscopic ablation of the ureteral stump has been described after nephrectomy for ectopic ureters or ureteroceles. A common method is to fulgurate the epithelium of the ureteral stump with electrocautery. This can be performed prophylactically or later if clinically indicated. The procedure has been described primarily for use in children. Other conditions for which this approach may be applicable include megaureter after nephrectomy for nonfunction and destruction of the distal part of a ureterocele during an excisional procedure to preserve urinary continence.

Open surgical removal of the ureteral stump remains the most common surgical approach. It also may be used when laparoscopy is unavailable or is unsuccessful. Open surgery is required when periureteral inflammation and fibrosis are extensive, when urosepsis and pyoureter are present, or when there is a tumor in the ureteral stump.

The surgical technique may require two incisions if the entire ureter remains. Distal ureteral stumps may be approached through lower abdominal midline, Gibson, or Pfannenstiel incisions. The ureter generally can be excised by an extraperitoneal approach. The ureter is excised as closely as possible to the ureterovesical junction and ligated with 2-0 absorbable suture. If complete ureteral excision is required, a cystotomy is performed, with excision of bladder cuff and closure of the bladder with 2-0 absorbable suture. When infection is present or the bladder has been opened, a drain should be used. Results after excision of ureteral stumps find 67 per cent cured, but cystitis may persist and a few patients may have recurrent sepsis.

Suggested Readings

Ehrlich RM, Koyle MA, Shanberg AM: A technique for ureteral stump ablation. J Urol 140:1240, 1988

Kavoussi LR, Clayman RV, Brunt LM, et al: Laparoscopic ureterolysis. J Urol 147:426, 1992

Pollack HM, Banner MP, Popky GL: Radiologic evaluation of the ureteral stump. Radiology 144:225, 1982

Summers J, Wilkerson J, Foster S: Transitional cell carcinoma in a residual ureter after nephrectomy for infection. J Urol 108:246, 1972

URETEROVAGINAL FISTULA

GILBERT ROSS, Jr., M.D.

Columbia, Missouri

Ureteral injuries leading to a ureterovaginal fistula generally occur as a consequence of pelvic operations for benign or malignant disease, which include an abdominal hysterectomy. A smaller number of ureteral injuries (10 to 15 per cent) result from vaginal hysterectomy. During any pelvic operation, the ureter necessarily must be visualized to avoid injury by clamping, cutting, or ligation in the areas where it is most vulnerable to injury. Many ureteral injuries occur as a consequence of urgent attempts to obtain hemostasis without being able to visualize the ureter in a bloody surgical field. Other risk factors include distorted pelvic anatomy from prior surgical procedures or radiation therapy; large pelvic masses, particularly ovarian, which displace the ureter medially; and skeletonization of the ureter, which may occur with radical hysterectomy from damage to the ureteral sheath. Many intraoperative injuries occur at the pelvic brim, in attempts to remove large ovarian masses.

Loss in the continuity of the ureter may result from division or laceration, or from ischemic necrosis related to clamping, ligation, or damage to the blood supply of the ureter. The nature of the injury will determine the subsequent clinical presentation. There may be flank pain, an abdominal or pelvic mass, prolonged ileus, abdominal distention, or urine leakage through the abdominal incision or the vaginal cuff. Roughly 25 per cent of ureteral injuries lead to a ureterovaginal fistula. In this instance, the leakage may become apparent almost immediately or, more commonly, after a delay of a few days or even several weeks or longer. Urine may puddle in the pelvis, leading to urinoma formation, and the drainage may be skimpy or profuse, continuous or intermittent. Various combinations of ureterovaginal and vesicovaginal fistulas may be encountered, and ureteral injury with or without a ureterovaginal fistula may be unilateral or bilateral.

Although many patients may be singularly asymptomatic except for urine leakage, if there is sepsis and the patient is in a catabolic state, the initial treatment should consist of good nutritional support, often including parenteral hyperalimentation, and prompt temporary urinary diversion.

PREVENTION

There is no general agreement on the need for preoperative excretory urography, but if there is a large pelvic mass, malignancy, or prior radiation therapy or surgery, there is a clear need for imaging studies of the urinary tract to determine the course of the ureters. Despite the very low incidence of unintentional injuries to the ureter during gynecologic procedures (0.5 per cent), injuries do occur. If recognized and dealt with immediately, a subsequent ureterovaginal fistula and possible reconstructive surgery will be avoided. Some surgeons find the preoperative placement of ureteral catheters helpful for ureteral identification on a case-by-case basis. At the very least, if they are easily removed at the end of the procedure, a tight ureteral ligation can be excluded. Should ureteral repair be necessary, only absorbable sutures should be used, either chromic catgut or one of the synthetics such as polyglycolic acid in a size commensurate with the tissue strength and tension required.

During the operative procedure, if there is even a hint that the ureter has been lacerated, and direct inspection cannot resolve the issue, indigo carmine dye and furosemide should be administered intravenously so that a small leak might be identified. Small lacerations may be closed with interrupted 4-0 chromic catgut sutures and drained extraperitoneally. Larger lacerations should be stented for 2 to 3 weeks as well as being drained. Occasionally, uncertainty about ureteral integrity, when there is the possibility of either a ligation or laceration, can be resolved only by passing a catheter through the area in question. One may use cystoscopy and ureteral catheterization but, even in the era of flexible cystoscopy, it is often more expeditious to open the bladder and pass a ureteral catheter retrogradely, replacing it with a ureteral stent if needed.

If the ureter has been clamped or ligated without a substantial amount of periureteral tissue, it is best to assume that the ureter has a reasonable chance of becoming ischemic and deal with the problem definitively to avoid ureteral injury. In this instance, or in circumstances in which the ureter has been divided completely, the level of injury dictates the surgical approach. If the juxtavesical ureter is involved, a ureteroneocystostomy is easily performed. Sometimes, a pull-through reimplantation is both possible and convenient. This leaves the ureteral orifice in its normal position, because the distal ureter is pulled into the bladder through the bed of the old intravesical ureter. Alternatively, a combined extra- and intravesical variation of the Politano-Leadbetter procedure may be utilized, with the development of an intravesical submucosal tunnel.

Currently, we prefer a totally extravesical reimplantation on the anterolateral side of the bladder, as described by Barry. Advantages are its simplicity and the fact that it generally requires less ureteral length and avoids cystostomy. Its major shortcoming is the considerable difficulty that may be encountered in retrograde catheterization. Two 2-cm parallel incisions about 3 cm apart are made perpendicular to the anticipated course of the ureter and deepened to expose the mucosa, which is then dissected free from the overlying flap of muscle and adventitia. The ureter is drawn distally beneath this flap, the distal mucosa is opened, and a direct anastomosis between the full thickness of the ureter and the mucosa of the bladder is performed using running 4-0 chromic catgut. During the anastomosis, a feeding tube should bridge the ureterovesical junction until the last stitch or two is taken to eliminate any possibility of mechanical obstruction. The distal portion of the isolated myoadventitial flap is then approximated to the adjacent bladder wall on top of the ureteral anastomosis using 3-0 chromic catgut, taking care to avoid compression. Uncomplicated ureteroneocystostomy does not require ureteral stenting, but the bladder should be drained with a catheter for 3 to 4 days.

If the ureteral injury is some distance above the bladder, precluding a tension-free anastomosis, any form of reimplantation may be augmented with a psoas hitch using heavy, long-lasting, absorbable polydioxanone suture. If the injury is high in the pelvic ureter without any substantial ureteral loss below that level, ureteroureterostomy is the treatment of choice. It is a simple matter to débride the ends of the proximal and distal ureteral segments, spatulate them, and perform an elliptical anastomosis with fine 4-0 chromic catgut in an interrupted fashion. The anastomosis should be drained and stented for 2 to 3 weeks using a double-J stent. Alternatively, if there has been extensive loss of the pelvic ureter below the level of injury, a bladder flap repair or transureteroureterostomy may be necessary.

INITIAL MANAGEMENT

When suspected urine leakage is first encountered, the surgeon should exclude the possibility of a vesicovaginal fistula by forcefully filling the bladder with dilute methylene blue or indigo carmine and noting the failure to subsequently obtain bluish-tinged fluid on a vaginal tampon. Excretion of such discolored urine after a subsequent injection of 5 ml of indigo carmine intravenously is prima facie evidence of a ureteral-vaginal communication. However, this maneuver does not define whether the injury is unilateral or bilateral, and a vesicovaginal fistula does not exclude the possibility of a concomitant ureterovaginal fistula. Excretory urography may show virtually any degree of hydronephrosis and delay in excretion, as well as extravasation in the pelvis and contrast in the vagina. Paradoxically, the injured side actually may show less dilation than the presumably normal contralateral side, if there is free drainage from the site of injury.

Although the success rate of retrograde catheterization in bypassing the site of fistulization is low, it should be attempted following ureterograms to define the site and extent of the injury and to exclude ureteral ligation. Unless there is absolute certainty that the contralateral side is normal, it is best to do bilateral ureterograms. If retrograde stenting with a guidewire and double-J stent is successful, this is all for the best, but often percutaneous nephrostomy will be required to obtain proximal drainage. Alternatively, exploration and a definitive repair may be undertaken at that time.

There are no hard or fast rules with regard to the exact timing of such an early definitive repair. It should perhaps be most strongly considered in instances in which there is a suspected total loss of ureteral continuity on one or both sides, which is identified in a patient who is in good general condition within 72 hours of the original procedure. If the patient is in tenuous condition, or if there is some uncertainty regarding the extent of the injury, percutaneous nephrostomy will relieve any urgency about dealing with the matter definitively. There is a natural tendency toward procrastination, because such injuries may be partial, permitting antegrade stenting after the establishment of a percutaneous nephrostomy. The nephrostomy and/or stent may permit spontaneous closure of the fistula in a number of such patients, avoiding a reconstructive surgical procedure.

Regrettably, it is impossible to anticipate which partial ureteral injuries with a fistula will heal while stented, and for that matter, in whom a stricture will develop. Nonetheless, if the patient is dry with a percutaneous nephrostomy alone, or a nephrostomy and stent, it appears reasonable to persist for about 4 weeks before removing the stent and clamping the nephrostomy tube. If there is persistent leakage, or evidence of obstruction manifested by flank pain or high renal pelvic pressures, surgical correction will be necessary. If the patient is not dry despite a functioning percutaneous nephrostomy and/or stent, there is little reason to wait longer than 3 weeks before proceeding with repair, because much of the early postoperative reaction will have subsided by that time.

SURGICAL OPTIONS

Most ureteral injuries with a ureterovaginal fistula can be managed by simple ureteral reimplantation or ureteroureterostomy. Working through an extraperitoneal approach, the surgeon should begin the dissection above the level of the injury and trace the ureter distally until it disappears into the necrotic mass or is inexorably entrapped in fibrous reaction. If ureteral length is inadequate for a tension-free intravesical reimplantation, an extravesical procedure still may be possible, or a psoas hitch may be included with either procedure. Although our past experience suggests that a direct, and potentially refluxing anastomosis, which perforce requires less ureteral length, is well tolerated if the kidney, ureter, and bladder are intrinsically normal, it is best to avoid reflux if at all possible by the use of a tunnel.

In an unirradiated field, the use of a bladder flap can compensate for more extensive ureteral losses on one or both sides. In most instances, bladder capacity is generally adequate to replace the entire pelvic ureter. If there is a substantial loss of lower ureter on both sides, the side of the longest residual segment of viable ureter should be bridged with the bladder flap and the opposite ureter swung across to create a transureteroureterostomy.

In performing a bladder flap repair, the dome of the bladder is extraperitonealized using the posterolateral aspect of the bladder as a base for about a 4-cm bladder flap, which is outlined running toward the anterior contralateral side of the bladder, narrowing slightly at the tip. If greater length is required, the flap may be made in a spiral circumferential fashion. The flap should be fixed to the psoas muscle to relieve potential tension. It is best to do an antireflux anastomosis with a submucosal tunnel placed near the tip of the flap if possible. The ureter is drawn through the flap wall and advanced through a 3-cm submucosal tunnel, where it is then spatulated and sutured down with interrupted 4-0 chromic catgut. If a submucosal tunnel cannot be developed, the ureter should be advanced into a 3-cm trough and sutured to adjacent bladder mucosa (and a bit of muscle) with 3-0 or 4-0 chromic catgut. A ureteral stent is left in place, and the flap closed in two layers with two 3-0 chromic catgut sutures contiguous with the closure of the bladder. A suprapubic tube and urethral catheter both should be used to drain the bladder, with the area drained and, although admittedly imperfectly, extraperitonealized as much as feasible.

If the injury is unilateral, the fistula occurs on a substrate of pelvic surgery following prior radiation therapy, or the bladder is so fixed, diminutive, or deformed that it precludes the use of a Boari flap, transureteroureterostomy may be the best alternative. In that procedure, it is best to use a midline transperitoneal incision for easy access to both ureters. The ureters are closest together near the aortic bifurcation, which is the usual level for the anastomosis. The surgeon must be sure that there is an adequate length of donor ureter, because tension may lead to anastomotic disruption, with disastrous results. After identifying both ureters, the end of the donor ureter is trimmed back to viable tissue at an angle of 45 degrees. The recipient ureter is exposed through an incision in the posterior peritoneum and mobilized just enough to permit easy juxtaposition of two ureters at the level of the anastomosis. The donor ureter is drawn beneath the peritoneum, the recipient ureter is opened medially for 2 cm, and the anastomosis is performed using running or interrupted 4-0 chromic catgut sutures. The recipient ureter should be stented with a double-J stent.

If both lower ureters have been lost, radiation is not implicated, and the bladder is too small to permit any type of bridging procedure, we prefer either an ileal substitution or, if bladder capacity requires enhancement, a patch ileal cystoplasty with a tail for ureteral replacement.

Where there has been extensive loss of both lower ureters in previously irradiated tissue and where fistulization has occurred, either with or without concomitant vesicovaginal involvement, supravesical diversion may be the only option, at least on an interim basis.

The extension of laparoscopic surgery in urology has recently raised a number of exciting possibilities. In one case, a ureteral laceration was recognized at the time of a laparoscopic procedure for endometriosis and closed laparoscopically over a ureteral stent. Whether or not such procedures will become commonplace remains to be seen. However, over the past decade, the widespread availability of simple percutaneous nephrostomy, guidewires, and stents has added immeasurably to the initial management of ureterovaginal fistula.

Suggested Readings

Dowling RA, Corriere JN, Sandler CM: Iatrogenic ureteral injury. J Urol 135:912, 1986

Gomel V, James C: Intraoperative management of ureteral injury during operative laparoscopy. Fertil Steril 55:416, 1991

Mann WJ: Intentional and unintentional ureteral surgical treatment in gynecologic procedures. Surg Gynecol Obstet 172:453, 1991

Tarkington MA, Dejter SW Jr, Bresette JF: Early surgical management of extensive gynecologic ureteral injuries. Surg Gynecol Obstet 173:17, 1991

SECTION 4

THE BLADDER
Congenital Disorders

BLADDER EXSTROPHY

MONEER K. HANNA, M.D.

New York, New York

Bladder exstrophy is included in the spectrum of abnormalities involving the ventral midline. The essential defect is an abnormally extensive cloacal membrane; instead of being restricted to what will be the perineal region, it extends onto the anterior abdominal wall. At one end of the spectrum, an epispadiac glans penis represents the mildest form; the other extreme is exemplified by cloacal exstrophy or vesicointestinal fissure. It is estimated that bladder exstrophy occurs in 1: 10,000 to 1:40,000 live births, and males are twice as likely to be affected as females.

Bladder exstrophy is not simply an abnormality of the bladder; there are equally serious skeletal, rectal, and genital defects as well, which may acquire importance during later life and adulthood. Thus the surgeon who assumes the responsibility of caring for a baby who is born with an exstrophic anomaly must have a clear policy for its management.

Historically, reconstruction was the first form of surgical treatment for exstrophy. This method was abandoned in favor of urinary diversion by transplanting the ureters to the sigmoid colon and relying on the rectal sphincter to provide continence. Recently, however, interest in reconstruction has been revived. The results of surgical reconstruction depend on the severity of the anomaly, but a significant portion also depends on the degree of technical skill and commitment of the surgeon.

EMBRYOLOGIC CONSIDERATIONS

The cloacal membrane, composed of outer ectodermal and inner endodermal membranes, extends over the infraumbilical region of the fetus. Mesodermal ingrowth from either side results in the formation of the abdominal wall musculature; thus the cloacal membrane must retreat caudally. Marshall and Mueke proposed that the under-regression of the cloacal membrane prevents mesodermal invasion, resulting in an unstable embryonic state. Because the cloacal membrane must rupture eventually, the pelvic viscera become exstrophied. Cloacal exstrophy represents the outcome of earlier breakdown of the cloacal membrane at the 5-mm stage, long before the formation of the urorectal septum. It is therefore conceivable that the disorderly conduct of the cloacal membrane, by initially producing a wedge, holds apart the developing mesoderm and subsequently ruptures, leaving behind a ventral midline defect that is likely to involve the bladder and genital tubercles. Indeed, Mueke and Marshall reproduced the abnormality by placing a foreign body on the developing abdominal wall of chick embryos to act as a mechanical obstruction, similar to a persistent cloacal membrane, and as a deterrent to mesodermal ingrowth. However, the precise mechanism of the sequence of events remains unclear.

ANATOMY

There is a ventral midline defect with the bladder open on the surface, separating the recti muscles. The size and quality of the protruding bladder may vary from a small polypoid patch to a pliable, sizable, and invertible bladder. The potential size of the bladder and the degree of intrinsic changes in the mucosa and muscle play a major role in the decision making for surgical reconstruction. Frequently, however, the detrusor muscle is thin and partially fibrotic and the mucosa may be ulcerated or polypoid, or show a variable degree of metaplasia. These pathologic changes are partly inherent in prenatal development, but postnatal secondary changes caused by exposure and rubbing of the mucosa against the diaper can contribute to the problem. The ureterovesical mechanisms are invariably deficient and reflux is likely to result once the bladder is closed. The penis appears to be short, broad, flat, and tethered upward by the dorsal urethral strip. The crura are pulled apart by the separated pubic bones and may give the impression that the penis is totally inadequate. In the female, the urethra is almost invisible, and the bladder merges into the vaginal mucosa between the bifid clitoris, but the uterus and the fallopian tubes are normal.

The anus is displaced anteriorly, but, in some babies, the weakness of the pelvic floor, coupled with constant crying, may result in rectal prolapse. Intrinsic deficiencies of the anorectal muscles occur in some cases and warrant serious concern if one contemplates ureterosigmoidostomy.

In cloacal exstrophy, the cecum lies between the exstrophied halves of the bladder. As one probes the various openings, the caudal one is that of the terminal ileum, and the other leads to the blind colonic pouch. Because the abnormality represents an early faulty embryogenesis, often the müllerian ducts and genital tubercles fail to fuse, causing duplication of the genital tract in the majority of cases. This may result in a double vagina and clitoris in the female. In the male, however, the penile crura and glans are completely separated, one half on either side, making the reconstruction of an acceptable phallus almost impossible. Furthermore, the anus is imperforate, the kidneys frequently are malformed, and in 40 per cent of cases meningomyelocele also occurs.

CLINICAL EVALUATION AND INITIAL MANAGEMENT

The diagnosis of bladder exstrophy can be made antenatally. Absence of bladder filling on sequential ultrasound examinations coupled with the low position of the umbilicus are strong indications of the abnormality. At birth the plastic umbilical clamp should not be used because it rubs and traumatizes the mucosa of the exstrophied bladder. Instead, the umbilical cord should be ligated with nylon suture and the bladder covered with Saran Wrap. The traditional use of Vaseline gauze or saline soaks should be avoided. They are apt to become dry at some point and cause mucosal bruising.

The eventual success of functional closure depends on the size and potential capacity of the bladder. These can be determined by an experienced observer. The bladder is stimulated by a few drops of cold saline and observation of the detrusor contractility is made. The bladder elasticity then is assessed by inverting it with the examiner's gloved finger. The interpubic space also is determined by palpation. In our experience it ranges between 2 and 8 cm. Evaluation of the upper urinary tract can be completed within a few hours of birth. Renal ultrasound and radionuclide studies should be obtained prior to surgical repair; however, intravenous pyelography is not recommended because it is uninformative during early life.

DEFINITIVE MANAGEMENT

The approach to bladder exstrophy is either functional closure or urinary diversion. The former requires multiple operations, and it has been demonstrated that selection and staged repair are definite factors leading to success. The ideal case for reconstruction is a female with a sizable bladder, relatively healthy and polyp-free mucosa, and normal kidneys. In contrast, a boy with an exstrophied small and scarred bladder, with an abnormal upper urinary tract, is best suited for permanent urinary diversion. Reconstruction of the genital tract is necessary regardless of whether one opts for functional closure or urinary diversion. Although penile lengthening and repair of chordee in males and pubic-clitoral repair in females may be incorporated in the primary surgery, subsequent follow-up at puberty and adulthood may show an unsatisfactory appearance, which can be improved significantly by a secondary or tertiary repair.

Various authors have advocated a number of approaches and made several contributions to the management of bladder exstrophy. It has become clear, however, that no single code can be applied to all cases.

Neonatal closure in the first 72 hours may obviate the necessity for iliac osteotomy, and the soft elastic pelvis of the neonate is relatively easy to approximate. After 72 hours, osteotomies facilitate closure of the abdominal wall and pubic bones, and they may be regarded as release incisions to avoid tension on the ventral repair. Furthermore they may contribute to achieving urinary continence by placing the urethra within the pelvis between the approximated pelvic floor muscles.

The main argument against osteotomy is the retraction of the penis toward the pubic bones, resulting in apparent shortening. Nevertheless, we have performed osteotomy when the bladder closure is done after 72 hours and in all cases where the pubic bones are widely separated.

There are three types of osteotomy. Traditionally, vertical iliac osteotomy, with which we have the greatest experience, can be done immediately prior to functional closure. Changing from prone to supine position is a slight disadvantage, but this can be avoided by performing innominate or the more simple and less demanding pubic osteotomy. The superior pubic ramus is divided at the point lateral to the insertion of the rectus abdominus and medial to the pubic attachment of the inguinal ligament. The obturator vessels and nerves are protected while the bone is cut. Approximation of the symphisis is relatively easy because of the cartilagenous nature of the ischiopubic junction. In older children the inferior pubic ramus is fractured during symphyseal approximation.

Protocol for Management

A personal series of 61 children and young adults born with epispadias-exstrophy anomalies constitutes the basis of the following recommendations.

Bladder Exstrophy

If the bladder is pliable and can be inverted and the kidneys are normal, functional reconstruction is recommended. At 24–48 hours after birth bladder closure, penile lengthening, and repair of the abdominal wall defect are performed. If inguinal hernias are present, they are repaired simultaneously and the child is placed in modified Bryant traction for 4 weeks. Thus phase one aims at the conversion of a bladder exstrophy to an epispadias. At 1 year of age, the epispadiac urethra is repaired and the umbilicus reconstructed. This creates outflow resistance, which increases the bladder capacity. Furthermore, the baby's genitalia look normal to the parents, which spares them the psychological trauma of an abnormal penile appearance during diaper change.

When the bladder capacity reaches at least 75 ml, bladder neck reconstruction is performed. Sphincteroplasty and ureteroneocystostomy are carried out in one sitting unless the child develops recurrent urinary infections, in which case ureteral reimplantation is performed at an early age. Horizontal submucosal tunnels are created well above the future bladder neck area.

We prefer to delay continence surgery until the child is older and more cooperative (5 to 6 years of age). Twenty-seven children under the author's care completed staged reconstruction and are available for evaluation of their urinary continence. We have utilized the Young-Dees-Leadbetter method in 15 children; 8 of the 15 achieved dryness for 3 hours or more during the day. The artificial urinary sphincter was implanted in four children, with eventual failure in all four. The gracilis muscle was raised, rotated as a pedicle flap, and wrapped around the scarred bladder neck as a sling. The result was gratifying in this group. An impressive continence rate was achieved when the modification of the cinch procedure described by Koff was utilized in six children. A 3 × 7-cm flap of detrusor muscle is raised, denuded of mucosa, and then wrapped around the bladder neck area. This procedure was successful in all six children. Ten of the 27 children required bladder augmentation because of small bladder capacity. Poor bladder compliance and elevated intravesical pressure resulting in upper urinary tract dilation was recorded in four children. All renal units improved following augmentation cystoplasty.

If the exstrophied bladder is small, bilateral osteotomies and tubularization of the bladder to form a urethra are performed simultaneously with urinary diversion, by transplantation of the ureters into a colonic conduit using an antirefluxing technique. In males, penile lengthening also is performed. One year later, the epispadias and umbilical defects are reconstructed. At 3 years of age, the rectal sphincter is evaluated. If this is adequate and the parents are judged to be unable to cope with multiple operations and possible failure, internal diversion by colosigmoidostomy, as described by Hendren, is performed. If the rectal sphincter is compromised and the parents are agreeable, the colonic conduit is anastomosed to the tubulized bladder, the former being a urine reservoir and the latter being a sphincteric mechanism, in the manner described by Arap. Further surgery for continence by tightening and reconstruction of the outlet or implantation of the artificial urinary sphincter may be required at a later date.

It can be concluded that reconstructive surgery is an essential part of the management, and functional closure is likely to be more rewarding in females with adequate bladder capacity and healthy mucosa. Disappointments occur, but the attempt is worthwhile if proper attention is given to surgical details, control of infection and reflux, and avoidance of urethral obstruction. Nonetheless, in some children there will be failure to achieve an acceptable degree of dryness, or upper urinary tract deterioration will ensue. For these "failures," ureterosigmoidostomy, in which adequate anorectal sphincters must be relied on, provides a satisfactory alternative on the understanding that lifelong follow-up by colonoscopy and barium enema are mandatory, because of the increased risk of colonic cancer. During the past 10 years we have performed continent urinary diversion in 17 children born with bladder exstrophy; Kock pouch, Indiana pouch, and Mitrofanoff procedures were utilized successfully. In this group, eight children failed staged reconstruction and nine were referred with ileal or colon conduit seeking urinary undiversion.

Cloacal Exstrophy

Babies who are born with cloacal exstrophy present an even more difficult problem, both ethically and surgically. If they remain untreated, they are likely to die, but surgical repair probably will be formidable and unlikely to result in a semblance of normality. We have encountered four cases, and each proved to be a surgical challenge. If surgical repair is warranted, the exomphalos is excised and ileostomy is performed. The ectopic bowel is separated but not excised from the hemibladders, which are then sutured together. This converts cloacal exstrophy to a classical exstrophy with an ileostomy. The ectopic bowel is dissected from the hemibladders and used in continuity with gastrointestinal tract. It should not be part of the urinary tract. The hemibladders are mobilized and joined together. In the male with severely defective genitalia, sex rearrangement, with removal of the gonads and corporal bodies, is recommended.

Subsequently, the two treatment options are continent urinary diversion and staged reconstruction, as in classical exstrophy. About half of such bladders are neuropathic. If bladder augmentation is deemed necessary, the stomach is used in preference to small bowel.

Epispadias

Epispadias is a lesser abnormality and can be repaired more successfully. The penile deformity may be corrected by release of the chordee and tubularization of the urethra, using the principles of hypospadias repair. In many cases the bladder neck is deficient and the bladder has a small capacity. Their correction can be achieved in well over 70 per cent of cases. As previously noted, the child with an epispadias generally has better prospects for an acceptable reconstruction, although repeated surgery may be necessary to achieve continence.

EPISPADIAS REPAIR IN MALES WITH CLASSIC BLADDER EXSTROPHY

ROBERT D. JEFFS, M.D.

Baltimore, Maryland

Bladder exstrophy, occurring once in 40,000 births, results from defective development of the infraumbilical abdominal wall, resulting in exposure of the bladder cavity and shortening of the surface structures from the umbilicus to the end of the urethra. Treatment in the male usually is directed toward conversion of the exstrophy condition to that of complete epispadias, with later repair of the penile epispadias and reconstruction for continence.

EXSTROPHY RECONSTRUCTION

In staged exstrophy reconstruction, consideration is given to penile repair at first presentation of the exstrophy patient. Pelvic osteotomy is beneficial in many instances not only in closure of the bladder but also in reducing the divergence of the corporal attachment to the inferior ramus of the pubis. Early decisions are based on (1) degree of pubic diastasis, (2) penile length, (3) length of urethral plate from veru to glans, (4) dorsal chordee and, (5) known potential for penile growth.

The decisions to be made at the time of closure are best based on experience. Osteotomy should be performed at birth when pubic separation is wide and apposition difficult to obtain. Osteotomy should be performed in most cases when presentation is delayed beyond 72 hours.

Penile management at birth involved three choices: (1) urethral plate to remain intact while reducing penile suspension, (2) lengthening of urethral plate with para exstrophy skin, and (3) sex reassignment.

The more recent use of the Cantwell-Ransley technique has made it possible to repair epispadias in exstrophy using the intact urethral plate. An extremely short plate may require interposition of paraexstrophy skin, although misuse of this tissue may lead to urethral and outlet strictures later. In rare cases of very short penis and plate, a change in sex of rearing should be considered.

In the interim between bladder closure and epispadias repair at 2 to 3 years of age, the penis receives a stimulus from first of all the testosterone surge in the first four months of age. Further stimulation should be given by testosterone injection at 1 and 2 years of age. Preoperative stimulation of 2 mg/kg is given 5 weeks and 2 weeks prior to epispadias repair. The caliber of the bladder outlet, bladder drainage, and urinary infection should be monitored frequently. Renal ultrasound at 3 months and one year of age will confirm upper track integrity.

EPISPADIAS REPAIR

Cystoscopy at 2 to 2½ years of age will allow measurement of bladder capacity, the degree of reflux, and the potential of the bladder and bladder neck. Resistance created by the penile repair usually provides the tension required for additional bladder growth and capacity.

The Cantwell-Ransley technique of epispadias repair frees the urethral plate from the veru to the glans, tubularizes it, and places it ventrally between the separated corporeal bodies, which then are approximated dorsally. A well-vascularized urethral plate is needed in this repair, which may not be present when lengthening by paraexstrophy skin has occurred initially.

The steps and advantages of this repair are: (1) full release of suspensory tissue at the pubis, (2) creation of ventral tilt to the penis, (3) dorsal lengthening of the corporeal bodies by incision and side-to-side anastomosis or patch graft, (4) ventral meatotomy (IPGAM) provides a good end meatus with glans closure, (5) excellent appearance of the glans, and (6) fewer fistulas at the coronal junction.

Penile cover is achieved by use of lateral flaps of penile skin and prepuce. Alternatively, ventral prepuce may be transferred by the "bucket-handle" maneuver or by island transfer to a deficient area on the dorsum of the penis.

Late presentation, prior failure, and short urethral plate may require special measures, such as: (1) excision of scar, (2) staged repair, (3) preputial pedicle graft to lengthen the urethra from the proximal extent to the meatus, and (4) free graft to the urethra from the prepuce, full-thickness skin, or mucosa from either the bladder or buccal areas. Penile cover in these cases is obtained from local flaps, temporary scrotal flaps, scrotal burial, or appropriate full-thickness or split-thickness grafts.

Caudal anesthesia with continuous infusion for 3 or 4 days is ideally suited to this repair. Not only is pain relieved but bladder spasms are controlled. Ditropan, Valium, and narcotics are used in addition.

A soft Silastic tube sutured at the meatus drains the bladder; other multiple openings are made in the short intravesical portion of the tube. Suprapubic drainage is used in addition in complicated cases in which prolonged drainage is required or in patients known to be prone to bladder spasms. Broad-spectrum antibiotics are used to convert a contaminated area to a clean surgical wound and should be continued for 5 to 7 days.

PROGNOSIS

Late adjustment to the epispadias repair may be required at puberty when the growth spurt has occurred. Revision of the resulting scars, and of recurrent suspensory tissue, may be needed. The Koff ventral medial rotation may be helpful in relieving residual dorsal chordee. Care in planning and execution from birth to puberty should provide a satisfactory penis for urinary and sexual function. Counseling and psychological support should be provided throughout the growing years.

Suggested Readings

Gearhart JP, Jeffs RD: Exstrophy of the bladder, epispadias, and other bladder anomalies. *In* Walsh PC, Retik AB, Stamey TA, et al (eds): Campbell's Urology, 6th ed. Philadelphia, WB Saunders, 1992, pp 1772–1821

Gearhart JP, Leonard MP, Burgers JK, et al: The Cantwell-Ransley technique for repair of epispadias. J Urol 148: 851, 1992.

IMPERFORATE ANUS, PERSISTENT CLOACA, AND UROGENITAL SINUS OUTLET OBSTRUCTION

R. LAWRENCE KROOVAND, M.D.

Winston-Salem, North Carolina

Failure of complete separation of the cloaca into a ventral urogenital sinus and posterior rectum at some time between the 4th and 12th weeks of gestation produces a broad spectrum of anorectal anomalies, including imperforate anus, urogenital sinus anomalies, and persistent cloaca. Anorectal anomalies occur approximately once in every 4000 to 5000 newborns and are more common in males. The embryologic defect responsible for the anorectal anomaly, coupled with the close association between development of the gastrointestinal and genitourinary systems, would imply frequent coexistence of developmental abnormalities in both systems, as is recognized in up to 48 per cent of investigated neonates with an anorectal anomaly. The frequency of recognition of genitourinary anomalies in these neonates is directly related to a high index of suspicion and to the thoroughness of the uroradiographic evaluation conducted. The incidence and severity of the accompanying genitourinary anomalies correlates well with the severity of the anorectal anomaly as defined by the level of the rectal fistula. The close relationship of an anorectal malformation with the VATER or VACTERRL associations mandates evaluation for all other components of these associations if two or more components are identified. This article provides a reasoned approach for urologic evaluation and management of the child with an anorectal malformation.

INITIAL CONSIDERATIONS

The initial surgical management of the newborn with an anorectal anomaly is directed by the pediatric surgeon. Initial management involves two decision parameters: (1) is a diverting colostomy necessary, and (2) are there any associated anomalies (urologic, nonurologic) that may represent a serious risk to the infant's life?

In 80 to 90 per cent of *male neonates* with an anorectal anomaly, a physical examination and a urinalysis provide sufficient information to determine the need for a colostomy. A perineal subepithelial midline raphe with a fistula passing meconium, a midline skintag below which an instrument can be introduced, or the finding of anal stenosis or an anal membrane all suggest a low defect, which most often can be managed with a minimal posterior sagittal anoplasty without the need for a protective diverting colostomy. The absence of a midline gluteal groove or anal dimple (flat bottom) suggests a high rectal pouch. Plain abdominal radiographs may demonstrate air in the urinary tract, suggesting a high lesion with a rectourinary fistula. Urinalysis in this situation most often will demonstrate meconium or squamous cells in the urine. These findings provide an absolute indication for a divided diverting colostomy as part of initial management. A uroradiographic evaluation (abdominal/pelvic ultrasound, voiding cystourethrogram [VCUG]) prior to creation of the colostomy may disclose a variety of urologic anomalies, so common in this group of neonates, and may indicate a need for additional evaluation (i.e., renography, endoscopy). With the information obtained from these uroradiographic studies, the urologist can direct necessary management of any accompanying genitourinary anomalies at the time of colostomy, sparing the patient a second operative procedure.

The initial decisions regarding surgical management of the *female neonate* with an anorectal anomaly are easier. In 90 per cent of female neonates with an anorectal anomaly, simple perineal inspection determines the need for a colostomy. The presence of a cutaneous or perineal fistula suggests a low defect that can be managed with a minimal posterior sagittal anoplasty or simple cutback procedure during the neonatal period, without a need for a colostomy. Careful inspection of the genitalia may reveal a fistula located just outside the hymen or that the posterior ring of the hymen is deficient; meconium may be seen within the vagina. These neonates have a high defect and require a protective divided diverting colostomy prior to definitive repair. Only 10 per cent of females with an anorectal malformation will not have a fistula. Absence of a recognizable fistula indicates a high lesion and the need for a colostomy.

If only a single orifice is identified, the baby has a persistent cloaca. Severe primary or secondary urologic malformations are found in up to 90 per cent of these neonates, necessitating a careful, complete urologic (uroradiographic) and possibly endoscopic evaluation prior to creation of a divided diverting colostomy. The necessity for a divided diverting colostomy in neonates with anorectal anomalies, especially those with persistent cloaca, cannot be overemphasized, because the divided diverting colostomy minimizes contamination of the urinary tract by fecal organisms and greatly reduces the risk of sepsis.

ASSOCIATED GENITOURINARY ANOMALIES

The incidence and severity of associated genitourinary anomalies in the neonate with an anorectal anomaly appears related to the level of the rectal fistula. The timing and extent of initial urologic (uroradiographic) evaluation depends on the clinical determination of the fistula level. Patients with a probable high-level fistula and the need for emergent uroradiographic evaluation include: (1) any female with a single perineal orifice; (2) neonates with a poorly formed sacrum or flat perineum; and (3) males with meconium or squamous cells in their urine, pneumaturia, or air within the urinary tract as demonstrated on plain abdominal radiographs.

All neonates thought to have a high-level fistula and all those with an abdominal or flank mass should undergo abdominal and pelvic ultrasonography and, ideally, VCUG, prior colostomy, or anoplasty. If the ultrasound is normal, delaying the VCUG until after colostomy or anoplasty appears appropriate. Children with low-level anomalies also should undergo renal ultrasonography prior to any surgical procedure; the VCUG may be delayed if the ultrasound is normal.

In the female with a persistent cloaca, genitography also should be done to define the anatomy of the malformation. Genitography is performed by placing an occlusive syringe against the perineal orifice and injecting contrast material into the cloaca under fluoroscopic monitoring. A simultaneous distal limb colostogram may assist further in defining the anatomy of the cloacal anomaly. Endoscopic examination of the cloaca, performed at the time of colostomy or prior to definitive repair, may provide additional useful anatomic information, thus assisting in planning the most appropriate management.

Renal agenesis-dysplasia, vesicoureteral reflux, and renal ectopia are the most commonly encountered urologic abnormalities in children with an anorectal anomaly. Neurogenic bladder may be encountered in 7 to 18 per cent of children with an anorectal anomaly. Malformations of the lumbosacral spine (partial or complete sacral agenesis and hemisacrum also are seen with increased frequency in these neonates (13 to 45 per cent) and are more common the higher the rectal lesion, mandating careful evaluation of the neonatal spine. Unsuspected lesions are frequent, often producing progressive bowel, bladder, and musculoskeletal dysfunction later in childhood, if uncorrected. Because of incomplete ossification of the lower spine in the neonate, plain radiographs frequently are unsatisfactory for defining the lumbosacral spine. Fortunately, this lack of ossification provides an ultrasonographic window into the lower spine, permitting excellent ultrasonographic evaluation of this area. The presence of a lumbosacral malformation increases the risk of a concomitant genitourinary anomaly, which may be encountered in up to 70 per cent of those evaluated.

Primary abnormalities of the müllerian duct system frequently occur in females with an anorectal anomaly. Vaginal duplication and vaginal septa are recognized in 35 to 45 per cent of girls with a persistent cloaca. Such anomalies require identification because of their potential early secondary obstructive effect on the urinary tract (i.e., obstruction by hydroscolpos, sepsis) and their implications related to future sexual function and reproduction. Genitography and endoscopy are most useful in evaluating for such anomalies.

UROLOGIC MANAGEMENT

The associated anomalies involving the genitourinary tract in the neonate with an anorectal anomaly represent some of the most devastating and technically demanding problems in pediatric urology. The goals in management are age related; some genitourinary anomalies require immediate management at birth, whereas others are best managed later in childhood.

The Newborn Period

Upper or lower urinary tract obstruction, vesicoureteral reflux, and urinary infection are the most common urologic problems requiring treatment that are encountered during the newborn period. In many instances, the urologic anomalies may be more life-threatening than the anorectal anomaly, thus requiring emergent treatment.

Unilateral renal agenesis/dysplasia is the most commonly identified genitourinary abnormality in patients with an anorectal anomaly. Although ultrasonography may suggest renal agenesis/dysplasia, accurate identification requires a radionuclide renal scan. The neonate with renal agenesis or dysplasia requires little treatment, if any, for the renal anomaly. Isolated obstruction of the upper urinary tract is managed similarly to that in an otherwise healthy newborn, bearing in mind the high risk of urinary infection in neonates and infants with anorectal anomalies.

Lower urinary obstruction with bilateral hydronephrosis may occur because of a congenital urethral stricture or neuropathic bladder or may be the consequence of compression of the lower urinary tract by distended bowel, hydrocolpos, or pooling of urine in a dilated, obstructed vagina. The critical combination of bladder outlet obstruction, urinary tract infection resulting from the presence of an intestinal fistula, and vesicoureteral reflux poses a significant threat to the life of these neonates, as well as to ultimate renal function, and must be dealt with emergently. A cutaneous vesicostomy or cutaneous vaginostomy may be necessary to relieve lower urinary obstruction and reduce the chance for sepsis. Sepsis in the neonate or infant with an anorectal anomaly must be considered urologic until proven otherwise.

Vesicoureteral reflux is the second most frequently identified genitourinary anomaly in these patients, affecting up to 35 per cent of patients overall and approaching 65 to 70 per cent in girls with a persistent cloaca, and is potentially the most common to require surgical intervention. In the newborn with severe bilateral vesicoureteral reflux, control of infection coupled with provision for adequate bladder drainage by intermittent catheterization or cutaneous vesicostomy may be necessary. A totally defunctionalized divided colostomy that prevents fecal spillover will help to minimize bacterial contamination of the urinary tract and reduce the risk of sepsis. Continuous antibiotic prophylaxis is mandatory until the reflux has resolved or has been corrected. Repair of severe bilateral reflux usually is performed after definitive repair of the anorectal anomaly, unless appropriate urinary drainage cannot be maintained and/or antibacterial prophylaxis cannot be provided. In such a situation, it may be prudent to correct the reflux prior to repair of the anorectal anomaly.

The First Year of Life

Urologic problems encountered in the first year of life are related to urinary tract infection, persistent vesicoureteral reflux, complications of a neuropathic bladder, and electrolyte imbalances. The divided diverting colostomy generally prevents symptomatic urinary tract infection. Antibacterial prophylaxis still may be necessary.

Although vesicoureteral reflux may resolve spontaneously, such an event is uncommon; most often, ureteroneocystostomy is necessary. Ureteroneocystostomy performed after repair of the anorectal anomaly may be technically difficult because of postsurgical scarring behind the bladder. A combined intravesical-extravesical approach is recommended for ureteral reimplantation. Prior to ureteral reimplantation, appropriate and effective bladder emptying must be established.

Boys with anorectal anomalies may develop recurrent epididymitis for uncertain reasons. Epididymitis is not limited to boys with a patent rectourinary fistula, because epididymitis occurs both before and after repair of the anorectal anomaly.

Hydronephrosis or symptomatic urinary infection in the child with a neuropathic bladder is managed in the same manner as for the child with myelodysplasia, employing clean intermittent catheterization coupled with antibacterial prophylaxis. Difficulty may be encountered when performing intermittent catheterization in males who have a urethral diverticulum or a remnant of the rectourethral fistula because the catheter tends to curl in these pouches. Fortunately, most of these problems are historical now that most anorectal anomalies are corrected employing the posterior sagittal technique, permitting accurate identification and resection of the rectourinary fistula while minimizing the potential for ureteral injury. Problematic pouches, especially those associated with recurrent infection or stone formation, may require surgical repair. Genital anomalies (hypospadias and cryptorchism) are repaired near the end of the first year of life.

LONG-TERM PROBLEMS

Long-term problems include management of the neuropathic bladder and urinary incontinence, difficulties related to urethral strictures, a persistent rectal pouch or diverticulum in the prostatic urethra, and long-term functional and reproductive problems in females with persistent cloaca.

The incidence of neuropathic bladder is reported as 7 to 18 per cent, appears related to the severity of the sacral abnormality, and often can be predicted on newborn examination by the finding of a flat bottom or a palpably abnormal sacrum. As noted, ultrasonography may provide the most valuable diagnostic modality for recognition of sacrolumbar anomalies. Most neuropathic bladders do not empty efficiently and are best managed with intermittent catheterization. Bladder outlet reconstruction, a bladder neck sling procedure, periurethral collagen injection, or placement of an artificial urinary sphincter may be necessary to establish urinary continence. As previously mentioned, associated abnormalities of the spinal cord may not be static and require careful long-term follow-up, especially during growth spurts when the risk of developing symptoms of a tethered cord are increased.

Because of the high risk for difficulty in emptying the bladder in girls with a persistent cloaca, care must be taken at the time of anorectoplasty to provide a urethra that will be suitable for intermittent catheterization. This is best accomplished at the time of posterior sagittal anorectoplasty by preservation and reconstruction of the common cloacal channel as the urethra. Vaginoplasty using a pull-through technique with or without rotation of skin flaps is also necessary at this time.

Adolescent males who have a large diverticulum or a remnant of the rectal pouch left behind because of incomplete dissection of the rectal fistula at the time of their anorectal pull-through procedure may encounter significant difficulty with intermittent catheterization. The catheter tends to enter these pouches preferentially. Stones may form in these poorly draining urethral/rectal stumps; poorly draining pockets may be a source of recurrent urinary tract infection. Secondary reconstruction and elimination of these pouches and stumps may be necessary. Urethral strictures must be treated prior to institution of intermittent catheterization. Fortunately, with the near-universal use of the posterior sagittal anorectoplasty, the abovementioned problems now are encountered far less frequently than in the past.

One of the more difficult long-term problems encountered in girls with a persistent cloaca who have undergone isolated treatment of the anal malformation by prior pull-through without attention to the associated vaginal and urethral anomalies is functional reconstruction of the urogenital sinus. Such secondary reconstructions are often technically difficult and prone to complication and unsatisfactory outcome.

UROLOGIC COMPLICATIONS AFTER ANORECTAL SURGERY

Urethral stricture, the result of injury to the male urethra during division of the rectourethral fistula, is the most commonly reported complication of anorectal malformation repair. Ureteral or vasal injury may occur during mobilization of the rectum when repairing high lesions. Fortunately, since popularization of the posterior sagittal anorectoplasty, such postoperative urologic complications are now uncommon. Development of a secondary neuropathic bladder and fistula recurrence are also recognized postoperative complications.

Suggested Readings

McLorie GA, Sheldon CA, Fleisher M, et al: The genitourinary system in patients with imperforate anus. J Pediatr Surg 22:1100, 1987

Parrott TS: Urologic implications of imperforate anus. Urology 10:407, 1977

Pena A: Posterior sagittal approach for the correction of anorectal malformations. *In* Mannick JA (ed): Advances in Surgery. Chicago, Year Book Medical Publishers, 1985, pp 69–100

Rich MA, Brock WA, Pena A: Spectrum of genitourinary malformations in patients with imperforate anus. Pediatr Surg Int 3:110, 1988

CONGENITAL BLADDER DIVERTICULA

ALAN B. RETIK, M.D.

Boston, Massachusetts

A bladder diverticulum represents herniation of vesical mucosa through points of deficiency in the bladder muscle. It is always a little confusing to distinguish a saccule from a diverticulum. For practical purposes, a saccule or protrusion larger than 2 cm is considered a diverticulum. Bladder diverticula represent different entities in children and adults. In the adult, diverticula are usually secondary to outlet obstruction, primarily benign prostatic hypertrophy. In the child, most diverticula are congenital and are not secondary to distal obstruction. Congenital diverticula are much more common in males than in females.

The etiology of bladder diverticula in children is far from clarified. It is our opinion that diverticula are secondary to a congenital weakness in the muscular wall, whether or not there is distal obstruction, and that this weak area is a potential source of diverticulum formation. Most diverticula originate at or near the edge of the trigone. We propose that this position of the diverticular mouth probably is caused by the following features: (1) the trigone is of different embryologic origin than the remainder of the bladder, and its continuity with the bladder may lead to points of weakness; and (2) the pressures of normal micturition may produce the greatest stress in the trigone area. This could result in an outpouching at a specific place along this potentially weak area. Reflux often is seen if the ureteral orifice is adjacent to the mouth of the diverticulum or a part of its wall. When the ureteral orifice becomes intimately involved in the rim of the diverticulum or actually within the sac wall, distortion of the ureteral orifice configuration takes place in addition to shortening of the intramural tunnel. The mechanism for ureterovesical competency thus is destroyed, and reflux ensues.

Bladder diverticula are detected radiologically. They sometimes are seen by excretory urography and are defined by voiding cystourethrography. At cystoscopy, one can usually identify the diverticulum just above and slightly lateral to the ureteral orifice, which is the usual location. Although diverticula more often are associated with vesicoureteral reflux, they may cause ureteral obstruction. On rare occasions, a posteriorly located diverticulum may fill with voiding and extend inferiorly, compressing the prostatic urethra and elevating the bladder neck, causing acute obstruction.

The treatment of bladder diverticula is surgical. They may be excised intravesically, extravesically, or by a combination of both techniques. In almost all instances, even with very large diverticula, excision can be done intravesically, which I believe is simpler and preferable. If the wall of the diverticulum is adjacent to the ureteral wall, ureteral reimplantation will have to be performed as well. I place fine traction sutures circumferentially around the diverticulum and ureteral orifice, and incise the mucosa with cautery. Then, using sharp dissection with tenotomy scissors, a proper plane can be established and the diverticulum and ureter dissected out. During the dissection, care should be taken to identify the vas deferens. The defect in the bladder wall is reapproximated with chromic catgut sutures, and the mucosa is reapproximated with fine chromic catgut sutures. It is sometimes helpful to dissect on an inflated Fogarty or Foley catheter balloon placed within the diverticulum.

Suggested Readings

Barrett DM, Malek RS, Kelalis PP: Observations of vesical diverticulum in children. J Urol 116:234, 1976

Johnston JH: Vesical diverticula without urinary obstruction in childhood. J Urol 84:535, 1960

Levard G, Aigrain Y, Ferkadji L, et al: Urinary bladder diverticula and the Ehlers-Danlos syndrome in children. J Pediatr Surg 24:1184, 1989

Lione PM, Gonzales ET: Congenital bladder diverticula causing ureteral obstruction. Urology 25:273, 1985

Taylor WN, Alton D, Toguri A, et al: Bladder diverticulum causing posterior urethral obstruction in children. J Urol 122:415, 1979

URACHAL ANOMALIES

ALAN B. RETIK, M.D.

Boston, Massachusetts

Anomalies of the urachus are quite rare. They may become manifest in childhood as well as in later life. The urachus is a three-layered, tubular structure that courses upward between the peritoneum and the transversalis fascia, from the anterior portion of the dome of the bladder toward the umbilicus. Failure of the urachal lumen to close and completely obliterate causes one of several anomalies. These are patent urachus (48 per cent), urachal cyst (31 per cent), urachal or alternating sinus (18 per cent), and vesicourachal diverticulum (3 per cent). Males are affected more than twice as often as females. Patent urachus and vesicourachal diverticulum sometimes are associated with obstructive disorders of the lower urinary tract or the prune-belly syndrome.

A *patent urachus* results when there is a communication between the urachus and both the bladder and umbilicus. This occurs when the urachal lumen fails to close. As mentioned above, a small percentage of these lesions may be associated with urethral obstruction. This entity usually presents shortly after birth, but not until the cord separates from the umbilicus and urinary drainage is noted from the cord. The diagnosis is confirmed by cystography with lateral films or by injecting methylene blue transurethrally or indigo carmine intravenously and observing a color change in the draining fluid. An injection of the fistulous tract also will differentiate this condition from a patent omphalomesenteric duct. The treatment of choice is complete excision of the urachus and umbilicus with a cuff of bladder. Treatment by cauterization of the urachal lumen is not satisfactory. Obviously, if lower urinary tract obstruction is present, it also should be treated. If the patent urachus is not excised, umbilical excoriation results, and this must be differentiated from omphalitis.

When the epithelial lining of the urachal remnant does not obliterate completely, there is the potential for development of a *urachal cyst*. The lining of the cyst usually is composed of transitional cell mucosa, but intestinal-type mucosa with goblet cells has been reported. Serous and mucinous secretions from these cells and cellular debris can collect and lead to the formation of a cyst, which occurs primarily in the lower third of the urachus. These cysts usually remain small and asymptomatic. However, they may enlarge on occasion, and a palpable mass may be detected in the lower midline abdominal wall. Urinary tract symptoms also may develop, with external bladder compression. The differential diagnosis consists of a bladder diverticulum, vitelline cyst, omphalocele, hernia of the abdominal wall, and ovarian cyst. The diagnosis of urachal cyst can be made by cystography, which will demonstrate an external mass compressing the dome of the bladder. Ultrasonography and direct injection of the cyst with contrast material also may be helpful diagnostically. If the cyst becomes infected, local and constitutional symptoms may result. Pain, tenderness, redness, and local swelling below the umbilicus may be accompanied by fever or by gastrointestinal and urinary symptoms. If an infected cyst is not treated, the resultant abscess may drain to the umbilical region or bladder. Initial treatment of an abscess consists of incision and drainage. However, this is only temporary and inadequate treatment, as evidenced by the high rate of recurrence of infection and because adenocarcinoma has been reported to be a late occurrence. Therefore, the recommended therapy for the urachal cyst is adequate treatment of the infection followed by complete excision of the urachus with a cuff of bladder.

A *urachal sinus* is usually the sequela of a small infected urachal cyst that has dissected to the umbilicus. The usual symptoms are umbilical drainage, periumbilical erythema, tenderness, intermittent fever, and uncommonly, the formation of a granuloma. In rare instances, it may dissect to the bladder through a very small communication and cause urinary symptoms. An alternating urachal sinus also can result, with intermittent drainage via the umbilicus or bladder. The diagnosis of a urachal sinus may be made by a fistulogram or cystogram. Cystoscopic examination will reveal an elevated area of erythema at the dome of the bladder, and, if an alternating sinus is present, purulent material may be seen emerging from that area. Treatment of a urachal sinus consists of complete excision of the tract and removal of a cuff of bladder and umbilicus.

A *vesicourachal diverticulum* is the least common urachal anomaly. It occurs when a communication exists between the urachal lumen and the bladder. It most often is seen in association with urethral obstruction or the prune-belly syndrome. This entity is often asymptomatic, but urinary infection and stone formation can occur. Specific therapy is not indicated unless symptoms are present. Excision of the urachus and diverticulum and relief of the lower urinary tract obstruction, if present, are necessary.

Suggested Readings

Bauer SB, Retik AB: Urachal and related umbilical disorders. Urol Clin North Am 5:195, 1978

Blichert-Toft M, Neilsen OV: Congenital patent urachus and acquired variants. Acta Chir Scan 137:807, 1971

Hinman F Jr: Surgical disorders of the bladder and umbilicus of urachal origin. Surg Gynecol Obstet 113:605, 1967

Rees HI: Infected urachal cysts. BMJ 2:184, 1953

Retik AB, Bauer SB: Bladder and urachus. *in* Kelalis PP, King LR, Belman AB (eds): Clinical Pediatric Urology. Philadelphia, WB Saunders, 1976, pp 544–571

SACRAL AGENESIS

STUART B. BAUER, M.D.

Boston, Massachusetts

Agenesis of the sacrum is a rare congenital anomaly that involves absence of part or all of two or more vertebrae. When the condition affects lumbar vertebrae, it is called the caudal regression syndrome.

Most cases of sacral agenesis are discovered during a newborn examination. In some children the anomaly is not detected until the child is referred for evaluation of day and nighttime urinary and/or fecal incontinence or, rarely, orthopedic deformities of the lower extremities. All children with incontinence should have their lower back inspected and the sacral spine palpated. Absence of the gluteal cleft extending craniad and flattening of the buttocks are sine qua non signs of sacral agenesis.

Any suspicion of this abnormality should be confirmed by anteroposterior and lateral radiographic views of the lower spine. Often gas in the bowel obscures adequate visualization of the sacral spine on the anteroposterior projection. Recently, computerized tomography has shown a sharp cutoff to the spinal cord, with sacral nerve roots streaming caudally, and absence of the cauda equina.

One per cent of insulin-dependent diabetic mothers have offspring with sacral agenesis; conversely, 16 per cent of children with this anomaly have an insulin-dependent diabetic mother, including those who had the disease during gestation only. It has been theorized that maternal antibodies to bovine insulin can cross the placenta and enter fetal tissues; this may be the cause of the defects noted in children of diabetic mothers (i.e., sacral agenesis, macroglossia). Thus, a family history of diabetes should be ascertained in all children with suspected agenesis of the sacrum. Sometimes, sacral agenesis is found in conjunction with other abnormalities such as imperforate anus, as part of the VATER syndrome (*v*ertebral defects, imperforate *a*nus, *t*racheo*e*sophageal fistula, and *r*adial and/or *r*enal dysplasia).

Neurourologic testing reveals that the degree of nerve root injury is variable and cannot be predicted from the number of affected vertebral bodies. It was originally thought that at least two vertebral bodies had to be affected for neurogenic bladder dysfunction to be present, but this has not been found to be true. In a review of 16 patients with sacral agenesis, 9 had detrusor contractions and 7 had an areflexic bladder. Of the nine with bladder contractions, three had normal sphincter activity and voluntary control with no apparent neurologic deficit, and six (37 per cent of the total group) had exaggerated sacral reflexes without voluntary control (upper motor neuron–type dysfunction). The seven patients with an areflexic bladder (43 per cent of the total) also had evidence of a lower motor neuron lesion in the sphincter; four had complete lesions with no electrical activity in the sphincter, whereas three had incomplete lesions. The type of lesion—upper motor neuron versus lower motor neuron—could not be predicted by the number of affected vertebrae. Seventy-five per cent of the children had normal sensation involving the sacral dermatomes. Thus, sensory afferents do not appear to be affected as commonly as motor efferents.

Urodynamic studies are needed to define accurately the level of denervation involving the vesicourethral unit. Such studies should be coupled with either renal ultrasonography or excretory urography and voiding cystography, to determine the status of the upper urinary tract, the presence of reflux and the competency of the bladder neck and urethra, respectively. The findings from these studies can guide the physician in appropriately treating the child's urinary incontinence.

Anticholinergic medication (i.e., oxybutynin [0.2 mg/kg twice a day] and probanthine [0.5 mg/kg three times a day]) will abolish uninhibited contractions in children with upper motor neuron lesions. If such children cannot empty their bladder because of incoordination between the detrusor and the external urethral sphincter (an upper motor neuron–type lesion), medication is combined with intermittent catheterization to empty the bladder and maintain continence. If drug therapy is unsuccessful in controlling this hyperreflexia, augmentation cystoplasty using a segment of intestine or stomach is advocated.

Children with lower motor neuron lesions and low urethral resistance require alpha-adrenergic drugs to increase urethral tone (i.e., phenylpropanolamine [2.5 mg/kg twice a day], ephedrine [1.0 mg/kg three times a day], or pseudoephedrine [0.5 mg/kg three times a day]) and anticholinergics to maintain low pressure during filling of the bladder in order to achieve continence. When urethral resistance cannot be raised sufficiently with medication, bladder neck reconstruction or placement of an artificial urinary sphincter is advised.

Vesicoureteral reflux is treated in the same way it is in children with other forms of neurogenic bladder dysfunction. The bladder must be emptied efficiently and with low pressure. Intermittent catheterization has been used successfully without increasing the risk of recurrent infection. If high pressure is present during filling, anticholinergic medication is added to reduce the hypertonicity. Indications for antireflux surgery include recurrent urinary infection, progressive pyelonephritic changes, persistent hydroureteronephrosis despite adequate emptying of the bladder, and severe reflux with a definitive anatomic abnormality at the ureterovesical junction. Trabeculation of the bladder is not a contraindication to ureteral reimplantation, but a cross-trigonal procedure is preferred over the Politano-Leadbetter technique because the trigone is less affected by trabeculation than the rest of the bladder. Bilateral reimplantation is not required for unilateral disease. In order for surgery to be successful, however, intermittent catheterization and anticholinergic agents (if necessary) must be continued postoperatively to ensure complete bladder emptying with low filling and emptying pressures.

Urinary diversion almost never is performed for sacral agenesis, but, when it is, it can be in the form of a continent catheterizable stoma. Manual dexterity is not an issue in these children. Intractable incontinence, inability to be catheterized, and a bladder that is not usable after other procedures to achieve continence have failed are the only reasons for this type of urinary diversion. The Mitrofanoff principle of creating a continent catheterizable stoma by employing the antirefluxing mechanism of the ureterovesical junction, or using the appendix or a similar narrow-tubed organ implanted into the bladder (or bowel reservoir if need be) in an equivalent manner, and closing off the bladder neck (in children with intractable incontinence) is quite applicable here.

Suggested Readings

Bauer SB: Neuropathology of the lower urinary tract. *In* Kelalis PP, King LR, Belman AB (eds): Clinical Pediatric Urology, 3rd ed. Philadelphia, WB Saunders, 1992, pp 419–422

Duckett JW, Snyder HM III: Use of the Mitrofanoff principle in urinary reconstruction. Urol Clin North Am 13: 271, 1986

Gotoh T, Shinno Y, Kobayashi S, et al: Diagnosis and management of sacral agenesis. Eur Urol 20:287, 1991

Guzman L, Bauer SB, Hallett M, et al: Evaluation and management of children with sacral agenesis. Urology 22:506, 1983

Menon RK, Cohen RM, Sperling MA, et al: Transplacental passage of insulin in pregnant women with insulin-dependent diabetes mellitus. N Engl J Med 323:309, 1990

Infections and Inflammatory Lesions

BACTERIURIA: PREVENTION AND TREATMENT

ANTHONY J. SCHAEFFER, M.D.

Chicago, Illinois

The urinary tract normally is sterile, and, hence, identification of bacteriuria should be considered an important observation. Not all bacteriuria is clinically significant, however. For example, patients with indwelling urethral catheters or asymptomatic bacteriuria may remain free of clinically significant urinary tract infection for long periods. Asymptomatic bacteriuria, however, is not necessarily benign, as evidenced by the sudden development of systemic symptoms of fevers and chills associated with bacteremia that frequently plague patients with catheter-associated bacteriuria.

Patients with asymptomatic bacteriuria caused by urea-splitting organisms, such as *Proteus mirabilis*, may rapidly form struvite infection stones that act as a focus for recurrent bacteriuria, pyelonephritis, and renal functional impairment. In most cases, bacteriuria is associated with symptoms attributed to either lower urinary tract infection (dysuria, urgency, frequency) or upper urinary tract infection (chills, fever, flank pain). Recent evidence suggests that the symptoms do not always adequately delineate the source of bacteriuria but probably do indicate the severity of the infection.

It has been well established that urinary tract symptoms and urinalysis alone are not adequate to diagnose and treat bacteriuria. The diagnosis of significant bacteriuria—that is, urinary tract infection—traditionally has been based on quantitative urine cultures demonstrating 100,000 or more colony-forming units per milliliter. It is now clear, however, that less than 100,000 colony-forming units/ml can be associated with significant urinary tract infection. In most cases, a count of 100 or more colony-forming units per milliliter of voided or catheterized urine should be considered indicative of urinary tract infection. The patient should receive appropriate therapy unless, for example, an indwelling urethral catheter or urinary conduit is associated with asymptomatic bacterial colonization and there are no urea-splitting organisms capable of forming infection stones. The major objections to performing a urine culture (i.e., patient inconvenience and excessive cost) can be overcome by the use of dip slides or other such devices that provide accurate quantitative urine cultures at relatively low cost.

Our assessment and management of culture-documented urinary tract infections are based on the classification of three infection patterns: isolated infection (symptomatic), unresolved bacteriuria during therapy, and recurrent urinary tract infections comprising reinfections and bacterial persistence. Isolated infections generally are caused by common gram-negative organisms (*Escherichia coli* in approximately 85 per cent of cases), although gram-positive staphylococci and streptococci are not uncommon. The source of the pathogens is usually the patient's bowel flora. A variety of antimicrobials are effective, and recurrent infections are rare. Antimicrobial sensitivity testing is necessary in only 5 to 10 per cent of patients to delineate effective alternative drug therapy because the pathogen was naturally resistant or acquired resistance to the first drug selected.

The increased susceptibility to recurrent infections in some women appears to be predisposed by a biologic defect that permits frequent colonization of the vaginal vestibule by bacteria from the rectal flora. Women with a history of recurrent urinary tract infections have vaginal and uroepithelial cells to which large numbers of *E. coli* attach in adherence assays in vitro. This finding suggests that women prone to recurrent infection may have an increased number of receptors and/or a particular type of receptor on their epithelial cells that contributes to their enhanced susceptibility to infection. The number and types of receptors on uroepithelial cells may be genetically determined. A patient's intrinsic susceptibility to infection also may vary because of increased or decreased ability of her uroepithelial cells to support adherence of uropathogenic bacteria, perhaps in response to hormonal or other influences. Such women characteristically have clusters of symptomatic infections (two thirds will have reinfections within 6 months), followed by 6- to 12-month infection-free intervals. A much smaller group of women and most men have infections resulting from bacterial persistence within the urinary tract, usually a stone, anatomic abnormality, or prostatic focus. These recurrences always are caused by the same organism and usually occur within several days of stopping antimicrobial therapy. Identification of the structural or functional cause is mandatory for effective management of these patients.

Before individual therapeutic regimens are discussed, three general therapeutic principles deserve emphasis. First, the fecal flora compose the ultimate reservoir for most urinary tract pathogens, and antimicrobial therapy—whether for urinary tract or other infections—can rapidly and significantly alter bacterial susceptibility either to the original drug (chromosomal resistance) or to other antimicrobials (R-factor resistance). When patients recently have been exposed to or are likely to require antimicrobial therapy, antimicrobial agents that are least likely to produce bacterial resistance should be used. Second, the cure of urinary tract infection depends on whether or not the infecting strain can be killed by the antimicrobial concentration in the urine, rather than in the serum. Because achievable levels of antimicrobials in urine are generally 100 times greater than those in the serum, it is important to note whether in vitro antimicrobial sensitivities reflect urine concentrations achievable in vivo. Renal failure may impede concentrating ability and reduce the achievable effect of urinary concentration. Finally, in vitro sensitivity testing is based on the assumption that the organisms tested are representative of those causing infection. In fact, the population is not homogeneous; some organisms are more or less sensitive to the reported minimal inhibitory concentration. The therapeutic implication is clear; in order to minimize selection of resistant mutants, one should choose the drug that can achieve urinary concentrations that exceed the minimal inhibitory concentration by the widest margin.

ISOLATED INFECTION

Isolated infections almost always are responsive to various oral antimicrobial agents. I generally manage such infections as described below unless the infection is complicated by an underlying functional or structural urinary tract abnormality (see High-Risk

Patients). Although pretherapy culture is not essential, I usually obtain one to document the infection. Antimicrobial sensitivity testing is not ordered unless I suspect that the pathogen is resistant (as a result of a history of previous antimicrobial therapy) or the patient has fever, flank pain, and/or chills, suggesting pyelonephritis. I generally continue therapy for 3 days. Although single-dose therapy appears to be effective, many patients continue to have symptoms for several days after initiating therapy and prefer continued antimicrobial therapy. I rarely obtain a culture during therapy unless persistent symptoms suggest unresolved bacteriuria. I believe that a follow-up urinalysis or culture 7 to 10 days after stopping therapy is mandatory. If the culture is positive, further therapy is based on the antimicrobial sensitivity testing, and repeat cultures are obtained during therapy. If the culture is negative and these patients are still symptomatic or the urinalysis continues to show pyuria, patients are re-evaluated several weeks later for other urologic diseases, such as stones, tumors, or tuberculosis.

Generally, I use the following drugs:

1. Nitrofurantoin, 100 mg orally four times daily. Nitrofurantoin usually is active against *E. coli, Streptococcus faecalis*, and *Staphylococcus aureus*. Some strains of *Enterobacter* species and *Klebsiella* species are resistant, and nitrofurantoin is not active against most strains of *Proteus*.
2. Penicillin G, 250 mg (400,000 units) orally four times daily. Ampicillin, 250 mg orally four times a day, is slightly more potent, but the difference in cost in my opinion does not warrant its use in most instances. Penicillin G achieves urinary levels that are remarkably effective against most strains of *E. coli, P. mirabilis, S. faecalis*, and *S. aureus*, and about 25 per cent of *Klebsiella*. The drug should be taken on an empty stomach so that complete absorption and full therapeutic urinary levels are achieved.
3. Sulfonamides: sulfamethoxazole (Gantanol), 1 gm orally twice daily; sulfisoxazole (Gantrisin), 500 mg four times daily orally. Sulfisoxazole produces about half the urinary concentration of biologically active drug as the same dose of sulfamethizole (Thiosulfil Forte). *E. coli* is the most susceptible species, followed by *Klebsiella* species, *P. mirabilis, Pseudomonas* species, and *S. aureus; S. faecalis* is resistant.
4. Trimethoprim-sulfamethoxazole (Bactrim or Septra), two tablets regular strength or one tablet double strength orally twice daily.
5. Fluoroquinolones: ciprofloxacin (Cipro), 250 to 500 mg orally twice daily; enoxacin (Penetrex), 200 to 400 mg orally twice daily; lomefloxacin (Maxaquin), 400 mg orally once daily; norfloxacin (Noroxin), 400 mg twice daily; ofloxacin (Floxin), 200 to 400 mg orally twice daily.

The dosage schedule probably increases patient compliance. These drugs are active against most uropathogens and are particularly attractive choices in patients with febrile urinary tract infections or recurrent urinary tract infections because they do not favor development of resistant strains (see below). Fluoroquinolones are not associated with multiple-drug (R-factor) resistance, so I use them when the patient is likely to be infected with a resistant strain as a result of recent exposure to sulfonamides, tetracycline, or penicillin.

Other drugs, such as oxytetracycline or tetracycline (250 to 500 mg orally four times daily) and cephalexin (Keflex, 250 to 500 mg four times daily) usually are reserved for therapy based on antimicrobial sensitivity testing. Tetracycline is very effective against *Pseudomonas* species. Cephalexin is not effective against some strains of *S. faecalis* but is quite effective against *Klebsiella*.

RECURRENT INFECTION

Reinfection

Recurrences at long intervals (usually longer than 2 weeks) and with different bacterial strains are characteristic of reinfection; however, reinfections at shorter intervals and even with the same species and serotype of *E. coli* are not uncommon. In my opinion, most men with initial urinary tract infection and all men with recurrent infections deserve a thorough urologic evaluation, which should include intravenous urography and cystoscopy. Because most recurrent infections in men are not reinfections but rather bacterial persistence, repeated segmental cultures of the urethra, bladder, urine, and expressed prostatic fluid are mandatory.

A thorough urologic evaluation is warranted in women with evidence of upper urinary tract infections, hemorrhagic cystitis, or other risk factors, such as a history of unexplained hematuria, obstructive symptoms, neurogenic bladder dysfunction, renal calculi, analgesic abuse, and severe diabetes mellitus. In the absence of these risk factors, intravenous urography may be deferred. We perform cystoscopy on all women with recurrent infections, because it has essentially no risk under local anesthesia and occasionally yields information about such conditions as enterovesical or vesicovaginal fistula, ectopic orifices, or ureterocele, or findings suggestive of neurogenic bladder dysfunction, which may be helpful in future management. Whether urethral stenosis contributes to reinfections in women remains controversial. It is apparent that, without vaginal colonization with fecal organisms, reinfection is unlikely to occur no matter how stenotic the urethra. However, it is possible that urethral stenosis in susceptible women can contribute to reinfections. Dilations of the stenotic urethra may be appropriate in such patients. There is little evidence, however, that urethral dilation or reconstruction is useful in the routine management of the majority of females with reinfections.

The primary goal of antimicrobial therapy should be to eliminate or reduce reinfections in the most convenient and inexpensive way. Reinfections in men are infrequent and best treated by intermittent therapy. We usually discuss three forms of management with the female patient. The first alternative is simply to treat each reinfection as it occurs. The patient is given a dip slide container and is instructed to culture her urine at the first symptoms of urinary tract infection. She then empirically starts antimicrobial therapy if the symptoms are severe enough. Because each infection is caused by bacteria from the fecal reservoir, it is important to minimize the impact of antimicrobial therapy on the bowel flora and prevent development of transferable drug resistance. Fluoroquinolones are the best choice because of their broad spectrum of activity and because they have not been associated with transferable drug resistance. Nitrofurantoin does not produce fecal resistance because of its complete absorption in the upper intestinal tract and is excreted in high concentrations in the urine. Likewise, trimethoprim-sulfamethoxazole rarely causes development of resistant strains. Broad-spectrum antimicrobial agents (such as ampicillin, tetracycline, cephalosporin) and sulfonamides (such as sulfisoxazole and sulfamethoxazole) should be avoided. If the initial culture is positive, we usually continue therapy for 3 days and then obtain a culture 7 to 10 days after therapy has been discontinued. It is mandatory to establish that the urine culture is negative after therapy. This is particularly true for patients who have been diagnosed by home dip slide culture and treated themselves initially. If symptoms persist, we obtain a repeat culture and perform sensitivity tests. The cost of treatment of each episode of bacteriuria is thus limited to two or three inexpensive dip slide cultures and a short course of antimicrobial therapy. This technique is particularly attractive to women who have infrequent infections and are willing to play an active role in their diagnosis and management.

If the patient's history suggests that reinfections are preceded by intercourse, we often suggest that she take a single antimicrobial tablet routinely before or after intercourse or at both times. Many patients will have a minimal number of reinfections when using this form of preventive therapy.

The most effective form of therapy is continuous, low-dosage prophylaxis. We favor this regimen as the initial form of therapy for all women who have frequent reinfections and also use it if intermittent therapy or therapy after intercourse proves to be impractical or ineffective. Once we have established that the urine culture shows no bacterial growth (most frequently as the patient is completing a 3-day course of antimicrobial therapy for antecedent infection), we institute nightly therapy with either 50 mg of nitrofurantoin, a half tablet of regular-strength trimethoprim-sulfamethoxazole, or one tablet of a fluoroquinolone. These agents are particularly desirable for long-term continuous therapy because, as noted earlier, they do not affect the fecal flora adversely in terms of selection of resistant mutants the way many antimicrobial agents do. The majority of patients will not have a urinary tract infection on these regimens. Infections can occur, however, and may not necessarily be associated with symptoms. Cultures should be performed at regular intervals.

We usually discontinue low-dosage continuous therapy after approximately 6 months and then simply follow the patient with frequent cultures to determine whether reinfections will occur. After a 6-month course of preventive therapy, approximately 30 per cent of women will have spontaneous remission for at least 6 months. Unfortunately, a remission is not a cure. Long infection-free intervals often are followed by reinfections, and intermittent or continuous therapy must be reinstituted. It also has been our impression that institution of oral contraceptives commonly is associated with onset of recurrent urinary tract infections. Many patients have reinfections that are associated with use of vaginal spermicidal agents, such as Encare Oval, which have been shown to increase vaginal colonization with uropathogens. Reinfections cease when the patients stop using the vaginal suppositories. If possible, therefore, we suggest that patients with recurrent infection avoid using spermicidal agents.

Bacterial Persistence

In some patients, infections tend to recur rapidly and are caused by the same species. Thus an infection usually is followed by a second within days of stopping therapy. It is important to establish whether the first infection actually was eradicated by antimicrobial therapy—that is, a negative culture on therapy. Thorough urologic evaluation is mandatory to identify whether the urinary tract is the focus of bacterial persistence that antimicrobial agents cannot reach or eradicate. The most common cause of bacterial persistence in men is chronic bacterial prostatitis. In women, the most common cause is infection stones resulting from urea-splitting organisms, such as *P. mirabilis.* A congenital or acquired anomaly, such as a calyceal diverticulum or a nonrefluxing urethral stump that has become secondarily infected, is a less common cause.

Surgical therapy plays a pivotal role in management of women with recurrent urinary tract infections. When the focus of bacterial persistence has been localized, it should be removed or the responsible defect should be corrected. Although the surgical procedure will cure the patient of the focus of recurrent infection, susceptibility to new infections frequently remains and can lead to further episodes of bacteriuria. If surgical removal of the focus is not possible, long-term suppressive antimicrobial therapy may be required.

Bacterial Prostatitis

Acute bacterial prostatitis is usually dramatic in presentation, easy to diagnose on physical examination, and associated with large numbers of bacteria in the prostatic secretions or bladder urine. Identification of bacteria in the expressed prostatic secretion or in voided bladder urine after prostatic massage at concentrations 1 log or more greater than that observed in the urethral (first-voided) urine specimen is diagnostic of bacterial prostatitis, a frequent cause of bacterial persistence. Patients with acute bacterial prostatitis respond dramatically to antimicrobial agents normally effective for acute urinary tract infections. I usually use either trimethoprim-sulfamethoxazole, one double-strength tablet two times a day or a fluoroquinolone.

Chronic bacterial prostatitis may respond to trimethoprim-sulfamethoxazole in a dosage of two regular-strength tablets or one double-strength tablet twice a day for 12 weeks. Approximately half the patients with chronic bacterial prostatitis caused by trimethoprim-sensitive organisms will be cured by this regimen. If the organism is resistant to trimethoprim, or if it persists in cultures of prostatic secretions obtained during the first 2 weeks of therapy, further trimethoprim-sulfamethoxazole therapy is pointless. Recent success has been reported with fluoroquinolone administered for 2 to 4 weeks. Approximately 70 per cent of patients who previously had failed long-term trimethoprim-sulfamethoxazole or carbenicillin therapy were cured.

Patients who are not cured by drug therapy may be managed by continuous low-dose suppressive therapy to prevent recurrent bladder infections. Trimethoprim-sulfamethoxazole (half a tablet nightly) or nitrofurantoin (50 mg nightly) is a suitable choice. When *Pseudomonas aeruginosa* is the pathogen, tetracycline hydrochloride (250 mg nightly) is recommended. It should be emphasized that discontinuation of therapy eventually results in recurrent bacteriuria.

HIGH-RISK PATIENTS

Any situation that predisposes to bacterial contamination of the urinary tract risks infection. Patients at increased risk of infection include those with renal failure, obstructive uropathy, or nephropathy caused by diabetes, analgesic abuse, or sickle cell disease, in whom there is a tendency toward papillary necrosis and secondary ureteral obstruction. Additionally, patients at increased risk of infection include those with neurogenic disorders of the urinary tract, those with urea-splitting bacterial infections that can lead to formation of infection stones, and those with indwelling catheters.

Women who are pregnant require careful monitoring for and treatment of bacteriuric episodes. I generally treat infections during pregnancy with a short course of cephalexin or nitrofurantoin. If recurrences are frequent, I may institute preventive therapy with nitrofurantoin, 50 mg at bedtime, for the remainder of the pregnancy. I avoid tetracycline, sulfonamides, and fluoroquinolones because of their potential effects on the fetus.

We do not treat patients who become bacteriuric as a result of indwelling urethral catheters unless they become symptomatic. If the catheter is to be removed, I obtain a urine culture, start the patient on the appropriate antimicrobial therapy, and then remove the catheter. A culture always should be obtained to document that the antimicrobial therapy is effective once the catheter has been removed.

Suggested Readings

Hooton RM, Hillier S, Johnson C, et al: *Escherichia coli* bacteriuria and contraceptive method. JAMA 265:64–69, 1991

Stamm WE, McKevitt M, Roberts PL, et al: Natural history of recurrent urinary tract infections in women. Rev Infect Dis 13:77–84, 1991

INTERSTITIAL CYSTITIS

PHILIP M. HANNO, M.D.

Philadelphia, Pennsylvania

Interstitial cystitis is a chronic, possibly inflammatory bladder condition of unknown etiology. It is a condition that is treatable but not curable. Its cardinal symptoms, pain on bladder filling relieved by emptying and urinary frequency, are really exaggerations of the normal perceptions of discomfort prompting urination that all persons experience. With no pathologic findings specific for interstitial cystitis, diagnosis of the condition can be extremely difficult. It is essential to rule out all known infectious and inflammatory conditions that can result in a similar symptom complex. Numerous attempts to find abnormalities associated with the symptoms to support the diagnosis have been made, but it remains essentially a diagnosis of exclusion. Unlike the vast majority of organic illnesses, one cannot diagnose interstitial cystitis on the basis of corroborative findings alone in a patient who is asymptomatic, because the diagnosis is fundamentally grounded in the symptomatology.

Interstitial cystitis, although reported in children and the elderly, most often afflicts middle-aged women, with a peak incidence in the fourth decade and a slightly higher prevalence in Jewish women and a lower incidence in black women. The disease onset is more commonly subacute than insidious, and full development of the classical symptom complex occurs in a short time. As a rule, the disease reaches its final stage rapidly and then stabilizes at that symptom level. Once the symptoms plateau, major deterioration is uncommon. The prevalence of diagnosed interstitial cystitis in the United States approximates 44,000 cases. If one calculates the number of patients with "painful bladder syndrome" who have not been evaluated for interstitial cystitis, the prevalence could be 5 to 10 times that figure. Interstitial cystitis patients are 10 to 12 times more likely than controls to report childhood bladder problems and twice as likely as controls to report a history of urinary tract infection. Quality of life indicators are somewhat lower than in patients on chronic renal dialysis for renal failure.

DIAGNOSTIC CRITERIA

To be diagnosed as having interstitial cystitis, patients must have either glomerulations on cystoscopic examination under anesthesia after bladder distention to 80 cm H_2O pressure or a classic Hunner ulcer, and they must have either pain associated with the bladder or urinary urgency. The diagnosis is unlikely in patients with a bladder capacity of greater than 350 ml on awake cystometry, an absence of sensory urgency with the bladder filled to 100 ml of gas or 150 ml of water during cystometry, and involuntary bladder contractions. An absence of nocturia and daytime frequency less than eight times also makes the diagnosis suspect.

There appear to be three groups of patients who show symptoms without an obvious cause. One group develops lower tract symptoms that resolve before any formal evaluation can be instituted. These are patients we would diagnose as suffering from the urethral syndrome. A second group of patients has the symptom complex long enough to be referred to a urologist, who elects to perform an evaluation including cystoscopy under anesthesia with hydrodistention of the bladder and biopsy. Those patients with glomerulation or Hunner ulcer are considered to have interstitial cystitis. Those without these "typical findings of interstitial cystitis" are in a twilight zone, but generally are treated as if they have interstitial cystitis. The specificity of the findings of bladder glomerulations and the percentage of the normal population that would be found to have glomerulations if the bladder were distended under anesthesia to 80 cm H_2O pressure are unclear. The number of patients with urethral syndrome who would have findings of interstitial cystitis if they were evaluated with bladder distention under anesthesia is also unknown.

ETIOLOGY

Although there is no lack of theories, the etiology of interstitial cystitis remains obscure. This is not necessarily surprising in a disease as difficult to categorize objectively as this one is. Today, the general opinion is that the etiology is multifactorial and that we may be dealing with a syndrome rather than a specific disease.

THERAPEUTIC MANAGEMENT

A disease with a multitude of therapies is generally a condition for which no truly effective treatment exists. Although the symptoms of interstitial cystitis can be controlled with one of a variety of treatments in the overwhelming majority of patients, there is little evidence that treatment accomplishes anything more than influencing the symptomatic expression of the disease rather than curing the condition.

Conservative Measures

Hydraulic distention is generally the initial therapeutic modality used in the treatment of interstitial cystitis because it is an initial part of the diagnostic process. Approximately 30 per cent of patients experience some symptomatic relief following distention, although we have been impressed that an almost equal number experience some exacerbation of their symptoms. Both effects seem to be short lived. At initial cystoscopy, we distend the bladder for 1 to 2 minutes at 80 cm H_2O pressure, empty it, refill it to establish the diagnosis, and let it remain distended for another 8 to 10 minutes.

Attempts at conservative, self-help regimens have much to recommend them and little in the way of side effects. Because 50 per cent of patients will experience spontaneous symptomatic relief for varying lengths of time, this can be a useful strategy in patients with mild to moderate symptoms. It is useful to have patients keep a voiding diary, recording their frequency for 2 weekdays and 1 weekend day every week. Any improvements will become apparent in the diary. Although some tend to overestimate the effect of certain foods and beverages on the symptoms of patients with interstitial cystitis, there is no doubt that many patients find their symptoms aggravated by specific foods and these should be eliminated. I always tell patients that there are no hard and fast rules with regard to diet, and to avoid whatever makes their symptoms worse. This often includes acidic beverages (citrus juices), caffeine, alcohol, and spicy foods. Bladder training (trying to increase the interval between urinations by a fixed amount every week) can decrease voiding intervals, but often at the expense of increased pain and discomfort. Decreasing stressful life-styles is often helpful.

Our next line of treatment is a trial of the antidepressant amitriptyline. It is the most potent tricyclic antidepressant in terms of blocking H_1 histaminergic receptors, stabilizes mast cells in vitro, and has actions that might tend to stimulate predominantly beta-adrenergic receptors in the bladder-body smooth musculature, an action that would further facilitate urinary storage by decreasing the excitability of smooth muscle in that area. It has analgesic actions that are not clearly understood and sedative properties that can be potentially beneficial to interstitial cystitis sufferers. In a dosage gradually increasing to 75 mg (always given before bed) over 3 weeks, responses have been over 50 per cent with little tachyphylaxis.

Experimental oral medications purported to show some efficacy include sodium pentosanpolysulfate (Elmiron), a synthetic glycosaminoglycan excreted in the urine; and nalmefene, an opiate antagonist capable of preventing mast cell degranulation in some experimental models. As of the spring of 1993, neither has received Food and Drug Administration approval in the United States. Results of a multicenter double-blind study of nalmefene have yet to be reported. Numerous studies of Elmiron have shown either no benefit or a marginal benefit in interstitial cystitis, with an excellent safety profile. Presently, Elmiron is available from the manufacturer (Baker-Norton, Miami, FL) on a compassionate use basis.

Small, uncontrolled series have reported efficacy with the old antihistamine hydroxyzine and the calcium channel antagonist nifedipine. The latter drug is known to inhibit smooth muscle contraction and cell-mediated immunity. Hydroxyzine can be administered at a dosage of 25 to 50 mg daily in divided doses. Nifedipine is administered in an extended release form at a dosage of 30 mg daily. The dosage can be doubled if symptoms do not respond after several weeks. Medical treatment of interstitial cystitis generally takes time to show results, and changes in therapy should not be undertaken until side effects warrant them or an adequate trial of several months has been completed.

In our practice, when distention and amitriptyline have failed, we move on to intravesical dimethylsulfoxide (DMSO). This is a product of the wood pulp industry and a derivative of lignum. Its pharmacologic properties include membrane penetration, enhanced drug absorption, anti-inflammatory and analgesic effects, collagen dissolution, muscle relaxation, and mast cell histamine release. For theoretical reasons we administer the 50-ml DMSO (Rimso-50) with 10,000 units of heparin, 10 mg triamcinolone acetonide (Kenalog), and 44 mEq bicarbonate. Treatments are weekly for 6 to 8 weeks. The response rate is about 60 per cent in most series and duration of response can be many months. Some patients can be placed on a monthly maintenance protocol and many patients can learn to administer the medication themselves at home. Silver nitrate has been used as a bladder instillation with good success by others. Chlorpactin (WWCS-90) in a 0.4% concentration is also an effective intravesical treatment with a success rate similar to DMSO. It is painful and requires anesthesia to administer. Nevertheless, we have used it in some patients refractory to all other therapies with surprisingly good results.

The rare patient with a discreet Hunner ulcer or a dominant area of ulceration can be treated with transurethral resection, fulguration, or laser irradiation. Transcutaneous electrical nerve stimulation (TENS) is effective in some patients, although it is used more frequently in Scandinavia than in the United States. The stimulation is delivered by suprapubic electrodes, and the rationale is to block afferent noxious impulses from the bladder. The generally recommended regimen is stimulation for 2 hours twice daily, although it would seem logical that longer periods of use would produce better results. The best results have been reported after treatment periods ranging up to 6 months. TENS has a negligible risk and is extremely noninvasive, and therefore can be considered as isolated or concomitant treatment, especially in patients whose main complaint is discomfort.

Surgical Therapy

It is certainly worthwhile to exhaust all reasonable conservative measures before proceeding to surgical therapy in a disease such as interstitial cystitis, which is chronic, not life threatening, and subject to spontaneous remission of symptomatology. Augmentation cystoplasty with supratrigonal cystectomy can be considered in unresponsive patients with a small-capacity bladder as measured under anesthesia. Patients with large-capacity bladders and intractable symptoms may be treated best with urinary diversion, with or without cystectomy. Continent diversion should be considered with caution in view of reports of pain developing in the pouch in some patients with a history of interstitial cystitis.

In most patients who cannot be managed conservatively (less than 10 per cent in our experience), we recommend urinary conduit diversion rather than substitution cystoplasty, because good results with the latter procedure are anything but assured, and the need for clean intermittent catheterization in about 15 to 25 per cent of women after cystoplasty turns what would still be considered a success for other disease processes into a failure, because intermittent catheterization may be excruciating for an IC patient.

SUMMARY

Interstitial cystitis is a difficult condition to manage and requires a tremendous amount of time from physician and his or her staff to successfully treat. The results of therapy can range from spectacular to awful and may change over a short period of time. Nevertheless, most patients with interstitial cystitis can be helped to live relatively normal lives and, with the aid of various forms of treatment modalities, including self-help, to tolerate their disability. Patients should be encouraged to contact the Interstitial Cystitis Association in New York (PO Box 1553, Madison Square Station, New York, NY 10159) for information and helpful programs.

Suggested Readings

Batra AK, Wein AJ, Hanno PM: Interstitial cystitis. A.U.A. Update Series 8:66–72, 1993

Hanno PM, Staskin D, Krane R, et al (eds): Interstitial Cystitis. Springer-Verlag, London, 1990

Koziol JA, Clark DC, Gittes RF, et al: The natural history of interstitial cystitis: A survey of 374 patients. J Urol 149:465–469, 1993

CYTOXAN CYSTITIS

GABRIEL P. HAAS, M.D.

Detroit, Michigan

PATHOPHYSIOLOGY

Cyclophosphamide (Cytoxan) is a commonly used alkylating agent for the treatment of a variety of malignancies, including solid tumors, lymphoproliferative diseases, and non-neoplastic diseases, such as rheumatoid arthritis, systemic lupus erythematosus, and Wegener granulomatosis. Cancer patients generally receive high-dose intravenous cyclophosphamide, whereas low-dose, long-term oral regimens are the treatment of choice for autoimmune diseases and other *benign* (relatively speaking) conditions. Treatment with cyclophosphamide, and related cytotoxic agents such as ifosfamide, is associated with major short- and long-term urologic complications. Patients treated with cyclophosphamide have an increased risk (up to ninefold) for developing urothelial malignancies, particularly transitional cell cancer of the bladder. A more common complication, hemorrhagic cystitis, is seen in up to 40 per cent of patients on low-dose therapies, and even more frequently in patients on high-dose IV therapy, such as required for bone marrow transplantation. Although the malignancies usually develop many years after exposure to the chemotherapy, hemorrhagic cystitis is more likely to be an acute complication during or shortly after therapy. Occasionally, symptoms may present years after the treatment.

The clinical manifestations of hemorrhagic cystitis vary from asymptomatic, intermittent microscopic hematuria to recurrent episodes of life-threatening hemorrhage accompanied by severe irritative symptoms, suprapubic pain, and hemodynamic instability. Patients can develop clot retention and upper tract obstruction, and, despite aggressive management, a 4 per cent mortality rate has been reported with intractable bladder hemorrhage. Occasionally, the renal pelvis is the source of the bleeding. Some patients have chronic irritative voiding symptoms and, less frequently, urge incontinence as the primary manifestation of their disease.

Acute findings of cyclophosphamide cystitis include an edematous bladder containing punctate hemorrhagic areas, mucosal ulcerations, and diffuse telangiectasia. The mucosa is friable and bleeds readily on manipulation. The long-term sequelae include fibrosis, reduced bladder capacity, and, occasionally, vesicoureteral reflux and hydronephrosis.

Cyclophosphamide is metabolized in the liver, and a high concentration of the metabolites can be found in urine. It is believed that is is not actually the cyclophosphamide, but rather its metabolic product, acrolein, that is responsible for the toxic side effects. Urothelial damage occurs through direct contact with this metabolite, and the severity of the effects may be related to the length and frequency of the exposure. Therefore, attempts to prevent the onset of hemorrhagic cystitis aim to reduce the exposure of the urothelium to the toxic compound(s) and to neutralize their effects.

PROPHYLAXIS AGAINST CYCLOPHOSPHAMIDE-INDUCED CYSTITIS

The best treatment of hemorrhagic cystitis is prevention of its onset. Patients undergoing therapy with cyclophosphamide or related chemotherapeutic agents should be well hydrated and alkalinized, and encouraged to void frequently. Patients undergoing brief, intensive high-dose regimens should have a urethral catheter placed and undergo saline bladder irrigation.

Recent success has been achieved in the prevention of cyclophosphamide cystitis with 2-mercaptoethane sodium sulfonate (Mesna). Mesna forms a nontoxic congener with acrolein and neutralizes the toxic effects on the urothelium. In order to be effective, concomitant administration with cyclophosphamide is indicated. There is mounting evidence in the chemotherapy literature that Mesna is highly effective in diminishing the risk and severity of hemorrhagic cystitis secondary to the administration of cyclophosphamide and related compounds. It is not known at this time if the use of Mesna diminishes the effectiveness of cyclophosphamide therapy or if it reduces the risk of subsequent transitional cancer.

TREATMENT

Management of cyclophosphamide cystitis depends on the severity of the symptoms. Patients whose major manifestation is urgency/frequency syndrome may respond to anticholinergic therapy. Patients with hemorrhagic cystitis require rapid and aggressive intervention. If the onset of symptoms occurs while the patient is on cyclophosphamide therapy, the drug should be discontinued. Patients should be cystoscoped for clot evacuation, establishment of the diagnosis, and fulguration of isolated bleeding points. Instrumentation may have an increased risk because of the patient's underlying immunosuppressed and myelosuppressed state.

A variety of intravesical irrigation solutions have been promoted to interrupt the hemorrhage. Cold saline irrigation may be tried as the first step. Silver nitrate (1%) or potassium aluminum sulfate (Alum) (1%) irrigation is a relatively safe option that can be administered without anesthesia and is effective in reducing bleeding. Both methods act by forming salt-protein precipitation over the bleeding surface. Precipitation from silver salts in the renal pelvis with consequent obstruction has been reported in association with ureteral reflux. The dense precipitate may also clog the Foley catheter and must be evacuated if the therapy is unsuccessful and alternate measures are indicated.

Prostaglandins E_2 and F_2 also have been used with some success in selected case reports. Prostaglandins are synthesized naturally by many organ systems, including the urinary tract, but the full scope of their activity is yet to be elucidated. It is believed that their beneficial effect in the treatment of hemorrhagic cystitis is derived from their ability to stabilize membranes and to improve healing of the microvascular epithelium, and from their effect on detrusor contractility. Several types of prostaglandins currently are available commercially, and further analogues are under development.

Formalin installation has been used as an effective means of controlling bleeding when less toxic alternatives have failed. Formalin is the aqueous solution of formaldehyde and works by cross-linking proteins over the bleeding surface. Administration is painful, so it should be given under anesthesia and only after vesicoureteral reflux has been either ruled out or prevented by ureteral catheterization and balloon obstruction. Administration of formalin in the presence of reflux has resulted in severe upper tract complications, including ureteral fibrosis and obstruction, hydronephrosis, and papillary necrosis. The incidence of lower tract complications proportionally depends on the concentration of formalin used. A 1% solution is relatively safe but less effective than higher concentrations. A 10% formalin solution is significantly more effective in controlling bleeding but has a much higher morbidity. This includes severe pain, bladder fibrosis, and reduction of both capacity and compliance, and perforation and peritonitis have been reported as well. Most authors recommend the use of a 5% solution. A cystogram should be performed prior to administration to rule out reflux.

Another substance with treatment precautions and toxicity similar to those of formalin, phenol (carbonic acid), has been used with some success, but the cumulative experience is more limited. The adverse side effects of phenol may be less extensive and permanent.

In conjunction with intravesical treatment, systemic pharmacotherapy may have a role in the management of severe cases. Intravenous epsilon-aminocaproic acid (Amicar), vasopressin, or conjugated estrogens have been tried with variable success. Aminocaproic acid inhibits plasminogen activation and fibrinolysis, and promotes clot formation over bleeding surfaces. Vasopressin diminishes bleeding secondary to capillary constriction. The mechanism of action of conjugated estrogens is not known, but they have been shown to diminish bleeding time and improve hemostasis.

Cystostomy, open bladder packing, urinary diversion, and angiographic embolization or ligation of the hypogastric arteries or their branches have been tried as last-resort intervention, with cystectomy as the ultimate method of controlling severe, life-threatening bleeding.

CONCLUSION

The risk of hemorrhagic cystitis and the development of urothelial cancer should be considered in all patients scheduled for cyclophosphamide therapy, particularly in those who are being treated for benign disease. Long-term survivors should have regular urologic follow-up, and patients with irritable voiding symptoms or microscopic hematuria should be evaluated for the presence of a malignancy rather than simply attributing these symptoms to mild cystitis alone.

Suggested Readings

Andriole GL, Yuan JJJ, Catalona WJ: Cystotomy, temporary urinary diversion and bladder packing in the management of severe cyclophosphamide-induced hemorrhagic cystitis. J Urol 143:1006, 1990

Brock N, Stebar J, Pahl J, et al: Acrolein, the causative factor of urotoxic side effects of cyclophosphamide, ifosfamide, trofosfamide, and sulfosfamide. Drug Res 29:659, 1979

DeVries CR, Freiha FS: Hemorrhagic cystitis: A review. J Urol 143:1, 1990

Donahue LA, Frank IN: Intravesical formalin therapy for hemorrhagic cystitis: Analysis of therapy. J Urol 141: 809, 1989

Jerkins GR, Noe NH, Hill D: Treatment of complications of cyclophosphamide cystitis. J Urol 139:923, 1988

Levine AL, Richie JP: Urological complications of cyclophosphamide. J Urol 141:1063, 1989

Liu YK, Harty JI, Steinbock GS, et al: Treatment of radiation or cyclophosphamide induced hemorrhagic cystitis using conjugated estrogen. J Urol 144:41, 1990

O'Keane JC: Carcinoma of the urinary bladder after treatment with cyclophosphamide. N Engl J Med 319:871, 1988

Plotz PH, Klippel JH, Decker JL, et al: Bladder complications in patients receiving cyclophosphamide for systemic lupus erythematosus or rheumatoid arthritis. Ann Intern Med 91:221, 1979

Santos GW, Tutschka PJ, Brookmeyer R, et al: Marrow transplantation for acute nonlymphatic leukemia after treatment with busulfan and cyclophosphamide. N Engl J Med 309:1347, 1983

CROHN'S DISEASE AND THE URINARY TRACT

MICHEL A. PONTARI, M.D.

Philadelphia, Pennsylvania

Crohn's disease, also called regional enteritis, is an inflammatory bowel disorder of unknown etiology. Lesions characteristically produce transmural inflammation of the bowel, and are often discontinuous, with skip areas of normal bowel in between. About one third of cases involve the ileum, one third the colon, and one third affect both areas. Rarely, the more proximal small bowel, and even the stomach or mouth, may be involved. The first reported complication of Crohn's disease involving the genitourinary tract appeared soon after the original description of the disease in 1932. The most common of these processes are cystitis, periureteral fibrosis with ureteral obstruction, fistula formation, and urinary tract calculi. Retroperitoneal and psoas abscesses and amyloidosis also occur. Complications such as these are more common in patients whose Crohn's disease is relatively severe, and usually of long duration. Approximately one quarter of patients with Crohn's disease will have symptoms referable to the urinary tract at some time during the course of their disease.

CYSTITIS

The most common urologic problem in patients with Crohn's disease is cystitis. Nocturia and dysuria are the most frequently reported symptoms. Bouts of cystitis in Crohn's disease patients are often recurrent. Repeated episodes can produce a bladder that, on cystogram, can appear to be fixed, spiculated, or have nodular filling defects of the dome. In the absence of an anatomic abnormality such as a stone or a fistula, bladder symptoms will decrease with successful treatment of the bowel disease.

URINARY TRACT CALCULI

Urinary tract calculi occur in 0.09 per cent of all patients admitted to general hospitals, whereas the incidence of stones in patients with inflammatory bowel disease ranges from 8 to 19 per cent. Most stones are calcium oxalate. Uric acid calculi are less common than oxalate stones in this population, but are found far more frequently than they would be in the general population. The great number of calcium oxalate stones can be explained on the basis of enteric or acquired hyperoxaluria, in which there is increased absorption of dietary oxalate. Normally, dietary calcium combines with dietary oxalate in the gut to form calcium oxalate, which is insoluble and eliminated in the feces. In patients with ileal dysfunction, such as in Crohn's disease, fatty acids cannot be absorbed normally in the ileum and are free to combine with calcium. Oxalate is then left unbound, and is able to be absorbed in the colon. Unabsorbed fatty acids also enter the colon and make the colonic mucosa more permeable to oxalate. Absorbed oxalate is excreted in the urine, resulting in hyperoxaluria. The situation is exacerbated by poor water absorption, dehydration, and oliguria in patients with ileostomies, making conditions even more favorable for stone formation.

Conditions that favor the formation of uric acid calculi include diarrhea and the presence of an ileostomy, both of which lead to the loss of large amounts of alkaline intestinal fluid. In both instances, the kidneys then will secrete a urine that is both more concentrated and more acidic than normal. Other factors that have been implicated in stone formation in Crohn's disease patients are urinary tract infection, urinary tract obstruction, steroid administration, prolonged bed rest, and decreased intestinal absorption of sodium with a resultant decrease in urinary sodium.

URETERAL OBSTRUCTION

Ureteral obstruction is more common on the right side because of the anatomic proximity of the right ureter to the terminal ileum, the most frequent site of bowel involvement by Crohn's disease. Right side obstruction occurs almost exclusively at the pelvic brim. Obstruction of the left ureter usually is due to involvement of the colon if distal, whereas proximal left ureteral obstruction more often is caused by involvement of the jejeunum. Bilateral distal ureteral obstruction is rare in Crohn's disease, but may occur in the setting of a pelvic abscess. Grossly, the spectrum of disease producing ureteral involvement ranges from mild periureteral fibrosis with mild ureteral dilation to encasement of the ureter in dense fibrosis. The origin of the periureteral fibrosis is thought to be extraperitoneal extension of an intestinal inflammatory process by way of the lymphatics. Microscopic examination of the periureteral process shows collagen, edema, and pseudomyxomatous changes consistent with lymphedema.

Urinary tract symptoms frequently are absent with ureteral obstruction. Symptoms related to bowel disease often have been present for years. Usually the urinalysis is benign and urine cultures are negative. On urography, the opacified ureteral lumen tapers symmetrically and appears cone shaped, suggestive of the cicatrical periureteral process. The mucosa is smooth and uninvolved by the fibrosis. With long-standing obstruction, the ureter may deviate toward midline. The ureteral obstruction resolves in the majority of cases after a surgical procedure to remove diseased segments of bowel. Cases also have been reported in which the ureteral obstruction was temporized with a stent or percutaneous nephrostomy, and resolved after treatment with steroids and/or antibiotics. In cases of long-standing ureteral obstruction, the ureter is surrounded by dense periureteral fibrosis, and ureteral dilation may not respond solely to conservative treatment or bowel resection alone. In these cases, a ureterolysis may be necessary as well. This decision must be made at the time of the bowel procedure. Ureteral strictures that persist after bowel surgery often respond to balloon catheter dilation.

ENTEROVESICAL FISTULA

Bladder involvement in Crohn's disease is by direct extension of the inflammatory process of an adjacent loop of bowel, or as the spread of an abscess. This process has various stages. Initial symptoms may include urinary frequency, urgency, dysuria, and hematuria. As a rule, bladder processes in Crohn's disease produce more symptoms than involvement of the ureter. With the development of an enterovesical fistula, pneumaturia and fecaluria may develop. The most common site for an enterovesical fistula in Crohn's disease is between the ileum and bladder. Colovesical fistulas also are seen. In women, the uterus acts as a natural barrier to protect much of the back of the bladder, and as a result enterovesical fistulas are much less common than in men.

The most sensitive test to diagnose an enterovesical fistula is a computerized tomography (CT) scan. In the absence of recent instrumentation or a gas-producing urinary tract infection (usually only seen in diabetics), the presence of air in the bladder is pathognomonic for an enterovesical fistula. CT can pick up much smaller amounts of air than can a plain film, and also will give more information about surrounding structures, which is valuable information in planning treatment. Cystoscopy is required in all patients with an enterovesical fistula, because this is the only modality that can evaluate the bladder mucosa directly and rule out bladder carcinoma as a cause of the fistula. Common findings at cystoscopy include bullous edema at the site of the fistula, generalized inflammation, or polypoid epithelial proliferation, which has been called the "herald sign" because it may be the initial presentation of a clinically silent extravesical inflammatory process. Frequently, the site of the fistula is not identified at cystoscopy. A good, cheap, easy, and sensitive first test is the administration of oral charcoal; the presence of charcoaluria will make the diagnosis.

In the age of antibiotics and good perioperative nutrition, most enterovesical fistulas can be treated by one operation that separates the bowel from the bladder, resects the involved bowel, re-establishes bowel continuity, and repairs the bladder defect. Two-stage procedures involving a temporary diverting colostomy are reserved for cases of enterovesical fistula associated with a frank abscess or a sick patient whose condition must be temporized. There is no indication in the modern era for a three-stage procedure.

OTHER GENITOURINARY COMPLICATIONS

Amyloidosis

A secondary form of amyloidosis that affects the kidneys and, rarely, the adrenal glands has been observed in Crohn's disease. Complications include the nephrotic syndrome and renal failure. The diagnosis rarely is made antemortem, but, if identified, is an indication for resection of the diseased bowel.

Retroperitoneal Abscess Formation

Transmural extension of Crohn's disease may result in bowel perforation and abscess formation. Depending on the location of the perforation, a retroperitoneal, perinephric, or psoas abscess may develop. Retroperitoneal abscess can cause renal displacement, ureteral deviation and obstruction, or bladder deformity, possibly even leading to an enterovesical fistula.

Other Fistulas

Much less commonly than enterovesical fistulas, Crohn's disease will produce fistulas between the rectum and male urethra (usually the bulbar segment) or vagina. Fistulas also have been noted between the ileum and ureter, vagina, uterus, or fallopian tube.

Suggested Readings

Banner MP: Genitourinary complications of inflammatory bowel disease. Radiol Clin North Am 25:199, 1987

Kyle J: Urinary complications of Crohn's's disease. World J Surg 4:153, 1980

Pontari MA, Garvey R, Ballantyne G, et al: The diagnosis and management of enterovesical fistulae. Am Surg 58: 258, 1992

Shield DE, Lytton B, Weiss RM, et al: Urologic complications of inflammatory bowel disease. J Urol 115:701, 1976

Siminovitch JMP, Fazio VW: Ureteral obstruction secondary to Crohn's disease: A need for ureterolysis? Am J Surg 139:95, 1980

LEUKOPLAKIA OF THE URINARY TRACT

RALPH C. BENSON, Jr., M.D.

Nashville, Tennessee

Leukoplakia was first described in 1861 and usually is characterized as cornification of a normally noncornifying membrane. Although leukoplakia of the upper and lower urinary tracts has been known for a long time and in excess of 300 cases have been described, its pathogenesis, malignant potential, and treatment continue to be enigmatic.

PATHOGENESIS AND HISTOPATHOLOGY

There is ongoing debate regarding the pathologic criteria for the diagnosis of leukoplakia. Many investigators require only the presence of squamous metaplasia of the transitional epithelium associated with keratinization. This description is probably inadequate in that it does not distinguish leukoplakia from squamous metaplasia with normal squamous epithelium as seen on the trigone of premenopausal women. I believe that the features for diagnosis of leukoplakia should include (1) squamous metaplasia and hyperkeratosis, (2) down growth of rete pegs (or acanthosis), and (3) dysplastic squamous maturation.

A number of theories exist as to the possible cause of leukoplakia, and one can fit most of these into the following categories: (1) embryologic dispersal of ectodermal cells, (2) spontaneous transformation, (3) epithelial response secondary to appropriate stimuli, and (4) vitamin A deficiency.

Embryologic contamination of misplaced cells from the primitive ectodermal layer is possible because the wolffian duct develops near the ectodermal tissues. Although several investigators have found no evidence of squamous cell rests in examining urinary tracts, others have found squamous epithelium in up to 8 per cent of bladders sectioned at autopsy. In many patients, including children and newborns, leukoplakia of the upper and lower urinary tracts has been found in the absence of any obvious inciting cause, thereby lending credence to the possibility of spontaneous transformation. In addition, studies of the various proliferative and metaplastic changes in bladder urothelium indicate that most of the changes are variations of normal cellular growth. It even has been suggested that transitional cell epithelium is a misnomer and that the bladder is normally lined by modified squamous epithelium.

It is known that vitamin A deficiency will produce leukoplakia-like changes in the urinary tract mucosa in rats, but such changes do not appear to have occurred in most vitamin A deficient patients, although two such cases have been reported. In these patients the deficiency did not appear to be the cause of the disease, because a trial of vitamin supplements changed neither the signs of vesicle leukoplakia nor the irritative clinical symptoms.

The most generally held theory, and the one to which the author ascribes, is that leukoplakia occurs as a reactive process secondary to exposure of transitional cells to appropriate stimuli. The proliferative, metaplastic, and neoplastic capabilities of the transitional cell are well documented and they occur in response to chronic irritation, chronic infection, or hormone imbalance. The reasons for patient presentation and the associated diagnoses in most series appear to substantiate the concept that leukoplakia occurs as a response to noxious stimuli.

DIAGNOSIS

The literature records approximately 502 cases of leukoplakia of the urinary tract (102 upper tract, 384 bladder, and 16 urethra). Although the incidence of this disorder previously was thought to be higher in men than in women, that is probably not the case. The most frequent complaint involving patients with leukoplakia of both the upper and lower tracts is irritative bladder symptoms, often secondary to chronic infection. Other frequently encountered reasons for evaluation are stone disease, hematuria, and urinary obstructive symptoms. Therefore, although an unusual disease, leukoplakia should be included in the differential diagnosis of common urologic complaints.

The diagnosis of leukoplakia of the renal pelvis or ureter (or both) usually is not made exclusively. Although it may be expected, leukoplakia is usually diagnosed secondary to exploration performed because of associated conditions. The classic findings of flank pain and passage of desquamated keratinous material are unusual. Although the diagnosis of upper tract leukoplakia in patients without a pathology is an extremely difficult one to make, it should be considered in the differential diagnosis of lucent filling defects of the renal pelvis and ureter.

Leukoplakia of the bladder may be diagnosed with relative ease at cystoscopy, although the condition rarely is suspected before the examination. The whitish-grey-yellow lesions often appear to be floating on an inflamed urothelium. The borders may be sharply demarcated or may appear to blend imperceptibly with the surrounding mucosa. Leukoplakia may be located anywhere within the bladder, but it characteristically spares the ureteral orifice. Biopsy easily will distinguish leukoplakia from similar-appearing alkaline incrustation, yeast cystitis, malakoplakia, or squamous metaplasia of the trigone in females.

Leukoplakia of the urethra is rare. It appears to be more common in males than in females, with only three female patients having been reported to date. Patients with urethral leukoplakia will present with a pattern of chronic, nonspecific, irritative complaints.

RELATIONSHIP TO UROTHELIAL MALIGNANCY

There appears to be a strong association between leukoplakia and cancer of the urinary tract. Although the concomitant cancer is usually of the squamous cell type, transitional cell carcinoma and the mixture of the two have been recorded in both upper tract and lower tract cancers. The literature suggests the simultaneous association of leukoplakia and malignancy in 8 to 13 per cent of upper tract lesions, 10 to 22 per cent of bladder lesions, and 15 per cent of urethral lesions.

No amount of documentation of the association between the simultaneous existence of leukoplakia and carcinoma can confirm cause and effect. The urologist's concern, however, is whether leukoplakia is a premalignant lesion. Although the definition of a premalignant lesion is debatable, the largest series of patients with leukoplakia thus far reported indicates that it frequently heralds frank malignant disease. No reported patients thus far have had documented progression of leukoplakia of the upper tract to carcinoma. The probable reason for this is that the vast majority of patients with leukoplakia of the upper tract have had the diagnosis made at nephrectomy for associated pathologic conditions. As many as 26 per cent of carefully followed patients with leukoplakia of the bladder have been reported to develop bladder cancer at a later date (latent period 3 months to 30 years, with a mean of 11 years). No patients with leukoplakia of the urethra have been noted to progress to carcinoma.

Because of the rarity of this disease, there is no consensus as to how upper and lower urinary tract leukoplakias should be treated. Initial treatment in most all patients is directed at the associated disease. Antibiotic therapy should be administered if the usual infection is present and anticholinergic drugs are often helpful for reduction of bladder spasms and associated irritative voiding symptoms. Transurethral treatment, such as fulguration, resection, or laser photoradiation, on the whole have been only modestly successful, and it is doubtful whether a cure has been achieved in any significant number of patients.

Urinary diversion in order to alleviate symptomatology may be effective; however, it is important to underscore the fact that malignant change can occur in the defunctionalized bladder and in the prostatic urethra if the bladder and prostate are not removed. If the decision is made not to perform cystectomy or cystoprostatectomy, these patients should be followed very carefully for the possibility of malignant transformation. Certainly nephrectomy, ureterectomy, cystectomy, cystoprostatectomy, or urothrectomy should be performed if there is concomitant carcinoma. Although the risk of subsequent malignant tranformation is very real and is in excess of 20 per cent, radical extirpation probably is not warranted in all patients at the time of diagnosis. The evidence is overwhelming that leukoplakia is a premalignant disease, and therefore these patients deserve careful and frequent follow-up examinations.

Suggested Readings

Benson RC Jr, Swanson SK, Farrow GM: Relationship of leukoplakia to urothelial malignancy. J Urol 131:507, 1984

Mueller SC, Thueroff JW, Rumpelt HJ: Urothelial leukoplakia: New aspects of etiology and therapy. J Urol 137: 979–989, 1987

O'Flynn JD, Mullaney J: Vesical leukoplakia progressing to carcinoma. Br J Urol 46:31, 1974

SCHISTOSOMIASIS OF THE URINARY BLADDER AND URETERS

ROBERT O. PETERSEN, M.D.

Philadelphia, Pennsylvania

The magnitude of the health problem of schistosomiasis commonly is unrecognized in the United States by virtue of the rarity of affected patients in this part of the world. However, the worldwide prevalence, primarily resulting from the frequency observed in North Africa and areas of the Middle East, has produced estimates of 200 to 300 million infected people. Only malaria exceeds the prevalence of this disease worldwide. Occasional patients immigrating from the above geographic locations, and Puerto Rico, where it is also endemic, are encountered in medical practice in the United States.

Urinary schistosomiasis (bilharziasis) is caused by the trematode genus *Schistosoma*, with five medically important species, the most frequently implicated being *S. haematobium*, *S. mansoni* and *S. matthei.*

Human infection is the result of direct penetration of intact skin by free-swimming cercariae subsequent to their release from the intermediate host, freshwater snails. Children and adults bathing or recreating in freshwater ponds and streams inhabited by the snails are at risk. The cercariae enter the venous system, traverse the pulmonary circulation, and ultimately migrate to the visceral and, in particular, the perivesical veins, where they mature into adults. Paired adults in this location produce approximately 100 eggs/day per female adult worm. The eggs released initiate a granulomatous response mediated by T lymphocytes, most prominently in the microvasculature and interstitium of the lamina propria of the vesical wall. Ulceration of the overlying urothelial mucosa results in the shedding of viable eggs into the bladder lumen, ultimately to be excreted in the urine. The urine containing the viable eggs, in the circumstance of suboptimal sanitary facilities, contaminates local freshwater streams containing the intermediate host snails, thus completing the cycle and perpetuating the conditions for future human infection.

Studies of the past two decades have improved greatly our understanding of both the clinical and pathological evolution of schistosomiasis infection. One direct result of this increased knowledge is a more accurate assessment of the magnitude of the worldwide health problem posed by schistosomiasis.

STAGES OF SCHISTOSOMIASIS

Schistosomiasis demonstrates a clinically active stage followed by a prolonged chronic inactive stage. During the initial infection (the active stage), adult worms are producing eggs that produce the granulomatous lesions in the bladder wall, and that are excreted in the urine in numbers proportional to the tissue density of organisms in the bladder wall. Propagation of the disease in a community is perpetuated by all those individuals with active infection excreting eggs into the local freshwater sites harboring the intermediate host snails. Clinically silent infections in the early active phase of disease are not uncommon. Conversely, some patients demonstrate the clinical features of ureteral obstruction and its consequences. Commonly, health programs designed to identify cases of active schistosomiasis address the demonstration of eggs in urine samples, with the therapeutic goal of administration of appropriate anti-schistosomal antibiotics to eradicate adult worms, reverse ureteral obstructive lesions, and arrest their development into lesions requiring surgical intervention.

Smith and Christie have analyzed the factors contributing to the severity of the clinical manifestations and found correlation with (1) the duration of infection, and (2) the intensity of infection (worm burden and tissue egg burden) to be the most important. Patients with high egg density in the vesical and ureteral walls tend to have larger granulomatous lesions in these sites, with corresponding higher probability of obstructive complications.

The clinically inactive stage is characterized by absence of adult worms and, therefore, cessation of egg production, dissemination, and resultant granuloma formation. Patients in this stage are either children or adults previously diagnosed and appropriately treated during the active stage, or adults in whom the adult worms have died without medical intervention. All patients in this stage, by virtue of no longer being a source of viable ova excreted in the urine, cease being a contribution to the dissemination of the disease.

BLADDER LESIONS

The hallmark lesion of schistosomias involving the lower urinary tract is the perioval granuloma. This lesion is most frequently observed in the lamina propria of the urinary bladder and is characterized by centrally clustered ova surrounded by a mixed population of acute and chronic inflammatory cells, including eosinophils, lymphocytes, plasma cells, and histiocytes, some with multinucleation. Lymphocytes predominate in these lesions. Such granulomas may be centered by a cluster of ova within small veins, the vascular structure being destroyed in the inflammatory lesion. The location of these characteristic granulomas varies from case to case, but they tend to affect the nontrigone areas of the bladder. The number of granulomas varies also, correlated with the intravascular worm burden. These early lesions are characteristically very cellular, with minimal fibroblastic response. The typical progression of the lesion is a quantitative reversal of the cell composition and the lesional fibrosis with a virtual extinction of inflammatory cells and increasing prominence of the fibrosis, which, in time, shows increasing calcification.

Thus, the early cellular infiltration around the clustered ova produces an inflammatory polypoid lesion that may persist, with progressive stromal fibrosis, or retract, with concurrent local muscle destruction and confluence of the fibrosis and the enveloped nonviable ova. This lesion evolution has been described as polyposis progressing to fibrous patches to "sandy" patches, the last lesion so named because the prominent granular dystrophic calcification confers a "sandy" texture to the cut surface.

Finally, it is common for affected urinary bladders to contain multiple granulomas with histologic features showing all phases of evolution; these are most prominent in patients in the clinically active phase of the disease. This variability is not observed in long-standing infections with protracted inactive phases, in which fibrosis, calcification, and nonviable ova constitute the uniform histologic features of the disease.

In addition to the above-described lesions, mucosal ulcerations, characteristically small and more common in the late or inactive stages, with prominent intramural fibrosis and calcification, are observed. Such ulcerations are the underlying cause for the high frequency of hematuria observed in bilharziasis.

Accompanying the granulomas are a spectrum of proliferative, metaplastic, and occasionally dysplastic changes of the urothelium, including cystitis cystica, cystitis grandularis, so-called mucinous or colonic metaplasia, squamous metaplasia, or simple urothelial hyperplasia of variable prominence. On occasion, the above proliferative and metaplastic urothelial changes are observed to have dysplastic features, possibly reflecting a morphologic step in the progression of neoplasia—here occurring in the context of schistosomiasis (refer to discussion on Schistosomiasis and Vesical Carcinoma, below).

URETERAL LESIONS

An integral component of bilharziasis is the commonly observed ureteral obstruction accompanying the lesions in the urinary bladder. Sharfi and Rayis reported ureteral involvement in 55 of 176 patients with urinary bladder schistosomiasis. A spectrum of lesions are observed that contribute to the anatomic or functional ureteral obstruction, including strictures, polyps, associated lithiasis and urothelial hyperplasias, and metaplastic changes similar to those noted in the infected urinary bladder.

When strictures are present, 90 per cent are located in the distal ureter and are accompanied by dilation of the more proximal ureter. In long-standing cases, hydroureter is accompanied by hydronephrosis, with a spectrum of severity from loss of renal parenchyma up to and including end-stage kidney(s) with complete loss of renal function. Indeed, death in renal failure has been observed if the ureteral obstructive nephropathy is bilateral. In many cases, evidence of superimposed pyelonephritis further contributes to the acceleration of renal function loss.

Ureteral involvement is indicative of patients who have had a major infection with a high egg tissue burden, with resulting inflammation and fibrosis in the lamina propria and destruction of the muscularis. If the fibrosis with granulomas predominates, the resultant lesion is a segmental stenosis of the ureter and proximal ureteral dilation. Nonstenotic obstructions are the result of preponderant loss of muscle, with adynamic segment(s) of the ureter producing functional impairment. Accompanying the intramural lesions are metaplastic urothelial changes, including ureteritis cystical and glandularis and squamous metaplasia. Lithiasis superimposed on the above morphologic changes is common.

Treatment of the above spectrum of ureteral lesions in schistosomiasis and the possible accompanying renal complications may require surgical excision of affected segments, with gratifying reversal of the obstructive complications in the proximal tract reported in some patients.

SCHISTOSOMIASIS AND VESICAL CARCINOMA

Abundant literature has accumulated over the years linking vesical schistosomiasis and cancer of the urinary bladder. The details of this relationship are still evolving. Studies in endemic areas have demonstrated a significantly different frequency distribution of histologic types of bladder carcinoma than that observed elsewhere. Squamous cell carcinoma is the most common type, followed by adenocarcinoma, with relatively few cases of transitional cell carcinoma; the last-mentioned histologic form comprises over 90 per cent of all vesical carcinomas observed in the United States. Additionally, it should be mentioned that virtually all examples of verrucous carcinoma, a variant squamous cell carcinoma rarely observed in the urinary bladder, have been reported in bilharzial bladders.

These frequency differences may be attributed to the high frequency of metaplastic changes observed in the urothelium in bladders with long-standing schistosomal infection. Also, dysplastic changes of the metaplastic urothelium are observed in schistosomiasis. However, the observations of high frequency of metaplasias, occasionally with dysplastic features, and a frequency of bladder carcinomas with histologic features reflecting this spectrum of metaplasias does not link schistosomiasis infection per se, in a causal manner, to the vesical malignancy. To this point, published autopsy studies from areas of endemic schistosomiasis failed to find higher frequencies of bladder cancer in patients with documented infection than in the noninfected population. Other studies suggest that the infected bladder is indeed at greater risk of development of carcinoma. The matter remains unsettled, and the role of *S. haemotobium* infection in the cause of bladder carcinoma awaits further clarification.

Suggested Readings

Cheever AW, Kamel IA, Elwi AM, et al: *Schistosoma mansoni* and *Schistosoma haematobium* infections in Egypt. III. Extrahepatic pathology. Am J Trop Med Hyg 27:55, 1978

Edington GM, von Lichtenberg F, Nwabuelo I, et al: Pathologic effects of schistosomiasis in Ibadan, Western state of Nigeria: I. Incidence and intensity of infection:

Distribution and severity of lesions. Am J Trop Med Hyg 19:982, 1970
El-Bolkainy MN, Ghoneim MA, Mansour MA: Carcinoma of the bilharzial bladder in Egypt: Clinical and pathological features. Br J Urol 44:561, 1972
El Sebai I, Sherif M, El-Bolkainy MN, et al: Verrucous carcinoma of the urinary bladder. Urology 4:407, 1974
Khafagy NM, El-Bolkainy MN, Mansour MA: Carcinoma of the bilharzial urinary bladder: A study of the associated mucosal lesions in 86 cases. Cancer 30:150, 1972
Sharfi AR, Rayis AB: The continuing challenge of bilharzial ureteric stricture. Scand J Urol Nephrol 23:123, 1989
Smith JH, Christie, JD: The pathobiology of *Schistosoma haematobium* infections in humans. Hum Pathol 17:333, 1986
Smith JH, Kamel IA, Elwi AM, et al: A quantitative postmortem analysis of urinary schistosomiasis in Egypt. I. Pathology and pathogenesis. Am J Trop Med Hyg 23: 1054, 1974
Von Lichtenberg F, Edington GM, Nwabuelo I, et al: Pathologic effects of schistosomiasis in Ibadan, Western state of Nigeria: II. Pathogenesis of the lesions of the bladder and ureters. Am J Trop Med Hyg 20:244, 1971

MALACOPLAKIA OF THE BLADDER

HUGH A.G. FISHER, M.D., F.A.C.S.

Albany, New York

Malacoplakia of the bladder is an inflammatory process. The bladder is the most common site of urinary tract involvement. The term "malacoplakia" is derived from the Greek words *malakos* (soft) and *plakos* (plaque). It was von Hanseman who first used this term in 1903 to describe the gross appearance of the bladder lesion. Since that time, malacoplakia of the bladder has been recognized as an uncommon clinical entity, and approximately 200 cases of this disease have been reported in the world literature. Malacoplakia remains an important consideration when evaluating lesions of the lower urinary tract.

Malacoplakia occurs in patients of all ages, with a peak incidence in individuals over 50 years. There is a 4:1 female-to-male ratio. Presenting symptoms of bladder irritability and hematuria suggest cystitis. Rarely, lower urinary tract involvement will cause obstructive hydronephrosis. Symptoms may be acute or chronic. A clear association between malacoplakia and urinary tract infection currently is widely recognized. Eighty to 90 per cent of urine cultures yield bacilliform organisms, most commonly *Escherichia coli.*

Malacoplakia of the bladder produces smooth, discrete raised lesions that appear as filling defects on an intravenous pyelogram or cystogram. On cystoscopy, only 25 per cent of malacoplakic lesions fulfill the classic description of being yellow, raised, and soft. Lesions may be gray, tan, red, or brown in color, and can appear ulcerated, hemorrhagic, firm, or plaque like. Lesions are most often multiple and range in size from 0.3 to 2.5 cm. Multiple small lesions are inseparable on radiographic and cystoscopic inspection from cystitis cystica. Lesions that are solitary or few in number and lack yellow color mimic papillary transitional cell neoplasm and are distinguished only by biopsy. When the lesions are multiple and of large size, differentiation from bullous cystitis is difficult. Finally, the differential diagnosis must include localized amyloid plaques, which are yellow in color on cystoscopy, and endometrioma of the bladder when lesions are found in the premenopausal woman.

Histologic examination reveals aggregates of large histiocytic cells (von Hanseman cells) admixed with an infiltrate of lymphocytes, plasma cells, and interspersed well-defined bundles of fibroblasts and collagen. Often a granulomatous reaction with giant cell formation is seen. This process is limited to the epithelium and superficial subepithelial connective tissue and typically does not involve the muscularis. The von Hanseman histiocytes contain Michaelis-Gutmann bodies, concentrically laminated calcific inclusions that are pathognomonic of malacoplakia.

The Michaelis-Gutmann inclusions are von Kossa stain positive and contain adsorbed inorganic calcium, which gives them their characteristic concentric lamination on microscopy. Electron microscopic studies have shown bacteria in various states of morphologic integrity to be present within the Michaelis-Gutmann inclusions, and acidic bacterial lipid polysaccharide has been identified within the Michaelis-Gutmann bodies by immunohistochemistry.

Recent studies suggest that the primary disorder in malacoplakia is abnormal bacterial digestion by tissue macrophages. Electron microscopy has demonstrated residues of bacteria in various stages of degradation inside the phagosomes of these macrophages. Leukocyte function in patients with malacoplakia has been studied and, although monocyte chemotaxis is normal, the percentage of intracellular bacterial killing is significantly less than that of normal control monocytes.

Monocytes in patients with malacoplakia have an abnormally low ratio of cyclic guanosine monophosphate (cGMP) to cyclic adenosine monophosphate (cAMP).

Treatment of malacoplakia of the bladder requires accurate tissue diagnosis. Lesions can be fulgurated or removed by superficial transurethral resection, and the patient is treated with antibiotics to eradicate infection. Antibiotic therapy should be culture specific, and a sterile urine should be documented at the conclusion of therapy. Cholinergic agonists such as bethanecol chloride (40 mg daily) may be used to increase monocyte cGMP levels. Ascorbic acid (0.5 to 1.0 gm daily) can be used to decrease monocyte intracellular cAMP. Healing usually is complete without scarring, but may be accompanied by appearance of new lesions in other bladder sites.

Suggested Readings

Elliott GB, Path FRC, Maloney PJ, et al: Malacoplakia of the urinary tract. Am J Roentgenol 116:830, 1972

Long JP, Althausen AF: Malacoplakia: A 25-year experience with a review of the literature. J Urol 141:1328, 1989

Stanton MJ, Maxted W: Malacoplakia: A study of the literature and current concepts of pathogenesis, diagnosis and treatment. J Urol 125:139, 1981

FOREIGN BODIES IN THE URINARY BLADDER AND URETHRA

WILLIAM BIHRLE, III, M.D.

Burlington, Massachusetts

The urethra and, by extension, the urinary bladder, like other body orifices, is the occasional repository for a vast array of foreign objects, large and small, incidentally or intentionally placed. Historical attempts to catalog the variety of materials and bodies entrapped in the lower urinary tract, although revealing in number and diversity, indicate that sexual gratification, abnormal psychology, and experimentation under the influence of mind-altering substances are the major motivations for insertion. Iatrogenic causes for retained foreign bodies may be assuming greater importance in an era of endourologic manipulation, although this remains unclear. The accidental placement of objects in the urethra is clearly of minor significance.

While it is intuitive that most foreign bodies in the female population are found in the bladder and in men remain in the urethra, a significant number of objects introduced through the male meatus pass into the bladder. This phenomenon may reflect ill-considered attempts by the patient to retrieve the object or, perhaps, a poorly understood antiperistaltic propulsive action of the male urethra.

The signs and symptoms of lower urinary tract foreign bodies in general are reflective of the location and size of the device. Irritative and obstructive symptoms, specifically urinary frequency, dysuria, hematuria or bloody discharge, and difficulty in voiding, occasionally with strangury or pain, are indicative of urinary tract irritation and blockage. Symptoms may be acute and immediate, in which case the patient presents early on for diagnosis and treatment. Unfortunately, in many instances the absence or nonurgent nature of the symptoms combines with a natural reticence on the part of an embarrassed patient to result in a delay in seeking treatment. Late symptoms, weeks to years following manipulation, are due to urinary obstruction from an enlarging, encrusted object or, more commonly, severe infection or abscess formation. Treatment requirements and subsequent morbidity obviously escalate in these situations.

The evaluation of the patient with a urinary tract foreign body is generally straightforward, provided the individual provides an accurate, honest history. In the unreliable historian, the presence of an unexplained chronic urinary tract infection should alert the clinician to this possibility. The physical examination, although often negative or nonspecific, revealing little more than suprapubic or perineal tenderness, may be fairly diagnostic. This is obviously the case in situations in which a portion of the object is visible at the meatus. However, an attempt to extract the body should be delayed until radiologic evaluation defines the specific nature, shape, and location of the device in the lower urinary tract. Examination of the pendulous urethra and perineum frequently will identify palpable objects lying distal to the urogenital diaphragm.

Plain film radiographs taken in the anteroposterior, oblique, and lateral positions generally will localize and define radiopaque objects in the urethra and bladder. The excretory urogram is an essential study, indispensable in identifying radiolucent bodies as filling defects, and extravasation resulting from a bladder injury. In cases of urinary retention or in the presence of a urethral object, the retrograde urethrogram will aid in delineating the point of obstruction as well as any associated injuries. It is axiomatic that urethral catheterization must await the outcome of urethrography to avoid compounding an existing injury. It always should be assumed that the frightened, embarrassed patient has attempted various maneuvers to dislodge the entrapped body, thereby potentially complicating the extraction process. Adjunctive imaging (i.e., ultrasonography, computerized tomography) is reserved for situations in which general evaluation of the pelvis (e.g., in the suspicion of abscess) is required. Some combination of these modalities almost always will accurately define the shape, location, size, and number of foreign bodies.

Cystoscopy remains the linchpin of diagnosis and treatment of urinary tract foreign bodies. Endoscopic inspection of the urethra and bladder almost uniformly defines the nature and extent of the problem. As a general rule, endoscopic manipulation and extraction is the preferred and most successful treatment for offending objects lodged within the anterior urethra. However, safe, nontraumatic removal of the body often will demand some ingenuity and access to a variety of forceps, baskets, snares, and the occasional magnet. Meatotomy, although somewhat disfiguring, is rarely necessary to accommodate particularly bulky objects. More extensive dissection of the urethra or perineum should be limited to the treatment of complications of imbedded objects, urethral tears, or abscess. Special attention to the intact removal of glass objects will avoid the tedious, frustrating, and traumatic extraction of multiple fragments. Soluble materials, such as wax or paraffin, have been eradicated successfully through dissolution with one or more organic solvents (i.e., Xylol or kerosene).

Foreign bodies of the proximal urethra and bladder, although usually successfully managed endoscopically, on occasion require a suprapubic cystotomy for safe removal. Objects in the urethra usually are manipulated or pushed into the bladder, where they can be accurately assessed, manipulated to allow nontraumatic transurethral removal, or fragmented and removed piecemeal. Long-standing bladder bodies often grow to significant size as a result of the formation of stone encrustation. Electrohydraulic or mechanical lithotripsy of the calculus uncovers the original material, permitting safe endoscopic extraction. Very large, awkward, or particularly fragile objects (i.e., glass) preferentially are removed through cystotomy. The incredible variety of objects and materials ultimately finding their way into the bladder should encourage the urologist to use his or her ingenuity and array of instruments to, at times, develop his or her own procedure.

Iatrogenic foreign bodies of the bladder are of particular concern in the era of heightened medicolegal awareness. These objects fall into two categories: (1) bits of catheter or stent material accidentally left during removal, and (2) erosion of drains or suture material placed in proximity to the bladder. The erosion of suture material and pledgets is a well-documented complication of the Stamey procedure. In general, these situations present chronically, sometimes months to years following the initial procedure, and usually as an unexplained recurrent urinary tract infection. Typically, the retained object has become encrusted, making simple endoscopic removal problematic. As a general rule, the lower urinary tract always should be endoscopically inspected to exclude other objects and associated urothelial injuries.

The incidence of urethral and bladder foreign bodies, although indeterminate, is at least stable and likely increasing as a result of the increase in lower urinary tract endoscopic manipulation and stent placement. The diagnosis always should be entertained in the presence of a recurrent and refractory urinary tract infection. The rate of recidivism is disturbingly high in the psychiatric and senile population, mandating psychological or medical evaluation in this group. The astounding catalog of reported lower tract foreign bodies militates against a proscribed, standard treatment, making each case different and individual. The only unpardonable sin, however, is a missed diagnosis in a high-risk patient with unexplained urinary tract symptoms.

Suggested Readings

Aliabadi H, Cass AS, Gleigh P, et al: Self-inflicted foreign bodies involving lower urinary tract and male genitals. Urology 26:12–16, 1985

Eckford SD, Persad RA, Brewster SF: Intravesical foreign bodies: Five year review. Br J Urol 69:41–45, 1992

Khan SA, Kaiser GW, Dailey B, et al: Unusual foreign body in urethra. Urol Int 39:184–186, 1984

Prasad S, Smith AM, Uson A, et al: Foreign bodies in urinary bladder. Urology 2:258–264, 1993

Schnall RI, Baer HM, Seidmon EJ: Endoscopy for removal of unusual foreign bodies in urethra and bladder. Urology 34:33–35, 1989

BLADDER CALCULI

NELSON N. STONE, M.D.

New York, New York

The history of bladder calculi dates back to ancient times. Examples such as an Egyptian skeleton over 7000 years old found with a stone in the pelvis are well known. Hippocrates clearly had recognized the contribution of calculus disease by his statement, "I will not cut, even for the stone . . . ." Practitioners of the day became known as lithotomists, and formalized treatment eventually evolved with the development of instruments to either crush or remove the bladder stones. With the onset of the industrial revolution, the high incidence of bladder stones gave way to an increase in the number of upper urinary tract stones. Despite the changes brought on by industrialization, in certain parts of the world where agrarian influences predominate, bladder calculi remain an important health concern.

Most bladder calculi in the United States are composed of calcium oxalate or uric acid. A single stone is more common than multiple ones, although in 25 to 30 per cent of patients more than one stone may be present. The most common factor predisposing a patient today to develop a bladder stone is the presence of outlet obstruction. In a review of 100 patients with bladder calculi, Douenias et al. found 88 with some form of outlet obstruction. In 17 of these cases the stones apparently had formed in the upper tracts and found their way into the bladder. This latter scenario is becoming more common today as an increasing number of patients undergo extracorporeal lithotripsy for renal stones. Causes of outlet obstruction that might lead to the formation of bladder calculi include prostate hypertrophy (72 to 81 per cent), urethral stricture (3 to 16 per cent), prostate cancer (<9 per cent), and neurogenic bladder. Other structural anomalies encountered with bladder calculi include bladder diverticulum and ureterocele.

CLINICAL FINDINGS AND DIAGNOSIS

Patients with bladder stones may or may not present with symptoms specifically from the stone. If the patient has significant benign prostatic hypertrophy symptoms, urgency and frequency may bring the patient to evaluation. Further history may reveal additional symptoms of painful voiding and intermittent hematuria. A urinalysis usually will demonstrate erythrocytes and leukocytes with or without bacteria. A recurrent urinary tract infection with the same organism, suggesting bacterial persistence, often can be caused by a urinary tract calculus.

Most radiographic studies are capable of demonstrating a bladder calculus. An intravenous pyelogram, often done to evaluate the hematuria associated with the stone, may demonstrate the vesical calculus, which commonly is seen lying transversely across the bladder. However, because up to one third of bladder stones may be composed of uric acid, visualization by roentgenography is not always guaranteed. Thus, in certain cases bladder sonography can be utilized to document the presence of a stone and will give the characteristic acoustic shadowing typically seen with a calculus.

The single most accurate exam for documenting the presence of a bladder stone is cystoscopy. The endoscopic exam not only will demonstrate the stone but also will aid in helping to determine the best route to removing the calculus. Any associated findings, such as an enlarged prostate (benign prostatic hypertrophy), bladder diverticulum, or urethral stricture, also can be identified and corrected prior to or in conjunction with the treatment of the stone.

TREATMENT

In most cases successful treatment of a bladder stone will require surgical removal or mechanical disruption. Only in select cases will medical therapy be indicated. Patients with chronic urinary catheter drainage, either urethral or suprapubic, are susceptible to formation of calcium phosphate stones around and on the ends of the catheters. In such cases a solution of Renacidin may be irrigated into the bladder to dissolve these encrustations and prevent recurrences. In addition, some cases of pure uric acid calculi may be managed by alkalinization of the urine with the hope of dissolving the stone.

The surgical treatment of bladder calculi has evolved significantly during the last 50 years. The techniques have changed from "blind" insertion of a crushing forceps into the bladder to open surgical removal or extracorporeal fragmentation. The procedures available today to remove bladder calculi include open surgical excision, percutaneous incision, endoscopic removal with or without fragmentation, and extracorporeal shockwave lithotripsy (ESWL). The choice of which procedure is most appropriate will depend on the individual circumstances of each case.

Open surgical excision is best reserved for very large stones less amenable to extraction by the other techniques. An incision is made, vertically or transversely, above the pubis down to the rectus fascia. The fascia is separated in the midline and the incision is carried down through the transversalis fascia until the extraperitoneal perivesical space is reached. A small incision is made in the wall of the bladder and the stone is extracted. The incisions are closed individually and the perivesical space is drained. Alternately, smaller stones may be removed by gaining percutaneous access to the bladder and then dilating the tract to remove the stone.

Two thirds of patients with bladder calculi have some form of outlet obstruction, and therefore may benefit from an endoscopic procedure that both corrects the infravesical obstruction and removes the stone. The decision to simultaneously treat both conditions must be weighed against the higher complication rate of 21 per cent when both procedures are combined. Thus, a patient with a large prostate who requires a transurethral resection and who, in addition, has several bladder stones may be treated best by two separate procedures. The techniques for cystolitholapaxy include mechanical crushing with a lithotrite and electrohydraulic or ultrasonic lithotripsy. The lithotrite is inserted under direct vision through the urethra, and the stone is grasped between the jaws and crushed. The smaller fragments then can be removed through the urethra. Difficulties with this procedure include poor visualization, bleeding, inadvertently grabbing bladder mucosa and causing a perforation, and encountering a stone too large for the jaws of the lithotrite.

The electrohydraulic lithotriptor (EHL) utilizes electrical energy to produce short bursts (1 to 5 seconds) of electrohydraulic shock waves that cause stone fragmentation. The energy is delivered through a flexible probe that passes down a cystoscope, allowing for direct visualization of the calculus during the fragmentation. The EHL probe always must be positioned under direct vision because firing of the unit against the bladder wall will result in a perforation. In a series of 304 cases Bulow reported this complication in 1.9 per cent of patients undergoing this procedure. Electrohydraulic lithotripsy is particularly suited for hard stones such as uric acid and calcium oxalate monohydrate.

The ultrasonic lithotriptor converts electromagnetic energy to high-frequency sound waves to fragment the stone. The energy is delivered by a transducer down a hollow rigid probe, which also may be passed under direct vision through a cystoscope. In general, the ultrasonic lithotripsy takes longer to perform than the EHL and therefore is not particularly suited for large bladder stones. Its use is best saved for ureteral stones being removed by the ureteroscopic approach.

An intracorporeal lithotriptor recently has been introduced and has been used to treat bladder stones. This device uses compressed air to activate a solid probe to work like a jackhammer. Vincente treated 47 patients successfully with this device. The major advantage of this device is the relatively low cost of the equipment compared to the other devices.

Probably the most significant advance in managing bladder calculi has been the introduction of ESWL as a treatment option. The advantages of the modern-day lithotriptor include excellent localization (either by fluoroscopy or ultrasound), no requirement for anesthesia or instrumentation, and the ability to perform the procedure on an outpatient basis in most cases. Vandeursen reported successful treatment in 10 patients treated with ESWL, none of whom needed an ancillary procedure to be free of the stones. As more experience is gained with ESWL, it soon may supplant the other forms of bladder calculus removal.

SUMMARY

Bladder calculus disease has become less common in the United States as upper tract disease predominates. However, it still remains a relatively common health problem world wide and may be seen more frequently in certain areas because of changes in immigration patterns. Several options of treatment are available, ranging from open surgery to extracorporeal lithotripsy. The most appropriate treatment will depend on a variety of factors and is best decided on by the treating physician.

Suggested Readings

Bulow H, Frohmuller HGW: Electrohydraulic lithotripsy with aspiration of fragments under vision—304 consecutive cases. J Urol 126:454, 1981

Douenias R, Rich M, Badlaii G, et al: Predisposing factors in bladder calculi. Review of 100 cases. Urology 37:240, 1991
Nseyo UO, Merril DC: Modified TURP loop in the incision of bladder neck. Urology 37:168, 1991
Nseyo UO, Rivard DJ, Bennett AH, et al: Management of bladder stones: Should transurethral prostatic resection be performed in combination with cystolitholapaxy? Urology 29:265, 1987
Vandeusen H, Baert L: Extracorporeal shock wave lithotripsy monotherapy for bladder stones with the second generation lithotriptors. J Urol 143:18, 1990
Vincente J, Laguna P, Paloa J, et al: Intracorporeal lithotripsy by lithoclast. J Urol 148:1, 1993

Bladder Injuries and Related Disorders

BLADDER INJURIES WITH PELVIC FRACTURE

JOSEPH N. CORRIERE, Jr., M.D.

Houston, Texas

The overall incidence of urologic injuries associated with pelvic fractures is 13.5 per cent. It is equally divided between males and females, although urethral injuries occur almost exclusively in men. About 90 per cent of the injuries are ruptured bladders, 3.5 per cent are ruptured urethras, and 1 per cent are both a ruptured bladder and a ruptured urethra.

A full 80 per cent of bladder ruptures associated with pelvic fractures will be extraperitoneal ruptures and 20 per cent will be intraperitoneal. An occasional patient will have both an intra- and an extraperitoneal component. Virtually every case of an extraperitoneal bladder rupture caused by blunt trauma will be associated with a fracture of the pelvis.

MECHANISMS OF INJURY

As the pelvic ring distorts during fracture, the bladder is torn as it is stretched between its points of fixation. This action creates an extraperitoneal bladder rupture. Uncommonly, a spicule of bone may slice the bladder wall. Over 65 per cent of the time there will be a contrecoup extraperitoneal injury to the bladder opposite the site of the fracture, implying that a bursting type of injury to the full bladder has occurred.

The usual mechanism for an intraperitoneal bladder injury is a blow to the full bladder, which then ruptures at its weakest point, the dome. This is a common injury in a motor vehicle accident when a passenger wearing a seat belt has the focus of the force of the collision directed to the abdomen.

DIAGNOSIS

A retrograde static cystogram is the only study that will definitively diagnose a ruptured bladder. The cystogram from an excretory urogram or even a computerized tomogram will miss some injuries and cannot be relied on. Although virtually all urethral ruptures occur with anterior arch fractures, a good rule is always to perform a retrograde urethrogram in a male with a pelvic fracture, especially if there is blood at the urethral meatus. Other warning signs are a high-riding prostate on rectal examination or marked ecchymosis and edema of the perineum, scrotum, and/or penis. If a ruptured urethra is found, urethral catheterization is usually contraindicated and a suprapubic cystotomy should be performed. If a tube is placed percutaneously, a cystogram still must be done to rule out a concomitant bladder injury. The cystogram must include a fully distended bladder (250 to 300 ml of contrast) as well as a postevacuation film to be sure a bladder injury is not present.

Hematuria is present with all bladder injuries and is usually gross in nature. If the cystogram shows no extravasation, the bladder is considered contused. If contrast leaks into the peritoneal cavity, the injury is classified as an intraperitoneal rupture. If the extravasation is confined to the perivesical soft tissue, it is called a simple extraperitoneal bladder rupture, and, if the contrast enters the perineum, scrotum, penis, anterior abdominal wall, or perinephric space, it is a complex extraperitoneal bladder rupture.

THERAPY

Bladder contusions necessitate Foley catheter drainage for a few days or, if minor, no therapy at all. If there is a major injury to the sacrum, the patient may have neuropraxis and be unable to urinate. A cystometrogram before removing the catheter will be helpful to make this diagnosis. These patients then are best treated with intermittent catheterization until their bladder recovers.

All intraperitoneal bladder ruptures should undergo formal repair. A midline incision with inspection of the peritoneal cavity should be performed. Débridement of any devitalized tissue should be done, followed by a two-layer watertight closure with 3-0 absorbable suture material. A suprapubic tube can be placed, but, if there is not a lot of bleeding, a urethral catheter may be all that is needed. A drain is not necessary.

Extraperitoneal bladder ruptures can be managed by Foley catheter drainage alone. In 10 days, at least 85 per cent of even complex injuries will heal and the Foley can be removed. A formal cystogram must be performed and the bladder shown to be intact prior to catheter removal. If the patient is to be explored for associated injuries and is not gravely ill, it is best to open the dome of the bladder and repair the extraperitoneal rents intravesically with a one-layer 3-0 absorbable suture closure. The dome then can be closed as detailed above and a suprapubic tube placed through a separate stab wound. It is best to leave the pelvic hematoma undisturbed. Again, no drain is necessary unless the hematoma is entered.

Patients who have a bladder neck laceration, especially if it extends into the prostatic urethra in the male or there is a concomitant vaginal injury in the female, need immediate repair and meticulous reconstruction or incontinence, stricture, or vesicovaginal fistula may result. These virtually always are seen with extraperitoneal bladder ruptures and rupture of the urogenital diaphragm.

POSTOPERATIVE CARE AND FOLLOW-UP

Once the cystogram shows the bladder rent has healed, the urethral or suprapubic catheter can be removed. Antibiotics should be given at that time to sterilize the urine. Once the urine is clear and the patient has returned to a normal voiding pattern, no further follow-up is necessary.

Suggested Readings

Corriere JN Jr: Trauma to the lower urinary tract. *In* Gillenwater JY, et al (eds): Adult and Pediatric Urology, 2nd ed. St. Louis, Mosby Year Book, 1991, pp 499–521

Corriere JN Jr, Sandler CM: Management of the ruptured bladder: Seven years experience with 111 cases. J Urol 26:830–833, 1986

Corriere JN Jr, Sandler CM: Mechanisms of injury, patterns of extravasation and management of extraperitoneal bladder rupture due to blunt trauma. J Urol 139: 43–44, 1988

Palmer JK, Benson GS, Corriere JN Jr: Diagnosis and initial management of urological injuries associated with 200 consecutive pelvic fractures. J Urol 130:712–714, 1983

Sandler CM, Hall JT, Rodriguez MB, et al: Bladder injury in blunt pelvic trauma. Radiology 158:633–638, 1986

BLUNT AND PENETRATING BLADDER TRAUMA

STANLEY A. BROSMAN, M.D.

Los Angeles, California

Disruption of the bladder wall by blunt or penetrating trauma can be suspected by learning the history of the injury, conducting a physical examination, and examining the urine. Most of these patients are seen in the emergency room and have been given an initial trauma assessment. For those with blunt abdominal or pelvic trauma, it is useful to know the time interval between their last urination and the traumatic event. A full bladder is susceptible to blunt trauma and more likely to sustain an intraperitoneal rupture. The sensation of a full bladder prior to the injury and the loss of that sensation or the inability to urinate suggests the possibility of a ruptured bladder. A history of prior bladder disorders may be helpful in managing the patient.

The physical examination can reveal if the abdomen or pelvis is tender. The presence of urine in the peritoneal cavity produces signs of peritonitis, with pain, rigidity, and inactive or absent bowel sounds. However, these findings may not be present for several hours after the injury. Palpation and percussion of the pelvis are useful in detecting a distended bladder.

The presence of dried blood or a bloody discharge coming from the urethra generally indicates urethral trauma. In women, a bimanual pelvic exam can help in the detection of urine extravasation, because the tissue planes become obliterated. In men, a bimanual rectal exam can provide the same information.

Gross hematuria is a typical finding, but as many as 20 per cent of patients may have microscopic hematuria as defined by less than 50 red blood cells per high-power field. A history of blunt abdominal trauma and hematuria usually warrants a retrograde cystogram. This is the most reliable study for diagnosing and assessing the severity of a bladder injury.

If there is a concern about a urethral injury, the cystogram should be preceded by a retrograde urethrogram. A 20F Foley catheter is used in patients with gross hematuria because there may be blood clots that will need to be evacuated. The catheter is placed just inside the meatus and contrast is injected after inflating the balloon with 2 to 3 ml of water, which will help to hold it in place. With verification that the urethra is normal, the catheter can be advanced into the bladder. The bladder should be emptied and the catheter connected to a drip infusion containing contrast. Allergy to iodine or intravenously administered contrast does not preclude this study. After each 100 to 200-ml aliquot of contrast has been instilled, the bladder can be viewed by fluoroscopy or standard-size films of the abdomen and pelvis. In many instances of bladder rupture, it is necessary to fill the bladder with 300 to 500 ml of contrast before extravasation can be identified. Films also should be obtained in the oblique position and particularly after the bladder has been emptied. This last film may be the only one that will make the diagnosis, and is useful in distinguishing intraperitoneal rupture from extraperitoneal injuries. Some patients will have both types of injuries.

There is a diversity of opinion regarding the reliability of computerized tomographic scanning in detecting bladder injuries. A carefully performed scan may be just as good as cystography, but, in most situations, retrograde cystography is the diagnostic procedure of choice.

Patients with penetrating injuries require more assessment. The status of the upper urinary tract, ureters, retroperitoneum, and intestine must be evaluated. A penetrating rectal injury can be diagnosed by proctosigmoidoscopy. Failure to diagnose and properly manage such an injury can lead to serious consequences.

The management of blunt trauma to the bladder producing an extraperitoneal extravasation often can be limited to the use of urethral catheter drainage for 7 to 10 days. The integrity of the bladder wall can be evaluated with a cystogram prior to removing the catheter. There is no limitation of ambulation, and patients do not need to remain in the hospital once their condition has stabilized.

Patients with extensive bladder disruption or intraperitoneal extravasation and penetrating trauma should be treated surgically. The operative procedure consists of débridement and a two-layer closure of the lacerations with absorbable suture material, and maintaining an empty bladder with catheters placed urethrally and suprapubically. Drains in the pelvis will decrease the opportunity for a pelvic abscess. When the bladder is opened, the integrity of the ureters should be evaluated. Indigo carmine given intravenously should be seen entering the bladder through the orifices and not exuding into the perivesical tissues.

Particular attention should be paid to determining the presence of any rectal injuries in patients with penetrating trauma. Colostomy, either loop or end, and presacral drainage are essential components of rectal injury management. Irrigation of the rectum with antibiotic solution may be of value in these patients. Small and isolated rectal or rectosigmoid perforations from stab wounds may be repaired primarily without fecal diversion in some situations.

Suggested Readings

Horstman WG, McClennan BL, Heiken JP: Comparison of computed tomography and conventional cystography for detection of traumatic bladder rapture. Urol Radiol 12:188, 1991

Kalolanov D, Patrashkov T: The diagnosis and treatment of closed bladder injuries. Khirurglia (Sofial) 42:69, 1989

Rehm CG, Mure AJ, O'Malley KF, et al: Blunt traumatic bladder rupture: The role of retrograde cystogram. Ann Emerg Med 20:845, 1991

TREATMENT OF NONRADIATED VESICOVAGINAL FISTULA

SHLOMO RAZ, M.D.

Los Angeles, California

Vesicovaginal fistula (VVF) is one of the most socially and emotionally distressing complications encountered by patients seen by urologists. The social and medicolegal implications of persistent and uncontrollable leakage of urine should not be underestimated. Early diagnostic intervention and prompt successful closure are of paramount importance in minimizing these. This article presents a brief discussion of the etiology, evaluation, and treatment of VVF.

ETIOLOGY

In developing countries, the most common cause of VVF is obstetric trauma, whereas in developed countries, most VVF cases occur secondary to gynecologic surgery. Hysterectomy for both benign and malignant disease is the most common cause. Although careful surgical technique may minimize the risk of postoperative fistula, it seems to be an inevitable consequence of this type of surgery. Other antecedent procedures include anterior colporrhaphy, cesarean section, bladder diverticulectomy, bladder neck suspensions, and radiotherapy. Infection, ischemia, diabetes, cancer, and inflammation likely contribute to the development of VVF.

EVALUATION

Vesicovaginal fistulas typically present as total daytime and nighttime urinary leakage or, in the case of small fistulas, as a watery vaginal discharge in a patient with normal voiding. Such symptoms occurring after a recent pelvic operation should prompt an early investigation, which may limit patient misery. Initial investigation includes a thorough history and physical exam, including vaginal speculum exam, on which most commonly the fistula will be found at the suture line of the vaginal cuff after hysterectomy. The status of the vaginal and perivesical tissues should be assessed at this time. Significant inflammation warrants a delay in repair. Having the patient wear a vaginal tampon after receiving oral phenazopyridine hydrochloride may help to confirm fistulas in doubtful circumstances.

Cystoscopy and vaginoscopy typically will reveal a supratrigonal fistula draining near the apex of the vagina. The instillation of indigo carmine or other dye may improve diagnostic accuracy if the fistula is not obvious. It is important to rule out multiple fistulas as well, and to assess the proximity of the fistula to the ureteral orifices. Finally, any patient with a history of pelvic malignancy must have a biopsy of the fistula site. A voiding cystogram with oblique and lateral views will help to localize the fistula and rule out multiple fistulas. The combination of the above should allow the evaluator to rule out coexisting stress urinary incontinence, which may occur in 7 to 25 per cent of patients and should be repaired at the same time. Intravenous pyelography is essential to assess for associated ureterovaginal fistulas, which may occur in up to 12 per cent of patients, and to rule out ureteral obstruction. If any doubt exists, retrograde pyelography is more likely to demonstrate the presence and location of a ureterovaginal fistula.

SURGICAL CONSIDERATIONS

In considering repair of uncomplicated VVF, the following factors are important: preoperative medications, the timing of repair, the surgical approach, the need to excise the fistula tract, and the need for adjuvant measures. Any patient with a positive preoperative urine culture should be placed on appropriate antibiotics and treated until the culture is documented negative. All patients should be given broad-spectrum IV antibiotics perioperatively. Preoperative vaginal estrogen creme will help to improve the vascularity of the vaginal tissues and is recommended.

The timing of operative repair has been a controversial area. Traditionally, authors recommended a waiting period of 3 to 6 months to allow appropriate resolution of the inflammatory response. During this time period, the patient is faced with continuous urine loss, social restriction or embarrassment, and emotional distress. Furthermore, no randomized trials exist to support late over early repair, and recent series have shown equivalent results with early intervention (1 to 10 weeks) in patients with uncomplicated iatrogenic fistulas. The most important consideration is the status of the vaginal and perivesical tissues, which in the case of iatrogenic fistulas frequently exhibit little inflammation that would interfere with the repair. Thus, we favor early intervention in instances in which the patient is in good general health and there is no cuff or pelvic infection.

The surgeon must consider whether an abdominal or transvaginal approach is appropriate. It is clear that the greatest likelihood of success is achieved with the first surgery, and therefore the procedure with which the surgeon is most comfortable is appropriate. Coincidental intra-abdominal pathology or vaginal pathology will dictate an abdominal or vaginal approach in some instances. The advantages offered by transvaginal closure include decreased postoperative morbidity, reduced hospital stay, decreased blood loss and operative time, and absence of cystotomy; also, in cases in which the fistula is close to the ureteral orifices, repair usually can be done without ureteral reimplantation. Thus, we favor this approach. In experienced hands the success rates are comparable for either technique.

The next important consideration is excision of the tract. Although classically the fistula tract has been excised to obtain healthy tissue for the repair, we have found this unnecessary. Excision of the tract leads to an enlarged fistula and increased blood loss, which can be avoided by including the tract in the repair without compromising results. Most simple fistulas do not require interposition of a vascularized graft, but this should be considered in complicated situations such as previous failed repair or large fistula.

TREATMENT

Treatment of vesicovaginal fistulas should begin with a conservative trial of Foley drainage for a period of 2 to 3 weeks. Small fistulas may respond to coagulation and drainage. Failure of conservative measures, however, necessitates operative repair. Fundamentals include watertight bladder closure, use of multiple layers, and tension-free nonoverlapping absorbable suture lines.

For transvaginal closure, the patient receives a Betadine douche and scrub the night before surgery and broad-spectrum IV antibiotics are administered perioperatively. The patient is placed in the exaggerated lithotomy position and repair begins with placement of a suprapubic tube with the aid of the Lowsley retractor, which is placed intravesically through the urethra and used to elevate the anterior bladder and abdominal walls. A small stab incision over the tip of the retractor allows it to be advanced through the abdominal wall, where it can be used to grasp the Foley catheter and draw it into the bladder. Fistulas in close proximity to the ureteral orifice necessitate insertion of a ureteral catheter, which can be removed at the end of surgery or the day following surgery. Placement of a small-caliber Foley catheter into the fistula through the vagina will aid in dissection and may require gentle dilation of the fistula tract with sounds.

For a high fistula, a J-shaped incision is made with its long arm directed anteriorly (Fig. 1). The convex portion of the incision circumscribes the fistula. This asymmetric incision will allow for advancement and rotation of the anterior flap over the repair without overlapping suture lines. The vaginal wall is dissected off the vesicopelvic ligament (perivesical fascia) by beginning away from the fistula where healthy tissue exists; this facilitates entrance into the proper plane and avoids bladder perforation. Dissection allows the creation of an anterior and posterior flap of vaginal wall extending 2 to 4 cm away from the fistula to allow tension-free closure of the vaginal wall (Fig. 2). Stay sutures are placed at the lateral margin of the fistula and the fistula is closed with 2-0 Vicryl or Dexon incorporating a partial thickness of the bladder wall and the vaginal wall in contact with the fistula. A second layer is inverted over the first at right angles and includes the perivesical fascia and bladder muscle (Fig. 3). These interrupted absorbable sutures are placed 1 cm away and are tied tension free. The short posterior flap is then excised and the anterior flap is advanced and rotated beyond the repair and closed (Fig. 4). Closure must include the perivesical fascia in order to obliterate the dead space.

For large fistulas or those that previously have failed repair, a peritoneal or labial fibrofatty flap should be considered. A peritoneal flap can be created easily by mobilizing the peritoneum off the posterior aspect of the

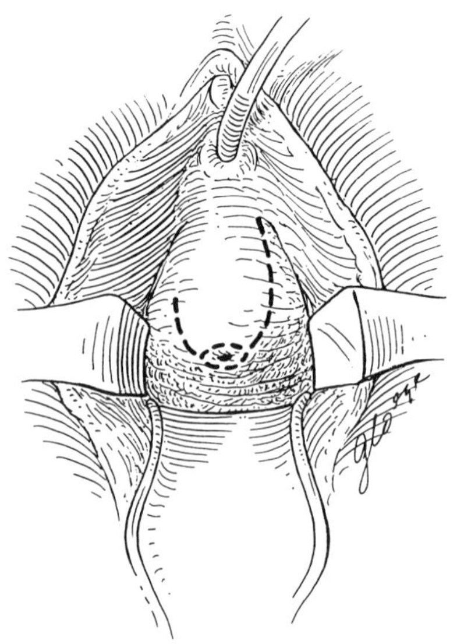

FIGURE 1. For high fistula, a J-shaped incision circumscribing the fistula is made in the anterior vaginal wall. (Reprinted with permission from Raz S: Atlas of Transvaginal Surgery. Philadelphia, WB Saunders, 1992.)

bladder and interposing it over the repair. Alternatively, a vascularized labial fibrofatty graft can be dissected from the labia majora and passed through a vaginal tunnel and used to cover the repair.

Transabdominal closure may be done through an extraperitoneal approach, or a transperitoneal approach if an omental flap is considered. Our preferred approach is intraperitoneal. The retrovesicle space is entered and the unopened bladder is dissected off the anterior vaginal wall, exposing the fistula. The fistula is circumscribed on the bladder side, completely freeing the bladder. The vaginal side of the fistula then is closed in two layers of Vicryl without fistula excision. The bladder then is closed in two layers. We prefer to interpose omentum or peritoneum between the vagina and bladder at completion of the repair. When used, the omental flap is based on the right gastroepiploic artery and is mobilized in a left-to-right direction.

An alternative method begins with an anterior vesicotomy. Once the bladder is open, ureteral catheters may be used to avoid injury to the ureters during the procedure and can be removed intraoperatively or the day following surgery. A Foley catheter may be placed through the fistula. Traction on the catheter with the balloon inflated improves exposure and aids in dissection. The fistula tract is circumscribed and the bladder then is

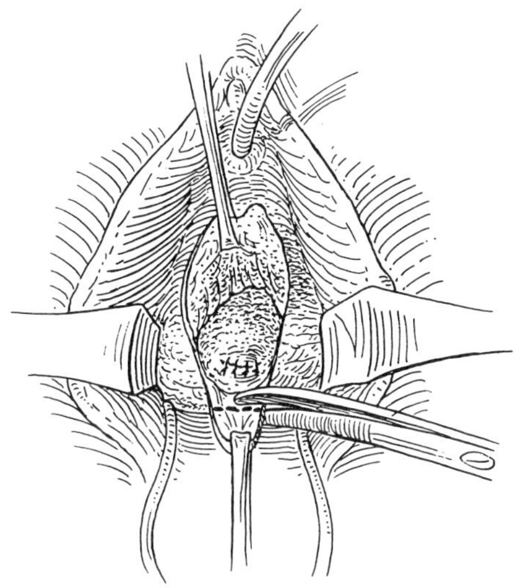

FIGURE 3. Closure of the fistula tract in two layers without débridement of the edges. (Reprinted with permission from Raz S: Atlas of Transvaginal Surgery. Philadelphia, WB Saunders, 1992.)

mobilized off the vaginal wall through this incision. Without excision, the fistula is closed with two layers of 2-0 absorbable suture. The vesicle wall is closed with a separate interrupted layer. Again an omental, fatty, or peritoneal flap may be interposed between the vagina and bladder repair if desired. A suprapubic tube is left prior to bladder closure.

Another popular technique involves ex-

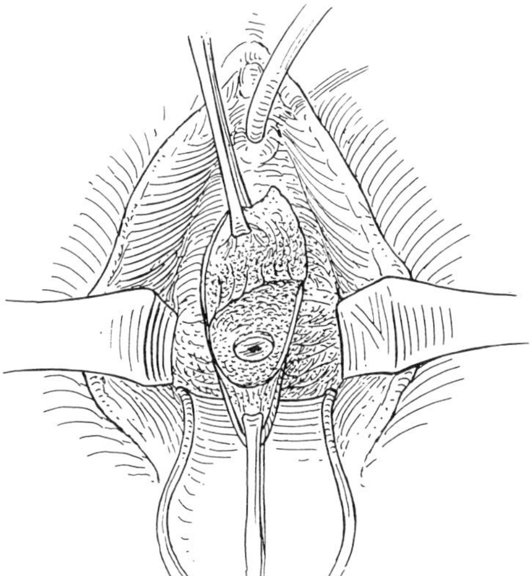

FIGURE 2. Creation of a vaginal wall flap anterior and posterior to the fistula. Dissection is begun away from the fistula in healthy tissue to facilitate entry into the proper plane. (Reprinted with permission from Raz S: Atlas of Transvaginal Surgery. Philadelphia, WB Saunders, 1992.)

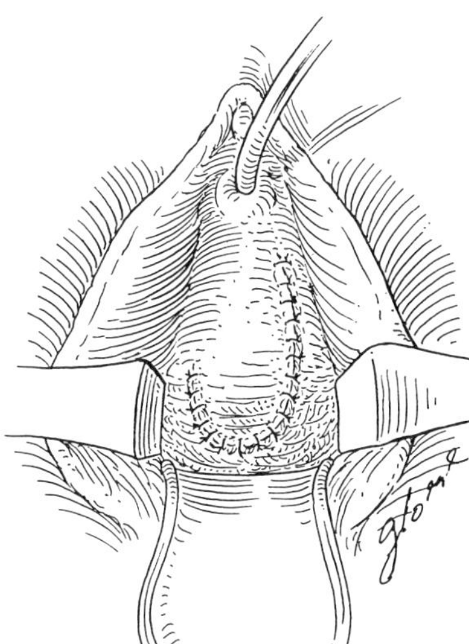

FIGURE 4. After excision of the posterior flap, the anterior flap is advanced and rotated beyond the repair and the vaginal wall is closed, with care taken to obliterate the dead space. (Reprinted with permission from Raz S: Atlas of Transvaginal Surgery. Philadelphia, WB Saunders, 1992.)

tending the anterior bladder incision posteriorly through the fistula, effectively bivalving the bladder in a sagittal plane. This aids in mobilization of the bladder off the vagina. Closure is as described above.

POSTOPERATIVE CARE

Postoperative care in all instances includes antibiotics until all catheters are removed and cholinolytic agents to prevent bladder spasm. Uninterrupted urinary drainage is essential for proper healing. The urethral Foley catheter is removed on the third to fifth day and the patient returns 10 to 14 days after surgery for a cystogram to document lack of extravasation and significant postvoid residual. At this time the suprapubic tube can be removed.

CONCLUSION

By adhering to the fundamentals described, a success rate of 90 per cent or better can be expected. Fundamentals of success include tension-free repair, nonoverlapping suture lines, and uninterrupted drainage. In addition, success will depend on the presence of infection, the underlying etiology, the presence or absence of cancer and radiotherapy, the number of previous repairs, the size of the fistula, and adequate blood supply. In most cases of iatrogenic fistulas, early repair will give results similar to those with delayed repair and will significantly reduce the patient's misery. Although we favor the transvaginal approach, the selected technique will depend on the surgeon's comfort and experience, and coexisting morbidity.

Suggested Readings

Goodwin WE, Scardino PT: Vesicovaginal and ureterovaginal fistulas: A summary of 25 years experience. J Urol 123:370, 1980

Little NA, Juma S, Raz S: Vesicovaginal fistulae. Semin Urol 7:78, 1989

O'Conor V: Review of experience with vesicovaginal fistula repair. J Urol 123:367, 1980

Tancer ML: Observations on prevention and management of vesicovaginal fistula after total hysterectomy. Surg Gynecol Obstet 175:501, 1992

Wang Y, Hadley HR: Nondelayed transvaginal repair of high lying vesicovaginal fistula. J Urol 144:34, 1990

Neurologic Urology

DIAGNOSTIC EVALUATION OF NEUROMUSCULAR DISORDERS OF THE BLADDER

ALAN J. WEIN, M.D.

Philadelphia, Pennsylvania

SIMPLIFICATION OF THE MICTURITION CYCLE—PATHOPHYSIOLOGY

Whatever disagreements exist regarding the anatomic, morphologic, physiologic, pharmacologic, and mechanical details involved in both the storage and expulsion of urine by the lower urinary tract, I have always believed that "experts" agree on certain points. First, the micturition cycle involves two relatively discrete processes: (1) bladder filling and urine storage, and (2) bladder emptying. Second, whatever the details involved, these processes can be summarized succinctly from a conceptual point of view. Bladder filling and urine storage require the following:

1. Accommodation of increasing volumes of urine at a low intravesical pressure and with appropriate sensation.
2. A bladder outlet that is closed at rest and remains so during increases in intra-abdominal pressure.
3. Absence of involuntary bladder contractions.

Bladder emptying requires the following:

1. A coordinated contraction of the bladder smooth musculature of adequate magnitude.
2. A concomitant lowering of resistance at the level of the smooth and striated sphincter.
3. Absence of anatomic (as opposed to functional) obstruction.

Any abnormality of bladder filling and urine storage, regardless of the exact pathophysiology, must result from a problem related to one or more of the pertinent factors listed. This is also the case for any problem with bladder emptying.

This division, with its implied subdivision

under each category into causes related to the bladder and to the outlet, provides a logical rationale for evaluation and classification of all types of voiding dysfunction and disorders related primarily to bladder filling and urine storage, or disorders related primarily to bladder emptying. This includes neurogenic and non-neurogenic causes. All aspects of urodynamic, radiologic, and video-urodynamic evaluation can be conceptualized as to exactly what they evaluate in terms of either bladder or outlet activity during filling/storage or emptying and whether they do so by acting primarily on the bladder or on one or more of the components of the bladder outlet. Finally, the individual disorders produced by various neuromuscular dysfunctions can be considered in terms of whether they produce primarily storage or emptying abnormalities or a combination.

Involuntary contractions most commonly are seen in association with neurologic disease or after neurologic injury, but also may be associated with inflammation or irritation of the bladder wall or bladder outlet obstruction or be idiopathic. Decreased compliance during filling may be secondary to neurologic injury or disease but also may result from any process that destroys the elastic or viscoelastic properties of the bladder wall. Decreased outlet resistance may result from any process that damages the innervation or structural elements of the smooth or striated sphincter. This may ultimately be the result of neurologic disease or injury, surgical or other mechanical trauma, or aging. Treatment of filling/storage abnormalities is directed toward increasing outlet resistance, either continuously or just during increases in intra-abdominal pressure.

Absolute or relative bladder contractility failure may result from temporary or permanent alteration in one of the neuromuscular mechanisms necessary for initiating and maintaining a normal detrusor contraction. Inhibition of the voiding reflex in a neurologically healthy person also may occur, either by a reflex mechanism secondary to painful stimuli, especially from the pelvic and perineal areas, or in cases when the inhibition is psychogenic in origin. Non-neurogenic causes also include impairment of bladder smooth muscle function, which may result from overdistention, severe infection, or fibrosis. Pathologically increased outlet resistance generally is seen in men. Although it is most often secondary to anatomic obstruction, it may be secondary to a failure of coordination of the striated or smooth sphincter during bladder contraction (dyssynergia). Treatment of failure to empty generally consists of attempts to increase intravesical pressure or facilitate the micturition reflex, decrease outlet resistance, or both. If other means fail or are impractical, intermittent catheterization is an effective way of circumventing emptying failure.

THE NEUROUROLOGIC EVALUATION

History

Incontinence is generally a primary symptom of filling/storage failure and may be bladder or outlet related; however, it also may result from ureteral ectopy and from congenital or acquired fistula. Leakage that is associated only with increases in intra-abdominal pressure implies stress urinary incontinence. Gravitational urethral incontinence implies a nonfunctional bladder neck and proximal urethra. Precipitous incontinence with a more sustained type of leakage similar to voiding is characteristic of involuntary bladder contractions and may occur in the absence of sensation or with urgency. Incontinence is not always, however, a primary symptom of filling/storage failure. Overflow or paradoxical incontinence may develop in a patient with insidious detrusor decompensation with emptying failure. The leakage in this case generally is most prominently associated with changes in position or sudden increases in intra-abdominal pressure, and therefore can mimic stress incontinence.

The impending sensation of micturition must be differentiated from the simple fear of leaking urine when one is exploring the meaning of "urgency." The former usually is associated with involuntary bladder contraction or decreased compliance, and the latter may be associated with leakage from simple sphincteric incontinence. Urgency that is associated only with pain is generally secondary to inflammatory disease. An increase in daytime urinary frequency may be psychogenic or may represent a response to pain on low-volume bladder distention (usually indicative of inflammatory disease), or may be due to detrusor hyperactivity. Increased frequency also may result from emptying failure, with a substantial residual urine volume and therefore a decreased functional bladder capacity, or it may exist in association with outlet obstruction–induced detrusor hyperactivity. Nocturia usually accompanies nonpsychogenic urinary frequency and may be associated, on the same basis as increased daytime frequency, with either storage or emptying failure. There is often no discernible voiding dysfunction in patients who complain of "pressure." This can be the result of an elevated intravesical pressure during filling, but one that is below the level necessary to elicit the sensation of distention or urgency. This symptom also may be representative of an accurate perception of inadequate emptying with a modest or large residual urine volume. Hesitancy and straining to void generally reflect a failure to empty adequately, but they can occur in an individual with frequency and urgency who, on toileting, simply has difficulty initiating a voluntary bladder contraction with a small intravesical urine content.

Physical and Neurologic Evaluation

Findings from a general physical examination are nonspecific and may simply provide confirmation of the presence and degree of voiding dysfunction.

The neurologic examination provides evidence of the presence or absence of a neurologic lesion and, if present, localizes it in an attempt to corroborate and explain a given voiding dysfunction. Mental status, cranial nerve function, motor and sensory function, and coordination are important. Evaluation of the deep tendon reflexes provides an indication of segmental spinal cord function as well as suprasegmental function. Hypoactivity of the deep tendon reflexes generally indicates a lower motor neuron (LMN) lesion, whereas hyperactivity generally indicates an upper motor neuron (UMN) lesion. Commonly tested deep tendon reflexes include the biceps (C5–C6), triceps (C6–C7), quadriceps or patellar (L2–L4), and Achilles (L5–S2). A pathologic toe sign (Babinski reflex) generally indicates a somatic UMN lesion but can be absent with a complete lesion and marked spasticity. A Babinski reflex may be present contralaterally with a unilateral lesion or may be present unilaterally with a bilateral lesion.

The generic term "bulbocavernosus reflex" (BCR) describes contraction of the bulbocavernosus and ischiocavernosus muscles (after penile glans or clitoral stimulation), or stimulation of the urethral or bladder mucosa (by pulling on an indwelling Foley catheter). Most would agree that the BCR reflects activity in S2–S4, but some believe that this may involve segments as high as L5. Motor control of the external anal sphincter (EAS) is variously described as being served by sacral cord segments S2–S4 or S3–S5. A visible contraction of the EAS after pinprick of the mucocutaneous junction constitutes the anal reflex, and its activity usually parallels that of the BCR. EAS tone, when strong, indicates that activity of the conus medullaris is present, whereas absent anal sphincter tone usually indicates absent conal activity. Volitional control of the EAS indicates intact control by supra spinal centers.

Radiologic Evaluation

Upper Tract

Many believe that the intravenous urogram is the optimal screening study of the upper tract in patients with significant voiding dysfunction. However, sonography can give adequate information about hydronephrosis, the presence of larger calculi, and occasionally hydroureter. Isotope studies may be useful to evaluate renal blood flow and function and to establish the presence of renal or ureteral obstruction.

Lower Tract

There are basic cystourethrographic patterns that relate directly to voiding dysfunction caused by neuromuscular disease. Their exact significance, however, often can be ascertained only by simultaneous urodynamic study. Specific details and illustrations of complications caused by such voiding dysfunction (reflux, trabeculation, cellules, diverticula) also are demonstrable by cystography and voiding cystourethrography.

Endoscopic Evaluation

This is valuable to exclude irritative, neoplastic, or preneoplastic changes in the bladder epithelium as a cause of voiding symptomatology. The presence or absence of trabeculation (which is compatible with obstruction, involuntary bladder contractions, or neurologic decentralization) also can be determined. Endoscopic examination likewise may be confirmatory of obstruction at a particular site, but it should be recognized that not everything that appears obstructive endoscopically is obstructive urodynamically, and a lack of a visually appreciated obstruction does not exclude functional obstruction.

Urodynamic/Video-Urodynamic Evaluation

Ideally, the urodynamic/video-urodynamic evaluation should be able to answer the implied questions regarding the normality or abnormality of each of the components of the two phases of micturition. Combined video-urodynamic or separate cystourethrographic study also provides information regarding the presence or absence of vesicoureteral reflux.

FLOWMETRY

Flowmetry is a way of integrating the activity of the bladder and the outlet during the emptying phase of micturition. The flow rate and pattern represent the recorded variables; if these are both normal, it is unlikely that there is any significant disorder of emptying. A normal flow, however, does not entirely exclude obstruction, which is defined strictly on the basis of a relationship between detrusor pressure and simultaneous flow. Consistently low flow rates with adequate volumes generally indicate increased outlet resistance, decreased bladder contractility, or both. Flow rates considerably in excess of normal may indicate decreased outlet resistance. Abnormal flow patterns come in only a few varieties. An abnormally broad plateau with a low mean and peak rate generally indicates outlet obstruction or decreased detrusor contractility. Intermittent flow is generally secondary to abdominal straining or sphincter dyssynergia but in rare instances may be due to undulating low-amplitude detrusor contractions.

In comparisons of flow rates in a given individual from one time to another, either for the purposes of evaluating treatment or for following a given condition, it is very important to standardize the rates to a given volume. Volume/rate nomograms may be useful in this regard. Most data in the literature cite norms of 15 and 25 ml/sec for mean and maximum flow rates. However, flow rates really should be standardized in terms of the minimum acceptable flow rates for given sex and age groups. Most "normal" data relate to flowmetry in patients below the age of 55.

RESIDUAL URINE VOLUME

Residual volume likewise integrates the activity of the bladder and outlet during emptying. It can be measured directly or estimated by cystography or ultrasonography. A consistently increased residual urine volume that reflects the usual status of that patient generally indicates increased outlet resistance, decreased bladder contractility, or both. Generally, a significant residual urine volume is considered to be indicative of relative detrusor failure, with or without outlet obstruction.

FILLING CYSTOMETRY

Cystometry refers to the method by which changes in bladder pressure are measured. The first sensation of bladder filling and the first sensation of fullness, as well as the urge to void and the feeling of imminent micturition, are important data to record. When a phasic involuntary detrusor contraction occurs, it is important to note whether this coincides with a sensation of urgency and whether suppression is possible. The pressure measured within the bladder is composed of that contributed by the detrusor plus intra-abdominal pressure. Thus, any pressure increment recorded on a simple cystometrogram may at least partially, and sometimes totally, reflect intra-abdominal pressures. To eliminate such artifactual problems, it is desirable to measure intra-abdominal pressure simultaneously, as reflected by a catheter-mounted intrarectal pressure balloon or by a catheter inserted next to the bladder. It is true that an experienced operator very often can tell the difference between a true detrusor contraction and an increase in bladder pressure caused by an increase in intra-abdominal pressure—by the configuration of the curve and by observation of the patient. However, if there is any question about this or if a significant decision is to be based on these data, electronic subtraction of the intra-abdominal pressure from the total bladder pressure (yielding detrusor pressure) is desirable.

The normal adult cystometrogram is divided into four phases:

Phase 1—The initial pressure rise represents the initial response to filling, and the level at which the bladder trace stabilizes is known as the initial filling pressure. This is contributed to by the initial myogenic response to filling and by the elastic and viscoelastic response of the bladder wall to stretch.

Phase 2—Phase 2 is called the tonus limb, and compliance (volume/pressure) is normally high and uninterrupted by phasic rises. In practice, the compliance seen in the urodynamic laboratory is always lower than that existing during physiologic bladder filling. Normally, in the laboratory, the rise is less than 6 to 10 cm of water. It is difficult to find stated values for normal compliance.

Phase 3—Phase 3 is reached when the elastic and viscoelastic properties of the bladder wall have reached their limit. Any further increase in volume generates a substantial increase in pressure. This increase in pressure is not the same as a detrusor contraction. If a voluntary or involuntary contraction occurs, phase 3 may be obscured by the rise in pressure so generated.

Phase 4—Ideally, involuntary bladder contractions do not occur during either phase 2 or phase 3, and phase 4 consists of the initiation of voluntary micturition. Many patients are unable to generate a voluntary detrusor contraction in the testing situation, especially in the supine position. This should not be called detrusor areflexia but, simply, absence of a detrusor contraction during cystometry, a finding that is not considered abnormal unless other clinical or urodynamic findings are present that substantiate the presence of neurologic or myogenic disease.

Involuntary bladder contractions during filling are always significant. "Detrusor hyperreflexia" and "detrusor instability" are both terms that relate to the generic term "involuntary bladder contraction." Detrusor hyperreflexia refers to an involuntary contraction that is the result of associated neurologic disease; detrusor instability refers to such an involuntary contraction seen in the absence of neurologic disease. Thus, a spinal cord injury patient with involuntary bladder contractions is said to have detrusor hyperreflexia, whereas an elderly male with such a finding and prostatic obstruction is said to have detrusor instability.

One of the most important concepts to be put forth in recent years is that "adequate storage at low intravesical pressure" will avoid deleterious upper urinary tract changes in patients with bladder outlet obstruction and/or neuromuscular lower urinary tract dysfunction. McGuire and coworkers have clearly shown that upper tract deterioration is apt to occur when storage, even though adequate in terms of continence, occurs at sustained urodynamically generated intravesical pressures of greater than 40 cm of water. Application of this concept to patients with storage problems caused by decreased compliance also has resulted in the concept of the passive "leak point" as a very significant piece of urodynamic data. This leak point is very simply measured during filling cystometry.

Voiding Cystometry/Combined Pressure Studies/Video-Urodynamic Studies

Intravesical pressure, intra-abdominal pressure (generally reflected by intrarectal pressure), and flow often are measured simultaneously. The purpose of pressure/flow studies is to be able to define better whether obstruction is present and to be able to assess detrusor contractility more precisely. By assessing patterns of detrusor pressure and flow, thereby inferring resistance and patterns of increased resistance, one often can ascertain the exact pathology. The normal adult male generally voids with a detrusor pressure of between 40 and 50 cm of water, and the normal adult female voids at a much lower pressure. Urodynamically, obstruction is defined only by the relationship between detrusor pressure and flow—high pressure and low flow.

Once obstruction is diagnosed, it is necessary to determine the site, and, in order to do this, simultaneous fluoroscopy often is used. This "video-urodynamic" study combines the cystourographic imaging described previously with simultaneous urodynamic studies, permitting, generally, an accurate determination of the site of obstruction at the time high pressure and low flow coexist. The video-urodynamic study is also extremely useful in assessing the etiology of complex cases of incontinence, because the precise pressure relationships existing in the bladder and urethra can be correlated with the cystourethrographic radiologic patterns, and a judgment thereby made as to why involuntary leakage occurs at a particular time. Here, the issue is generally whether the fluoroscopic demonstration of leakage occurs with detrusor hyperactivity or in the absence of detrusor hyperactivity or whether the incontinence is due in part to both detrusor and outlet-related causes.

Electromyography

For the vast majority of urologists, electromyography is a urodynamic study that permits evaluation of the striated sphincter during the emptying phase of micturition. Kinesiologic electromyography is the term that describes this application—that is, the study of the activity of one group of muscles (in this case, the striated musculature of the outlet) with respect to another (in this case, the bladder). Normally, as the bladder fills with urine, there is a gradual and sustained increase in electromyographic activity recruited from the pelvic floor muscles. This reaches a maximum just before voiding. Compositely, this is known as the guarding reflex. The lack of a guarding reflex suggests neural pathology, as does the inability to produce a sphincter "flare" when given the command to "stop voiding." Voluntary voiding is normally preceded by complete electrical silence—relaxation of the striated sphincter.

There is a marked increase in electromyographic activity in response to a number of stimuli, including cough, Credé and Valsalva maneuvers, and the BCR, and in response to the request to stop voiding, a maneuver accomplished by most through forceful contraction of the pelvic floor musculature. A simultaneous increase of electromyographic activity with an increase in intravesical pressure during filling cystometry is not always indicative of detrusor striated sphincter dyssynergia. Abdominal straining or attempted inhibition of a bladder contraction will yield an identical pattern.

All of these circumstances represent types of "pseudodyssynergia" and are extremely difficult to differentiate from true dyssynergia on the basis of any type of urodynamic study done solely during bladder filling. The term "detrusor-striated sphincter dyssynergia" should refer to obstruction to the outflow of urine during bladder contract caused by involuntary contraction of the striated sphincter. This is seen most often in patients with discrete neurologic disease, such as suprasacral spinal cord transection after spinal shock has passed. Individuals suspected of having detrusor-striated sphincter dyssynergia but who are without identifiable neurologic disease always should be investigated further with sophisticated video-urodynamic evaluation during a full micturition study. True detrusor-striated sphincter dyssynergia is extremely uncommon (some say it does not exist) in patients without neurologic disease, and such a diagnosis deserves exhaustive study before it is in fact confirmed.

FORMULATION

Once the neurourologic evaluation is completed, functional classification of a voiding dysfunction is possible. After consideration of other practical matters (e.g., prime risk factors, disease prognosis, patient/family ability/resources), treatment is able to proceed according to "menu" of treatment, from the simplest to the most complicated (see "Drug Therapy for Neurogenic and Non-Neurogenic Bladder Dysfunction").

Suggested Readings

Krane RJ, Siroky MB (eds): Clinical Neurourology, 2nd ed. Boston, Little, Brown, 1991, pp 161–318

Mundy AR, Stephenson TP, Wein AJ: Urodynamics: Principles and Application. Edinburgh, Churchill Livingston, 1984

Wein AJ: Neuromuscular dysfunction of the lower urinary tract. *In* Walsh PC, Retik AB, Stamey TA, et al (eds): Campbell's Urology, 6th ed. Philadelphia, WB Saunders, 1992, pp 573–642

Wein AJ, Barrett DM: Voiding Function and Dysfunction: A Logical and Practical Approach. Chicago, Year Book Medical Publishers, 1988

Yalla S, McGuire E, Elbadawi A, et al: Neurourology and Urodynamics: Principles and Practice. New York, Macmillan, 1988, pp 147–236

DRUG THERAPY FOR NEUROGENIC AND NON-NEUROGENIC BLADDER DYSFUNCTION

ALAN J. WEIN, M.D.

Practical application of the current interest in the neurophysiology and neuropharmacology of the bladder and bladder outlet has resulted in the successful clinical use of drug therapy to alleviate or improve many types of voiding dysfunction, both neurogenic and non-neurogenic in etiology. The clinical urologist should easily be able to incorporate into his or her everyday practice the use of many of these agents and should not be frightened off from their use by complicated pharmacologic and physiologic jargon and data that often have little clinical relevance. To rationally and effectively utilize pharmacologic therapy for the treatment of voiding dysfunction, it is necessary to understand a few basic principles. First, the actual therapy usually is directed not toward the level of the primary pathology, but rather toward the end organ structures involved; it is therefore not necessary to understand totally the physiology of normal and abnormal voiding function to treat the clinical manifestations of voiding dysfunction. Second, all the pharmacologic agents that affect voiding do so by facilitating or inhibiting urine emptying or urine storage by an effect on the bladder, the outlet, or both.

To help us decide which drugs (or other manipulations) might be helpful in a given situation, we have adopted a very simple, functional classification of voiding disorders (Table 1) and of treatment for these disorders (Tables 2 and 3). All varieties of voiding dysfunction can be classified according to whether these two functions (emptying and storage) are performed normally. Some dysfunctions appear to share deficits of both storage and emptying (such as the voiding dysfunction seen in the typical paraplegic). In our experience, these usually can be converted pharmacologically or surgically to predominantly one or the other deficit, which then can be treated or circumvented. This classification is not meant to supplant other more detailed classification schemes from which one can infer both etiology and treatment. However, one has only to attend the case presentation sessions of any current seminar in neurology to see that the "experts" often disagree significantly as to the etiologic significance of many of the relevant urodynamic, radiologic, and neurologic data.

FAILURE TO EMPTY URINE PROPERLY

Failure to empty can occur because of a temporary or permanent impairment of nerve or reflex function, a temporary or permanent impairment of bladder contractility, or anatomic or functional bladder outlet obstruction. Whatever the etiology, excluding spontaneous recovery, there are only a finite number of possible therapeutic options (see Table 3). Pharmacologic treatment includes measures designed to increase intravesical pressure by increasing bladder contractility,

TABLE 1. The Expanded Functional Classification

FAILURE TO STORE
- Because of the bladder
  - Detrusor hyperactivity
    - Involuntary contractions
      - Suprasacral neurologic disease
      - Bladder outlet obstruction
      - Idiopathic
    - Decreased compliance
      - Fibrosis
      - Idiopathic
  - Sensory urgency
    - Inflammatory
    - Infectious
    - Neurologic
    - Psychologic
    - Idiopathic
- Because of the outlet
  - Stress incontinence
  - Nonfunctional bladder neck/proximal urethra

FAILURE TO EMPTY
- Because of the bladder
  - Neurologic
  - Myogenic
  - Psychogenic
  - Idiopathic
- Because of the outlet
  - Anatomic
    - Prostatic obstruction
    - Bladder neck contracture
    - Urethral stricture
  - Functional
    - Smooth sphincter dyssynergia
    - Striated sphincter dyssynergia

TABLE 2. Therapy to Facilitate Urine Storage

INHIBITING BLADDER CONTRACTILITY/DECREASING SENSORY INPUT/INCREASING BLADDER CAPACITY
1. Timed bladder emptying
2. Pharmacologic therapy
   a. Anticholinergic agents
   b. Musculotropic relaxants
   c. Calcium antagonists
   d. Potassium channel openers
   e. Prostaglandin inhibitors
   f. Beta-adrenergic agonists
   g. Tricyclic antidepressants
   h. Dimethylsulfoxide (DMSO)
3. Biofeedback, bladder retraining
4. Bladder overdistention
5. Electrical stimulation (reflex inhibition)
6. Acupuncture
7. Interruption of innervation
   a. Central (subarachnoid block)
   b. Peripheral (sacral rhizotomy, selective sacral rhizotomy)
   c. Dorsal
   d. Perivesical (peripheral bladder denervation)
8. Augmentation cystoplasty

INCREASING OUTLET RESISTANCE
1. Physiotherapy, biofeedback
2. Electrical stimulation of the pelvic floor
3. Pharmacologic therapy
   a. Alpha-adrenergic agonists
   b. Tricyclic antidepressants
   c. Beta-adrenergic antagonists
   d. Estrogens
4. Vesicourethral suspension (SUI)
5. Bladder outlet reconstruction
6. Surgical mechanical compression
   a. Sling procedures
   b. Artificial urinary sphincter
7. Nonsurgical mechanical compression
   a. Periurethral Polytef injection
   b. Periurethral collagen injection
   c. Occlusive devices

CIRCUMVENTING PROBLEM
1. Antidiuretic hormone–like agents
2. Intermittent catheterization
3. Continuous catheterization
4. Urinary diversion
5. External collecting devices
6. Absorbent products

measures to decrease outlet resistance, or both.

Increasing Intravesical Pressure

A physiologic bladder contraction is mediated primarily by nerve impulses traveling in the postganglionic parasympathetic (pelvic) nerves. Although other contractile neurotransmitters may exist, no one would argue that acetylcholine is the primary one in the normal bladder, and agents that imitate or enhance its action would be expected to cause or facilitate bladder contraction. Agents that inhibit the enzymatic degradation of acetylcholine (anticholinesterases), such as physostigmine and neostigmine, are available but seldom are used for urologic purposes.

Of all the acetylcholine-like drugs, only bethanechol chloride (Myotonachol, Urecholine, Duvoid) is said to exhibit a relatively selective action on the urinary bladder and gut with little or no action on ganglia or on the cardiovascular system at therapeutic dosages. It has been recommended in a single subcutaneous dose of 5 to 10 mg for the treatment of postoperative or postpartum urinary retention in awake and alert patients. It has been used in the "rehabilitation" of atonic or hypotonic bladders. The regimen involves an initial dose schedule of 7.5 to 10 mg of the drug subcutaneously every 4 to 6 hours. This regimen may be initiated with an indwelling catheter in place, with the catheter being removed after a few doses have been administered. When the residual urine on a timed voiding schedule has decreased to an acceptable level, the subcutaneous dosage is decreased to 5 mg four times daily and then changed to an oral dose of 50 to 100 mg four times daily. In a case of partial but incomplete bladder emptying, a therapeutic trial of the oral agent in a dosage of 25 to 100 mg four times daily can be used in conjunction with attempted voiding every 4 hours. In order to stimulate or facilitate the development of reflex bladder contractions in patients with spinal cord injuries, bethanechol has been used in dosages similar to those employed in the rehabilitation regimen or in lower doses (2.5 to 5 mg subcutaneously or 25 to 50 mg orally).

Our own experience and that of others with bethanechol alone in the treatment of all types of patients with inadequate bladder emptying generally has been disappointing. Although a subcutaneous dose of 5 mg does increase the intravesical pressure at all points along the accommodation curve of the cystometrogram and does decrease the bladder capacity threshold, its ability to stimulate a physiologic bladder contraction in a patient who cannot normally initiate one, as well as its ability to

TABLE 3. Therapy to Facilitate Bladder Emptying

INCREASING INTRAVESICAL PRESSURE/ BLADDER CONTRACTILITY

1. External compression, Valsalva maneuver
2. Promotion or initiation of reflex contractions
   a. Trigger zones or maneuvers
   b. Bladder training, tidal drainage
3. Pharmacologic therapy
   a. Parasympathomimetic agents
   b. Prostaglandins
   c. Blockers of inhibition
      i. Alpha-adrenergic antagonists
      ii. Opioid antagonists
4. Reduction cystoplasty
5. Electrical stimulation
   a. Directly to the bladder or spinal cord
   b. To the nerve roots
   c. Transurethral intravesical electrotherapy

DECREASING OUTLET RESISTANCE

1. At a site of anatomic obstruction
   a. Prostatectomy
   b. Balloon dilation
   c. Intraurethral stent
   d. Decrease prostate size or tone
      i. Luteinizing hormone–releasing hormone agonists
      ii. Antiandrogens
      iii. 5-alpha-reductase inhibitors
      iv. Alpha-adrenergic antagonists
   e. Urethral stricture repair/dilation
2. At the level of the smooth sphincter
   a. Transurethral resection or incision of the bladder neck
   b. Y-V–plasty of the bladder neck
   c. Pharmacologic therapy
      i. Alpha-adrenergic antagonists
      ii. Beta-adrenergic agonists
3. At the level of the striated sphincter
   a. Surgical sphincterotomy, botulinum A toxin
   b. Urethral overdilation
   c. Urethral stent
   d. Pudendal nerve interruption
   e. Pharmacologic therapy
      i. Skeletal muscle relaxants: benzodiazepines, baclofen, dantrolene
      ii. Alpha-adrenergic antagonists
   f. Psychotherapy, biofeedback

CIRCUMVENTING THE PROBLEM

1. Intermittent catheterization
2. Continuous catheterization
3. Urinary diversion

augment a "weak" detrusor contraction, is questionable. In addition, urethral resistance actually may be increased by a pharmacologically active dose of the drug. The effectiveness of the currently recommended oral dosages of bethanechol is even more questionable. It is difficult to find reproducible urodynamic data that support a general recommendation for the usage of bethanechol in any specific category of patients. Most, if not all, long-term studies in such patients are neither prospective nor double blind and do not exclude the effects of other simultaneous regimens. Short-term studies in which the drug was the only variable generally have failed to demonstrate significant efficacy in terms of flow and residual urine volume data. Whether repeated doses of any cholinergic agonist can achieve a clinical effect that a single dose cannot is speculative. It is generally agreed that, at least in a denervated bladder, an oral dose of 200 mg is required to produce the same effect as a subcutaneous dose of 5 mg. The question of whether bethanechol may be efficacious in a particular patient can be answered by a brief urodynamically controlled trial in which institution of therapy is the only variable.

When used for testing or for therapy, bethanechol should never be given intramuscularly or intravenously. When used as recommended, bethanechol may cause flushing, nausea, vomiting, diarrhea, gastrointestinal cramps, bronchospasm, headache, salivation, sweating, and difficulty with visual accommodation, all as a consequence of its peripheral acetylcholine-like effects. Its use is contraindicated in patients with anatomic or functional bladder outlet obstruction. It is also contraindicated in patients with bronchial asthma, peptic ulcer, hyperthyroidism, enteritis, partial or complete bowel obstruction, cardiac arrhythmia, or a history of recent gastrointestinal surgery. Because it may lower blood pressure, it should not be given to patients with hypotension, bradycardia, or coronary artery disease.

Other agents, such as histamine, serotonin, adenosine triphosphate, metaclopromide, and prostaglandins, have been shown to stimulate the smooth muscle of the bladder. No consistent clinical success has yet evolved from these observations or from efforts to inhibit the tonic inhibitory effect exerted by opioids on the micturition reflex.

One of the presumed effects of the sympathetic nervous system is to promote urine storage by exerting an inhibitory effect, during filling, on the parasympathetic ganglia of the bladder via an alpha-adrenergic receptor. It is possible, therefore, that alpha-adrenergic blocking agents may facilitate the micturition reflex on this basis. Anecdotal experience with alpha-adrenergic blockers in successfully treating nonobstructive urinary retention in patients with reactive bladders appears to substantiate such an effect, although an alternate mechanism has been postulated—simply decreasing outlet resistance rather than a facilitatory effect on PS ganglionic transmission.

Decreasing Outlet Resistance

Smooth Sphincter

Alpha-adrenergic receptor sites (causing contraction) exist in the smooth muscle of the bladder neck and proximal urethra. Functional obstruction may occur at this level and should be considered when incomplete or high-pressure emptying occurs despite an adequate bladder contraction in a patient without anatomic obstruction or detrusor–external sphincter dyssynergia. Additional evidence in such a patient is a voiding cystourethrogram that shows poor opening of the vesical neck and proximal urethra following bladder contraction. In such a situation, alpha-adrenergic blockade may improve emptying, and a therapeutic trial is warranted. Functional obstruction at the level of the bladder neck and proximal urethra often occurs as a part of the syndrome of autonomic hyperreflexia and is similarly susceptible to alpha-adrenergic blockade. Some studies with alpha-adrenergic blockade have been interpreted as showing an inhibitory effect on the external striated sphincter as well. Such effects, if they do occur, probably result from central (spinal cord or brain) actions. Before giving up pharmacologically in a patient with proven or suspected striated sphincter dyssynergy, a trial of alpha blocker is worthwhile.

Phenoxybenzamine was the most commonly utilized alpha blocker until reports appeared of gastrointestinal tumors in rats with large doses. Prazosin (Minipress; 2 to 10 mg daily in three divided doses), terazosin (Hytrin; 2 to 10 mg at bedtime), and doxazosin (Cardura) are now the most commonly utilized. Potential side effects caused by alpha-adrenergic blockade include orthostatic hypotension, reflex tachycardia, nasal congestion, diarrhea, miosis, inhibition of seminal emission, and retrograde ejaculation. Side effects unrelated to the alpha-adrenergic blocking properties of phenoxybenzamine include nausea, vomiting (probably due to gastric irritation), and a generalized feeling of weakness and tiredness, which may disappear after prolonged therapy.

Alpha-adrenergic blocking agents also have been used to treat both bladder and outlet abnormalities in patients with so-called autonomous bladders—such as those with myelodysplasia, sacral spinal cord or infrasacral neural injury, and voiding dysfunction following radical pelvic surgery. Parasympathetic decentralization has been reported to lead to a conversion of the usual beta (relaxant) response of the bladder body in response to sympathetic stimulation into an alpha (contractile) effect. Decreased bladder compliance is a common clinical problem in such patients, and this, along with a fixed urethral sphincter tone, results in the paradoxical occurrence of both storage and emptying failure. In these patients, alpha blockade is capable of increasing bladder compliance and decreasing urethral resistance.

Striated Sphincter

Functional obstruction also can occur at the level of the striated sphincter. There is no class of pharmacologic agents that selectively relaxes the striated musculature of the pelvic floor. Three different types of drugs have been used to treat voiding dysfunction secondary to outlet obstruction at the level of the striated sphincter: (1) the benzodiazepines (diazepam [Valium] is the most common), (2) baclofen (Lioresal), and (3) dantrolene (Dantrium), all of which have been characterized under the general heading of antispasticity drugs. Baclofen and the benzodiazepines exert their actions predominantly within the central nervous system, whereas dantrolene acts directly on skeletal muscle. Unfortunately, there is no completely satisfactory form of therapy for alleviation of skeletal muscle spasticity. Although these drugs are capable of providing variable relief of spasticity in some circumstances, their efficacy is far from complete, and this, along with troublesome muscle weakness, adverse effects on gait, and a variety of other side effects, may minimize their overall usefulness.

Besides diazepam, the benzodiazepine derivatives include chlordiazepoxide (Librium, others) oxazepam (Serax), lorazepam (Ativan), prazepam (Centrax), alprazolam (Xanax), and halazepam (Paxipam). Although pharmacologically these groups can be classified as centrally acting muscle relaxants, they often are categorized under the heading of drugs used in the treatment of anxiety. Effective total daily oral doses of diazepam, the most widely used agent of this group, range from 4 to 40 mg.

The most common side effects of all members of this group are oversedation and impairment of higher cerebral function. Few references are available that look specifically at any of the diazepines in the treatment of functional obstruction at the level of the striated sphincter. In general, I have not found the recommended oral doses of diazepam to be effective in controlling classic detrusor-striated sphincter dyssynergia that is secondary to neurologic disease. If the etiology of incomplete emptying in a neurologically normal patient is obscure and the patient has what appears to be inadequate relaxation of the pelvic floor striated musculature (i.e., what Hinman describes as the "non-neurogenic neurogenic bladder"), a trial of such an agent may be worthwhile.

Dantrolene sodium (Dantrium) is a skeletal muscle relaxant that directly affects skeletal muscle by acting on excitation-contraction coupling. The drug has been used by others with some success in patients with neurologic disease and classic detrusor–external sphincter dyssynergia, but our own results have been less than satisfactory. We do *not* recommend a trial of this agent in the patient with presumed external sphincter dyssynergia but no other neurologic findings. Although no inhibitory action on bladder smooth muscle occurs, the generalized weakness that may be induced by dantrolene often is significant enough to compromise its therapeutic effects. Other potential side effects include euphoria, dizziness, diarrhea, and hepatotoxicity. Fatal hepatitis has been reported in approximately 0.1 to 0.2 per cent of patients treated with the drug for 60 days or longer, and symptomatic hepatitis may occur in 0.5 per cent of patients treated with dantrolene for more than 60 days; chemical abnormalities of liver function are noted in up to 1 per cent.

Baclofen (Lioresal) is an agent that inhibits the transmission of monosynaptic and polysynaptic spinal cord reflexes and has been found useful in the treatment of skeletal spasticity resulting from a variety of causes (especially multiple sclerosis and traumatic spinal cord lesions). It also may depress involuntary bladder contractions secondary to a spinal cord lesion. Determination of optimal dose in individual patients requires careful titration. Treatment is started at an initial dose of 5 mg three times daily, and the dose is doubled every 3 days until a daily total dose level of 60 mg is reached. The manufacturer's recommended maximum daily dose is 20 mg four times daily.

Potential side effects include drowsiness, insomnia, rash, pruritus, dizziness, and weakness. It may impair the ability to walk or stand, and is not recommended for the management of spasticity in rheumatic disorders, stroke, cerebral palsy, or the muscular rigidity of parkinsonism for that reason. Sudden withdrawal has been shown to provoke hallucinations. Drug delivery and not lack of pharmacologic action is often what frustrates pharmacologic therapy. Intrathecal administration of baclofen via an implanted infusion pump has shown initial promising results for not only spasticity but sphincter and bladder hyperactivity as well.

Benign Prostatic Hypertrophy

Although other endocrine factors are doubtless involved, the androgenic influence on prostatic growth and function is obviously central. Free plasma testosterone enters prostatic cells by diffusion, and is rapidly metabolized to other steroids. More than 90 per cent is irreversibly converted to the main prostatic androgen, dihydrotestosterone (DHT) by the enzyme 5-alpha reductase. DHT or testosterone is bound to specific androgen receptors in the nucleus, where activation of the steroid receptor occurs. Although much remains to be elucidated regarding the hormonal interaction and necessities for the induction and maintenance of benign prostatic hypertrophy (BPH), it is clear that, clinically, a reduction in prostatic size of approximately 20 to 30 per cent can be induced either by interfering with the conversion of testosterone to DHT or by interfering with androgen receptor binding and metabolism.

Finasteride (Proscar) is a 5-alpha reductase inhibitor. The finasteride study group has reported a total symptom score improvement of 21 per cent at 1 year compared to 2 per cent with placebo. Peak flow rate improved by 22 per cent as opposed to 8 per cent for placebo. Prostatic volume decreased by 19 per cent as opposed to 3 per cent with placebo. The mean serum DHT concentration decreased during the first 2 weeks of treatment to levels present after castration. Serum testosterone and luteinizing hormone concentrations increased slightly and remained within normal ranges throughout the study. Approximately 50 per cent of men who received the drug had a decrease of 20 per cent or more in the size of the prostate, and the median decrease of prostate-specific antigen concentration was 50 per cent; and this seemed to be stable beginning with month 3 of treatment. In the finasteride group, 4.4 per cent of patients complained of an ejaculatory disorder and 3.4 per cent of impotence, compared to 1.7 per cent incidence of these in the placebo group. There were no other significant side effects.

It is important to understand the concept of two prostatic components contributory to the bladder outlet obstruction caused by BPH. The static component refers to the mechanical obstruction of the prostatic urethra caused by the bulk of the enlarging prostatic adenoma. The dynamic component of obstruction refers to the resistance contributed to by the tone of the prostatic smooth muscle. Smooth muscle is present in hyperplastic stromal nodules, mixed epithelial/stromal nodules, the bladder neck, and the prostatic capsule. The contractile properties of prostatic smooth muscle are mediated primarily by $alpha_1$-adrenergic receptors. Using a selective $alpha_1$ antagonist, terazosin hydrochloride (Hytrin), symptom score improvements of up to 44 per cent versus 23 per cent for placebo have been recorded, along with peak flow improvements up to 34 per cent versus 10.4 per cent for placebo. Potential side effects include orthostatic hypotension, fatigue, dizziness, and nasal stuffiness.

FAILURE TO STORE URINE PROPERLY

Urinary incontinence falls under this category and may result primarily from a detrusor or sphincter component. Incontinence with or without urgency usually results from involuntary bladder contractions or decreased compliance. These may be secondary to neurologic disease, bladder outlet obstruction, or inflammatory disease or may be idiopathic. Pharmacologic attempts at treatment of this type of disorder utilize agents that decrease bladder smooth muscle contractility. For classic stress urinary incontinence and intrinsic sphincter dysfunction, pharmacologic therapy is directed primarily at increasing outlet resistance.

The "urgency-frequency symptom complex," a term applied to the frequent strong desire to void or the frequent feeling of imminent micturition in an uninfected patient without anatomic outlet obstruction, is an extremely distressing and problematic complaint. Assuming no obvious reversible cause exists, the treatment usually consists of one or a combination of the agents used to inhibit bladder contractility. Often, however, this symptom complex is not associated with urodynamic abnormalities, a fact that most likely accounts for the generally less than optimal results achieved with this type of treatment. Certainly it would seem that the ideal treatment for this type of urgency, which seems to be more sensory than motor in origin, would be an agent that produces topical anesthesia or hypesthesia of the bladder and urethral mucosa.

Inhibiting Bladder Contractility

Atropine and atropine-like agents therefore depress true involuntary bladder contractions of any etiology. In such patients, the volume to the first involuntary contraction generally will be increased, the amplitude of the contractions decreased, and the total bladder capacity increased, with a proportionate reduction in symptomatology. Although the threshold volume for an unsuppressible involuntary contraction may be increased, the "warning time" may not, and thus urgency and incontinence still may occur unless therapy is combined with a timed voiding or toileting regimen. The effect of the antimuscarinics or intravesical pressure during filling in patients who exhibit only decreased compliance has not been well studied. Propantheline bromide (Pro-Banthīne, others) is the oral agent most commonly used to produce an antimuscarinic effect in the lower urinary tract. The usual adult oral dosage is 15 to 30 mg every 4 to 6 hours, although higher doses are sometimes necessary and well tolerated. Oral administration in the fasting state rather than with or after meals is preferable from the standpoint of bioavailability. There seems to be little difference between the antimuscarinic effects of propantheline on bladder smooth muscle and those of other antimuscarinic agents, such as glycopyrrolate, isopropamide, hyoscyamine, anisotropine, methylbromide, and others. Some of these agents (e.g., glycopyrrolate) have a more convenient dosage schedule (two or three times daily), but their clinical effects on the lower urinary tract seem to be indistinguishable.

The potential side effects of all antimuscarinic agents include inhibition of salivary secretion (dry mouth), blockade of the ciliary muscle of the lens to cholinergic stimulation (blurred vision for near objects), tachycardia, drowsiness, and inhibition of gut motility. Those agents that possess some ganglionic blocking activity also may cause orthostatic hypotension and impotence at high doses. Antimuscarinic agents generally are contraindicated in patients with narrow-angle glaucoma and should be used with caution in patients with significant bladder outlet obstruction because complete urinary retention may be precipitated.

Musculotropic relaxants fall under the general heading of direct-acting smooth muscle depressants, whose "antispasmodic" activity reportedly is directly on smooth muscle at a site that is metabolically distal to the cholinergic receptor mechanism. Although all three of the agents to be discussed do relax smooth muscle in vitro by a papaverine-like activity, all have been found in addition to possess variable anticholinergic and local anesthetic properties.

Oxybutynin hydrochloride (Ditropan) is a moderately potent anticholinergic agent with a strong independent musculotropic relaxant activity and local anesthetic activity as well. This agent has been used successfully to depress detrusor hyperreflexia in patients with neurogenic bladder dysfunction. The recommended oral dose of oxybutynin in adults is 5 mg three to four times daily. The potential side effects are those of antimuscarinic agents. Topical application of oxybutynin to normal or intestinal bladders has been mentioned. This conceptually attractive form of alternative drug delivery awaits further clinical trials and the development of a preparation specifically formulated for that purpose.

Dicyclomine hydrochloride (Bentyl) also is reported to possess a direct relaxant effect on smooth muscle in addition to an antimuscarinic action. An oral dose of 20 mg three times daily in adults has been reported to increase bladder capacity in patients with detrusor hyperreflexia. I have used 10 to 20 mg three to four times daily. The potential side effects are antimuscarinic ones.

Flavoxate hydrochloride (Urispas) is another compound that has been reported to have a direct inhibitory action on smooth muscle in addition to anticholinergic and local analgesic properties. The recommended adult dosage is 100 to 200 mg three or four times daily. As with all agents in this group, a short clinical trial may be worthwhile. Reported side effects are rare and primarily anticholinergic.

The dependence of contractile activity on changes in cytosolic calcium varies from tissue to tissue, but interference with calcium inflow, intracellular calcium release, or concentration is a potential mechanism of bladder smooth muscle relaxation.

Terodiline is an agent with both calcium antagonist and antimuscarinic properties in vitro. It has been marketed in Europe since 1986 for the treatment of bladder instability and hyperreflexia. There have been a number of randomized and blinded studies on the inhibitory action of terodiline on bladder hyperactivity, and these have shown clinical effectiveness. Terodiline was withdrawn from clinical investigation in the United States after reports of cases of a rare ventricular arrhythmia in 1991. With new precautions and exclusions, it may reappear on the clinical scene.

Many clinicians have found tricyclic antidepressants, particularly imipramine hydrochloride (Tofranil and others), to be especially useful agents for facilitating urine storage, by both decreasing bladder contractility and increasing outlet resistance. Imipramine has prominent systemic anticholinergic effects, but it has only a weak antimuscarinic effect on bladder smooth muscle. A strong direct inhibitory effect on bladder smooth muscle exists, however, that is neither anticholinergic nor adrenergic. One might postulate a further decrease in bladder body contractility if in fact a peripheral blockade of norepinephrine reuptake actually occurs as a result of the increased concentration of beta-adrenergic over alpha-adrenergic receptors in this area. An enhanced alpha-adrenergic effect in the smooth muscle of the bladder base and proximal urethra, where alpha receptors outnumber beta receptors, generally is considered to be the mechanism whereby imipramine increases outlet resistance. Our usual adult dose for voiding dysfunction is 25 mg four times daily; half that dose is given in elderly patients. Imipramine elimination half-life has been shown to be prolonged in both the elderly male and the elderly female. In our experience, the effects of imipramine on the lower urinary tract are often additive to those of atropine-like agents and, consequently, a combination of imipramine and an antimuscarinic or an antispasmodic is sometimes especially useful for decreasing bladder contractility. If imipramine is used in conjunction with an atropine-like agent, it should be noted that the anticholinergic side effects of the drugs may be additive.

When tricyclic antidepressants are used in the generally larger doses, the most frequent side effects are those attributable to their systemic anticholinergic activity. Allergic phenomena, including rash, hepatic dysfunction, obstructive jaundice, and agranulocytosis, also may occur, but rarely. Central nervous system side effects may include weakness, fatigue, parkinsonian effect, a fine tremor noted most in the upper extremities, a manic or schizophrenic picture, and sedation, probably from its antihistaminic effect. Postural hypotension also may be seen, presumably on the basis of selective blockade (a paradoxical effect) of alpha$_1$-adrenergic receptors in some vascular smooth muscle. Antidepressants can be shown electrophysiologically and hemodynamically to have a depressant effect on the myocardium shortly after their institution. However, it has been pointed out that, in the animal studies showing a direct myocardial depressant effect, plasma concentrations in the toxic range for humans were present. Whether cardiotoxicity will prove to be a legitimate concern in patients receiving smaller doses for lower urinary tract dysfunction remains to be seen and is potentially a matter of concern. Consultation with an individual patient's internist or cardiologist is always helpful before instituting such therapy in questionable situations. The onset of significant side effects (severe abdominal distress, nausea, vomiting, headache, lethargy, irritability) following abrupt cessation of high doses of imipramine in children suggests that the drug should be discontinued gradually, especially in patients receiving high doses. Tricyclic antidepressants also can cause excess sweating of obscure etiology and a delay of orgasm and orgasmic impotence, whose cause is likewise unclear. The use of imipramine is contraindicated in patients receiving monoamine oxidase inhibitors, because severe central nervous system toxic effects, including hyperpyrexia, seizures, and coma, can be precipitated. The potential side effects of the antidepressants—specifically weakness, fatigue, and postural hypotension—may be especially significant for elderly persons.

Increasing Outlet Resistance

Stimulation of the alpha-adrenergic receptors of the smooth musculature of the bladder neck and proximal urethra can increase outlet resistance sufficiently to improve some cases of mild to moderate sphincteric incontinence. Improvement has been correlated with changes in objective urodynamic parameters, most commonly an increase in maximum urethral closure pressure. Various pharmacologic agents that produce alpha-adrenergic stimulation when administered orally are available. Generally, outlet resistance is increased by a variable degree by such an action. Potential side effects of all of these agents include blood pressure elevation, anxiety, and insomnia caused by stimulation of the central nervous system, headache, tremor, weakness, palpitations, cardiac arrhythmias, and respiratory difficulties. All drugs should be used with caution in patients with hypertension, cardiovascular disease, or hyperthyroidism.

Ephedrine is a noncatecholamine sympathomimetic agent that owes part of its peripheral action to the release of noradrenaline but that also directly stimulates both alpha- and beta-adrenergic receptors. The adult dosage is 25 to 50 mg orally four times daily. Some tachyphylaxis develops to its peripheral actions, probably as a result of depletion of norepinephrine stores. Pseudoephedrine (Sudafed, others) is a stereoisomer that is used for similar indications with similar precautions. The adult dosage is 30 to 60 mg four times daily, and the 30-mg dose form is available as an over-the-counter drug in the United States. Phenylpropanolamine hydrochloride shares the pharmacologic properties of ephedrine and is approximately equal in peripheral potency while causing less central stimulation. It is available in 25- and 50-mg doses and in 75-mg time-release capsules and is a component of numerous proprietary mixtures marketed as appetite suppressants and for the treatment of nasal and sinus congestion (usually in combination with an H_1 antihistamine drug).

The effects of imipramine on the bladder have been discussed. On a theoretical basis, an increase in urethral resistance might be expected if an enhanced alpha-adrenergic effect were produced at this level because of an inhibition of norepinephrine reuptake. Many clinicians, myself included, have noted improvement in sphincteric incontinence in patients who were treated with imipramine primarily for reasons related to bladder hyperactivity but who had, in addition, some component of sphincteric incontinence.

Although some clinicians have reported spectacular cure and improvement rates for sphincteric incontinence with agents that produce an alpha-adrenergic effect in the urethra, my own experience coincides with those who report that treatment with such agents often produces some improvement, but rarely total dryness in cases of severe or even moderate stress incontinence. A clinical trial, when possible, is certainly worthwhile, however, especially in conjunction with pelvic floor physiotherapy/biofeedback.

Although many studies in the literature lack objective evidence of a positive effect of estrogen therapy on stress incontinence in the female, such therapy certainly seems potentially capable of facilitating urinary storage in some postmenopausal patients by increasing the sum total of factors contributing to urethral outlet resistance. The clinical experience of many supports an augmentative or perhaps additive effect with alpha-adrenergic therapy in this regard. Whether this effect is related to changes in the autonomic innervation, changes in receptor content or metabolism of the smooth muscle, or changes in estrogen-binding sites or in the nonmuscular elements of the urethral wall or "mucosal seal" mechanism has not been settled. Caution must be exercised with respect to the potential oncologic risks (uterine cancer), and a potential prescriber is encouraged to consult a larger reference text in that regard.

Suggested Readings

Wein AJ: Neuromuscular dysfunction of the lower urinary tract. *In* Walsh PC, Retik AB, Stamey TA, et al (eds): Campbell's Urology, 6th ed. Philadelphia, WB Saunders, 1992, pp 573–642

Wein AJ: Non-surgical management of bladder dysfunction. *In* Webster G, Kirby R, King L, et al (eds): Reconstructive Urology. Boston, Blackwell Scientific Publications, 1993, pp 403–420

Wein AJ, Barrett DM: Voiding Function and Dysfunction: A Logical and Practical Approach. Chicago, Year Book Medical Publishers, 1988

Wein AJ, Van Arsdalen KN, Levin RM: Pharmacologic therapy. *In* Krane RJ, Siroky MB (eds): Clinical Neuro Urology. Boston, Little, Brown, 1991, pp 523–558

TREATMENT OF THE NONFUNCTIONING URETHRA IN FEMALES

RODNEY A. APPELL, M.D., F.A.C.S.

Cleveland, Ohio

The failure to store urine may be simplified by considering the problem to be located either at the level of the bladder or at the level of the urethra. The choice of the appropriate therapeutic approach for treating urinary incontinence depends to a large degree on the underlying cause of the problem. When the problem originates in the urethra, the difficulty often is related to incompetence of the urethral sphincteric mechanism at the neck of the bladder. Although this incompetence may be the result of some defect in anatomic support, it also may be related to a problem in the intrinsic urethral closure mechanism itself as a result of sympathetic neurologic injury, surgical trauma, or myelodysplasia. Urodynamically, in these cases, the bladder neck and the proximal segment of the urethra are open at rest without a detrusor contraction; however, it must be kept in mind that intrinsic sphincter deficiency (ISD; formerly type III stress urinary incontinence) may exist in association with an anatomic abnormality of the position of the bladder neck and urethra (urethral hypermobility, or type II stress injury incontinence). Nearly all procedures developed to restore urinary control in this type of outflow disorder of intrinsic sphincter deficiency are based on the principle of enhancing urethral pressure to resist the flow of urine.

The treatment of urinary incontinence related to the incompetent urethra has been a challenging problem and frequently involves surgical augmentation of intraurethral pressures by the use of slings made of analogous or synthetic materials, implantation of an artificial sphincter, or periurethral injection of bulk-enhancing agents. Attempts to treat this problem with pharmacologic agents have not been consistently efficacious. The choice of which treatment modality to use with which patient is quite controversial and depends on the physician's skills with the various techniques, patient motivation and specific needs, and the availability of support for the physician and patient alike.

PHARMACOLOGIC AGENTS

Alpha-Sympathetic Agonists

Theoretically, because of the preponderance of alpha-adrenergic receptor sites in the bladder neck and proximal urethra, alpha-sympathetic agonists have been tried, but improvements in urethral closure pressure demonstrated urodynamically have not been translated into long-term clinical success because of side effects and tachyphylaxis.

Estrogens

Estrogen therapy seems capable of facilitating urinary storage in some women. Whether this effect is related only to changes in the autonomic innervation, to the function of the smooth muscle, or to changes in nonmuscular components of the urethral wall has not been determined. Estrogen certainly stimulates and supports urethral and trigonal smooth muscle and epithelium and can influence certain factors related to the maintenance of urethral pressure, such as the smooth muscle of the urethra and bladder neck, the connective tissue of the urethra and periurethra, the vascular bed of the urethra, and the urethral mucosal seal (referring to the plasticity of the epithelium and lamina propria, which allows for aposition of the folds of epithelium supported by the vascularity of the submucosa acting as a framework). In addition, the sensitivity to alpha-adrenergic stimulation, the alpha-adrenergic receptor content and autonomic innervation of the bladder outlet are estrogen dependent, and some have attempted dual pharmacologic treatment with estrogens followed by alpha agonists, again with limited long-term success.

SURGICAL INTERVENTION

Slings

Many different techniques are described for performance of sling surgery. The differences in technique can be classified by the surgical approach and the material employed as the sling. The placement of autologous, heterologous, or synthetic material beneath the urethra provides an increase in urethral compression and a plate for receiving the transmission of intra-abdominal pressure to the bladder neck and proximal urethra. The technical demands on the surgical approach are accurate placement of the sling beneath the bladder neck and proximal urethra with a broad base of compression, and a simple and safe passage of the ends of the sling through the retropubic, extravesical space for attachment to the rectus fascia or pubic bone without excessive tension that could provoke permanent urinary retention or intractible detrusor instability resulting from obstruction to the outlet. The aim is coaptation of the urethra, not obstruction. The optimal surgical approach should minimize the risk of damage to the bladder, bladder neck/proximal urethra, and vagina. An abdominovaginal approach combines dissection into the retropubic space abdominally with a vaginal incision that aids in accurate perforation for the arms of the sling and accurate placement of the body of the sling beneath the urethra. More recently, many surgeons have been reducing the total surgical endeavor by using needle techniques (modifications of standard suspension procedures) to facilitate the placement of the sling, even so much as to use a portion of the anterior vaginal wall as an in situ sling.

The Artificial Urinary Sphincter

In the treatment of urinary incontinence resulting from ISD, one of the goals is to establish a normal voiding pattern while allowing the patient to become dry between voidings. Treatment is designed to close the outflow channel; however, this may result in the inability of the patient to empty the bladder completely or at all. Of the treatments designed for ISD, only implantation of the artificial urinary sphincter (AUS) allows for the obstruction to be relieved at the time of voiding so that the actual voiding pattern is normalized and the desired state of dryness is accomplished. It is not sufficient to state that women with ISD are natural candidates for the AUS. They must also have adequate manual dexterity, mental capacity, and motivation to manipulate the labial pump mechanism each time they need to urinate.

The sphincter has four components: a pump mechanism, a cuff that encircles the bladder neck/proximal urethra, a pressure-regulating balloon, and tubing connectors. The most difficult part of the surgery is negotiating around the bladder neck/proximal urethra, because the urethovaginal septum is not a true surgical plane, but this appears to be facilitated by a transvaginal placement of the cuff. The AUS provides continence without pressure necrosis or fibrotic contraction of the bladder neck/proximal urethra. The AUS is intended to permit intermittent urethral compression, thus allowing the patient to reduce urethral resistance voluntarily during voiding, as opposed to other compressive procedures in which the patient is voiding against a relative obstruction.

Periurethral Injections

Autologous fat and blood, heterologous collagen, and synthetics have been used to treat ISD. The best results with periurethral injections occur in those females who have no detrusor problems, have an adequate bladder capacity, and have little or no anatomic abnormality. Many patients for whom the sling or AUS is indicated are unsuitable surgical candidates, and therapy with injectables is less invasive than open surgery. A significant number of patients who have no options available for resolving their incontinence would benefit from periurethral injection therapy. Submucosal injection with cross-linked collagen has been safe, effective, and easy to perform under local anesthesia in clinical trials. Currently, only cross-linked collagen has been approved by the U.S. Food and Drug Administration, and injection with autologous fat or blood is unproven.

CONCLUSION

Of the alternative treatments available or under study for females with ISD, sling surgery is successful in 81 to 98 per cent, implantation of the AUS (either by abdominal or transvaginal approach) in over 90 per cent, and injection therapy in between 64 and 95 per cent of patients. The primary goal in treatment of women with ISD is to allow coaptation of the mucosa of the proximal urethra without obstruction. In theory, this goal is best attained by using the AUS, but the difficulty in the surgery has caused the search for alternative forms of management, especially simpler sling techniques and the use of injectables. More important than the choice of therapy is the identification of the proper patient for treatment. Correction of an anatomic abnormality by one of the many resuspension procedures will be inadequate for correction of those patients with ISD. Current urodynamic, radiographic, and endoscopic techniques must be employed to properly select those patients who require augmentation of outlet function.

Suggested Readings

Appell RA: Artificial sphincter and periurethral injections. *In* Benson JT (ed): Female Pelvic Floor Disorders. New York, WW Norton, 1992, pp 257–268

Blaivas JG, Klutke G, Raz S, et al: Symposium: When sphincter failure is the cause of female stress incontinence. Contemp Urol 5:33–54, 1993

Staskin DR: Sling surgery for the treatment of female stress incontinence. Probl Urol 5:106–122, 1991

STRESS URINARY INCONTINENCE IN FEMALES

CHRISTOPHER K. PAYNE, M.D.

Stanford, California

Although the problem of urinary incontinence is as old as civilization, only recently has it received extensive publicity. The National Institutes of Health (NIH)–sponsored conference on the topic in 1988 was a catalyst for change, focusing attention on a subject that had previously been largely ignored and even considered taboo. Today, increasing numbers of patients are seeking treatment for incontinence. This has sparked the health care industry to make significant investments to research and develop new treatments. It is an exciting time for the clinician with new weapons in the therapeutic arsenal; however, the excitement is tempered by the realization that little is known about the long-term effectiveness of most treatments and there are very few data available to guide in selection of treatment for an individual patient. This article reviews the current options for treating incontinence and provides some practical guidelines that will help the clinician to individualize treatment of a particular patient. Although only stress urinary incontinence (SUI) in females is discussed here, this accounts for approximately half of the total problem of urinary incontinence in the United States.

PATIENT EVALUATION

It is helpful to separate the stress-incontinent population into two categories, those with anatomic incontinence (AI) and those with intrinsic sphincter dysfunction (ISD). Considering the bladder neck and proximal urethra together as the primary sphincter unit, patients with AI are incontinent because the sphincter unit is malpositioned and/or hypermobile. The sphincter is functionally normal but poorly supported. Increases in intra-abdominal pressure thus are inappropriately transmitted to the bladder but not to the urethra, so urine is forced out of the bladder. Patients with ISD have a damaged or incompetent sphincter unit in a normally supported anatomic position. The sphincter is functionally ineffective because of fibrosis, scarring, and neurologic or vascular injuries that prevent proper coaptation of the walls of the urethra.

Unfortunately, the true physiology of stress incontinence is more complex. Many women without incontinence are observed to have urethral hypermobility. Hypermobility and sphincter dysfunction can coexist, making classification difficult. Nonetheless, the awareness of ISD as a clinical entity is one of the major advances in the evaluation and management of SUI of the past decade. Although surgeons long have known that the "lead-pipe" urethra from radiation or surgical scarring responds poorly to standard bladder suspension operations, only recently have the more subtle manifestations of ISD been appreciated.

This article cannot review fully the evaluation of the incontinent female. However, the distinction between AI and ISD is so critical to proper therapy that a few caveats must be mentioned. The history and physical exam usually provide most of the information necessary to make the differentiation. Patients with AI have mild to moderate incontinence that clearly is related to strenuous physical activity. The urethra is markedly mobile with cough and Valsalva maneuver. In contrast, patients with ISD have severe incontinence that occurs with minimal activity. They complain that they leak "constantly" and leak "like a dripping faucet." On physical exam the urethra may not move at all with cough and strain but the incontinence is severe. The degree of stress incontinence reported by the patient and observed by the physician is the single best clue to the presence of ISD. All patients with severe incontinence must be suspected of having ISD. Urodynamics, radiologic and video studies, and cystoscopy may be helpful to confirm clinical suspicions or to evaluate borderline cases but are primarily adjuncts to history and physical exam.

Other factors that impact on treatment decisions that must be assessed in the initial evaluation include:

1. Degree of pelvic prolapse (bladder, rectum, uterus, or vault)
2. Presence or absence of urgency and urge incontinence
3. Other diseases affecting the patient, her overall medical condition
4. Impact of incontinence on the patient's life-style
5. Patient's wishes and goals for her future

We will return to these considerations in the final section on treatment planning. It is presumed that other urologic problems such as hematuria, infections, and urinary retention are evaluated and treated prior to undertaking a work-up of SUI.

THERAPEUTIC OPTIONS—OVERVIEW

The following discussion organizes the methods of treating SUI into three basic categories—pharmacologic treatment, surgical treatment, and "conservative" or nonpharmacologic, nonsurgical therapy. The physiologic rationale behind each treatment is presented and published results are summarized. It is beyond the scope of this article to discuss specific techniques in detail, particularly with regard to the various surgical options. The suggested readings listed at the end of the article provide more details.

It is important to realize that the results of therapy for SUI are not easy to compare. Reports often fail to define the type and degree of incontinence at entry. Specific treatment regimens may be quite different in the hands of different investigators. Results typically are reported at the end of the intervention, and follow-up is rarely as long as 1 year. Because of the nature of the disease, success is largely subjective and the definitions used vary considerably from one study to the next. There are not enough studies that compare treatment within the same category (i.e., one drug against another) and very few that compare treatments across categories (i.e., pharmacologic treatment against surgery). Thus, the interpretation of the literature necessarily reflects the biases and opinions of the author.

"CONSERVATIVE THERAPY"

The beginning of conservative therapy for SUI is making the proper diagnosis and explaining the problem to the patient. It is important to reassure the patient that the problem is not life threatening, that good therapy is available, and that the patient does not need to simply accept the limitations on her lifestyle. Many patients associate incontinence with terminal illness, and some simply seek an endorsement of their health. Many patients with infrequent, minor degrees of incontinence are happy with reassurance and will continue to lead a normal life, occasionally wearing a protective pad for important occasions. After eliminating this small group, the majority of patients who present for evaluation of incontinence want to be treated. For the majority of patients with SUI it is appropriate to consider some form of conservative therapy.

Pelvic Floor Exercises

Pelvic floor exercises (PFEs) are the standard to which all other methods of conservative therapy should be compared. Dr. Arnold Kegel, a California gynecologist, popularized the exercises that often bear his name by systematically studying their use in a large number of patients. He taught patients to contract the pubococcygeus muscles vigorously, without contracting the abdominal or buttock muscles. One of the first medical uses of biofeedback was his "perineometer," which provided patients immediate information about the strength of their contractions. In papers on the subject from the late 1940s and early 1950s, he reported an 84 per cent cure rate in over 500 patients. These exercises, at least in theory, increase the bulk of the levator musculature. They may increase the resting tone of the urethra, improve the support of the sphincter unit during stress, and strengthen the reflex contraction of the pelvic floor that occurs with increases in intra-abdominal pressure. Clinical improvement does seem to correlate roughly with improved strength of contraction when some form of biofeedback is used to monitor therapy.

For a variety of reasons Kegel exercises have never been popular in this country. They are time and labor-intensive and have been poorly reimbursed. There has been a feeling in the medical community that PFEs are something "good to do" but not a serious treatment. Whereas Kegel emphasized the importance of the initial instruction period, in which patients learn to isolate the appropriate muscles, patients often simply are given brief verbal instructions with no opportunity to practice and master the exercises. Whereas enthusiastic support of the therapist and frequent follow-up evaluations were considered by Kegel to be crucial to the success of the program, patients often have no follow-up after the initial visit until they have completed the prescribed treatment program. It is not surprising that many surgeons feel that PFEs rarely make a significant impact on the problem.

When the results of PFEs for SUI are appraised critically, it is clear that a majority of patients respond to the therapy. Whether incontinence diaries, pad tests, or subjective measures are used as the end-point, investigators generally report from 60 to 90 per cent of patients as either "cured or improved." However, beyond being able to say that most patients receive at least some benefit from the treatment, there are far more questions about PFEs than there are answers. There is no agreement about how best to teach the exercises, about the optimal frequency or duration of the therapy, about how to select patients who are most likely to benefit from therapy, about the potentially additive benefit of biofeedback to an exercise program, or about the durability of the response to therapy.

As mentioned above, Kegel originally employed biofeedback in teaching PFEs. One interesting and simple method of providing biofeedback at home is weighted vaginal cones. Tactile biofeedback occurs when the patient senses the cone slipping out of the vagina and is thus encouraged to strengthen her contraction. In the event that the cone falls out, biofeedback is immediate. The patient progresses to higher weights as tolerated. Cones were found to be superior to PFEs alone in Jonasson's randomized trial of postpartum incontinence. In Peattie's study, 63 per cent of women awaiting surgery for SUI decided to cancel the operation after completing a course of treatment with vaginal cones. However, 23 per cent of the patients originally enrolled in the study dropped out and were not included in the results. Other studies also show high dropout rates. Many patients will not accept the idea of inserting the cone into the vagina and others are frustrated when they are unable to reach the end of the series of cones. The advantage of vaginal cones is that they are relatively inexpensive and can be used at home. This might reduce the dependence on a therapist to monitor treatment and thus reduce cost. There are several randomized studies comparing office-based biofeedback to PFEs alone; the results are contradictory. There are as yet no conclusive data proving that the results of PFEs, performed under the supervision of an enthusiastic and qualified therapist, are improved by any form of biofeedback.

Electrical Stimulation

Electrical stimulation of the pelvic floor by vaginal or anal probes was designed as a therapy for detrusor instability and urgency incontinence. Initial success rates are 50 to 90 per cent. Stimulating the sacral nerves of the pelvic floor induces reflex relaxation of the motor input to the bladder; this is the rationale for using electrical stimulation to treat detrusor instability. It is less clear how the technique works in treating SUI, and there has been much less reported about the use of electrical stimulation for SUI. Eriksen and Eik-Nes used electrical stimulation to treat 55 women awaiting surgery for SUI. The average course of treatment was 5 months. Two thirds of the patients improved enough to cancel their surgery and most maintained the improvement over 2 years of follow-up. These excellent results have not yet been reproduced in other studies, and some investigators have had very little success with electrical stimulation for any form of incontinence. There is no consensus as to the best way of delivering the stimulation or the optimal characteristics of the wave form. Nonetheless, there is currently a wave of enthusiasm for this treatment modality, and several companies have developed units for home therapy. However, these units are quite expensive compared to PFEs and have not been proven to be superior. It is likely that any improvement attained with electrical stimulation will require some form of chronic maintenance therapy.

Behavioral Modification Techniques

The other commonly used method of conservative therapy is behavioral modification. This is a relatively simple form of therapy that combines fluid restriction, timed or prompted voiding and PFEs. Here, however, PFEs are taught as a technique for suppressing urgency rather than as the primary therapy. Biofeedback is employed via a voiding diary. Anticholinergic medication often is used as a supplement. This form of therapy is referred to as bladder drill in the British literature and usually has been employed to treat urgency and urge incontinence. However, in a recent study sponsored by the National Institute on Aging study these techniques were equally effective in reducing incontinent episodes when applied to patients with SUI as to those with urgency incontinence.

Summary

There are more questions surrounding conservative therapy than there are answers. Few studies directly compare any of these treatments to each other, to pharmacologic therapy, or to surgery. Few studies have enough patients or characterize them well enough to allow conclusions to be drawn regarding which patients are most likely to benefit from the therapy. It does appear that conservative therapy is not likely to cure, and may not significantly improve, patients with severe degrees of incontinence and/or ISD. However, there is clear evidence that conservative therapy reduces the number and severity of incontinent episodes in most patients with AI. The available data suggest that the best candidates are younger, highly motivated patients with low-grade incontinence and without prior surgery. There is a role for these treatments in the therapy of SUI. It is now crucial to develop the criteria to match a patient with the most appropriate therapy. Treatment should be delivered in as simple, inexpensive, and effective a way possible, and in the most expedient fashion.

MEDICAL THERAPY

Alpha Agonists

The primary medical therapy of SUI is based on the premise that the resting tone of the smooth muscle fibers in the bladder neck and urethra can be increased through stimulation of alpha-adrenergic receptors in the area. A variety of alpha agonists are available for the treatment of SUI. All have similar side effects and efficacy. Ephedrine (25 to 50 mg qid), pseudoephedrine (30 to 60 mg qid), and phenylpropanolamine (50 to 75 mg tid) have been used with some success. None of the drugs are specific to the lower urinary tract and all have significant systemic side effects, including anxiety, hypertension, insomnia, cardiac arrythmias, and tremors. Phenylpropanolamine may cause fewer central side effects and is available without a prescription in over-the-counter appetite suppressants. Another commonly used drug is Ornade (a fixed combination of 75 mg of phenylpropanolamine with 12 mg of chlorpheniramine). Because it is prepared in a timed-release formulation it can be given every morning, but it has the disadvantage of the drying, sedating, and constipating side effects of the antihistamine. For mild incontinence, alpha agonists may cure up to 20 to 35 per cent of patients, and response rates as high as 75 per cent have been reported. It is rare that a patient with significant incontinence is both markedly improved and able to tolerate the side effects chronically. Patients who respond to medical therapy must continue the medication indefinitely in order to maintain the improvement.

Estrogen

The idea of estrogen therapy for the treatment of urinary incontinence always has seemed attractive. All forms of incontinence are more common with aging, and estrogen receptors have been demonstrated in the vaginal wall muscles, urethra, bladder, ureters, and pelvic floor musculature. Estrogen replacement therapy is postulated to increase the mucosal seal effect of the urethra and thus facilitate urine storage.

In clinical practice, use of estrogens for SUI has been somewhat disappointing. Urodynamic parameters are little changed and subjective response is rarely dramatic. Three placebo-controlled, double-blinded trials showed no difference between study groups. There is evidence in an animal model that estrogens increase the alpha receptor content of the lower urinary tract and some suggestion in human studies that the effects of estrogens and alpha agonists may be additive. However, any benefits from either estrogens or alpha agonists are contingent on indefinite continuation of therapy. Finally, estrogen therapy must be considered in terms of the patient's overall medical condition. Estrogen may have beneficial effects on the genitourinary system, the skeletal system, and the patient's emotional status and sense of well-being. These benefits must be weighed against an increased risk of endometrial cancer and/or resumption of menses as well as a possible increased risk of other cancers. The risk-benefit ratio tilts in favor of estrogen use when the patient has had a hysterectomy.

Estrogens are beneficial as a preoperative treatment for the patient with atrophic vaginitis. Here, a course of estrogen therapy for several weeks prior to surgery can make the tissues more pliable and improve healing. Topical preparations (vaginal creams) usually are preferred, although equivalent results can be achieved with oral therapy. It seems that treatment of stress incontinence requires higher doses than treatment of atrophic vaginitis; usual daily doses for short-term therapy are one-half an applicator (2 gm) of the vaginal cream or 1.25 mg of Premarin orally. The dose can be doubled if necessary. For long-term therapy, the lowest dose that achieves the desired effect should be employed.

Tricyclic Antidepressants

Tricyclic antidepressants are the final category of drugs used to treat SUI. Because these drugs primarily are used for the treatment of depression, their pharmacologic effect on the urinary tract must be extrapolated from research on the central nervous system. Imipramine is the most commonly used, but the entire family of drugs possesses the following properties: they inhibit the reuptake of norepinephrine at the presynaptic nerve terminal, they are major sedatives (central nervous system action) and they have antihistaminic properties. Imipramine in particular, and related drugs to varying degrees, have significant anticholinergic properties, although they are thought to have weak anticholinergic effects on the bladder. In treating SUI, the principle effect probably is due to alpha stimulation of the bladder neck and urethra. In general, the anticholinergic side effects and sedation prevent the wide use of these drugs for SUI.

SURGICAL THERAPY

The standard for treatment of SUI is surgery. Since the anterior colporrhaphy was popularized by Howard Kelley in 1914, there have been numerous descriptions of new operative procedures and modifications of previous ones. One group of the operations, the bladder neck suspension (BNS) procedures, has as a common goal the repositioning of the sphincter unit in a well-supported retropubic position. Most of the BNS procedures, if done properly, will result in cure of the patient properly diagnosed with AI. It has become clear in recent years that no BNS procedure can reliably cure ISD. This has led to a resurgence in the popularity of various pubovaginal sling procedures. Sling procedures are intended to provide compression and coaptation of the proximal urethra to restore the integrity lost from withdrawal of hormones, trauma, radiation, and other causes. Most of these procedures can cure the patient who had been properly diagnosed with ISD. Finally, there has been a growing interest in periurethral injection of bulking agents to treat all forms of SUI. Currently there is no perfect agent, but intensive efforts are underway to develop an ideal substance and this may be realized within the next few years. These classes of operations are summarized briefly below.

Anterior Repair (Colporrhaphy)

Designed primarily to treat anterior vaginal wall prolapse, this operation consists of dissecting the plane between the bladder and vaginal wall and then closing the hernia by placing mattress sutures that reapproximate the pubocervical fascia in the midline. Although some sutures are placed at the level of the bladder neck and proximal urethra, this procedure cannot, by its very nature, significantly elevate the sphincter unit. Good results are obtained in repair of cystoceles, but cure rates for SUI are only about 60 per cent. At this time there are no satisfactory criteria to select those patients who will be cured.

Bladder Neck Suspension

Retropubic BNS Procedures

Although a plethora of individual variations have been described, most surgeons perform one of two standard operations. In the Marshall-Marchetti-Krantz (MMK) procedure (1949) the space of Retzius is dissected and the periurethral fascia and vaginal wall are secured to the periosteum of the pubis using absorbable sutures. It is safe to say that, in experienced hands, this operation is as likely to cure SUI caused by hypermobility of the sphincter unit (AI) as is any other. SUI should be cured in better than 90 per cent of cases when patients are properly selected. The disadvantages of the MMK procedure include the possibility of producing urethral obstruction by placing the sutures too close to the urethra, inability to correct pelvic prolapse, the risk of osteitis pubis, and the morbidity of an abdominal operation.

When an abdominal approach is indicated for a BNS, the author prefers the suspension introduced by Burch in 1961. Here, absorbable sutures are placed into the fascia at the vaginal fornix lateral to the bladder neck and urethra. This tissue is suspended laterally to Cooper's ligament. When the tissues will not easily reach Cooper's ligament, the obturator fascia may be used as the supporting structure. Some surgeons prefer this modification in all cases, but the obturator fascia is not as reliable a structure as Cooper's ligament. Because the sutures are placed more laterally than in the MMK procedure, obstruction is uncommon. Mild cystoceles can be corrected, although one must be careful not to leave a defect behind the bladder where an enterocele can form. Enterocele rates in excess of 20 per cent have been reported; however, if the surgeon is aware of this potential complication, the pouch of Douglas can be closed at the time of BNS using pursestring sutures. The morbidity of an abdominal operation is a disadvantage.

TRANSVAGINAL (NEEDLE) BNS PROCEDURES

Since the first needle suspension procedure was described by Pereyra in 1959 there have been numerous refinements. Currently, most surgeons use one of two approaches—the Stamey operation (1973) or the Raz procedure (1981 and 1984). Both operations provide support and elevation of the sphincter unit via vaginally placed sutures that then are tied over the anterior abdominal wall fascia. Stamey is credited with introducing the concept of using endoscopy as a guide for suture placement and to evaluate bladder neck elevation and closure. He was also the first to use a synthetic "bolster" to secure the vaginal end of the sutures. Raz introduced the "inverted-U" incision with lateral dissection into the retropubic space. The urethropelvic ligament is identified and dissected, allowing suture placement under direct vision. Based on our current understanding of the anatomy of pelvic support, this is the critical structure for cure of AI. The sutures include bites of the periurethral and pubocervical fascias as well as the vaginal wall without epithelium, thus providing maximal support for the sphincter unit. By entering the retropubic space, the needle can be passed under finger control and injuries to the bladder neck and urethra are rare.

The Stamey operation essentially accomplishes an MMK suspension vaginally. The sphincter unit is supported by medially placed sutures, primarily in the periurethral fascia. Therefore, many of the same problems seen in the MMK procedure are evident in the Stamey. Mid-urethral obstruction can occur from sutures not placed directly at the bladder neck. In addition, because the needle is passed blindly through the retropubic space, there is a higher likelihood of injury to the urethra and bladder neck as well as perforation of the urethral envelope. This can lead to fibrosis and ISD or severe irritative symptoms. Pelvic prolapse is not corrected. The immediate morbidity is considerably less than with a retropubic BNS, and the cure of SUI is approximately the same. The sutures in a Raz procedure are placed laterally, in a position analogous to that in a Burch procedure. Because the sutures are placed under direct vision, optimal anatomic results should be achieved in almost every case. Although the Raz procedure involves more dissection and thus somewhat more immediate postoperative morbidity than the Stamey, it offers several important advantages. The operation is easily modified to treat all degrees of anterior vaginal wall prolapse, including Grade 4 cystoceles. It is applicable to redo procedures in which urethrolysis must be performed to free the urethra from local scar tissue. Obstruction and urethral or bladder neck injury are rare. The immediate perioperative morbidity is still considerably less than with any of the retropubic procedures.

SUMMARY

A variety of operations have been devised to treat SUI. An experienced surgeon can achieve excellent results using any of the above BNS procedures for properly selected patients with AI. A cure rate of 90+ per cent should be expected. Many of the failures in older series are due to undiagnosed ISD. At best, suspension procedures will cure ISD in 60 per cent of cases. Long-term results of BNS operations are less well documented. Some authors have argued that the cure rate of BNS procedures is only 50 per cent at 5 years; others believe that delayed failure is rare. More data are needed before a satisfactory answer to this question can be given.

Although the excellent success rates establish surgery as the gold standard for treatment of SUI, there are several disadvantages. Mortality is rare with any of the suspension procedures, but all the risks of surgery and anesthesia are present. The typical hospitalization is 1 to 3 days for vaginal procedures and 3 to 5 days for retropubic operations. It takes 3 weeks for a patient to recover fully from a vaginal operation, and longer for a retropubic procedure. Thus, the expense of surgical therapy, measured both in direct costs and in time away from work, is a major consideration given the magnitude of the clinical problem. Another problem common to all BNS procedures is the de novo development of detrusor instability. Although coexistent urge incontinence or idiopathic bladder instability usually will resolve when SUI is treated with a BNS, some patients with little or no urgency inexplicably develop instability postoperatively. In most cases this will resolve within 3 to 6 months and the patient can be supported through this period with anticholinergics and behavioral therapy. In about 8 to 10 per cent of patients there will be persistent instability beyond 6 months. These patients should be carefully evaluated with urodynamics to rule out obstruction, and in severe cases urethrolysis should be considered even in the absence of definite evidence of obstruction.

Pubovaginal Sling Procedures

The first sling procedures were developed at the turn of the century, but it was not until the 1940s that the operation was popularized by Aldridge and others for treating all types of SUI. However, the operations never gained the wide popularity of BNS procedures because of a higher incidence of complications, primarily urinary retention, and detrusor instability. There has been a renewed interest in the sling procedures beginning with McGuires' report in 1978 and gaining momentum as ISD has become recognized as a subtype of SUI that responds poorly to BNS procedures. The pendulum continues to swing in the direction of more sling procedures, with some authors recommending a sling as primary therapy for SUI, even for patients with AI.

The standard sling is composed of a strip of fascia placed underneath the urethra with each end secured to the anterior abdominal wall fascia. The fascial strip usually is harvested from the anterior abdominal wall when making a Pfanensteil incision; however, fascia lata, dura mater, and synthetic materials (Dacron, Mersilene) have been used. With synthetic materials the risk of erosion, infection, and fistula formation is substantial. Although the entire operation originally was done from a retropubic approach, the dissection of the plane between the urethra and vagina can be quite difficult from above. Today, most surgeons use a vaginal approach to dissect the plane between the urethra and vaginal wall and then pass the fascial strip using a long clamp without dissecting the retropubic space.

It is now clear that it is not necessary to use such a long strip of fascia. A shorter segment may be extended with permanent sutures. Good results can be obtained using a 3 × 5-cm "postage stamp" of fascia with a suture in each corner. The four sutures are passed into a suprapubic stab incision using a double-pronged needle just as in a BNS. This allows for a very small suprapubic incision, minimizing morbidity. When any shorter length of fascia is used, it is critical to suture the fascial strip to the periurethral fascia so that it will not slip to one side when the sutures are passed into the abdominal incision. The latest sling modification by Raz (1989 and 1990) employs an in situ flap of vaginal wall as the sling material. The periurethral fascia and urethropelvic ligaments are used to create an elastic compression of the urethra. The entire operation is done vaginally. Early results are equivalent to those with any of the other published operations.

Nearly all authors agree that the sling should not be tied under significant tension, regardless of the technique employed in construction. In fact, some have advised simply positioning the sling under the urethra and leaving it under no tension whatsoever. Although this is probably important to prevent erosion when synthetic materials is used, it seems likely that at least some patients will fail this type of operation who might be cured if the sling is secured to provide a modest degree of compression.

Any of the sling procedures should cure SUI in 90 to 95 per cent of cases. The overall rate of urinary retention ranges from 5 to 20 per cent; however many of the patients with permanent retention have underlying neurologic problems or chronic obstruction or have had a prior bladder augmentation. Nonetheless, there is clearly a higher rate of retention requiring intermittent catheterization with a sling procedure than with a BNS. Similarly, the rate of detrusor instability after a sling is about 15 per cent, perhaps double the rate after a BNS. For these reasons, careful consideration should be given before using slings in patients with AI.

Periurethral Injections

The concept of injecting bulking agents periurethrally to treat SUI was popularized by several reports from Politano and associates during the 1970s and 1980s. Teflon paste was the initial agent used. It seems logical that a permanent substance injected into the correct area of the bladder neck and urethra could promote coaptation and compression of the urethral mucosa and thus restore continence. As might be expected, these and subsequent studies have shown that periurethral injections work best in patients with ISD. Just as the procedure seemed to be gaining momentum in the United States, Malizia and associates discovered the migration of the Teflon particles to distant sites, including brain and lung, in an animal model. This complication has never been reported in human subjects, despite many years of use in ear, nose, and throat (ENT) procedures. However, the possibility of migration, together with scattered reports of local inflammatory problems including sterile abscesses and sinus tract drainage, and the difficult medicolegal climate, has dampened enthusiasm for using Teflon to treat SUI.

Attention now is focused on glutaraldehyde cross-linked bovine collagen (GAX collagen). The material is much easier to inject and has not been shown to migrate, and cross-linking has reduced allergic reactions to a minimum. However, some resorption of the material does occur and long-term results are not well documented. This is apparently the reason the material has not been approved for general use by the Food and Drug Administration (FDA). Teflon is available (approved for ENT applications) but is not approved for use in the urinary tract.

Studies are underway examining the use of autologous fat, bioglass, silica particles, and other synthetics. It is likely that some type of injectable material eventually will fill an important niche in the treatment of female SUI. The ideal material will be an easy-to-inject paste; be completely biocompatible, causing no inflammatory response; be neither degraded nor phagocytized; and be inexpensive. Until such a material is developed or GAX collagen becomes available, Teflon should be used only with careful informed consent and with the patient's understanding that it is not FDA approved. Even so, there are frail, elderly patients with severe incontinence for whom a Teflon injection might be the preferred therapy. Most investigators agree that the ideal candidate for injections has ISD with little or no hypermobility. In these patients, cure rates of 75 to 90 per cent can be expected, although multiple injections may be required. Although injectables have been used in other types of patients, the results, even in the short term, do not approach the results of BNS and sling procedures.

The key to the procedure is in injecting the material directly below healthy unscarred urethral mucosa. When this is accomplished there is a dramatic elevation and coaptation of the mucosa after only a few cubic centimeters have been used. When the mucosa is very scarred (as in a patient with incontinence after a radical prostatectomy), it is much more difficult to affect proper coaptation. Urinary retention can be expected in the patient with a poorly contractile, neurogenic bladder; however the overall incidence of retention and instability appear to be less than with sling procedures. In females, the injection is easily performed under local anesthesia with or without mild sedation.

Artificial Sphincter

Although excellent results have been reported in selected female patients with SUI, the risks of infection and erosion are much more significant in the female patient than in the male. If erosion occurs, reconstruction may be difficult and urinary diversion required. It is a mechanical device and as such has a definite failure rate over time. Long-term ischemic atrophy of the urethra also can lead to failure and recurrent incontinence. The artificial sphincter offers an advantage to the surgical options outlined above only for the patient with the combination of ISD and a noncontractile bladder. These patients generally remain on self-intermittent catheterization after a sling procedure but might be able to void adequately by Valsalva and crede with a sphincter. Even in this unusual situation, the operation should be undertaken with some trepidation and only after a full explanation of the possible complications.

SELECTION OF THERAPY FOR AN INDIVIDUAL PATIENT

In May 1992, the U. S. Department of Health and Human Services published Clinical Practice Guidelines for the treatment of urinary incontinence in adults. The guidelines state that, "surgery, except in very specific cases, should be considered only after behavioral and pharmacologic interventions have been tried." This is a broad statement encompassing all types of incontinence. The standard treatment for SUI, whether caused by AI or ISD, is surgery. Despite this fact, the rationale behind the guidelines is still appropriate. Stress incontinence is not a life-threatening or inevitably progressive disease; a failure with one form of therapy does not preclude use of another form. For this reason it has been argued that the least invasive form of therapy always should be tried first. Many patients will be satisfied with therapy that improves, but does not cure their incontinence.

The patient's wishes always must be considered in treatment selection.

A flow chart encompassing many of the individual patient factors to be considered in treatment planning is presented in Figure 1. The first step in the decision-making process is to document the presence of SUI and to classify properly the cause as AI or ISD. Although some will argue that all patients with SUI should be offered a trial of conservative therapy before surgery, there are no good data to suggest that any nonsurgical therapy will make a significant impact on ISD. Therefore, it is reasonable to offer a sling (or peri-

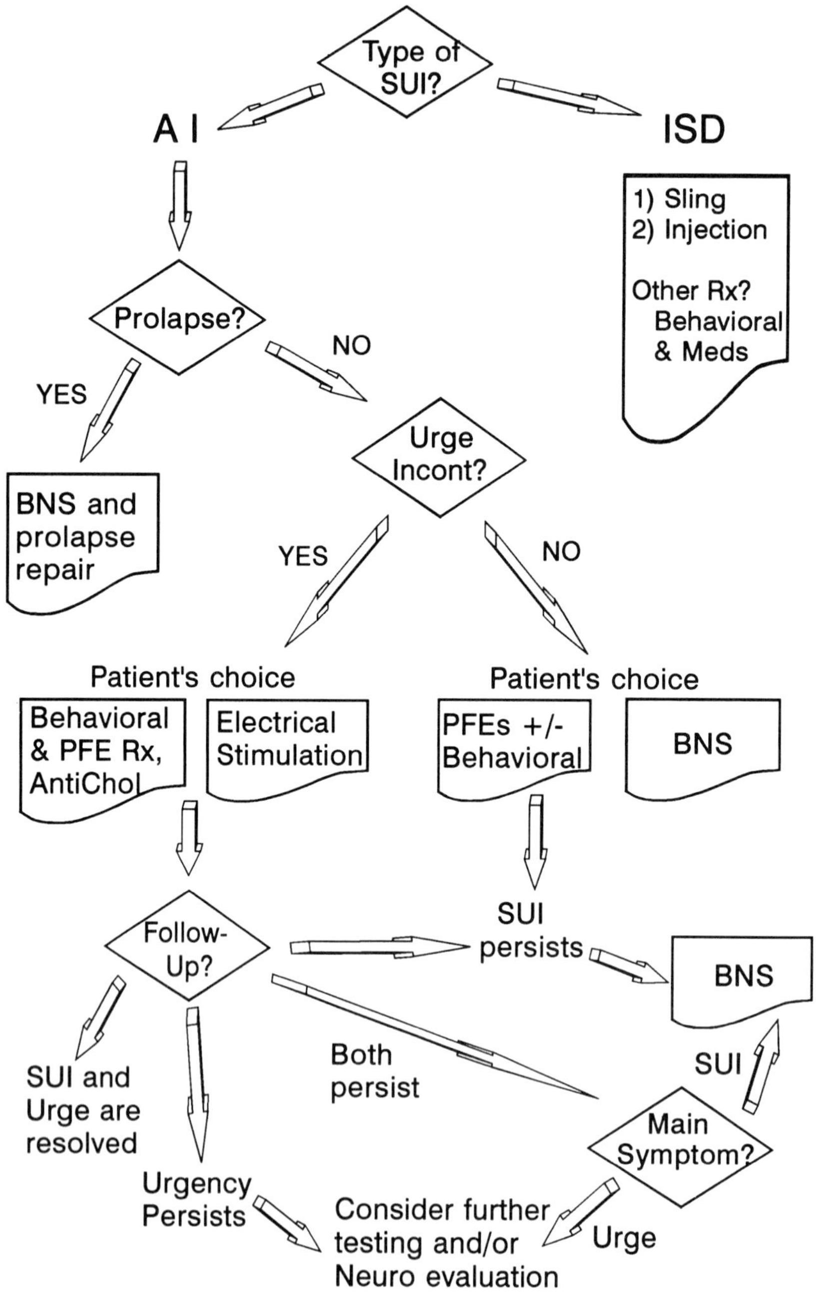

FIGURE 1. An algorithm for the treatment of stress incontinence in females. Decision and evaluation points are marked by diamonds; options therapeutic are marked by the document symbol. Any such algorithm must allow for considerable individualization of therapy based on the combination of subjective symptoms, objective findings, and personal goals that is unique to a particular patient. See text for full discussion.

urethral injection therapy in some cases) as first-line therapy to patients with ISD who are in reasonable and medical condition. Conservative therapy with a combination of estrogens, alpha agonists, and behavior modification is clearly second best. Some of these patients may be best served by an indwelling catheter.

Moving on to the larger group of patients with AI, the next decision point is evaluation of vaginal prolapse. Patients with symptomatic vaginal prolapse and AI can reasonably be offered surgery to repair both conditions as initial therapy providing they are in satisfactory overall health. Neither conservative therapy nor medication will relieve high-grade prolapse. Included in this category are patients with moderate to severe cystoceles associated with residual urine, recurrent cystitis, and irritative voiding symptoms, as well as patients with any other type of prolapse causing significant local symptoms. These patients ideally are treated with a transvaginal BNS and simultaneous repair of the prolapse, although a combined retropubic and vaginal procedure, usually done by a urologist-gynecologist team, is another acceptable approach. For those patients who prefer conservative therapy or are not candidates for surgery, PFEs can be combined with a pessary to relieve the prolapse. When the prolapse is due to cystocele, however, a pessary will often aggravate SUI.

Patients with AI in the absence of symptomatic prolapse next are evaluated for coexistent urge incontinence. It should be noted that, regardless of the findings on a cystometrogram, when a patient gives a clear history of urgency and urge incontinence she is presumed to have detrusor instability. If urge incontinence is present, the two nonsurgical options presented in Figure 1 may be offered, and other combinations of treatment are possible. These patients should be given a fair trial of nonsurgical therapy before a BNS is performed. It is possible that electrical stimulation will find an important niche in this group of patients. The final category of patients have AI, no significant prolapse, and no urge incontinence. Conservative therapy should be presented as an option to all of these patients. Pelvic floor rehabilitation undoubtedly can make an impact on the quality of life of these patients by reducing the frequency and severity of incontinence. It also is reasonable to discuss surgery as initial therapy. Factors that favor surgical therapy are young and vigorously active patients, moderate degree of incontinence, completion of childbearing, and a strong desire to be totally dry. Factors that favor nonsurgical therapy include sedentary life-style, significant medical problems, mild incontinence, and plans for further childbearing. No treatment other than BNS has been demonstrated to be superior to PFEs, and most patients in this group will have a significant improvement in urinary control with a 6- to 12-week trial of PFEs. Whether or not the patient is satisfied with the treatment depends largely on the individual factors listed above.

This represents only one of several reasonable approaches for managing female SUI. Stress incontinence is not one disease and there is no one best treatment. Therapeutic success and patient satisfaction can be achieved by any algorithm that is based on individual patient characteristics and a thorough knowledge of the treatment alternatives. Despite considerable recent publicity, most lay people and many health professionals remain unaware of the wide variety of treatments available for the incontinent population. Almost all patients with incontinence can achieve significant improvement, and in most cases SUI is a curable condition. It is our charge to educate and inform our colleagues and the public about the many tools at our disposal.

Suggested Readings

Fischer-Rasmussen W: Treatment of stress urinary incontinence. Ann Med 22:455, 1990

Jeter JF: Pelvic muscle exercises with and without biofeedback for the treatment of urinary incontinence. Probl Urol 5:72, 1991

Raz S: Atlas of Transvaginal Surgery. Philadelphia, WB Saunders, 1992

Urinary Incontinence Guideline Panel: Urinary Incontinence In Adults: Clinical Practice Guideline. AHCPR publ no 92-0038. Rockville, MD, Agency for Health Care Policy and Research, Public Health Service, U.S. Department of Health and Human Services, 1992

Wein AJ: Voiding function and dysfunction. *In* Gillenwater JY, Grayhack JT, Howards SS, et al (eds): Adult and Pediatric Urology, 2nd ed. St. Louis, Mosby Year Book, 1991, pp 933–1100

FEMALE INCONTINENCE AND THE ARTIFICIAL URINARY SPHINCTER

IRVING J. FISHMAN, M.D.

Houston, Texas

Urinary incontinence is believed to affect between 10 and 15 million Americans. In most patients, this potentially debilitating problem can be addressed with either pharmacotherapy, bladder retraining, or conservative surgical approaches such as cystourethropexies, sling procedures, or injection therapy. In patients who have failed conservative management, the artificial urinary sphincter (AUS) prosthesis has become a reasonable alternative.

In 1973, Dr. F. Brantley Scott developed and implanted the first AUS. Since then, over 2550 incontinent patients worldwide have benefited from this device. The AS 800 model was implanted in 1799 of these patients. The majority of these women suffered from urethral sphincter incompetence of varying etiologies, including myelomeningoceles, pelvic floor weakness with stress incontinence, and neurogenic bladders. In all of them, more conservative attempts at restoring urinary continence had failed.

Two hundred thirty-nine females have undergone implantation of the AUS by the author and associates since 1973. Of these, 108 received the AUS 791/792 model and 68 received the AS 800 device. Among the latter, patient ages ranged from 5 to 84 years. Table 1 lists the various etiologies of urinary incontinence in these 68 patients.

THE AUS DEVICE

The basic objective of the AUS is to allow patients to have dynamic control of the outflow from their bladders, as opposed to simply obstructing the outflow, as with a sling procedure. The AUS components are made of medical-grade silicon elastomer, and the cuff has a Dacron-reinforced backing with a snap-like closure. In the initial devices, the pressure in the cuff was generated by the patient squeezing the inflate pump, which transferred fluid from the abdominal reservoir into the cuff. One of four unidirectional valves (V4 valve) built into the system then determined the actual pressure in the cuff. This device proved to be unreliable and prone to repeated failures (721 cases). The introduction of a pressure-controlling balloon and resistor systems to control rate of cuff refill was a major step forward (models 742, 761, and 791/792). As a result of the experience that was gleaned by the implanting surgeons and improvements in biomaterials and engineering, the design, quality, and reliability of the device improved greatly over the years. The latest device is the American Medical System (AMS) AS 800 (Fig. 1), which consists of an occlusive cuff of variable length, a pump with a locking mechanism, and a dip-coated pressure control balloon that reliably delivers the preset pressures. The surgeon has the option of deciding what pressure is most appropriate for the individual patient. The new cuff has a narrower backing (1.7 cm) and an additional coating of silicon on the inside to improve the occlusive efficiency (to offset pressure tissue atrophy) and to decrease the wear at the fold sites of the cuff. With these improvements, the

TABLE 1. Etiologies of Incontinence

ETIOLOGY	NUMBER OF PATIENTS
Myelomeningocele	18 (26%)
Pelvic fracture	2 (2%)
Spinal cord injury	1 (1%)
Stress incontinence	14 (20%)
Neurogenic bladder	7 (10%)
Exstrophy-epispadias	3 (4%)
Posturethroplasties	8 (11%)
Sacral dysgenesis	2 (2%)
Other	13 (19%)

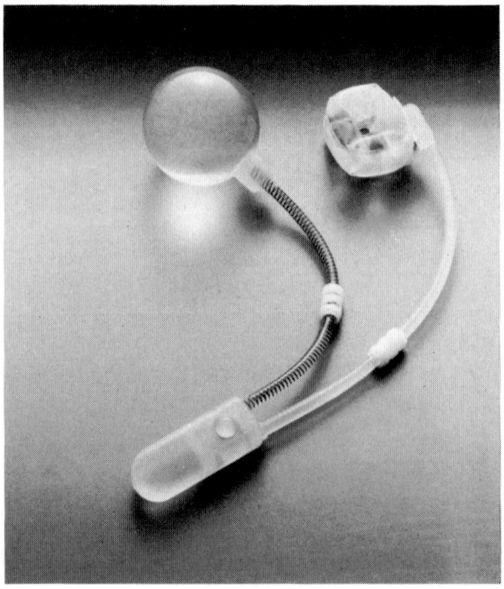

FIGURE 1. American Medical System AS 800. (Courtesy of American Medical Systems, Inc., Houston, Texas.)

reliability of the device has improved tremendously.

PATIENT CANDIDATES

Females with urinary incontinence of multiple etiologies are potential candidates for the AUS implant. Among these are girls with neurogenic bladders resulting from myelomeningoceles, sacral agenesis, spinal trauma, or peripheral neuropathies and women with stress incontinence that has not responded to more conservative measures. The most typical patient is a woman who has adequate bladder compliance and capacity but whose bladder neck and urethral sphincter are nonocclusive, as in type III stress incontinence.

Potential candidates for the AUS are evaluated with extensive urodynamic testing, which includes simultaneous pressure-flow and electromyographic studies, voiding cystourethrography, and cystoscopy. The bladder compliance and associated capacity should be adequate to make the patient socially continent with the AUS implanted. In some women with small bladder capacity or poor compliance despite anticholinergic medication, implantation of the AUS has resulted in increased bladder capacity. However, if there is persistent elevated intravesical pressure with small bladder capacity, augmentation cystoplasty is a very beneficial option. Patients with evidence of outflow obstruction resulting from detrusor sphincter dyssynergia or anatomic obstruction are either managed with a bladder flap urethroplasty at the time of AUS implantation or treated with intermittent self-catheterization postoperatively.

In addition, a careful evaluation of the patient's past surgical or pelvic trauma is essential to ascertain the amount of scarring that may be present, especially in the area of the urethrovaginal septum. The patient is apprised of the risk of the surgery and the possibility of device failure at any time subsequent to the surgery. Patients must be highly motivated to have the surgery, and they must have the manual dexterity as well as the mental competence and initiative to operate the device. Young girls who refuse to pump the device in order to urinate may cause significant deterioration of their renal function.

IMPLANTATION TECHNIQUES

Proper positioning of the sphincter cuff is the most challenging part of the operation. The plane between the bladder neck and the vagina is not very distinct, even in females who have not previously had surgery in that area. Patients who have undergone multiple conventional anti-incontinence procedures and young girls who have had bladder neck reconstruction offer the surgeon very few anatomic landmarks with which to work. Two basic approaches have been advocated for implantation of the cuff. The original approach, as described by Scott, was retropubic. More recently, a transvaginal perineal approach has been used in combination with a suprapubic inguinal incision for placement of the other components.

In the retropubic approach, the patient is placed in a lithotomy position with the thighs parallel to the abdomen in order to maximize room for the surgeon and the assistants. In addition, this makes feasible an intraoperative cystoscopy to assess urethral patency. A 10-minute surgical scrub of both the abdomen and the vagina is performed.

The retropubic space is entered via a Cherney incision that transects both rectus muscles and optimizes pelvic exposure. The pelvic fascia is incised on either side of the bladder neck. The latter is usually well defined with the help of an intravesical Foley catheter balloon, but if there is any doubt about the anatomy because of extensive local scarring, the bladder should be opened from above to facilitate visualization of the bladder neck and the ureteral orifices. Bilateral blunt and careful sharp dissection with angled scissors with simultaneous transvaginal palpation allow one to develop a space through the proximal urethrovaginal septum. An instrument that was developed specifically to expedite this portion of the operation is the Cutter clamp (Lone Star Medical Products, Houston, TX), which consists of two hollow, detachable arms that fit together at the level of a clamp proximally and at the distal curved ends. The latter are configured into male and female tips that fit together (Fig. 2).

Once the endopelvic fascia is incised and the bladder neck is identified, the Cutter clamp is positioned in the area of the proposed cuff site. The arms are tightened in the clamp, and cystoscopy as well as vaginal examination allows the surgeon to rule out excess tissue entrapment of either the bladder or the vagina. Appropriate adjustments then can be made. Once its is determined that the correct plane has been chosen, the cutting blade is advanced from the male clamp into the hollow of the female end, thereby cutting through the urethrovaginal plane. The female arm is then unclamped and removed to expose the cutting blade. A 1-0 polypropylene suture is advanced through a hole in the blade and the latter then is gently removed, pulling the attached suture through this newly created space. A right-angle clamp then is attached to the suture and is guided gently along the new track. The space is carefully stretched to approximately 2 cm to accommodate the cuff.

The required cuff length is determined by measuring the loose circumference around the bladder neck. (The length of the BN cuff ranges from 7 to 10 cm.) The cuff then is positioned into this space and snapped closed. Care must be exercised to avoid twisting of the cuff in the course of positioning it around the bladder neck. The pressure-regulating balloon then is implanted in a paravesical space, assuring that there is no contact between it and the cuff. Rubbing of two silicon components can ultimately lead to thinning of the silicon and leakage. The balloon and cuff tubings are brought through the abdominal muscles and fascia in order to help fix them in place. The deactivation pump is advanced into a space created in one of the labia majora with the help of an extended nasal speculum. The latter minimizes local trauma. After the balloon is filled with an appropriate amount of saline or contrast plus water solution, the redundant tubing is amputated and Quick connectors are used to connect the appropriate tubes. The wounds are checked for hemostasis, irrigated with copious amounts of antibiotic solution, and closed securely in multiple layers. Drains are avoided to minimize the risk of infection. The cuff is left deactivated for approximately 4 to 6 weeks. If, in the course of the cuff placement, the urethra or bladder was entered, the longer deactivation period may better allow for adequate healing.

Recently, Appell has popularized the transvaginal placement of the cuff around the bladder neck using a technique similar to that described by McGuire for the sling procedure. The theoretical advantage of this approach is simplification of the positioning of the cuff around the bladder neck under direct vision. The main concern, however, is that of increasing the risk of infection by the transvaginal approach. Surprisingly, infection has not been a major problem. In a series of 34 women with type III stress urinary incontinence, no infections, erosions, or bladder instabilities were noted. Nineteen of these women had been followed for at least 3 years. Four were emptying their bladders with intermittent self-catheterization.

RESULTS

The 239 patients in our series were followed for as long as 9 years. A total of 12 patients required revisions—3 because of mechanical failures and 9 because of surgical problems. Five devices (7 per cent) were lost because of infections. Ten devices (14 per cent) were total failures because of infection and erosion of the cuff. Of the remaining patients, 86 per cent continue to be socially continent.

Sexual activity is not compromised by the presence of an AUS, and seven of the patients ultimately delivered nine healthy children. The mode of delivery was left to the discretion of the obstetrician, but four were vaginal deliveries without any adverse effects on the mother or baby.

In summary, women suffering from total

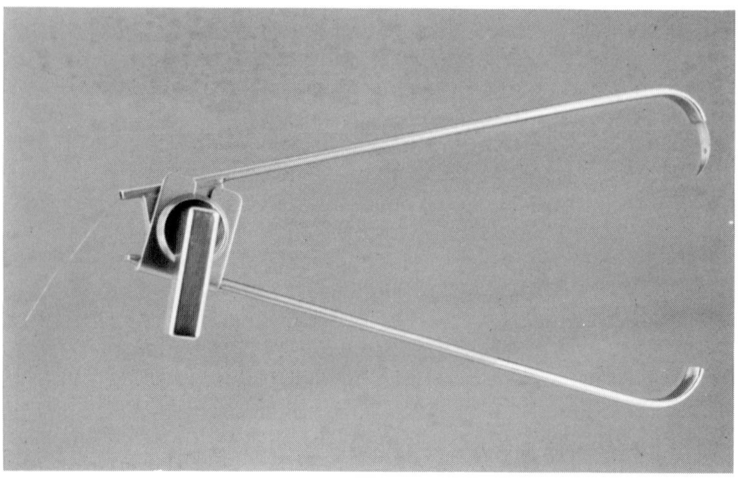

FIGURE 2. Cutter clamp with blade exposed.

urinary incontinence, unresponsive to conventional therapy, can regain continence via implantation of the AMS AS 800 and still go on to lead normal productive lives. As urologists, it behooves us to be familiar with this therapeutic option.

Suggested Readings

Appell RA: Techniques and results in the implantation of the artificial urinary sphincter in women with type III stress urinary incontinence by a vaginal approach. Neurourol Urodynam 7:613–619, 1988

Donovan MG, Barrett DM, Furlow WL: Use of the artificial urinary sphincter in the management of severe incontinence in females. Surg Gynecol Obstet, 161:17–20, 1985

Light JK, Scott FB: Management of urinary incontinence in women with the artificial urinary sphincter. J Urol 134:476–478, 1985

Raz S, McGuire EJ, Ehrlich RM, et al: Fascial sling to correct male neurogenic sphincter incompetence: The McGuire/Raz approach. J Urol 139:528, 1988

Scott FB: The use of the artificial sphincter in the treatment of urinary incontinence in the female patient. Urol Clin North Am 12:305, 1985

ENDOSCOPIC INJECTION OF TEFLON, FAT, AND COLLAGEN FOR FEMALE URINARY INCONTINENCE

RODNEY A. APPELL, M.D., F.A.C.S.

Cleveland, Ohio

Urethral sphincteric incontinence implies that the resistance to urinary outflow has been lowered to the point that it does not adequately protect the patient from urinary loss. The treatment of female urinary incontinence caused by the incompetent urethra has been a challenging problem. Treatment frequently involves surgical augmentation of intraurethral pressures. Another technique to treat this type of incontinence is by the injection of bulk-enhancing agents into the periurethral tissues. This bulk compresses the urethral lumen and increases the resistance to the outflow of urine.

Attempts to treat urinary incontinence by the use of injectables have been considered for decades; the technique was first described by Murless in 1938 and since has been investigated by others using a variety of materials. Most investigators have concluded that the basic approach is effective, but they have been daunted by problems with the bulking agents themselves. One example is an agent known as Polytef (Urethrin), an extremely thick paste that is a sterile mixture of polytetrafluoroethylene (PTFE) micropolymer particles, glycerin, and polysorbate (which is identical in its chemical makeup to Teflon) that has been studied for two decades by researchers at the University of Miami, where it showed considerable promise. However, there have been reports of mild reactions to injection of the material, and of greater concern has been the demonstration that injected particles may migrate to other organ systems, setting up granulomatous reactions. Even though no adverse sequelae have been documented, concerns have thwarted clinical acceptance of the material and stimulated the search for safer and easier-to-handle substances.

Glutaraldehyde cross-linked collagen (GAX-collagen or Contigen) has completed a multicenter efficacy and safety study. This biocompatible and biodegradable substance is a sterile, nonpyogenic purified bovine dermal collagen that is cross-linked with glutaraldehyde and dispersed in phosphate-buffered physiologic saline. As a substance for injection into humans, this has the additional positive attribute of not eliciting a foreign body reaction. Although a minimal inflammatory response results from this noncytotoxic material, there has been no evidence of particle migration. The fact that Contigen is biodegradable is both its strength and its weakness. There is no concern regarding migration and granuloma formation because Contigen begins to degrade in 12 weeks and is completely degraded in 9 to 19 months, but there is a concern over the durability of the substance and the subsequent need for repeated injections over time to sustain its efficacy. This has led to attempts to use autologous substances such as fat and blood and synthetic substances such as silicone microspheres. However, early reports with fat and blood have demonstrated very short periods of efficacy and studies with injected silicone microspheres have ceased in the United States because of the overriding concern for safety in using silicone in the human.

PATIENT SELECTION

A good candidate for the procedure is the female with low urethral closure pressure in the most proximal portion of the urethra. Decreased urethral resistance may be due to a problem with anatomic support (genuine stress urinary incontinence or urethral hypermobility) or to a deficit in the intrinsic urethral closure mechanism (so-called type III stress urinary incontinence). In the latter, the proximal urethra no longer functions as a sphincter. The bladder neck and proximal urethra are open at rest in the absence of a detrusor contraction, which may be determined radiographically and/or urodynamically. If the proximal portion of the urethra fails to close, the patient is a suitable candidate. Conversely, a good closure of the urethra at rest suggests the patient would benefit from a standard resuspension procedure.

SURGICAL TECHNIQUE

Materials may be injected transurethrally or periurethrally. The possible complications of bleeding and extrusion of the injectable substance are eliminated by using a periurethral rather than a transurethral approach. Local anesthesia can be used, with the added advantage of having the patient stand and perform a few provocative maneuvers in an attempt to cause urinary leakage. When both the patient and the physician are satisfied, the procedure is officially terminated. Some substances, such as Teflon, expand after injection and may result in urinary retention, whereas other substances, such as Contigen, lose some of their bulk as a result of resorption of water and local anesthetic, thus requiring more than one session to render the patient continent.

EFFICACY AND SAFETY OF INJECTABLES FOR FEMALE INCONTINENCE

Of the alternative treatments available for patients with urinary incontinence related to outlet incompetence, periurethral injections must be compared with slings and the artificial sphincter. Sling surgery is successful in 81 to 98 percent of patients and artificial sphincter surgery is successful in more than 90 per cent of patients regardless of whether the abdominal or transvaginal approach is used. Injection with PTFE is successful in 70 to 95 per cent of women and injection with GAX-collagen is successful in 64 to 95 per cent. Because the results are comparable and therapy with injectables is less invasive than the open surgical procedures of slings and artificial sphincters, the question of why injectables have not been universally accepted and approved arises. The answer involves two objectionable aspects: (1) the inability to quantify the amount of material needed in any given women and (2) the safety of the injected substance.

With respect to the quantity of material needed, studies with PTFE have demonstrated that the ability to render continence in a single treatment varies between 50 and 63 per cent, and that with GAX-collagen is 55 per cent. As stated, PFTE expands after injection, resulting in retention of urine in some patients, whereas GAX-collagen bulk is reduced by water resorption, explaining the likely need for repeated injections to gain full continence with this substance. However, once continence has been attained with GAX-collagen, 80 per cent of patients will remain continent for at least 2 years.

The safety issue, especially with regard to migration of particles and foreign body granuloma formation with PTFE and immunogenicity with GAX-collagen, has delayed approval of injectables for incontinence. With GAX-collagen, the cross-linking with gluaraldehyde not only enhances durability of the substance but also reduces the potential to produce local immune-type reactions. None of the patients in the multicenter trials (many of whom have been followed for greater than 5 years) has had an adverse event related to immunogenicity.

CONCLUSION

The goal of treatment in women with an intrinsic urethral deficiency as the etiology of their incontinence is to compress the proximal aspect of the urethra, allowing for coaptation of the mucosa without obstruction, meaning that the pressure necessary to open the urethra (leak point pressure) is increased while there is no significant change in the closure pressure of the urethra. Periurethral injections have the potential to accomplish this compression. The etiology of the defect, tissue condition at the injection site, and plane of placement of the injectable affect the degree of correction. The best results are in those patients who do not have detrusor problems, have an adequate bladder capacity, and have minimal anatomic abnormality (urethral hypermobility). Because therapy with injectables is less invasive than open surgery, a significant number of these patients will benefit when injectables are an approved modality of treatment, especially elderly patients with other significant medical problems that make them unsuitable surgical candidates.

Suggested Readings

Appell RA: Commentary: Periurethral polytetrafluorethylene (Polytef) injection. *In* Whitehead ED (ed): Current Operative Urology 1990. Philadelphia, JB Lippincott, 1990, pp 63–66

Appell RA: Injectables for urethral incompetence. World J Urol 8:208–211, 1990

Appell RA: Periurethral injections. *In* Hurt WG (ed): Urogynecologic Surgery. Gaithersburg, MD, Aspen Publishers, 1992, pp 139–145

Politano VA: Periurethral Teflon injection for urinary incontinence. Urol Clin North Am 5:415–422, 1978

TREATMENT OF URINARY INCONTINENCE IN THE MALE

J. KEITH LIGHT, M.D.

Syracuse, New York

Urinary incontinence is a common and often devastating condition that has severe psychosocial and physiologic repercussions. An estimated 1 to 2 per cent of males between 15 and 64 years of age have some degree of incontinence, yet only 5 per cent of them seek medical advice. The incidence of incontinence among elderly men is even greater; 17 per cent of noninstitutionalized men over 65 years of age and a staggering 55 per cent of male nursing home patients are incontinent.

With proper physician evaluation and counseling, the vast majority of incontinent men can be treated successfully. Physician awareness of the proper sequence of evaluation and treatment is important.

CAUSES OF INCONTINENCE

Urinary incontinence occurs whenever intravesical pressure exceeds outlet resistance. The problem therefore may involve the bladder, the sphincter mechanism, or both.

Bladder

Problems of the bladder resulting in urinary incontinence usually involve abnormalities in detrusor contractility. Abnormalities in detrusor contractility that result in urinary incontinence most often are secondary to uncontrolled contractions (i.e., detrusor instability, which is defined as an involuntary rise in intravesical pressure during filling). These involuntary contractions may be symptomatic or asymptomatic and often are associated with urinary leakage. When a neurologic cause for detrusor instability is obvious, the term "hyperreflexia" is preferred. Detrusor instability becomes progressively more common as the male ages, reaching an estimated incidence of approximately 70 per cent in males over 70 years of age. The development of detrusor instability currently is thought to be independent of the presence of bladder outflow obstruction. Typical symptoms of detrusor instability include frequency, nocturia, urgency, and urge incontinence, whereas the symptoms of outflow obstruction are decreased force of stream, hesitancy, and intermittency. The two conditions of detrusor instability and outflow obstruction may coexist.

Neurologic lesions resulting in detrusor hyperreflexia include multiple sclerosis, stroke, and impaired cognitive function. Frequently, however, no cause can be found, and the term "idiopathic" is used. The increase in intravesical pressure from uncontrolled contractions is often sufficient to overcome sphincter resistance, because of either associated reflex relaxation or actual weakness. Urinary incontinence results. Detrusor hypocontractility has been stated to be the most common cause of incontinence in elderly patients. This hypocontractility may be associated with detrusor instability or outflow obstruction. The end result frequently is impaired urination, resulting in varying degrees of postvoid residuals. These two abnormalities, impaired contractility and elevated postvoid residuals, may predispose to urinary incontinence, especially if associated instability is present. Because the symptoms associated with detrusor hypocontractility are identical to those of bladder outflow obstruction, the former condition frequently is underdiagnosed unless urodynamic testing is performed.

Sphincter

Sphincter function, both the proximal and distal components, may be compromised secondary to congenital or acquired causes. Causes of congenital sphincter insufficiency include urethral malformations and neurologic disorders resulting in sphincter denervation (e.g., meningomyelocele). Causes of acquired insufficiency include traumatic injury to the posterior urethra, prostatic cancer, infrasacral neurologic abnormalities, irradiation, and postsurgical changes. Sphincter insufficiency in men occurs most often as a result of prostatectomy. Although fewer than 1 per cent of patients become incontinent following transurethral resection of the prostate, the incidence of varying degrees of sphincter insufficiency after radical prostatectomy has been reported to be as high as 87 per cent. The number of these patients requiring surgical intervention, however, is estimated at approximately 3 per cent.

DIAGNOSIS OF INCONTINENCE

The primary goal in evaluating male urinary incontinence is to determine accurately the cause of the problem. This necessitates a thorough history and physical examination. Special attention is required in dealing with elderly and debilitated patients. Urodynamic evaluation can be extremely helpful and must be tailored to the individual patient. Useful information can be obtained with simple determinations of flow rate and postvoid residual urine, together with the voiding volume chart. A normal flow rate tends to exclude significant outflow obstruction. A voided volume chart often provides information regarding the severity of the symptoms and may suggest underlying detrusor instability as the cause for the urinary incontinence. Cystometry frequently will reveal the presence of detrusor instability, whereas pressure-flow studies are necessary to confirm the presence of detrusor hypocontractility as opposed to outflow obstruction as the cause of increased postvoid residuals.

TREATMENT

Treatment of male urinary incontinence must address the specific cause.

Bladder

OVERACTIVITY

Pharmacologic therapy is the mainstay in controlling detrusor instability. Agents used to inhibit detrusor contractility include anticholinergics and antispasmodics (e.g., propantheline, oxybutynin chloride). In general, these agents act by increasing the volume to the first involuntary contraction and decreasing the force of this contraction, thus increasing the functional bladder capacity and improving control. Caution is required when these agents are used in the presence of severe outflow obstruction because urinary retention may occur. For patients who remain incontinent despite pharmacologic manipulation, particularly those with neuropathic bladder dysfunction, augmentation cystoplasty may be required.

UNDERACTIVITY

Clean intermittent catheterization is now the mainstay in achieving bladder drainage where failure of emptying occurs because of detrusor hypocontractility or areflexia, because there is no reliable pharmacologic agent to achieve this.

Sphincter Insufficiency

The smooth muscle component of both the proximal and distal sphincter contain an abundance of alpha receptors, stimulation of which results in muscle contraction with an increase in outlet resistance. Alpha-1-adrenergic agonists, such as terazosin and prazosin, may be tried with minor degrees of urinary incontinence secondary to sphincter insufficiency. Severe insufficiency, however, such as occurs following prostatectomy, usually requires more aggressive treatment. Options include injection of foreign substances such as Teflon or collagen, reconstruction of the bladder neck, or implantation of an artificial urinary sphincter. Teflon and collagen currently are awaiting Food and Drug Administration approval for general release.

The most commonly utilized and successful surgical option is currently the AS800 artificial urinary sphincter. Mechanical reliability of the device has improved significantly following various manufacturing changes, including nonkinkable tubing, surface treatment of the cuff, a narrow back design, and the ability to deactivate the device utilizing the poppet valve located in the pump. Complications associated with the surgery include a 2 per cent incidence of device infection, a less than 1 per cent incidence of urethral erosion, and pressure atrophy of the tissue beneath the cuff. The cuff always is placed around the bulbar urethra because of previous surgical intervention at the bladder neck area. An overall continence rate of 90.5 per cent is achieved. A certain degree of stress urinary incontinence may occur, however, requiring the use of one or two small pads per day. With few exceptions, however, patients are satisfied with the postoperative result and enjoy normal activities.

Suggested Readings

Hu T: The economic impact of urinary incontinence. Clin Geriatr Med 2:673–687, 1986

Marks JL, Light JK: Male urinary incontinence—what to do? Postgrad Med 83:121–127, 1988

Marks JL, Light JK: Management of urinary incontinence after prostatectomy with the artificial urinary sphincter. J Urol 142:302–304, 1989

MYELOMENINGOCELE

ISRAEL FRANCO, M.D.

Valhalla, New York

Management of the patient with bladder dysfunction resulting from myelodysplasia in the newborn period has changed significantly over the years. Management in the older child and in the adult tends to be geared more toward a symptomatic approach. Ideally, aggressive treatment of the newborn patient could help prevent the deleterious effects of increased intravesical pressure on the upper and lower urinary tract, which in turn would make the management of the older patient easier.

EVALUATION

All patients with myelodysplasic disease should have a basic evaluation when first seen. This should include a complete history and physical examination. The history should contain a detailed outline of the bowel and voiding pattern. For children on clean intermittent catheterization, this requires information regarding frequency of catheterization and the length of dry intervals between catheterizations. A history of urinary tract infections, particularly infections associated with a febrile episode, is also essential. A past surgical history is important to help elucidate whether there may be postsurgical tethering of the cord. In the newborn patient with myelodysplasia, it is important to know if the child has a ventriculoperitoneal shunt or if there are any Chiari malformations.

The physical examination should include a detailed exam of the abdomen, genitalia, and lower extremities. Lower extremity reflexes should be recorded, as well as the bulbocavernosus reflex and perianal sensation and reflexes. In some children, abnormalities of their sacral nerve roots are all that may be present. The examination should include mild abdominal and suprapubic pressure to determine if any urine leakage occurs. The degree of pressure required gives the examiner an idea of the status of the outlet resistance mechanisms. One should look for evidence of fasciculations of the lower extremity muscles. This hyperactivity of the muscles can be an early indicator of tethering of the spinal cord.

The next step in the evaluation of the myelodysplastic patient is to evaluate the urinary tract radiologically and urodynamically. Ultrasound evaluation of the upper and lower urinary tract is the mainstay of the management of the myelodysplastic patient. In the newborn myelodysplastic patient, the evaluation should be done immediately at birth and prior to surgical closure of the back. Follow-up ultrasounds should be performed 1 to 6 weeks after back closure, 3 months later, and then at least every 6 months in the first 2 to 3 years of life. A renal *and bladder* ultrasound should be done on each occasion during the follow-up. Subtle ultrasonographic changes of the upper urinary tracts are harbingers of impending lower tract dysfunction. These minor changes must be investigated further with voiding cystourethrography and with urodynamic studies. Increasing intravesical pressure and vesicoureteric reflux are important signs of deterioration. A baseline voiding cystourethrogram is mandatory in all children and should be repeated as indicated by changes on the ultrasound. Some authors prefer nuclear cystograms for follow-up. Our preference is to use contrast for the voiding cystourethrogram because, in this patient population, anatomic detail of the bladder is important in gauging progressive bladder dysfunction.

Urodynamic evaluation should be performed prior to closure of the back and then subsequently 3 to 6 months after closure. The majority of myelodysplastic patients will have bladder and sphincter dysfunction in one form or another. The findings on cystometry may include uninhibited bladder contractions or areflexia, although a normal detrusor sometimes is seen. Electromyography of the external urinary sphincter may reveal complete or partial denervation, hyper-reflexia, or normal activity of the sphincter. Any combination of detrusor and sphincter function is possible. The most dangerous sphincter and bladder signs are the hyperactive sphincter with a hyper-reflexive bladder. This combination can lead to rapid deterioration of the upper urinary tracts as well as to progressive destruction of the bladder. The unrecognized hyper-reflexive bladder with a denervated sphincter can deteriorate quite rapidly post-surgically after sphincter placement or after a sling procedure. The patient's bladder can change rapidly from a smooth, high-capacity reservoir to a trabeculated, low-capacity, high-pressure reservoir.

The introduction of the term "leak point pressure" (pressure at which urine leaks around a catheter during water cystometry) represents a landmark in the management of the myelodysplastic patient. The recognition that the leak point pressure should be kept below 40 cm of water pressure has changed the approach to these patients. Studies have shown clearly that elevated leak point pressures above 40 cm of water pressure will lead to deterioration of the upper urinary tracts, whereas pressures that are below 40 cm usually will not damage the upper urinary tracts unless vesicoureteral reflux and urinary tract infections supervene. The leak point pressure should be used as a guide in determining what form of treatment therapy is to be prescribed for the myelodysplastic patient.

MANAGEMENT

The management of the older patient with myelodysplasia tends to be problem-directed, except in the newborn. In the case of the newborn, management should be based on a prophylactic philosophy. Continence is not important early on in life, it is the maintenance of low intravesical pressures that is paramount. The neonate with a low leak point pressure does not require intervention. It is when the leak point pressure is elevated that one needs to tailor management toward lowering the pressure. In all patients, three factors generally dictate management; urinary tract infections, upper tract deterioration, and incontinence.

An important aspect of the management of these patients is to define the patient's needs as well as those of the caregivers. Older patients who have been incontinent of urine and stool and who are not overly concerned about their appearance generally lack sufficient motivation to achieve total stool and urinary continence. In these cases, imposing rigid clean intermittent catheterization requirements may not be feasible. In contrast, the needs of the parents and caregivers may be just as important in determining the mode of management in the individual patient. Those patients who are unable to be catheterized as frequently as is required to maintain low intravesical pressures in the presence of a normal urinary sphincter or a hyperactive one are not good candidates for intermittent catheterization. Diversion or bladder autoaugmentation is a better alternative in these children. In some cases, patients who have been rendered completely continent of urine have gone on to renal failure following neglect on their part or by their caregivers in providing adequate decompression of the reservoirs.

Clean Intermittent Catheterization

The introduction of clean intermittent catheterization by Lapides has had a dramatic impact on the management of the patient with myelodysplastic disease. Reduction or elimination of residual urine is the key to elimination of recurrent urinary tract infections in patients with myelodysplasia. Intermittent catheterization is indicated in the child with high intravesical pressures with high leak point pressures, and in patients with incomplete emptying or urinary retention. Clean intermittent catheterization can also be utilized in any patient in an attempt to achieve urinary continence. It usually is used in combination with antispasmodics and/or α-adrenergic stimulators.

Pharmacologic Therapy

The use of anticholinergic agents in the myelodysplastic patient is an integral part of the therapy for these patients. Reduction of intravesical pressure can be achieved with the use of oxybutynin (Ditroypan) 5 mg tid, propantheline (Pro-Banthīne) 7.5 to 15 mg qid, or hycosamine (Levsin). Recent reports in the literature on the use of intravesical instillation of oxybutynin have shown it to be quite effective in children who cannot tolerate oral anticholinergics because of side effects (dry mouth, facial flushing, dizziness, tachycardia, and hallucinations).

Valium has a limited role in the patient with myelodysplasia and, if required, the patient should be considered for untethering of the spinal cord or for a rhizotomy.

α-Adrenergic agents such as ephedrine and phenylpropanolamine are also quite useful in the management of the myelodysplastic patient. The α-adrenergics tend to have their greatest effects at the level of the bladder neck, and this leads to increased outlet resistance. These agents lend themselves best to the patient with partial denervation of the external urinary sphincter. They rarely are effective in the patient with complete denervation of the sphincter. Imipramine's mode of action is a combination of α-like activity and anticholinergic-like activity at the level of the sphincter and detrusor respectively. It can be used in conjunction with either anticholinergics or α-adrenergics.

Electrical Stimulation of the Bladder

Stimulation of the bladder detrusor transurethrally has been used with some success by Kaplan in Chicago as well as by other investigators in different locations throughout the country. The technique has resulted in significant increases in bladder capacity as well as in the ability of the patients to sense bladder fullness. It has produced a limited number of patients who have been able to void spontaneously after these treatments. Other benefits include improved bowel function in the myelodysplastic patient. Clearly, this mode of therapy is not a replacement for direct stimulation of the sacral nerve roots. Direct stimulation of the dorsal nerve roots presently is being evaluated in several centers in the United States. The best results appear to be in patients with spinal cord injuries although successes have been reported in patients with myelodysplastic disease as well. The long-term results of this form of stimulation are as yet unavailable.

Spinal Cord Injury

Tethering of the spinal cord commonly is seen in patients with myelodysplastic disease. The question is, in which patient is it clinically significant? The deleterious effects of tethering generally occur about the time that major growth spurts occur. This is usually between 2 and 5 years of age and in adolescence. Subtle changes in the bladder can and should be picked up by routine monitoring. Once the diagnosis of tethering has been made, the cord should be surgically untethered. In some instances, selective dorsal rhizotomies can be performed at the time of untethering. Our results with this procedure have been quite encouraging. We have seen dramatic changes in bladder capacity in the young child, with total elimination of uninhibited bladder contractions in all patients.

Urinary Diversion

The most commonly used form of diversion in the newborn myelodysplastic patient is the vesicostomy. The procedure should be reserved for the patient in whom clean intermittent catheterization is not a viable alternative as well as for those patients in whom the upper tracts are severely hydronephrotic and who require prolonged urinary diversion. The use of bowel segments for urinary diversion should be confined to those cases in which no other reasonable alternative is available for preservation of the upper tracts. Urinary diversion as the treatment of choice has been replaced almost entirely by clean intermittent catheterization with or without bladder autoaugmentation or bladder augmentation with bowel patches.

The introduction of clean intermittent catheterization has made bladder augmentation possible in the treatment of the myelodysplastic patient. The small hyper-reflexive bladder now can be converted into a capacious low-pressure reservoir with the use of a detubularized patch of either ileum or colon or with a stomach patch. Augmentation alone or in combination with an incontinence procedure has improved the lives of many myelomeningocele patients. The Mitrofanoff procedure, which provides a catheterizable abdominal stoma, has further improved our approach to the myelodysplastic patient. The wheelchair-bound patient or obese patient now can be catheterized easily through an abdominal stoma while using less bowel than with other comparable continent diversions. As with any treatment method that is seen as a panacea, there is always a downside. Recent reports indicate that bladder augmentations are more prone to calculi formation, more so than had been reported in the prior literature. Also, smaller stature in children augmented early on in life has been attributed to the inherent metabolic acidosis associated with bowel segments placed within the urinary tract. There also have been reports of spontaneous rupture of the augmented bladder as well as catheter-induced injuries.

Autoaugmentation involves removal of large segments of the bladder muscle and is another means of reducing intravesical pressure. This procedure should be limited to the patient who has a good bladder capacity but who has high intravesical pressures. This procedure can lend itself ideally to a laparoscopic approach.

Prosthesis Surgery

The use of the artificial urinary sphincter has seen its zenith. Like any mechanical device, it is prone to malfunction and infection in the long term. When it works well, it is capable of rendering the patient who is incontinent of urine dry for extended periods of time. The use of this device is limited to the older patient and to those who have adequate dexterity to manipulate the pump mechanism. Most of the recent literature has leaned toward the use of fascial slings in both males and females to increase outlet resistance, rather than, toward the artificial urinary sphincter.

The use of Teflon or collagen injections at the level of the bladder neck can be a valuable adjunct in the management of urinary incontinence. The key factors in selecting patients for this operation are low intravesical pressure associated with a high-capacity reservoir bladder. The utility of these agents has been mired in controversy and bureaucracy. They generally have a limited role in the management of the myelodysplastic patient, but at times can be all that is needed to render the patient dry.

CONCLUSION

The patient with myelodysplasia requires early and close monitoring of the urinary tract by ultrasound and urodynamics. The goal is to preserve the native bladder and maintain it as a high-capacity, high-compliance reservoir that empties completely. Achievement of this goal by the use of any combination of the aforementioned modalities is clearly in the best interests of the patient, thereby obviating the need for bladder augmentation with its inherent problems. Bladder preservation and reduction of the potential for urinary tract infections clearly protects the upper urinary tract from hydronephrosis and from pyelonephritic scarring. A wide array of procedures now are available for rendering the patient continent, provided that he or she is a candidate for clean intermittent catheterization. Continued vigilance is the essence of management in the patient with a myelomeningocele.

Suggested Readings

Bauer S, Hallett N, Koshbin S, et al: Predictive value of urodynamic evaluation in newborns with myelodysplasia. JAMA 252:650, 1984

Ducket J, Snyder HM: Continent urinary diversion and variations on the Mitrofanoff principle. J Urol 136: 1158–1162, 1986

Franco I, Storrs B, Firlit CF, et al: Selective sacral rhizotomy in patients with high pressure neurogenic bladders: Early results. J Urol 148:648–650, 1992

Kaplan W, McLone D, Richards I: Urologic manifestations of tethered cord. J Urol 140:1285–1288, 1988

McGuire EJ, Woodside JR, Borden TA, et al: The prognostic value of urodynamic testing in myelodysplastic patients. J Urol 126:205, 1981

CLEAN INTERMITTENT CATHETERIZATION IN CHILDREN AND ADULTS

ANANIAS C. DIOKNO, M.D.

Royal Oak, Michigan

Clean intermittent catheterization (CIC) is now accepted worldwide. Review of the literature during the last 10 years will attest to the popularity of CIC among urologists as well as other specialists dealing with bladder emptying problems. Reports emanating not only from North America but also from Europe, Scandinavia, South America, and Asia attest to the safety and effectiveness of this form of treatment. This treatment modality, introduced by Lapides in 1972, has revolutionized our methods of treating neurogenic and non-neurogenic bladder dysfunction and allowed us to develop other methods of treatment, such as continent diversion, because of the availability of CIC. Although the exact mechanism of the effectiveness and safety of CIC has not been completely elucidated, it is safe to say that prevention of bladder overdistention and high bladder pressures and frequent, regular, complete bladder emptying are essential keys to a successful program. Lapides theorized that bladder resistance is reduced by bladder ischemia resulting from bladder overdistention and high pressures on the bladder wall. Hinman and Cox postulated that bacterial multiplication and bladder invasion is prevented if the bladder is emptied completely with frequent regularity.

INDICATIONS

CIC should be considered in all patients who are unable to empty the urinary bladder completely or partially. Urinary retention may be a manifestation of neurogenic and sphincter dysfunction secondary to spinal cord injury, multiple sclerosis, myelodysplasia, spinal cord tumor, peripheral neuropathy, and other neurologic disorders. It also may be observed following certain surgical procedures, such as vaginal or suprapubic bladder neck suspension, anterior colporrhaphy, hysterectomy, hemorrhoidectomy, laminectomy, abdominoperineal resection, and other pelvic and abdominal operations. Urinary retention also may occur on a psychogenic basis, or it may be the presentation of men with an obstructing prostate gland, patients with a hypotonic or underactive detrusor, or in women postpartum.

Other candidates for CIC include patients with continent intestinal pouches. Another indication is the prevention of urethral strictures following internal urethrotomy, to maintain the patency of the urethral canal during the healing process. Similarly, CIC is now used for prophylaxis among myelodysplastic infants with detrusor-sphincter dyssynergia (DSD) to prevent deterioration of the upper tracts that will be observed in a high proportion of these children if allowed to void reflexly or drain by crede maneuver.

Many patients in urinary retention will present with inability to urinate or difficulty emptying the bladder with or without urinary incontinence. Patients may present with an indwelling urethral or suprapubic tube. Attempts should be made to determine if these patients are candidates and, if so, they should be switched to CIC.

CONTRAINDICATIONS

Intermittent catheterization is contraindicated in patients with restricted hand function as well as patients with severe mental incompetency unless there is a significant other who cares for the patient and will be available to do the intermittent catheterization regularly and frequently all the time. Patients with a small contracted bladder who are unresponsive to bladder relaxants or unable to have augmentation cystoplasty should not be considered for CIC. It is not recommended for men with urethral strictures or false passages unless these are corrected prior to institution of CIC. Using a significant other to perform the task should be considered thoughtfully, because it may create a situation of total dependence. The quality of the relationship should be evaluated thoroughly prior to instituting the program. Age alone is not a contraindication to this technique.

CIC can be used in patients with genitourinary prostheses. CIC is appropriate for patients with an artificial sphincter, although catheterization appears safer if the cuff is located in the bladder neck rather than the bulbous urethra. In patients with a penile prosthesis, the inflatable prothesis appears to be safer than the semi-rigid, although safety has been shown for either type. CIC also is reported to be safe for patients with renal transplants.

PRETREATMENT EVALUATION

Evaluation of prospective candidates for the CIC program is mandatory. Initial success is based on the status of the urethra and bladder as well as patient compliance. Urethral strictures and false passages should be identified by cystourethroscopy or retrograde urethrography and treated prior to initiation of CIC. The baseline assessment of the upper tracts should be accomplished using either excretory urography, renal scan, or ultrasonography. A voiding cystourethrogram should be performed to detect the presence of vesicoureteral reflux. In patients with neurologic dysfunction, assessment of the bladder and sphincter function is important to determine the bladder capacity, the intravesical pressure at capacity, and the presence or absence of detrusor hyperreflexia and DSD.

Urinary incontinence in patients on the CIC program usually is due to detrusor hyperreflexia, urethral sphincter insufficiency, or overflow from a distended bladder. The involuntary detrusor contractions can be controlled in most cases with anticholinergic-antispasmodic agents (Table 1). The most commonly used agent is oxybutynin at a dose of 5 mg orally tid. In intractable cases, the dose can be increased to 10 mg orally three or even four times a day. Children and adults can tolerate this preparation without significant side effects. However, in the elderly, caution should be used; the usual initial dose in the elderly is 2.5 mg orally twice to three times per day. The dose can be increased if incontinence persists and the patient is able to tolerate the low dose. Urethral sphincteric insufficiency may be combated with the use of an alpha-adrenergic agent Phenylpropanolamine at a dose of 50 to 75 mg orally twice a day. In intractable cases, bladder neck suspension or urethral sphincter augmentation procedures, such as sling procedures or artificial sphincter implantation, may be necessary in conjunction with self-catheterization to effect complete continence.

For those patients with chronic urethral or suprapubic indwelling catheters who are to be switched to CIC, every effort should be made to identify and remove all pre-existing calculi inside the bladder. Otherwise these calculi will continue to grow, forming a nidus for infection and trauma to the bladder wall.

When the patient is dependent on a significant other, compliance is improved by instructing everyone involved not only in the technique but on the rationale for frequent, regular catheterization and the need for long-term surveillance. All of the alternative treatments should be thoroughly explained to the family, so that they will be well informed and confident about their choice of therapy.

TABLE 1. Drugs Used To Promote Urine Storage

INHIBIT DETRUSOR CONTRACTILITY
Anticholinergics
Propantheline bromide (Pro-Banthīne)*
Methantheline bromide (Banthīne)
Dicyclomine hydrochloride (Bentyl)
Belladonna alkaloids (atropine)
Hyoscyamine (Cystospaz)
Glycopyrrolate (Robinul)
Anisotropine methylbromide (Valpin)
Emepronium bromide (Cetiprin)
Ganglionic blockers
Direct Smooth-Muscle Relaxants
Oxybutynin chloride (Ditropan)*
Flavoxate hydrochloride (Urispas)
Imipramine (Tofranil)*
Beta-Adrenergic
Terbutaline (Bricanyl)
Prostaglandin Inhibitors
Indomethacin (Indocin)
Aspirin
Spinal Cord Reflex Inhibitors
Baclofen (Lioresal)
Hydramitrazine (Lisidoril)
Calcium Antagonists
Flunarizine
Nifepidine
INCREASE OUTLET RESISTANCE
Alpha-Adrenergics
Phenylpropanolamine hydrochloride (Propadrine)*
Imipramine (Tofranil)*
Ephedrine sulfate
Pseudoephedrine (Sudafed, Actifed)
Beta Blocker
Propranolol

Courtesy of Dr. William Brock.
* Drugs of choice in children.

CIC INSTRUCTION

The specific details of the instructions have been presented elsewhere and will not be repeated. However, several important points are worth mentioning. The instructor should be well grounded in the basic principles of the technique and have had considerable experience. Teachers are often nurses, enterostomal therapists, physicians, physician assistants, and physical therapists. Of importance is the instructor's degree of enthusiasm for the program. A strong endorsement by the caregiver increases the chance for success by increasing the patient's enthusiasm to learn and be successful.

It is important to introduce the patient and the family to the technique prior to the actual teaching. An illustrated handout, a slide presentation, or a teaching videotape is useful if reviewed before the teaching session.

The catheter of choice for adults and older children is the 14F plastic catheter. For younger patients, especially male infants, an 8F or 10F plastic feeding tube usually is adequate. For older men with previous prostatic resection, a coudé-tip catheter may be preferrable to the straight-tip catheter. In general, a plastic catheter is preferred to a rubber or latex catheter, because plastic catheters are slightly stiffer and their transparent walls make it possible for the patient to see the urine. The plastic catheter is also easier to clean and lasts longer, usually 3 to 6 months. The catheter can be carried dry in a plastic bag, compact, paper towel, or any convenient container. No sterilizing solution is used, and lubricant is provided only for males. For the sake of cleanliness and prevention of malodor, the patient, when possible, washes his or her hands and then rinses the inside and outside of the catheter with clear water. The patient must be warned not to forego catheterization when soap and water are not available, but to catheterize at the prescribed time regardless of circumstances.

For ambulatory patients, catheterization can be accomplished in the standing, sitting, or squatting position, draining the urine directly into the toilet bowl. For the wheelchair-bound patient, disposal is accomplished by using either a catheter extension, which can be used to drain the urine directly into the toilet bowl, or a clear plastic liquid-detergent container with a hanger attached to the wheelchair as a temporary receptacle.

In general, catheterization should be done every 4 hours during the waking hours and once at night, although the frequency will be determined by the volume of residual urine. The goal for an adult patient is to drain no more than 400 ml with each catheterization. For children, the guidelines are 150 ml for 1- to 5-year-olds, 250 ml for 6- to 9-year-olds, and 300 ml for children 9 years and older.

It is important to place the patient on an antimicrobial agent at least a day prior to teaching intermittent catheterization. It is also the author's practice to keep the patient on an antimicrobial preparation for at least 2 to 3 weeks following the initiation of the program. Long-term prophylaxis will depend on the subsequent clinical course of the patient. Generally, asymptomatic bacteriuria is not treated unless the patient is undergoing a bladder or urethral operation or is to undergo procedures that require sterile urine (e.g., hip replacement). Patients having recurrent symptomatic urinary tract infections should be investigated thoroughly to determine the reason for such recurrent infections. Most commonly, the reason is bladder overdistention resulting either from infrequent catheterization, extreme overhydration, or a small-capacity, noncompliant bladder. Efforts to prevent infection should be directed to reduce recurrent high intravesical pressure with the use of bladder relaxants, frequent catheteriyzation, augmenting the bladder, and similar techniques. Any attempt to prevent recurrent infections with the use of antibacterials will be effective only while the patient is on antibacterial therapy. In the long term, the patient will develop resistant strains and more symptomatic infections that will be increasingly difficult to treat. Again, the philosophy is to eradicate the abnormal physiology (high bladder pressure) rather than chasing the bacterial contaminant.

Patients with vesicoureteric reflux are at high risk for acute upper tract infection. These patients deserve a prophylactic antimicrobial preparation unless the reflux disappears or is corrected surgically. Low-grade reflux usually subsides while the patient is on an intermittent catheterization program, whereas high-grade reflux usually persists. If persistent high-grade reflux is associated with recurrent infections or worsening of the upper tracts, reimplantation should be advised.

Recently a nonreusable prelubricated catheter was introduced in Europe and appears to be gaining popularity in that part of the world. At present, it appears that it is an excellent alternative for males with increased sensitivity along the urethra during catheterization. The prelubricated catheter reduces the friction and enhances the ease of catheterization. Fortunately, discomfort and difficulty with male catheterization has not been a significant problem. The advantage of the nonreusable prelubricated catheter is overshadowed by the significant cost of the single-use catheter.

Teaching of CIC may be hampered by poor hand function, as in the case of severe arthritis of the hand or among quadriplegic patients. Fortunately, innovative therapists have introduced mechanical devices for use by quadriplegics who otherwise would be excluded because of poor hand function. Occasionally, hand motion can be improved with arthroplasty procedures.

When access to the urethra is difficult or impossible, intermittent catheterization can be performed by creating a continent stoma in the abdomen, using either the bladder, the ileum, or even the appendix. For those with small-capacity, noncompliant bladders who are able and willing to catheterize intermittently, the bladder can be enlarged by an augmentation enterocystoplasty procedure, utilizing the cecum, the ileum, or even the stomach. This procedure can be done in conjunction with the creation of an abdominal neourethra, with or without closure of the urethra or bladder neck. A problem with the use of a bowel segment is the overproduction of mucus by the intestinal mucosa, and periodic irrigation may be required.

POTENTIAL COMPLICATIONS

Bacteriuria and Urinary Sepsis

One of the hardest concepts to accept in the CIC program is that clean, unsterile self-catheterization is safe and actually reduces rather than causes urinary tract infection. This misconception stems from medical and nursing school teachings that automatically equate bacteriuria with urinary tract infection. There is now mounting evidence that asymptomatic bacteriuria alone is of limited significance in a patient on CIC. Although prophylactic antimicrobial therapy has been shown to reduce the incidence of bacteriuria in patients on CIC, there is no convincing evidence that long-term prophylaxis reduces the incidence of symptomatic infection or urinary sepsis. Our present practice is not to attempt to eradicate the bacteria in patients on CIC unless the patient is to undergo instrumentation or other procedures that require temporarily sterile urine.

The significance of pyuria in patients using a CIC program has not been studied to any great extent. Menon and Tan reported in 1992 a comparison between the pyuria count of patients with an indwelling Foley catheter and patients who are voiding and on intermittent catheterization. They reported a significantly lower pyuria count and a lower incidence of urinary tract infection among the group who were not constantly catheterized. They also concluded that a low pyuria level of less than 30 white blood cells per high-power field was associated with a nil or low incidence of bacteriuria and urinary tract infection.

Kass and associates reported a 56 per cent incidence of bacteriuria in 255 myelodysplastic children treated with CIC. Febrile urinary tract infection was observed only in 3 per cent of 190 children without vesicoureteric reflux, whereas it was observed in 37 per cent of 65 children with reflux. Among the refluxers, the highest incidence was observed in those with high-grade reflux.

Genital infection associated with CIC has been reported. One report showed that 4 of 50 men developed acute epididymitis. All responded well to antibiotic therapy. In most patients who developed genital infection, it was preceded by previous indwelling urethral catheterization.

Urethral Trauma

Long-term follow-up has shown that patients with normal and impaired urethral sensation can successfully catheterize at frequent intervals for many years with little risk of harming the urethra. Lapides and associates reported a 2 per cent incidence in 100 patients, and Maynard et al. reported 1 case in 63 patients. All trauma was minor and reversible.

On occasion, difficulty may be encountered by a male patient in passing the catheter at the region of the posterior urethra as a result of external sphincter spasm or a tight bladder neck. In these cases, the use of a coudé-tip catheter may be necessary.

Renal Deterioration

The two major factors that predispose to renal deterioration are pre-existing vesicoureteric reflux and high intravesical pressures resulting from uncontrolled, uninhibited bladder contractions, bladder overdistention from infrequent catheterization, or the presence of a small noncompliant bladder.

Hilwa and Perlmutter reported no deterioration in their patients using CIC and actually observed improvement in 7 of 10 patients with pre-existing hydronephrosis. Maynard and Diokno reported that none of 28 spinal cord patients followed for 3.7 years developed hydronephrosis, hydroureter, or radiographic evidence of pyelonephritis. In the author's series of 60 patients placed on an intermittent catheterization program 10 years earlier, no deterioration of the renal function or architecture was noted. Barnett and associates reported their experience using a CIC program rather than urinary diversion in eight patients with neurogenic bladder and requiring renal transplantation. They concluded that CIC is a reasonable alternative to urinary diversion in these groups of patients requiring renal transplant.

A newer concept in the use of intermittent catheterization is the prophylactic program in preventing renal deterioration in myelodysplastic infants who are identified as having DSD with preserved upper tracts. Kasabian, Bauer, et al., in 1992, reported that newborns with high bladder pressure and DSD treated with oxybutynin and CIC attained preservation of the normal upper tracts in 92 per cent of the cases followed for 5 years, whereas infants treated expectantly had changes in their upper tracts in 48 per cent of the population followed. The authors concluded that expectant therapy can no longer be advocated for these high-risk infants because the prophylactic therapy of oxybutynin and CIC is so effective.

Urolithiasis

Bladder calculi have been reported to occur in adult and pediatric patients while on CIC. Solomon and associates reported four male patients on intermittent catheterization who developed bladder calculi with a pubic hair nidus. It is believed that the pubic hair was inadvertently introduced into the bladder during catheter insertion.

Maynard and Diokno reported nephrolithiasis in 3 of 63 spinal cord patients on a CIC program. All stones were small and were passed spontaneously. Hypercalciuria and immobilization were suspected to be the major factors in the development of these upper tract calculi.

Urinary Incontinence

The use of a CIC program for the express purpose of alleviating urinary incontinence is effective for patients with urinary incontinence secondary to overflow urinary incontinence and in patients with DSD. The overflow urinary incontinence may be due to a neurogenic areflexic bladder or to a non-neurogenic atonic bladder secondary to obstruction or bladder overdistention. For those with DSD, use of bladder relaxants in conjunction with CIC is of utmost importance to prevent the overactive bladder from contracting and pushing the urine past the spastic urethral sphincter.

Diokno et al. reported achieving an 88 per cent continence rate among 43 myelodysplastic patients treated with CLC with and without the use of a pharmacologic adjunct. De la Hunt and associates reported 84 per cent dryness or minor stress incontinence among 86 children treated with CIC.

SUMMARY

A clean intermittent catheterization program is a well-accepted method of treating patients with bladder emptying dysfunction. It can be used as either a temporary or a permanent method of bladder emptying and can be used by the patient, family members, hospital or nursing home staff, or other day care–type caregivers. It can be used to relieve urinary retention, prevent upper tract deterioration, reverse upper tract deterioration, control urinary incontinence, and prevent recurrent urethral strictures. It has been established to be safe and effective. Complications are few, and most are preventable or manageable.

Suggested Readings

Diokno AC, Sonda LP, Hollander J, et al: Fate of patients started on clean intermittent self-catheterization therapy ten years ago. J Urol 129:1120–1122, 1983

Hinman F, Cox C: The voiding vesical defense mechanism: The mathematical effect of residual urine, voiding interval and volume on bacteriuria. J Urol 91:491–498, 1966

Kasabian NG, Bauer SB, Dyro FM, et al: The prophylactic value of clean intermittent catheterization and anticholinergic medication in newborns and infants with myelodysplasia at risk of developing urinary tract deterioration. Am J Dis Child 146:840–843, 1992

Kass EJ, Koff SA, Diokno AC, et al: The significance of persistent bacilluria in children on long term intermittent catheterization. J Urol 126:223–225, 1981

Lapides J, Diokno AC, Silber SJ, et al: Clean intermittent self-catheterization in the treatment of urinary tract disease. J Urol 107:458–461, 1972

Wyndaele JJ, Maes D: Clean intermittent self-catheterization: A 12-year followup. J Urol 143:906–908, 1990

DIABETES, MULTIPLE SCLEROSIS, AND PARKINSON'S DISEASE

JERRY G. BLAIVAS, M.D.

New York, New York

Lower urinary tract symptoms in patients afflicted with neurologic diseases usually are attributed to the underlying condition, yet this is not necessarily the case. Urologic disorders such as cystitis, bladder and prostate cancer, and benign prostatic hypertrophy are probably as common in these patients as in the general population and require the same kind of diagnostic evaluation. Once urologic conditions are excluded, the diagnosis and treatment of neurogenic bladder is accomplished best when there is a clear understanding of the underlying pathophysiology. This, in turn, requires knowledge about the neurophysiology of micturition and the effect of specific neurologic lesions on normal physiology.

NEUROPHYSIOLOGY OF MICTURITION

Normal voiding is accomplished by activation of the micturition reflex. This is a coordinated event characterized by relaxation of the striated urethral sphincter, contraction of the detrusor, opening of the vesical neck and urethra, and onset of urine flow. The micturition reflex is integrated in the pontine micturition center, which is located in the rostral brain stem. Interruption of the neural pathways connecting the pontine micturition center to the sacral micturition center usually results in detrusor–external sphincter dyssynergia. Detrusor–external sphincter dyssynergia commonly is seen in patients with multiple sclerosis, but is never due to Parkinson's disease or diabetes mellitus. Patients with untreated detrusor–external sphincter dyssynergia are at high risk for developing urologic complications such as vesicoureteral reflux, hydronephrosis, urolithiasis, and urosepsis.

Neurologic lesions above the pons leave the micturition reflex intact. When micturition is affected, it usually is characterized by loss of voluntary control. This usually is manifest as detrusor hyperreflexia, but loss of awareness of bladder events or concern about the consequences of incontinence are also common. Although these patients are usually incontinent, they are at little risk for developing urologic complications unless they are treated with an indwelling vesical catheter, or have other urologic abnormalities.

Neurologic lesions that interfere with the sacral reflex arcs, although uncommon, are seen most often in patients with diabetic cystopathy, which is discussed in detail below.

TREATMENT OVERVIEW

Although the ultimate goal of therapy is the restoration of normal voiding, this usually is not possible unless the neurologic condition is cured or remits, or if the symptoms are caused by a coincidental urologic condition such as benign prostatic hypertrophy. The social and emotional consequences of urinary bladder symptoms, particularly incontinence, always must be weighed against the risks to the patients' general health imposed by the proposed therapy. For example, women with mild, yet uncontrollable incontinence resulting from refractory detrusor instability may be managed better with incontinence pads (which pose no threat to their health) than with an indwelling vesical catheter (which predisposes to urinary infection).

On the basis of clinical and urodynamic findings, urinary bladder symptoms may be classified as filling/storage abnormalities, emptying abnormalities or combinations of the two (Table 1). Treatment should be directed at the underlying urodynamic abnormality that is responsible for the symptom (Table 2).

TABLE 1. Classification of Voiding Dysfunction

STORAGE PROBLEMS
Bladder Related
- Involuntary detrusor contractions
  - Detrusor instability (idiopathic)
  - Detrusor hyperreflexia (suprasacral neurologic lesions)
- Low bladder compliance
  - Neurogenic (myelodysplasia)
  - Fibrosis (indwelling catheter, tuberculosis)
- Sensory urgency
  - Infection/inflammation
  - Tumor
- Fistula

Sphincter Related
- Urethral hypermobility
- Intrinsic sphincter deficiency

EMPTYING PROBLEMS
Bladder Related
- Detrusor areflexia (neurogenic)
- Impaired detrusor contractility (myogenic)
- Psychogenic

Outlet Related
- Vesical neck obstruction
- Prostatic obstruction
- Urethral stricture

STORAGE AND EMPTYING DISORDERS
- Detrusor–external sphincter dyssynergia
- Bladder outlet obstruction and involuntary detrusor contractions
- Impaired detrusor contractility and sphincteric incontinence

TABLE 2. Treatment Overview

INVOLUNTARY DETRUSOR CONTRACTIONS
- Pharmacologic (intermittent self-catheterization may be necessary)
  - Anticholinergics
  - Tricyclic antidepressants
- Behavior modification
- Electrical stimulation
- Biofeedback
- Denervation procedures
- Augmentation enterocystoplasty (intermittent self-catheterization may be necessary)
- Urinary diversion

LOW BLADDER COMPLIANCE
- Pharmacologic (intermittent self-catheterization may be necessary)
  - Anticholinergics
  - Tricyclic antidepressants
- Augmentation enterocystoplasty (concomitant intermittent self-catheterization is usually necessary)
- Urinary diversion

DIABETES MELLITUS

Involvement of the lower urinary tract by diabetes mellitus is thought to be due to an autonomic neuropathy caused by a metabolic derangement of the Schwann cell. This results in segmental demyelinization and impairment of nerve conduction. The resulting clinical syndrome is called diabetic cystopathy (Frimodt-Moller). The most prominent clinical features of diabetic cystopathy are its insidious onset and gradual progression. The first symptom is usually impairment of bladder sensation, which results in a gradual increase in the time interval between micturitions. As the condition progresses, the patient may void only once or twice a day and require abdominal straining to initiate and maintain micturition. Eventually, the strength and force of the stream become impaired and urinary retention occurs.

The incidence of diabetic cystopathy is not well documented, but approximately 25 to 50 per cent of unselected diabetics recount the classic symptoms when specifically queried. Urodynamic studies have documented diabetic cystopathy in 27 to 85 per cent of patients. In Frimodt-Moller's study, diabetic cystopathy correlated with the duration of diabetes (generally occurring approximately 10 years after onset) but not with the severity. Diabetic cystopathy almost always coexists with other signs of peripheral neuropathy.

Urodynamic Findings

The principal urodynamic findings include impaired bladder sensation, increased cystometric bladder capacity, decreased detrusor contractility, and impaired uroflow. Impaired sensation is characterized by increased bladder volumes at the first awareness of bladder filling, and the first urge to void, and an increased bladder capacity. Increased bladder capacity in patients with diabetes has been documented in many studies, but, like assessment of bladder sensation, quantitative data are difficult to extrapolate from one series to another. Frimodt-Moller compared bladder capacity and micturition volume in normal volunteers and unselected diabetics. He found that there was a significant difference in both bladder capacity (913 ml for diabetics, 625 ml for normal controls) and micturition volume (655 ml for diabetics, 513 ml for normal controls.) However, large-capacity bladders are not necessarily pathologic. Weir and Jaques found that, of 3500 patients referred for urodynamic evaluation, 109 had cystometric bladder capacities in excess of 800 ml, but one third of these were urodynamically normal despite the large capacity.

Impaired detrusor contractility is considered to be one of the manifestations of diabetic cystopathy, but there has been little documentation of this in the literature. In Frimodt-Moller's series there was no statistical difference in voiding pressure between normal age- and sex-matched controls and unselected diabetic patients. Norlen et al, in contrast, reported that 6 of 12 diabetics awaiting renal transplantation because of diabetic nephropathy had impaired detrusor contractility.

Detrusor instability has not been reported in any of the series on diabetic cystopathy; however, unpublished data from our laboratory suggest that as many as 25 per cent of symptomatic diabetics may have detrusor instability.

Differential Diagnosis

The classic symptoms of diabetic cystopathy are fairly pathognomonic; however, most patients with diabetes do not have these symptoms. Much more commonly, diabetic men have vague symptoms of prostatism and, in fact, the two conditions often coexist. In the series of Frimodt-Moller, diabetic cystopathy was found in 38 per cent and bladder outlet obstruction (mostly benign prostatic hypertrophy) in 26 per cent of 124 patients. Because both diabetic cystopathy and bladder outlet obstruction usually result in impaired uroflow, screening uroflowmetry is of little help in making this distinction. However, simultaneous measurement of detrusor pressure and uroflow usually is definitive. Bladder outlet obstruction is documented by measuring a high or normal detrusor pressure in the presence of an impaired urinary flow rate. In patients with impaired detrusor contractility, both detrusor pressure and uroflow are low. Occasionally, patients with poor detrusor contractility as a result of diabetic cystopathy also have bladder outlet obstruction. This is a difficult diagnosis to confirm. It requires either sophisticated computer analysis of detrusor pressure/uroflow plots or videourodynamics with a micturitional static urethral pressure profile as decribed by Yalla et al.

Treatment

Treatment of lower urinary tract symptoms in patients afflicted with diabetes is best accomplished when there is a clear understanding of the underlying pathophysiology. Of particular importance is the distinction between diabetic cystopathy, impaired detrusor contractility, and bladder outlet obstruction. Surgical treatment of prostatic obstruction usually is curative, but empiric outlet-reducing surgery may cause worsening of symptoms in patients with impaired detrusor contractility or diabetic cystopathy.

Autopsy studies have demonstrated that chronic pyelonephritis occurs at a rate four to five times higher than that in the nondiabetic population. Moreover, the incidence of bacteriuria and urinary tract infections is much higher in diabetics. Whether the increased rate of urinary tract infection is due to diabetic cystopathy or other manifestations of diabetes is not known. Nevertheless, the association of a large postvoid residual urine volume, bacteriuria, and urinary tract infection is well known, and, if these risk factors are present, they demand treatment.

To date, there have been few meaningful studies of therapeutic trials in patients with diabetes and bladder symptoms. Accordingly, most of the remaining recommendations are based on personal observations.

Asymptomatic Patients with Diabetic Cystopathy

The natural history of untreated asymptomatic diabetic cystopathy is not known. However, because there appear to be few short-term sequelae from this condition, either no treatment at all or conservative, reversible, noninvasive therapy seems a most reasonable approach. Scheduled, timed voiding is a simple and effective means for dealing with the sensory abnormality that leads to infrequent voiding. Double voiding may permit emptying of a bladder that otherwise leaves a large residual. Straining to void may be helpful in some patients but harmful in others. To test the efficacy of straining, a simple uroflow and postvoid residual urine measurement may be obtained with and without straining. If the flow and postvoid residual urine improve, straining should be recommended; if it causes a fall in uroflow or an increased residual urine, the patient should be specifically instructed not to strain.

Patients with excessively large bladder capacities or residual urine should have urodynamic studies performed to determine whether there are other risk factors that need treatment. Of particular importance is the presence of bladder outlet obstruction and bladder compliance, because of the danger of upper urinary tract damage.

Asymptomatic bacteriuria is common in patients with diabetes, but no clear-cut treatment guidelines have been formulated. A reasonable approach is to treat asymptomatic bacteriuria with culture-specific antibiotics whenever it is detected. If bacteriuria recurs after the antibiotics are discontinued, urologic investigation should be undertaken to exclude urologic risk factors such as bladder outlet obstruction, low bladder compliance, vesicoureteral reflux, and urolithiasis. If no risk factors are found, further treatment of the bacteriuria may be unnecessary.

Symptomatic Patients with Diabetic Cystopathy

The mainstay of treatment for symptomatic diabetic cystopathy is institution of clean intermittent self-catheterization. If infection is present, it should be treated with culture-specific antibiotics. A number of other treatment regimens have been recommended over the years and many have gained both popularity and credibility, but in our judgment none of these are successful, nor are they worth trying. These therapies include parasympathetic agonists such as bethanechol chloride; alpha-adrenolytic agents, alone or in combination with cholinergic agonists; transurethral prostatectomy or vesical neck incision; reduction cystoplasty; and vesicoplication. Another "time-honored" treatment is the Credé maneuver. However, in a prospective urodynamic evaluation of the Credé maneuver, we found that, even on theoretical grounds, it would be effective in only about 1 per cent of patients.

Symptomatic Men with Prostatism

Diabetic men with prostatism present very difficult diagnostic and therapeutic problems. In our judgment, the sine qua non of treatment is an accurate diagnosis, which requires sophisticated urodynamic studies to distinguish prostatic urethral obstruction, impaired detrusor contractility, diabetic cystopathy, and detrusor instability. Treatment should be dictated by the underlying condition.

Symptomatic Women with Incontinence

Treatment of women with incontinence also requires sophisticated urodynamic studies not only to define accurately the underlying condition, but also to prognosticate about the dangers of urinary retention after surgery to alleviate sphincteric incontinence. Women with diabetic cystopathy or impaired detrusor contractility are more likely to have voiding difficulty or urinary retention after surgery.

MULTIPLE SCLEROSIS

Multiple sclerosis (MS) is most common in the third to fifth decades of life and has a female-to-male ratio of about 3:1. Pathologically, it is characterized by focal demyelination that results in impairment of nerve conduction. The course of the disease process is very variable, but the great majority of patients have mild neurologic abnormalities that tend to exacerbate and remit over time. The most severe cases are characterized by gradual progression that ultimately may lead to quadriplegia. The demyelinating plaques have a predilection for the white matter of the cervical spinal cord, particularly the posterior and lateral columns. Because these are the pathways that subserve vesical and urethral function, bladder symptoms are prominent in the majority of patients.

Urodynamic Findings

Detrusor hyperreflexia is seen in over 50 per cent of patients with MS and detrusor–external sphincter dyssynergia is found in about half of these. Detrusor areflexia is much less common. Bladder symptoms and urodynamic findings are subject to the same exacerbations and remissions as the underlying disease process.

Treatment

Because the course of MS is so variable, treatment of bladder symptoms requires careful consideration and a highly individualized approach in each patient. We believe that the most effective treatment is predicated on a clear understanding of the underlying pathophysiology as determined by urodynamic studies. In general, therapy should commence with the least invasive treatment; ablative or irreversible surgery should be reserved for patients with stable or progressive disease who have no reasonable hope for recovery and in whom conservative therapy has failed. Most patients with exacerbating and remitting forms of MS will continue in that pattern for long periods of time; these patients are best managed conservatively for as long as possible.

PARKINSON'S DISEASE

Parkinson disease is a degenerative neurologic disorder that usually is characterized by a slowly progressive course. The classic symptoms consist of the clinical triad of bradykinesia, tremor, and skeletal rigidity. The annual prevalence of Parkinson's disease is estimated at 100 to 150 cases per 100,000 population. Pathologically there is degeneration of the pigmented neurons of the substantia nigra. This results in a relative dopamine deficiency and a predominance of cholinergic activity on the corpus striatum.

Urinary bladder symptoms occur in approximately 25 per cent of patients. The most common symptoms are urinary frequency, urgency, and urge incontinence. Urodynamic studies confirm detrusor hyperreflexia in the majority of these patients. Voluntary control of the external urethral sphincter is preserved in about half of the patients. Several investigators have documented electromyographic abnormalities characterized by a delayed or incomplete relaxation of the external sphincter during the detrusor contraction, but the clinical significance of this is uncertain. Parkinson's disease does not cause clinically significant detrusor–external sphincter dyssynergia; treatment of the electromyographic abnormalities is not indicated.

Men with Parkinson's disease pose a considerable diagnostic and therapeutic challenge. The majority of men have diminished urinary flow rates, detrusor hyperreflexia, and a clinical picture consistent with both prostatism and neurogenic bladder. Because arteriosclerotic cerebrovascular disease is also common in Parkinson's disease, it is most difficult to determine whether the detrusor hyperreflexia is due to Parkinson's disease, other supraspinal neurologic lesions, or benign prostatic hypertrophy. In most instances, prostatic obstruction can be diagnosed accurately by videourodynamics. However, when there is concomitant symptomatic detrusor instability, there are no prognostic indicators that will predict the likelihood of persistent detrusor instability after prostatectomy. The usual clinical adage is to recommend prostatectomy when the patient is clearly obstructed and treat persistent postoperative instability pharmacologically. In our experience this has been almost uniformly unsuccessful.

In men with detrusor instability who do not have prostatic obstruction, we find the urodynamic study to be most useful in predicting the outcome of behavioral therapy. If the patient perceives involuntary detrusor contractions as an urge to void and is able to contract the sphincter, abort the stream, and abolish the detrusor contraction, we believe that there is an excellent chance that behavioral therapy will be effective. If the patient has no awareness or is unable to contract the sphincter, anticholinergics are prescribed. In our experience, anticholinergics are effective in only about one third to one half of patients.

Suggested Readings

Blaivas JG: Neurologic dysfunctions. *In* Yalla S, McGuire E, Elbadawi A, et al (eds): Principles and Practice of Urodynamics and Neurourology. New York, Macmillan, 1988.

Blaivas JG: The neurophysiology of micturition: A clinical study of 550 patients. J Urol 127:958–963, 1982

Blaivas JG: Urinary problems in Parkinson's disease. Curr Opin Neurol Neurosurg 1:284, 1988

Blaivas JG, Barbalias GA: Detrusor-external sphincter dyssynergia in men with multiple sclerosis: An ominous urologic condition. J Urol 131:94, 1984

Frimodt-Moller C: Diabetic cystopathy. Dan Med Bull 25: 49–60, 1978

Bladder Tumors

TREATMENT OF SUPERFICIAL BLADDER TUMORS

PRAMOD C. SOGANI, M.D.
New York, New York

Bladder cancer is the third most prevalent malignant disease among male patients and the 10th among female patients in the United States. Approximately 50,000 new cases of bladder cancer, mostly transitional cell carcinoma, are recorded annually. The majority of these patients (75 to 80 per cent) have superficial bladder tumors at the time of initial presentation. The superficial tumors include papillary tumors that involve only the mucosa (Stage T_a) or submucosa (Stage T_1) and flat carcinoma in situ (CIS).

The natural history of superficial bladder cancer is unpredictable because of tumor heterogeneity. The majority of patients develop tumor recurrences following endoscopic resection. The rates of recurrence after initial transurethral resection vary from 30 per cent with a solitary papillary tumor to more than 90 per cent in some cases of multiple tumors. Most tumors recur within 6 to 12 months with the same stage and grade, but 10 to 15 per cent of patients with superficial tumors subsequently develop invasive or metastatic cancer. Most recurrences are probably new tumors arising from other areas of dysplastic urothelium, but a significant proportion may be true recurrences resulting from inadequate treatment or from tumor cell implantation.

CIS of the bladder is defined as high-grade flat cancer confined to the urothelium. It may occur in association with superficial or muscle-invasive transitional cell carcinoma, but it also can occur alone. It may be localized or diffuse. It may be asymptomatic or it may produce severe symptoms of bladder irritability. Some patients have a protracted course lasting for more than a decade without developing invasive bladder cancer. Others progress rapidly to invasive bladder cancer that has a poor prognosis despite definitive treatment.

The most clinically useful prognostic parameters for tumor recurrence and subsequent cancer progression in a patient with superficial bladder tumors are: tumor grade, depth of tumor penetration, multifocal tumors, frequency of recurrence, tumor size, presence of CIS, lymphatic invasion, and papillary or solid tumor configuration. Tumor recurrence and progression rates are higher in patients with larger or multifocal tumors, high-grade tumors (grade 3 versus grades 1 and 2), tumors with lamina propria invasion (Stage T_1 versus Stage T_a), those invading lymphatic spaces, and those associated with severe dysplasia or CIS. In patients with Stage T_a, grade 1 tumors, fewer than 2 per cent will have tumor progression, whereas in those with Stage T_1, grade 3 tumors, approximately 40 per cent will have cancer progression. Another important factor is the extent of involvement with CIS: Those patients with only focal involvement have a more indolent course than those with diffuse involvement.

MANAGEMENT

The minimal requirements for clinical staging of bladder cancer per se are:

1. A complete history concerning prior urothelial tumors.
2. Cystoscopy and biopsy of existing lesions to define tumor grade and extent.
3. Random biopsies (from randomly selected sites) to identify other possibly uninvolved areas.
4. Bimanual examination under anesthesia to evaluate depth of bladder wall infiltration.
5. Intravenous pyelography to detect other possible urinary track lesions or intramural ureteral obstruction.
6. Possible biopsy of the prostatic urethra in some cases to seek early transitional cell neoplasm at that site.

If the diagnosis of superficial tumor is established, more elaborate staging techniques, such as those using computerized tomography of the abdomen and bone scan, are not indicated.

SURGICAL TREATMENT

Surgical treatment of superficial bladder tumors depends on the reliability of clinical staging and on the possibility of removing the tumor completely with conservative or radical procedures. At this time, basic procedures for bladder cancer surgery are transurethral resection (TUR) or fulguration with the resectoscope or Neodymium:yttrium-aluminum-garnet crystal (Nd-YAG) laser, partial cystectomy, and total cystectomy.

Transurethral Resection

Although the initial diagnosis of bladder cancer may be made during outpatient cystoscopy under local anesthesia, the definitive evaluation, including endoscopic resection, should be performed under anesthesia producing complete bladder relaxation. TUR is the primary modality for removal of Stages T_a and T_1 tumors and focal CIS. Most patients with superficial bladder cancer can be treated adequately with transurethral resection or fulguration of the tumor. Such a procedure saves bladder function, entails minimal morbidity and can be performed repeatedly. The overall survival rate for these patients is excellent (approximately 70 per cent 5-year survival). About 10 to 15 per cent ultimately require more aggressive therapy. A TUR removes the existing tumor but does not prevent the development of new tumors. Therefore patients should be closely followed.

Patients generally are followed with urinary cytology examinations and surveillance cystoscopy on a 3-month basis for the first 2 years after the treatment of initial tumor. The risks of recurrence are highest within this period. If no recurrences are noted within 2 years, the interval is increased to 6 months for the next 2 years, then yearly.

The Nd:YAG laser has been used in the treatment of superficial bladder tumors with good local tumor control. However, this has not been adopted for general use because of its limitations in obtaining material for staging and grading of tumor.

Partial Cystectomy

This procedure is reserved for patients whose tumors are not amenable to adequate endoscopic resection because of their location at sites that are inaccessible to the resectoscope. Operative mortality is low, and bladder function and sexual potency are preserved. It cannot be performed more than once in a given patient. After partial cystectomy, the patient should be kept on surveillance cystoscopy.

Total Cystectomy

Total cystectomy generally is not performed for superficial bladder tumors. The indications for total cystectomy are:

1. Unusual large tumors not amenable to complete transurethral resection, even on repeated occasions.
2. Some high-grade tumors.
3. Multiple tumors and frequent recurrences that make TUR impractical.
4. Symptomatic, diffuse CIS that does not respond to intravesical therapy.
5. Involvement of the prostatic urethra.
6. Irritative bladder symptoms with deterioration of upper tracts.

Cystectomy has a mortality rate ranging from 3 to 5 per cent and involves the sacrifice of normal urinary and sexual functions. Such "radical treatment" has a major advantage over the "conservative methods" of surgical management in providing absolute prophylaxis against new tumor formations.

Choice of Surgical Procedures

Besides characteristics of the tumor such as stage and polychronotropism, selection of operative procedures for bladder cancer should take into account such factors as morbidity, mortality, and functional loss, because more than 40 per cent of bladder cancer patients are more than 70 years old. Allowing for the aforementioned limitations, TUR seems to be the best method for treating superficial bladder tumors—localized CIS or Stage T_a or T_1 tumors.

INTRAVESICAL THERAPY

The treatment of superficial bladder tumors has three objectives: (1) to eradicate existing disease, (2) to inhibit tumor recurrence, and (3) to prevent progression to muscle invasion or metastasis. As already elucidated, TUR removes the existing tumor but does not prevent tumor recurrence. This provides the rationale for adjuvant therapy. Many patients with grade 1 papillary T_a tumors derive little benefit from adjuvant therapy following TUR. However, adjuvant intravesical chemotherapy or immunotherapy is indicated in patients who are at high risk for tumor recurrence. These include patients with Stage T_1 tumors (especially if multiple), multifocal papillary Stage T_a cancers (grade 2 or 3), or diffuse CIS.

Intravesical therapy brings a high concentration of drugs in contact with tumor-bearing mucosa. Tumor implantation after resection may be inhibited by reducing the number or viability of free-floating malignant cells. Residual carcinoma or precursor mucosal lesions may be destroyed, thus preventing tumor recurrence. The relative impermeability of the bladder wall inhibits the absorption of the drug, thus limiting toxicity to local rather than systemic problems.

Intravesical therapy is divided into three major categories:

1. Prophylactic or adjuvant. Prophylactic therapy is given after a presumed complete transurethral resection as an adjunct to prevent true recurrences.
2. Therapeutic, designed to eradicate the established papillary tumors.
3. Therapeutic, for patients having CIS either as a primary disease or in association with a papillary or sessile carcinoma that has been resected.

Several agents have been used for instillation therapy of superficial bladder cancer. Of these, the most commonly used agents in the United States are thiotepa, doxorubicin (Adriamycin), mitomycin-C, and Bacillus Calmette-Guérin (BCG). Thiotepa is an alkylating agent that acts by cross-linking nucleic acids and proteins. Doxorubicin and mitomycin-C are antibiotic chemotherapeutic agents that act by inhibition of DNA synthesis. BCG is an attenuated strain of *Mycobacterium bovis* that has stimulatory effects on immune responses.

Individual drug doses and schedules vary widely. The induction treatment usually consists of four to eight weekly treatments. This may be followed in the event of a response by monthly treatments for up to 1 year and, in some cases, for 2 years. Average chemotherapy doses are 30 to 60 mg for thiotepa, 40 to 80 mg for doxorubicin, and 20 to 40 mg for mitomycin-C. The BCG product is a biologic response modifier, and dose varies with strain; 120 mg (Armand Frappier and Pasteur), 50 mg (Tice), and 60 mg (Connaught). The optimal dose, concentration, contact time, interval between instillations, and total duration of the treatment have not been defined and still are controversial.

The principle side effect of thiotepa is myelosuppression, related to absorption consequent to its relatively low molecular weight. Therefore, monitoring of white blood cell and platelet counts is mandatory. Systemic toxicity from Adriamycin is less than that from thiotepa because of the former drug's higher molecular weight and thus less extensive absorption. Mitomycin-C is not absorbed from the bladder and bone marrow depression does not occur. The most common side effect of mitomycin-C is bladder irritation, which occurs in 10 to 15 per cent of patients. BCG produces an intense local inflammatory reaction in most patients. This is manifested as dysuria, frequency, urgency and passing shreds of tissue lasting from 6 to 24 hours after instillation. Serious systemic complications with BCG are uncommon but may occur; 25 per cent of patients may have a flu-like syndrome lasting from 12 to 24 hours.

Results of Intravesical Therapy

All of the four most commonly used agents for intravesical therapy—thiotepa, mitomycin-C, doxorubicin, and BCG—have been effective in reducing the frequency of tumor recurrence when compared with transurethral resection alone and can eliminate existing tumors (Table 1). The most effective of these agents appears to be BCG. Numerous studies conducted in the United States and Europe regarding the effectiveness of BCG as a prophylactic agent have demonstrated a complete response rate ranging from 63 to 100 per cent after a minimum follow-up of 1 year. The recurrence rate for individuals treated with thiotepa is 45 per cent, with doxorubicin is 40 per cent, with mitomycin-C is 30 per cent, and with BCG is 20 per cent. It also has been shown that BCG significantly reduces tumor progression and improves survival; however, clinical trials with other agents suggest that intravesical chemotherapy does not reduce disease progression or improve survival.

The results of intravesical instillation used for therapeutic reasons in eradication of existing papillary tumors (Stages T_a and T_1) reveal that complete response is seen in 60 per cent of patients treated with BCG, 50 per cent of those treated with mitomycin-C, 30 per cent of those treated with doxorubicin, and 35 per cent of those treated with thiotepa.

Perhaps one of the areas of greatest value for the use of BCG has been in the treatment of CIS. Approximately 72 per cent of patients will have their cancer permanently eradicated from the bladder following BCG therapy, 40 per cent following mitomycin-C, 25 per cent following doxorubicin, and 15 per cent following thiotepa. BCG appears to be the agent of choice for initial therapy of CIS. The management of the nearly 30 per cent of patients who continue to have CIS after BCG therapy remains a problem. The options include intravesical mitomycin-C or other chemotherapy, alpha-interferon, hematoporphyrin therapy, and cystectomy.

Other agents have been used against superficial bladder tumors. These include interferon (IFN), keyhole limpet hemocyanin, interleukin-2 (IL-2), maltose tetrapalmitate, transfer factor, and tumor necrosis factor. None has approached the response rate achieved with BCG. Alpha-2-interferon (alpha-IFN) may play a role in the management of CIS and deserves further investigations.

Suggested Readings

Brosman SA: BCG immunotherapy—techniques and results. Urol Clin North Am 19:557, 1992

Herr HW: Transurethral resection and intravesical therapy of superficial bladder tumors. Urol Clin North Am 18:525, 1991

Herr HW, Pinsky CM, Whitmore WF, et al: Experience with intravesical BCG therapy for superficial bladder tumors. Urology 25:119, 1985

Herr HW, Pinsky CM, Whitmore WF, et al: Long term effect of intravesical BCG on flat carcinoma in situ of the bladder. J Urol 135:265, 1986

BACILLE CALMETTE-GUÉRIN INTRAVESICAL THERAPY FOR SUPERFICIAL BLADDER TUMORS AND CARCINOMA IN SITU

DONALD L. LAMM, M.D.

Morgantown, West Virginia

Intravesical chemotherapy, as previously reviewed, results in significant reduction of the rate of bladder tumor recurrence and completely eradicates carcinoma in situ in about 40 per cent of patients. Unfortunately, current intravesical chemotherapy does not alter the long-term course of bladder cancer. In general, fewer than 20 per cent of patients with carcinoma in situ (CIS) will remain disease free for 5 years following chemotherapy, and in patients with Stage T_a or T_1 transitional cell carcinoma the 5-year incidence of tumor recurrence, disease progression, and patient survival is not significantly different from that for patients treated with transurethral re-

TABLE 1. Response Rates (%) in Superficial Bladder Cancer

	Recurrence Rate after Prophylaxis	Elimination of Existing Disease	Eradication of CIS
BCG	20	60	72
Mitomycin-C	30	50	40
Doxorubicin	40	30	25
Thiotepa	45	35	15

From Brosman SA: BCG immunotherapy techniques and results. Urol Clin North Am 19:557, 1992, with permission.

section alone. Fortunately, intravesical bacille Calmette-Guérin (BCG) immunotherapy has a completely different mechanism of action than cytotoxic chemotherapy, and the notable limitations of chemotherapy often do not apply to immunotherapy. Specifically, increasing data suggest that BCG immunotherapy provides superior long-term protection from tumor recurrence, reduces the incidence of muscle invasion and the consequent need for cystectomy, and improves patient survival.

BACKGROUND

Following reports of the successful local application of BCG in the treatment of melanoma and other skin cancers, Morales and associates, in 1976, reported the first significant clinical experience with BCG in bladder cancer. In nine patients, 120 mg of Armand Frappier BCG given weekly for 6 weeks with percutaneous sensitization resulted in a 12-fold reduction in tumor recurrence. This trial prompted National Institutes of Health funding of two controlled clinical trials. In the first reported controlled BCG trial, we observed a significant reduction in tumor recurrence, from 46 per cent in controls to 22 per cent with BCG instillation. At the Memorial Sloan-Kettering Cancer Center, Herr and associates had similar results in a higher risk population. Median time to recurrence was reduced from 3 months in controls to 18 months with BCG treatment. Overall, tumor recurrence was reduced from 100 per cent in controls to 63 per cent with BCG treatment. These studies, plus the controlled demonstration of the superiority of BCG over thiotepa reported by Brosman, prompted the enthusiastic evaluation and endorsement of BCG treatment of bladder cancer in the United States.

BCG VERSUS CHEMOTHERAPY

To date, randomized controlled studies have failed to show that any of the commonly used intravesical chemotherapies are superior to the old standby, thiotepa. Of all controlled comparisons, only the EORTC comparison of Epodyl and Adriamycin has achieved statistical significance, with Epodyl winning out. In contrast, three comparisons of BCG with thiotepa and two comparisons of BCG with Adriamycin found BCG to be significantly better. Only with mitomycin-C has the advantage of BCG not been clearly apparent. Although the Finnish study headed by Alfthan found Pasteur BCG to be superior to mitomycin-C, two Dutch studies failed to find RIVM or Tice BCG superior to mitomycin-C and Rubben in Germany found neither BCG nor mitomycin-C to be superior to transurethral resection alone, with only a 7 per cent reduction of recurrence with each treatment. These negative comparisons may relate to the preparation of BCG used, the schedule of treatment, or the low-risk nature of the patients studied. It is clear, however, that in the United States when patients at high risk for tumor recurrence are studied using an appropriate BCG treatment schedule, BCG is far superior to mitomycin-C. The Southwest Oncology Group study that the author directed comparing Tice BCG with 20 mg mitomycin-C using the same six weekly and then monthly treatments schedule had to be terminated at the first interim analysis because of the highly significant ($p<.006$) advantage of BCG. Overall recurrence was reduced from 32.6 per cent with mitomycin-C to 19.5 per cent with BCG, and the median time to recurrence was prolonged from 20 to more than 36 months.

TUMOR PROGRESSION

Although controlled studies unfortunately have failed to demonstrate that chemotherapy reduces stage progression in superficial bladder cancer, increasing evidence suggests that BCG immunotherapy favorably alters the natural history of this disease. We were the first to report a reduction in progression in 90 nonrandomized patients, and further experience has confirmed our observation. Three randomized studies have demonstrated reduction in progression with BCG treatment. Herr et al. evaluated 86 patients and found the time to progression to muscle invasion or metastasis to be prolonged significantly following BCG treatment. In this study, stage progression occurred in 35 per cent of patients not receiving intravesical therapy and 28 per cent of patients treated with BCG. Mortality in this study was reduced from 32 to 14 per cent with BCG use, and cystectomy was required in 42 per cent of controls compared to 26 per cent of patients given BCG treatment. In a subsequent report with 3 years additional follow-up, cancer deaths were reduced from 37 to 12 per cent (significant at $p<.01$). The Southwest Oncology Group compared BCG with Adriamycin and found an increase in stage or extent of disease occurred in 37 per cent of patients receiving Adriamycin compared to 15 per cent of those receiving BCG. Pagano et al. studied 133 randomized patients and found progression to Stage T_2 or higher in 17 per cent of control patients versus 4 per cent of those treated with BCG. In summary, all of these studies show significant reduction in disease progression with the use of intravesical BCG, with the mean rate of progression being 28 per cent for controls and 14 per cent for those receiving BCG.

CARCINOMA IN SITU

The malignancy most susceptible to BCG, and the only malignancy to date for which BCG is specifically approved by the Food and Drug Administration (FDA), is CIS. More than 700 patients with CIS around the world have been treated with BCG, and the average complete response rate is 70 per cent. In the first Southwest Oncology Group study, 70 per cent of patients treated with BCG had complete response and 65 per cent maintained complete response for at least 5 years. In a second Southwest Oncology Group study, the overall complete response rate was increased to 87 per cent when patients received an additional 3-week course of BCG at 3 months. Maintenance BCG therapy with three weekly treatments every 6 months for 3 years has yielded an estimated 4-year disease-free rate of 83 per cent. This remarkable long-term success with BCG in the treatment of CIS exceeds that reported in early cystectomy series, and therefore BCG has replaced cystectomy as the initial treatment of choice for CIS.

TREATMENT TECHNIQUES

Two FDA-approved preparations of BCG are commercially available in the United States, and many others have been found to be effective and are in use in other countries. Connaught BCG (Theracys) is used in a dose of 120 mg and Tice BCG in a dose of 40 mg. The viability or "colony forming units" (CFU), rather than milligrams wet weight, is the important measure of potency, and both preparations provide in excess of 2×10^8 CFU. The initial six weekly induction treatments conceived by Morales are so remarkably effective that it has been very difficult to find significantly better regimens. Controlled and uncontrolled trials have demonstrated that percutaneous sensitization is not necessary. Rodrigues-Netto and others have reported oral BCG to be highly effective, but we were unable to confirm the local antitumor activity of oral BCG in a controlled trial.

Although a single 6-week induction course of BCG can provide long-term protection from tumor recurrence in perhaps 40 per cent of patients, additional treatment is needed in some patients. Catalona et al. found 34 per cent of 104 patients responded to a 6-week course of BCG, whereas 53 per cent of 60 patients showed response only after a second 6-week course of therapy. It is important to realize that a continuous 12-week course of BCG is counterproductive in most patients. Ratliff and associates observed a suppression of immune response and a high recurrence rate in patients given 12 continuous weeks of BCG. My current recommendation for optimal induction therapy, as discussed in the section on CIS, is six weekly instillations followed by a rest period of 6 weeks and three additional weekly treatments.

MAINTENANCE BCG

In our early experience, we observed that quarterly maintenance BCG immunotherapy, using a single instillation, reduced the rate of tumor recurrence fourfold, from 1.9 to 0.49 tumors per 100 patient months. In the murine bladder cancer model, we have confirmed that BCG treatment without maintenance provides long-term (9-month) protection from subsequent tumor challenge, but further BCG treatments significantly reduced tumor growth in animals when challenged at 15 months. Subsequent clinical trials, however, were unable to demonstrate any benefit of maintenance BCG immunotherapy over a single 6-week induction course. Badalament et al. found no difference in outcome of prophylactic therapy when comparing standard 6-week induction with the addition of monthly BCG therapy.

To evaluate maintenance therapy, 660 Southwest Oncology Group patients with rapidly recurring Stage T_a or T_1 lesions or CIS received the standard 6-week induction using 120 mg of Connaught BCG. Patients were then stratified by prior therapy, disease type (papillary versus CIS), and tuberculin skin test and randomized to observation versus three weekly BCG instillations at 3 months, 6 months, and every 6 months to 3 years. After an average follow-up of 3.2 years, the time to biopsy-confirmed recurrence revealed a dramatic and highly significant advantage of maintenance therapy. Considering only those patients who had complete response and were disease free at 3 months after induction therapy, maintenance BCG resulted in an increase in long-term disease-free status: from 65 per cent in the observation group to 83 per cent in the maintenance group in patients with CIS and from 50 to 83 per cent in patients with rapidly recurrent Stage T_a or T_1 transitional cell carcinoma. This difference is statistically significant at a *p* value of less than .000001, and therefore leaves no remaining question about the superiority of continued maintenance treatment in patients with bladder cancer rendered disease free after induction therapy. More importantly, this maintenance therapy has resulted in statistically significant improvement of patient survival compared with induction only. In 391 randomized patients, the excellent 86 per cent survival at 4 years observed with induction therapy was improved to 92 per cent in patients receiving maintenance BCG.

COMPLICATIONS

BCG now is used widely around the world and generally is associated with few significant side effects. Because BCG works by inducing an inflammatory and immune response, symptoms such as cystitis are expected, and occur in up to 90 per cent of patients. Dysuria and frequency usually occur after the third instillation. Systemic symptoms of low-grade fever and malaise also are seen at this time in about one third of patients. These responses are usually self-limited, last about 24 hours, and require only symptomatic treatment. Such symptoms are best viewed not as an adverse reaction, but rather as an anticipated response of the desired immune stimulation. Hematuria also occurs in about one third of patients, but is more problematic because it raises concern about increased risk of systemic BCG absorption. I recommend delay of treatments, if possible, until gross hematuria has resolved but do treat in the presence of microhematuria. If irritative bladder symptoms, malaise, or fever persist or progress, isoniazid 300 mg daily is given until symptoms resolve. Treatment then is reinstituted the day prior to BCG instillation and continued for 3 days. Prophylactic isoniazid is not indicated for asymptomatic patients, and recently has been shown to decrease the antitumor effect of intravesical BCG in animals.

Significant reactions to intravesical BCG occur in only 5 per cent of patients. Fever greater than 103°F is the most common reaction, occurring in 3 per cent of all patients. The febrile period usually is limited to 48 hours or less, but unfortunately cannot be distinguished from the onset of systemic BCG infection or hypersensitivity sepsis. Hence patients developing a high fever should be hospitalized for observation and treated with isoniazid 300 mg and rifampicin 600 mg daily. BCG sepsis has been observed in approximately 0.4 per cent of patients treated with intravesical BCG, and to date 10 deaths may be attributed to intravesical BCG. Fortunately, with increased awareness of the need to postpone BCG treatments in patients with recent resection, hematuria, traumatic catheterization, or cystitis, the incidence of sepsis appears to have dropped. Patients typically present with high fever, shaking chills, and hypotension, and may develop confusion, disseminated intravascular coagulopathy, and respiratory failure. BCG sepsis cannot be distinguished immediately from gram-negative sepsis, so broad-spectrum antibiotic treatment for potential gram-negative sepsis as well as isoniazid 300 mg and rifampicin 600 mg daily is required. BCG hypersensitivity is observed in animal models and may occur simultaneously with systemic infection. Therefore, prednisolone 40 mg daily is recommended in addition to isoniazid and rifampin. The addition of prednisolone to isoniazid and rifampin (but not prednisolone alone) reproducibly improves survival in the animal model of BCG sepsis, and has resulted in 100 per cent survival in five patients so treated.

CONCLUSIONS

BCG immunotherapy heralds a new era in the successful management of superficial bladder cancer. The grave prognosis of grade 3 transitional cell carcinoma has been dramatically and in most patients permanently altered with modern optimal BCG treatment regimens. Previous dogma regarding the early application of radical cystectomy made in the era of intravesical chemotherapy no longer apply, and must be re-evaluated. Although fear of BCG toxicity is common, those familiar with BCG know that the benefits of treatment far exceed the risks. BCG immunotherapy is the clear treatment of choice for CIS and aggressive superficial transitional cell carcinoma, and urologists presented with such patients should learn to use BCG or refer these patients to those who have mastered this treatment.

Suggested Readings

Catalona WJ, Hudson M, Gillen DP, et al: Risks and benefits of repeated courses of intravesical BCG. J Urol 137: 220, 1987

Herr HW, Laudone VP, Badalament RA, et al: Bacillus Calmette-Guérin therapy alters the progression of superficial bladder cancer. J Clin Oncol 6:1450, 1988

Lamm DL: Carcinoma in situ. Urol Clin North Am 19: 499–508, 1992

Lamm DL: Long-term results of intravesical therapy for superficial bladder cancer. Urol Clin North Am 19:573–580, 1992

Lamm DL, Blumenstein BA, Crawford ED, et al: A randomized trial of intravesical doxorubicin and immunotherapy with bacille Calmette-Guérin for transitional-cell carcinoma of the bladder. N Engl J Med 325: 1205, 1991

Lamm DL, van der Meijden APM, Morales A, et al: Incidence and treatment of complications of bacillus Calmette-Guérin intravesical therapy in superficial bladder cancer. J Urol 147:596, 1992

Morales A, Eidinger D, Bruce AW: Intracavitary bacillus Calmette-Guérin in the treatment of superficial bladder tumors. J Urol 116:18, 1976

PHOTORADIATION FOR SUPERFICIAL BLADDER TUMORS AND CARCINOMA IN SITU

RALPH C. BENSON, Jr., M.D.

Nashville, Tennessee

BIOLOGY AND INSTRUMENTATION

Photodynamic therapy (PDT) represents a new and unique approach to the treatment of malignant disease. The past decade of investigation has produced slow but relentless progress establishing PDT to the point that it is now being employed in Phase III trials against standard and approved drugs for the treatment of noninvasive transitional cell carcinoma of the bladder.

Many compounds have been and currently are being evaluated as potentially valuable photosensitizers; these include a number of porphyrins, naphthalocyanines, purpurins, chlorins, and bacteriochlorins. Historically, the photosensitizers most commonly used for this purpose include hematoporphyrin derivative (HPD, or Photofrin-I) and porfimer sodium (Photofrin-[R]), formally known as dihematoporphyrin ether/ester; (DHE, or Photofrin-II). Photofrin is the drug that is under clinical investigation at the present time and it is the purified form of hematoporphyrin derivative, which includes a mixture of non-metalloporphyrins, primary dimers, and oligomers. In addition to being a potent photosensitizer, Photofrin will emit a brick-red fluorescence (600 and 700 nm) when excited with low-energy ultraviolet (400 nm) or blue (510 nm) light. This property has led to the use of Photofrin as a tumor localization aid and as a means of early cancer detection. It was this property of fluorescence that initially led investigators to observe that HPD tended to localize in rapidly proliferating tissues such as malignant tumors.

After intravenous injection, the majority of the highly lipophilic components of Photofrin-II are transported in the blood by lipoproteins. After 24 to 48 hours, Photofrin is concentrated primarily in the liver, spleen, and kidneys because of increased dye binding by reticuloendothelial cells. It also is bound to skin in mast cells, macrophages, and Langerhans cells. The preferential localization and prolonged retention by tumor tissue may be attributable to Photofrin's chemical properties, including lipophilicity, hydrophobicity, and molecular charge. In addition, it is known that Photofrin binds to vascular endothelium and therefore tumor characteristics such as increased neovascularity, enhanced vascular permeability and altered collagenous stroma may play a part in the preferential retention of the agent by tumors. In order for Photofrin to produce cytotoxicity in the tissue in which it resides, it must be activated by light corresponding to one of its spectral absorption bands. There are a number of visible wavelengths that can activate the drug (400 to 630 nm), but red light at a wavelength of 630 nm is used most commonly clinically. This wavelength gives maximal tissue penetration up to a depth of 1 cm.

The mechanisms of action of Photofrin-mediated photodynamic destruction of tumor is probably multifactorial. Photodynamic action begins with the absorption of light by a sensitizer (Photofrin), followed by a cascade of photochemical reactions resulting in generation of singlet molecular oxygen. Singlet oxygen is toxic to the cell wall, membrane organelles, and DNA. In addition to the destructive effects of singlet oxygen, PDT indirectly causes tumor damage via effects on vascular endothelium leading to vascular stasis, hypoxia, and tumor death. Also, an immunologic effect may occur resulting in the release of cytokines such as interleukin-2 and tumor necrosis factor–alpha, which in turn results in prolonged tumor remission. In summary, Photofrin-II, after intravenous injection, appears to localize in rapidly dividing tissues such as cancer, where it subsequently can be identified because of its brick-red fluorescence if the tissue is exposed to ultraviolet or blue light. It also has the propensity to destroy the tissue in which it resides if it is exposed to light that corresponds to one of its spectral absorption bands.

Unfortunately, there are no conventional light sources that will allow sufficient delivery of light to the interior of the bladder to activate the photosensitizing reaction. It is for this reason that the current primary source of light for PDT is the laser, because of its high power density, small beam diameter, and high coupling efficiency to optical fibers, which allow light to be conveniently delivered to many areas. An argon ion pumped-dye laser system is the instrument most often used in the clinical setting. These systems are similar and use a 5- to 20-watt argon ion laser to pump a laser with a circulating dye (rhodamine B, DCM, or Kiton red) to produce light near 630 nm. The distal end of the fiber can be varied to accommodate the particular therapeutic situation: an optically flat end to produce an expanding cone of light, a rounded tip to further expand the spot, a cylindrical tip to diffuse the light within a narrow beam, or a "light bulb" tip for use in large, hollow organs such as the bladder.

CLINICAL APPLICATION OF PDT FOR SUPERFICIAL BLADDER CANCER

It long has been this author's contention that transitional cell carcinoma in situ (CIS) remains the best indication for the use of PDT in the bladder. However, there are other patients who might benefit from this therapy, including those with noninvasive papillary transitional cell carcinoma that is extremely diffuse or perhaps even those with lesions limited to the submucosa (Stage T_1) that recur after conventional therapy. At the present time, PDT does not appear to be indicated for frankly invasive tumors.

Focal Therapy

Patients are given intravenous Photofrin at a dose of 2 mg/kg body weight. The previously documented tumor-bearing area then is exposed to laser light 2 to 3 days after injection. Although focal therapy rarely is indicated for the management of papillary superficial bladder cancer, there have been several reports employing this therapeutic modality for recurrent lesions. Front surface illumination with either a cleaved fiber or a microlens (more even illumination) can be carried out using either a rigid or a flexible cystoscope and a 400-μ fiber. The light dose should range from 100 to 200 J/sq cm at a power density no greater than 150 mW/sq cm. It may be necessary to overlap illumination fields to cover the entire tumor adequately. Although the overall response rate for such treatments has been reported to be from 70 to 100 per cent, response rates vary with the size of the tumor treated. For tumors over 2 cm, response rates of less than 50 per cent generally are obtained.

Our group originally directed treatment attempts primarily at patients with resistant CIS in whom all conservative treatment measures, including electrofulguration and various intravesicle chemotherapeutic agents, had failed. Fifteen patients with focal resistant CIS were treated and followed up for at least 6 months. All patients had biopsy and cytologic evidence of disappearance of the lesion in the treated area at the 3-month follow-up cystoscopic examination. Eight patients had one or more recurrent lesions, either in the treated area or at a remote site, during follow-up that ranged from 6 to 38 months. One patient underwent cystectomy and urinary diversion because of progression to Stage T_1 disease after multiple recurrences. Metastatic disease did not develop in any patient.

The problem with focal PDT in the treatment of either papillary superficial bladder cancer or CIS is that it does not address the reality of recurrence, which usually occurs at a distant site. Bladder mapping studies have confirmed the fact that the photosensitizer appears to be present in all frankly malignant or dysplastic areas. If recurrences may be due, at least in part, to existing dysplastic cells, it may be possible to diminish recurrence rates by delivering adequate light to the entire bladder. Several groups have investigated ways to deliver light of an appropriate dosage to the entire bladder in hopes of reducing recurrence. The methods employed include a lipid-diffusing medium, a laser light–scattering optic coupled with a driving instrument that irradiates the bladder in sequential strips, and modification of the distal end of the fiber resulting in a spherical or bulb tip that will deliver reasonably even light doses to the entire bladder.

Whole Bladder Phototherapy

PDT originally was employed for the treatment of CIS and more recently has been used for prophylaxis of superficial transitional cell carcinoma. In whole-bladder photoillumination, the quartz fiber is coupled to the argon pumped-dye laser and passed cystoscopically into the bladder. A quantity of normal saline necessary to unfold the bladder mucosa is instilled and is recorded as the treatment volume. This volume subsequently is used to calculate the surface area, treatment time, and power density that should be used. The fiber is placed in the middle of the bladder either visually or with the assistance of transabdominal ultrasonography. Dosage appears to be critical in whole bladder PDT, and therefore any volume change during treatment mandates calculation of a new treatment time.

The majority of patients who have undergone whole-bladder PDT are those with resistant diffuse CIS. Data from six studies treating similar patients from 1983 to 1988 are available. All patients were reported to receive either HPD or Photofrin. Light doses varied from 10 to 45 J/sq cm and methods of determining fluence were not standardized. Of the 47 patients with refractory CIS reported in the literature, 46 (97.8 per cent) were noted to have a complete response (negative cytology and/or biopsy) with follow-ups from a median of 3 to 12 months. Because of these initially encouraging pilot studies, a Phase II trial in North American and in Europe presently is underway employing whole-bladder PDT as an alternative to cystectomy in patients with resistant CIS. All patients receive 2 mg/kg Photofrin, followed in 40 to 48 hours by whole-bladder PDT using a spherical diffuser-tipped fiberoptic and a total light dose of 15 J/sq cm.

In addition to the treatment of CIS with whole-bladder PDT, a Phase III clinical trial of whole-bladder PDT for the prophylaxis of recurrent superficial bladder cancers has been initiated. After transurethral resection of bladder tumors (up to Stage T_1/grade 3), patients are randomized to either a single course of PDT using Photofrin and a whole-bladder light dose of 15 J/sq cm or to observation. Follow-up cytologies and cystoscopies are rigorously carried out every 3 months. An unscheduled 1-year follow-up interim analysis performed on a cohort of 24 patients well matched demographically has revealed that the median time to recurrence for the observation group was 93 days, but it had not yet been reached for patients receiving PDT. Although these initial results were very encouraging, this study subsequently has been closed because of the observation of significant bladder contraction in two patients. This very significant adverse effect most probably is dose related, and efforts are underway at the present time to attempt to redefine an appropriate drug and/or light dose for whole-bladder PDT for the prophylaxis of recurrent superficial bladder cancer.

ADVERSE REACTIONS

Although the incidence of side effects in bladder cancer PDT is not always reported, there appears to be a general "post-PDT syndrome" characterized by the irritative bladder symptoms of urinary frequency, urgency, and dysuria. This symptomatology is transient but may vary in duration from a few days to several weeks. Reports of irreversible bladder contracture from extensive fibrosis have appeared occasionally, and this reaction appears to be due to high light dosing, bladder overdistention, or vigorous treatment of patients already having fibrosis as a result of prior radiation therapy. The most common systemic adverse effect is cutaneous phototoxicity (primarily mild sunburn), which has been reported in 20 to 50 per cent of patients. The problem, although troublesome, resolves without sequelae. Often patients are counseled to remain out of direct sunlight and intense indoor light for 4 to 6 weeks after drug administration. A second-degree burn, which rarely occurs, is the most serious skin reaction that can result from accidental solar exposure. Proper perioperative patient education and counseling can prevent this problem.

CONCLUSION

For a new and relatively complex modality, PDT appears to have tolerable toxicity. There have not been any deaths reported secondary to adverse reactions in more than 10,000 patients with various cancers undergoing PDT.

Suggested Readings

Benson RC Jr: Treatment of diffuse transitional cell carcinoma in-situ by whole bladder hematoporphyrin derivative photodynamic therapy. J Urol 134:675–678, 1985

Benson RC Jr, Farrow GM, Kinsey J, et al: Detection and localization of in-situ carcinoma of the bladder with hematoporphyrin derivative. Mayo Clin Proc 57:548–555, 1982

Marcus SL, Dugan MH: Global status of clinical photodynamic therapy: The registration process for a new therapy. Laser Surg Med 12:318–324, 1992

Nseyo U: Photodynamic therapy. Urol Clin North Am 19: 591–599, 1992

Prout GR, Lin C, Benson RC Jr, et al: Photodynamic therapy with hematoporphyrin derivative in the management of superficial papillary transitional cell carcinoma of bladder. N Engl J Med 317:1251–1255, 1987

LASER TREATMENT OF BLADDER CANCER

JOSEPH A. SMITH, Jr., M.D.

Nashville, Tennessee

Laser energy has been used as endoscopic treatment for transitional cell carcinoma of the bladder for over a decade now. The efficacy of treatment is well established and the advantages and disadvantages as an alternative to electrocautery resection have been demonstrated. Continuing changes in laser technology and instrumentation are likely to expand the use of lasers for the treatment of bladder cancer.

RELEVANT PHYSICS AND TISSUE EFFECTS

Lasers emit a coherent, monochromatic, unidirectional beam of light. The observed tissue effects are primarily from thermal transformation of the light and are partially dependent on the wavelength. The greater the tissue absorption for a particular wavelength, the more the coagulative properties. However, strongly absorbed wavelengths result in tissue vaporization. Hemostasis is greatest in lasers with primary coagulative tissue effects.

The neodymium:yttrium-aluminum-garnet (Nd-YAG) laser (wavelength 1060 nm) has been used most often in urologic surgery for treatment of bladder cancer. This wavelength is poorly absorbed by body tissues and penetrates some 4 to 5 mm into the tissue. Excellent hemostasis is observed, and the laser energy is readily transmitted by a small flexible fiber. Argon (514 nm) and potassium titanyl phosphate (532 nm) lasers are strongly absorbed by body pigments and have more superficial penetration than a Nd:YAG laser. The carbon dioxide laser (wavelength 10,600 nm) is strongly absorbed by water and there are no commercially available flexible fibers for transmission of CO_2 laser energy.

The primary determinant of laser tissue effect is the energy density (the amount of total energy delivered for a given area of tissue). Noncontact laser fibers have a beam divergence of 5 to 7 degrees. Therefore, the distance between the fiber tip and the bladder wall is important in determining energy density. Contact laser fibers greatly increase the energy density by decreasing the spot size. This increases the vaporization characteristics of the laser. Most clinical series of laser treatment of bladder cancer have used noncontact fibers.

New fiber design has resulted in right-angle emitting tips that operate either by reflection or refraction. This has facilitated laser treatment of both benign and malignant disease of the prostate. There are no reported data on use of right-angle–emitting laser fiber probes for treatment of bladder cancer.

SUPERFICIAL BLADDER CANCER

Some of the initial enthusiasm surrounding laser treatment of superficial bladder cancer was based on the premise that noncontact thermal coagulation would result in a decreased overall recurrence rate. Clinical series have not supported this contention, although they have demonstrated the effectiveness of laser treatment on the local disease process. In most series, overall recurrence rate does not appear to have been favorably affected by laser treatment but local recurrence rates have been quite low. In fact, a randomized prospective study from Scandinavia showed a statistically significant decrease in local recurrence rate for laser treatment of superficial bladder cancer compared to electrocautery resection alone.

Laser therapy of bladder cancer can be performed with either a rigid or a flexible cystoscope. Often, anesthesia is not required. Patients are able to perceive the laser energy but the thermal coagulation is less painful than the sensation associated with the irregular propagation of electrical energy through the bladder wall. Obturator nerve spasm does not occur as a consequence of laser treatment. Tumors within diverticula also can be treated satisfactorily, and the risk of stenosis of the ureteral orifice appears to be quite low. The singular advantage of laser treatment is the lack of associated bleeding.

There are some drawbacks to laser treatment of superficial bladder cancer. First of all, tissue is not retrieved for histologic examination in the customary manner. Cold-cup biopsies taken before laser therapy can establish the diagnosis and determine tumor grade. In addition, the thermally coagulated tumor can be removed after treatment and submitted for histologic examination. The tissue usually maintains sufficient architectural detail for pathologic examination.

A complication unique to laster treatment, especially with a Nd:YAG laser, is perforation of adjacent viscera, usually the small bowel. Some 30 per cent of the laser energy occurs in the form of forward scatter beyond the bladder wall. Small bowel perforation may occur even in the absence of bladder perforation. Performing treatment with the bladder in a relatively collapsed state and limiting the energy density to only the amount necessary to obtain thermal coagulation of the tumor should make bowel perforation a rare (<1 per cent of cases) complication.

INVASIVE BLADDER CANCER

The ability of a Nd:YAG laser to produce deep thermal injury without significant vaporization forms the basis for its use in the treatment of invasive bladder cancer. After Nd:YAG laser irradiation, thermal changes deep within the bladder wall may occur with little visible effect on the tissue surface. The maximal coagulation temperature can be reached in the deep muscle of the bladder without superficial tissue ablation or vaporization. Thus, when white discoloration of the bladder surface is evident, the associated zone of coagulation necrosis may extend some 4 or 5 mm into the bladder wall.

Selection of patients for laser therapy depends on accurate staging. Unfortunately, traditional methods for staging of invasive bladder cancer are notoriously inaccurate. Up to one third of patients with invasive disease are understaged. Viewed simplistically, laser treatment is capable of extending the margin after electrocautery resection some 5 mm. Therefore, control or cure of tumors extending beyond that distance is unlikely. Logically, then, an aggressive transurethral resection of the tumor should be performed prior to laser therapy. This serves to debulk the lesion as well as to provide tumor tissue for histologic examination.

Because transmural coagulation of the bladder wall is the aim of therapy, higher energy densities are used for treatment of invasive cancer than for superficial disease. A characteristic white discoloration indicative of adequate thermal necrosis is observed. These changes may be less characteristic in treating invasive bladder cancer than they are in the treatment of superficial disease. The contrast between treated areas and the irregular surface created by electrocautery resection is sometimes difficult to perceive. Because of this, energy should be applied in a systematic fashion.

After a deep thermal injury from a Nd:YAG laser, bladder healing is delayed, and complete re-epithelization may not occur for several months. If complete healing of the bladder occurs with a pale white scar but epithelium that is otherwise normal, we have not seen residual tumor at the site of laser treatment either on biopsy or with long-term follow-up. In all of the patients in our series who were considered treatment failures, the area treated by the laser has not healed and follow-up cystoscopy has shown either gross residual tumor or poor healing.

Recently, a combined laparoscopic and transurethral endoscopic approach has been used for treatment of invasive bladder cancer. Animal studies have shown the ability to obtain transmural coagulation of the bladder wall reliably by this method. In addition, laparoscopy allows displacement of loops of bowel from the dome of the bladder, intraoperative monitoring of treatment depth, and application of energy to the serosal or intraperitoneal surface of the bladder wall.

Local recurrence of tumor has been uncommon in patients with Stage T_2 lesions treated definitively with a Nd:YAG laser. With the increasing depth or penetration, results are less impressive. For the most part, laser therapy should be restricted to selected patients with stage T_2 tumors or those who are not candidates for radical surgery. Whether a combined laparoscopic approach will extend the indications for laser treatment of bladder cancer is uncertain.

Suggested Readings

Beer M: Adjuvant laser treatment of bladder cancer: Eight years experience with the neodymium:YAG laser. Br J Urol 63:476–479, 1989

Beisland HO, Seland P: A prospective, randomized study on neodymium:YAG laser irradiation vs. TUR in the treatment of urinary bladder cancer. Scand J Urol Nephrol 20:209–212, 1986

Hofstetter AG: Laser treatment of bladder cancer. *In* Smith JA Jr (ed): Lasers in Urologic Surgery. Chicago, Mosby Year Book (in press)

Smith JA Jr: Laser treatment of invasive bladder cancer. J Urol 135:55–57, 1986

Smith JA JR: Landau S: Neodymium:YAG laser specifications for safe intravesical use. J Urol 141:1238–1240, 1989

INVASIVE BLADDER CANCER

JOHN A. FREEMAN, M.D.

Los Angeles, California

Invasive bladder cancer implies tumor cells penetrating through the lamina propria to involve the muscularis with or without extension into the perivesical fat. The depth of muscularis involvement is not important, merely its presence. Interestingly, most patients who develop invasive bladder cancer present with an invasive lesion. Only about one third have a history of prior superficial disease. Over the last three decades it has become increasingly clear that the therapeutic modality that offers the best chance for cure in patients with invasive bladder cancer is radical cystectomy. Five fundamental observations have led to this conclusion.

First, the morbidity and mortality associated with radical cystectomy have decreased in the last three decades as a result of medical, surgical, and anesthetic advances. Currently perioperative complications occur in 10 per cent and surgical mortality in less than 2 per cent of patients, with an average hospital stay of 9 days following cystectomy. The decrease in perioperative morbidity, altered body image, and life-style impairments has made surgical intervention a more appealing therapeutic option.

Second, bladder cancer tends to spread progressively from its origin in the mucosa into the lamina propria, muscularis, and perivesical fat, and subsequently to contiguous pelvic structures, with an increasing incidence of pelvic lymph node metastases at each site. Wide, en bloc resection of the bladder and pelvic lymph nodes provides negative surgical margins and low local recurrence rates.

Third, transitional cell carcinoma is very resistant to even high doses of radiation therapy. Only 11 to 38 per cent of patients with invasive transitional cell tumors treated by radiation therapy alone survive 5 years, and local failure can occur in 33 to 68 per cent. Employing high-dose short-course or standard fractionation regimens followed by radical cystectomy has all but been abandoned because neither has resulted in lowering the pelvic recurrence rates or improving the long-term survival of patients treated with combined therapy.

Fourth, chemotherapy alone or in combination with bladder-sparing surgery has not yielded long-term survival comparable to radical cystectomy. Recent trials have demonstrated the efficacy of MVAC (methotrexate, vinblastine, Adriamycin, cisplatin) combination chemotherapy in patients with bladder cancer. Significant downstaging occurs in up to two thirds of patients with clinical Stage T_2 to T_4 lesions; however, up to half of patients restaged as clinical T_0 following neoadjuvant MVAC are subsequently found to have P_2 or higher lesions on examination of the pathologic bladder specimen. Although bladder sparing appears feasible in some patients, it is not yet possible to identify which patients are ideal candidates for this therapy and which patients will fail conservative therapy and die from a potentially curable lesion.

Finally, modern surgical reconstruction of the genitourinary tract can return the individual patient to a satisfactory and functional life-style. Continent urinary diversion, particularly using the orthotopic neobladder, has revolutionized urinary diversion following cystectomy. The use of an inflatable penile prosthesis and construction of a myocutaneous neovagina has facilitated sexual rehabilitation of these patients and addresses the psychological component of radical surgery that these patients fear.

DIAGNOSIS AND STAGING

The diagnosis of invasive bladder cancer generally is made by biopsy at the time of transurethral resection (TUR) of bladder tumor. Staging of the malignancy then is undertaken according to the TNM system. The T stage is determined by the TUR pathology, which establishes depth of bladder wall invasion, cell type, growth pattern, involvement of remaining urothelium, presence or absence of carcinoma in situ (CIS), and status of the prostatic urethra, and by physical examination. Bimanual examination under anesthesia is an important component, because a palpable mass is generally at least a T_{3a} lesion and fixation implies pelvic wall involvement, raising the clinical stage to T_{4b}.

Clinical staging is not complete until the lymph nodes and potential sites of distant metastases (lung, liver, and bone) have been evaluated. Pelvic adenopathy can be evaluated grossly by computerized tomography scan, magnetic resonance imaging, or lymphangiography, but these tests are not sensitive or specific enough on an individual basis to base therapeutic decisions on their results. Chest radiographs are obtained routinely. Bone scans are obtained only in the setting of elevated alkaline phosphatase levels; similarly, no evaluation of the liver is performed if liver function tests are normal.

PATIENT SELECTION

Potential candidates for radical cystectomy with en bloc pelvic lymph node dissection include: (1) any patient with a muscle-invading tumor, regardless of grade; (2) patients with high-grade, lamina propria invasive tumors with evidence of lymphovascular invasion, with or without CIS; and (3) patients with diffuse CIS or recurrent superficial cancer who fail intravesical therapy. Advanced age alone is not a contraindication to surgery.

PRESURGICAL ADJUVANT THERAPY

Both radiation and chemotherapy have been attempted prior to planned radical cystectomy to decrease the incidence of local recurrence and improve survival. From 1971 to 1978, patients undergoing radical cystectomy were treated preoperatively with 1600 cGy of irradiation in a high-dose, short-course regimen over 4 days; no significant survival advantage or decrease in pelvic recurrence was noted in these patients. Other trials of preoperative radiation therapy have demonstrated mixed results and no clear survival advantage or decrease in local recurrence. We have not routinely used preoperative radiation for transitional cell tumors of the bladder since 1978, except in the case of pelvic spill of tumor by perforation at the time of TUR or open cystotomy where decreased tumor implantation in the scar has been shown.

Neoadjuvant chemotherapy utilizing MVAC is considered for patients with Stage T_{3A} lesions or higher and patients with suspected pelvic nodal metastases. Significant downstaging does occur as stated above, with better responses noted for the lower clinical stages, which may facilitate surgery. However, no randomized trial has demonstrated a delay to progression or survival advantage.

PREOPERATIVE AND POSTOPERATIVE CARE

Modern surgical therapy, which has diminished morbidity and mortality to acceptable levels, inherently includes appropriate preoperative and postoperative care. Our routine includes hospital admission the day prior to surgery for a standardized, well-tolerated mechanical and antibiotic bowel prep, intravenous hydration, evaluation by the enterostomal therapist, and administration of digitalis to prevent perioperative cardiac dysrythmias. Controlled hypotensive anesthesia minimizes blood loss during the operation, and intensive care monitoring postoperatively has diminished the morbidity and mortality that formerly discouraged application of radical cystectomy in the treatment of invasive bladder cancer. Warfarin anticoagulation is used routinely postoperatively to diminish the risk of deep venous thrombosis and subsequent pulmonary embolism.

PATIENT SURVIVAL

Survival following radical cystectomy depends on the pathologic stage of the primary bladder tumor and the status of the pelvic lymph nodes. Survival at 5 years for stages P_0, P_{IS}, P_1, P_2, P_3, and P_4 node-negative tumors is 95, 85, 80, 75, 44, and 36 per cent, respectively. The incidence of pelvic lymph node metastases increases incrementally with increasing P stage: 1 per cent for P_{IS}, 13 per cent for P_1, 20 per cent for P_2, 24 per cent for P_{3a}, 42 per cent for P_{3b}, and 45 per cent for P_4 tumors, in our experience. Survival in this node-positive population is markedly reduced, with only 50 per cent 5-year survival for all patients with Stages P_{3a} or lower (primary tumor confined to the bladder specimen) and less than 20 per cent 5-year survival for patients with Stages $_{3b}$ or higher (extravesical spread of the primary tumor).

GENITOURINARY RECONSTRUCTIVE TECHNIQUES

Since the re-emergence of radical cystectomy as the therapeutic modality of choice in invasive bladder cancer, emphasis has shifted to reconstruction of the genitourinary tract following this ablative surgery. The psychological importance of urinary reconstruction to as normal a system as possible in the cancer patient cannot be overstated. Prior to the era of continent urinary diversion, the ileal conduit was the standard form of urinary diversion following cystectomy. The complications of ileal conduit diversion, including reflux pyelonephritis, nephrolithiasis, and impairment of renal function, and the social implications of an external collecting device made this form of diversion less than ideal. Attempts were made to fashion urinary diversions that more closely duplicated the bladder's inherent functions.

Beginning in 1982, the Kock principles were applied to the formation of a large-capacity, low-pressure, nonrefluxing, continent ileal urinary reservoir. Since that time, more than 700 continent cutaneous urinary reservoirs have been constructed by the faculty in the Department of Urology at the University of Southern California (USC) School of Medicine. Since the last modification of the Kock pouch was made, early complications have occurred in 14 per cent and late complications in 20 per cent of patients.

The majority of reoperations in this group are accounted for by cutaneous incontinence and procedures to remove stones that have formed on staples within the pouch. Problems associated with the afferent antireflux valve have been rare and include ureteroileal anastomotic strictures in 3 per cent and stenosis of the antireflux nipple in 2 per cent. Patient satisfaction with continent urinary diversion has been tremendous.

Nonrefluxing orthotopic ileal neobladders anastomosed to the urethra (Kock urethra) have been constructed in appropriate male and female patients at USC since May 1986, and represent the next major advance in continent urinary diversion. Over 300 ureteroileal urethrostomy procedures have been performed, and over 90 per cent of males currently requiring urinary diversion after cystectomy are candidates for this type of procedure. To date, 98 per cent of patients void spontaneously; only 2 per cent require intermittent catheterization. Nocturnal enuresis occurs in 20 to 30 per cent unless the patient arises at night to void. Even those with persistent nocturnal incontinence, however, prefer to void per urethra rather than be completely continent and have a cutaneous stoma. Incontinence, manageable with an artificial urinary sphincter, has occurred in 4 per cent of patients. Typically this happens following salvage procedures after pelvic irradiation that damages the external sphincter. Because the Kock urethra patients are spared complications associated with the continence nipple mechanism and the cutaneous stoma, we anticipate that these patients should have a much lower long-term complication rate.

Nerve-sparing surgery generally is not performed at the time of cystectomy for bladder cancer because of our concerns of an increased incidence of local recurrence, which uniformly portends a fatal outcome in our experience. Rehabilitation of male sexual function is managed with an inflatable penile prosthesis. The reservoir and pump mechanism are implanted at the time of cystectomy when the pelvis is open, the corporal cylinders are placed later during an overnight hospitalization. Patient satisfaction is dependent on libido and sensation in the glans penis, which generally remains good unless a urethrectomy is necessary as well. Construction of a neovagina in female patients formerly utilized a small bowel segment; however, a persistent mucoid discharge made this undesirable. Recently, a rectus myocutaneous neovagina has been utilized in appropriate patients with excellent results. Satisfaction following this important aspect of cancer patient care has been encouraging in both males and females.

POSTSURGICAL CHEMOTHERAPY

Adjuvant chemotherapy delivered after radical cystectomy was undertaken in a prospective, randomized fashion at USC in 1980. A significant delay in time to progression was demonstrated in the chemotherapy arm, and a survival advantage was seen, although follow-up was short and many patients in the chemotherapy arm did not complete therapy. The efficacy of adjuvant chemotherapy, however, awaits the results of more trials before its routine use can be advocated.

URETHRECTOMY

Urethrectomy is included routinely in the anterior exenteration performed in female patients. In male patients, urethrectomy is performed if tumor grossly involves the anterior urethra or involves the prostatic stroma during random biopsy at the time of TUR. Tumor involvement of the transitional lining of the periurethral ducts without stromal invasion does not mandate urethrectomy. The issue of the retained urethra has taken on added significance since the advent of orthotopic neobladders, and we routinely obtain frozen section analysis of the prostatic apical urethral margin during surgery for any patient undergoing orthotopic diversion to the urethra. Urethral recurrence following cystectomy is estimated to be 9 per cent at 5 years and 17 per cent at 10 years for patients without CIS; if CIS is present, the risk of urethral recurrence may be as high as 40 per cent at 10 years. Urethral cytologic washes are performed annually on all patients with CIS and immediately on any patient who experiences blood at the meatus. To date, there have been no urethral recurrences in Kock urethra patients after 7 years' experience.

PATIENT FOLLOW-UP

Follow-up after radical cystectomy and urinary diversion is designed to evaluate the patient for evidence of tumor recurrence and deterioration of the upper tracts. Four months after surgery, the patients are evaluated with pouch-o-grams and intravenous pyelography to monitor the urinary system, chest radiographs, a biochemical liver profile, and physical examination. They are then followed every 4 months the first year, every 6 months the second year, and yearly thereafter. Urinary cytologies are obtained if CIS was present in the ureters, and the urethra is monitored as described above. Long-term follow-up is essential to identify complications of diversion or tumor recurrence in the upper tracts, which occurs in 3 to 5 per cent of patients.

Suggested Readings

Lieskovsky G, Boyd SD, Skinner DG: Cutaneous Kock pouch urinary diversion. Prob Urol 5(2):256, 1991

Logothetis CJ, Johnson DE, Chong C, et al: Adjuvant cyclophosphamide, doxorubicin, and cisplatin chemotherapy for bladder cancer: An update. J Clin Oncol 6: 1590, 1990

Skinner DG, Boyd SD, Lieskovsky G, et al: Lower urinary tract reconstruction following cystectomy: Experience and results in 126 patients using the Kock ileal reservoir with bilateral ureteroileal urethrostomy. J Urol 146: 756, 1991

Skinner DG, Lieskovsky GL: Management of invasive and high-grade bladder cancer. *In* Skinner DG, Lieskovsky G (eds): Diagnosis and Management of Genitourinary Cancer. Philadelphia, WB Saunders, 1988, pp 295–312

Wallace DM, Bloom HJG: The management of deeply infiltrating (T3) bladder carcinoma: Controlled trial of radical radiotherapy vs. preoperative radiotherapy and radical cystectomy. Br J Urol 48:587, 1973

DEFINITIVE RADIOTHERAPY IN THE TREATMENT OF INVASIVE TRANSITIONAL CELL CARCINOMA OF THE BLADDER

CRAIG L. SILVERMAN, M.D.

Philadelphia, Pennsylvania

Present surgical management of invasive transitional cell carcinoma (ITCC) yields excellent local and pelvic control rates. There is an associated small operative risk as well as the need for reconstructive surgery to devise a reservoir that serves as a pseudobladder. The role of definitive radiotherapy in ITCC has been relegated mainly to those patients considered to be inoperable because of overlying medical illnesses, patients who refused surgery, or patients with disseminated disease but with symptomatic bladder disease requiring palliation. For radical radiotherapy to be considered as an alternative to radical surgery in patients, it must eradicate the disease, prevent late relapse in the bladder, and leave the bladder functional.

Standard radiotherapy for the treatment of ITCC of the bladder usually entails treatment not only of the bladder itself but also of the regional lymph nodes. Shipley et al. routinely gave patients 5040 cGy to the entire pelvis and then boosted coverage of the areas of known disease to 6800 to 7200 cGy, but were very careful to avoid irradiating the entire bladder. Such a technique of irradiating the entire pelvis followed by a boost to the bladder itself is fairly common. It is believed that a four-field boost is the safest technique, leading to the lowest gastrointestinal complication rate, as opposed to rotational arc therapy or two-field boost using only a low-energy accelerator or cobalt.

PROGNOSTIC FACTORS

Shipley et al. evaluated their experience and determined several prognostic factors. Stage is very important; a higher stage indicates a worse prognosis. In addition, initial hemoglobin level was found to be important, with patients having hemoglobin levels of greater than 12 gm/dl improving significantly more than those with levels below that value. This finding has been noted by other groups as well. Also, the presence of hydronephrosis prior to treatment was found to be a significant indicator of poor prognosis. Finally, the extent of transurethral resection of the bladder was found to be significant (greater resection indicating a worse prognosis), as was a papillary morphology of the tumor as opposed to a solid morphology (the former indicating a poor prognosis).

Results of Radiotherapy

In order to evaluate more fully the efficacy of radiotherapy, certain parameters should be compared. First is the ability of the radiotherapy to eradicate the tumor completely (i.e., complete response by cystoscopy and biopsy). Jahnson et al. evaluated their extensive 20-year experience. Eighteen per cent of their patients never completed radiotherapy because of deterioration of their general medical condition, development of distant disease, severe cystitis, or death. Of 177 evaluable patients, 73 per cent achieved a cystoscopically complete response. Analysis by initial T stage demonstrated that 40 of 47 patients with T_1 lesions, 39 of 47 patients with T_2 lesions, 40 of 67 patients with T_3 lesions, and 11 of 18 patients with T_4 lesions achieved complete response. However, 43 patients (33 per cent of responders) later relapsed, evenly spread throughout all four initial T stage groups (i.e., T_1 lesions recurred as often as T_3 or T_4 lesions).

In the Toronto series of Gospodarowicz et al., the complete response rate was much lower, on the order of 46 per cent overall. Early T_2 and T_{3a} lesions responded 50 to 70 per cent of time. Survival in complete responders naturally was improved significantly over that in those patients achieving no response. The 5-year survival rate of complete responders was approximately 50 to 60 per cent, versus less than 8 per cent in the nonresponder group. Five-year corrected survival after complete response was 57 per cent in patients with T_1 lesions, 31 per cent in those with T_2 lesions, 16 per cent in those with T_3 lesions, and 6 per cent in those with T_4 lesions.

COMPLICATIONS

High-dose irradiation to the bladder is not without significant potential risk. Jahnson et al. noted that 58 of 262 evaluable patients had Grades II through IV complications. The urinary complications included seven Grade IV complications. A total of 8 per cent of patients experienced significant urinary complications; gastrointestinal complications were more frequent, with a 23 per cent complication rate at 5 years and a 34 per cent rate at 10 years. The Toronto group noted much less incidence of significant urinary or gastrointestinal complications, with only 1 of 30 patients who received 6000 cGy developing significant complications.

PRESERVATION OF BLADDER FUNCTION

Not only is eradication of the disease important, but the patient must be left with a functioning intact bladder in order to advocate the use of definitive radiotherapy in this setting. To merely eradicate the disease but leave the patient with a nonfunctioning bladder is not to the patient's benefit, and the patient would probably have been served best by a cystectomy at the onset of treatment. In the Toronto series, of the original 121 patients, 26 (21.5 per cent) had both freedom from bladder relapse and preserved bladder function. This included 6 of 41 patients with a T_{3b} lesion. Shipley et al. reported that 33 of their original 55 patients had good to fair function after treatment, but no long-term data were available.

It is also important to determine whether or not salvage surgery is possible for patients who undergo definitive radiotherapy and then recur. It must be noted that a minority of patients failing radiotherapy are suitable for salvage cystectomy, even those patients for whom the pelvis is the first site of recurrence. It is technically difficult for the surgeon to do a salvage cystectomy, and there can be considerable mortality and morbidity associated with such surgery, although there have been positive experiences reported at M. D. Anderson Hospital.

CONCLUSION

At the present time, radical radiotherapy for bladder cancer can yield fair results, especially with earlier T stage tumors. However, even in patients who initially respond completely, recurrence rates are fairly significant and salvage cystectomy difficult. Preservation of bladder function remains a difficult but achievable objective in a minority of patients. Newer protocols now are evaluating the use of cis-platinum in conjunction with radiotherapy. The hope is to increase the initial complete response rate as well as the durable response rate such that the dose to the bladder can be lowered to ensure better bladder function.

Suggested Readings

Gospodarowicz MK, Hawkins NV, Rawling GA, et al: Radical radiotherapy for muscle invasive transitional cell carcinoma of the bladder—failure analysis. J Urol 142:1448–1454, 1989

Jahnson S, Pedersen J, Westman G: Bladder carcinoma—a 20-year review of radical irradiation therapy radiotherapy. Radiother Oncol 22:111–117, 1991

Shipley W, Rose MA, Perrone TC, et al: Full dose irradiation for patients with invasive bladder carcinoma—clinical and histological factors prognostic of improved survival. J Urol 134:679–693, 1985

M-VAC THERAPY FOR TRANSITIONAL CELL CANCER OF THE BLADDER

MITCHELL C. BENSON, M.D.

New York, New York

In 1991, approximately 52,000 cases of bladder cancer were diagnosed in the United States, accounting for 4.6 per cent of all malignancies. Superficial lesions (papillomas, papillary tumors, carcinoma in situ, and with or without mucosal involvement) account for 70 per cent of bladder cancers, with muscle-invasive disease accounting for the remainder of cases. Superficial bladder carcinoma can be controlled adequately with intravesical therapy; approximately 3 per cent of cases progress to invasive disease. Standard treatment for muscle-invasive disease is radical cystectomy; unfortunately, despite aggressive surgical therapy, patients may relapse in the liver, lung, bone, and central nervous system. In patients with positive lymph nodes at radical cystectomy, the prognosis is particularly dismal: only 7 to 36 per cent will survive 5 years. Recurrence of superficial or invasive tumors correlates with vascular and lymphatic invasion, tumor grade, stage, aneuploidy, and lack of ABH blood group isoantigens.

Because micrometastases can be present at the time of cystectomy, effective systemic treatment as well as local surgical management are necessary for cure. Systemic treatment of metastatic and locally advanced urothelial tract tumors has evolved over the last 15 years from single-drug to multidrug regimens; only recently has the superiority of combination therapy been demonstrated. The most active combinations include M-VAC (methotrexate + vinblastine-Adriamycin-cisplatin), CISCA (cisplatin, Adriamycin, and cyclophosphamide), and CMV (cisplatin, methotrexate, and vinblastine). This article focuses on the M-VAC regimen, discussing its development; efficacy in the metastatic, neoadjuvant, and adjuvant settings; randomized trials comparing M-VAC to combinations/single agents; and future directions of M-VAC treatment.

SINGLE-AGENT TRIALS AND DEVELOPMENT OF THE M-VAC REGIMEN

Phase II single-agent studies provided the foundation for the M-VAC regimen. In previously untreated patients, the most active agents were cis-platinum (complete response plus partial response [CR + PR] rate = 40 per cent), methotrexate (CR + PR = 38 per cent), Adriamycin (CR + PR = 20 per cent), and vinblastine (CR + PR = 22 per cent). Complete responses were rarely observed even with the most active of single agents. Additionally, the duration of response was often short, generally 3 to 5 months. Durable complete and partial response rates in pretreated patients often are significantly lower, in part because of the inability to administer full doses of drug (e.g., nephrotoxicity causing inadequate platinum dosages). In a study by Tannock et al., no responses were observed when cisplatin was used as a single agent for salvage after treatment with methotrexate, Adriamycin, and cyclophosphamide.

The most active agents (methotrexate, vinblastine, Adriamycin, and cisplatin) were combined in the M-VAC regimen. Table 1 outlines the dosing schedule of the original M-VAC regimen of Sternberg et al. Of the 113 patients with metastatic disease treated with

TABLE 1. The M-VAC Regimen

	Day 1	Day 2	Day 15	Day 22
Methotrexate	30		30	30
Vinblastine		3	3	3
Adriamycin		30		
Cisplatin		70		

the M-VAC regimen between 1983 and 1985, 83 were evaluable. Complete response was attained in 31 (37 per cent) patients; another 31 (37 per cent) attained a partial response, and 23 per cent of patients progressed on treatment. Further analysis demonstrated that only those patients attaining a complete response realized a survival advantage.

RANDOMIZED TRIALS: THE SUPERIORITY OF M-VAC

Entry requirements and selection factors in single and combination chemotherapy Phase II trials can vary significantly and, as a result, produce invalid conclusions. Efficacies of regimens can be assessed only through prospective randomized studies. Valid comparisons of regimens require: (1) adequate sample size, (2) equal distributions of prognostic factors, and (3) adequate dosing schedules. Three randomized trials have compared M-VAC to either single-agent or combination regimens in patients with advanced urothelial tract tumors. Table 2 summarizes the response rates and the dosage schedules of trials.

The Intergroup Study by Loherer et al. randomized 239 patients to cisplatin 70 mg/m^2 q3 weeks or M-VAC. A statistically significant difference was seen in the CR + PR rate, as well as overall survival (13.5 months for the M-VAC–treated patients versus 7.4 months for cisplatin-treated patients). It is important to note that the overall response rates observed in both the cisplatin and M-VAC arms were lower than in the single-institution studies previously reported. Logothetis et al. randomized 110 patients to either M-VAC or CISCA (cyclophosphamide 650 mg/m^2, Adriamycin 50 mg/m^2, and cisplatin 100 mg/m^2). M-VAC demonstrated a statistically significantly higher CR + PR rate than CISCA (65 versus 45 per cent, $p < .05$). Median survival was longer in the M-VAC–treated group (62.5 weeks) than the CISCA-treated group (36.1 weeks). Pizzocaro et al. randomized 28 patients to M-VAC or cisplatin (100 mg/m^2) and methotrexate (300 mg/m^2) plus leucovorin rescue. Although the numbers of patients in each arm are too small for meaningful statistical comparisons, a higher response rate was demonstrated with M-VAC (CR + PR = 71.4 per cent) than cisplatin and methotrexate (CR + PR = 50 per cent).

M-VAC RESPONSE DATA

Neoadjuvant Therapy

M-VAC has been studied extensively in the neoadjuvant setting. Advantages of neoadju-

TABLE 2. M-VAC Versus Single-Agent or Combination Regimens

Trial	No. Patients	%CR	%PR	p (CR +PR)
Loherer et al. (1990)				
Cisplatin (70 mg/m^2/q3wk)	117	3	7	
				.02
M-VAC	122	18	18	
Logothetics et al. (1990)				
CISCA*	55	25	21	<.05
M-VAC	55	35	30	
Pizzocaro et al. (1991)				
Cisplatin (100 mg/m^2) + Methotrexate	12	8.3	41.7	
				NA
M-VAC	14	28.5	42.9	

*CISCA= cisplatin, Cytoxan, and Adriamycin, recycle q3 weeks.

vant therapy over adjuvant treatment include the possibility of downstaging the primary lesion, allowing for surgical cures in otherwise unresectable patients, and the treatment of micrometastatic disease. A recent multi-institution analysis of 147 patients receiving neoadjuvant therapy (90 per cent of whom were treated with M-VAC) demonstrated an increased survival in patients who attained a major pathologic response (as defined by final P stage of P_0, PIS, P_a, or P_1).

A recent randomized trial by Logothetis et al. evaluated three cycles of neoadjuvant M-VAC + cystectomy + two cycles of adjuvant M-VAC versus cystectomy + five cycles of adjuvant M-VAC. No survival advantage was detected between the two groups. The overall survival in both groups appeared higher than would be expected from surgery alone. Until randomized trials are complete, neoadjuvant therapy should be considered investigational. Currently, the Southwest Oncology Group is performing a randomized trial of neoadjuvant M-VAC (three cycles) versus cystectomy. This trial is important to determining whether neoadjuvant therapy can and should be considered standard treatment.

Adjuvant Setting

The prognosis of patients who have node-positive disease is poor. Although the staging performed prior to radical cystectomy often includes pelvic imaging, this is a less-than-perfect technique, and microscopic lymph node metastases still may be detected in the final pathology.

A randomized trial by Skinner et al. demonstrated a survival advantage with adjuvant cisplatin, doxorubicin, and cyclophosphamide over observation after radical cystectomy, but the role of M-VAC as adjuvant treatment is less clearly defined. A recent retrospective study by Fradet et al. has shown a survival advantage to M-VAC–treated patients with node-positive disease. Stockel et al. randomized 26 patients with pT_{3b}, pT_{4a}, or node-positive disease to observation or systemic treatment with M-VAC or M-VEC (epirubicin substituted for Adriamycin). A significant disease-free survival advantage (p = .0015) was detected in the treated group. Because the median follow-up in this small group of patients is short (24 months), definitive conclusions about the efficacy of M-VAC in the adjuvant setting cannot be made at this time. Large prospective randomized trials would help to answer these questions in the future. At this time, adjuvant M-VAC should be considered to be standard treatment.

M-VAC TREATMENT TOXICITIES

Toxicities encountered by patients treated with M-VAC can be severe and sometimes fatal. Prevention of common M-VAC toxicities includes: (1) reduction of the duration and severity of white blood cell count nadir through growth factor support, and (2) substitution of one or more components of M-VAC with analogues to prevent renal and cardiac toxicity. Critical analysis of these modifications is essential to determining whether reduction in toxicity can be achieved without compromising response.

In the initial M-VAC study by Sternberg et al. nadir white blood cell count ranged from 2600 to 3000/mm^3; 17 per cent of patients required hospitalization for nadir sepsis. Other studies have observed similar or higher rates of neutropenia and sepsis (e.g., Tannock encountered neutropenic sepsis in 41 per cent of patients). The recent Intergroup study reported rates of neutropenia and sepsis of 24 and 10 per cent, respectively, with fewer than 25 per cent of patients receiving treatment without dose modifications. Both granulocyte (G-CSF) and granulocyte/macrophage (GM-CSF) colony-stimulating factors have been effective in alleviating the depth and duration of neutropenia. Gabrilove et al. administered G-CSF to 27 patients receiving M-VAC and reduced the number of days of absolute neutropenia and days of antibiotic treatment, and increased the number of patients who were able to receive Day 14 of M-VAC. Mucositis also was reduced in the G-CSF–treated patients. Similarly, Aso et al. compared the white blood cell count nadirs of 26 patients treated with M-VAC without G-CSF (Cycle 1) to their respective nadirs in a M-VAC + G-CSF cycle (Cycle 2). Thus, the patients served as their own controls. A significant rise in the median white blood cell count nadir from Cycle 1 to Cycle 2 (2100 versus 3200), as well as decreases in the period of neutropenia, were observed. It is clear that administration of growth factor can both decrease neutropenia and increase treatment delivery; whether this translates into increased complete response rates and more durable responses cannot yet be answered.

The hydration requirements necessary for

the safe administration of cisplatin can make M-VAC administration difficult, especially in elderly patients with cardiac or renal dysfunction. Substitution of carboplatin for cisplatin would shift the dose-limiting toxicity from renal tubular damage from cisplatin to myelosuppression by carboplatin. Unfortunately, response rates of carboplatin as a single agent are significantly lower than those seen with other platinum analogues.

Special care must be taken in those patients who have an ileal conduit or another form of intestinal diversion. Methotrexate normally is excreted through the kidney but can be reabsorbed through the terminal ileum. Fossa et al. observed that methotrexate levels 43 to 48 hours after administration were elevated in 8 of 11 patients, and were particularly high in those patients who had an ileal conduit 2 years or less before chemotherapy. Thus, to avoid severe and potentially lethal toxicity, patients with any intestinal diversion must be catheterized before and during methotrexate administration.

DOSE-ESCALATED M-VAC REGIMENS

The response patterns of M-VAC–treated patients demonstrate the necessity of attaining a complete response for long-term survival. Strategies for improving overall response could focus on intensifying dose to overcome resistance mechanisms, or using agents to reverse resistance. Dose intensity, or the amount of drug delivered to a patient per unit time (milligrams per square meter of body area per week), has been found to correlate with response in ovarian cancer, breast cancer, and lymphoma. Unfortunately, Scher found no relationship between response and the cumulative dose intensity of M-VAC. One possible explanation for this failure is the low individual dose intensities for Adriamycin (5.1 to 4.5 mg/m^2 per week) and cisplatin (14 to 12.6 mg/m^2 per week) utilized in the M-VAC regimen. Two trials have escalated one or more M-VAC components. Arap et al. increased the dose of methotrexate to 1000 mg/m^2 on Day 1, followed by leucovorin 24 hours later. Overall response rates were not improved over conventional M-VAC (CR + PR rate = 56 per cent [95 per cent confidence limits, 36 to 78 per cent]). Logothetis et al. intensified the Adriamycin (60 mg/m^2), cisplatin (100 mg/m^2), and vinblastine (4.5 mg/m^2) in the M-VAC regimen and used growth factor support with GM-CSF. In this study of 30 evaluable patients refractory to standard M-VAC or CISCA, a response rate of 30 per cent could be observed with some complete responders.

BIOLOGIC CORRELATES OF RESPONSE

Analysis of M-VAC response patterns in patients has identified the following groups of patients as having a lower probability of attaining complete response:

1. Those with hepatic metastases.
2. Those with non–transitional cell histologies (i.e., adeno/squamous cell carcinoma).
3. Those undergoing retreatment of disease that has relapsed within 1 year after complete response.

Although several in vitro mechanisms for acquired and intrinsic drug resistance have been identified, only recently have attempts been made to correlate biologic parameters to response. Urothelial cells can develop resistance by several mechanisms (Table 3). One such mechanism responsible for resistance to two M-VAC drugs (Adriamycin and vinblastine) is P-glycoprotein, a 170 to 180-kD inte-

TABLE 3. Potential Resistance Pathways for Patients Treated with M-VAC

	Decreased Drug Accumulation	Changes in Drug Target
Methotrexate	Folate transport proteins	Altered dihydrofolate Reductase (DHFR) Increased DHFR
Vinblastine	P-glycoprotein	Altered Microtubules
Adriamycin	P-glycoprotein	Altered topoisomerase II
Cisplatin	Unknown	Glutathione, metallothionene, platinum adducts

gral membrane protein responsible for the efflux of hydrophobic natural product chemotherapeutic agents. Benson et al. have demonstrated that P-glycoprotein is expressed at a low rate in untreated urothelial tract tumors (<6 per cent expression). However, two M-VAC–treated tumors have shown increased expression. Similarly, Petrylak et al., using an immunohistochemical technique, found low positive rates (13 and 0 per cent) in nonconsecutive primary and metastatic urothelial tumors, respectively; these increased (39 and 55 per cent, respectively) after M-VAC treatment. These results imply that either P-glycoprotein expression is induced in these tumors, or that treatment is selecting those cells that are adapted to survive treatment.

CONCLUSIONS

The M-VAC regimen has proven effective in treating metastatic urothelial transitional cell cancer. Two randomized clinical trials have shown it to be superior to single-agent cisplatin or CISCA. Toxicities at times can be severe; however, all efforts must be made to deliver the proper dosages, and not substitute platinum analogues.

Future studies will focus on the role of dose intensification with growth factor support in increasing the CR + PR rate in the neoadjuvant, adjuvant, and metastatic settings. Elucidation of the mechanisms responsible for M-VAC resistance might guide future trials in tailoring treatment around resistance phenotypes.

Acknowledgments: I would like to express my thanks to Dr. Daniel Petrylak and Dr. Alan Yagoda. Were it not for the Instructions to Authors, their names would be listed as coauthors.

Suggested Readings

Benson MC, Giella J, Whang IS, et al: Flow cytometric determination of the multidrug resistant phenotype in transitional cell cancer of the bladder: Implications and applications. J Urol 146:982–986, 1991

Loehrer PJ, Elson P, Kueber JP, et al: Advanced bladder cancer: A prospective trial comparing single agent cisplatin vs MVAC combination therapy (INT 0078). Proc Assoc Clin Oncol 9:132, 1990

Logothetis C, Dexus F, Finn L, et al: A prospective randomized trial comparing MVAC and CISCA chemotherapy for patients with metastatic urothelial tract tumors. J Clin Oncol 6:1050–1055, 1990

Logothetis C, Dexus FH, Sella A, et al: Escalated therapy for refractory urothelial tumors: Methotrexate-vinblastine-doxorubicin cisplatin plus unglycosylated recombinant human granulocyte-macrophage colony stimulating factor. J Natl Cancer Inst 82:667–672, 1990

Pizzocaro G, Milani A, Piva L, et al: Methotrexate, vinblastine, adriamycin and cisplatin versus methotrexate and cisplatin in advanced urothelial cancer. A randomized study. Eur Urol 20:89–92, 1991

ADENOCARCINOMA OF THE BLADDER

GABRIEL P. HAAS, M.D.

Detroit, Michigan

Adenocarcinoma of the bladder is extremely rare, constituting less than 1 per cent of bladder cancers. These lesions can be subdivided into primary bladder adenocarcinomas, generally arising from the base of the bladder; adenocarcinomas of urachal origin, found predominantly at the dome; and secondary tumors, usually invading directly from adjacent organs such as the rectosigmoid, ovaries, endometrium, or cervix. Secondary tumors, in fact, are the most common adenocarcinomas found in the bladder.

The etiology of urachal carcinomas is poorly understood. The urachus, an embryonic remnant that courses as a peritoneal fold in the midline from the dome of the bladder to the umbilicus, is associated with variable benign and malignant abnormalities. Inappropriate closure may result in a patent urachal sinus, there may be urachal cysts present, and these may become infected in both pediatric and adult patients. The cord is lined by enteric, glandular epithelium, and it is from this element that adenocarcinomas may arise. These tumors are most common in the 40- to 70-year age groups and are twice as common in men as women.

Primary adenocarcinomas of the bladder more often are found in elderly men, 60 to 80 years of age. Although most originate from the base, they may arise from any part of the bladder, including the dome. These lesions often are associated with a history of mucosal irritation, and cystitis glandularis is believed to represent a predisposing state for malignant transformation. Although the defunctionalized bladder, schistosomiasis, and chronic infections are most likely to result in the development of squamous cell cancer of the bladder, the prevalence of adenocarcinoma also is increased under these circumstances. The strongest association, however, is with a history of bladder exstrophy, even if successfully closed in early childhood. Such patients have a 400-fold increased risk for developing adenocarcinoma, compared to the general population.

The usual presentation is that of hematuria. Irritable voiding symptoms, dysuria, and urgency/frequency are less common. Patients occasionally will complain of passing mucus in their urine. Unfortunately, the lesion usually becomes symptomatic late in the course of the disease; therefore, most patients present with deeply invasive, advanced tumors of poor prognosis.

The diagnosis is established at the time of cystoscopy and biopsy. Urachal carcinomas generally are very well demarcated from normal epithelium; primary bladder adenocarcinomas display more infiltration along the mucosa. Ten per cent of urachal carcinomas arise from deeper layers of the urachal tract and may not be visible during cystoscopy.

Histologically, the lesion appears as a typical glandular epithelial malignancy often indistinguishable from tumors with gastrointestinal sources. Goblet cells resembling colonic epithelium, atypical, multilayer glandular elements containing mucus, and mucus secreting cells are typical findings. Less common histologic findings include signet cell elements, an even worse prognostic sign, or clear cell adenocarcinoma, an entity more common in women and thought to arise from urethral sites. Flow cytometric analysis demonstrates frequent abnormalities in DNA content. Very few patients display a diploid pattern, but those who do have a better prognosis. Some urachal tumors have been shown to express the CA 125 tumor marker, and this serum marker may be helpful in following therapy.

The tumor spreads by aggressive local invasion and by both hematogenous and lymphatic metastases. Staging studies should include computerized tomography, chest radiography, and bone scan. Localized disease should be managed by aggressive surgical intervention to offer the best chance of remission. Historically, urachal adenocarcinomas were thought not to represent panepithelial disease, and therefore they often were managed by partial cystectomy with wide excision of normal bladder cuff—unfortunately this procedure is wrought with a very high rate of local recurrence (>50 per cent) and cannot be recommended. Primary adenocarcinoma of the bladder should be treated with radical cystectomy, pelvic lymph node dissection, and urinary diversion. Urachal adenocarcinomas should be treated with a radical cystectomy and en bloc excision of the entire urachal tract, including the anterior peritoneum and abdominal wall surrounding the umbilicus.

Only successful surgery yields the hope of effective extirpation, but, unfortunately, the tumor is often deeply invasive by diagnosis, so local recurrence, as well as metastases, are common. Advanced disease is refractory to radiation therapy and most chemotherapy. Combinations of 5-fluorouracil, methotrexate, mitomycin-C, doxorubicin, and platinum demonstrated very limited efficacy. Five-year survival rates of up to 33 per cent have been reported after successful surgical intervention; however, these figures drop to less than 10 per cent in the face of recurrent or metastatic disease. Poor prognosis the consequence of advanced disease at the time of diagnosis and the lack of effective therapy.

Suggested Readings

Anderstrom C, Johanson LS, Von Schultz L: Primary adenocarcinoma of the bladder: A clinicopathologic and prognostic study. CA 52:1273–1280, 1983

Badalament RA, Cibas ES, Reuter VE, et al: Flow cytometric analysis of primary adenocarcinoma of the bladder. J Urol 137:1159–1162, 1987

Choh H., Lamb S, Pintar K, et al: Primary signet-ring cell carcinoma of the urinary bladder. CA 53:1985–1990, 1984

Guarnaccia S, Pais V, Grous J, et al: Adenocarcinoma of the urachus associated with elevated levels of CA 125. J Urol 145:140–141, 1991

Sheldon CA, Clayman RV, Gonzales R, et al: Malignant urachal lesions. J Urol 131:1–8, 1984

Song J, Farrow GM, Lieber MM: Primary adenocarcinoma of the bladder: Favorable prognostic significance of deoxyribonucleic acid diploidy measured by flow cytometry. J Urol 144:1115–1118, 1990

SQUAMOUS CELL CARCINOMA OF THE URINARY BLADDER

ZEV WAJSMAN, M.D.

Gainesville, Florida

Squamous cell carcinoma (SCC) of the bladder is relatively infrequent in western society (1.6 to 8 per cent of bladder tumors), whereas it is the most common cancer in patients with endemic schistosomiasis. The tumor frequently is associated with chronic inflammation; it is found in patients with indwelling catheters, bladder calculi, and neurogenic bladders with suprapubic tubes. However, it is also found in patients without any pre-existing conditions. The bladder epithelium has the ability to undergo metaplasia in response to irritating stimuli. In addition to the most frequently found transitional cell carcinoma (TCC), SCC, adenocarcinoma, and other conditions may be seen simultaneously.

Some pathologists use the terminology of epidermoid tumors when describing transitional cell carcinoma of the bladder, which sometimes has led to unnecessary confusion. SCC is characterized by aggregates of keratinized cells, usually in sheets, containing concentric groups of keratinized cells. When these cells are well differentiated, they may cause a diagnostic problem. To unexperienced pathologists, these findings may be confused with severe squamous metaplasia. When a biopsy of a "white plaque" is performed, cells with squamous metaplasia with keratinization are seen under the microscope, and, indeed, may be confused with well-differentiated SCC. In females, this entity is seen quite frequently in the bladder neck or trigone, and it is usually benign. However, in male patients and female with chronic irritative symptoms, such findings of severe metaplasia and keratin formation should raise the index of suspicion and alert the pathologist to the possible existence of SCC.

INCIDENCE AND CLINICAL PRESENTATION

Bladder cancer is highly prevalent in some areas of Africa and the Middle East. It is the most common cancer in Egypt. The incidence of SCC in bilharzial bladders is about 20 per cent. The presenting symptoms usually are associated with a history of urinary infections and irritations. A higher frequency of dysuria and urgency is noted. In some female patients without pre-existing factors, the only symptom may be severe frequency. Such rather nonspecific complaints may, and indeed frequently do, cause delay in diagnosis. White flakes and debris may be seen in the urine.

DIAGNOSIS

Usually the SCC is a solid lesion, rarely exophytic, and seen most frequently at the trigone, and rarely at the dome of the bladder. The majority of patients will be diagnosed with deep invasion. Deep transurethral resection (TUR) of an abnormal lesion will help to obtain an adequate specimen. The highly differentiated form of SCC is recognized by the presence of cell containing keratin pearls. Poorly differentiated forms may be difficult to distinguish from anaplastic type of TCC. This distinction, however, may be of value, because patients with invasive TCC may benefit from systemic chemotherapy. Cytologic examination of the urine may show typical keratinized cancer cells; however, many of these tumors are necrotic, and the yield for cytology is low. Cystoscopy reveals white flakes and debris obstructing the view.

In this country, SCC most commonly is diagnosed in patients with neurogenic bladders, usually in association with chronic indwelling catheters or suprapubic tubes. With commonly utilized self-catheterization, the frequency of malignancy in the neurogenic bladder should be reduced. However, in many of the patients with neurogenic bladders SCC is recognized late. Such patients should be monitored at least once a year with cystoscopic examinations, with cytology and biopsy of any suspicious lesion. A history of hematuria and any abnormal endoscopic findings should be pursued aggressively with deep and, if necessary, repeated biopsies.

TREATMENT

An aggressive surgical approach is the only effective treatment of SCC of the bladder. Very rarely, SCC will be present as a small superficial, well-defined lesion and a TUR may be sufficient. SCC is usually not a multifocal disease, and segmental cystectomy can be used for a small, well-localized tumor located at the dome (rare). However, in the vast majority of cases SCC will be invasive, and even superficial tumors show evidence of intramural, lateral lymphatic extension. Very low-grade, well-differentiated tumors occasionally may have a low malignant potential and grow slowly, but metastatic deposits of these well-differential cells are not uncommonly seen in regional lymph nodes at the time of cystectomy.

The primary treatment of choice in SCC of the bladder is radical cystectomy. In spite of their rather poor prognosis in general (similar to that of TCC stage for stage), some cases of SCC are unpredictable and, even when spread to regional lymph nodes, they should be treated aggressively. Cystectomy frequently will be indicated for palliation, because many patients may present with severe local symptoms, severe frequency, hematuria, pain, or a foul, intolerable smell.

In the female, anterior pelvic exenteration, with pubectomy when indicated, should be performed. Ileal conduit or continent-type diversion can be considered. Bilateral radical pelvic lymph node dissection is done routinely. In males, radical cystectomy, usually without en bloc urethrectomy, should be sufficient. Because pure SCC is not a multifocal disease, the urethra is not at risk and neobladder formation is a reasonable alternative. However, in view of the invasive nature of SCC and the high chance of local pelvic recurrent disease, ileal conduit or continent diversion is a safer alternative to the neobladder.

The role of preoperative or postoperative radiation therapy is not well established in SCC of the bladder. Systemic adjuvant chemotherapy frequently is used now in patients with invasive TCC of the bladder, especially in cases of regional lymph node metastasis and in tumors with vascular invasion and perivesical fat infiltration. SCC of the urinary tract is not known to respond well to chemotherapy. However, because anaplastic SCC may not be distinguished from high-grade TCC easily, patients with such tumors should be given the benefit of the doubt and treated with one of the regimens used in platinum-based chemotherapy.

SUMMARY

SCC of the bladder is a rare, well-defined malignancy with a usually poor prognosis. A high index of suspicion in diagnosis of clinical symptoms, careful pathologic evaluation, and aggressive radical surgery may benefit some patients even with local and regional spread.

Suggested Readings

Droller MJ: Transitional cell cancer: Upper tracts and bladder. *In* Walsh PC, Gittes RF, Permutter AD, et al (eds): Campbell's Urology, 5th ed. Philadelphia, WB Saunders, 1986, p 1406

Olsen S: Vesical leukoplakia and squamous carcinoma. *In* Olsen S (ed): Tumors of the Kidney and Urinary Tract. Philadelphia, WB Saunders, 1984, pp 174–178

Scher HI: Systemic chemotherapy in regionally advanced bladder cancer. Urol Clin North Am 19:747, 1992

TREATMENT OF GENITOURINARY RHABDOMYOSARCOMA IN CHILDREN

ROBERT E. STECKLER, M.D.

Camden, New Jersey

Rhabdomyosarcoma is a solid malignant tumor of mesenchymal origin that resembles striated muscle. Nonetheless, it may develop in sites devoid of striated muscle, such as the bladder and prostate. Rhabdomyosarcomas are the most common soft tissue sarcomas in children less than 15 years old and comprise the sixth most common solid tumor in children, accounting for 5 to 8 per cent of all childhood malignancies. Approximately 250 new cases are seen annually in the United States. There is a familial association, albeit fairly weak, in which there is a greater incidence of sarcomas in the siblings of probands, as well as an increased incidence of breast cancer, brain tumors, and adrenal carcinomas in relatives.

CLINICAL PRESENTATION

The mode of presentation largely reflects the primary site of the tumor and the associated pattern of dissemination. Prostatic origin is the most common, and these tumors generally present as large pelvic masses palpable on abdominal and rectal examinations. Strangury may or may not exist, although some degree of bladder outlet obstruction is present in virtually all children. Just as the mass may extend into the bladder and urethral lumens, the tumor may encroach on the rectum and cause obstipation.

Bladder rhabdomyosarcomas commonly arise from the bladder neck or trigone, which understandably may make them difficult to distinguish from a mass arising primarily from the prostate. The tumors tend to grow into the bladder cavity, so in addition to the symptoms of outlet obstruction, the children may experience hematuria or passage of mucosanguineous material.

Tumors arising from the vagina occur almost exclusively in the very young, whereas cervical or uterine rhabdomyosarcomas occur more commonly in older girls. There may be an associated bloody or mucosanguineous discharge not unlike that seen secondary to foreign bodies. The mass itself may protrude through the introitis.

Paratesticular rhabdomyosarcomas generally present as painless testicular or inguinal enlargement, and may be indistinguishable from primary testis tumors.

DIAGNOSIS

Complete physical examination is imperative, with special attention given to the rectal and pelvic examinations. Voiding cystourethrography (VCUG) often is performed at initial presentation in the evaluation of obstructive symptoms, and will reveal a filling defect in the bladder or prostatic urethra. Intravenous pyelography often reveals upper tract dilation secondary to bladder outlet obstruction and/or elevation of the bladder base. Once a pelvic rhabdomyosarcoma is suspected, a biopsy must be performed to obtain a tissue diagnosis. Biopsy may be performed during cystourethroscopy/vaginoscopy, or by a transrectal or transperineal approach.

Regarding scrotal or inguinal masses, an ultrasound examination is recommended and testis tumor markers should be drawn because testis tumors are far more common. Radical inguinal orchiectomy should follow.

Blood samples should be obtained for a complete blood count and serum chemistries, including electrolytes, urea and creatinine, liver function studies, and calcium, phosphorus, and uric acid levels (in anticipation of chemotherapy). Clinical staging is gained via computerized tomography (CT) of the chest, abdomen, and pelvis with or without ultrasonography. Retrograde filling of the bladder with contrast can help define the involvement of the bladder wall. Bone marrow aspirates and biopsies are necessary even in the absence of obvious metastases or an abnormal blood count/smear. A bone scan or skeletal survey is recommended as well.

Pathologic confirmation of rhabdomyosarcoma can be based on finding cross striations reminiscent of skeletal muscle; however, this is often difficult with the standard stains. Immunocytochemical diagnosis currently provides the most valuable and reliable means to identify rhabdomyosarcomas, the most common of which use antibodies directed against desmin or muscle-specific actin.

The rhabdomyosarcoma then must be classified as to subtype, which is of utmost clinical importance because subtype predicts clinical behavior and response to therapy. There are basically four subtypes: embryonal, botryoid, alveolar, and pleomorphic. Embryonal tumors present considerable cytologic variability, are characterized by abundant myxoid stroma with a dominant spindle cell component, and mimic the various stages of striated muscle morphogenesis. Botryoid rhabdomyosarcomas occur less commonly and represent an embryonal variant. The embryonal and botryoid tumors carry intermediate and good prognoses, respectively, and together comprise the category of favorable histology. Alveolar tumors have a macroscopic honeycomb appearance akin to the lung, which is the result of interlacing strands of fibrovascular stroma. These tumors represent an unfavorable histology and carry a poor prognosis. The pleomorphic tumors occur almost exclusively in adults and are discussed no further.

Treatment and prognosis are strongly influenced by the clinical group or extent of disease at the initiation of chemotherapy. The site of the primary tumor will determine the clinical presentation, pattern of dissemination, surgical resectability, and the locoregional tolerance for radiotherapy. As stated above, alveolar histopathology bodes poorly for the patient as well.

TREATMENT

Significant progress has been made in the treatment of rhabdomyosarcomas since the organization of the Intergroup Rhabdomyosarcoma Study (IRS) in 1972. Current treatment algorithms are based on the cumulative work of IRS, I, IRS II, and IRS III. The most consistent and successful results generally are seen when employing a multimodal approach, starting with chemotherapy, followed by radiotherapy and surgery thereafter. Chemotherapy is based on the premise of multiagent therapy combining as many drugs as possible to avoid multidrug resistance.

Vincristine, actinomycin D, and cyclophosphamide in combination (VAC) are the mainstay of current chemotherapy. Current recommendations are as follows, with modifications as determined by clinical group, primary site, and histology. Confirmatory incisional or cystoscopic biopsy is followed by pulse VAC for 8 weeks. Tumor response to primary chemotherapy is monitored closely by CT, VCUG, and cytoscopy/vaginoscopy.

Interval biopsies of residual tumor are obtained as necessary. A complete or partial response to induction chemotherapy mandates another 8 weeks of pulse VAC, which is to be followed by repeat biopsy or surgical excision. If no residual tumor is found, a 2-year course of pulse VAC is completed. If residual disease is confirmed, the 2 years of pulse VAC is supplemented by age-adjusted radiotherapy. If the initiating 8-week cycle of VAC fails to produce better than 50 per cent tumor regression, one should proceed to a partial cystectomy when possible. In the event that bladder-sparing surgery is impossible, radiotherapy should be initiated followed by a repeat biopsy at 6 months. Anterior exenteration or partial cystectomy when feasible then is performed. Nerve-sparing techniques can be applied to both the prostatectomy and the cystectomy when the tumor anatomy permits. Complete excision with clear margins warrants 2 years of pulse VAC. The persistence of gross or microscopic disease demands additional radiotherapy plus 2 years of pulse VAC.

Children with nonmetastatic bladder and prostate sarcomas had overall 73 per cent 3- and 5-year survival rates according to IRS-II. Treatment of nonbladder and prostate genitourinary tumors yielded 83 and 80 per cent 3- and 5-year survival rates, respectively. A major objective of IRS-II was to preserve a functional bladder without compromising survival. Despite comparable 3-year survival rates between IRS-I and IRS-II, the 3-year disease-free survival rate in IRS-II was 52 per cent versus 70 per cent in IRS-I. By protocol design, bladder salvage rates initially were much higher in IRS-II (97 per cent) than in IRS-I (58 per cent); however, IRS-II failed to show any improvement in bladder salvage rates at 3 year compared to IRS-I (22 per cent in IRS-II and 23 per cent in IRS-I). The need for more effective treatment in children with rhabdomyosarcomas of the bladder or prostate is obvious if progress is to be made in the fight to retain the bladder. Radical cytoprostatectomy currently is deferred until induction chemotherapy and radiotherapy have clearly failed and viable cancer remains that is not amenable to partial cystectomy.

IRS-IV currently is investigating the efficacy of VAC versus vincristine and actinomycin D combined with ifosfamide (VAI) versus vincristine and ifosfamide combined with etoposide (VIE) in an effort to replace cyclophosphamide. The search for an improved multiagent front-line therapy is continuing to evolve through the efforts of the IRS. Tremendous room for improvement remains regarding therapies for children who escape initial control or suffer recurrences.

Paratesticular rhabdomyosarcomas are best considered as a separate entity from other genitourinary sarcomas. The mainstay of treatment for paratesticular rhabdomyosarcomas remains radical inguinal orchiectomy. These paratesticular tumors are more likely to spread via the lymphatics, with retroperitoneal nodal disease occurring in approximately 30 per cent of cases. The pattern of spread to retroperitoneal nodes is identical to that which occurs with germ cell tumors of the testis. The IRS recommends performing an ipsilateral retroperitoneal node dissection, which should preserve ejaculatory function; however, there is increasing controversy regarding the necessity of node dissections with localized disease when clinical staging is negative for nodal involvement.

Patients with low-stage disease currently are treated with retroperitoneal node dissection and 2 years of adjuvant VAC chemotherapy. Patients with gross nodal disease in the retroperitoneum or distant metastases receive primary cytoreductive VAC chemotherapy, which is followed by lymphadenectomy and radiotherapy.

Suggested Readings

Maurer HM, Gehan EA, Beltangady M, et al: The Intergroup Rhabdomyosarcoma Study-II. Cancer 71:1904–1922, 1993.

Raney RB, Gehan EA, Hays DM, et al: Primary chemotherapy with or without radiation therapy and/or surgery for children with localized sarcoma of the bladder, prostate, vagina, uterus, and cervix: A comparison of the results in Intergroup Rhabdomyosarcoma Studies I and II. Cancer 66:2072–2081, 1990

Raney RB, Hays DM, Tefft M, et al: Rhabdomyosarcoma and the undifferentiated sarcoma. *In* Pizzo PA, Poplack DG (eds): Principles and Practice of Pediatric Oncology, 2nd ed. Philadelphia, JB Lippincott, 1993, pp 769–794

Shapiro E, Strother D: Pediatric genitourinary rhabdomyosarcoma. J Urol 148:1761–1768, 1992

NEPHROGENIC ADENOMA

DONALD E. NOVICKI, M.D.

Scottsdale, Arizona

Nephrogenic adenoma is a benign tumor usually found in the urinary bladder but occasionally encountered in the urethra and ureter. There is a single report of the tumor developing in an ileal conduit. The term "nephrogenic adenoma," which is somewhat a misnomer, was coined by Friedman and Kuhlenbeck because of the histologic similarity of the lesion to renal tubules. Early authorities postulated that the lesions represented redifferentiation of bladder epithelium derived from mesoderm of the caudal portion of the mesonephric duct. Subsequent reports of lesions occurring throughout the lower urinary tract and the strong association of the disease with external irritative factors shed considerable doubt on the embryologic theory of pathogenesis. Mostofi's theory of metaplastic transformation of urothelium better fits the current concept of the process.

INCIDENCE

Cases have been reported in individuals ranging from the first to the eighth decades of life, but most commonly the disease occurs in mid-life. There is a male predominance in adults, but in children females outnumber males by about a 3:1 ratio. Approximately 300 cases have been reported; the bladder trigone and posterior and lateral walls most commonly are involved.

Presentation

The lesions have been discovered occasionally in asymptomatic individuals, but irritative bladder symptoms and hematuria are the most common presenting symptoms. Infrequently, the disease is discovered during evaluation for a bladder filling defect, which rarely may cause ureteral obstruction. The clinical presentation most often suggests a diagnosis of urinary tract infection or bladder malignancy. A key historical factor is the association of nephrogenic adenoma with external or surgical trauma, recurrent urinary tract infections, prolonged catheter drainage, and bladder calculi. The recent literature suggests an association with renal transplantation, possibly implicating compromised immunity as a causative factor. The lesions usually are discovered by cystoscopy. Their appearance varies from yellow-tan to pink polypoid or papillary structures that often mimic transitional cell carcinoma. Sometimes flat to slightly raised erythematous patches with a velvety appearance resembling carcinoma in situ are present. The lesions may be solitary or multiple and occasionally are widespread. Biopsy provides a definitive diagnosis.

HISTOPATHOLOGY

The histopathologic findings are characteristic. The surface epithelium is often cuboidal but may be transitional. Tubular or glandular structures resembling renal tubules are within an edematous stroma. These structures are lined by cuboidal epithelium with a granular, eosinophilic cytoplasm and have a hyalinized basement membrane. In mesonephric carcinoma, basement membrane hyalinization is absent, and this feature serves to distinguish these entities. Surface urothelium adjacent to the lesions often shows changes of chronic cystitis or cystitis cystica.

TREATMENT

The usual management is transurethral biopsy and resection of all visible lesions. Long-term follow-up suggests that recurrent tumors develop in about one half of patients and multiple recurrences will be manifest in about 25 per cent. Most authorities suggest periodic surveillance cystoscopy similar to the follow-up provided for individuals with bladder cancer. Aggressive surgery, including partial and total cystectomy, has been employed in unusual cases when multiple bulky lesions, frequent recurrences, or incapacitating symptoms are present. Nephrogenic adenoma has been associated with transitional cell carcinoma of the bladder three times, with adenocarcinoma of the bladder twice, and with squamous cell carcinoma once. There is no convincing evidence in any of these cases that the malignancy developed as a result of transformation of the nephrogenic adenoma. Careful and prolonged follow-up is suggested because of this association.

SUMMARY

Nephrogenic adenoma is a curious, benign neoplasm most likely arising as a metaplastic transformation of urothelium secondary to chronic irritation or as a result of an immunocompromised host. All ages and sexes are affected, and the clinical presentation most often mimics bladder malignancy. Endoscopic removal of the lesions provides diagnosis and in most cases definitive treatment. Because of an uncertain long-term natural history and because of a weak association with bladder malignancy, periodic indefinite follow-up is advised.

Suggested Readings

Gonzalez JA, Watts JC, Alderson TP: Nephrogenic adenoma of the bladder: Report of 10 cases. J Urol 139:45, 1988

Mostofi FK: Potentialities of bladder epithelium. J Urol 71:705, 1954

Ritchey ML, Novicki DE, Schultenover SJ: Nephrogenic adenoma of bladder: A report of 8 cases. J Urol 131: 537, 1984

CARE OF PATIENTS FOLLOWING URINARY DIVERSION

KATHERINE F. JETER, Ed.D., E.T.

Spartanburg, South Carolina

There are now several options available for patients whose diseased or defective bladder requires urinary diversion. The choice of which diversion offers optimal quality of life to the patient will be based on a variety of factors, including the patients' diagnoses, gender, age, mental and physical abilities to understand and perform the self-care requirements of the procedure, and access to a particular operation. In some areas of the country, an adult with bladder cancer has only one option—an ileal conduit—because that is the only procedure being performed by urologists in that locale. Conversely, in a large university setting, patients may be presented with two or three options and require extensive instruction and counsel before making a choice. It is usually helpful for prospective patients to meet someone of the same sex and within the same age range who has had the proposed operation. There are questions of a practical nature that can be answered best by someone who has experienced living with a new and different method of urinary excretion. Clinical experience has demonstrated that patients usually ask different questions of physicians, nurses, and fellow patients or lay people. All of the questions are equally important to the patient, so it is desirable to provide information from each of these resources.

PRINCIPLES OF TEACHING

Whether the patient will have a conventional urostomy, continent urostomy, or continent reservoir to the urethra, perioperative teaching principles are the same. Most lay people are unfamiliar with normal urinary function. To facilitate their understanding of how they will function postoperatively, it is imperative to clarify how the normal kidneys and bladder make, store, and eliminate urine. This is easily presented with simple line drawings. The diversion or choice of diversions then can be illustrated. The changes in life-style and the care requirements are easier to explain in terms of comparison to the normal, healthy process. As an example, without explanation and demonstration, patients are likely to be very alarmed by the presence of threads of mucus in the urine which will occur when intestinal segments are used for any of the diversions. Once normal function has been reviewed, the details of the newly created system and the reason for the presence of mucus will be easier to understand.

How and when information is presented is critical to learning. Booklets, videotapes, and preoperative instruction in the home or in an outpatient setting are useful adjuncts to the surgeon's initial explanation. Research has shown that the average American reads at the fifth to seventh grade level. Illiteracy in some parts of the country is fairly common. Thus, all printed patient education materials should be screened carefully to ascertain that they will be understandable. Video has become an increasingly popular means of teaching because it is a familiar medium for patients, and it allows patients to view programs with family members who may not be available when the doctor is making explanations. Furthermore, the versatility of computer graphics in video programs has made it easy to show how the urinary system will be revised and the postoperative care that will be needed without showing actual surgical procedures or frightening pictures.

The stressors associated with the diagnosis of cancer, the effects of general anesthesia, and postoperative pain combine to interfere significantly with knowledge acquisition and retention. Instruction periods should be kept brief and information should be repeated frequently. Patients and families should be required to demonstrate some self-care skills prior to discharge, and instruction must be continued postoperatively in the patient's home, the physician's office, or a clinic setting. Patients need to know what supplies they will be required to purchase, where they can be obtained, and when to reorder. Arrangements must be made for them to pay for their equipment or for it to be provided. Reimbursement varies from state to state. Medical social workers, discharge planners, medical supply stores, enterostomal therapy nurses, and members of the United Ostomy Association are usually the best sources of information about products, retail outlets, and reimbursement issues.

CARE OF AN ILEAL CONDUIT

Stoma Site Selection

Vital to patients' acceptance and a satisfactory quality of life with a conventional urostomy is the placement and configuration of the stoma. The site should be selected prior to surgery with the patient examined in all postural positions. Ideally, the stoma is situated well below the belt line and far enough from the ileac crest, the midline incision, and the pubic bone or pubic hair that there is a smooth surface on which the pouching system can be seated. Skin folds and pre-existing scars must be avoided. A stomal bud that protrudes ¼ to ½ inch will ensure that urine flows from the tip of the stoma directly into the collecting pouch, rather than seeping out onto the skin, causing pouch leakage and skin irritation. The use of subcuticular or removable monofilament nylon sutures at the mucocutaneous junction is another detail that makes stomal care easier in the early postoperative period and prevents troublesome scarring in the extended postoperative period.

Pouching Selection

The most common type of management system used today is a one- or two-piece pouch with a pectin-based wafer that adheres to the skin (Fig. 1). The stomal opening is precut or is fashioned with scissors to the exact size of the base of the stoma. The tacky, water-soluble pectin amalgam is safe for most skin types and the incidence of allergy or reaction is rare. However, contact with urine melts the amalgam, and the pouching system should be changed regularly, every 3 to 7 days, to prevent leakage and maceration of the peristomal skin.

Other options are a disposable pouch with an adhesive surface ready for application and a nonadhesive urostomy appliance held in place with a waist belt and a soft silicone O-ring encircling the stoma (Fig. 2).

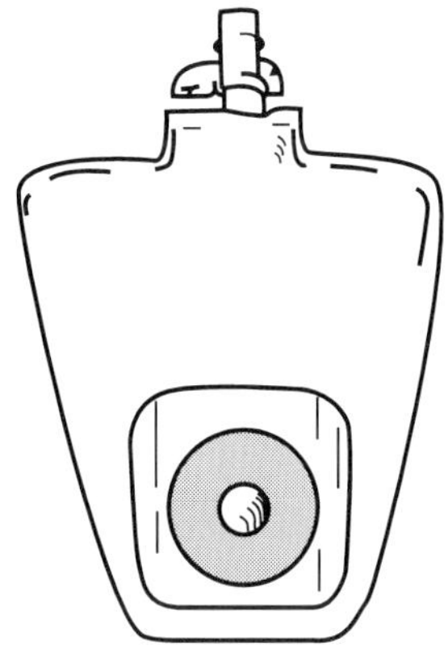

FIGURE 1. One or two-piece pouch with pectin amalgam.

Stomal Care

Patients who wear a urostomy appliance should use gravity drainage during extended periods of recumbency to direct urine away from the stoma and into a leg or bedside drainage bag. This protects the stoma from the damaging effects of prolonged contact with urine, which often results in urine crystal

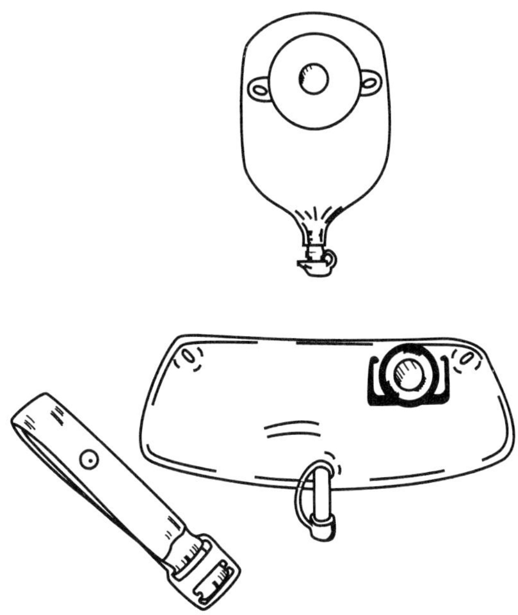

FIGURE 2. Disposable pouch with (*A*) adhesive surface (*B*) nonadhesive urostomy appliance held in place with a waist belt.

formation, stomal irritation and bleeding, and stomal stenosis.

The importance of maintaining a dilute urine should be emphasized. Highly concentrated, alkaline urine is more irritating to the stomal mucosa. Ample fluid intake, including cranberry juice, will help maintain a dilute urine. In a novel study in the United Kingdom, daily intake of cranberry juice also was shown to reduce mucus formation in the conduit urine. If the conduit urine remains alkaline, ascorbic acid may be indicated. For adults, as much as 1 gm four times daily may be required and for children as much as 250 mg three or four times daily may be needed to acidify the urine to the desired pH of 6.0. Patients should be instructed to check their urine pH with Nitrazene paper. The Nitrazene strip should be put into a droplet of urine and not directly on the stomal mucosa to assure accuracy of the test.

When patients are scheduled for routine examinations that include urinalysis and culture, or when an infection is suspected, the urine pouch should be removed and the stoma and skin should be cleansed gently. The stoma should be catheterized using aseptic technique. When urine is collected directly from the pouch, as happens frequently in doctors' offices, in emergency rooms, and on general hospital units, the bacterial count will be unreliable.

During warm weather and when patients are on antibiotics, fungal rashes under the pouch and around the stoma are a common occurrence. A prescription-strength antifungal powder or cream should be prescribed to be applied sparingly each time the pouch system is changed. Ointments and creams used too liberally will interfere with adhesion of the pouch.

Patients should be taught to recognize the signs and symptoms of urinary tract infection, such as flank pain, malodorous urine, nausea, vomiting, fever, and fatigue, and to report them to their urologist immediately. They should go to the office or clinic prepared to remove their pouch to give a specimen and replace a new pouch.

Resuming preoperative activities and hobbies becomes of paramount importance as patients recover from their operation. Bathing, swimming, sports, sexual intimacy . . . how to treat the stoma and the pouch system during these activities is an understandable question. Normally patients shower and bathe without any stomal covering on the days they are changing their pouch. They wear their pouch during bathing on other days. A collection device always is worn when swimming. The majority of males will be impotent after cystectomy. As their interest in intimacy increases in the months following surgery, the use of injections or a vacuum device, or the implantation of a penile prosthesis, can be discussed with the man and his partner.

CARE OF A CONTINENT UROSTOMY

Patient Selection

It would seem reasonable to assume that a continent urinary diversion offers numerous advantages over a conventional ileal or colon conduit and that an internal continent reservoir would always be aesthetically preferable. However, some patients find routine catheterization every 4 to 6 hours and pouch irrigation once or twice daily to clear the pouch of accumulating mucus to be unacceptable requirements. It sounds preferable to live without an abdominal collection device, and for many patients it definitely is, but for some, the trade-offs are more bothersome than changing a pouch once or twice a week, draining it regularly into the toilet during the day, and connecting it to bedside drainage when sleeping.

All facets of each treatment alternative should be delineated carefully and each patient's personality type, emotional resources, and life-style should be matched to the operation's requirements.

Stoma Site Selection and Construction

A urostomy that will not require continuous use of a pouch may be flush with the skin and situated lower on the abdomen, but no less precision is required in selecting the optimal location and in constructing the stoma. The patient must be able to see the stoma to easily insert a catheter into it to drain the urine from the reservoir. Furthermore, in the early postoperative period, and occasionally when the continence mechanism fails, there will be the requirement for a pouching system; thus, preoperative marking of the optimal stoma site is just as important to the patient with a continent urostomy as it is to the patient with a conventional diversion.

Postoperative Care

When all tubes and stents are removed, usually several weeks after surgery, the patient will be required to learn how to catheterize and irrigate the internal pouch. Initially, the reservoir capacity is fairly small and catheterization will be required every 2 to 3 hours while awake and once or twice at night. A 14F to 18F red rubber catheter usually is recommended. A coudé-tip catheter may be helpful to patients who have difficulty inserting a straight catheter. Patients are instructed to wash their hands and the catheter and to moisten the catheter with water or a water-soluble lubricant. They should be instructed to direct the large end of the catheter into a receptacle or the toilet or sink and insert the lubricated tip into the reservoir until urine begins to flow. If they meet resistance as they pass the catheter, they should take several deep breaths, perhaps change position, and continue with gentle pressure. In the first few weeks, the pouch must be irrigated with normal saline every 2 to 3 hours or after each pouch emptying to clear the reservoir of mucus plugs. As the reservoir capacity increases over a span of 3 to 4 weeks, intervals between catheterization are increased. Ultimately, patients with continent urostomies drain their pouch every 3 to 5 hours while awake and irrigate it in the morning and at bedtime or more often when mucus plugs occur.

Catheters are washed and reused. After they have been allowed to air dry, they are stored in Saran bags or a convenient plastic-lined cosmetic or tobacco pouch. Catheters should be replaced with new ones when they become spongy or brittle.

With the Kock pouch, intubation may be more difficult with a full pouch because of the pressure on the nipple valve. Patients should be advised of this. When they cannot successfully intubate their reservoir, they must seek medical attention. Slippage of the nipple associated with the Kock continent diversion has been a problem in up to 20 per cent of patients with this type of diversion. When it becomes difficult or impossible to intubate and drain the reservoir, revision of the nipple is required.

CONTINENT RESERVOIRS TO THE URETHRA

Because continent reservoirs to the urethra often are referred to as a "neobladder" or orthotopic bladder replacement or substitution, this terminology, combined with the surgeon's enthusiasm for the procedure and the patients' limited understanding and their desire to "be normal," can be misleading. Some patients are gravely disappointed that they do not urinate just as they did prior to their surgery. Sometimes they must catheterize to empty their internal reservoir. Incontinence during sleep is not uncommon. Preoperative patient evaluation and thorough instruction are required to ascertain that the patients' expectations are realistic, and that they understand the limitations and differences between a surgically created intestinal bladder and a normal bladder.

FOLLOW-UP CARE

During the early postoperative period, regardless of the type of urinary diversion, patients are followed closely by their urologist. They also need ready access to a nurse specialist who will reinforce pre- and postoperative instruction and be available to answer questions, dispel fears, and resolve management difficulties. In the extended postoperative period, many changes may occur that will impact management and quality of life but may not require surgical consultation or intervention. Skin changes associated with aging, fluctuation in weight, divorce, marriage or remarriage, new sports interests, equipment failure, financial problems—each of these influences may potentiate a crisis for the patient. Patients should be referred to an enterostomal therapy nurse or a medical-surgical nurse clinician with experience in urostomy care. Because far fewer urinary diversions than fecal diversions are performed, not all of these nurse specialists have experience in the management of the various urinary diversion. Occasionally, patients will be required to travel to another center for assistance and should be helped to find the care they need.

ADDITIONAL RESOURCES

In addition to nurses who specialize in rehabilitation of persons with stomas, the American Cancer Society (1559 Clifton Road NE, Atlanta, GA 30329-4251), the United Ostomy Association (36 Executive Park, Suite 120, Irvine, CA 92714), and some of the product sales representatives and medical suppliers can provide information and assistance.

Children with urinary diversions may derive great benefit from attending a summer Youth Rally especially for young people with ostomies. This event is sponsored cooperatively by the United Ostomy Association and the Wound, Ostomy and Continence Nurses Society (National Office, 2755 Bristol Street, Suite 110, Costa Mesa, CA 92626). Youngsters are supervised by counselors who have ostomies and nurse specialists. They are encouraged to learn or improve self-care, and draw from school and social experiences of other young people with similar conditions.

SUMMARY

Care and rehabilitation of adults and children who require urinary diversion is a continuing process that should be shared by urologists, nurse specialists, and the patients themselves to minimize postoperative complications and maximize quality of life. Use this checklist to ensure that all perioperative needs have been anticipated and met:

1. Do the patient and the family understand the diagnosis and the proposed operation?
2. Is the patient mentally, physically, and emotionally competent to manage the requirements of a conventional or continent urostomy or a neobladder?
3. If there will be an abdominal stoma, have provisions been made for the stoma site to be marked prior to surgery with the patient in all postural positions?
4. Are the patient and the patient's family prepared for all of the tubes and drains and what will happen in the immediate postoperative period?
5. Is someone designated to teach the patient and the patient's family prior to hospital discharge?
6. Does the patient know what supplies are required and where to get them? Have financial arrangements been made for their purchase?
7. Has a visiting nurse or nurse specialist been scheduled for home and outpatient follow-up?
8. Has a referral been made to the United Ostomy Association?
9. Does the patient know which signs and symptoms to report to the urologist and which ones to report to the nurse specialist?
10. Have individualized written instructions and supplemental educational materials been provided for each patient prior to discharge and did those materials actually accompany the patient into the home?

Finally, patients now have several options when a diseased or dysfunctional bladder must be removed or bypassed. No single method of diversion has yet been shown to be ideal for all patients. The key to patients' acceptance of their treatment and their return to a satisfactory life-style depends on the course of their disease and in large part on the manner in which they are prepared for and followed after their diverting procedure.

Suggested Readings

Hampton BG, Bryant RA: Ostomies and Continent Diversions: Nursing Management. St. Louis, Mosby-Yearbook, 1992

Klein EA: Options in the surgical treatment of bladder cancer. J ET Nurs 19:122, 1992

SECTION 5

THE PROSTATE AND SEMINAL VESICLES

Prostate Inflammation and Infections

PROSTATITIS

LINDA M. DAIRIKI SHORTLIFFE, M.D.

Stanford, California

The term "prostatitis" has been used to describe vague symptoms of perineal aching, ejaculatory and voiding disturbance, and low back pain. With knowledge of special fractionated urine specimens, microscopic examination of the prostatic fluid, and prostatic immunology, prostatitis may be divided into at least three separate categories: acute and chronic bacterial prostatitis, nonbacterial prostatitis, and prostatodynia. Patients with acute or chronic bacterial prostatitis have documented bacterial infections of the prostate, which are usually caused by gram-negative organisms—*Escherichia coli, Enterobacter, Serratia, Klebsiella, Pseudomonas,* or *Enterococcus.* Those with nonbacterial prostatitis have evidence of prostatic inflammation but no signs of bacterial infection. Those with prostatodynia have complaints associated with prostatitis without signs of bacterial infection or true prostatic inflammation. Because treatment of these three entities differs, differentiation among them is important. Fractionated urine specimens and microscopic examination of prostatic fluid usually will distinguish among these syndromes.

Fractionated urine specimens as originally described by Meares and Stamey remain the hallmark of the diagnosis of true bacterial prostatitis. In the circumcised patient, the urine specimens are collected without special skin preparation; in the uncircumcised man, the foreskin is taped back and the meatus is cleaned with soap and dried. In either case, after the patient thinks that he has a full bladder, he is asked to void, and the examiner collects four specimens for quantitative bacterial cultures:

1. The first 5 to 10 ml voided to show urethral organisms (voided bladder-1; VB_1).
2. A midstream specimen to show bladder specimens (voided bladder-2; VB_2).
3. Prostatic fluid obtained by prostatic massage for culture and microscopic examination to show prostatic organisms (expressed prostatic secretions; EPS).
4. The first 5 to 10 ml voided after prostatic massage to show a combination of prostatic and urethral organisms (voided bladder-3, VB_3).

For adequate interpretation of growth, 0.1 ml of each specimen (and at least 0.01 ml of prostatic fluid) must be plated for quantitative bacterial colony counting.

Bacterial infection is localized to the prostate if the number of bacterial colonies cultures from the EPS or VB_3 is at least 10 times greater than that found in the urethral VB_1 specimen. The bladder urine (VB_2) should be sterile at the time of localization. Isolated examination and culture of prostatic fluid alone (or even cultures of prostatic fluid and bladder urine) cannot be used to diagnose bacterial prostatitis because urethral organisms may contaminate the prostatic fluid specimen during collection and cause misleading results. In particular, urethral and skin commensals such as staphylococcus, streptococcus, diptheroids, and possible *Ureaplasma* and *Chlamydia* may contaminate these specimens.

Microscopic examination of the prostatic fluid will define patients with prostatic inflammation. In patients with nonbacterial prostatitis and acute and chronic bacterial prostatitis, prostatic inflammation usually is shown by the presence of more than 15 leukocytes and occasional oval fat macrophages per high-power microscopic field (magnification 400 to 450 times) of prostatic fluid. It has been reported that as many as 20 per cent of new patients presenting to a general urology office have evidence of prostatic inflammation as defined by increased numbers of leukocytes in the prostatic fluid. The majority of these cases are not caused by bacterial prostatitis, and patients with prostatodynia usually do not have abnormal numbers of leukocytes in the prostatic fluid.

In confusing and complicated situations, quantitation of prostatic fluid or VB_3 immunoglobulins and detection of prostatic fluid antibodies against common infecting bacteria can be used to diagnose bacterial prostatitis. These tests are performed in research situations, however, and may not be available routinely.

ACUTE BACTERIAL PROSTATITIS

Men with acute bacterial prostatitis usually complain of a sudden onset of malaise, low back and perineal pain, chills, fever, and obstructive and irritative voiding symptoms, such as dysuria, urinary frequency, and intermittent urinary stream. On rectal examination, there may be a nodular, boggy, or normal-feeling gland that is painful to palpation. A gram-negative bacterial pathogen usually can be cultured from the prostatic fluid and urine. Because of the prostatic pain and risk of disseminating bacteria from an acutely infected prostate into the systemic circulation, however, prostatic massage to obtain fluid should not be performed acutely. The organisms usually can be cultured from the voided urine specimens. When the bladder urine is infected, moreover, the results of EPS cultures are uninterpretable.

These men are usually acutely ill and may need to be admitted to a hospital for treatment with parenteral antimicrobials such as aminoglycosides and ampicillin. Once cultures and sensitivities are obtained, treatment with an orally administered antimicrobial agent that reaches systemic levels to which the organism is sensitive should be continued at full dosage for 2 to 4 weeks to prevent the development of chronic bacterial prostatitis. The severe prostatic inflammation in acute bacterial prostatitis allows many antimicrobial agents that would ordinarily be excluded from the prostate gland to enter it in concentrations sufficient to cure the infection. In fact, perhaps as a result of this, acute bacterial prostatitis is the most successfully treated of the prostatitis syndromes.

Any bladder outlet obstructive symptoms caused by the inflammation and swelling of the infected prostate probably are treated best with a temporary percutaneous suprapubic drainage catheter. A suprapubic catheter prevents further irritation and bacterial colonization of the prostate and urethra that a urethral catheter will cause.

CHRONIC BACTERIAL PROSTATITIS

Men with chronic bacterial prostatitis have a variety of symptoms. Some have chronic perineal aching or low back pain with intermittent bladder irritative symptoms and voiding difficulties; others are almost asymptomatic even when bacteriuric. Prostatic examination usually reveals a gland that feels normal. The most common characteristic of such patients is a history of recurring urinary infections caused by the same organism, because the prostate acts as a nidus for the bacteria. Routine courses of antimicrobial therapy clear bladder infections only temporarily while the patient is taking the drug; when the antimicrobial agent is stopped, the prostatic bacteria reinfect the bladder. Men who have bacteriuria must have their urinary infection treated before lower tract fractionated urinary specimens for quantitative bacterial localization are collected. This may be done by treating with antimicrobial agents such as nitrofurantoin, tetracycline, and other agents that do not ordinarily enter the prostatic fluid in significant concentrations. After the patient has taken the drug for several days and a midstream urine culture shows no growth, the fractionated urinary specimens may be collected. To make a diagnosis of bacterial prostatitis, both prostatic fluid leukocytosis and bacterial localization to the prostate must be found. When prostatic fluid is difficult or inconvenient to obtain after transurethral resection of the prostate or other urethral surgery, VB_3 culture (compared with VB_1 culture) or antibody levels against commonly infecting organisms may be diagnostic.

Over the last few years the number of antimicrobial agents that may be useful for treating chronic bacterial prostatitis has increased. To be effective, an antimicrobial agent must diffuse into the prostate gland and prostatic secretions in concentrations adequate to eradicate the organism responsible for the infection. Few drugs have been demonstrated to be actively secreted into the prostatic fluid, but trimethoprim is one. Trimethoprim-sulfamethoxazole (160 mg/800mg twice a day), carbenicillin indanyl sodium (764 mg four times a day), and the fluoroquinolones (ciprofloxacin and norfloxacin) taken for 30 to 40 days have been reported to cure some patients when the bacteria is sensitive to the drug. If these drugs fail, a parenteral course of aminoglycoside (gentamicin or tobramycin) for 10 days occasionally has been successful. Because therapeutic failure may be due to infected prostatic calculi, daily low-dose antimicrobial therapy with a drug to which the organism is sensitive (such as nitrofurantoin 50 or 100 mg a day or trimethoprim-sulfamethoxazole 40 mg/200 mg a day [half a single-strength tablet] may prevent relapse of bladder infections and render the patient asymptomatic by suppressing bacteriuria.

If infected prostatic calculi as demonstrated on radiograph or prostatic ultrasound are responsible for chronic infection, radical transurethral resection of the prostate or total prostatectomy may cure the infection if the calculi are in areas that may be removed. Unfortunately, these calculi are often in locations incompletely removed with transurethral surgery, and the side effects of surgery and suboptimal success rate may render this therapeutic option unacceptable to many men with bacterial prostatitis. Oral zinc has not been proven to be useful for treating either bacterial or nonbacterial prostatitis, even though zinc levels in prostatic fluid of men with bacterial prostatitis have been found to be decreased.

NONBACTERIAL PROSTATITIS

Men with nonbacterial prostatitis may present with complaints indistinguishable from those of chronic bacterial prostatitis, but without documented episodes of bacterial cystitis. They usually complain of perineal discomfort and ejaculatory and voiding abnormalities; they have a normal prostatic examination. No single organism has as yet been identified as causing this problem, but elevated prostatic fluid immunoglobulin levels and some data implicating various organisms suggest that some substance or organism may be responsible. *Chlamydia, Ureaplasma,* and various gram-positive organisms have been implicated but no conclusive data have been found. The insignificant prostatic fluid antigen-specific antibody levels against *C trachomatis, U. urealyticum,* gram-positive organisms, and *Bacteroides* in men with nonbacterial prostatitis, however, make a major role for these organisms unlikely. In these men fractionated urinary collections for bacterial localization document no prostatic bacteria, but microscopic examination of the prostatic fluid shows a leukocytosis. It is important in these men, however, to be certain that unusual or fastidious systemic organisms, such as *Mycobacterium tuberculosis,* or fungi, such as *Coccidioides, Histoplasma* or *Candida,* or not causing a pyuria misinterpreted as nonbacterial prostatitis.

Because the etiology of this problem is unknown, therapy is often unsatisfactory. Because chlamydiae and mycoplasmas are difficult to culture and are not routinely sought by most bacteriology laboratories, a therapeutic trial with a tetracycline (doxycycline 100 mg twice a day for 2 or 3 weeks) or erythromycin (500 mg four times a day for 2 or 3 weeks), to which most of these organisms are sensitive, is reasonable. If no improvement occurs, anti-inflammatory agents such as indomethacin or ibuprofen sometimes give symptomatic relief. Complaints of voiding dysfunction may be handled symptomatically. Finally, the patient should be counseled that his prostatic symptoms and inflammation are unrelated to known infections, cancer, or venereal diseases.

PROSTATODYNIA

Men with prostatodynia suffer from a variety of perineal ejaculatory and voiding complaints often indistinguishable from the other syndromes. The prostate feels normal and fractionated urinary collections reveal no prostatic source for bacteria. In addition, there is no history of recurrent bacteriuria. Microscopic examination of the prostatic fluid reveals no inflammation; hence this is not a true "prostatitis." The cause of the symptoms in such patients is not understood. There are some data indicating that psychological disturbance, pelvic and perineal muscle spasm, and abnormal spasm of the urethral sphincter during voiding contribute to the symptoms. Although these patients may have a primary voiding dysfunction, it is important, nevertheless, to evaluate their bowel habits, and perform careful perianal and rectal examination to be certain that their symptoms are not caused by fistulas or other rectal problems.

Because there may be multiple causes for the findings in prostatodynia, no single therapy is effective. Most treatments for the other prostatic syndromes are unsuccessful when applied to patients with prostatodynia because neither inflammation nor infection is present. For patients who demonstrate abnormal sphincter spasm during voiding, a short trial with an alpha-adrenergic blocking agent such as prazosin (1 mg three times a day), phenoxybenzamine hydrochloride (10 mg at bedtime or twice a day), or low doses of a muscle relaxant such as diazepam may produce symptomatic relief. If relief occurs, however, a trial of stopping the drug therapy should occur after awhile, because symptoms in this syndrome tend to be intermittent. These men must be told, moreover, that the symptoms may disappear or reappear without warning. Other symptomatic therapies such as sitz baths and elimination diets also may be useful. Patients with persistent complaints of frequency, voiding discomfort, and suprapubic pain may need cystoscopy to evaluate for the presence of a bladder tumor, carcinoma in situ, or interstitial cystitis or sigmoidoscopy.

Suggested Readings

Barbalias GA, Meares EM, Sant GR: Prostatodynia: Clinical and urodynamic characteristics. J Urol 130:514–517, 1983

Meares EM Stamey TA: Bacteriologic localization patterns in bacterial prostatitis and urethritis. Invest Urol 5:492, 1968

Shortliffe LD, Sellers RG, Schachter J: The characterization of nonbacterial prostatitis: Search for an etiology. J Urol 148:1461, 1992

Shortliffe LD, Wehner N: The characterization of bacterial and nonbacterial prostatitis by prostatic immunoglobulins. Medicine 65:399, 1986

Shortliffe LD, Wehner N, Stamey TA: The use of a solid-phase radioimmunoassay and formalin-fixed whole bacterial antigen in the detection of antigen-specific immunoglobulin in prostatic fluid. J Clin Invest 67:790, 1981

PROSTATIC CALCULI

GRANNUM R. SANT, M.D.

Boston, Massachusetts

PREVALENCE

Prostatic calculi, although infrequent in young men, are common in middle-aged and older men. Plain pelvic radiographs show radiopaque prostate stones in 10 to 15 per cent of men over 50 years of age. However, small stones not visible on radiographs frequently are uncovered during transurethral prostatic resection, and this suggests a much higher incidence of prostatic calculi in elderly men. Indeed, prostatic ultrasound reveals calculi and calcifications in over 50 per cent of men undergoing transrectal ultrasound examination. This finding is confirmed by careful examination of surgical and autopsy tissue, which reveals tiny calculi in nearly all adult prostates.

SIGNIFICANCE

Most prostatic calculi are clinically silent and insignificant. Stones may elicit an inflammatory reaction, and the resulting induration may raise the specter of prostate carcinoma on digital rectal examination. Transrectal ultrasound with ultrasound-guided biopsy may be needed to exclude prostatic adenocarcinoma in such patients. A more significant aspect of prostatic calculi is their association with chronic bacterial prostatitis (CPB) and relapsing urinary tract infections in men. As with infected renal calculi, stones in the prostate can become infected and serve as a nidus for recurrent urinary infections. Infected prostatic calculi can serve as a source of bacterial persistence and relapsing urinary tract infection. Such calculi harbor bacterial pathogens within the stone interstices and, consequently, they cannot be sterilized by antibiotics. Permanent cure of infection can be achieved only by the successful surgical removal of all infected calculi.

Proof that a prostatic stone is infected requires specialized cultures of the crushed stone. Localization of infection to the prostate is accomplished by simultaneous quantitative cultures of urine from the urethra (first voided bladder specimen; VB_1), midstream bladder urine (VB_2), expressed prostatic secretions (EPS), and post–prostatic massage bladder urine (VB_3). These bacteriologic localization cultures confirm the diagnosis of bacterial prostatitis. In the aggregate, men with CBP who also have prostatic stones are less responsive to oral antibiotic treatment than those with CPB but without calculi.

ETIOLOGY

Obstruction of prostatic ducts, especially by nodules of benign prostatic hyperplasia, can lead to ductal dilation, stasis, accumulation of prostatic secretions, and formation of corpora amylacea and prostatic stones. However, intraprostatic urinary reflux now is considered to be the major pathogenetic mechanism for the formation of stones in the prostate. Carbon dye studies of men undergoing transurethral resection of the prostate (TURP) unequivocally demonstrate the presence of such reflux. This is corroborated by the observation that, on crystallographic analysis, many prostate stones contain mineral constituents that are present in the urine rather than prostatic secretions. The current consensus suggests that intraprostatic urinary reflux into the prostatic ducts is important in the formation of prostatic calculi from corpora amylacea.

NONINFECTED PROSTATIC CALCULI

Most prostatic stones are incidental findings discovered by radiography or ultrasound or during prostatectomy. In the absence of infection or bacterial prostatitis, no special treatment is indicated. The prostatic expressate and semen in such patients typically harbor greater than normal numbers of white cells, macrophages, and red blood cells. Hematospermia occasionally can be caused by prostatic calculi.

Prostatic stones do not influence the performance of transurethral prostatectomy. Clusters of stones are not infrequently uncovered during the posterior apical resection on either side of the verumontanum. If these stones are uninfected, no adverse postoperative sequelae occur even if some are left behind in the prostatic tissue.

INFECTED PROSTATIC CALCULI

As with "infection" ("struvite") renal calculi, prostatic stones can become infected and be a source of bacterial persistence and relapsing urinary tract infection. Although urine and prostatic secretions can be sterilized with suitable antibiotic therapy, the sequestered bacterial pathogens within the calculi inevitably reinfect the prostatic fluid and urine. Infected calculi cannot be sterilized completely by antibiotic drugs. The vicious cycle of recurrent infections can be interrupted only if all infected calculi are surgically removed.

A number of options are available for treatment of men with infected prostatic calculi and CBP. Oral antibiotic therapy, especially with the fluoroquinolones, effects clinical and bacteriologic cure in 60 to 70 per cent of patients with CBP. Treatment failure after an appropriate course of antimicrobial therapy (usually 4 to 6 weeks) should alert the clinician to the possibility of infected prostatic stones. For such patients who fail standard therapy, chronic antimicrobial suppression with trimethoprim-sulfamethoxazole (TMP-SMX) (one regular-strength tablet orally each day) or nitrofurantoin (50 to 100 mg orally once daily) is particularly useful in young men who want to avoid transurethral or open prostatectomy. Long-term administration of these antibiotics prevents the development of bladder infections and symptoms, although the prostatic calculi themselves remain infected.

Total prostatectomy seldom is indicated, although it does remove all calculi and is curative. The risks of incontinence and impotence as well as the surgical risks of the operation preclude its widespread application.

TURP can be curative if all infected calculi are removed. To achieve the latter, the resection must extend beyond the false "surgical" capsule to the "true" capsule to remove the infected calculi and tissue from the posterior prostate lobes. Such a "radical TURP" for infected prostatic calculi requires an aggressive resection down to the true capsule and the gland apices—areas with a predilection for stone occurrence.

The risks of bacteremia are real, and appropriate, culture-specific serum levels of antibiotics should be established preoperatively (usually given ½ hour before the resection) and continued for 24 hours postoperatively. The use of an O'Connor drape placed in the rectum is helpful as the resection proceeds to the true capsule. It is obvious that an experienced endoscopic resectionist is critical to the safety and success of a radical TURP. If all infected stones are removed, as documented by plain radiograph or ultrasound, symptomatic and bacteriologic cure can be achieved in upward of 80 per cent of patients. Following a radical TURP, the urine should be sterilized for 3 to 4 weeks with oral administration of an appropriate antibiotic (e.g., TMP-SMX, fluroquinolone). The recovered prostatic calculi should be cultured (by washing and after crushing) to confirm the presence of bacteria within the calculi. The bacteria in the stones are usually identical to the organisms localized to the prostate or cultured from the urine.

Suggested Readings

Barnes RW, Hadley HL, O'Donohue EPN: Transurethral resection of the prostate for chronic bacterial prostatitis. Prostate 3:215, 1982

Kirby RS, Lowe D, Bultitude MI, et al: Intraprostatic urinary reflux: An aetiological factor in abacterial prostatitis. Br J Urol 54:729, 1982

Meares EM Jr: Infection stones of the prostate gland: Laboratory diagnosis and clinical management. Urology 4:560, 1974

Meares EM Jr: Prostatitis syndromes: New perspectives about old woes. J Urol 1123:141, 1980

Sutor DJ, Wooley SE: The crystalline composition of prostatic calculi. B J Urol 46:533, 1974

Prostate Tumors

TREATMENT OF BENIGN PROSTATIC HYPERPLASIA

A. RICHARD KENDALL, M.D.

Philadelphia, Pennsylvania

Although the exact etiology and pathogenesis of benign prostatic hyperplasia (BPH) is unknown, it is obvious that the aging process and the presence of testes are requirements. It has long been recognized that this benign tumor of the prostate does not occur in the male castrated prior to puberty, regresses after castration, and can be hormonally reproduced in animal models. Testosterone is essential for the development of this condition, but BPH may be triggered by growth factors produced by the stroma. Testosterone acts as a prohormone for the formation of dihydrotestosterone (DHT), which is the principal androgen (90 per cent) found in the prostate. Thus, testosterone diffuses into the stromal and epithelial cells and is changed to DHT by 5-alpha-reductase. DHT binds to androgen receptor protein, and this hormone-receptor complex binds to specific DNA sites in the nucleus, resulting in the stimulation of protein synthesis and cell growth. Conversely, androgen withdrawal results in a decrease in protein synthesis and cell death. As the prostate ages, tissue DHT may decrease but there is increased metabolism of androgens toward DHT and increase in nuclear androgen receptors. Thus, as the prostate ages, it becomes more sensitive to androgens that maintain the abnormal size.

Once established, BPH does not grow rapidly, and the size of the prostate is maintained by a combination of cell proliferation and a decrease in the rate of cell death. Prostatic hyperplasia is a combination of stromal and glandular hyperplasia, and it is postulated that, whereas the fibromuscular stromal component of a normal prostate may be 45 per cent, it is increased to over 60 per cent in the hyperplastic gland. Thus, stromal hyperplasia may outstrip that of the glandular cells. There appear to be growth spurts in the prostate from puberty until age 20 and after the age of 40.

Marco Caine postulated that there were two different components involved in BPH. The first was mechanical and was essentially a basic anatomic obstruction that was slowly progressive as the gland enlarged. The second was a dynamic component that varied with sympathetic stimulation. It has been well documented by numerous authors that alpha receptors generally are found in the area of the bladder neck as well as the capsule and smooth muscle of the prostate, and their stimulation or inhibition may alter the dynamic component.

NONINTERVENTIONAL (MEDICAL) THERAPY

At the current time, treatment for BPH can be classified as noninterventional (medical) and interventional (surgical). This first section deals solely with the noninterventional aspects of treatment, which include: (1) alpha-1-adrenergic blockers to reduce tone, (2) antiandrogen therapy to reduce bulk, and (3) observation.

In 1968, Lytton, in a study that has been quoted widely over the years, stated that a 40-year-old man had a 10 per cent chance of needing a prostatectomy by the age of 80. It became apparent over the years that closer to 20 per cent of those individuals may have a prostatectomy, some requiring the operation and an increasing number of patients having undergone transurethral resection for too few symptoms.

The medical treatment of benign prostatic hyperplasia is in its infancy. The obstructive and irritative symptoms of BPH are well known to the reader. Various score systems have been developed that rate symptoms in various categories from 0 to 3 or 5. These categories include urinary hesitancy, intermittency, terminal dribbling(?), decrease in size and force of stream, sensation of incomplete vesical emptying (a symptom heard every day from women), nocturia, daytime frequency, urgency, and dysuria, which by itself is rarely a symptom of prostatism. The American Urological Association has addressed this issue in the November 1992 issues of the *Journal of Urology* and has determined a symptom index.

Once a patient is determined to have significant symptomatology, the decision for interventional or noninterventional therapy must be made. All patients appreciate a conservative physician, and the lesser number of transurethral resections being performed today may not be totally due to the effect of alpha blockers and it is certainly far too early to indict finasteride. We may have simply learned that this disease may stabilize and the symptoms may not be too bothersome or harmful, so that the patient can continue to be observed. Patients have become wiser, and far fewer unnecessary 5-gm transurethral resections are being performed.

When evaluating symptomatology, we must be mindful that there are other causes for irritative symptoms than simple BPH. Thus, carcinoma in situ, urinary tract infections, carcinoma of the prostate, neurogenic bladder disease, and prostatitis all must be excluded. There is no question in my mind that, with aging and prostatic enlargement, there may be a decreased functional capacity of the bladder and increased detrusor irritability, but beware of the assumption that all symptoms are due to BPH, especially in the presence of a strong urine flow.

Alpha-Adrenergic Blockers

Based on the finding of a predominance of alpha-1-adrenergic receptors in the area of the vesical neck and the smooth muscle of the stroma and capsule, the concept of alpha-adrenergic blockade was developed mainly as a result of the pioneering work of Marco Caine. He postulated that variations in tone could result from variations in autonomic stimulation. His original studies were with phenoxybenzamine, which is a nonselective blocker, and more recently we have utilized selective alpha-1 blockers such as prazosin, terazosin, and doxazosin. It is of course difficult to evaluate objectively the results of medical treatment in patients who state they are better from almost the first tablet and yet their flow rate remains unchanged. The placebo effect in medicine may be 15 per cent, but it may be closer to 40 per cent in evaluating patients with voiding symptomatology. Regardless, I believe it is universally accepted that there is significant improvement in over 50 to 60 per cent of patients. It is somewhat easier to explain the improvement in flow than the reduction in irritative symptoms.

At the present time, I begin patients on terazosin 2 mg at bedtime. A very rare patient is highly sensitive and will complain of hypotensive symptomatology. Otherwise, I slowly progress the patient to a maximum dose of 5 mg (some advocate 10 mg) and select a final dose that is the least amount necessary to improve symptomatology. Besides the highly sensitive individual with tachycardia and palpitations, there has only been an occasional complaint of easy fatigability. Discontinuation of medication has mainly been for lack of beneficial effect and in only a very small percentage because of side effects. Thus, I believe that Caine was correct when he spoke of the dynamic component and the ability of alpha blockers to improve symptomatology in many patients. Until now, this has been the successful first-line therapy in patients who require some form of intervention short of operation. Other specific blockers are being developed and should be at least as successful.

Antiandrogen Therapy

For years, research in the medical treatment of BPH has been directed toward some form of hormonal therapy. The long-held hope was that androgen withdrawal would reverse the development of BPH. Over the years, many agents have been tried and most found to have too little value considering the side effects, including hot flashes, loss of libido, impotence, and gynecomastia. Various attempts at androgen ablation to reduce bulk have included:

1. Operative castration, which produced limited improvement and was a tough sell.
2. Medical castration utilizing luteinizing hormone–releasing hormone, which after 4 to 6 months produced a significant decrease in prostatic volume and some symptomatic relief but too many side effects.
3. Antiandrogens such as flutamide, a nonsteroidal antiandrogen that competes with testosterone and DHT for androgen re-

ceptor sites. Several studies reported some improvement in a small number of patients, but too many patients had either gastrointestinal or breast complications. Cyproterone acetate is another antiandrogen that may inhibit pituitary luteinizing hormone secretion as well.

4. Progestational agents such as megesterol acetate, which may inhibit the production of androgens and also produce androgen blockade.

5-Alpha Reductase Inhibitors

All of the above treatments had limited beneficial effects and numerous side effects, and the elderly population as well as urologists anxiously awaited clinical trials of finasteride. A 5-alpha-reductase deficiency had been described clinically in the 1960s, and these males, although virilizing at puberty, had an undeveloped prostate. Thus, it was hoped that finasteride, the 5-alpha-reductase inhibitor, would impair prostatic growth without affecting sexual function. Amidst great publicity, Merck finally released Proscar during 1992. The long-awaited study was multicentered, double-blinded, and placebo-controlled, involving 895 men thought to have urinary obstruction secondary to prostatism. Following the administration of 5 mg of finasteride daily, the initial results can be summarized as follows:

1. Serum testosterone concentrations increased approximately 8 to 10 per cent after approximately 2 weeks of treatment and remained increased thereafter.
2. A significant reduction in prostate-specific antigen occurred, with a mean decrease of approximately 50 per cent. This alarmed many who fervently believed that prostate-specific antigen determination will lead to early diagnosis of prostatic carcinoma and produce improvement in mortality rates.
3. The mean obstructive score decreased from a baseline of 7 to approximately 5.
4. The maximum urinary flow rate after 12 months of treatment increased 3 cc/sec or more in 31 per cent of patients.
5. During the first 6 months, the prostate size decreased progressively, after which it did not significantly change, and at the end of 12 months, the prostatic volume had decreased approximately 19 per cent in the average patient.

At the present time, finasteride is being used widely. It is not yet clear whether it should be begun prior to the onset of symptomatology in the hope of preventing this disease and thus treating 100 per cent of the male population or the physician should await the onset of significant symptomatology and hope that the medication will work as well at this later date and, it is hoped, treat less than 50 per cent of the American population. At the cost of at least $600/year, someone is going to have to answer the question of how much is it worth to improve the flow rate by several milliliters per second and shrink the prostate by 19 per cent. Unfortunately, if this is left to the medical profession, newspapers, and general hysteria of our population, we will have every male on finasteride, and society cannot afford the luxury or expense. At the time of this writing, probably more primary care physicians are prescribing Proscar than urologists.

There may be an alternative, inasmuch as Permixon has been widely utilized in Europe and has been found not only to be a 5-alpha-reductase inhibitor but also to inhibit the binding of DHT to the cell receptors in the prostate, block the uptake of DHT into the cell's nucleus, and inhibit the enzyme 3-alpha-reductase, which also can play a role in prostatic enlargement. It has been reported recently that the berry of the saw palmetto (*Serenoa repens*), a small palm tree indigenous to the Atlantic seaboard from South Carolina to Florida, has the same effects on testosterone metabolism as Permixon. Many men have utilized extracts of *Serenoa repens* purchased as herb medications at health food stores.

Aromatase Inhibitors

It is popular at present to believe that BPH is primarily a disease of the stroma. Estrogen appears to increase stromal growth and, by estrogen inhibition, there is hope that resolution of BPH may occur.

Observation

At the present time, a combination of alpha-1-adrenergic blockers to inhibit the dynamic component and a 5-alpha-reductase agent to potentially decrease the mechanical component appears to be popular among urologists. The medical treatment of BPH is just beginning and, until it is improved vastly, patients with progressive prostatism will continue to be treated with operative intervention. However, *observation* without any therapy is a distinct option in patients with milder symptomatology and no obviously harmful complications. This disease will stabilize in many, thus avoiding long-term "pill-taking" or unnecessary operation. I personally have more patients on observation than any medication, and they are appreciative.

INTERVENTIONAL (SURGICAL) TREATMENT

The medical treatment of BPH is indeed in its infancy, and it is doubtful at this point in time that medications available today will be successful in encouraging patients to take drugs the remainder of their lives. Therefore, various interventional (operative) techniques can be offered to the patient with BPH, including prostatectomy, transurethral incision of the prostate, balloon dilation, microwave hyperthermia or thermotherapy, cryosurgery, prostatic stents, and laser irradiation.

Transurethral Resection

As Nesbit pointed out, transurethral resection became possible with the development of the incandescent lamp by Edison in 1879, the development of the cystoscope by Nitze in 1887, and the development of the high-frequency current by Hertz in 1888. Probably 90 to 95 per cent of men undergoing prostatectomy in the United States have a transurethral resection, with the remainder undergoing enucleation by the suprapubic or retropubic approach.

INDICATIONS

Indications for operation may be absolute, such as urinary retention and hydronephrosis with azotemia. Strong indications include recurrent urinary tract infections with residual urine, and moderate indications include increasing obstructive and irritative symptoms and vesical changes with increasing trabeculation. There remain some questionable indications that are utilized at times for advising prostatectomy; these include increase in size of the prostate, cystoscopic examination revealing a visually obstructing large prostate, decreased flow without significant irritative symptoms, postmicturitional dribbling, and the presence of a hernia or hemorrhoids, which one may misinterpret as secondary to straining to void. A Foley urethral catheter, suprapubic drainage, or intermittent catheterization are all options in poor-risk patients. As noted previously, BPH may cause detrussor irritability with urinary frequency, urgency, and nocturia. One should be leery of advising operation in patients whenever the irritative far exceed the obstructive symptoms.

There are many complications of prostatism that may be prevented by early transurethral resection, but the prophylactic prostatectomy is to be condemned. Vesical decompensation with residual urine, vesical diverticulum, vesical calculi, azotemia with hydronephrosis, and detrussor hyperreflexia all may be secondary to obstructing prostatism.

PREOPERATIVE EVALUATION

There has always been some question of how much evaluation is necessary in the patient with clear-cut prostatism. Obviously a history and physical with an observed or measured urine flow and urinalysis is essential. An intravenous urogram is probably unnecessary in the patient with a normal urinalysis and normal renal function. Cystoscopic examination may be necessary at times to confirm the diagnosis in patients with questionable symptomatology. Urodynamics are unnecessary in the work-up of patients with prostatism unless irritative symptoms are predominant. It is important to realize that one can have true prostatic obstruction without residual urine that represents vesical decompensation. If one is going to check residual urine by catheterization, a simple cystoscopy might provide more information. Ultrasonic determination of residual urine is also useful and noninvasive. In the average patient, the history, physical examination, flow rate, and urinalysis may be all that is absolutely necessary.

The preoperative evaluation should include:

1. Stabilization of renal function.
2. Prevention or awareness of venous disease.
3. Control of infection. The tendency is to overutilize antibiotics. The patient with sterile urine does not profit from prophylactic antibiotics, although the urine can be sterile and prostatic chips culture positive. Patients with documented infected urine must be treated pre- and perioperatively.
4. Routine blood work, including complete blood count, creatinine, prothrombin time, partial thromboplastin time, and bleeding time. These latter tests of the intact he-

mostatic mechanisms may not be essential but are obtained in our institution.

Stool softeners are administered to all patients preoperatively and an enema the night before. Complete medical evaluation is essential inasmuch as these are older individuals, and patients should not take aspirin or any nonsteroidal antiinflammatory drug for preferably 1 week prior to operation. The adjustment to same-day admission has been difficult but doable. It is obvious that the risk factors are presence of renal failure, infection, and a prostate greater than 45 gm.

Prior to operation, *informed consent* is essential. Each surgeon has his or her own descriptive way, but the possibilities of bleeding, urinary tract infection, incontinence, stricture, sexual dysfunction, and retrograde ejaculation should be explained to the patient. Certainly if a vasectomy is to be performed, this should be so noted.

Choice of Operative Technique

The choice of operation depends on many factors.

1. Size of the gland. Today, far fewer truly large glands are seen, and I have believed strongly that the resident finishing his or her training should have experience with over 100 transurethral resections and must feel comfortable resecting at least 80 gm of tissue. This may no longer be achievable.
2. If the bladder capacity is markedly diminished, resection is more difficult, but this can be obviated by a continuous-flow resectoscope of a suprapubic trocar.
3. Calculi can be fractured by electrohydraulic lithotripsy or a lithotrite and the operation still can be performed transurethrally. If the stone is extremely large or hard, the resection still can be performed transurethrally in conjunction with a small incision cystolithotomy.
4. In the presence of a diverticulum, a transurethral resection can be performed and later a diverticulectomy only if there are problems postoperatively. Invariably, even in the presence of a small-mouthed large diverticulum, the patient will have improved voiding with the outlet resistance reduced and have no significant symptoms. With a large narrow-mouthed diverticulum and poor emptying, a diverticulectomy combined with retropubic or suprapubic prostatectomy may be indicated.
5. Urethral strictures can be dilated, incised, or bypassed by a perineal urethrostomy and still a transurethral resection can be performed.
6. There are some who believe that, if an older patient has a hernia, he must have some degree of prostatism and a prostatectomy should be performed prior to a herniorrhaphy. This may lead to a great number of unnecessary transurethral resections. However, an elderly person with an inguinal hernia certainly should be evaluated to see if he has significant prostatism, which, if present, should be corrected prior to the hernia repair. With an extremely large prostate gland, herniorrhaphy can be performed at the time of enucleative procedures.
7. If the hips are immobile, transurethral positioning may be impossible, but this is quite rare and usually one can approach the prostate via a perineal urethrostomy.

Anesthesia

The anesthesia of choice for a prostatectomy is spinal. During a transurethral resection, it allows for relaxation, immobilizes the patient, and yet allows evidence of early perforation and dilutional hyponatremia. Also, spinal anesthesia provides a good 2-hour period of relaxation in the recovery room.

Operation

It has been noted by the Mayo Clinic that 65 per cent of patients have a urethral caliber less than 28F. At the onset of operation, the urethra should be calibrated and dilated, initially by passing a 26F sound and then progressively passing sounds increasing through 30F. If there is a meatal stricture or narrowing, a dorsal meatotomy can be performed with the curved knife blade, producing an excellent cosmetic result. Internal urethrotomy can be performed to provide a urethra adequate for resection, and, in a large gland with or without any narrowing of the urethra, a perineal urethrostomy should be performed. Routinely, a 26F resectoscope should be utilized.

The surgeon must have a game plan, and it is not in the provence of this discussion to teach the reader how to perform a transurethral resection. Having been trained by Reed Nesbit, I personally believe that, with modern optics, resectoscopes, and coagulation units, one should begin at 11:00 to 12:00, isolate the lateral lobes, and totally resect tissue down to the surgical capsule from the vesical neck to apex. In larger glands, one might resect the subvesical, midvesical, and apical regions and then the floor. Water should not be used for irrigation; glycine 1.5% (200 mOsm) is an ideal irrigation solution. During resection, one should fulgurate only individual bleeders, and the resection should be smooth to avoid devascularized tissue. After termination of the procedure, all chips must be evacuated and a 24 Foley urethral catheter inserted. Today, many urologists prefer to use continuous bladder irrigations, with the catheter being removed by the second postoperative day.

COMPLICATIONS

Intraoperative.

Prolonged erection can limit the ability to reach the vesical neck and interfere with the resection. In the past, perineal urethrostomy was the procedure of choice and, at times, Ketamine, nerve blocks, or ice compresses were advocated. At the present time, an intracavernous injection of dilute epinephrine (1:100,000) is most efficacious.

If the *current does not cut*, check to be sure that nonelectrolyte solution is being utilized.

Bleeding is usually arterial, which can be controlled once tissue is resected down to the capsule. Occasionally one must be aware of the ricochet and this is one of the main reasons for having a game plan and not jumping from area to area. Arterial bleeding is bright red and pulsatile, as contrasted to venous bleeding secondary to sinusoids being entered.

An *obturator reflex* more often occurs while resecting bladder tumors, but, when working on the lateral prostatic wall, one may encounter the sudden obturator reflex, which can lead very quickly to perforation. When an overactive obturator reflex is noted, it is best to avoid the area, decrease the current, and use short bursts for fulguration.

Perforation can occur for many reasons but is most common when undermining the trigone or resecting too deep on the roof or lateral prostatic walls. Minor perforations need not trouble the skilled resectionist, but, with deep perforations, one should consider hemostatis and cessation of operation with insertion of a catheter. A cystogram is not always essential and may be positive even when the perforation is minimal and insignificant. When the capsule is widely thinned with probable perforation, antibiotic therapy should be utilized postoperatively. Evidence of perforation includes restlessness, abdominal pain, and nausea and may be similar to the symptoms found in the transurethral resection syndrome.

The *transurethral resection syndrome* is essentially a hypervolemic dilutional hyponatremia secondary to increased absorption of nonelectrolyte fluid (glycine) through sinusoids or areas of capsular thinning. When water was utilized as an irrigant, hemolysis was an additional problem. Cerebral edema leads to increased intracranial pressure with increase in blood pressure, bradycardia, confusion, nausea, vomiting, and visual disturbances. (Sodium is usually below 118 mg/liter at the time of symptoms.) It has been estimated that, during the average resection, 1000 ml of fluid may be added to the vascular compartment. If the irrigation fluid is kept at 60 cm H_2O, allowing adequate visualization, and then raised to 70 cm H_2O, the amount of absorption has been estimated to double. It is now thought that some of the symptomatology may not be due to just hypervolemia and hyponatremia but may be related to the metabolism of glycine, with some aspects of ammonia intoxication. There is no question that there is increased risk of this syndrome in patients with glands over 50 gm and resection time over an hour and a half. The treatment is to immediately decrease intravenous fluids to a keep-open rate and administer diuretics, which suffice in most cases. In some patients with confusion, oliguria, and other more severe symptomatology, the administration of 200 to 300 ml of 3% to 5% hypertonic saline also may be required. It has been our practice for over 35 years to induce diuresis at the time of anesthetic induction. Originally, mannitol was our choice, but Lasix is now used routinely.

Immediate Postoperative (Recovery Unit) Complications.

Ninety-eight per cent of uncontrolled *bleeding* is due to a missed vessel, and the patient should not leave the operating room until the urine is essentially clear. If the bleeding is dark in nature and there are open sinusoids, this venous bleeding usually can be controlled by insertion of a Foley catheter with the balloon distended to at least 50 ml and held on traction against the vesical neck for 3 minutes longer than the bleeding time. If bleeding continues in the recovery room, prothrombin time, partial thromboplastin time, and bleeding time are obtained and, if these are normal, one might consider a re-examination of the prostatic fossa while the spinal anesthesia is still in effect. Almost invariably when endoscopy is repeated, one finds either an arterial pumper, which can be controlled producing immediate clear urine, or clots, which when evacuated result in a satisfactory color to the irrigation fluid.

If one cannot control the bleeding, serum fibrinogen and fibrin degradation products should be obtained. It is very rare to have to explore the patient through a suprapubic approach and pack the prostatic urethra. The causes of bleeding might be local fibrinolysis, which may be treated with Amicar; systemic fibrinolysis, which is more unusual; or disseminated intravascular coagulation, which one can hope to prevent or control by treatment of pre-existing problems such as prostatic carcinoma or urinary tract infection and replacement of clotting factors.

Later Postoperative Complications.

Inability to void usually responds to reinsertion of the catheter for 24 to 48 hours. Retained chips may be a cause. Cystoscopy need not be performed immediately inasmuch as there may be so much edema of the prostatic fossa one would be somewhat visually confused as to the further needs of the patient. Certainly, if there is further difficulty in voiding, urodynamics may be in order unless the patient was known to have a decompensated bladder, necessitating a longer period of drainage. Occasionally resection of residual tissue is necessary.

Delayed bleeding may occur and usually responds to reinsertion of the catheter and evacuation of clots. Occasionally cystoscopy with fulguration may be necessary.

The patient may develop *urinary tract infection.* Sepsis after catheter removal should arouse suspicion of incomplete vesical emptying. The availability of antibiotics has significantly reduced the incidence of epididymitis. Vasectomy is still a valid option prior to instrumentation but is utilized far less than in the past.

Foot drop may be due to improper positioning on the table, with pressure on the peroneal nerve by the stirrups.

Late Complications.

Impotence should be unusual in the patient previously sexually active. The etiology may be damage to the neurovascular bundle in proximity to the prostatic fossa. At times, a definite explanation may be difficult in the elderly patient with infrequent sexual activity preoperatively. The true incidence of this complication is unknown but is probably less than 5 per cent.

Retrograde ejaculation occurs in probably 75 per cent or more of patients and is not a problem when explained preoperatively.

In cases of *recurrent obstruction,* there may be a 7 to 8 per cent need for a second transurethral resection up to 10 years later. The incidence varies with the skill of the surgeon.

Urinary tract infection may be secondary to residual urine, stricture, or an incomplete resection with devascularized tissue.

It is hoped that *urethral stricture* can be prevented by the operative measures discussed, postoperative meatal care, and early removal of the catheter.

Vesical neck contracture frequently is due to too deep resection at the vesical neck, especially in a small gland. The typical presentation is a patient voiding well for 2 to 3 weeks and then experiencing marked dimunition in the force of the stream. This can be treated by dilation or incision and rarely requires an open vesical neck plasty. Intermittent self catheterization may aid in keeping the vesical neck open.

Incontinence may be secondary to vesical hyper-reflexia (urge incontinence) or, more unfortunately, due to vesicosphincter imbalance (stress incontinence). Most incontinence clears within 3 months, but a very small percentage of cases may persist. Quite frequently, one can visually examine the sphincter area and find that it appears perfectly normal, and stress incontinence may be enhanced by a high intravesical pressure. There are times when one can view a defect in the area of the distal internal sphincter (distal to the verumontanum) and yet there is no incontinence.

Other Interventional Techniques

Transurethral resection and prostatectomy have come under great scrutiny because of the large numbers of these operations (400,000) being performed and the subsequent high cost to society. There have been alternatives in the past, but, over the last few years, many newer options have been suggested. However, be the truth known, nothing has so far come close to equaling a properly performed transurethral resection.

It was believed that *transurethral incision of the prostate* would reduce cost and morbidity. This technique essentially involves a Collings knife incision from the area of the trigone just distal to the ureteral orifices through the vesical neck to the verumontanum. The incision should be deep into the prostatic capsule. The indications have been the same as for transurethral resection, but with a gland less than 20 gm and the absence of prostatitis or hematuria. In the younger individual (who very well may not need operative intervention), this may be considered by some because of the lesser incidence of retrograde ejaculation. It is an excellent procedure for treatment of a vesical neck contracture.

Balloon dilation of the prostate exploded onto the scene several years ago and is still searching for a role. Originally, a 70F, then a 90F, and now a 125F balloon has been utilized. There are numerous different technologies, and I believe this will never find a permanent or major role in the urologists' armamentarium.

There are several *permanent epithelializing prostatic stents* on the market, made of stainless steel and titanium, that have various lengths and lumens. At best these will be advocated in extremely poor-risk patients who do not respond to drug therapy or intermittent catheterization.

Microwave hyperthermia (40° to 44° C) or *thermotherapy* (>45° C) initially was performed rectally and now is used transurethrally as technology has developed. It is far too early to judge this technique, and time will tell.

Transurethral laser-induced prostatotomy, vaporization by direct contact, and *visual laser ablation of the prostate* all are in their infancy, and it is far too early to justify the claims of their individual proponents.

Summary

Interventional therapy for prostatic hyperplasia should be avoided when unnecessary. However, in the patient with true symptomatology and potential damage to his health, transurethral resection is still the gold standard to which all alternatives will have to be compared and it has withstood all challenges and the test of time.

Suggested Readings

Dixon CM, Lepor H: LASAR ablation of the prostate. Semin Urol 10:173, 1992

Lepor H, Walsh PC (eds): Benign Prostatic Hyperplasia. Urol Clin North Am 17(3), 1990

Mebust WK: Transurethral surgery. *In* Walsh PC, Retik AB, Stamey TA, Vaughn ED, Jr (eds): Campbells Urology, 6th ed. Philadelphia, WB Saunders, 1992, pp 2900–2922

CARCINOMA OF THE PROSTATE—STAGES A_1 AND A_2

JOSEPH A. SMITH, JR., M.D.

Nashville, Tennessee

According to an American College of Surgeons survey performed in 1982, 26 per cent of patients with adenocarcinoma of the prostate presented with Stage A disease. With the increasing use of alternative treatment for bladder outlet obstruction, the frequency with which Stage A prostate cancer has been diagnosed is diminishing. In addition, many patients who otherwise are candidates for transurethral prostatectomy have a serum prostate-specific antigen level obtained preoperatively. Abnormalities in prostate-specific antigen with subsequent biopsy confirmation of adenocarcinoma identify preoperatively some patients who otherwise would have been diagnosed as having Stage A prostate cancer.

By definition, Stage A tumors are nonpalpable. Increasingly, however, transrectal ultrasonography and prostate-specific antigen levels identify patients with nonpalpable prostate tumors. It is a misclassification to include these patients under the category of "Stage A" lesions. There is no evidence that the tumors identified via prostate-specific antigen abnormalities are the same as those historically detected through transurethral resection of the transition zone of the prostate. Newer staging systems include a category for tumors detected by ultrasound or prostate-specific antigen as opposed to the classic Stage A lesions.

Undoubtedly, some patients with Stage A prostate cancer suffer disease progression and tumor-related death. However, the majority of patients have a tumor that is likely to remain clinically insignificant during their lifetimes. Ideally, a method is needed to predict tumor behavior in an individual patient so that appropriate therapy can be recommended on a case-by-case basis. Although certain features, including tumor grade, volume, ploidy pattern, and serum prostate-specific antigen levels are of some value, none accurately predicts the prognosis in an individual patient. A rational treatment policy should be based on an attempt to spare morbidity for the substantial majority of patients not in need of therapy while selectively applying definitive treatment to those with clinically significant disease.

NATURAL HISTORY OF STAGE A CARCINOMA

The most important factor influencing the management of Stage A carcinoma of the prostate is the predicted natural history of untreated disease. Although there is little information available about the natural history of untreated Stage A_2 carcinoma, a relatively poor prognosis if left untreated is implied by several findings. Some 25 per cent of patients undergoing pelvic lymph node dissection for clinical Stage A_2 carcinoma of the prostate are found to have histologic evidence of nodal metastasis. Also, in patients with Stage A_2 tumors who undergo radical prostatectomy, the significant majority are found to have residual cancer present within the prostate. The tumor diffusely involves the prostate in most of these patients and nearly one third are found to have margin-positive disease.

In contrast, there are several studies suggesting a low rate of progressive disease and an even lower rate of death from carcinoma of the prostate in Stage A_1 disease. Some studies have shown a progression rate with prolonged follow-up of up to 20 per cent of untreated patients with Stage A_1 disease. It should be emphasized, however, that progressive disease does not necessarily equate with death from prostate cancer or even significant disease-related morbidity. Most studies have shown a death rate from prostate cancer of only 1 or 2 per cent in patients with Stage A_1 disease.

DETECTION OF RESIDUAL DISEASE

A frequent concern in patients with Stage A carcinoma of the prostate is that the transurethral prostatectomy may have only sampled the lesion, leaving behind undetected diffuse carcinoma. A clinical concern, then, is how to detect significant residual tumor in patients with Stage A_1 disease. Frequently, a repeat transurethral resection has been used to sample residual tissue. However, our study in 55 patients showed no further tumor in 82 per cent of patients undergoing a repeat transurethral resection for Stage A_1 disease, whereas isolated foci of cancer were found in 14 per cent of patients. None of these patients was reclassified as having Stage A_2 disease. Only 4 per cent of patients had diffuse foci of carcinoma detected, resulting in reclassification as Stage A_2. On the basis of this series, it was concluded that repeat transurethral resection was not a useful procedure in most patients.

Transrectal ultrasound can give information about the internal architecture of the prostate that is not necessarily obtained by digital rectal palpation and may be capable of identifying residual cancer in some patients with Stage A_1 disease. Patients with benign prostatic hyperplasia have enlargement of the transition zone, which compresses the peripheral zone of the prostate, sometimes making it more difficult to interpret by transrectal ultrasound. After transurethral resection, there is an expansion of the peripheral zone. One month after transurethral resection, there is minimal scarring or distortion of the prostate on transrectal ultrasound, although the periurethral defect is apparent. The mixed echo appearance of the transition zone is difficult to interpret either before or after transurethral resection, but hypoechoic areas may be identified that are characteristic of significant residual disease. Furthermore, these patients may have coexistent peripheral zone cancers.

After Stage A_1 disease is detected in an otherwise young and healthy patient, transrectal ultrasound seems indicated. Although there are no good data to support the contention that transrectal ultrasound is able to identify the small number of patients with significant residual carcinoma, representative transrectal core biopsies that sample multiple areas of the prostate should identify carcinoma in the small number of patients with diffuse residual disease.

RESULTS OF DEFINITIVE THERAPY

As with other stages of apparently localized prostate cancer, the primary treatment options for Stage A carcinoma are radical prostatectomy and external beam irradiation. Typically, variations in patient selection, staging, treatment method, and duration of follow-up vary, making comparison of different series difficult. A particular problem is that most radiation series do not distinguish between Stage A_1 and Stage A_2 or, sometimes, between A and B lesions.

Radical Prostatectomy

Important information about Stage A carcinoma of the prostate after radical prostatectomy is determined by calculation of disease-free survival rates but also by examination of the histologic specimen. In our series of 41 patients undergoing pelvic lymph node dissection for Stage A_1 carcinoma, none had histologic nodal metastasis identified. Although the majority of patients do have at least microscopic evidence of residual cancer as well as tumor in the peripheral zone, rarely is significant residual disease left behind after a transurethral resection shows A_1 carcinoma.

The differing prognosis for Stage A_2 cancer compared with Stage A_1 is reflected in the results and findings after radical prostatectomy. A significant number of patients have capsular penetration and up to 25 per cent have margin-positive disease. Even though most of the tumors arise in the transition zone, there frequently is associated tumor in the peripheral zone.

Survival data after radical prostatectomy seemed to justify the procedure in patients with A_2 carcinoma. Nearly two thirds of patients remain alive and free of disease 10 years after radical prostatectomy and cancer death is observed in only around 10 per cent. These results appear to be significantly better than those obtained with expectant management alone.

External Irradiation

There are few studies reporting a minimum of 10 years of follow-up of patients with Stage A_2 prostate cancer treated by irradiation. Also, in many series, adequate staging of the pelvic lymph nodes was not performed, which may adversely affect the results, because patients with positive nodes usually are excluded from radical prostatectomy series. Surprisingly, a recent review showed little difference in survival between patients segregated into Stage A_1 and A_2 categories. This most likely is a consequence of limited follow-up, given the acknowledged differing prognosis between these two groups.

SUMMARY AND RECOMMENDATIONS

Stage A carcinoma of the prostate historically encompasses disease causing no palpable abnormality of the prostate that is discovered incidentally after a transurethral prostatectomy. Transrectal ultrasonography has defined a new group of patients with nonpalpable tumors diagnosed by needle biopsy. How these two groups of patients interrelate remains unclear, and new issues regarding the biologic significance of low-volume disease have emerged.

It is important and pertinent to understand exactly what has occurred when a transurethral resection for presumed benign prostatic hyperplasia shows adenocarcinoma on histologic examination. At autopsy, almost 30 per cent of men over the age of 65 will have microscopic evidence of carcinoma of the prostate if careful examination is performed. A transurethral resection of the prostate is merely an extended sampling of tissue that, by virtue of these figures, is likely to discover incidental cancer in some patients. The sheer weight of numbers suggest that the overwhelming majority of these patients will not die from cancer of the prostate even in the absence of any treatment.

Unfortunately, there is no reliable method to determine the prognosis in an individual patient or to distinguish the small number of patients with incidentally discovered, nonpalpable prostate cancer who are destined to develop disease progression and die from the majority who have biologically and clinically insignificant disease. Emerging recommendations that careful surveillance be employed in some of these patients seem valid and logical, but the success of such a policy in identifying disease progression at a point when intervention is still potentially curative has not been demonstrated. Carcinoma of the prostate is a progressive disease, even when detected at an early stage and with a low volume. Therefore, in a select subgroup of young patients, aggressive treatment is indicated. For the substantial majority, however, a policy of careful evaluation and follow-up seems appropriate.

Suggested Readings

Bagshaw MA, Cox RS, Ramback JE: Radiation therapy for localized prostate cancer: Justification by long-term follow-up. Urol Clin North Am 17:787–802, 1990

Epstein JI, Walsh PC, Eggleston JC: Prognosis of untreated stage A_1 prostate carcinoma: A study of 94 cases with extended follow-up [Abstract]. J Urol 135:242A, 1986

Lowe BA, Listrom MB: Incidental carcinoma of the prostate: An analysis of the predictors of progression. J Urol 140:1340–1344, 1988

Parfitt HE Jr, Smith JA Jr, Gleidman JB, et al: Accuracy of staging an A_1 carcinoma of the prostate. Cancer 51: 2346–2350, 1983

Smith JA Jr, Cho Y: Management of stage A prostate cancer. Urol Clin North Am 17:769–777, 1990

ADENOCARCINOMA OF THE PROSTATE—CLINICAL STAGES B_0, B_1, AND B_2 (T1c, T2a & b, and T2c)

JOSEPH E. OESTERLING, M.D.

Ann Arbor, Michigan

EARLY DETECTION AND DIAGNOSIS

Adenocarcinoma of the prostate is the most common malignancy in men in the United States and the second most frequent cause of cancer deaths. In 1994, it is estimated that approximately 200,000 new cases will be diagnosed and about 38,000 men will die of this condition. Thus, prostate cancer *kills*. At some point in time, each of these life-taking cancers began as a focus in the prostate gland and was organ confined. Because there is no curative therapy for advanced prostate cancer, it is necessary to detect these lesions before extracapsular spread has occurred if we are to have an impact on the mortality rate. Indeed, Jewett has demonstrated that men with organ-confined disease who undergo radical prostatectomy have a survival equivalent to that of age-matched men without prostate cancer.

How, then, do physicians identify clinically significant prostate cancer at an early, organ-confined stage? Based on all data available to date, it appears that the most effective method for detecting early prostate cancer is through the combined use of digital rectal examination (DRE) and serum prostate-specific antigen (PSA). The American Cancer Society, the American Urological Association, and the American College of Radiology recommend that men 50 years of age or older undergo an annual prostatic evaluation consisting of *both* a DRE and a serum PSA determination. However, it is reasonable that this prostatic evaluation be restricted to men with a life expectancy of ten years or more. Given the fact that many prostate cancers are slow growing, there is no value to subjecting an elderly person to either a serum PSA determination *or* a DRE for the detection of early prostate cancer. On the other hand, there are some men who are at high risk for the development of prostate cancer and may benefit from these diagnostic tests earlier than age 50 years. These individuals include African-American men and men with a family history of prostate cancer. There are no definitive data to date to indicate that a previous vasectomy is a risk factor for the subsequent development of prostate cancer. As a result, a recent National Institute of Health (NIH) panel has concluded that "screening for prostate cancer should not be any different for men who have had a vasectomy than for those who have not."

If the serum PSA level (as determined by Tandem-R PSA assay or the IMx PSA assay) is less than or equal to the age-specific reference range (0.0–2.5 ng/ml for men aged 40 to 49 years, 0.0–3.5 ng/ml for men aged 50 to 59 years, 0.0–4.5 ng/ml for men aged 60 to 69 years, and 0.0–6.5 ng/ml for men aged 70 to 79 years) and the DRE is unremarkable, the patient should be followed with annual evaluations; the prostate gland should be assessed for the development of palpable abnormalities, and the serum PSA concentration should be monitored with regard to the "rate of change." If the serum PSA level is greater than the age-specific reference range and the DRE is benign, a transrectal ultrasound should be performed. After assessing the echogeneity of the gland, any visible lesion should be biopsied. In addition, a *systemic*, sextant biopsy of the remaining prostatic tissue should be carried out. If none of these cores contain tissue from the transition zone, two additional specimens, one from each side, from the anterior part of the prostate should be taken in order to completely sample the gland. In the setting of an abnormal DRE, irrespective of the serum PSA level, the patient should undergo a transrectal ultrasound. Using ultrasound guidance, the palpable abnormality should be biopsied as should all hypoechoic lesions. In addition, a *systematic*, sextant biopsy of the remaining prostate gland should be performed. Using this approach to decide whom to subject to a prostatic examination and how to carry out this evaluation should allow the practicing clinician to detect more clinically significant, life-threatening prostate cancers at an early, potentially curable stage.

STAGES OF CLINICALLY LOCALIZED PROSTATE CANCER

When cancer is identified, the patient is assigned a clinical stage on the basis of the findings. This chapter addresses patients with clinically localized prostate cancer that was diagnosed on the basis of a DRE and/or serum PSA determination. Clinical Stage B_0 (T1c) refers to a nonpalpable prostate cancer associated with an elevated serum PSA value; it was the elevated serum PSA level that prompted the subsequent work-up and diagnosis. A clinical Stage B_1 (T2a or T2b) tumor is a cancer that involves less than one entire lobe of the prostate gland by DRE. Clinical Stage B_2 (T2c) denotes a lesion that occupies both lobes of the prostate but is still organ confined.

Stage B_0 (T1c) tumors have pathologic characteristics that are very similar to those of Stage B_1 (T2a or T2b) lesions. In a recent study by Stormont and colleagues, 70 percent of the Stage B_0 (T1c) prostate cancers were organ confined at the time of surgery as compared to 67 percent for the Stage B_1 (T2a or T2b) tumors. The mean tumor volume was 7.4 ml (range: 0.3 to 56 ml) for Stage B_0 (T1c) lesions and 5.1 ml (range: 0.2 to 42 ml) for Stage B_1 (T2a or T2b) cancers. Twenty per cent of the nonpalpable cancers were associated with positive surgical margins as compared to 23 per cent for the palpable tumors. Thus, Stage B_0 (T1c) cancers appear to be of clinical significance and warrant therapeutic consideration, just as do Stages B_1 (T2c) and B_2 (T2a or T2b) prostate cancers.

TREATMENT

The treatment options available for these clinically localized prostate cancers are: (1) expectant therapy, (2) radiation therapy, and (3) radical prostatectomy. Which of these is most efficacious, however, is not known. As of this time, no prospective, randomized clinical trial with adequate follow-up has been completed that compares these three treatments in men with an additional life expectancy of 10 years or more. Until the results of such an investigation become available, it is of utmost importance to inform the patient of the benefits and risks of each treatment option and allow him to be actively involved in deciding on the appropriate therapy.

Expectant Therapy

Because some prostate cancers are slow growing and behave in an indolent manner, it has been suggested that a prudent approach to management is no initial therapy. With this approach, the morbidity and mortality associated with either radiation therapy or radical prostatectomy can be avoided and quality of life preserved. Johansson and colleagues recently reported on 117 patients with Stages B_1 and B_2 prostate cancer who were followed expectantly until symptomatic disease developed; palliation therapy was initiated at that time. The 10-year overall survival rate was 40 per cent, and the progression-free survival rate was 43 per cent. Whitmore and associates, in another study of patients with Stage B prostate cancer who were followed expectantly for greater than 8 years, observed similar findings. In yet another report by Adolfsson and Carstensen on 61 patients with Stage B prostate cancer who received no initial therapy, the probability at 10 years for progressing to Stage C disease was 72 per cent, for developing skeletal metastases was 23 per cent, and for dying of prostate cancer was 8 per cent.

These studies demonstrate that some patients with clinically localized prostate cancer do well without initial treatment. They also serve to emphasize the steady but slow progression of early prostate cancer to advanced, life-threatening disease. Thus, a patient with a limited life expectancy (<10 years) because of advanced age or poor health should be managed in this manner. If local, obstructive symptoms subsequently develop in the absence of systemic disease, a transurethral resection of the prostate can be performed. If symptomatic, systemic disease occurs eventually, androgen deprivation therapy should be initiated. In the interim, the patient can be monitored periodically with DRE, serum PSA, and radionuclide bone scan when indicated.

Radiation Therapy

The first report of using ionizing radiation to treat clinically localized adenocarcinoma of the prostate was by Paschkis and Tittinger in 1910. Since then, a variety of types of radiation therapy have been developed and utilized for this malignancy.

EXTERNAL BEAM RADIATION THERAPY

External beam radiation therapy, utilizing high-energy photons, has enjoyed the most widespread clinical use in recent years. The largest experience with this treatment modality comes from Bagshaw and associates at Stanford University. In a series of more than 900 patients and employing approximately 7000 cGy, they observed a 15-year overall survival rate of 33 per cent for Stage B prostate cancers; the disease-specific survival rate was 45 per cent for all Stage B tumors. Other investigators have reported similar results. However, it must be kept in mind that comparing results of various radiation therapy series is difficult because of the (1) tremendous variation in the treatment regimens utilized at different cancer centers; (2) random, concomitant use of androgen deprivation therapy; (3) lack of accurate pathologic staging, because pelvic lymph node status is not always known; and (4) lack of standardized criteria for determining persistent/recurrent disease in follow-up.

Recently, there has been much enthusiasm for using "fast" neutrons in external beam radiation therapy. Neutron therapy is associated with a more predictable dosimetry, a greater and more immediate impact on cellular DNA, and an improved efficacy in the presence of tissue hypoxia. Preliminary results in patients with locoregionally advanced (Stages C and D_1) prostate cancer showed greater survival and reduced local recurrence rates for the neutrons as compared to conventional photons. Nevertheless, additional properly designed studies with large numbers of patients and extended follow-up will be necessary to delineate the true role of "fast" neutrons in the treatment of prostate cancer.

Complications associated with external beam radiation therapy are most frequently related to the gastrointestinal tract or the lower urinary tract. Approximately 30 to 40 per cent of patients will experience gastrointestinal tract symptoms while undergoing treatment. They are rarely disabling, because 95 per cent of the patients are able to continue the treatment protocol without interruption. Approximately 10 per cent of patients undergoing definitive external beam radiotherapy will have long-lasting gastrointestinal symptoms; these include chronic diarrhea, mucosal ulcers of the rectum, anorectal fistulas, and anal stenosis. Nevertheless, a diverting colostomy is rarely indicated (in less than 1 per cent of the patients), because conservative measures usually are effective in controlling these untoward effects. Genitourinary symptoms also occur in 10 per cent of patients and include urinary frequency, urgency, dysuria, and occasional hematuria. Some degree of urinary incontinence develops in 3 to 5 per cent of patients, and impotency occurs in up to 50 per cent of potent patients on extended follow-up. Finally, the postirradiation incidence of urethral stricture disease is approximately 5 per cent.

INTERSTITIAL RADIATION THERAPY

A variety of radioactive sources have been used for interstitial radiation therapy. These include ^{125}I (iodine), ^{198}Au (gold), and ^{191}Ir (iridium). This treatment modality was explored initially by Whitmore and colleagues at Memorial Sloan-Kettering Cancer Center beginning in 1972. After performing a limited bilateral pelvic lymphadenectomy, ^{125}I seeds were placed in the parenchyma of the prostate gland. At 5-year follow-up, the overall survival rate was 95 per cent for Stage B_1 tumors and 64 per cent for Stage B_2 disease; the 5-year tumor-free survival rate, however, was 66 per cent for Stage B_1 lesions and 30 per cent for the larger B_2 cancers. By 10 years, more than 40 per cent of the patients with Stage B_1 lesions and 70 per cent of the men with B_2 prostate cancers had evidence of tumor progression. These percentages are higher than for similar-stage patients who are treated with radical prostatectomy.

Carlton and colleagues combined ^{198}Au brachytherapy with external beam radiotherapy in an attempt to improve the overall efficacy of radiation therapy; all patients underwent a bilateral pelvic lymphadenectomy prior to receiving the irradiation. The overall and disease-free survival rates at 10-year follow-up were 84 and 54 per cent for Stage B_1 cancers and 52 and 26 per cent for Stage B_2 tumors, respectively. When these results are compared with the findings from series using external beam radiotherapy alone, there is no discernable advantage for the combination therapy.

Most recently, iridium and palladium have been utilized as radioactive sources. After a limited bilateral pelvic lymphadenectomy is performed, these isotopes are positioned in the prostatic parenchyma from the perineum using a template and ultrasound guidance to ensure accurate placement. No long-term results with these radioactive isotopes and technique of placement are yet available.

Complications with any type of interstitial radiation therapy include those routinely associated with pelvic lymphadenectomy and the effect of radiation therapy on adjacent pelvic structures. Although the overall complication rate is minimal and the therapy is technically straightforward to carry out (pelvic lymphadenectomy and placement of radioactive implants into the prostate gland), the long-term efficacy of interstitial radiation therapy has not been demonstrated. As a result, it is not considered a viable treatment option for the younger patient with a clinically significant prostate cancer.

Radical Prostatectomy

Radical prostatectomy was first pioneered as a treatment for prostate cancer by Hugh Hampton Young in the early 1900s. Although considered by many to be the most effective therapy available for localized prostate cancer, it has been associated with significant morbidity. Impotence, some degree of urinary incontinence, and significant blood loss were universal phenomena for patients undergoing this procedure until the recent advancements by Walsh. By more precisely defining the pelvic anatomy, Walsh has been able to modify the technique of radical prostatectomy such that the dorsal vein complex from the penis can be controlled with minimal blood loss, the autonomic innervation to the corpora cavernosa can be preserved to maintain potency, and a direct, mucosa-to-mucosa urethrovesical anastomosis can be accomplished for complete urinary continence. This anatomic approach is applicable to both retropubic prostatectomy and perineal prostatectomy.

For patients with organ-confined prostate cancer, radical prostatectomy is a most effective treatment in terms of both local control and long-term survival. In a report by Walsh and Jewett, the 15-year disease-free survival rate for Stage B_1 prostate cancer was 51 per cent. Gibbons and colleagues at the Mason Clinic reported a 50 per cent disease-free survival rate in patients with clinically localized prostate cancer and treated with radical prostatectomy; for large Stage B_2 prostate cancer, the 15-year disease-free survival rate was 25 per cent. Although direct comparison of these results with those of external beam and interstitial radiation therapy series is not possible, it is believed that the survival rates obtained with radical prostatectomy are as good as or superior to irradiation in the properly selected individual.

It is the opinion of this author that radical prostatectomy should be reserved for the healthy man with an additional life expectancy of 10 years or more who has a clinically localized prostate cancer by all preoperative parameters (local clinical stage from DRE, tumor grade from the biopsy specimen, and the serum PSA concentration). In these men, the procedure should be performed according to the technique of Walsh. With this anatomic approach and excellent visualization deep into the pelvis and under the pubic symphysis with the aid of a halogen headlight and magnification (surgical loupes), the radical prostatectomy can be "tailored" to the specific needs of each patient. For men with a low serum PSA concentration and a low-grade, low-volume cancer, a bilateral nerve-sparing procedure can be performed. However, if a large apical lesion is present, the autonomic innervation to the corpus cavernosum on both sides should not be preserved in order to ensure adequate surgical margins. If the cancer lies in close proximity to the posterolateral aspect of the prostate gland as determined at the time of surgery, the neurovascular bundle on that side should be widely excised. Also, there is no need to preserve the neurovascular bundles in patients who are impotent preoperatively. By utilizing these principles, the radical prostatectomy becomes an excellent cancer operation without compromising routine body functions and quality of life.

In Walsh's series of 600 patients undergoing radical prostatectomy, it was possible to preserve potency in 68 per cent of those men who were sexually active preoperatively. The return of erectile function, however, was dependent on the patient's age, the clinical and pathologic stage of the tumor, and whether or not one or both neurovascular bundles were excised. Younger men (<50 years of age) with organ-confined tumors in whom both neurovascular bundles were preserved had the best outcome; 90 per cent of such individuals were potent at 1-year follow-up. Urinary incontinence is another potential complication of radical prostatectomy. In the Walsh series, 92 per cent of the patients achieved complete urinary control (no need for protection) at 1-year follow-up; 8 per cent had some degree of stress urinary incontinence. Of these latter patients, two men have required placement of an artificial external urinary sphincter. Other long-term untoward effects reported by various investigators include bladder neck contracture in 3 to 12 per cent of patients, thrombophlebitis in 3 to 12 per cent, and pulmonary embolus in 2 to 5 per cent. Intraoperative complications include hemorrhage requiring a blood transfusion in 5 to 10 per cent and rectal injury in approximately 1 per cent of the men undergoing radical prostatectomy.

SUMMARY

Clinical Stage B refers to those prostate cancers identified by an elevated serum PSA concentration (Stage B_0) or a palpable abnormality on DRE (Stages B_1 and B_2) and no evidence of extracapsular spread. Treatment options include expectant therapy, external beam or interstitial radiation therapy, and radical prostatectomy via either the retropubic or the perineal approach. Because no data are available to definitively conclude that one therapy is superior to the other, it is most important to inform the patient of the various treatments and consider his opinion when making the final management decision. Although the treatment of prostate cancer must be *individualized,* the following general guidelines for the management of clinical stage B prostate cancer may be useful: (1) radical prostatectomy or external beam radiation therapy for healthy men less than 70 years of age, (2) external beam radiation therapy for men between 70 and 75 years of age and older men if their health is sufficiently good and they desire treatment, and (3) expectant therapy for older men and patients with other significant, comorbidities.

Suggested Readings

Bagshaw MA, Cox RS, Ramback JE: Radiation therapy for localized prostate cancer: Justification by long-term follow-up. Urol Clin North Am 17:787, 1990

Johansson JE, Adami HO, Andersson SO, et al: High 10-year survival rate in patients with early, untreated prostatic cancer. JAMA 267:2191, 1992

Oesterling JE: Prostate-specific antigen: Improving its ability to diagnose early prostate cancer. JAMA 267: 2236, 1992

Oesterling JE, Jacobsen SJ, Chute CG, et al: Serum prostate-specific antigen in a community-based population of healthy men: establishment of age-specific reference ranges. JAMA 270:860, 1993

Oesterling JE, Suman VJ, Zincke H, et al: PSA-detected (clinical stage T1c or B_0) prostate cancer. Urol Clin North Am 20:687, 1993.

Paulson DF: Perineal prostatectomy. *In* Walsh PC, Retik AB, Stamey TA, et al (eds): Campbell's Urology, 6th ed. Philadelphia, WB Saunders, 1992, pp 2887–2899

Russell KJ, Laramore GE, Krall JM, et al: Eight years experience with neutron radiotherapy in the treatment of stage C and D prostate cancer: Updated results of the RTOG 7704 randomized trial. Prostate 11:183, 1987

Stormont TJ, Farrow GM, Myers RP, et al: Clinical stage B_0 or T_{1c} prostate cancer: Nonpalpable disease identified by elevated serum prostate-specific antigen concentration. Urology 41:3, 1993

Walsh PC: Radical retropubic prostatectomy. *In* Walsh PC, Retik AB, Stamey TA, et al (eds): Campbell's Urology, 6th ed. Philadelphia, WB Saunders, 1992, pp 2865–2886

Walsh PC, Donker PJ: Impotence following radical prostatectomy: Insight into etiology and prevention. J Urol 128:492, 1982

Whitmore WF Jr: Experience with ^{125}iodine implantation in the treatment of prostate cancer. *In* Skinner DG (ed): Urological Cancer. New York, Grune & Stratton, 1983, pp 37–39

Whitmore WF Jr, Warner JA, Thompson IM: Expectant management of localized prostate cancer. Cancer 67: 1091, 1991

CARCINOMA OF THE PROSTATE—STAGE C

PHILIP M. HANNO, M.D.

Philadelphia, Pennsylvania

Prostate cancer is being diagnosed at a higher rate than ever before. In 1990, the most recent year for which national data are available, detection of prostate cancer grew by 16 per cent over the previous year, making it the largest increase ever reported for a cancer in a single year. Preliminary data from 1991 indicate that the rate may increase by an additional 30 per cent or more. It is estimated by the National Cancer Institute that, in 1993, prostate cancer will be diagnosed in 165,000 American men and 35,000 men will die from it.

At the present time, the death rates from prostate cancer have remained virtually the same for decades. If diagnosis and treatment make a difference, we should see a dramatic drop in the death rate from prostate cancer in the years ahead given the explosive growth in the use of prostate-specific antigen, transrectal ultrasound–guided biopsy, general prostate cancer screening, and radical treatment. If they do not make a difference, things will change little.

The treatment of Stage A and Stage B carcinoma remains controversial in the medical community in this country and around the world. Specialists naturally tend to favor the discipline in which they are trained. As every urologist knows, assessing the life expectancy of patients with prostate cancer prior to treatment is far more important than such assessments for virtually any other potentially curable malignancy. If it is hard to be dogmatic with regard to treatment of disease localized within the prostate, it is even more difficult when one is discussing Stage C disease. In the Veterans Administration Cooperative Urological Research Group studies, there was an approximately 50 per cent 5-year survival and 20 per cent 10-year survival rate in 1050 cases of Stage C disease. Of note, however, only 17.2 per cent of the deaths reported were attributed to cancer of the prostate.

How is clinical Stage C carcinoma defined? Although it may have different meanings to different physicians, essentially it denotes tumors producing unequivocal palpable evidence of extraprostatic tumor extension, but no clinically detectable evidence of metastases. In C_1 disease extraprostatic extension is minimal and in C_2 disease there is extensive extraprostatic tumor invasion. The Whitmore system of staging is essentially based on prior American criteria but uses the UICC (TMN) broad designations: Stage C_1 is extension beyond the capsule unilaterally and may include the seminal vesicles; Stage C_2 is bilateral extension; and Stage C_3 denotes extension into bladder, rectum, levator muscles, or pelvic side walls.

Certain problems arise in dealing with Stage C_1 tumors. It is extremely hard to diagnose them clinically. In addition, extension into the capsule clearly has a different prognosis than extension through it. Treatment decisions for C_1 disease based on clinical staging are subject to a number of errors. It has been estimated that 25 to 50 per cent of cases will be clinically overstaged. Up to 50 per cent of these patients may have positive lymph nodes. Finally, up to 60 per cent of this group of patients may have positive margins after radical prostatectomy.

We stage these patients with PSA, multiple transrectal ultrasound–guided prostate biopsy cores to help to determine the extent of tumor in the gland, bone scan, and endorectal surface coil magnetic resonance imaging. We have found the latter study to be very helpful in determining advanced local spread and seminal vesicle involvement. Patients with no other evidence of spread and an equivocal magnetic resonance image can be given the benefit of the doubt in terms of consideration for curative therapy depending on their wishes and life expectancy.

The question of whether to go ahead with laparoscopic pelvic lymph node dissection in this group of patients is a philosophical one. Few believe that this group of patients are potentially curable with radical prostatectomy. If one is inclined to believe that radiation therapy is preferable to immediate hormonal therapy and/or watchful waiting with delayed hormonal therapy, a case can be made for sampling the pelvic nodes. The corollary, of course, is that the potential morbidity of anesthesia and node dissection must be less than the morbidity of a course of radiation therapy confined to the prostate. If the radiation therapist intends to treat regardless of nodal status, it is harder to justify sampling the nodes. If the nodal area would be included in the radiation field regardless, a similar argument can be made.

There are numerous therapies proposed for Stage C carcinoma of the prostate, but none currently is considered curative. They include limited-field radiation therapy combined with pelvic lymphadenectomy, interstitial radiation therapy (now generally guided by transrectal ultrasound), external beam radiation therapy without lymphadenectomy, primary surgical excision, immediate endocrine therapy, delayed endocrine therapy initiated at the onset of local or systemic symptoms, and transurethral prostatectomy.

Because there is no proven "right" or "wrong" way to treat Stage C prostate cancer, one must read the extensive literature on the subject and combine the findings with his or her own experience. The results of radiation therapy in treating large prostate cancers are not encouraging. If one accepts that Stage C cancers are incurable, the issue becomes how best to deal with local growth and metastatic disease. Reports in the literature note local tumor recurrence in 53 per cent of patients treated with external beam radiation; no difference in local progression when irradiated patients are compared with nonirradiated controls; and no difference in the time to first evidence of distant metastases in patients randomly assigned to external beam irradiation and those expectantly treated with delayed hormonal therapy at the time of metastases. We therefore tend to agree with Stamey that judicious use of transurethral prostatectomy for obstructive symptoms and hormonal therapy for both local and distant disease is a far less morbid, simpler, and less expensive way to proceed. It also eliminates the need for node dissection, except perhaps in research centers. This is certainly to some extent a nihilistic approach, but until data demonstrates a better way, it seems reasonable. Because current evidence suggests that early hormonal therapy may increase patient survival in comparison to delayed hormonal therapy, we encourage this unless sexual potency is a major quality of life issue.

Recently two other approaches have sparked interest. Large local tumors have been treated with hormonal therapy for several months followed by radical prostatectomy. Only time will tell if survival is improved, but preliminary data suggest that the incidence of positive margins is diminished when hormonal therapy is given prior to surgery. Transperineal prostate cryotherapy under ultrasound guidance currently is being tested at medical centers around the country. The morbidity of the procedure appears to be low, and the possibility for good local control of Stage C disease certainly exists.

We eagerly await the results of future treatment trials for clinical Stage C prostatic cancer. Presently the long-term prognosis is dismal in patients with an otherwise long life expectancy. However, older patients often will succumb to other maladies. With the current "epidemic" of radical prostatectomy, we are likely to learn quite a lot about the natural history of microscopic (*pathologic*) Stage C disease and whatever benefits accrue from local control. Long-term follow-up of these patients, many of whom are treated with different adjuvant therapies, is likely to yield important information relative to the best therapies for *clinical* Stage C disease.

Suggested Readings

Chelsky MJ, Schnall MD, Seidmon EJ, et al: Use of endorectal surface coil magnetic resonance imaging for local staging of prostate cancer. J Urol 150:391–395, 1993

Cohen JK, Onik G, Miller R: Treatment of localized carcinoma of the prostate using percutaneous transperineal cryosurgical ablation: A preliminary report. J Urol 149:232A, 1993

Fair WR, Heston WDW: Is combined modality therapy appropriate for apparently localized carcinoma of the prostate? Urol Clin North Am 18:477–480, 1991

Fallon B, Williams RD: Current options in the management of clinical stage C prostatic carcinoma. Urol Clin North Am 17:853–866, 1990

Schellhammer PF, Kuban DA, Eli-Mahdi AM: Local failure after definitive radiation or surgical therapy for carcinoma of the prostate and options for prevention and therapy. Urol Clin North Am 18:484–499, 1991

Stamey TA, McNeal JE: Adenocarcinoma of the prostate. *In* Walsh PC, Retik AB, Stamey TA, et al (eds): Campbell's Urology, 6th ed. Philadelphia, WB Saunders, 1992, pp 1180–1221

Whitmore WF: Management of clinically localized prostatic cancer. JAMA 269:2676–2677, 1993

CARCINOMA OF THE PROSTATE—STAGE D

BARRY S. STEIN, M.D.

Providence, Rhode Island

Carcinoma of the prostate is the most common malignancy by incidence and second most common cause of death in men. There will be 165,000 new cases of prostatic cancer with 35,000 deaths resulting from this disease expected for 1993. Historically, up to 75 per cent of men are incurable at the time of diagnosis, although with earlier detection it is hoped that this percentage will decline. In fact, however, given our improved imaging techniques (computerized tomographic scan, magnetic resonance imaging) and increased attention to nodal status (particularly with the advent of laparoscopic lymph node dissection), the number of Stage D_1 patients actually is increasing in our hands.

TIMING OF TREATMENT

The initial treatment of the patient with Stage D carcinoma of the prostate should be hormonal. Controversy exists as to when that initial treatment should be instituted. Advocates of immediate (or early) hormone therapy maintain that rapid treatment may provide a longer interval before ultimate relapse. Advocates of delayed hormonal therapy believe that early treatment increases cost and patient morbidity and does not significantly prolong time to progression or survival time.

Several studies have examined this issue without yielding a definitive answer. The original Veterans Administration Cooperative Urological Research Group (VACURG) study appeared to demonstrate no difference between early and late hormone therapy in terms of survival. Re-examination of this study, excluding the cases of cardiovascular death resulting from diethylstilbestrol complications, questions the original conclusion and suggests fewer cancer-related deaths in the initially treated men. Several recent studies seem to support a longer survival in patients treated at the time of diagnosis.

Academics aside, and practically speaking, I find it difficult for the patient to accept no treatment as an option. Patients with extensive bony metastasis, especially spinal, should be treated with prompt hormone therapy to prevent the complication of spinal cord compression resulting from vertebral collapse. In these cases, the resultant paraplegic may well not respond to surgery and subsequent hormone therapy, and this should be prevented if possible in high-risk patients.

RATIONALE FOR THERAPEUTIC CHOICES

Androgen production, necessary for prostatic cell growth, can be interrupted in several locations. The hypothalamus produces luteinizing hormone–releasing hormone (LHRH), which stimulates the pituitary to increase release of luteinizing hormone (LH). LH, in turn, stimulates the Leydig cells in the interstitial space of the testis to produce testosterone. Free, unbound testosterone can diffuse passively into the cytoplasm of prostate cells, where it is converted by 5-alpha-reductase to dihydrotestosterone (DHT). DHT can bind to receptor proteins, and this complex can translocate into the prostatic cell nucleus, where DNA binding, and ultimately messenger RNA production, can take place. Negative feedback loops exist by which the levels of circulating testosterone and LH can influence secretion of LHRH and LH.

In addition to the testicular androgens, which are under LH control, the adrenal cortex, stimulated by adrenocorticotropic hormone, can produce the weaker androgens androstenedione and dehydroepiandrosterone (DHEA). These adrenal androgens thus are not under control by LHRH or LH, and attempts to hormonally treat the pituitary-testicular axis will not affect their production.

Reduction of testicular androgens can be accomplished by a variety of actions aimed at varying target organs. Estrogens provide much stronger negative feedback to the hypothalamus and pituitary gland than testosterone itself. Thus administration of exogenous estrogens, such as diethylstilbestrol (DES), will reduce circulating LH levels and thereby reduce testosterone levels. Estrogens also appear to have a direct inhibitory effect on prostate cancer cells. LH secretion also can be inhibited by the administration of LHRH superanalogues, such as leuprolide. The superanalogues, for the first 4 to 7 days of treatment, actually cause a rise in serum testosterone levels, as may be surmised. Chronic administration of these agents, however, causes down-regulation of the pituitary receptors as a result of overstimulation. The pituitary ceases production of LH, and testosterone production by the testis ceases. Circulating testosterone levels fall to "castrate range." The remaining measurable androgens are produced by the adrenal gland as discussed above. Cessation of therapy will lead to return to normal levels of testosterone.

CURRENT HORMONE THERAPY CHOICES

Currently, the following choices are available for hormone therapy: DES, orchiectomy, LHRH analogues, antiandrogens, and combined therapy. DES, orchiectomy, and LHRH analogues all are equally efficacious as single-"agent," first-line, hormone therapy.

Estrogen therapy can lead to reductions in serum testosterone levels to castrate range in approximately 5 to 7 days. Estrogens, however, have attendant complications that may make DES therapy a poor choice. The VACURG-I study showed that, for Stage C patients treated with DES 5 mg/day, the cardiovascular deaths exceeded the cancer deaths. In the same study, the Stage D patients treated with DES had about equal chances of dying of cardiovascular disease or cancer. As the VACURG-II study demonstrated, the cardiovascular risks are reduced at the 1 mg/day dose, but this dose may not suppress testosterone levels in all men. Doses of 3 mg/day and above will completely suppress testosterone levels in virtually all males; however, even at this dose, the risk of cardiovascular complications may outweigh the benefits. If using DES as initial therapy, I would recommend a 1 mg/day dose and would follow testosterone levels to ensure that the patients remain in the castrate range.

Orchiectomy, of course, reduces testicular androgen production by removing the site of its production. Three hours after orchiectomy, serum testosterone levels are reduced by 90 per cent. Orchiectomy is equally effective as hormonal therapy, and ensures lifelong patient compliance as well. It is a short outpatient procedure and may be performed under local anesthesia. This remains the most commonly performed method of hormone treatment. For some patients, however, psychologically this is not acceptable.

LHRH analogues (there are now several that are approved by the Food and Drug Administration [FDA]) also can provide excellent hormonal management. There are fewer side effects, largely comprised of hot flashes, and no cardiovascular toxicity. These agents cause down-regulation of pituitary receptors, driving LH levels to zero, and thereby decrease serum testosterone levels to castrate range. Cessation of therapy will lead to a prompt rebound in serum testosterone levels. In a large, randomized series comparing leuprolide 1 mg daily and DES 3 mg daily, no significant difference was noted in regard to tumor response. Cardiovascular toxicity was much greater in the DES group. Because of the initial increase in circulating testosterone levels during the first 4 to 7 days of therapy, symptoms may temporarily worsen. This is known as the "flare" effect, and can be prevented by a 1-week pretreatment with either DES or flutamide. Monthly preparations now are commonly available.

Currently, the only FDA-approved nonsteroidal antiandrogen is flutamide. Flutamide is a competitive inhibitor for testosterone and DHT receptors. Flutamide is not useful as monotherapy because it has a weaker affinity for the receptors than testosterone or DHT, and a buildup of testosterone proximal to the receptor eventually will overcome the inhibition.

Whatever method is utilized for hormone therapy, approximately 85 per cent of patients will respond favorably, with significant tumor regression. This response will last approximately 18 to 24 months on the average. Because most prostate cancer contains both hormone-dependent and hormone-independent clones of cells, ultimate progression of disease is presumed to be on the basis of the hormonally independent cells. Of the 15 per cent nonresponse, some will be due to the initial tumor being comprised largely of hormonally independent cells. However, studies reveal that approximately 10 per cent of what is diagnosed as prostate cancer may be other poorly differentiated tumors, most significantly transitional cell carcinoma of the prostate. Immunostaining is essential in weeding these out of the differential diagnosis in patients with poorly differentiated tumors.

Recent studies have examined the role of initial dual hormone therapy treatment. The theory supporting dual therapy is that any of the aforementioned hormone treatments is effective in reducing testosterone levels to "castrate" range, but not to zero. This is because a small amount (approximately 5 per cent) of testosterone is made in the adrenal gland, and is not under LH/Leydig cell control. Antiandrogens can, as a second agent, effectively block the action of the adrenal androgens peripherally, giving total androgen blockade. Dr. Labrie from Quebec published studies showing that the time to progression was approximately twice as long with dual therapy as with monotherapy. Despite initial skepticism, several randomized trials have shown at least some improvement in survival with dual therapy compared to monotherapy plus placebo. In a National Cancer Institute–sponsored study reported on by Crawford and associates, men with limited metastatic disease had a significantly prolonged survival when treated initially with dual therapy. Thus, in a subset of patients, those with minimal metastatic disease, there may in fact be advantages to dual therapy. This comes at a price, however, because antiandrogen therapy alone is approximately $300 a month.

HORMONE FAILURE OPTIONS

Once a patient escapes hormone therapy control, no proven curative treatment exists. Therapy may be palliative, chemotherapeutic regimens, or experimental. Problems requiring palliative therapy most often surround bone pain, although anemia, urinary retention, renal obstruction, and hematuria also may be present challenging problems.

The great majority of prostate cancer patients fail hormone therapy as a result of bone pain. If there are localized areas of bone pain, radiotherapy to these sites is possible. Larger areas may be treated with half-body or even total-body radiation for pain control. Phosphorus-32 also has been used for pain control. Further bone pain may be controlled with long-acting analgesics such as MS-Contin. Anemia, another common complication, may be managed with blood transfusions as needed, and hematocrits should be followed closely in the hormonal failure patient. Urinary retention may require local therapy such as repeated transurethral resection of the prostate or radiotherapy, or an indwelling catheter (at times a suprapubic tube) may be required. Upper tract obstruction is a complication that may require assessment of the patient's wishes regarding invasive treatment. In my experience, it is often difficult, if not impossible, to insert ureteral stents retrogradely. Percutaneous tubes, once inserted, usually cannot be removed because significant tumor regression is unlikely. Great thought must be undertaken before this treatment is initiated. Gross hematuria resulting from prostate cancer can be very difficult to control. A combination of transurethral fulguration and oral Amicar may control this problem.

Standard chemotherapy agents provide insufficient responses in carcinoma of the prostate, but on occasion may be helpful in at least temporarily alleviating widespread bone pain. I have most frequently recommended cis-platinum, but results are not outstanding.

Several experimental protocols are currently in use. These include new looks at multichemotherapeutic agents such as combinations of estracyt and vinblastine, or new agents such as suramin. Early trials look encouraging, but more work is needed for these agents to move into mainstream treatment.

Finally, very recent evidence suggests that some patients initially treated with dual hormone therapy may experience regression of disease with cessation of the antiandrogenic arm. In these patients, the testicular component of treatment (i.e., LHRH analogues) must be continued. Prostate-specific hormone levels, if they are going to decrease, will do so within the first 4 weeks of antiandrogen deprivation.

Suggested Readings

Catalona WJ: Prostate Cancer. New York, Grune & Stratton, 1984

Schultz MJ, Crawford ED: Advanced carcinoma of the prostate. *In* Stein BS, Caldamone AA, Smith JA Jr (eds): Practice of Urology. New York, Norton Medical Books, 1992

Stamey TA, McNeal JE: Adenocarcinoma of the prostate. *In* Walsh PC, Retik AB, Stamey TA, et al (eds): Campbell's Urology, 6th ed. Philadelphia, WB Saunders, 1992, pp 1159–1221

RADIATION THERAPY AFTER RADICAL PROSTATECTOMY

CRAIG L. SILVERMAN, M.D.

Philadelphia, Pennsylvania

For men who elect to undergo a radical curative surgery for early prostate cancer, there exists the potential for local tumor bed recurrence. Analysis of surgical specimens has demonstrated several findings that have been shown to increase the likelihood of local prostatic bed recurrence. These include capsular perforation, the presence of tumor at the surgical margins, involvement of the seminal vesicles, bladder neck involvement, and increased acid phosphatase levels postprostatectomy. A review of the recent urologic literature demonstrates that a fairly consistent percentage of patients (30 to 35 per cent) undergoing radical prostatectomy have one or more such pathologic characteristics indicative of spread outside the prostate itself and increased chance of local recurrence. Eggleston analyzed his experience and demonstrated a progressive increase in the incidence of all patterns of extraprostatic extension and especially seminal vesicle involvement with increasing clinical stage. It is estimated that 6 to 20 per cent of patients with Stage A_2 disease, 20 to 30 per cent of those with Stage B_1 lesions, and as many as 60 per cent of those with Stage B_2 lesions may indeed have one or more pathologic findings indicative of extraprostatic extension.

The presence of pathologic involvement of the seminal vesicles carries a much worse prognosis than mere capsular extension or perforation. Bladder neck involvement also has been found to be a very negative prognostic factor. Gibbons et al. have developed a pathologic staging system that denotes more precisely the pathologic extent of tumor by extent of periprostatic extension and have demonstrated an increase in local recurrence for increasing C substage (Fig. 1).

For patients who fall into these high-risk groups, adjuvant postoperative radiotherapy offers an opportunity to reduce local recurrence and, it is hoped, increase if not the length, then the quality of survival.

ADJUVANT RADIOTHERAPY

There recently have been several studies concerning the use of routine postoperative radiotherapy following radical prostatectomy. Most patients were selected on the basis of the

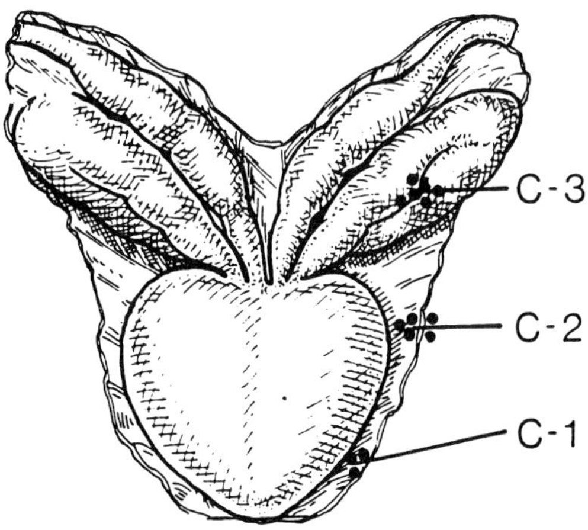

FIGURE 1. Pathologic staging system for Stage C carcinoma of the prostate. Stage C_1: invasion through prostatic capsule into extra prostatic tissue, no tumor at surgical margins, and no seminal vesicle involvement. Stage C_2: tumor at surgical margins, with or without capsule penetration, and no seminal vesicle involvement. Stage C_3: invasion of seminal vesicles, with or without tumor at surgical margins or capsular penetration. (From Gibbons RP, Code BS, Richardson RG, et al: Adjuvant radiotherapy following radical prostatectomy: Results and complications. J Urol 135:65–68, 1986, with permission.)

following: extracapsular spread, incomplete resection (enucleation only) for what was suspected to be benign disease, involvement of the seminal vesicles, or positive margins.

Table 1 lists the results of several series evaluating adjuvant radiotherapy. There is excellent local control, approaching 100 per cent in patients for almost all series. Even patients who had gross recurrences had excellent salvage rates. There are improved local control and disease-free survival rates for irradiated patients compared to patients in the same series who had similar pathologic findings but did not have radiotherapy. It must be pointed out, however, that patients were selected for treatment based on the individual surgeon's preference, and additional biasing factors may play a part in interpreting these results. The notable exception is the recent series by Paulson that reanalyzed the original data by Anscher and Prosnitz published 3 years earlier. Paulson concluded that the original data were tainted by the inclusion of inappropriate patients, and his new analysis containing only appropriate patients showed no significant improvement in local control or survival.

It is unclear from these data whether or not the 5- and 10-year disease-free survival or actuarial survival is significantly affected by adjuvant radiotherapy. The incidence of distant disease does not seem to be affected in several series that evaluated it. Gibbons tried to investigate the effect on local control by periprostatic extension, capsular perforation, positive margins, or seminal vesical involvement (pathologic C substage), but too few patients per group were available to make a significant conclusion.

COMPLICATIONS

Aggressive irradiation of the prostatic bed or bed plus pelvic node areas is not without potential for serious long-term complications. A review of recent series show a fairly consistent incidence of complications following radical prostatectomy and irradiation. Approximately 20 to 25 per cent of patients will experience chronic complications, including proctitis, urethral stricture, lymphedema, or cystitis, with a small percentage of patients requiring permanent colostomy or urinary diversion. Fortunately, most complications are mild to moderate in severity (Table 2).

RADIATION TECHNIQUE

Technique is very dependent on the suspected volume of tissue at risk. Inclusion of the pelvic lymph nodes after a lymphadenectomy will increase the chance of lymphedema and should be done only in the presence of residual disease or with a high preponderance of positive nodes in the pelvic node dissection specimen.

When only the bed is believed to be at risk, the treatment volume should be kept as small as possible, usually a 7 × 7-cm field using either rotational arc technique, four-field box technique, or conformal therapy. Extensive treatment planning will help minimize the dose to the anterior rectal wall and bladder neck, which should reduce the incidence of both acute and chronic complications. Barium in the rectum and a Foley catheter at the time of simulation will help identify those vital tissues and should be used in conjunction with a computerized tomography scan or magnetic

TABLE 1. Results of Studies of Adjuvant Radiotherapy

AUTHOR	NO. OF PATIENTS	DOSE (GY)	LOCAL CONTROL (%)	5-YEAR DISEASE-FREE SURVIVAL (%)	OVERALL SURVIVAL (%)
Jacobson	26	54–70	100	69	89
	24*	—	83	71	92
Gibbons	22	49–70	95	59	73
	23*	—	70	35	39
Meier	19	45–65	94	68	60
	39*	—	70	42	57
Paulson	46	55–70	64	85	92
	113*	—	59	87	95
Forman	34	60–70	100	72	82
Lange	45	60	100	79 C lesions 72 D_{1a} lesions	

*Surgery-only patients with similar high-risk pathologic characteristics.

TABLE 2. Complications of Combined Radical Prostatectomy and Adjuvant Radiotherapy

Author	No. of Patients	Complications	Incidence of Complications (%)
Meier	19	Lymphedema	3 (5 surgery alone)
		Temporary incontinence	11 (23 surgery alone)
		Chronic incontinence	11 (21 surgery alone)
		Urinary stricture	27 (18 surgery alone)
Gibbons	22	Chronic proctitis	27
		Chronic cystitis	27
		Fistula	14
		Rectal incontinence	5
		Urinary diversion	5
		Surgery alone	6
Ray	32	Incontinence	3
		Proctitis	9
		Stricture	6
		Lymphedema	3
Lange	45	Lymphedema	2
		Hematuria	2
Pilepich	28	Proctitis	18
		Cystitis	4
		Stricture	8
		Ostomy placement	4
Anscher	46	Cystitis	17 Grade 1, 4 Grade 2, 7 Grade 3
		Proctitis	26 Grade 1, 11 Grade 2, 0 Grade 3
		Incontinence	17 Grade 1, 2 Grade 2, 2 Grade 3

resonance imaging to minimize the dose to these tissues.

DOSE CONSIDERATIONS

Patients who have extraprostatic extension but negative margins should receive 55 to 60 Gy in 6 weeks. There are few data on dose response, and this dose range should be effective. For patients who have positive margins or involvement of the seminal vesicles, a dose of 65 to 70 Gy is recommended. In these instances the tumor burden is larger and should require additional dosing for control. This may increase the chance of complications, but the increased tumor burden justifies increasing the dose by 500 to 1000 cGy.

CONCLUSION

For patients undergoing radical prostatectomy for early-stage prostate cancer, there still exists the potential for local tumor bed recurrence. As preoperative staging becomes more sophisticated with magnetic resonance imaging, prostate-specific antigen levels, and ultrasonography, the likelihood of encountering clinically unsuspected extraprostatic extension should decrease, but there always will be occasions where such extension is found. Particularly poor prognostic findings include bladder neck involvement, seminal vesicle involvement, and positive surgical margins. Also, as the urological surgeon attempts to maintain potency, sparing of the neurovascular bundle may increase the chance of local recurrence in patients with more diffuse glandular disease. The addition of planned adjuvant radiotherapy is very effective in reducing the incidence of local recurrence, with results nearing 100 per cent control, but the effect on survival and incidence of distant disease is minimal. There is approximately a 20 per cent chance of complications following both procedures; most of these are mild, but more severe complications requiring surgical intervention can result. Careful treatment planning should reduce this complication rate significantly.

Suggested Readings

Eggleston J, Walsh P: Radical prostatectomy with preservation of sexual function: Pathological findings in the first 100 cases. J Urol 134:1146–1148, 1985

Gibbons RP, Cole BS, Richardson RG, et al: Adjuvant radiotherapy following radical prostatectomy: Results and complications. J Urol 135:65–68, 1986

Jacobson GM, Smith JA, Stewart JR: Postoperative radiation therapy for pathologic stage C prostate cancer. J Radiat Oncol Biol Phys 13:1021–1024, 1987

Meier R, Mark R, St Royal L, et al: Postoperative radiation therapy after radical prostatectomy for prostate carcinoma. Cancer 70:1960–1966, 1992

Paulson DF, Moul JW, Robertson JE, et al: Postoperative radiotherapy of the prostate for patients undergoing radical prostatectomy with positive margins, seminal vesicle involvement and/or penetration through the capsule. J Urol 143:1178–1182, 1990

SARCOMAS OF THE PROSTATE

BETTE LAZZARO, M.D.

Philadelphia, Pennsylvania

Sarcomas of the prostate are unusual entities, accounting for 0.1 to 0.2 per cent of all prostatic neoplasms. Thirty per cent are observed in the first decade of life. The most common prostatic sarcoma is embryonal rhabdomyosarcoma, seen predominantly in infants and children. A few cases have been documented in adults. Rhabdomyosarcoma of the prostate may arise in patients with a history of neurofibromatosis.

Histologically, the embryonal form consists of relatively small cells with dark, even nuclei and scant cytoplasm. The tumor is microscopically similar to other "small blue-cell tumors" such as Ewing's sarcoma, neuroblastoma, and lymphoma. Electron microscopy or immunohistochemistry may be of help in making the diagnosis.

Clinically, the tumor is characterized by rapid growth, a large pelvic mass, and hematuria or urinary obstruction. If untreated, dissemination to lungs, bone, liver, regional lymph nodes, and serosa is the rule. A computerized tomographic scan may show an enlarged, inhomogeneous prostatic mass with invasion of perirectal fat or pelvic tissues. Ultrasound and magnetic resonance imaging (MRI) also may show the presence of prostatic tumor, with periprostatic extension. MRI in the sagittal plane and/or lateral films of intravenous pyelograms and cystograms may demonstrate the relation of the tumor to the bladder.

Recently, treatment for rhabdomyosarcomas of the prostate using a combined-modality approach (surgery, radiation, and chemotherapy) has markedly improved prognosis, with a survival rate of 60 to 90 per cent in children with apparently localized disease. Initially, chemotherapy may be used to shrink the tumor prior to surgical excision. There is some evidence that there may be increased survival using combined-modality therapy with intensified pulse chemotherapy as opposed to ordinary-dose pulse chemotherapy. In addition to combination chemotherapy and radiation, the surgical approach includes radical cystectomy with continent diversion to the urethra, feasible even in a small child. Partial cystectomy also may be considered, depending on the extent of disease, especially with newer high-dose and combined-modality chemotherapy regimens. Approaches to combined-modality treatment remain somewhat controversial, at issue being the value of extirpative surgery as opposed to initial treatment with chemotherapy and subsequent conservative surgical excision.

Sarcomas of the prostate in adults are extremely rare. In patients older than 40 years, malignant fibrous histiocytomas, leiomyosarcomas, osteogenic sarcomas, pleomorphic liposarcomas, rhabdomyosarcomas, hemangiopericytomas, and angiosarcomas have been observed.

The average survival time in adults with prostatic sarcomas other than rhabdomyosarcomas is 32 months. True rhabdomyosarcomas in adults may carry a worse prognosis. Leiomyosarcomas show a peak frequency in the seventh decade, and may present with dysuria, urinary retention, hematuria, and prostatic enlargement. In tissue sections, whorls and bundles of smooth muscle cells are seen, with mitoses and frequently hemorrhage and necrosis. Invasion of periprostatic tissues may be seen. Immunohistochemistry may show the tumor cells to be positive for desmin and vimentin, and electron microscopy may show smooth muscle filaments within cells. It is critical to distinguish a reactive postoperative spindle cell nodule of the prostate from a true sarcoma, the diagnosis being based primarily on light microscopic appearance.

Therapy for leiomyosarcomas and other prostatic sarcomas includes radical surgery, chemotherapy, and radiation. Although survival beyond 5 years is unusual, multimodality therapy recently has increased survival time.

A cystosarcoma phylloides–like tumor of the prostate has been seen in adults in which the glands are benign but the stromal component shows a potentially malignant spindle cell proliferation. The majority of cases have shown benign clinical behavior.

The issue of a mixed malignancy, "carcinosarcoma" or metaplastic carcinoma, is an important one. This entity should be distinguished from pure prostatic sarcoma. Carcinosarcoma, or metaplastic carcinoma, contains malignant glands as well as a malignant stromal component. The stromal component may consist of chondrosarcoma, fibrosarcoma, osteogenic sarcoma, or another histologic subtype. Light microscopic, immunohistochemical, or electron microscopic identification of an epithelial component characterizes the tumor as metaplastic adenocarcinoma. The issue of whether the stromal component arises from the glandular component or synchronously with it probably is not relevant to the overall biology of such lesions. Metaplastic carcinomas should be considered variants of prostatic adenocarcinoma, and tend to be clinically aggressive, with recurrence and visceral metastases. Bony metastases may be absent, and the tumor may show resistance to antiandrogen therapy, unlike typical prostatic adenocarcinomas.

Suggested Readings

Hays D, Raney RB, et al: Improved survival and bladder preservation among patients with bladder/prostate primary tumors in Intergroup Rhabdomyosarcoma Study III (IRS). Proc Annu Meeting Am Soc Clin Oncol 10:A1119, 1991

Herr HW: Sarcomas of the urinary tract. *In* deKernion JB, Paulson DF (eds): Genitourinary Cancer Management. Philadelphia, Lea & Febiger, 1987, pp 259–270

Mietinnen M: Rhabdomyosarcoma in patients older than 40 years of age. Cancer 62:2060–2065, 1988

Petersen RO: Urologic Pathology. Philadelphia, JB Lippincott, 1992

Raney RB, Gehan EA, et al: Primary chemotherapy with or without radiation therapy and/or surgery for children with localized sarcoma of the bladder, prostate, vagina, uterus, and cervix. A comparison of the results in Intergroup Rhabdomyosarcoma Studies I and II. Cancer 66:2072–2081, 1990

ENDOMETRIAL CARCINOMA OF THE PROSTATE

GERALD SUFRIN, M.D.

Buffalo, New York

Carcinoma of the prostate commonly originates from the acinar epithelium of this organ, although other histologic types, including transitional cell carcinoma, adenocarcinoma of ductal origin, and endometrial carcinoma of the prostate, also have been identified. Endometrial carcinoma of the prostate originally was reported in a patient with a prostatic malignancy composed of cells that phenotypically resembled those found in endometrial carcinoma of the uterus.

Endometrial carcinoma of the prostate tends to arise in the region of the veru, and its histologic appearance has suggested that the prostatic utricle, a structure of müllerian duct origin, provides the site of origin of the lesion. The prostatic utricle consists of a layer of basal and columnar cells embedded in a smooth muscle and connective tissue stroma, separated from the prostate by a pseudocapsule.

Endometrial carcinoma of the prostate usually presents as an exophytic tumor composed of polypoid fronds; less commonly, a sessile tumor may be observed. The tumor grows into the urethral lumen as well as into the substance of the prostate gland. Microscopically, the tumor is composed of columnar cells with clear to eosinophilic cytoplasm containing basal nuclei and prominent nucleoli. The term "endometrial carcinoma of the prostate" is a descriptive term based on morphology, and it is unclear whether or not developmental, molecular, or biochemical significance also can be given to this variant of prostate cancer.

Endometrial carcinoma of the prostate arises "centrally" (i.e., adjacent to the prostatic urethra), in contrast to the more peripheral origin of acinar carcinoma, and therefore hematuria and obstructive voiding symptoms are found in 58 and 84 percent, respectively, of patients with this lesion. This contrasts to patients with acinar carcinoma, in whom the above symptoms occur in only 5 and 44 per cent of cases, respectively. In further contrast to acinar carcinoma, rectal examination is suggestive of malignancy in only one third of cases, whereas cystoscopy is positive in over 85 per cent. Finally, and because of the urethral or "central" location of origin of this lesion, transperineal or transrectal prostatic biopsy has been diagnostic in less than 20 per cent of cases as contrasted to an accuracy of over 85 per cent in patients with acinar carcinoma.

At diagnosis, over 80 per cent of patients with endometrial carcinoma of the prostate present with organ-confined disease, in contrast to acinar carcinoma, with which this occurs in only about 35 per cent of cases. In addition, although transurethral resection of the prostate is relatively insensitive as a biopsy technique for the early detection of prostatic acinar carcinoma, it is highly accurate in the early diagnosis of endometrial carcinoma because of the urethral or "central" site of origin of this lesion. In contrast to prostatic acinar carcinoma, neither prostatic serum acid phosphatase nor prostate-specific antigen appears to be a reliable or predictable marker for the early detection or subsequent clinical monitoring of patients with prostatic endometrial carcinoma.

Endometrial carcinoma of the prostate metastasizes to lymph nodes and to bone, where it produces osteoblastic lesions. This is of some relevance because approximately 50 per cent of patients with endometrial carcinoma of the prostate also have been found to have coexisting foci of acinar prostatic carcinoma.

Previous approaches to the treatment of endometrial carcinoma of the prostate have included transurethral prostatectomy, radiotherapy, and suprapubic prostatectomy, but, surprisingly, radical prostatectomy has been used in only approximately 10 per cent of cases. The limited number of reported cases of endometrial carcinoma of the prostate and the rather limited follow-up make conclusive comments regarding survival difficult, although 75 per cent of patients have remained free of disease for at least 2 years following treatment.

Although transurethral prostatectomy or suprapubic prostatectomy appear to offer satisfactory short-term, symptomatic local control, it is difficult to recommend either of these modalities as definitive or curative therapy. The proximity of the tumor to the external sphincter, the inability to assess accurately surgical margins, the relatively high incidence (50 per cent) of coexisting acinar carcinoma, and the tendency for local recurrence after resection or enucleation suggest that these limited approaches are not adequate as definitive forms of therapy in an otherwise fit patient. Moreover, the inherent limits of endoscopic or enucleative surgery and the low stage at diagnosis of most patients with endometrial carcinoma suggest that, in appropriately staged individuals, pelvic lymphadectomy and radical prostatectomy offer the optimal opportunity for cure. Patients with organ-confined disease but who are not candidates for, or who reject, radical prostatectomy can be offered radiotherapy.

Although the role of transurethral resection in the definitive management of patients with local (i.e., organ-confined and potentially curable endometrial carcinoma of the prostate) is questionable, endoscopic resection is of value in managing patients with disseminated disease who also manifest local symptoms such as hematuria or obstruction.

The value of orchiectomy or other therapies designed to inhibit or eliminate androgens in the treatment of disseminated endometrial carcinoma of the prostate is unclear. Based largely on morphologic criteria and extrapolating from the response of uterine carcinoma, it has been suggested that estrogens are contraindicated and that progestional agents might be of value in treating metastatic endometrial carcinoma of the prostate, although there is no conclusive evidence to support this belief.

The optimal treatment of disseminated endometrial carcinoma of the prostate remains to be defined, although a reasonable approach might involve the use of luteinizing hormone–releasing hormone analogues or bilateral orchiectomy and medroxyprogesterone acetate (1 gm IM every 14 days) or megesterol acetate (40 to 320 mg/day PO, in divided doses). However, if this is found to be ineffective or escape from hormonal manipulation becomes apparent, therapy with doxorubicin, cyclophosphamide, and 5-fluorouracil, because of its role in uterine carcinoma, should be considered. In patients with endometrial carcinoma of the prostate, the identification of hormone binding sites, including receptors for progesterone or androgen, may be important in the selection of rational systemic therapy.

Endometrial carcinoma of the prostate contrasts in its clinical, pathologic, and biochemical manifestations with the more common acinar carcinoma of the prostate. The tendency of this lesion to present at a lower stage and often in a more organ-confined fashion suggests that radical prostatectomy, in appropriately selected cases, may offer the optimal opportunity for definitive treatment and cure.

Suggested Readings

Aydin F: Endometroid adenocarcinoma of prostatic urethra presenting with anterior urethral implantation. Urology 41:91, 1993

Daugherty RK, Cos LR, Keller JW, et al: Nondetectable prostate-specific antigen in moderately differentiated adenocarcinoma of prostate. Urology 39:552, 1992

Epstein JI, Woodruff JM: Adenocarcinoma of the prostate with endometroid features. Cancer 57:111, 1986

Odom DG, Westphal KW, Hawksley VC, et al: Endometroid carcinoma of prostate. Urology 31:217, 1988

Perrapato SD, Shah PC, Huben RP, et al: Locally recurrent endometroid adenocarcinoma of the prostate after radical prostatectomy. J Urol 145:373, 1991

TRANSITIONAL CELL CARCINOMA OF THE PROSTATE

GERALD SUFRIN, MD

Buffalo, New York

Transitional cell carcinoma (TCC) of the prostate occurs as either a primary lesion originating from and limited to the prostate; (< 0.5 per cent of all cases of prostatic carcinoma) or, more commonly, synchronously or metachronously with bladder, ureteral, or renal pelvic TCC. Anatomically, TCC of the prostate, either primary or in association with other sites of urothelial carcinoma, may be limited to the prostatic urethral mucosa alone and/or may involve the periurethral glands, ducts, acini, or stroma of the prostate. Recent studies suggest that TCC of the prostate has a predilection for the veru and for the region adjacent to the veru.

TCC of the prostate excludes orthotopic bladder replacement because 40 per cent of patients with prostatic TCC will demonstrate simultaneous or delayed urethral carcinoma. In addition, TCC of the prostate may limit options in patients with bladder cancer who might otherwise be candidates for bladder-sparing surgery, and involvement of prostatic stroma by TCC is associated with nodal metastases in over 50 per cent of cases.

Diagnosis and staging of prostatic TCC requires a thorough transurethral resection (TUR) prostatic biopsy, particularly in the region of the veru, and in patients with palpable prostatic induration, core biopsies and/or fine-needle aspirates also are valuable. Although urinary cytology can help identify otherwise unsuspected cases of prostatic TCC, cup biopsy of the prostatic urethra is inadequate for diagnosis and may provide misleading information. In all patients in whom orthotopic bladder replacement is contemplated and patients who are at increased risk of TCC of the prostate, systematic TUR biopsy of the prostate is essential.

In primary TCC of the prostate, limited exclusively to the prostatic urethral mucosa, thorough TUR of the prostate with subsequent bacillus Calmette-Guérin (BCG) instillation is a reasonable option, provided no evidence of ductal, acinar, or stromal spread is detected. It is incumbent on the urologist embarking on such therapy, however, to instruct the patient in the need for careful periodic and meticulous follow-up, to include repeat TUR biopsies and cytologic studies, because of the tendency of TCC to multifocality, recurrence, early stromal invasion, and progression. Moreover, continued assessment of the distal urethra is also essential. Failure to control the lesion in this fashion should suggest cystoprostatectomy and urethrectomy as a definitive procedure.

If biopsy demonstrates ductal, acinar, or stromal invasion, TUR of the prostate with or without BCG is not appropriate as definitive therapy and cystoprostatectomy with urethrectomy is warranted. Moreover, the literature suggests that, for cure and in an otherwise fit patient, radiotherapy for TCC of the prostate is not as effective as cystoprostatectomy. Systemic chemotherapy including cis-platinum, methotrexate, and vinblastine (CMV) or methotrexate, vinblastine, doxorubicin, and cis-platinum (MVAC) in an adjunctive setting in appropriately selected cases (e.g., nodal dissemination or positive margins) may be rational even though data supporting the use of systemic chemotherapy in prostatic TCC are lacking.

In patients in whom TCC of the prostate is associated with bladder carcinoma, TUR of the prostate and BCG instillation seems logical only if all bladder and prostatic lesions are mucosal, there is no evidence of prostatic ductal, acinar, or stromal invasion, and follow-up is meticulous. However, because of the possibility of recurrence and early progression and dissemination, early cystoprostatectomy with urethrectomy may be the most effective option. If invasive TCC of the bladder occurs in a favorable location (i.e., the dome) in association with only mucosal involvement of the prostate, a theoretic case could be made, in selected patients, for bladder-sparing surgery in conjunction with TUR of the prostate and intravesical BCG, even though early radical cystoprostatectomy would appear to offer the optimal opportunity for cure. If ductal, acinar, or stromal invasion of the prostate occurs, cystoprostatectomy and urethrectomy is indicated. Additionally, either CMV or MVAC would be appropriate in individuals at risk for dissemination and relapse.

Despite current trends and strategies directed toward maintaining the integrity of the lower urinary tract in patients with TCC in general, the propensity of TCC of the prostate for multicentricity, rapid recurrence, early invasion, and dissemination dictates in many cases that consideration should be given to early extirpative surgery with appropriate systemic adjunctive therapy (when indicated) as offering the optimal chance for cure.

Suggested Readings

Bretton PR, Herr HW, Whitmore WF Jr, et al: Intravesical bacillus Calmette-Guérin therapy for in situ transitional cell carcinoma involving the prostatic urethra. J Urol 141:853, 1989

Matzkim H, Soloway MS, Hardeman S: Transitional cell carcinoma of the prostate. J Urol 146:1207, 1991

Montie JE, Wood DP, Mendendorp SV: The significance and management of transitional cell carcinoma of the prostate. Semin Urol 7:262, 1990

Reese JH, Freiha FS, Gelb AB, et al: Transitional cell carcinoma of the prostate in patients undergoing radical cystoprostatectomy. J Urol 174:92, 1992

Sakamoto N, Tusneyoshi M, Naito S, et al: An adequate sampling of the prostate to identify prostatic involvement by urothelial carcinoma in bladder cancer patients. J Urol 149:318, 1993

PERCUTANEOUS CRYOSURGERY OF THE PROSTATE USING TRANSRECTAL ULTRASOUND GUIDANCE

E. JAMES SEIDMON, M.D.

Philadelphia, Pennsylvania

Prostate cancer is now the most common cancer in men, with over 165,000 new cases diagnosed and approximately 35,000 deaths for 1993. If diagnosed early enough, surgical removal of the prostate generally is considered to be the best therapy. The number of cases is expected to increase dramatically over the next 5 years as a result of the aging of the population and improvements in the method of diagnosis. Increasing use of serum prostate-specific antigen and transrectal ultrasound in asymptomatic men is resulting in improved detection of the disease. In many cases the cancer is detected by ultrasound-guided biopsies because the tumor is not palpable.

The optimal management for early prostate carcinoma remains controversial. Some studies suggest that excellent survival is obtained for early well-differentiated tumors that are managed conservatively, achieving low 10-year disease-specific mortality with this approach and delayed therapy. Although local tumor progression occurs over time, the likelihood of dying from the disease may be less than 10 per cent over 10 years. Depending on the age and life expectancy of the patient, conservative management is a reasonable option for some patients. For many men, however, there may be a psychological barrier to leaving a cancer untreated once it has been discovered, even if the risk is small.

RADICAL PROSTATECTOMY AND RADIOTHERAPY

The conventional treatments for localized prostatic cancer are radical prostatectomy and external beam radiation. A consensus conference sponsored by the National Institutes of Health concluded that radiation therapy and radical prostatectomy offer similar survival rates 10 years after therapy. However, this has not been confirmed by a randomized controlled trial.

Radical prostatectomy, which is an attempt to eradicate prostate cancer totally, consists of a complete excision of the prostate and seminal vesicles. It generally is reserved as the treatment of choice for those patients with Stages A_2, B_1, and B_2 disease, but it also has been performed by some surgeons for local control of Stage C disease. The principle adverse effects of radical surgery include mortality in 1 to 3 per cent of patients, impotence in 30 to 70 per cent, incontinence in 3 per cent, urethral stricture in 7 per cent, and deep vein thrombosis in 7 per cent. Alternatively, external beam radiotherapy also has been used to provide local disease control for the same stages as mentioned above, and the complications include chronic diarrhea in 5 per cent of patients, bowel injury necessitating colostomy in 3 per cent, impotence in 30 to 50 per cent, and incontinence in 1 per cent. More disturbingly, recent studies demonstrate that positive surgical margins are found in 33 to 50 per cent of patients after radical prostatectomy. After radiation therapy, residual tumor has been found in ultrasound-guided biopsies in 80 to 93 per cent of patients.

Alternative treatments also are available. Interstitial radioactive seed implantation has been used extensively, and, although less severe side effects are observed, the local failure rate appears higher than that with the other two therapies. Hormone therapy also appears to provide good local control; however, it will not eradicate the disease entirely, and therefore is not usually recommended except for those men who have a short life expectancy. Often because of significant tumor bulk, advancing age, or mitigating medical problems, some patients are offered radiation therapy, interstitial seeds, or hormonal therapy as alternative treatment. Because of the morbidity, mortality, and high cost associated with these other treatment modalities, percutaneous cryosurgery under transrectal ultrasound guidance offers potentially a much less morbid and perhaps a more desirable treatment for Stage C disease.

ULTRASOUND-GUIDED PERCUTANEOUS CRYOSURGERY

Cryosurgery, the in situ destruction of tumor by the application of low temperatures, also has been used to treat localized prostate cancer (Stages A_2, B_1, and B_2). The advantages of cryosurgery are that it historically causes less impotence and incontinence than radiation or surgery and produces little blood loss. Although not previously compared to radiation or surgery in a randomized trial, the reported stage-for-stage survival following cryotherapy is comparable to that of other treatment modalities. The major limitation in the past has been the inability to monitor the freezing process adequately and thereby avoid injury to normal adjacent structures or ensure adequate freezing of the entire tumor. Thus, the complications of this treatment in the past have included urethral-rectal fistula in 10.7 per cent of patients. Importantly, however, impotence was seen in only 7.4 per cent of men in early studies.

An important advance in the use of cryotherapy is the simultaneous use of real-time ultrasound to monitor the freezing process in men with prostate cancer. Ultrasound permits more accurate placement of the cryosurgical probes. During the freezing process, a hyperechoic rim is observed emanating from the cryoprobe, accompanied by posterior acoustic shadowing. This allows documentation that the freezing has extended to sufficient tissue margins.

Using this technique, the procedure has been performed on over 100 patients with prostate cancer over the past 5 years. There was no reported mortality, incontinence, venous thrombosis, pulmonary embolus, proctitis, wound infection, or other complications associated with more traditional surgery or radiotherapy. Prostatic cryosurgery has the additional advantage of not limiting the patient's therapeutic options after treatment. Patients can be re-treated cryosurgically and have been shown to convert from positive to negative biopsies. Additionally, radiation therapy and radical prostatectomy remain viable treatment alternatives even after cryosurgery. Finally, cryosurgery may be effectively utilized even in patients who have undergone prior radiation therapy or radical prostatectomy.

Equipment and Technique

Prophylactic antibiotics are administered the day prior to the procedure. Antibiotics are continued during the procedure. The procedure is carried out under general or epidural anesthesia. Once anesthetized, the patient is placed in a modified dorsal lithotomy position and prepped and draped accordingly. Sterile surgical techniques are used.

The equipment used for the procedure includes a urethral warming device and a transrectal ultrasound probe with an attached transperineal needle insertion guide, a 3-mm liquid nitrogen cryoprobe, and a needle wire guide system with an introduction cannula. Flexible cystoscopy is performed and, under direct visualization, a suprapubic tube 10F Cope drainage catheter is placed. Through the flexible cystoscope, a 0.038-inch Amplatz wire is placed into the bladder and the flexible cystoscope is then removed. The urethral warming catheter is inserted into the bladder over the wire. The distal end of the urethral warming catheter is fixed to a Buchwalter retractor and the scrotum is elevated to the anterior abdominal wall.

The urethral warming device, a catheter that circulates heated saline at 44° to 45° C (measured at both the inflow and outflow), is necessary to protect the urethra. It poses no risk to the patient because the saline never comes in contact with the patient. In previous cryosurgical studies without a urethral warmer, urethral sloughing has been noted in a majority of patients. The urethral warming device reduces this incidence to 4.5 per cent. Although this device is not yet approved by the Food and Drug Administration it is believed that it does not present a potential for serious risk or harm to the health, safety, or welfare of the patient and it is critical to the continued success of the procedure.

Using the transrectal ultrasound transducer, the prostate is surveyed and the lesion defined. Using the longitudinal ultrasound plane and the attached needle insertion guide, five 18-gauge trocars are placed circumferentially into the prostate gland under ultrasound guidance. When appropriately placed as confirmed by ultrasound, a wire is inserted and a cannula and dilator are placed over the wire, again confirming placement by ultrasound. The cannula remains in place and the dilator and the wire trocar are removed. Then the cryoprobes are placed through the cannula. On confirmation by ultrasound that the cryoprobes are in the correct position, the liquid nitrogen is turned on and the procedure monitored using transrectal ultrasound. When the freezing is determined to include the entire gland as noted by the hyperechoic rim on ultrasound, the liquid nitrogen is halted.

In general, the probes are not long enough to freeze the whole prostatic length; therefore, to ensure that the apex is completely frozen, the probes are thawed, pulled back, and refrozen. Once the entire prostate has been treated, the probes are thawed, and removed. Occasionally, the probes will be placed in one or two additional positions to ensure complete freezing of the gland. The tracts then are closed with interrupted 3-0 chromic sutures. Antibiotics are continued for 5 days following the procedure. The suprapubic catheter is left until the patient is able to void and low post-void residual urines.

Hazards and Precautions

The known risks of cryosurgery include urethral-rectal fistula and urethral-cutaneous fistula. The chances of these complications occurring should be minimized by ultrasound monitoring and the use of the urethral warming device. Incontinence is a potential risk of the procedure if the external sphincter is completely frozen. The area of this structure is well visualized under transrectal ultrasound, which should enable the surgeon to avoid this complication. Impotence again is a potential complication. Also, sepsis and hemorrhage are potential complications. Sepsis can be minimized by using strict sterile technique and preprocedural antibiotic coverage. Bleeding is not anticipated to be a major problem with this procedure because of the small size of the probes. The technique used to control bleeding is to suture the cannula sites in the perineum with interrupted 3-0 chromic sutures.

Suggested Readings

Addonizio JC: Another look at cryoprostatectomy. Cryobiology 19:223–227, 1982

Onik GM, Cohen JK, Reyes GD, et al: Percutaneous radical cryosurgical ablation of the prostate under transrectal ultrasound guidance. CA 72:1291–1299, 1993

Trumble TE, Whalen JT: The effects of cryosurgery and cryoprotectants on peripheral nerve function. J Reconstr Microsurg 8:53–58, 1992

SECTION 6

THE URETHRA

Congenital Disorders

URETHRAL VALVES

W. HARDY HENDREN, M.D.

Boston, Massachusetts

Urethral valves occur in a wide spectrum of severity. At the mild end of this spectrum are boys who have voiding disturbances such as frequency, urgency, day wetting, and sometimes bed wetting. At the severe end of the spectrum are neonates, and sometimes older boys, who have high-grade obstruction of the bladder with bladder wall hypertrophy, cellules, and severe hydroureteronephrosis. In some there is massive vesicoureteral reflux. Others have widening and tortuousity of the ureters without reflux. In recent years, with the advent of maternal ultrasound examination of the unborn fetus, some cases are detected in utero.

Symptoms caused by urethral valves vary with the severity of urethral obstruction present. Small valves with minor urethral obstruction and minimal bladder hypertrophy may have minimal symptoms. When there is more severe obstruction, which often is associated with vesicoureteral reflux, urinary infection may be the first symptom noted. In severe cases with hydronephrosis, early clinical manifestations may include infection, uremia, discovery of an abdominal mass, failure to thrive, and, sometimes, hematuria. Occasionally, parents will notice a weak dribbling stream. In my experience, however, it is relatively rare that this has been noted by parents, although the same parents will volunteer that the stream is much improved when valves have been resected. Residual urine is not always present in boys with valves. The bladder, like any hollow viscus, can compensate for obstruction by muscular hypertrophy, emptying completely with high pressure and no residual up to a point where the bladder muscle decompensates. When obstruction is relieved, some very hypertrophied bladders will be noncompliant, exhibiting high pressure and small volume. Augmentation cystoplasty can be helpful in selected cases of that sort.

The anatomy of urethral valves was described by Young 74 years ago. Type I valves are the most common. They arise from the urethral crest just distal to the verumontanum. In severe cases the valve leaflets encircle dorsally to form a diaphragm at 12 o'clock as viewed through the endoscope. The endoscopic view may show a narrow vertical slit between the valve leaflets, much like a pair of vocal cords in the adducted position.

The diagnosis of urethral valves should be suspected in utero when ultrasound examination discloses a large bladder, hydronephrosis, and sometimes oligohydramnios. A male neonate with a large bladder should be suspected of having valves. Similarly, an older male with infection or abnormal voiding should be studied for valves. The upper tracts always should be screened by intravenous pyelogram or ultrasonography. A cys togram with multiple spot films while voiding should make the diagnosis if the clinician and/or the radiologist know how to recognize urethral valves. Awareness of the entity of valves is essential for their diagnosis! A motion picture film is available showing the wide spectrum of urethral valves.

Surgical ablation of urethral valves today should be straightforward. The endoscopic and video monitoring equipment now available allows an experienced teacher to monitor the endoscopic techniques of the pupil in the operating room. In 1919 Young resected valves with a cold punch. Later, some surgeons split the pubic symphysis, resecting the urethral valves under direct vision through the opened prostatic urethra. Then other blind techniques were used, passing a hooked electrode under fluoroscopic control to cut valves or avulsing them with a Foley balloon catheter or the Fogarty embolectomy balloon catheter. In my experience, valves almost uniformly can be resected under direct vision using a small (7.5-mm) endoscope through which a ureteral catheter is passed, using its metal stylette as a cutting electrode by attaching a Bovie cord to it. Accurate placement of the end of the wire against the valve leaflets while applying brief bursts of cutting current using a foot pedal can destroy valves without injury to important adjacent structures such as the urethral sphincter, the verumontanum, or the bladder neck. This technique is shown in Figure 1.

Some patients with urethral valves require no further treatment beyond resecting the valves. Usually voiding will improve immediately and lesser degrees of vesicoureteral reflux often will disappear. Impressive hydroureteronephrosis may disappear gradually. It is important to emphasize, however, that in some cases the secondary changes are too great to expect spontaneous improvement. If there is high-grade reflux and hydroureteronephrosis, ureteral reimplantation should be considered. Similarly, in some patients without reflux there is obstruction at the ureterovesical junction, which should be relieved. Reimplanting ureters into a hypertrophied bladder can be much more difficult than into a normal bladder. Severe obstructive uropathy secondary to urethral valves has been a common cause for establishing urinary diversion in males with severe valve pathology. This was the most common single cause for urinary diversion in a large group of patients whose urinary tracts I have reconstructed after longstanding urinary diversion. In most patients, diversion could have been avoided in retrospect.

Urethral valves are much more common

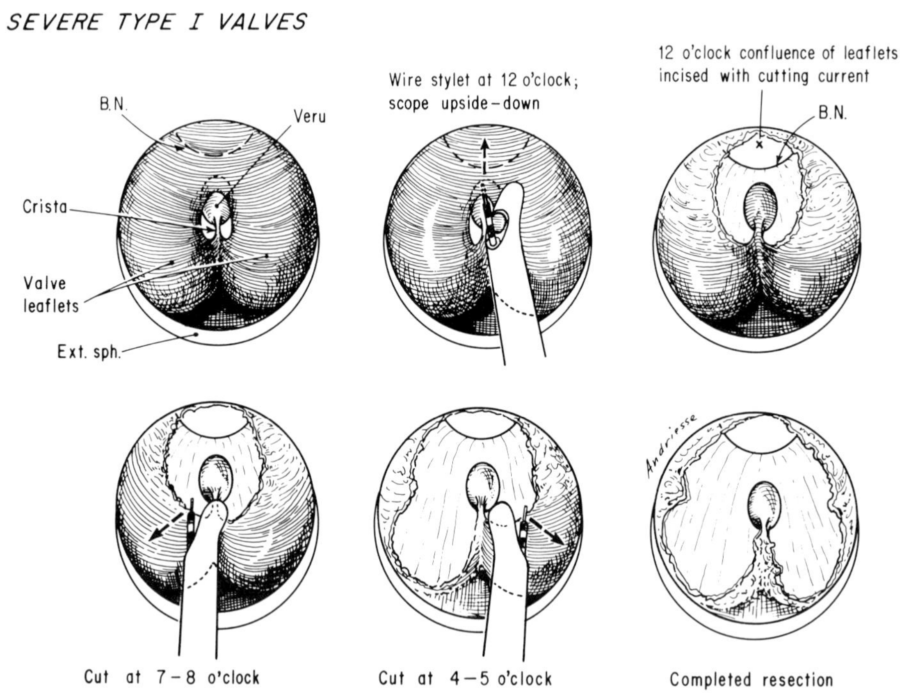

FIGURE 1. Technique for resecting severe type I urethral valves. Note that valves arise from the crista urethralis, just distal to the verumontanum. The crista may be short, as depicted above, or it may be quite long in some patients. Valve leaflets are an accentuation of normal folds that arise from the veru. They encircle dorsally to form a diaphragm at 12 o'clock. Valves are best seen with the bladder full and the irrigating reservoir about 3 feet above the level of the patient. Shown is a wire electrode made from a 3F woven ureteral catheter, using its wire stylette as the electrode. It is important to cut off the end of the sheath so that there are no side holes in the catheter, lest the current arc from a side hole to the lens, a costly mistake. The scope should be introduced fully into the bladder before advancing the electrode, to avoid inadvertently puncturing the side wall of the urethra. By turning the scope upside down, the electrode can cut the 12 o'clock confluence of valve leaflets accurately. Following this, the residual leaflet tissue is cut at 7 to 8 o'clock, and at 4 to 5 o'clock. Once the valves are resected, there is a cloverleaf deformity giving a clear view of the external sphincter, the bladder neck, and the veru. The 12 o'clock confluence of the leaflets is close to the external sphincter. This obviates using a cutting loop drawn toward the operator, lest the sphincter be cut. It is tempting to incise the greatly hypertrophied bladder neck (B.N.) in these cases, but that can cause stress incontinence and/or retrograde ejaculation in the future.

than generally appreciated. Any male patient with an abnormality in voiding should be suspected of having urethral valves until disproved by voiding cystourethrography and cystourethroscopy by an experienced observer.

Suggested Readings

Hendren WH: Posterior urethral valves. In Ashcraft KW (ed): Pediatric Urology. Philadelphia, WB Saunders, 1990, pp. 313–351

Hendren WH: Posterior urethral valves in boys: A broad clinical spectrum. J Urol 106:298–307, 1971

Hendren WH: "Urethral Valves: Diagnosis and Endoscopic Resection." A film available from Eaton Film Library, Norwich, CT.

Hendren WH: Urinary tract refunctionalization after long-term diversion. A 20 year experience with 177 patients. Ann Surg 212:478–495, 1990

Young HH, Frontz WA, Baldwin JC: Congenital obstruction of the posterior urethra. J Urol 3:289–292, 1919

URETHRAL MEATAL STENOSIS

HYMAN H. RABINOVITCH, M.D.

Philadelphia, Pennsylvania

Narrowing of the external urethral meatus (meatal stenosis) may be congenital or acquired. *Congenital meatal stenosis* in the uncircumcised male infant with a complete prepuce is exceedingly rare if it occurs at all. It may be seen occasionally in infants born with hypospadias, in whom the prepuce is almost invariably deficient ventrally. The diagnosis is made on physical examination by the finding of a rounded pinhole meatus and the observation of a thin, forceful urinary stream directed downward. Treatment consists of a lateral meatotomy.

Meatal stenosis in the female child was a common diagnosis in the 1960s and 1970s. It was mistakenly thought to be a cause of urinary tract infection and/or diurnal enuresis and was managed by cystoscopy and meatotomy. The true cause of the urethral obstruction, seen on voiding cystourethrography as a "spinning top urethra," now is believed to be due to inappropriate contraction of the external urethral sphincter at the time of voiding. Meatal stenosis in the female child has disappeared as a disease entity, along with bladder neck contracture (Marion disease).

Acquired meatal stenosis in the male child may be seen following hypospadias repair. The diagnosis is usually obvious on inspection of the meatus and confirmed by observation of the abnormal urinary stream, which may be accompanied by straining to void. Treatment by intermittent distal urethral dilation with a well-lubricated catheter of appropriate size may be sufficient. Alternatively, meatotomy may be required.

The most common cause of acquired meatal stenosis in the male is neonatal circumcision. Removal of the protective prepuce exposes the external urethral meatus to the wet diaper. The salt and acid (or alkaline ammonia) content of the urine incites a chemical meatitis frequently seen in the circumcised infant boy still in diapers. As a result of the fibroblast invasion of the area, there may be fibrosis with gradual (over a period of years) contraction and narrowing of the external urethral meatus. The incidence of clinical meatal stenosis in circumcised boys is unknown but would appear to be in the vicinity of 1 to 2 per cent.

The usual presentation of meatal stenosis is by the physical finding of a small meatus in an asymptomatic boy 2 to 10 years of age. Meatal stenosis is a spectrum disorder. The extremes (normal at one end and severe or moderate meatal stenosis at the other) are obvious, but the cases in between may present some difficulty in diagnosis. They represent the cases that could be categorized as small normal meatus or early meatal stenosis.

The normal size of the external urethral meatus in boys of different ages has been documented. Rather than calibration of the meatus with sounds, it would seem preferable to make the diagnosis of meatal stenosis on clinical grounds based on observation of the meatus (size and configuration) and of the urinary stream (caliber, force, and direction).

The normal meatus in a boy is a slit that can be opened by pressing with a thumb on either side, exposing the distal urethra. The normal stream at the point of exit from the meatus is a rectangle in cross section, with the greater distance of the rectangle directed longitudinally. The direction of the stream is normally in line with the shaft of the penis.

Significant meatal stenosis is characterized by a small (at times pinhole) round opening at the tip of the glans penis. The stream is fine (a small circle in cross section) and forceful and the time it takes to empty the bladder is prolonged. The stream typically is directed upward because of deflection by closure of the ventral aspect of the meatus. Difficulty in directing the stream into the toilet is a common complaint, as is urinary infrequency (twice a day). A complaint of dysuria and/or urinary frequency is uncommon unless there is an associated urinary tract infection.

Clinical meatal stenosis is treated by ventral meatotomy under general anesthesia on an outpatient basis. Older, more cooperative boys will tolerate meatotomy under local anesthesia. Questionable meatal stenosis is best managed by follow-up evaluations.

Meatal stenosis is rarely a cause of significant obstructive uropathy and, therefore, radiologic evaluation of the urinary tract is not warranted.

Suggested Readings

Litvak AA, Morris JD, McRoberts JW: Normal size of the urethral meatus in male children. J Urol 115:736, 1976

Noe HN, Dale GA: Evaluation of children with meatal stenosis. J Urol 144:455, 1975

MEGALOURETHRA

ANTHONY A. CALDAMONE, M.D.

Providence, Rhode Island

Megalourethra is a rare congenital anomaly of the anterior urethra. The dilation of the urethra is secondary to poor development of the corpus spongiosum and/or the corpus cavernosa rather than to distal obstruction. Megalourethra traditionally is divided into two types: scaphoid (incomplete) and fusiform (complete). These two forms can be distinguished by their clinical and radiographic appearance. The scaphoid type of megalourethra is the more common and the less severe form of this anomaly (Fig. 1). The scaphoid megalourethra is a localized deficiency of the corpus spongiosum in the anterior urethra that results in formation of a ventral saccular diverticulum that balloons during voiding. This diverticular appearance results because the dorsal urethral wall is fixed and supported by the corpus cavernosa. Generally the glanular urethra is normal. In the fusiform megalourethra, the corpora cavernosa as well as the corpus spongiosum are absent, resulting in an elongated sac-like penis that distends markedly when filled with urine. Several authors dispute the arbitrary distinction between the scaphoid and fusiform types of megalourethra, believing that the disorder is more appropriately viewed as a spectrum rather than two distinct entities.

Mesodermal dysplasia is the likely etiology of megalourethra because the disorder is associated with other mesodermal abnormalities of the genitourinary system. Generally, the more severe genitourinary and cardiac anomalies are found with the fusiform megalourethra.

ASSOCIATED ANOMALIES

Megalourethra frequently is associated with other congenital anomalies, particularly of the upper urinary tract and anterior abdominal wall. Fusiform megalourethra has been associated with other diffuse mesenchymal disorders including renal dysplasia-hypoplasia, vesicoureteral reflux, megacystitis, atresia or stenosis of the posterior urethra, imperforate anus with rectovesical fistula, and undescended testes. In addition, fusiform megalourethra commonly is seen with prune-belly syndrome. Generally, fusiform megalourethra is associated with more severe upper tract as well as nongenitourinary anomalies. Scaphoid megalourethra also has been reported to be associated with posterior ure-

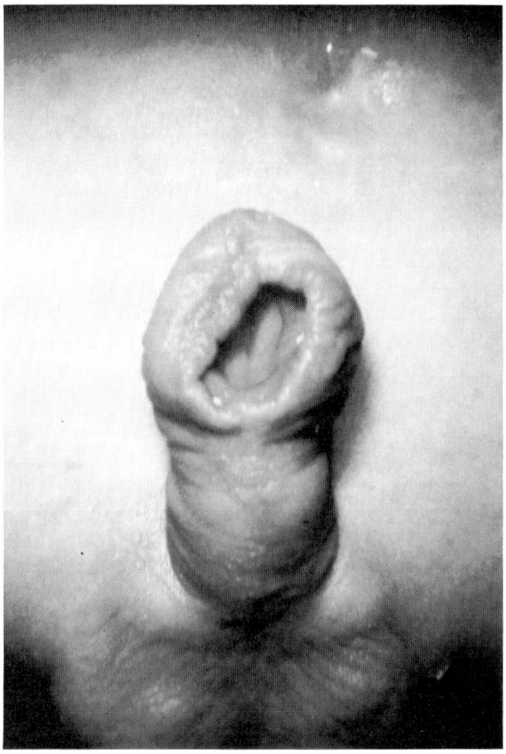

FIGURE 1. Scaphoid distal megalourethra in a child with prune-belly syndrome. (Courtesy of Howard McSnyder.)

thral valves, urethral duplication, and hypospadias (Fig. 2).

DIAGNOSIS

The diagnosis of megalourethra generally is made by physical examination. It most commonly is confused with urethral diverticulum. Voiding results in massive ballooning of the anterior urethra because of the lack of investment of the corpus spongiosum. With time this dilation becomes more progressive. The high incidence of associated upper urinary tract anomalies warrants full upper tract evaluation in all patients. An abdominal ultrasound including the kidneys and bladder should be the first diagnostic test. When indicated, an excretory urogram with a follow-up voiding film will delineate the upper and lower tracts and avoid catheterization.

Sepsis following urethral instrumentation has been well documented; therefore, it is recommended that antibiotic coverage accompany any instrumentation. The megalourethra is susceptible to bacterial colonization as a result of meatal contamination and stasis. Suppressive antibiotics are indicated, therefore, for long-term management, particularly if other genitourinary abnormalities are present.

MANAGEMENT

Prior to surgical correction of megalourethra, a thorough evaluation for other congenital anomalies is mandatory because of the high incidence of associated life-threatening anomalies.

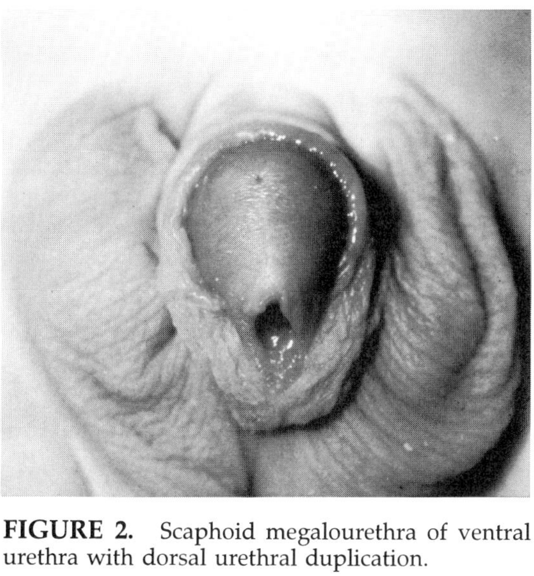

FIGURE 2. Scaphoid megalourethra of ventral urethra with dorsal urethral duplication.

Nesbitt originally treated a large scaphoid megalourethra by circumcision and excision of the redundant urethra, with reapproximate of the urethral skin over a catheter stent. After making a circumscribing incision at the level of the corona and degloving the penile shaft, a ventral incision is made in the midline of the redundant ventral aspect of the urethra. The excess urethra is excised from the lateral flaps and a new urethra created by suturing over an appropriately sized catheter based on the patient's age. A two-layered closure of the urethra using an inner running suture and outer interrupted sutures generally affords a water-tight closure. The redundant penile skin then is excised and tailored to the cylindrical form of the phallus. The skin then is resutured at the corona, thereby covering the urethroplasty in order to prevent urethrocutaneous fistula.

In the case of fusiform megalourethra, repair is complicated by lack of supporting structures and minimal corpora cavernosa as well as by excessive length of the penis. As a result of the lack of supporting structure, repair of fusiform megalourethra is most often unsatisfactory. The suggestion of gender reassignment in these cases has been proposed. Many of these patients do not come to repair because of the severity of associated anomalies and subsequent low survival rate. The most common cause of demise is renal failure resulting from renal dysplasia.

Suggested Readings

Appel RA, Kaplan GW, Brock WA: Megalourethra. J Urol 135:747, 1986

Lindner A, Jonas P, Hertz M, et al: Scaphoid megalourethra. Br J Urol 52:143, 1980

Mortensen PH, Johnson HW, Coleman GA, et al: Megalourethra. J Urol 134:358, 1985

Nesbitt TE: Congenital megalo-urethra. J Urol 73:839, 1959

Shrom SH, Cromie WJ, Duckett JW: Megalourethra. Urology 17:152, 1981

MODERN HYPOSPADIAS

JOHN W. DUCKETT, Jr., M.D.

Philadelphia, Pennsylvania

For successful results in hypospadias surgery, one must be equipped with: (1) a variety of techniques; (2) knowledge of past procedures; (3) experience with delicate, precise, optically enhanced surgical technique; and (4) full awareness of the pitfalls in order to avoid them. Either get into hypospadiology completely or stay out. Do not dabble!

CLASSIFICATION

The classification scheme of hypospadias is presented in Figure 1.

INCIDENCE

One in 300 boys have hypospadias. Their fathers have hypospadias in 8 per cent of cases and their male siblings are affected in 14 per cent of cases. Besides undescended testes (9 per cent of cases) and inguinal hydroceles or hernias (9 per cent of cases), the incidence of other anomalies is not significant in isolated hypospadias. When other systems are involved, evaluation of the upper tracts and bladder is indicated. Utricles may be present in perineal and penoscrotal varieties (15 per cent of cases).

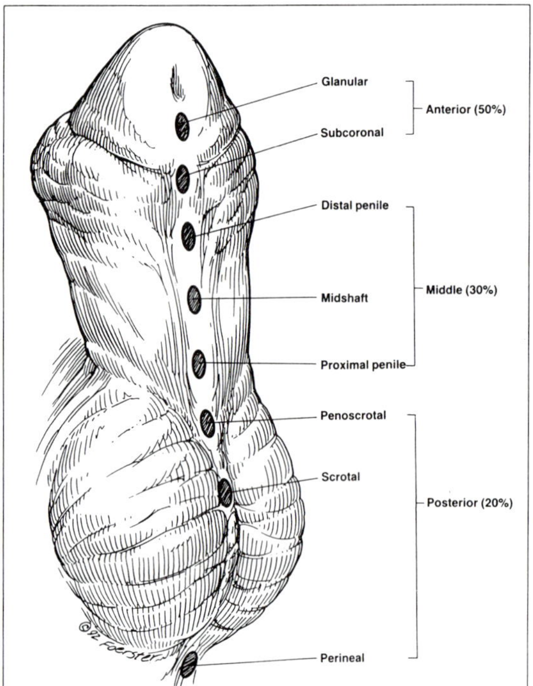

FIGURE 1. Classification of hypospadias. The location of the meatus *after* correction of curvature provides the most practical classification for hypospadias. The glanular and subcoronal locations make up the anterior class, representing 50 per cent of hypospadias cases. The distal penile, midshaft, and proximal penile locations make up the middle class (30 per cent), and the penoscrotal, scrotal and perineal locations make up the posterior class (20 per cent).

AGE AND PREOPERATIVE PREPARATION

The best age for surgical correction is between 6 and 18 months, when the babies are amnestic of the procedure. Management in a diaper is easier on the parents and permits outpatient surgery.

Instruments

Ophthalmologic instruments are necessary, including Castroviejo forceps and needle holders, and iris scissors. Optical magnification is essential, although low magnification will suffice (1× to 2×). Some prefer using operative microscopes. Sutures of 7-0 size are recommended.

Ancillary Procedures

The use of 1:100,000 epinephrine in 1 per cent lidocaine is helpful in diminishing operative and postoperative bleeding. A tourniquet is optional but should be released every 20 minutes. Hemostasis with cauterization must be more aggressive if a tourniquet alone is used. A compressive dressing is required for the first several hours after surgery to avoid hematoma and edema formation. This should be easily removed at home by the parents in 72 hours. We prefer to compress the penis on the lower abdomen with gauze and a bio-occlusive dressing. Urinary diversion is accomplished with a 6F stent (Kendall) placed into the bladder and sutured to the glans with 5-0 Prolene. This drips into the diaper at a continuous rate and is removed in 10 to 14 days. Oxybutynin or B & O suppositories cut into thirds are prescribed for bladder spasms.

SURGICAL TECHNIQUES

Meatal Advancement and Glanuloplasty (MAGPI) (Fig. 2)

The majority of cases of hypospadias are caused by canalization of the glans urethra. This leaves the meatus at the subcoronal area, frequently stenotic, with a dorsal lip that deflects the stream downward at 30 to 45 de-

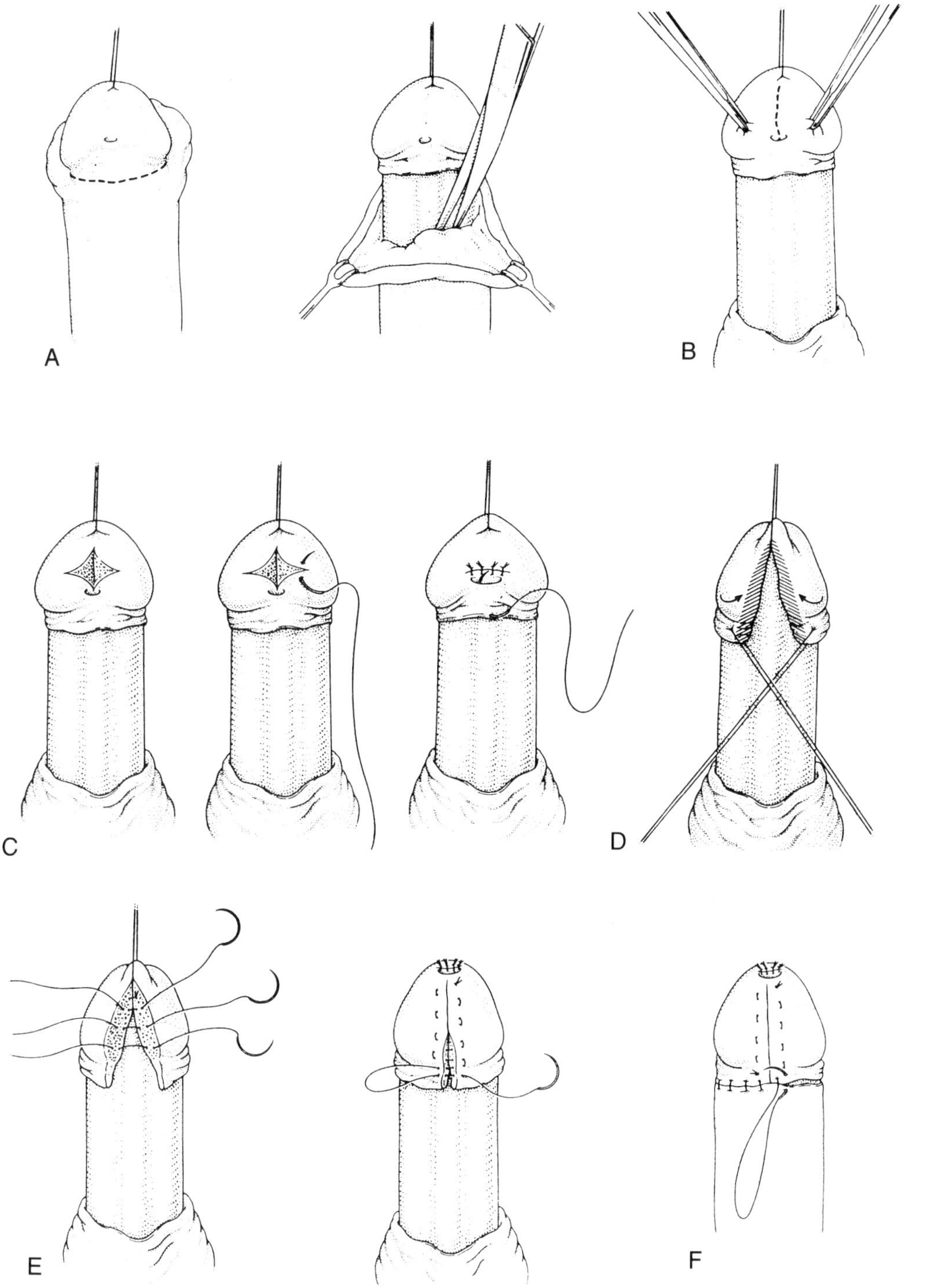

FIGURE 2. MAGPI procedure. *A*, The skin of the penile shaft is dissected away. *B*, A typical MAGPI meatus configuration has a coronal or subcoronal meatus deflected downward by a bridge of tissue at the coronal margin. A wedge of this bridge of tissue is excised all the way into the glanular groove and down into the dorsal meatus 1 to 2 mm. *C*, This creates a diamond-shaped defect that is closed transversely with interrupted sutures. This widens the meatus considerably. *D*, A traction suture on the ventral meatal edge is pulled forward while the two lateral glanular traction sutures are pulled downward, forming a conical-shaped glans. The medial edges of this redundant glanular tissue are excised. *E*, Deep glanular tissue, as well as the superficial epithelial layer, is brought together with interrupted sutures. *F*, A sleeve reapproximation of the skin of the penile shaft is made, excising redundant dorsal foreskin; dorsal-to-ventral skin cover may be required. No stent or catheter is necessary.

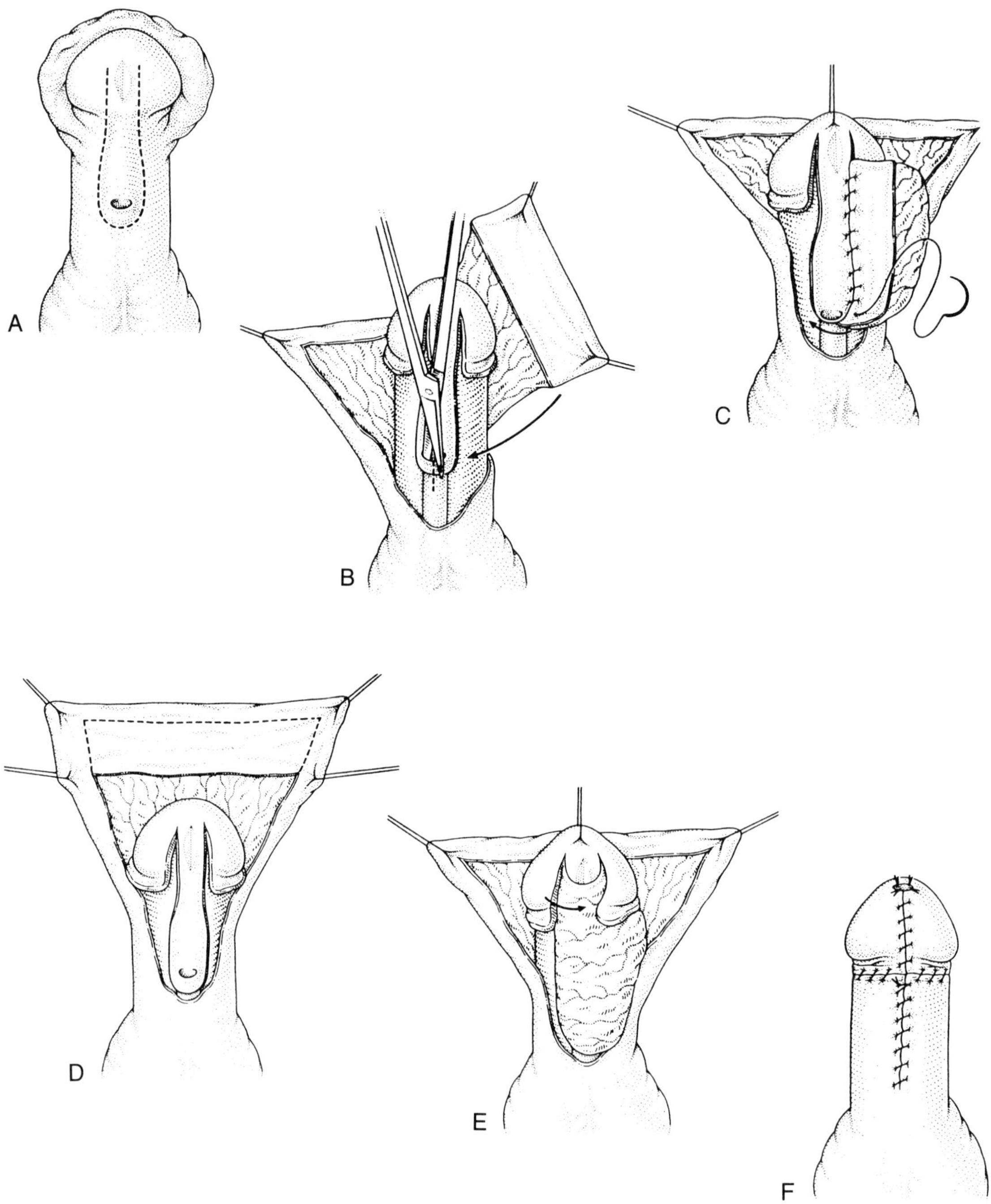

FIGURE 3. Onlay island flap procedure. This is most appropriate for the distal, middle, and proximal penile meatal locations, with preservation of the urethral plate when minimal curvature exists after skin takedown. *A,* Glanular wings are developed with parallel incisions onto the ventral glans, out to the tip of the glanular groove. *B,* The proximal meatus is cut back to good spongiosal tissue, excising the skin edges of the native meatus. The urethral strip is 4 to 5 mm in breadth. The proximal urethra is tailored, and a transverse preputial flap that is wider than is needed is taken from the ventral prepuce. *C,* The onlay flap is sutured to one side of the urethral plate and tailored to create a neourethra of 12F caliber. *D,* Approximately two thirds of the epithelial flap is discarded, leaving a broad pedicle for overlapping the suture lines. *E,* The glanular wings are reapproximated in the midline with interrupted sutures around the meatus and deep mesenchymal sutures to bring the glans proper together. The dorsal prepuce is split down the midline and rotated around to the ventrum to close in the midline for skin cover. *F,* Appearance of completed onlay island flap repair.

grees. The bridge of tissue distal to the meatus in the glanular groove must be wedged out. The dorsal meatal edge can be advanced up to the end of the urethral groove with fine sutures (meatoplasty).

The glanuloplasty is accomplished by elevating the ventral edge of the urethral meatus forward and rotating the flattened glanular wings around to the ventrum in a conical shape. Excess skin on the ventral "V" is excised in order to bring together the glanular wings. *It is most important to reapproximate glans tissue in a two-layer fashion with a deep closure of glans mesenchyme and a superficial layer of glans epithelium.* This exaggerated rotation of glans tissue on the ventrum prevents the meatus from regressing back to the subcoronal area.

Complications include a 1 per cent secondary surgical rate with meatal regression the most common complaint. Fistulas should not occur. Modifications of the MAGPI procedure include the Arap, Firlit, King, GAP, pyramid, and Mathieu procedures.

Onlay Island Flap (Fig. 3)

For the distal midshaft meatus without curvature, one may preserve the urethral plate with a parallel incision into the glans similar to that in the Mathieu procedure. Certainty of straightness is checked with artificial erection. Ventral urethral construction is made from a transverse preputial onlay flap. Sizing of the flap is done after one edge is sutured to the urethral plate, taking care that redundancy, which could lead to a diverticulum or ballooning of the neourethra, is avoided.

Tunica Albuginea Plication (Fig. 4)

Straightening of curvature may require several maneuvers. The urethral plate may be left intact while skin takedown proceeds and straightness is assessed with artificial erection. Many times, only minimal curvature will remain. The next step is to resect all fibrous tissue on the ventrum if it is tethering the penis ventrally.

Dorsal tucks, or plication of the dorsal tunica albuginea, may be done to straighten the penis. These are made with two parallel incisions about 8 mm apart at 10 and 2 o'clock on the dorsal lateral aspect of the corpora at the apex of maximal bend. The neurovascular bundles in Buck's fascia are elevated to avoid injury. The outer edges of these two parallel incisions are sutured together with permanent suture, tucking the midportion underneath. No ellipse of tunica albuginea is removed. The knots are buried beneath Buck's fascia.

Transverse Preputial Island Flap (Fig. 5)

When curvature must be released by excising the fibrous chordee, this leaves a gap between the proximal meatus (penoscrotal or perineal) and the tip of the glans. A full-tubed urethra may be formed from the transverse preputial island flap, dissected from the undersurface of the outer layer of dorsal prepuce. Holding sutures are placed in a rectan-

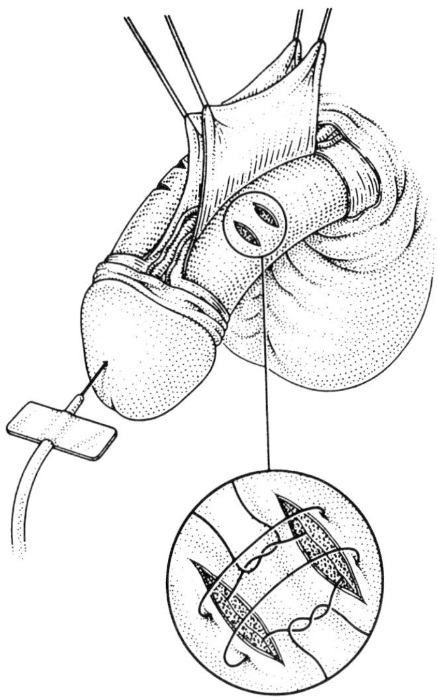

FIGURE 4. Tunica albuginea plication. The straightening procedure for curvature consists of a combination of excising ventral fibrous tissue and taking dorsal tucks as needed for final straightening. The curvature may be so severe that preservation of the urethral plate is impossible. With artificial erection, a 25-gauge butterfly needle is placed through the glans into the corporal tissue and injected with saline with a tourniquet at the base. At the point of maximal bend, parallel incisions are made through the tunica albuginea after elevating a layer of Buck's fascia, making sure that the neurovascular bundles on the dorsum are preserved. These parallel strips, about 8 mm apart, are approximated at their lateral edges using two permanent 5-0 Prolene stitches (inset). These tucks on either side achieve the final straightening.

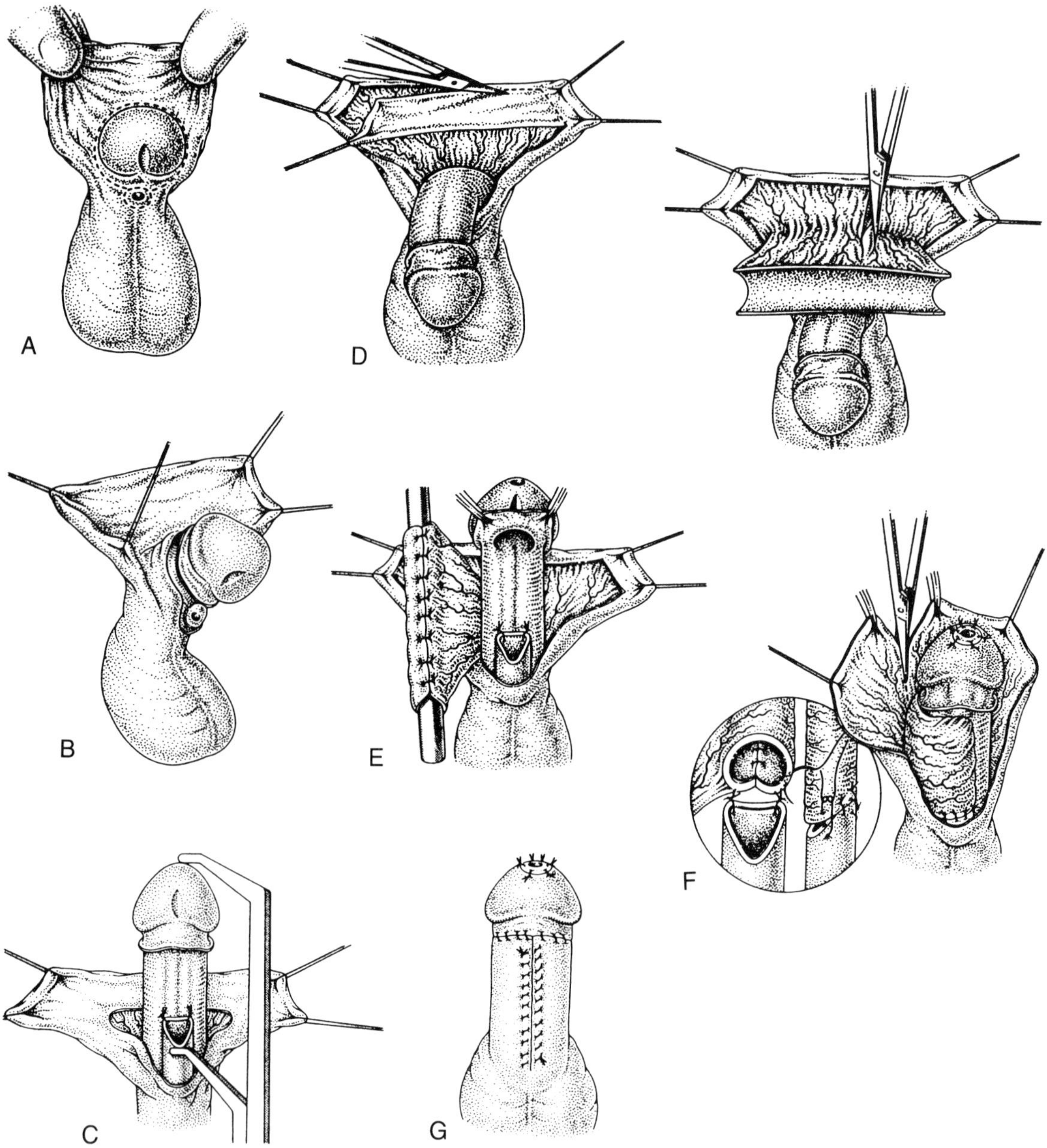

FIGURE 5. Transverse Preputial Island Flap Urethroplasty. For a severe curvature without preservation of the urethral plate, the straightening procedure proceeds as needed. *A,* The prepuce is incised in a horseshoe shape to obtain sufficient length for the flap. The proximal urethra is freed from the glans. *B,* Holding sutures are placed on the undersurface of the prepuce to form a 12- to 15-mm wide rectangle. *C,* The proximal urethra may drop all the way down into the scrotum unless it is fixed to the tunica albuginea with fine sutures. The required length of neourethra is measured. *D,* The transverse preputial flap is developed. The base of the flap must be freed up adequately to avoid torsion of the shaft during rotation to the ventrum. *E,* The preputial flap is tubularized to a caliber of 12F as confirmed with a bougie à boule. The distal edges of the tube are approximated with interrupted sutures so that the edges may be trimmed to fashion the appropriate length. A wide glans channel is made underneath the glans cap against the corporal bodies. (An alternative method is to split the glans and make glans wings.) *F,* A proximal oblique anastomosis is made fixing the urethroplasty to the tunica albuginea along its posterior edge (inset). The neourethra is tailored to fit the gap to avoid redundancy and trimmed for a meatoplasty at the apex of the glans. The dorsal preputial and penile skin is split in its midline in order to rotate the wings of tissue around to the ventrum for a midline closure with a horizontal mattress suture of chromic material. A 6F Kendall catheter is placed through the repair just into the bladder and sutured to the glans with 5-0 Prolene, allowing urine to drip into the diaper. *G,* Appearance of completed preputial island flap repair.

gular fashion on the undersurface of the prepuce, measuring to make the width 12 to 15 mm. The length, however, must suffice to bridge the gap, and sufficient flap tissue always can be obtained by cutting down along the penile skin in a horseshoe fashion on either side. The inner shiny skin with its blood supply is dissected free of the outer prepuce and penile skin by dissecting the axially oriented subcutaneous tissue free from the outer skin. The plane usually dissects very neatly and the vasculature is obvious in the pedicle.

The pedicle is rotated around the shaft in order to bring the rectangle of skin to the ventrum. This is tubularizd over an 8F catheter as a template and, after careful suturing, should calibrate at 12F with a bougie à boule.

A proximal oblique anastomosis is made to the native urethra after all of the skin is removed from the urethral meatus. The dorsal edge is fixed to the tunica albuginea.

The glans is channeled, staying close to the tunica albuginea of the corpora cavernosa. A tip of glans epithelium is excised. Glanular tissue must be removed in order to make this glans channel of adequate width (18F to 20F). Splitting the glans may be appropriate in certain cases, with approximation around the neourethra.

Buccal Mucosa Grafts (Fig. 6)

Redo cases may require excising the previous urethroplasty and replacing it with new epithelium. A free graft of buccal mucosa, depending on the length of the urethra to be replaced, has been our recent preferred urethral replacement. Because the graft must be revascularized, perfect cover of viable tissue must be assured and drainage must be appropriate so that no hematoma occurs. Bladder mucosa has a longer experience but the complications have been excessive.

Skin Cover

In all hypospadias cases, the skin of the shaft of the penis is dissected to the penoscrotal junction or below. In the MAGPI, it is often possible to reapproximate the cylinder of penile skin back to the glans, similarly to a circumcision, excising the redundant dorsal prepuce. It may be necessary to rotate the median raphe back to its ventral position in certain cases with torsion.

Alternately, the dorsal preputial skin may be split down the midline, permitting rotational flaps around each side, brought together in the midline on the ventrum and sutured up to the corona. The excess skin is excised obliquely.

COMPLICATIONS

Fistula is the most common reason for secondary surgery. One should wait a minimum of 6 months for complete healing to occur before attempting closure. This can be done

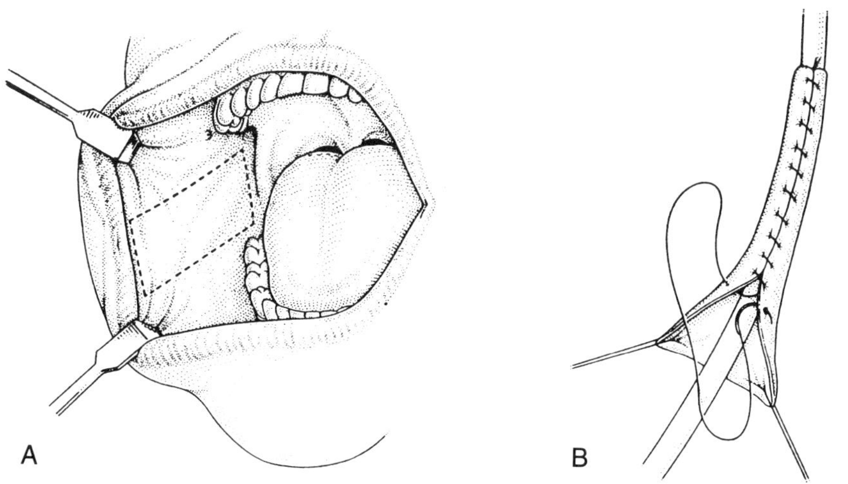

FIGURE 6. Buccal mucosa graft. In secondary cases when there is no penile skin for a flap procedure, a graft must form the neourethra. Buccal mucosa is thicker and more appropriate for urethral replacement than bladder mucosal tissue, although its length is limited to 4 to 5 cm. *A*, The inner check mucosa is harvested, avoiding Stensen's duct, to make an appropriate urethral replacement for age. *B*, The neourethra is formed over an appropriate sized catheter.

with a delicate excision of the epithelialized fistulous tract and reapproximation of the urethra and skin in two to three layers with fine sutures. No catheter is necessary. *Strictures* are next in the list of complications. They are due to poor vascularization or, more commonly, overlap of the two suture lines with a kink. These require open revision; internal optical urethrotomy is not successful over the long term. *Residual chordee* may be corrected with dorsal tucks. *Meatal stenosis* may be revised with a variety of meatoplasties. *Urethral diverticula* occur when urine leaks at the anastomosis, creating an epithelialized pocket. These can be quite large in size. Tapering of the urethra may be required. If a preputial flap is made too wide, it will distend over time and a fusiform diverticulum will form.

CONCLUSIONS

The author is prejudiced toward the use of vascularized tissue in hypospadias repair. Free grafts of penile or preputial skin may do well during the early years, but complications develop as the penis grows at puberty. It seems more logical to use vascularized skin, if possible, than to use the same skin as a graft. The buccal mucosal graft seems to be a better urethral substitute, but long-term results are not in yet. Delicate tissue handling, good plastic surgical principles, and attention to the many details should provide a secondary surgery rate of less than 5 per cent in hypospadias cases.

Suggested Readings

Duckett JW: Editorial Comment: Autologous buccal mucosa graft for hypospadias repair: An initial report. Dessanti, A. et al. J Urol 147:1081–1084, 1992

Duckett JW: Hypospadias. *In* Gillenwater JY, Grayhack JT, Howards SS, et al (eds): Adult and Pediatric Urology, vol 2. Chicago, Year Book Medical Publishers, 1991, p 2125

Duckett JW: Hypospadias repair. *In* Frank JD, Johnston JH (eds): Operative Paediatric Urology. London, Churchill Livingstone, 1990, p 202

Duckett JW, Keating MA: Technical challenge of the megameatus intact prepuce hypospadias (MIP) variant: The pyramid procedure. J Urol 141:1407–1408, 1989

Duckett JW, Snyder HM: Meatal advancement and glanuloplasty hypospadias repair after 1,000 cases: Avoidance of meatal stenosis and regression. J Urol 147:665–669, 1992

Keating MA, Duckett JW: Bladder mucosa in urethral reconstructions. J Urol 144:827–834, 1990

THE SUBCORONAL MEATUS

EDMOND T. GONZALES, JR., M.D.

Houston, Texas

Over the past 20 years, surgical techniques to repair hypospadias have become increasingly standardized. Today, most surgeons skilled in hypospadias surgery utilize a limited number of basic techniques, although among these surgeons many minor variations in technique exist. The incidence of major complications has tumbled, even for very proximal defects requiring complex reconstruction, and the emphasis now is to stress excellent cosmetic as well as functional results.

The child with a coronal or subcoronal meatus continues to present a limited surgical dilemma. If there is no chordee, the location of the meatus often presents no functional problem, although ventral deflection of the urinary stream could be a source of concern to the boy. If significant chordee is present, it may be difficult to know how much reconstruction will be necessary until the operative procedure is begun. Chordee may be a result of insufficient, inelastic ventral shaft skin; can result from thickened, fibrous, paraspongiosum bands; may be caused by a congenitally short urethra; or can be associated with a primary corporal disproportion. In this situation, the urologic surgeon who only does an occasional hypospadias repair may become involved with a defect that requires a major urethral reconstructive procedure with which he or she is not comfortable.

Horton and Devine initially emphasized the importance of a well-positioned glandular meatus and described a technique that placed the meatus at the tip of the glans with a minimal risk of meatal stenosis. Used originally in their major reconstructions, these principles soon were applied to repair more distal lesions with the popularization of the "flip-flap" technique. Other surgeons have described variations of this technique, all reporting excellent results with minimal morbidity and complications (Fig. 1).

When Duckett introduced the meatal advancement and glanuloplasty (MAGPI) technique for very distal defects, the cosmetic results were sufficiently satisfactory and the risks were sufficiently minimal to increase the enthusiasm of surgeons to recommend repair of even the most minor defects. From its original description the MAGPI procedure has been altered substantially (Fig. 2), and has spurred alternative techniques by Arap and Zaontz. These procedures can be done routinely through day surgery and require only a short-term or no indwelling urethral catheter. In our experience, the safe and effective application of these techniques, however, requires a careful preoperative assessment and a thorough understanding of the variations in development of the hypospadiac penis that make reconstruction of a distally placed meatus procedure of special concern.

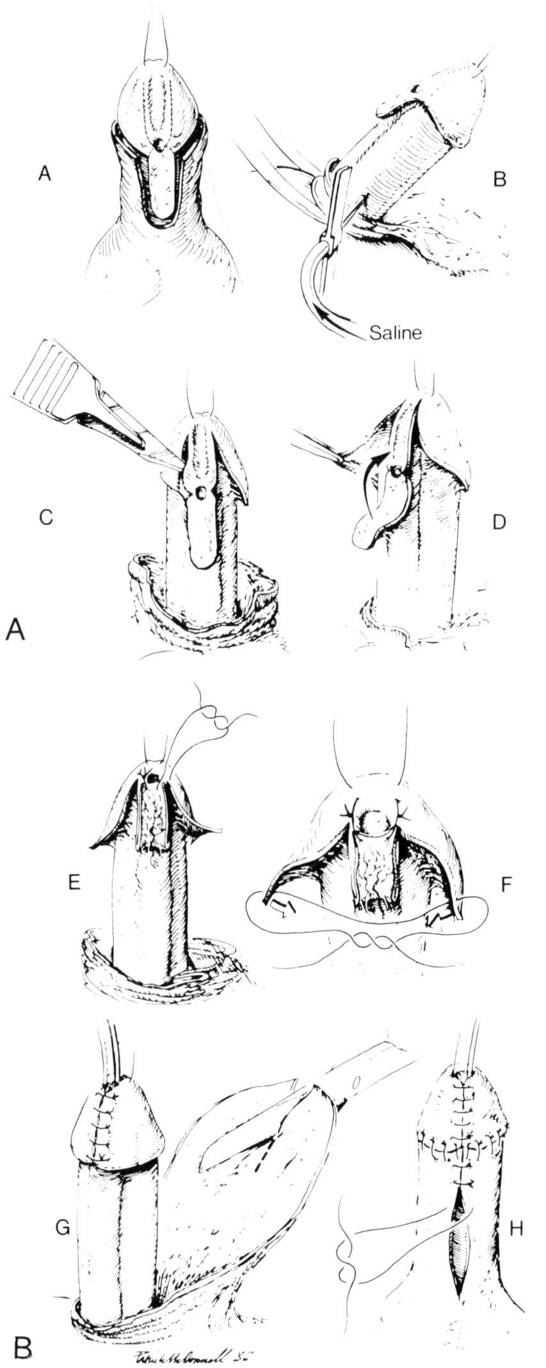

FIGURE 1. Meatal-based flap for repair of distal hypospadias. (From Gonzales ET, Veeraraghavan KA, Delaune J: The management of distal hypospadias with meatal-based, vascularized flaps. J Urol 129:119, 1983, with permission.)

From a clinical point of view, it is convenient to categorize the subcoronal meatus in one of three categories. In many cases, there is a small midline meatus that sits on or immediately proximal to the coronal margin. In this situation, there is little or no chordee and the ventral shaft skin is thick, elastic, and healthy. The corpus spongiosum usually extends right up to the meatus. In other cases, the meatus may be broad and flattened, usually placed slightly more proximal to the corona than described above. Careful inspection will identify that the corpus spongiosum begins to flare some distance before reaching the meatus itself. There may be varying degrees of chordee associated with these particular meatal anomalies, but, generally, the shaft skin on the ventrum of the penis is healthy and elastic. Finally, there may be a distally placed meatus that is associated with significant chordee and usually with identifiably deficient and dysplastic ventral skin. The corpus spongiosum flares widely and is often flattened and broad. An appreciation of these concepts is important in planning the appropriate surgical techniques for repair of the subcoronal meatus. In our experience, it is not always possible to know preoperatively what will be the most acceptable technique for managing the defect. Thus an organized approach has been developed and is based on the use of three common procedures available to every hypospadiac surgeon. Our experience is summarized in an article by Gibbons and Gonzales.

If the subcoronal meatus is pinpoint in nature, is on or close to the coronal margin, and is associated with no evident chordee and with healthy and elastic ventral shaft skin without evident bifurcation of the corpus spongiosum before the meatus, and the glans has a satisfactory ventral groove, a variant of the MAGPI procedure or a glans-approximating procedure (GAP) is chosen as the primary approach to repair this defect. If the meatus is somewhat more proximal and opened but with elastic shaft skin, or if there is mild chordee, a meatal-based flap is outlined and preserved as the shaft skin is dissected from the corpora cavernosa and urethra. In many situations, release of the tethered ventral skin will allow mild chordee to be released adequately. If some chordee persists, this often can be repaired by a dorsal plication of the tunica albuginea. In this situation, if the meatus remains elastic and the glans can be brought around the ventrum to allow adequate coverage, the meatal-based flap can be amputated and a MAGPI or GAP performed. If the meatus does not advance satisfactorily onto the glans, the meatus can be advanced by using the in situ flap.

If the meatus is slightly more proximal and very patulous, the MAGPI procedure does not work as well as the meatal-based flap procedures or the GAP because the broad, fish-mouthed urethral meatus cannot be advanced far enough out under the glandular tissue and tends to retract, so that the ultimate position of the meatus is less satisfactory. We have performed over 200 meatal-based flap procedures since the late 1970s with a fistula rate of less than 3 per cent and with almost no incidence of meatal stenosis (Fig. 3). An alternative procedure is a simple in situ tubularization of the wide urethral plate, as described by King many years ago. This approach affords excellent cosmetic results, but is associated with a slightly higher fistula rate in my hands.

When there is significant chordee present after release of all of the shaft skin, it may be necessary to transect the urethra and allow the meatus to fall into a more proximal position to correct this ventriflexion adequately. In this situation, the meatal-based flap can be discarded and a standard transverse preputial flap procedure undertaken. If there is no or only moderate chordee (correctable by dorsal plication), but the ventral shaft skin is very thin, one might consider a vascularized, inner preputial flap as an onlay rather than as a complete tubularized neourethra. Because there is no circumferential anastomosis, the risk of developing a urethral stricture is significantly less after an onlay as compared to a tubularized neourethra.

This summary emphasizes the variability that one might see with a coronal or subcoronal meatus and stresses the need for the surgeon who is interested in dealing with hypospadias to be familiar with all of the available principles for managing such lesions. In our experience, the majority of children with a subcoronal meatus now can be handled satisfactorily with a variant of the MAGPI procedure, and it has become our procedure of choice whenever possible. However, if we are to achieve optimal results in as many children as possible, we must be prepared to use any

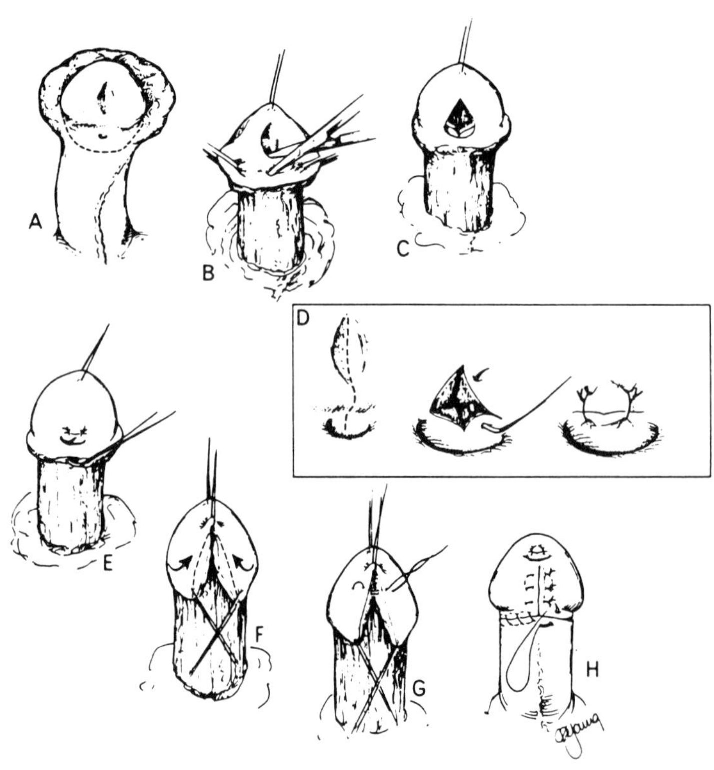

FIGURE 2. The MAGPI procedure as modified by Duckett and McSnyder. *A*, Subcoronal meatus. *B–D*, Circumferential subcoronal incision 8 mm proximal to meatus and corona; incision of bridge of tissue between meatus and glanular groove. Note the extent and depth of the incision (inset). Inset (*D*) shows transverse Heineke-Mikulicz closure of dorsal meatal edge to distal glanular groove. *E and F*, Three traction sutures placed at apex of ventral meatus and lateral glans where foreskin stops; glans edges are pulled together ventrally "V" fashion, and redundant edges excised. *G*, Vertical mattress approximation brings the glans beneath the meatus. *H*, Sleeve reapproximation of the penile skin, with excision of excess foreskin, completes the repair. Rotational flap closure is used if a ventral skin defect exists. (From Duckett JW: Hypospadias. *In* Gillenwater JY, Grayhack JT, Howards SS, et al [eds]: Adult and Pediatric Urology, vol 2. St. Louis, Mosby-Year Book, 1991, p 2114, with permission.)

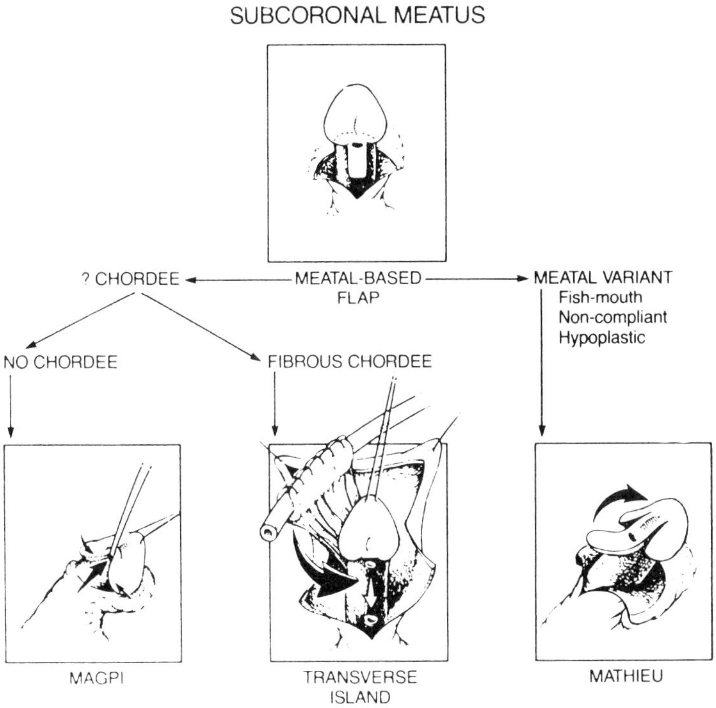

FIGURE 3. Use of meatal-based flap in management of distal hypospadias. (From Gibbons MD, Gonzales ET: The subcoronal meatus. J Urol 130:739, 1983, with permission.)

one of several techniques in order not to overlook the child with a subtle meatal variant.

Suggested Readings

Gibbons MD, Gonzales ET: The subcoronal meatus. J Urol 130:739, 1983

Gonzales ET, Veeraraghavan KA, Delaune J: The management of distal hypospadias with meatal-based, vascularized flaps. J Urol 129:119, 1983

Hollowell JG, Keating MA, Snyder HM, et al: Presentation of urethral plate in hypospadias repair: Extended applications and further experience with the onlay island flap urethroplasty. J Urol 143:98, 1990

Scherz HC, Kaplan GW, Parker MG: Modified meatal advancement and glanuloplasty (ARAP) hypospadias repair): Experience in 31 patients. J Urol 142:620, 1989

Zaontz MR: The GAP (glans approximation procedure) for glandular/coronal hypospadias. J Urol 141:359, 1989

Other Urethral Conditions

URETHRAL DIVERTICULA

JOSEPH C. CERNY, M.D., F.A.C.S.

Detroit, Michigan

Urethral diverticula are epithelial-lined pouches that communicate with the urethral lumen by a narrow neck. This often-misdiagnosed lesion of the lower urinary tract is common in the female urethra and causes persistent irritative symptoms. Such lesions frequently go unrecognized unless the astute clinician has a high index of suspicion. Urethral diverticula occur with a frequency of 1 to 6 per cent. They have been known to occur in girls, in whom they are considered congenital lesions. Their occurrence in infancy supports this theory. Congenital diverticula may be due to a cystic dilation of fetal ducts or meatal obstruction. There is often a spontaneous resolution of the congenital diverticulum.

Urethral diverticula in adult females are considered acquired lesions secondary to repeated infection and obstruction of the periurethral glands, with formation of suburethral cysts that subsequently rupture and drain into the urethral lumen. Calculi have been found in diverticula and probably develop because of stasis and infection. Thirty-five cases of carcinoma have been reported occurring within the urethral diverticulum. This could be the result of chronic inflammation, irritation, and infection. Women with urethral diverticula often suffer from chronic symptoms of frequency, urgency, irritative voiding, dysuria, dyspareunia, perineal pain, postvoid dribbling, and stress incontinence. They also may have obstructive symptoms if the diverticulum is large enough to occlude the urethra. Because these symptoms are seen in common disorders of the urinary tract, such as cystitis, the correct diagnosis often is not suspected, and patients with normal examinations often are mislabeled as complainers.

The differential diagnosis of urethral diverticula includes prolapsed urethra, ureterocele, urethral polyp, caruncle, suburethral cysts, and Skene duct abscess. The diagnosis is suggested in patients who have had frequent recurrent urinary tract infections or many of the irritative symptoms listed earlier. The physical examination is important. Special attention must be paid to the appearance of the urethra and the anterior vaginal wall. One should look for mass lesions protruding into the vagina. Next, the urethra should be palpated for masses or stones and stripped distally to look for a discharge of purulent material or urine. Because patients often will have normal cystoscopy, careful examination of the urethra is recommended. Simultaneously, stripping of the urethra often will identify the ostium of the diverticulum that might otherwise be missed. Positive-pressure urethrography after physical examination appears to be the most helpful diagnostic tool. It provides confirmation of diagnosis, along with identification of the location and the number of diverticula. This is best performed with the Trattner double-ballooned catheter. This catheter has proximal and distal balloons for occlusion of the meatus and vesical neck. A separate lumen opens between the occlusive balloons into the urethra, and contrast may be injected into the urethra, which should fill the diverticulum. Voiding cystourethrography often will achieve similar results. Transvaginal ultrasound recently has been shown to be useful in establishing the diagnosis, as well as clarifying orientation of the diverticulum relative to the urethra and bladder neck (e.g., circumurethral or subtrigonal).

The urethral diverticulum is treated best by complete excision. The diverticulum should be filled with a space-occupying material, such as the balloon of a Fogarty catheter placed cystoscopically, or an injected coagulant. This will allow dissection without deflating the lesion. A transvaginal approach with a flap incision overlapping the urethra is recommended. The periurethral fascia is incised transversely, and the diverticulum identified and dissected to its neck and *totally* excised. The urethral mucosa and submucosa are closed longitudinally with continuous absorbable suture over a 16 F Foley catheter, the periurethral fascia trimmed and approximated transversely, and the vaginal flap advanced and closed, care being taken to avoid overlapping suture lines. Postoperative bladder drainage by both urethral and suprapubic catheter for 7 to 10 days is advisable. Alternatively, it is possible to marsupialize a diverticulum by incising the urethra and the walls of the diverticulum and allow the tract to granulate. This should be reserved only for very small and very distal diverticula. Otherwise, the urethra becomes shortened, which may lead to stress incontinence. The occurrence of carcinoma in a diverticulum, although rare, would support the excision of these lesions even when asymptomatic. In those patients having both a urethral diverticulum and genuine stress urinary incontinence secondary to urethral hypermobility, a transvaginal suspension procedure followed by urethral diverticulectomy can be performed at the same operative session.

In males, the urethral diverticulum is seen even less often. A small number are found in boys 13 years old and under, and these also are considered congenital, particularly when they are located in the anterior urethra. These are thought to be caused by developmental defects similar to those producing hypospadias. Theories such as failure of fusion of the lateral urethral folds or failure of development in the spongiosum leading to herniation of the urethra through a defect in the floor have been proposed. Also, rupture of a congenital periurethral cyst into the urethral lumen is a possibility. Anterior urethral valves, which may cause obstruction, cause a saccular dilation similar to the diverticula, making it difficult to separate these lesions from urethral diverticula. Anterior valves, however, should present much earlier with obstruction.

Most of the diverticula found in adult males, as in females, are acquired. The symptomatology is similar to that in females and includes obstructive and irritative symptoms such as urgency, frequency, dysuria, purulent urethral discharge, postvoid dribbling, and incontinence. A palpable perineal bulge and hematuria are also common complaints. Patient even may notice a delayed or complete failure of emission or ejaculation. In the posterior urethra, symptoms of prostatitis are seen—perineal ache, low back pain, frequency, urgency, and dysuria. The acquired diverticulum commonly is related to trauma, infection, or instrumentation of the urethra and often occurs in the posterior urethra and at the penoscrotal junction.

Foreign bodies, such as urethral calculi, prostatic stones, and Foley catheters, may lead to erosion through the urethra, producing a cavity. Periurethral abscesses may erode into the urethra, and external trauma, such as a straddle injury, can create diverticula. Pressure injury from a urinal at the penoscrotal junction or from incontinence clamps leads to necrosis of supporting spongiosum and diverticula formation. This type of acquired diverticulum can be seen in the paraplegic who does self-catheterization or is on continuous catheter drainage, or in the postprostatectomy incontinent male. Infection and stasis of urine in the diverticulum may lead to stone formation.

The treatment of the male urethral diverticulum depends on the size and the amount of supporting structure. The smaller diverticula may be treated transurethrally with the resectoscope cutting stylet or may be left alone if asymptomatic and draining well. Larger diverticula will need surgical excision by single-stage or multistage procedure, depending on the amount of supporting tissue. A suprapubic urinary diversion may be required, although a urethral catheter is sometimes adequate. A perineal urethrostomy may be useful in anterior lesions. Although these lesions are uncommon, they must be considered in patients who have chronic recurrent urinary tract infections.

Suggested Readings

Benjamin J, Elliot L, Cooper JF, et al: Urethral diverticulum in adult female: Clinical aspects, operative procedures, and pathology. Urology 3:1, 1974

Houser LM, Von Eschenbach AC: Diverticula of female urethra. Diagnostic importance of postvoiding film. Urology 3:452, 1974

Huffman JW: The detailed anatomy of the paraurethral ducts in the adult human female. Am J Obstet Gynecol 55:86, 1948

Lapides J: Transurethral treatment of urethral diverticula in women. J Urol 121:736, 1979

Sholem SL, Wechsler M, Roberts M: Management of the urethral diverticulum in women: A modified operative approach. J Urol 112:485, 1974

Spence HM, Duckett JW Jr: Diverticulum of the female urethra: Clinical aspects and presentation of a simple operative technique for cure. J Urol 104:432, 1970

Spencer WF, Streem SB: Diverticulum of the female urethral roof managed endoscopically. J Urol 138:147, 1987

URETHRAL FISTULA

MARK HOROWITZ, M.D.

Seattle, Washington

Urethral fistulas to the skin, vagina, bladder, or rectum may be congenital or develop secondary to trauma, infection, neoplasm, radiation, or surgery. They develop in part because the urethra is very fragile and therefore, during surgery or instrumentation, must be handled with extreme care. Edema, infection, inadequate blood supply, bleeding, and inadequate skin flaps interfere with proper wound healing and increase the incidence of fistula formation. Furthermore, urethral fistulas can be very difficult to diagnose and challenging to correct.

All males with imperforate anus should be suspected of having a congenital urethrorectal fistula. These fistulas usually enter the proximal bulbar or prostatic urethra and are associated mostly with high imperforate anus. Division of the fistula is achieved at the time of rectal pull-through surgery. Complications may occur from a small stump that creates a diverticulum, causing infection or difficulty with catheterization. In the newborn, a urethrorectal fistula is best identified by observation of meconium in the urine or at the urethral meatus and, rarely, by air in the bladder. Other studies that may be helpful but not diagnostic in the work-up are retrograde urethrography, voiding cystourethrography, barium enema, and computerized tomography with contrast enema. However, in our experience, cystoscopy has been the most sensitive modality for diagnosis of recto-urethral or recto-vaginal fistulae. Some patients may go undiagnosed until they develop urinary tract infection, epididymitis, or hyperchloremic metabolic acidosis from urine absorption in the bowel.

In the female, a congenital fistula between the urethra and vagina is found in patients with "masculinization" of the urethra (i.e., adrenogenital and urogenital sinus syndromes). These patients may present with urinary infection, vaginal distention, and incontinence. Rectal-vaginal fistulas in females with imperforate anus and a single perineal opening often indicate a persistent urogenital sinus. Cystography and sinography are often diagnostic. Poor drainage from the urogenital sinus may result from a functional obstruction at the distal end of the urogenital sinus. If the fistula is distal, a simple cutback can be performed. With a more proximal fistula, exposure may be difficult, especially in the preadolescent child. The perineal approach is usually best. We advise preoperative bowel preparation and antibiotics. A sponge or laparotomy pad in the rectum can facilitate the dissection. We have found it helpful to position the patient in the prone position with the legs spread apart and knees bent (skydiver position). If the fistula is large or if the entire urethra requires reconstruction, a broad strip of vaginal mucosa is tubularized and closed in two layers with running absorbable suture. A large posterior pedicle flap based on the perilabial tissue and extending into the buttock then can be used to cover this repair with pliable vascularized tissue that can reach up to the cervix if necessary. The repair is left intubated for 10 to 14 days. Other options for urethral reconstruction are bowel, ureter, fallopian tube, bladder, and skin.

Cancer can cause fistulas by tumor necrosis, by direct invasion, or as a result of treatment (i.e., surgery, radiation therapy). Treatment of these fistulas should be individualized. Surgical repair depends on the extent of tumor, prognosis, overall condition and strength of the patient, and the need for further therapy. For example, a patient with poor peripheral vasculature who requires further radiation will not heal a fistula repair as well. These fistulas are best managed with strict adherence to the principles of fistula repair (listed below).

Infection causing urethrocutaneous fistulas often is associated with an indwelling urethral catheter, particularly in the patient with neurogenic bladder. Infection and fistula formation also is seen with distal scarring or stricture. Bunts reported the development of urethral fistula in 10 per cent of spinal cord injury patients, probably because of indwelling urethral catheters. Intermittent catheterization and new methods for diversion should lower this rate considerably.

The most common cause of urethrocutaneous fistula in children is surgical reconstruction of the urethra in patients with hypospadias and epispadias. Technical problems that cause fistula are thin flaps with poor vasculature, overlapping suture lines, distal urethral narrowing, and postoperative hematoma formation. Even if the principles of hypospadias surgery are followed carefully, the fistula complication rate is 15 per cent. Because of inadequate tissue and/or scarring, fistula repair can be very difficult and often disappointing, sometimes requiring multiple operations. These fistulas vary in size from a pinhole that require careful observation to diagnose to larger holes. Fistulas after hypospadias urethroplasty may cause dribbling and/or "side sprinkles" during voiding, and sometimes infection. In the case of a very small fistula, the diagnosis is made based on history. Stricture of the urethra distal to a fistula is not infrequent. If not treated at the time of fistula repair, the fistula will recur.

The most important principle in repair of the urethrocutaneous fistula following hypospadias surgery is patience. Fistulas in the acute period are associated with inflammation, which precludes acute repair. Usually 4 to 6 months are required to permit appropriate healing with the return of normal color, texture, and elasticity of the penile skin. At this point, surgical repair may be attempted with high potential for success.

Tiny fistulas may be repaired as outpatient procedures, without catheter drainage. The fistula should be carefully and completely excised and closed in several layers using fine absorbable suture. An adjacent pedicle flap then is used to ensure coverage without overlap of sutures. Larger fistulas usually require a more extensive procedure in which epithelialized adjacent tissue is turned in to the lumen as an island pedicle flap to construct a urethra and to prevent narrowing at the fistula site. A second flap then is used to provide skin coverage and prevent suture overlap. Any distal obstruction, such as meatal stenosis or strictures near the fistula, also must be corrected.

It may be necessary to stage a urethrocutaneous fistula closure when dealing with fistulas accompanied by periurethral abscess. This would be performed by first draining the purulent areas and marsupializing the remaining urethral mucosa to the overlying skin, followed several months later by formal reconstruction. When there is no other alternative, muscle and musculocutaneous flaps can be used as healthy, well-vascularized tissue to repair a fistula of unusual magnitude. Muscle provides mechanical protection for the underlying urethra and facilitates local wound healing. It also helps to avoid the direct apposition of mucosal and skin suture lines. The gracilis muscle and the inferior half of the rectus abdominis are the two muscle groups most commonly employed.

Successful surgical correction of a urethral fistula depends on strict adherence to basic principles:

1. Understand the etiology.
2. Never attempt a repair while inflammation persists.
3. Resect the fistula tract completely and make sure the urethral lumen is adequate.
4. Most errors are made by not doing enough rather than by doing too much. Difficult cases will require large flaps or mobilization of well-vascularized tissue.
5. Optical magnification is essential.
6. If necessary, use remote tissue either as a graft if there is a vascularized bed or, in more severe cases, as a flap.
7. Close in multiple layers.
8. Never overlap suture lines.
9. Close tissue without tension and void hematomas.
10. Use appropriate diversion and take steps to prevent infection.

Suggested Readings

Bunts RC: Management of urologic complications in 1,000 paraplegics. J Urol 79:733, 1958

Heckler FR, Aldridge JJ, Songcharoen S, et al: Muscle flaps and musculocutaneous flaps in the repair of urinary fistulas. Plast Reconstr Surg 66:94, 1980

Horton CE, Devine CJ, Graham JK: Fistula of the penile urethra. Plast Reconstr Surg 66:409, 1980

CONDYLOMATA ACUMINATA

AUGUST ZABBO, M.D.

Providence, Rhode Island

Condylomata are genital warts that result from infection of the anogenital area with certain types of the human papillomavirus (HPV). These lesions most commonly are transmitted sexually. The only symptoms are the unsightly nature of the lesions and occasionally some minor irritation from trauma during sexual activity. Recently, an association between infection with HPV and gynecologic malignancies has been made. Most of these malignancies are cervical intraepithelial neoplasia, which is discovered on Pap smears from the cervix, but these may be the precursors of invasive cervical carcinoma. For this reason, gynecologists now are referring the male partners of patients in whom they make the diagnosis of HPV infection for urologic evaluation. So far it has not been demonstrated that aggressively seeking and treating all HPV infections in the male partners of women with HPV infection results in a lowering of the recurrence rate among these women. Nevertheless, these patients seek an opinion as to whether there is evidence for male involvement and, once such evidence is found, generally demand treatment.

HPV has over 50 subtypes, only some of which have a predilection for infection of the genital skin. HPV types 6 and 11 generally are associated with the classic condylomata acuminata, with the typical vascular warty excrescences found in the mucocutaneous moist areas such as the urethral meatus, perianal area, or foreskin and also with the more typical cutaneous warts on the penile shaft. HPV types 16, 18, 31, and 33 more often are associated with the so-called flat warts or subclinical HPV infection, which is seen only after incubation of the genitalia with 3 per cent to 5 per cent acetic acid. These latter types are also those that are most associated with gynecologic malignancies. There also have been recent reports associating these types of viruses with penile intraepithelial neoplasia and possibly with invasive penile carcinoma. Latent infection—that is, the presence of viral particles in the genital skin without clinically detectable lesions—recently has been described.

HPV is probably the most prevalent sexually transmitted infection in the United States; however, exact numbers are not available because it is not among the diseases reportable to public health authorities. Depending on the aggressiveness and sophistication of the diagnostic methods used, the prevalence in the female population may be as high as 30 per cent. Given this high prevalence, the proclivity of this infection to recur, and the existence of latent infections, attempts to eliminate the reservoir of HPV by local destructive treatments of warts and subclinical lesions may be futile. Some gynecologists then have reverted to the position of closely following patients with evidence of dysplasia caused by these viruses rather than persisting in efforts to eradicate the virus. Among men who are referred for examination for HPV infection because their female sexual partners are found to be infected, approximately 60 per cent will be found to have HPV-associated lesions. It has been the recommended practice to aggressively treat all lesions found in these men in the hopes of eliminating the male reservoir of the virus. Recent studies, however, using sophisticated methods such as polymerase chain reaction, have found evidence of the virus in clinically uninvolved areas; therefore, until a systemic treatment is available, efforts at eliminating the male reservoir of HPV also may be futile.

UROLOGIC EXAMINATION AND DIAGNOSIS

Urologists who see patients referred for examination for HPV infection must explain fully the nature of the infection and the potential consequences, and temper the aggressiveness of therapeutic recommendations with this knowledge. There are now available clinical kits that pathologists can use to subtype the HPV infection, but, again, this knowledge as yet has no therapeutic implications until improved methods for clearing the virus are discovered. There may be some prognostic value in knowing that the subtype is not one associated with neoplastic changes. Children can become infected with HPV at the time of birth, by routine nonsexual familial contact, and as a result of sexual abuse. Therefore, children with genital warts deserve a thorough physical examination and social evaluation for sexual abuse.

The currently recommended routine for examination for condylomata acuminata follows. The individual urologist must decide for himself or herself, based on the foregoing information, how aggressively to treat the lesions that may be found. Patients nearly always insist on complete clearing of any visible lesions. The incubation period for condylomata acuminata is usually 3 to 6 weeks but can be as long as 9 months. For this reason, even patients with negative exams should be followed for possible late occurrence of lesions. There is an unknown incidence of spontaneous regression, but it is thought to be high and may take up to 2 years.

On arrival for the initial consultation, patients with suspected HPV lesions are given an information sheet on condylomata acuminata and HPV explaining the viral nature of their infection, the risks of malignancy for themselves and their partners, the mechanics of the examination, and the diagnostic and therapeutic procedures they are about to undergo as well as the follow-up care that will be required. This provides a reference for the patient's later use in understanding this infection and also educates them somewhat concerning control of potentially more serious sexually transmitted diseases. A urine specimen is obtained for routine urinalysis and also for urine cytology, in which the cytologist looks for the typical koilocytotic changes consistent with condylomata acuminata. Some examiners prefer sampling the urethra with a calcium alginate swab and preparing a Pap smear. If the cytology or smear is positive for condylomatous changes, the patient returns for urethroscopy. Because the incidence of bladder condylomata is very low, routine cystoscopy is not recommended; cystoscopy is reserved for cases in which there are signs and symptoms of possible bladder involvement. Approximately 5 per cent of men will be identified as requiring urethroscopy and, among these, approximately one half are found to have condylomatous involvement of the urethra.

The initial inspection of the genitalia is done, being sure to retract the foreskin fully and examine the entire penile surface. Inspection of the pubic and inguinal areas is carried out, as is a complete examination of the scrotum. Inspection of the perianal area is important to be sure there are not condylomata there. Many men will inquire about the risks of oral condylomata, and this is seen to occur occasionally. Although a cursory exam can be done in the urologist's office, a full examination would require inspection of the larynx by an otolaryngologist. Care must be taken not to confuse pearly papules of the glans penis, normal sebaceous glands of the penile skin, senile keratoses, fibroepithelial skin tags, and other sexually transmitted diseases such as the lesions of syphilis or molluscum contagiosum with condylomata.

After initial inspection, the genitalia are wrapped with two dressing sponges soaked with 3 per cent to 5 per cent acetic acid. These are left to incubate for 5 minutes. On removal of the acetic acid sponges, the entire penis, pubic, and inguinal area is re-examined with the aid of magnification (surgical loupes or colposcope). The so-called acetowhite areas can be identified by these methods. Condylomata are not the only cause of acetowhite changes, and nearly any area of inflammation will turn white with acetic acid incubation. If no obvious condylomatous lesions are identified, the areas of acetowhite staining are biopsied first and the results of the biopsy obtained before proceeding with treatment. Approximately 20 per cent of the acetowhite areas are found to be due to some other benign inflammation, not condylomatous in nature. If there is extensive acetowhitening, which is often associated with balanoposthitis or other minor skin inflammation, treatment with a combination steroid/antifungal cream may be advantageous, with the patient returning in 1 month to see if the acetowhite resolves. Biopsies are obtained using a 2-mm skin punch biopsy under local anesthesia and cauterizing the base with a silver nitrate stick.

TREATMENT OPTIONS

Multiple therapies have been described for condylomata acuminata, and a critical review of any therapy with sufficient follow-up shows that a 30 per cent or greater recurrence rate can be expected. Whether this recurrence rate is due to persistent HPV infection or reinfection is impossible to determine. Patients are counseled to use a condom until all lesions are cleared and also until their sexual partner has had all lesions cleared.

The fact that so many alternative therapies have been advanced for treatment of condylomata acuminata is evidence that none has been shown to be far superior in terms of recurrence rates. Treatment is based on the extent of condylomatous involvement as well as the location of the condylomata. Single small lesions can be removed with excisional biopsy using either the punch biopsy instrument or scissors. Extensive involvement of the foreskin usually is handled best by circumcision, with other locally destructive methods used to treat those lesions that are not removed with the circumcised skin. Cryotherapy using liquid nitrogen has been used extensively. This is accomplished by freezing the involved skin until it whitens. There is a moderate amount of pain associated with this therapy and control of the depth of destruction is limited. Electrodesiccation also has been popular because the instruments are commonly available. The major problems with this type of therapy are, again, the lack of control of the depth of penetration of electrical energy and the relatively extensive scarring that can be caused by electrosurgical techniques used on large lesions. Particular caution should be used when treating urethral or urethral meatal warts with electrocautery because urethral stricture or meatal stenosis may occur.

Podophyllin resin in a 20 per cent solution in benzoin also has been used widely. The lesions are painted with the solution with a cotton-tipped applicator and the patient then is instructed to wash the solution off in 4 to 6 hours. The treatment is repeated once or twice weekly until the warts have disappeared. Recently, a 0.5 per cent solution of purified podophyllotoxin has been marketed for patient self-application. Bichloracetic acid and trichloracetic acids have been used extensively by gynecologists in treating condylomata in their patients. These acids also can be used for self-application by the patients. The lesions are painted with the solution and an intense skin reaction develops. If the reaction is too intense or a wider area was painted than intended, neutralization with dilute sodium bicarbonate solution can be accomplished.

Five fluorouracil (5-FU) cream in a 5 per cent concentration has been used to treat external and urethral condylomata acuminata. In treating external lesions, the cream is applied carefully to include only the condylomatous lesion and to avoid normal skin. Interlesional injection of alpha-interferon recently has been approved for treatment of condylomata by the Food and Drug Administration. A self-limited flu-like illness is a commonly seen side effect but usually does not limit the therapy. However, the incidence of leukopenia may be as high as 26 per cent.

Laser therapy has been advanced as an efficient means of therapy with minimal scarring and ease of application. The current lasers that are used include the carbon dioxide (CO_2), neodymium:yttrium-aluminum-garnet (Nd:YAG), and potassium titanyl phosphate (KTP) lasers. Each of these can be used in an office setting utilizing local anesthesia. Because there have been found to be infectious viral particles in the plume of smoke that results from laser therapy, a smoke evacuator is mandatory. Extensive involvement of the genitalia or perianal region may necessitate regional or general anesthesia. Another approach to these extensive lesions is to have multiple sessions in the office under local anesthesia. Urethral meatal condylomata are treated very well with the lasers, and this also can be done as an office procedure under local anesthesia. Urethroscopy with lasering of intraurethral condyloma also can be done in an office that is equipped with either a Nd:YAG or KTP laser.

The lasers vary in their depth of penetration, which must be taken into account. The CO_2 laser is reserved for external condylomatous lesions as well as urethral meatal lesions that can be expressed outside of the urethral meatus. For internal urethral lesions, a laser fiber must be used and, because none currently is available for the CO_2 laser, the KTP or Nd:YAG laser would be needed.

Therapy of external condylomata with the CO_2 laser is done with a power setting of 2 to 5 watts and a focused beam. The visible condyloma and a surrounding 1 to 2-mm border of the lesion are treated. The treatment is accomplished by photocoagulating the surface of the lesion, which results in carbonization of the surface. The carbonized surface is wiped clean with a gauze sponge and the application repeated until the basal layer is reached. This is shown as an opalescent to shiny white area. When the treatment is completed, a small amount of bacitracin ointment is applied and the patient repeats application of the ointment three times a day until the eschar is healed. The patient is re-examined in 6 weeks for persistent or recurrent lesions.

If urethral meatal warts are treated, the patient is given a prescription for 5-FU cream, which is instilled intraurethrally once a day for 2 weeks. The cream should be inserted after voiding and allowed to remain in the urethra for 2 to 3 hours (until the next void). It should not be left indwelling overnight because marked urethral irritation can occur; it is also important to protect the scrotum from spillage of the urethral cream.

Intraurethral warts require either the KTP or Nd:YAG lasers. Because their depth of penetration is greater than that of the CO_2 laser, they also are preferred for large penile or perianal warts. The sapphire contact tip of the Nd:YAG laser limits the penetration of energy so that direct contact with surface warts can be accomplished. In treating intraurethral warts, a pediatric cystoscope is used. The lesions are visualized and treated with a focused beam at 1 to 2 watts for the KTP laser or 10 to 20 watts for the Nd:YAG laser. The lesions are photocoagulated, which results in complete whitish discoloration of the wart itself and its base. Again, adjunctive 5-FU cream is used whenever intraurethral warts are treated.

Healing after laser therapy takes 1 to 2 weeks, and patients are instructed to return every 6 weeks until the condylomatous lesions are cleared. At that time, a 6-month follow-up is scheduled because late recurrences are known. Using this approach has resulted in approximately 60 per cent elimination of condyloma with a single treatment and a greater than 90 per cent clearance of condylomata with multiple treatments.

Whether the complete clearance of clinical lesions has resulted in the elimination of HPV infection from the patient is unknown. Future developments in immunologic therapy of this infection may lead to more definitive treatment.

Suggested Readings

Breitenecker G, Gitsch G: What's new in diagnosis and treatment of HPV-associated cervical lesions. Pathol Res Pract 188:242–247, 1992

Brown DR, Fife KH: Human papillomavirus infections of the genital tract. Med Clin North Am 74:1455–1485, 1990

Reichman RC, Strike DG: Pathogenesis and treatment of human genital papillomavirus infections: A review. Antiviral Res 11:109–118, 1989

Syrjänen K, Syrjänen S: Epidemiology of human papilloma virus infections and genital neoplasis. Scand J Infect Dis Suppl 69:7–17, 1990

NONSPECIFIC URETHRITIS

EVAN BARRY KRISCH, M.D.

Camden, New Jersey

The causes of nonspecific urethritis have changed over the past few decades. Prior to accurate culturing for *Chlamydia* and *Ureaplasma,* these organisms were probably the main causes of idiopathic nonspecific urethritis. Presently, approximately 60 per cent of nonspecific urethritis is caused by *Chlamydia, Gonococcus,* or *Ureaplasma.* Additional etiologies have been suggested and include *Trichomonas vaginalis,* viruses, yeasts, multiple bacteria, foreign bodies, catheters, urethral instrumentation, soaps, and manual stimulation.

Signs and symptoms of nonspecific urethritis can include dysuria, urethral itching, watery or purulent penile discharge, and initial hematuria. When perineal or abdominal pain occurs concomitantly, cystitis and/or prostatitis usually are present.

LABORATORY EVALUATION

Laboratory evaluation must be performed to isolate the cause of urethritis. The three-glass urinalysis technique is a simple initial test. Specimen one (VB_1) is the first 10 ml of the patient's voided urine. The remainder of the voided urine is listed as specimen 2 (VB_2). For males, a VB_3 sample also is obtained by first massaging the prostate and then having the patient void. The VB_1 sample should be examined for white blood cells, and, in cases of pure urethritis, will show a larger number of white cells when compared with the VB_2 and VB_3 specimens. A urethral swab also should be utilized to obtain a specimen, which should be examined under microscopy. These samples should be sent for routine culture as well as for *Chlamydia, Ureaplasma,* and gonococcal cultures. If these are all negative, repeat cultures may be done, but other causes of urethritis must be considered.

TRICHOMONAS VAGINALIS

Trichomoniasis is a common sexually transmitted disease found in 30 to 50 per cent of women and 5 to 60 per cent of men presenting to sexually transmitted disease clinics. Males may suffer from prostatitis and epididymitis in addition to urethritis. Higher risk can be assigned to men with a previous history of sexually transmitted diseases, to men whose sexual cohort is positive for trichomonads, and to men who currently have gonococcal or nongonococcal urethritis (10 to 20 per cent).

Direct examination of the urine for trichomonads has a significant inaccuracy rate (50 per cent). Culturing for *T. vaginalis,* indirect hemagglutination titer for trichomonas, and recent development of polymerase chain reaction–based methods have improved detection rates. Once detection of *T. vaginalis* is noted, treatment should be given to both patient and cohort. Initial treatment should be with metronidazole (Flagyl), 250 to 500 mg three times a day for 7 to 10 days. If the sexual cohort is asymptomatic, a single 2-gm dose should eradicate the organism. Caution must be given to both patient and cohort regarding alcohol consumption during the treatment. Pregnant females also must be advised that Flagyl will cross the placental barrier as well as be present in breast milk. All patients should be cultured for other pathogens, as listed above. If improvement is noted, repeat examination by urethral swab and urinalysis should be performed 7 to 14 days after treatment. If *T. vaginalis* is isolated again, a second course of treatment is recommended. No unprotected intercourse should be occurring during the treatment and follow-up.

If no improvement is noted, repeat examination still must be performed, with repeat cultures for other possible pathogens. In males, chronic prostatitis must be considered and evaluation and treatment performed as indicated.

VIRUSES AND YEASTS

Certain viruses also have been implicated in nonspecific urethritis. Herpes simplex has been isolated in the urethra of approximately 30 per cent of men during a primary infection. Usually these patients have genital lesions, but some cases of urethritis have occurred without penile lesions. Among men with gonococcal or nongonococcal urethritis, herpes simplex has been isolated in 2 to 6 per cent. Condylomata acuminata have been found in the urethra as well but usually cause urethral symptoms and initial hematuria. This is an uncommon symptom with other causes of urethritis. Cytomegalovirus has been examined as well, and does not appear to play a significant role.

Yeast infections, beginning as a balantis, also have been implicated in nonspecific urethritis. Studies do not reveal yeast as a significant cause, although it may occur in association with other agents. Studies have also noted yeast in 2 to 4 per cent of patients without urethritis.

BACTERIA

Multiple bacteria have been noted to occur in the urethra of men and women with urethritis. In one study, *Haemophilus influenzae* and *Haemophilus parainfluenzae* were isolated from 10 per cent of men with urethritis. Additional studies have shown *Haemophilus* to be present in the genitourinary tract in men without urethritis. The percentage has varied from 0 to 9. This also casts doubt on the significance of *Haemophilus* as a cause for nonspecific urethritis.

Mycoplasma hominis and *Mycoplasma genitalium* infections have been examined as a potential source of nonspecific urethritis. In one study, 14 per cent of men with gonococcal urethritis had associated *Mycoplasma* detected, and 27 per cent of patients with recurrent nongonococcal urethritis had *Mycoplasma* detected. Interestingly, 12 per cent of patients without clinical signs of urethritis had *Mycoplasma* isolated. In a second study, *Mycoplasma* was noted to occur in 19 per cent of men with urethritis. This occurred most commonly in men with nongonococcal urethritis (19 of 28). *Mycoplasma* occurred alone in only 3 per cent. *Mycoplasma*, along with *Ureaplasma*, may play a role in potentiating other urethral infections as well.

Staphylococcus epidermidis, *Staphylococcus aureus*, *Corynebacterium* species, *Enterobacter* species, *Streptococcus* species, and *Gardinella vaginalis* also have been isolated, but appear either to be secondary to contamination from the physiologic microflora or play a minor role in the etiology of nonspecific urethritis.

NONINFECTIOUS CAUSES OF URETHRITIS

There are various noninfectious causes of urethritis. Chemical irritants such as soaps, shampoos, vaginal douches, and spermicidal jellies and foams have been implicated. Smoking, caffeine, alcohol, and chocolate also have been suggested as potential causes and enhancers of urethritis.

Traumatic causes of urethritis also occur and include placement of urethral latex catheters and self-insertion of foreign bodies into the urethra. Manual stimulation (i.e., stripping of the urethra) also has been implicated in nonspecific urethritis. Additional structural causes of urethritis include urethral diverticula, meatal stenosis, urethral strictures, and urethral tumors.

Urethritis also may occur with certain systemic diseases, including Stevens-Johnson syndrome, Wegener granulomatosis, and Reiter syndrome. Approximately 2 per cent of men with nongonococcal urethritis develop Reiter syndrome.

TREATMENT

The initial approach to urethritis should begin with a thorough history and physical examination. With the addition of a careful laboratory examination, as described earlier, greater than 80 per cent of urethritis can be diagnosed and treated as indicated. When urethritis is present and no specific etiology can be determined, empiric treatment is often necessary. Initial treatment should be with tetracycline 500 mg PO qid or doxycycline 100 mg PO bid. Treatment should continue for 14 days. During that time, culture results may assist in tailoring therapy. If an infectious etiology is suspected, all sexual cohorts should be tested and likewise treated. If the patient becomes clinically cured, a repeat laboratory evaluation to document bacteriologic cure should be performed approximately 1 week after treatment is completed. If no clinical response is noted, patient compliance, and new sexual contacts, should be considered as potential sources of failure. If these potential causes are excluded, *Ureaplasma* and *Mycoplasma* should be suspected, because they may be resistant to tetracycline. Empiric treatment with erythromycin 500 mg PO qid or trimethoprim-sulfamethoxazole, 2 tablets q 12 h, then should be utilized for a 1- to 2-week course of therapy.

Recurrent or persistent urethritis after therapy, if compliance is assured, requires further evaluation. These tests would include cystoscopy and urethroscopy, assessment of urinary flow rate, and upper urinary tract evaluation. It is not uncommon to find recurrence or persistence caused by prostatitis, which would require longer treatment (i.e., 4 to 6 weeks) and occasionally chronic suppressive therapy.

Suggested Readings

Fowler JE Jr: Urethritis in men. Semin Urol 9:15, 1991

Krieger JN, Verdon M, Siegel N, et al: Risk assessment and laboratory diagnosis of trichomoniasis in men. J Infect Dis 166:1362, 1992

Nacey JN, Delahunt B: Toxicity study of first and second generation hydrogel-coated latex urinary catheters. Br J Urol 67:314, 1991

Pec J, Straka S, Novomesky F, et al: Mechanical urethritis and ascendent genitourinary infections due to sexual stimulation of the urethra by inserted foreign bodies. Genitourin Med 68:399, 1992

Riley DE, Roberts MC, Takayama T, et al: Development of a polymerase chain reaction–based diagnosis of *Trichomonas vaginalis*. J Clin Microbiol 30:465, 1992

Saultz JW, Toffler WL: Trichomonas infections in men. Am Fam Physician 39:177, 1989

Stefanik M, Rychna K, Valkoun A: Microbial causative agents of male urethritis. J Hyg Epidemiol Microbiol Immunol 36:111, 1992

Sturm AW: *Haemophilus influenzae* and *Haemophilus parainfluenzae* in nongonococcal urethritis. J Infect Dis 153: 165, 1986

TREATMENT OF GONORRHEA AND CHLAMYDIA INFECTIONS

EVAN BARRY KRISCH, M.D.

Camden, New Jersey

Chlamydial and gonococcal infections are the most common sexually transmitted diseases in the world. These infections occur concurrently in 15 to 50 per cent of heterosexuals, with a slightly lower occurrence rate in homosexuals. It is for this reason that the current recommendations for treatment of these infections include regimens active against both pathogens.

Although gonococcal infections in the United States have decreased substantially in the 1980s, chlamydial infections have increased dramatically during this time. Chlamydial infections are now the most prevalent sexually transmitted disease in the United States. It is estimated that greater than 4 million cases occur annually. Although *Chlamydia trachomatis* first was isolated in 1907, it is only within the past 15 years that its importance in urethritis has been noted.

The most common cause of nongonococcal urethritis is *C. trachomatis. Ureaplasma urealyticum* is quite common as well, and can be isolated in 40 to 50 per cent of men with chlamydial or gonococcal infections. Although it may be abnormal, *Ureaplasma* may be a nonpathogenic organism. Other etiologies of nongonococcal urethritis may include *Trichomonas vaginalis, Candida albicans, Mycoplasma hominis,* and *Neisseria meningitidis.*

Nongonococcal urethritis may be difficult to differentiate from gonococcal urethritis because the symptoms are identical. Although urethral discharge and dysuria may occur in both, profuse and purulent urethral discharge is more common with gonococcal infections. Chlamydial infections can be associated in males with epididymitis, Reiter syndrome, proctitis, and infertility, and in females with cervicitis, endometritis, and salpingitis. Precise asymptomatic carrier rates for nongonococcal urethritis presently are unknown, but in males the rate approaches 15 per cent. This therefore explains the high risk of transmission noted within the general population. In field follow-up studies, chlamydial transmission appears to require more sexual exposure than gonococcal transmission. Also, transmission of both gonorrheal and chlamydial infections is more efficient from men to women.

Diagnostic evaluation for nongonococcal infections has become more important because of the high asymptomatic carrier rate and the increased prevalence in the general population. A urethral Gram stain is very helpful in differentiating gonococcal from nongonococcal urethritis. Enzymatic immunoassays, utilizing urethral swabs, now are used commonly. Direct immunofluorescence, nucleic acid probes, and antibody detection tests are beginning to be implemented as well. The results vary, but provide a sensitivity of approximately 50 to 75 per cent. The specificity of these tests approaches 95 per cent. These laboratory tests can help to avoid the increased morbidity of inadequate treatment of combined infections.

The treatment for coinfections has undergone a significant change in recent years. Gonorrhea no longer should be treated with penicillins or tetracyclines because of the high level of plasmid-mediated resistance to these drugs. The current recommendation for the treatment of gonorrhea is ceftriaxone 250 mg intramuscularly. An alternative regimen is spectinomycin, 2 gm intramuscularly, as a single dose (Table 1).

Recent studies comparing two third-generation cephalosporins, cefixime and cefotaxime, with ceftriaxone have been performed. It appears that a single 500-mg dose of intramuscularly administered cefotaxime is as effective as 250 mg of intramuscularly administered ceftriaxone. It is also apparent that 400 or 800 mg of a single oral administration of cefixime is equally effective in the eradication of gonorrhea. Alternatively, a single dose of cefuroxime axetil (1 gm), as a single dose, has been shown to be effective in combination with 1 gm of probenecid.

Single-dose regimens have not been effective against chlamydial infections in the past. Chlamydia persists inside the host cell and has a long life cycle. For this reason, eradication of chlamydia requires a longer course of treatment. The conventional treatment has been 7 days of tetracycline, 500 mg 4 times

TABLE 1. Gonococcal Infections

First Line
Ceftriaxone 250 mg IM single dose
+
Doxycycline 100 mg PO bid × 7 days
Second Line
Spectinomycin 2 gm IM single dose
+
Doxycycline 100 mg PO bid × 7 days
Alternative Regimens
Ofloxacin 400 mg PO single dose
or
Cefotaxime 500 mg or 1 gm IM single dose
or
Cefixime 400 or 500 mg PO single dose
or
Cefuroxime axetil 1 gm single dose
or
Azithromycin 1 gm PO single dose

daily, or doxycycline, 100 mg twice daily also for 7 days (Table 2). In patients unable to take tetracyclines because of intolerance or contraindication, a 7-day regimen of erythromycin base, 500 mg orally four times daily, is used.

Because of the frequency of coinfections, as well as the difficulty of culturing nongonococcal infections, the recommendation is for the treatment of gonococcal and nongonococcal infections at the time of presentation.

Multiple other options are now available for the treatment of concurrent infections. Recently, the fluorinated 4-quinolones have become available and exhibit excellent activity against *Neisseria gonorrhoeae* as well as *C. trachomatis* and *U. urealyticum*. Side effects with these drugs are quite minimal. Numerous studies with a single oral dose of ofloxacin 400 mg have shown equivalent clinical and microbiologic cure rates for *N. Gonorrhoeae* when compared with conventional treatment. Ofloxacin studies also have shown cure rates equivalent to those of tetracycline for nongonococcal infections when used as a 7-day course of 200 or 300 mg twice daily.

Recently, a single-dose regimen has become available for the treatment of gonococcal and nongonococcal urethritis. Azithromycin, an azalide (macrolide) antibiotic, provides low blood levels but high tissue levels. It is for this reason that this drug is released slowly into the blood system. Azithromycin has shown equivalent cure rates when compared to conventional treatments for nongonococcal urethritis and gonorrhea. The effective dose is 1 gm azithromycin administered orally.

A small proportion of patients will not respond to the conventional treatments. Reculturing and testing should be performed for a different etiologic agent. If one is noted, appropriate treatment should be instituted. If nongonococcal urethritis is documented after initial therapy, retreatment should be with erythromycin, although ofloxacin and azithromycin are excellent choices as well.

TABLE 2. Treatment of Chlamydia

FIRST LINE
Doxycycline 100 mg PO bid × 7 days
or
Tetracycline 500 mg PO qid × 7 days
SECOND LINE
Erythromycin 500 mg PO qid × 7 days
ALTERNATIVE REGIMENS
Ofloxacin 400 mg PO bid × 7 days
or
Azithromycin 1 gm PO single dose
or
Sulfisoxazole 500 mg PO qid × 10 days

Suggested Readings

Bowie WR: Effective treatment of urethritis: A practical guide. Drugs 44:207, 1992

Handsfield HH, McCormack WM, Hook EW III, et al: A comparison of single dose cefixime with ceftriaxone as treatment for uncomplicated gonorrhea. N Engl J Med 325:1337, 1991

Jones RB, Mogabgab WJ, McCormack WM, et al: Randomized comparison of cefotaxime and ceftriaxone in patients with uncomplicated gonorrhea. Clin Ther 13: 550, 1991

Maiti H, Chowdhury FH, Richmond SJ, et al: Ofloxacin in the treatment of uncomplicated gonorrhea and chlamydial genital infection. Clin Ther 13:441, 1991

Martin DH, Mroczkowski TF, Dalu ZA, et al: A controlled trial of single dose azithromycin for the treatment of chlamydial urethritis and cervicitis. N Engl J Med 327: 921, 1992

Mogabgab WJ, Holmes B, Murray M, et al: Randomized comparison of ofloxacin and doxycycline for chlamydia and ureaplasma urethritis and cervicitis. Chemotherapy 36:70, 1990

Ridgway GI: Advances in the antimicrobial therapy of chlamydial genital infections. J Infect 25(suppl 1):51, 1992

Zenilman JM: Update on bacterial sexually transmitted disease. Urol Clinics North Am 19:25, 1992

TRICHOMONAL INFECTIONS IN MEN

ROBERT M. MOLDWIN, M.D.

New Hyde Park, New York

Trichomonas vaginalis is the most common sexually transmitted pathogen, accounting for 180 million cases of infection worldwide. The pathology associated with this microbe has been described primarily in the gynecologic literature; however, trichomonal disease in the male is noteworthy. Its asymptomatic presence promotes the spread of this organism among sexual partners. Symptomatic trichomonal infections, although uncommon, usually present as nongonococcal urethritis. In either form, *Trichomonas* will go undetected unless physician awareness leads to evaluation of its presence and eradication.

THE ORGANISM

Trichomonas vaginalis is a motile organism possessing four anterior flagella and a fifth flagellum that runs the length of its body (Fig. 1). An axostyle traverses the organism's entire

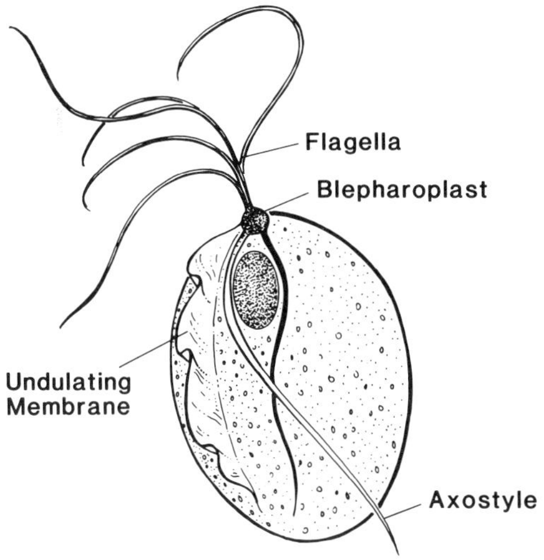

FIGURE 1. Trichomonas vaginalis. (From Moldwin R: Sexually transmitted protozoal infections. *Trichomonas vaginalis, entomoeba histolytica,* and *giardia lamblia.* Urol Clin N Am 19:93–101, 1992.)

length and protrudes through the cell membrane opposite the flagella. Trichomonads can vary from 10 to 30 μm in size and may be round or pyriform in shape. They are fastidious organisms requiring a complex formulation of nutrients and a moderately anaerobic environment to survive. Trichomonads are killed within several minutes at 60°C. Cooling significantly impairs their characteristic jerky motility.

EPIDEMIOLOGY

Although trichomonal infections commonly are seen and treated in the female patient, they are thought to cause less than 5 per cent of cases of urethritis in the male. However, in selected groups the incidence of trichomonal urethritis is much higher. For instance, trichomonads may be identified in 14 to 60 per cent of men with infected female partners. Conversely, female partners of males harboring the organism will be infected in 67 to 100 per cent of cases. These findings suggest that infected males rapidly clear trichomonads from their urethra. Kreiger and Rein have postulated that the high zinc concentrations of prostatic secretions may be an important host defense mechanism against these organisms.

CLINICAL FINDINGS

The high prevalance of trichomonal infection worldwide rests to a large degree on its asymptomatic carriage, which may be as high as 40 to 50 per cent in the female patient. In males, symptoms are seen in only 10 per cent of patients. Complaints in the male patient may include a mucopurulent urethral discharge, mild dysuria, or postvoid burning.

Trichomonal prostatitis, epididymitis, and balanitis are very uncommon. Persistent infections have been associated with meatal stricture disease. Several in vitro studies have demonstrated a decrease in sperm motility associated with *Trichomonas;* however, the clinical significance of these findings is unknown at this time.

LABORATORY FINDINGS

Patient complaints and physical findings are notoriously inaccurate when making the diagnosis of trichomonal urethritis. The wet mount examination has been the most widely used tool in the female population. This technique can be adapted to the male by examination of urethral swabbings or discharge. A wet mount can be performed by creating a suspension using 85% (physiologic) sodium chloride. Expressed prostatic secretions can be examined directly. The mount should be evaluated microscopically soon after the specimen is obtained because the organisms lose their characteristic jerky motility when cooling on the slide. Although the wet mount is certainly the most cost-effective method to diagnose a trichomonal infection, its sensitivity is only 50 to 70 per cent.

Culture of secretions remains the gold standard when diagnosing a trichomonal infection. Sensitivities of culture range from 86 to 97 per cent. The main drawback of culture is the usual 2- to 7-day waiting period for results. This problem has been offset somewhat by the introduction of in-office culture systems such as the InPouch (Biomed Diagnostics Inc., Santa Clara, CA). Using this method, inoculation with as few as four organisms per milliliter can be viewed microscopically within 24 hours. Another useful method to confirm the presence of *Trichomonas* is a monoclonal stain for the organism. The Direct Enzyme Amino Assay test (California Integrated Diagnostics, Venicia, CA) can be performed in 1 hour under a light microscope. The rapid latex agglutination test has a very high specificity and sensitivity (greater than 99 and 95 per cent, respectively) and can be performed in minutes without a microscope. The polymerase chain reaction (PCR) is a technique that has become increasingly useful in the identification of a wide variety of microorganisms. The technique is extremely sensitive and can detect both viable and nonviable organisms. PCR technology is presently under development for the identification of *T. vaginalis* in clinical isolates.

TREATMENT

Metronidazole is the mainstay of treatment for trichomonal infections, with resistance being a very rare event. Metronidazole's activity is due to its interaction with trichomonal nucleic acid synthesis.

Major adverse side effects of metronidazole include:

1. Nausea and vomiting. This effect is the most common problem, occurring in 2.6 to 26 per cent of patients.
2. Disulfiram-like reaction. Alcoholic beverages should not be consumed while being treated with metronidazole.
3. Headache, dizziness.
4. Metallic taste.
5. Darkening of urine.
6. Leukopenia, which generally resolves after drug discontinuation. This problem has not been reported with single-dose therapy (discussed below).
7. Other adverse reactions: pancreatitis, skin eruptions, pseudomembranous colitis, and hemolytic uremic syndrome.

Metronidazole can be administered in either of two therapeutically equivalent regimens: single dose and 7 day. A single dose of 2 gm is preferable because compliance is assured and side effects of the medication are uncommon. The 7-day course of therapy can be given as 500 mg twice daily.

The most common cause of treatment failure is reinfection from the patient's sexual partner. It is therefore imperative that both parties be evaluated and treated simultaneously. Rare cases of treatment failure unrelated to reinfection usually are treated effectively with larger oral doses or parenteral administration of metronidazole.

Suggested Readings

Borchardt KA, Smith RF: An evaluation of an InPouch™ TV culture method for diagnosing *Trichomonas vaginalis* infection. Genitourin Med 67:149, 1991

Drugs for parasitic infections. Med Lett Drugs Ther 32: 23, 1990

Krieger JN: Urologic aspects of trichomoniasis. Invest Urol 18:411, 1981.

Kreiger JN, Tam MR, Stevens CE, et al: Diagnosis of trichomoniasis: Comparison of conventional wet mount examination with cytologic studies, cultures, and monoclonal antibody staining of direct specimens. JAMA 259:1223, 1988

Lossick JG: Treatment of sexually transmitted vaginosis/vaginitis. Rev Infect Dis 12(suppl):S665, 1990

Riley DE, Roberts MC, Takayama T, Kreiger JN: Development of a polymerase chain reaction-based diagnosis of *Trichomonas vaginalis*. J Clin Microbiol 30:465, 1992

Saxena SB, Jenkins RR: Prevalence of *Trichomonas vaginalis* in men at high risk for sexually transmitted diseases. Sex Transm Dis 18:138, 1991

Schaaf VM, Perez-Stable EJ, Borchardt K: The limited value of symptoms and signs in the diagnosis of vaginal infections. Arch Intern Med 150:1929, 1990

Thomason JL, Gelbart SM: *Trichomonas vaginalis*. Obstet Gynecol 74(part 2):536, 1989

MANAGEMENT OF TRAUMA OF THE EXTERNAL GENITALIA AND URETHRA

JOHN W. WEIGEL, M.D.

Kansas City, Kansas

Injuries of the external genitalia frequently involve the anterior urethra and commonly include trauma to the bladder, pelvic organs, and rectum. In general, external genitalia injuries can be classified as either blunt or penetrating. The former include crush injuries, straddle injuries, and, in the case of the penis, fracture of the tunica albuginea and Buck's fascia of the corpora. These usually are "closed" injuries. Penetrating, or "open," injuries include lacerations, avulsion of skin, and amputation wounds.

PENILE BLUNT INJURIES

Crush injuries of the penis and blunt trauma often occur during sexual excitement or activity, at which time the corpora are engorged. The skin may be damaged, the erectile tissue may be injured, or the tunics may be torn or ruptured. The latter two injuries may result in sexual dysfunction. Urethral injury must be ruled out. Blood at the meatus or hematuria suggests urethral injury and must be investigated with urethrography. This should be done using sterile contrast diluted 50:50 with sterile saline. If a catheter is already in place, contrast may be injected through a small plastic infant feeding tube alongside the catheter, to delineate gross tears. Urine may extravasate into the penis if the urethra is torn and if Buck's fascia is intact. Extravasation outside the penis into the scrotum, upper thighs, and lower abdominal walls may occur if Buck's fascia is no longer intact. Crush injuries of the penis usually can be managed conservatively. Corporal fibrosis with erectile dysfunction and/or urethral stricture may develop if tissue damage is severe.

Fractured penis occurs during sexual activity and usually is accompanied by a cracking sound, extreme pain, and significant ecchymosis and hematoma. Some authorities advocate nonoperative therapy for fractured penis if there is minimal deformity. I believe that such injuries should be explored and the defect repaired to prevent subsequent chordee or penile deformity. It is important to examine patients carefully for any break in the skin that might signify a human bite injury, which must be considered infected and treated aggressively with broad-spectrum antibiotics.

An unusual but potentially severe form of trauma consists of a hair or other material being wrapped around the coronal area of the penis. This has been reported with some frequency in infants and children and may be a form of child abuse in some cases. This condition may be difficult to recognize because of edema obscuring the hair. The foreign body must be removed and the area examined under magnification.

PENETRATING PENILE INJURIES

Open wounds should never be closed if there is significant contamination or danger of infection. All such wounds can be cleansed, débrided, and closed secondarily after 3 to 5 days of dressing changes. All functioning tissue should be preserved; in general, these wounds are débrided as one would a wound of a hand or the face. Redébridement may be necessary.

Underlying urethral injuries must be looked for and repaired. It is important not to leave easily palpable knots beneath the skin when repairing the tunics. Knots can be inverted, and absorbable suture material no larger than 3-0 can be used to prevent problems. Antibiotics should be used both systemically and in the wound-irrigating solution. Avulsion of the penile or penoscrotal skin may occur in "power takeoff"* injuries. Such wounds should be irrigated and cleansed carefully and, if not badly contaminated, may be closed using split-thickness skin grafts obtained from the lower abdomen or thighs. Suture lines should be staggered, and one should avoid a ventral suture line that may cause a downward curvature or chordee. A traction suture in the penis is helpful, and the use of an external wire or other type of "frame" around the penis maintains some extension and prevents an "accordion effect" postoperatively from penile retraction, which can cause loss of the graft. An alternative method is that of burying the shaft of the penis within the scrotum and releasing it at a later date. Split-thickness grafts are probably the treatment of choice in most cases. It is important to excise skin remnants distal to the corona to prevent edema, and to remove preputial skin in the uncircumcised patient. This skin may be used for grafts.

Penetrating injury of the penis secondary to gunshot wounds may result in significant loss of tissue. Such wounds should be cleansed and conservatively débrided, and, if minor, may be closed primarily. If there is any question, the wound should be treated by delayed closure. Scrotal skin usually is available as replacement tissue and can be used either in the form of a pedicle graft or, occasionally, to bury the penis, as in a first-stage Cecil urethroplasty, with later release. Urethroplasty can be done at a later date if necessary.

Amputation wounds are uncommon. They may be treated successfully if the amputated portion can be retrieved, preserved in sterile cold Ringer solution or saline with heparin and possibly antibiotics, and reanastomosed using either macroscopic magnification or microscopic surgical techniques. The type of repair depends on the facilities available and the skill and experience of the surgeon. Microsurgical techniques are preferable if feasible. Vascular anastomoses should be done so far as possible, and the urethra and Buck's fascia reapproximated. Some authors advocate excising the penile skin and burying the amputated portion within the scrotum for later release using the Cecil technique. Psychiatric evaluation of these patients obviously is needed in many cases.

---

* Injuries associated with agricultural and other equipment; the clothing is engaged and the skin pulled off the penis or scrotum or both. The name refers to a device on the back of a tractor. Also known as "de-gloving" injuries.

Penile burns are treated as burns elsewhere in the body. The inner layer of preputial skin, if available, may be valuable in subsequent grafts.

Surgical repair of the penis done under local anesthetic should never involve the use of epinephrine in the anesthetic agent, and one must be careful to avoid constrictive dressings. It is wise to use absorbable sutures in penile repairs when possible, to avoid the often-difficult job of removing sutures over a sensitive area. Chromic catgut sutures are useful in this respect. Complex-reconstructive procedures can be done at a later date.

SCROTAL INJURIES

Most crush injuries of the scrotum do not result in testicular rupture. Patients who sustain a blow or injury of this sort and are able to walk around afterward usually do not have a ruptured testis. The scrotum is elastic, and any sort of bleeding can result in a great deal of swelling, hematoma, and ecchymosis. Intrascrotal injuries should be treated with bed rest, scrotal elevation, and ice bags, and, if infection is a possibility, antibiotics should be given. Injuries of the epididymis may result in a sperm granuloma at a later date and loss of sperm conduction. Testicular rupture is an extremely painful injury that does require repair if the testis is to be salvaged. Testicular sonograms and, if necessary, nuclear scans may be of some help in identifying such lesions. Intrascrotal lesions should be explored if rupture of the testicular tunics is suspected. Frequently, such lesions are stellate, and it may be difficult to salvage much of the testis and yet repair the injury. Tunica vaginalis may be of some use in the repair of these injuries. A soft compression dressing may be used after intrascrotal exploration; however, care must be taken not to force the testis up into the inguinal channel, where it may become stuck.

Lacerations of the scrotum are repaired as are lacerations in any other area of the body. Significant skin loss can occur with scrotal regeneration, and laxity of scrotal tissues often permits closure even with large skin defects. In total scrotal avulsions, the testes may be placed in subcutaneous thigh pouches and scrotal reconstruction done at a later date using skin from the medial aspect of the thighs. Penetrating injuries ordinarily are explored and débrided, and all nonviable tissue is excised. Clean wounds may be closed primarily. Contaminated or dirty wounds are left open, the patient is placed on dressing changes for 3 to 5 days, and delayed closure is done.

URETHRAL INJURIES

Urethral injuries are more common in the male than in the female. Fixation of the male urethra to the pubic bone by the suspensory ligaments of the penis and the puboprostatic ligaments prevents the mobility found in the adult female urethra. In childhood, there is more fixation of the female urethra, and injuries may occur and often involve the vagina as well. Urethrovaginal fistula is common, and attempts at repair often lead to vaginal stenosis. These injuries may be treated best from above, with omental interposition between the urethra and vagina.

Anterior Urethral Injuries

One can consider anterior urethral injuries in the male as either external or internal. External injuries include crush injuries, urethral injuries associated with fractured penis, penetrating injuries, amputations, and avulsions. Treatment often depends on the type of genital injury associated with urethral injury. As noted, urethrography is essential in the diagnosis of such injuries and should be done under fluoroscopy when possible. Sterile solutions that would be suitable for intravenous injection should be used. The patient should be positioned obliquely, with the dependent thigh flexed and with the penis pointed in a cephalad direction. Minor extravasation without evidence of infection can be treated with an indwelling urethral catheter for 10 to 14 days and antibiotic coverage. It is wise to obtain a urethrogram at the time of catheter removal.

Severe injuries are treated best with suprapubic diversion. Urethral lacerations should be repaired in a transverse direction to avoid narrowing of the lumen and to minimize stricture formation. Large wounds may require marsupialization and delayed reconstructive procedures. The urethra should be spatulated if reanastomosis is to be done to provide as wide a circumference as possible. The urethra must be mobilized adequately enough to prevent tension at the suture lines. Primary anastomosis after a large defect may result in shortening of the urethra and penis and in downward chordee or curvature.

Straddle injuries and perineal injuries from

blows, explosions, or blasts may injure the bulbous urethra in the male and any part of the urethra in the female. Urethral contusion or partial or complete tears may result. Nearly one third of urethral straddle injuries are complete and about two thirds are partial or incomplete. A suprapubic tube should be inserted, and, in the case of closed crush injuries, surgical treatment of the wound should be delayed if possible because it is difficult to determine the viability of the involved tissues and more accurate evaluation is possible later. Drainage is mandatory if infected urine is present. If urethral repair or anastomosis is indicated, absorbable suture should be used.

Patch graft urethroplasty ordinarily is reserved for reconstructive surgery. Secondary procedures for reconstructing genital and urethral injuries can be complex and often include skin and tissue flap techniques. Included are vascularized flaps, microvascular techniques, and myocutaneous flaps. Flaps from the groin supplied by the superficial circumflex vessels may be used and, on occasion, the vascular pedicles can be divided and anastomosed to recipient penile vessels if vascular length is not sufficient. Gracilis muscle myocutaneous flaps with overlying skin may be transferred to the perineum for reconstructive surgery involving this area, the vagina, the penis, and other sites.

Internal urethral injuries are common, and the majority are associated with lower tract instrumentation. Prevention must, of course, be stressed. Trauma to the infant male urethra frequently follows instrumentation with infant feeding tubes and other catheter devices. It is important to realize that nearly 10 per cent of normal newborns do not void in the first 24 hours, and a small number do not void until after 48 hours. Urine output for the first few days of life is only 50 to 60 ml/day, and unnecessary catheterization often is done. Infants with posterior urethral valves may be difficult to catheterize, and subsequent trauma and stricture formation may occur.

The female urethra may be damaged during various gynecologic surgical procedures and as a result of obstetric causes. Patients who are suffering partial urethral loss under such circumstances should be treated with reconstruction using vaginal tissue. If there is significant tissue loss, labial flaps with underlying fat and bulbocavernosus muscles may be used.

Urethral damage can occur subsequent to allergy to latex catheters and from sterilizing solutions. Infection secondary to instrumentation may contribute to scar and stricture formation and possibly tissue loss.

Posterior Urethral Injuries

Posterior urethral injuries are usually of a closed nature, and most of these occur in the male. Excluding injuries from urethral instrumentation, a large percentage are secondary to motor vehicle accidents. Most posterior urethral ruptures occur in the presence of pelvic fractures; nearly 10 per cent of all pelvic fractures have an associated urologic injury, either ruptured bladders or partial or complete urethral tears. It is unusual for partial or complete transection of the urethra to occur in females with pelvic fractures, but occasionally this occurs. In male infants and children, injuries usually occur higher in the bladder neck area because of lack of development of the prostate. It is important to do a proctoscopic examination in patients with massive crush injuries as part of the workup, to rule out colorectal trauma. Rectal bleeding or bony fragments found on digital examination of the rectum are diagnostic. Major neurologic damage can occur as well and usually is due to stretching and contusion rather than to severance of nerves.

The mortality in patients incurring open pelvic fractures approaches 50 per cent, as opposed to only about 10 per cent in closed fractures. Death generally results from bleeding, sepsis, or injury to other organ systems. Although the urologic injuries usually are not life threatening, they are the most common cause of long-term disability after such accidents. The degree of blood loss tends to parallel the amount of comminution and the number of pelvic fractures present. The greatest sources of continuing hemorrhage are normally the open venous ends at the fracture sites. Fractures into the greater sciatic notch may lacerate large branches of the hypogastric vessels, and fracture-dislocations of the sacroiliac joint may tear or disrupt the common iliac vessels or the external iliac and hypogastric vessels at the bifurcation. The resultant bleeding may rapidly become lethal unless adequately controlled.

There are several potential causes of urethral injury in patients with pelvic fractures. Diametric fractures with displacement (Malgaigne fractures) of the hemipelvis superiorly place traction on the hypogastric wing. Displacement of the symphysis superiorly may lead to rupture of the puboprostatic ligaments and to stretching and possibly incomplete or complete tearing of the prostatomembranous urethra. A guillotine-like effect may follow bilateral fractures of the superior and inferior pubic rami. Diastasis of the symphysis and avulsion of one puboprostatic ligament and a tear of the urogenital diaphragm from the contralateral bone may cause urethral tears, as can bony fragments. Possible urethral injuries secondary to pelvic fractures and dislocations include contusions, stretching, occlusions from pelvic hematoma, partial and complete tears, and avulsions. Various degrees of damage to the urogenital diaphragm may occur.

Management

Principles of management include control of hemorrhage, pelvic fracture stabilization, evaluation for possible damage to other organ systems, and the immediate treatment of life-threatening problems. Urologic evaluation frequently must be delayed until airway and hemorrhage assessment is done. Arteriographic evaluation and occasionally embolization may be necessary. Urologic treatment is aimed toward preservation of continence, the minimization of stricture formation, and avoidance of immediate and delayed treatment complications, including impotence. Signs and symptoms frequently present in patients with urethral injury associated with fractures of the pelvis include blood at the meatus. Voiding dysfunction or complete inability to void may be present secondary to urethral compression or disruption or possibly a ruptured bladder. One must assume a urethral injury in these patients until proven otherwise. The classic findings of a complete urethral tear include a palpable hematoma on rectal examination, with a high-riding prostate. These patients may have ecchymosis in a "butterfly" pattern over the perineum. The bladder neck ordinarily retains its sphincteric activity, and urine does not extravasate into the pelvis.

Uroradiographic Evaluation

It is important to perform intravenous pyelography (IVP), cystography, and urethrography in patients with pelvic fractures who are suspected of having urologic trauma. Arteriography, CT scanning, and, occasionally, magnetic resonance imaging may be indicated, especially if other organs—usually intraabdominal—are involved. An elevated bladder on the IVP implies total urethral disruption. A "teardrop" bladder results from hematoma. Large amounts of extravasated blood may be present in these patients. An IVP is unreliable in the evaluation of a ruptured bladder, and a cystogram is about 85 per cent accurate in these cases. Urethrography should be done under fluoroscopy if possible. If contrast medium passes into the bladder, there is at least partial continuity of the urethra. Animal studies have shown that urethral instrumentation may increase the severity of a partial injury significantly and cause a complete tear or disruption. Partial injuries may or may not lead to stricture formation whether treated with or without stents. Suprapubic bladder drainage is adequate and appropriate for a hematoma compressing and stretching the urethra.

Extravasation without passage of contrast into the bladder at the time of urethrography usually denotes complete urethral transection. Rupture may occur just above or below the urogenital diaphragm. However, in the majority of patients, there is disruption both above and below the urogenital diaphragm. Complete occlusion without extravasation implies urethral occlusion and stretching from hematoma.

Repair

As a rule, such injuries are best treated with insertion of a suprapubic tube, and delayed urethroplasty should be done 3 to 6 months after injury. This method now is recommended in treating these injuries in both male and female children as well as in adults, and there appears to be a significantly decreased incidence in subsequent impotence in males. This modality accepts the probable need for urethroplasty, the exception being in those patients with compression from hematoma without complete disruption. There is not universal agreement in this area, and some authorities believe that, if there is significant displacement of pelvic fractures, an open procedure may be indicated, and certainly if there are bony fragments within the urethra, these must be removed. There are significant medicolegal overtones regarding the treatment of these injuries, and deviation from the standard approach of suprapubic tube insertion without disturbance of the retropubic space could invite litigation.

The strictures resulting from these injuries usually can be repaired through a perineal route with either direct anastomosis or a patch graft or tube urethroplasty. Difficult strictures with severe pelvic distortion may require partial pubectomy and urethroplasty. These injuries may involve transection of the pudendal vessels and nerves and avulsion of the corpora cavernosa, resulting in impotence regardless of the method of treatment. Patients with such injuries frequently require as long as 1 year and occasionally up to 3 years to regain potency. The continence mechanism also may be damaged. There are numerous advantages to the initial management by suprapubic tube insertion. This procedure can be done by nonurologic surgeons and avoids possible damage from instrumentation of the urethra. Catheters passed up the urethra in these patients usually pass behind the prostate, and manipulation of the catheter plus catheter balloon inflation may further damage the parasympathetic nerves that mediate erections. One can expect impotence rates associated with an injury treated in this fashion to vary from 0 to 15 per cent and possibly higher. Patients normally will be continent after these injuries unless there has been damage to the bladder neck from prior surgery or other factors. Some authors believe that, in patients with highly distorted fractures, a suprapubic tube should be inserted initially but, once the threat of bleeding has been reduced over a few days, hematoma evacuation should be done and efforts made to realign the urethral ends.

I believe that external fixation techniques of pelvic fractures may improve the results in alignment considerably and decrease the hazards of delayed urologic reconstruction. Follow-up urethrography and urologic evaluation obviously are indicated in all cases.

Conclusion

A well-planned, thorough urologic evaluation of patients with genital and pelvic trauma is vital in order to preserve and restore function and to prevent the potentially crippling and sometimes fatal sequelae of such injuries. The urologist is an essential member of the treatment team and must be knowledgeable and prepared to manage both the initial and reconstructive phases of surgery in these patients.

Suggested Readings

Dixon CM, Hricak H, McAninch JW: Magnetic resonance imaging of traumatic posterior urethral defects and pelvic crush injuries. J Urol 148:1162–1165, 1992

Corriere JN Jr: Trauma to the lower urinary tract. *In* Gillenwater JY, et al (eds): Adult and Pediatric Urology, 2nd ed. Chicago, Mosby-Year Book, 1991, pp. 499–522

Penson DF, Seftel AD, Krane, RJ, et al: The hemodynamic pathophysiology of impotence following blunt trauma to the erect penis. J Urol 148:1171–1180, 1992

INJURY OF THE ANTERIOR URETHRA

STEVEN M. SCHLOSSBERG, M.D.

Norfolk, Virginia

Anterior urethral injuries commonly are caused by blunt trauma, such as a straddle injury of the bulbar urethra. The severity of injury may vary from a mild contusion that goes unrecognized to a severe disruption with extravasation into local tissues. The most minor injuries often present years later as an isolated short bulbar urethral stricture. More severe injuries are recognized because of bloody urethral discharge or, in some cases, perineal swelling caused by hematoma or urinary extravasation. The fluid may be confined to Buck's fascia or break through it and be limited by Colles' fascia. If suspicion of injury exists, a retrograde urethrogram should be performed. Using intravenous contrast, a gentle injection with 10 ml of contrast should be performed. If this is insufficient, more contrast should be injected and the radiograph repeated. Contrast is a tissue irritant, and, therefore, an attempt to limit extravasation into local tissues is important. The urethrogram will show if there is extravasation of contrast. If the radiograph is normal, injury to the corpus spongiosum still may be present, which could lead to future stricture disease.

Urinary diversion is the treatment of choice. The goals are to prevent infection, limit further injury, and promote healing. It is likely that formation of urethral stricture is determined mostly by the injury and not the type of urinary diversion. There are proponents of both suprapubic and urethral catheter diversion. If the injury is minor and catheter diversion is planned, a soft silicone catheter can be placed, if necessary, with the aid of a flexible cystoscope and a guidewire.

The more severe injuries should be managed by suprapubic drainage and, if urinary extravasation is present, periurethral drainage of the urinoma and hematoma. Immediate repair of blunt injuries should be condemned. The more minor injuries may heal without ever needing repair; in the more severe injuries, precise determination of the extent of the injury is difficult, making immediate repair uncertain.

Bulbar urethral injury by sharp penetrating trauma presents a different situation. Because tissue damage is not as extensive, immediate repair is possible and reliable. With minimal débridement, repair is completed with mobilization of the urethral edges and end-to-end anastomosis. A two-layer anastomosis is performed with fine chromic suture for the mucosa and slow-dissolving absorbable suture for the outer layer. Usually, a suprapubic tube and urethral catheter are placed.

Pendulous urethral injury is much less common. A blunt injury is possible and would be treated in a similar fashion. The pendulous portion of the anterior urethra also may be injured with a penile fracture. The integrity of the urethra should be evaluated and, if the urethra is injured, it should be repaired at the time of the operative repair of a penile fracture. Penetrating injuries are treated in a fashion similar to that for sharp bulbar injuries. If the wound is clean, a repair can be performed. If the wound is contaminated, the urethra should be débrided, the wound left open, and a suprapubic tube placed. The risk of developing significant infection, with its morbidity, should be avoided. If a fistula develops, it can be repaired at a later surgery.

The treatment of anterior urethral injuries depends on the experience and judgment of the treating physician. When in doubt, suprapubic diversion is indicated. More minor injuries can be managed with a urethral catheter. Acutely, surgery is indicated in severe blunt injury when drainage of periurethral fluid is necessary, in penetrating trauma when primary repair may be indicated, and in contaminated penetrating wounds when periurethral drainage and débridement are necessary.

Suggested Readings

Guerriero WG: Anterior urethral disruption. *In* Guerriero WG, Devine CJ Jr (eds): Urologic Injuries. Norwalk, CT, Appleton-Century-Crofts, 1984, pp. 133–141

Jordan GH, Devine PC: Immediate management of external urethral injury. *In* Cass AS (ed): Genitourinary Trauma. Cambridge, England, Blackwell Scientific Publications, 1988, pp. 195–207

Pierce JM Jr: Disruptions of the anterior urethra. Urol Clin North Am 16:329–334, 1989

Tumors

URETHRAL CARCINOMA

ERIC A. KLEIN, M.D.

Cleveland, Ohio

Primary carcinoma of the urethra is a rare but aggressive cancer and the only urologic neoplasm that occurs more frequently in women than men. Urethral cancers primarily are treated surgically, with recent emphasis on combined modalities incorporating surgery, radiation, and chemotherapy for more advanced tumors. These newer approaches have arisen because of the relatively poor prognosis of most tumors, which are typically locally extensive, prone to local recurrence, may present with regional lymph node involvement, and often are resistant to single-modality therapy.

Cancers of the male and female urethra have many similarities, including delays in diagnosis as a result of the nonspecific nature of symptoms, a propensity for aggressive local behavior, a similar pattern of nodal and hematogenous metastases, and clinical/anatomic divisions into proximal and distal tumors that dictate the extent of surgical therapy. Because of some differences in histology and anatomic relationships, tumors in the male and those in the female traditionally are considered separately.

CARCINOMA OF THE FEMALE URETHRA

The female urethra averages 3 to 5 cm in length and runs just deep to the anterior vaginal wall. It is surrounded by connective tissue and an inner longitudinal and outer circular muscularis. Proximally, it is lined by transitional epithelium contiguous with bladder epithelium, whereas the distal two thirds is lined by stratified squamous epithelium. The urethra also is surrounded by submucosal glands, which may give rise to cancers from their ducts or epithelium.

For various reasons the urethra is divided clinically into proximal and distal portions. Lymphatic drainage of the proximal urethra is to the pelvis, including external iliac, internal iliac, and obturator nodes, whereas the distal segment drains predominantly to inguinal lymph nodes. Furthermore, the continence zone in the female is located in the proximal portion of the urethra, which permits local excision of distal urethral tumors without affecting urinary control.

Female urethral cancers occur predominantly in the fifth to seventh decades with unknown etiology. Squamous cell carcinoma is the predominate histologic type (55 to 70 per cent), with adenocarcinomas accounting for 15 to 20 per cent, transitional cell carcinomas (TCCs) for 10 to 15 per cent, and melanoma, undifferentiated tumors, and metastatic tumors for the remainder. Except for melanoma, which has an extremely poor prognosis, the natural history, outcome, and surgical treatment of primary urethral carcinomas does not depend on histology. Urethral tumors may be confined to the mucosa or extend through underlying tissues to invade the lamina propria, muscularis, or surrounding tissues, including the bladder neck, vagina, vulva, and symphysis pubis. The presence of palpable or radiographically enlarged lymph nodes usually indicates metastases rather than infection or reactive lymphadenitis. Although up to 60 per cent of patients in older series presented with palpable nodes, less than 10 per cent present with evidence of distant metastases, typically of lung, liver, bone, or brain. Local recurrence is the most common cause of treatment failure and usually precedes the onset of metastases.

Symptoms, Diagnosis, and Staging

The nonspecific nature of symptoms arising from urethral cancers often results in a delayed diagnosis. Urethral or vaginal bleeding is the most frequent symptom, but may be attributed to dysfunctional menses, the onset of menopause, or urinary tract infection. Irritative symptoms, incontinence, and dyspareunia also may be seen, and large tumors near the bladder neck may result in urinary retention. Physical examination may reveal a localized area of induration, a mass extending into the vagina or bladder neck, or, in advanced cases, a perineal mass with palpable inguinal nodes. Cystoscopy and transurethral or transvaginal biopsy are necessary to confirm the diagnosis, and abdominopelvic computerized tomographic (CT) scan and chest radiograph are necessary for staging.

Although there are no universally adopted staging systems for cancer of the female urethra, most often stage is assigned by the extent of invasion into underlying tissue and surrounding organs, with higher stage tumors carrying a worse prognosis and a larger therapeutic burden. More than one half of the patients present with locally advanced disease. Although tumors confined to the mucosa are virtually all curable, long-term survival for tumors penetrating the submucosa or muscularis approximates only 40 to 45 per cent, and that for tumors involving the vagina, bladder, or lymph nodes only 15 to 25 per cent.

Treatment

Treatment of urethral tumors depends on whether the tumor is located in the proximal or distal portion. Tumors of the distal third confined to the mucosa or with superficial (submucosal) invasion can be cured by either wide local excision (partial urethrectomy) or interstitial radiotherapy (typical dose 50 to 60 Gy over 6 to 7 days). Good local control also has been reported with use of the CO_2 or neodymium:yttrium-aluminum-garnet laser, applying a power of 20 to 30 W in 0.5- to 2.0-second pulses. Because of the morbidity of inguinal lymphadenectomy, groin dissections are reserved for those patients with palpable lymph nodes.

Tumors that arise in the proximal two thirds of the urethra or that exhibit more extensive invasion require anterior pelvic exenteration with en bloc urethrectomy, and partial or total vaginectomy with or without vulvectomy. A less radical alternative for proximal *superficial* lesions is total urethrectomy with closure of the bladder neck and creation of a continent cutaneous catheterizable stoma by use of the Mitrofanoff principle or by bladder augmentation with an ileocecal cap. A full bilateral pelvic lymphadenectomy is indicated at the time of pelvic exploration. Some authors also have advocated partial excision of the inferior surface of the symphysis pubis in order to ensure a negative margin anteriorly. Following exenteration, an omental flap or synthetic mesh is required to prevent bowel herniation into the perineum. Depending on the extent of dissection, the perineal defect can be closed primarily or reconstructed with a musculocutaneous flap. Vaginal reconstruction may be considered in younger patients. The use of radiation therapy alone in advanced tumors is not warranted because of a limited capacity for local control.

Because of relatively poor long-term survival in high-stage tumors treated by single-modality therapy, some authors have advocated the use of preoperative or postoperative external radiotherapy in high-stage patients. One common regimen is 45 Gy given over 4 to 5 weeks followed by anterior exenteration. Similarly, there are a number of chemotherapeutic agents with activity against squamous carcinomas at other sites, including cis-platinum, 5-fluorouracil, mitomycin, and bleomycin, that may be successfully combined into an integrated therapeutic approach. At present, the role of these combined-modality approaches and their potential ability to result in an improved cure rate or organ-sparing surgery must be considered investigational.

Tumors found in urethral diverticula are more commonly adenocarcinomas, but otherwise have a presentation similar to that of other urethral cancers. The diagnosis and management of these tumors is also similar, and treatment by local or radical excision depends on stage and location. Primary urethral melanoma accounts for about 4 per cent of female urethral cancers, is treated by radical excision, and carries a poor prognosis. Benign mesenchymal tumors such as leiomyoma, lipoma, or hemangioblastoma can be cured by local excision; primary sarcomas of the urethra are rare and are treated by wide excision.

CARCINOMA OF THE MALE URETHRA

The male urethra averages 20 cm in length and can be divided into prostatic, membranous, bulbous, and pendulous portions. The urethra is surrounded by submucosa and, in the bulbous and pendulous portions, by the corpus spongiosum. The prostatic portion is lined by transitional epithelium, the bulbomembranous and pendulous portions by stratified columnar epithelium, and the fossa navicularis and meatus by squamous epithelium. The bulbous and pendulous urethra are lined by periurethral glands and, along with the Cowper glands of the urogenital diaphragm, may give rise to adenocarcinomas. The lymphatic drainage of the male urethra is similar to that of the female, with posterior (prostatic and bulbomembranous) urethral drainage to the pelvis and anterior urethral drainage to the inguinal nodes. However, there is some overlap in the lymphatic channels, and up to one quarter of posterior urethral cancers may have inguinal adenopathy.

Cancers of the male urethra occur most commonly in the sixth and seventh decades. About 80 per cent of male urethral cancers are squamous cell carcinomas, with TCC of the prostatic urethra accounting for 15 per cent and adenocarcinomas accounting for the remainder. Overall, 55 per cent of urethral tumors occur in the bulbomembranous portion, 36 per cent in the pendulous portion, and 9 per cent in the prostatic portion. Many patients with squamous cancers give a history of urethral stricture or instrumentation, leading to speculation that repeated trauma to the urethra may result in squamous metaplasia followed by tumor formation. Human papilloma viruses also have been proposed recently as an etiologic agent. TCC of the prostatic urethra almost always is associated with bladder cancer.

Symptoms, Diagnosis, and Staging

Like female urethral cancers, these tumors tend to invade locally and metastasize to regional lymph nodes long before systemic spread. Involvement of the corpus spongiosum is common in distal tumors, as is invasion of the deep structures of the perineum in bulbomembranous tumors. Symptoms typically include an obstructive urinary pattern, including retention and/or overflow incontinence, urethral mass, dysuria or pain, recurrent strictures, urethral bleeding, or fistula. Diagnosis requires cystoscopy and transurethral or percutaneous biopsy. Retrograde urethrography or voiding cytourethrography may be useful in defining the location and extent of the tumor and associated urinary fistulas. A CT scan of the abdomen and pelvis and a chest radiograph should be obtained to complete the staging evaluation.

Urethral tumors are staged according to the depth of invasion and extension to adjacent organs. Clinical stage predicts prognosis as well as determines the extent of surgical therapy. Long-term survival can be expected in 50 to 60 per cent of patients with distal tumors and, historically, in only 10 to 15 per cent of those with high-stage tumors.

Treatment

Standard treatment for *distal (pendulous) urethral tumors* is primarily surgical, with partial or total penectomy as necessary to obtain an adequate (2-cm) proximal tumor-free margin. If there is insufficient penile length for the patient to direct the urinary stream after partial penectomy, total penectomy with perineal urethrostomy should be performed. Partial or total urethrectomy with sparing of the corpora cavernosa but complete excision of the surrounding corpus spongiosum may be considered in selected cases with minimal invasion of the lamina propria. A few cases of small tumors managed successfully by one or more transurethral resections also have been reported, but these patients must be monitored more closely for the development of local recurrences. Patients with papillary TCC or those medically unable or unwilling to undergo more extensive procedures are the best candidates for this approach. Inguinal lymphadenectomy is reserved for patients with palpable or biopsy-proven inguinal metastases.

Management of *bulbomembranous tumors* is usually more arduous because these tumors tend to present late and at higher stages than distal urethral tumors. Adequate treatment usually requires cystoprostatectomy with en bloc urethrectomy and excision of the urogenital diaphragm. Resection of the penis, scrotum, and undersurface of the pubis may be necessary in selected cases. The role of pre- or postoperative chemotherapy in these patients is under study and not yet established. Pelvic lymphadenectomy is performed routinely at the time of pelvic exenteration, whereas inguinal dissections are reserved for those patients with palpable nodes.

The management of TCC of the *prostatic urethra* deserves special consideration. This occurs almost exclusively as a manifestation of TCC of the bladder, either as direct mucosal extension of tumors near the bladder neck in patients with diffuse carcinoma in situ, or in isolation following intravesical chemotherapy for superficial disease. In these instances a careful search for concomitant bladder tumors must be sought. Management depends on the stage of the associated bladder tumor, with those patients with invasive tumors typically undergoing cystoprostatectomy. In patients with bladder tumors not demanding cystectomy and only superficial involvement of the prostatic urethra, full transurethral resection of the prostate followed by intravesical bacillus Calmette-Guérin may be considered as primary therapy. Invasion of the prostatic stroma in association with a bladder tumor is a sign of aggressive disease and typically requires cystoprostatectomy with or without chemotherapy. Patients with prostatic involvement by TCC who undergo cystectomy are at high risk for urethral recurrence and also should undergo complete urethrectomy, including the fossa navicularis. There are a few instances of TCC invading the prostatic stroma in the absence of associated bladder tumors, and, although the experience is anecdotal, some of these patients have been successfully managed by systemic methotrexate-vinblastine-Adriamycin-cis-platinum chemotherapy followed by radical prostatectomy rather than by cystoprostatectomy. Patients with TCC of the bladder who undergo cystoprostatectomy without urethrectomy should be monitored for urethral recurrence by urethral wash cytology at 6 to 12-month intervals. Patients with documented recurrences should be treated by urethrectomy.

Suggested Readings

Forman JD, Lichter AS: The role of radiation therapy in the management of carcinoma of the male and female urethra. Urol Clin North Am 19:383, 1992

Grigsby PW, Corn BW: Localized urethral tumors in women: Indications for conservative versus exenterative therapies. J Urol 147:1516, 1992

Hussein AM, Benedetto P, Sridhar KS: Chemotherapy with cisplatin and 5-fluorouracil for penile and urethral squamous carcinomas. Cancer 65:433, 1990

Johnson DW, Kessler JF, Ferrigni RG, et al: Low dose combined chemotherapy/radiotherapy in the management of locally advanced urethral squamous cell carcinoma. J Urol 141:615, 1989.

Zeidman EJ, Desmond P, Thompson IM: Surgical treatment of carcinoma of the male urethra. Urol Clin North Am 19:359, 1992

SECTION 7

THE PENIS AND THE SCROTUM

CONGENITAL MICROPHALLUS

MARK R. ZAONTZ, M.D.

Camden, New Jersey

Microphallus (or micropenis) is a multispecialty challenge in the newborn period and a source of worry to both the family and physicians. Various investigators have measured standard penile stretch length. This refers to the distance between the pubis and tip of the glans on full stretch and closely correlates to the erect penile size. Feldman and Smith have shown that the average normal penile stretch length in the newborn is 3.5 cm, with a range of 2.8 cm (3rd percentile) to 4.2 cm (97th percentile). Micropenis is defined as a normally formed penis in the newborn period with a stretch length of less than 2.5 standard deviations from normal. Thus, any newborn male with a penis smaller than 2.5 cm on stretch falls into the category of micropenis.

Care must be taken in differentiating the neonate with a concealed but otherwise normal-size penis from the neonate with microphallus. A prepubic fat pad may mask the true size of an otherwise normal penis. Likewise, "dysgenetic bands" may cause partial or complete penile retraction beneath the abdominal wall, again hiding the identity of a normal penis. Manual expression of the hidden penis generally will resolve any lingering questions as to true penile size. Finally, some infants are born with significant penoscrotal webs, which may lead to confusion over actual size. Generally, palpation of normal-sized corporal bodies and glans in these infants are sufficient to declare them otherwise normal. The concealed penis usually will grow along normal lines.

ETIOLOGY

Microphallus is thought to represent an endocrinologic problem affecting genital growth. In order for the external genitalia to achieve normal development by the 12th week of gestation, placental human chorionic gonadotropin (hCG) must stimulate the normal fetal testes. Once penile development occurs, its growth will proceed only if luteinizing hormone–releasing hormone (LHRH), secreted by the hypothalamus, stimulates the pituitary to release luteinizing hormone (LH) to further stimulate the fetal testis. Fetal testosterone is necessary not only for normal penile development but continued penile growth in the second and third trimesters by directly stimulating androgen receptors at the local level. Hence, those factors regulating penile growth involve the hypothalamic-pituitary-gonadal (HPG) axis.

Not uncommonly, other findings in the newborn with microphallus include small, low-volume, possibly cryptorchid testes. As these males reach puberty, secondary male characteristics often are inadequately developed, the prostate remains small, and, although erections may be normal, ejaculation typically is absent. Additionally, bone age may lag behind chronologic age and gynecoid features may be seen.

Hypogonadotropic Hypogonadism

A functioning hypothalamic-pituitary axis is not needed for penile development because placental hCG provides this stimulus. Boys born with an anencephally frequently are noted to have a small but otherwise normally developed penis. Micropenis at birth thus frequently denotes deficient stimulation of LH antenatally. This may be secondary to primary hypothalamic dysfunction (absence of LHRH stimulation), as seen in Prader-Willi syndrome, Kallmann syndrome, a number of the dwarf syndromes, and DeMorsier syndrome. Other endocrinologic problems must be evaluated in primary hypothalamic failure because there commonly exist deficiencies in other releasing hormones, such as hypoglycemia resulting from adrenocorticotrophic hormone deficiency or retarded growth secondary to growth hormone deficiency.

Primary Testicular Dysfunction (Hypergonadotropic Hypogonadism)

The presence of androgen insensitivity, 5-alpha-reductase deficiency, and/or testicular dysgenesis may result in microphallus and, in other cases, an abnormally formed phallus, as in testicular feminization syndrome. In the "vanishing testis syndrome," the infant is genotypically and phenotypically male but without the presence of testes. These testes were thought to have "vanished" secondary to in utero testicular torsion or some other vascular accident. The phallus of such an infant typically is not a micropenis, but, for normal penile growth to continue, androgen replacement is necessary. Often, partial defects in 5-alpha-reductase and/or testicular responsiveness may be overcome with androgen replacement and adequate penile growth achieved.

Idiopathic Microphallus

Some infants defy any of the aforementioned etiologic causes of micropenis, and work-up reveals an intact HPG axis. Normal penile growth has been seen at the time of puberty in a number of these children without any treatment.

EVALUATION

Initial evaluation of the micropenis should include urologic, genetic (chromosomal analysis), and endocrine (serum levels of LH, follicle-stimulating hormone, testosterone, and dihydrotestosterone) work-ups. Also, both stretched penile size and testicular presence, location, and volume should be evaluated.

Diagnosis of hypogonadotropic hypogonadism can be made by measuring levels of testosterone before and after hCG treatment. If the testes respond by actively secreting significantly higher levels of testosterone, primary testicular failure is not the problem. If gonadotropin-releasing hormone (GnRH) is given and a rise in the basal LH level occurs, normal pituitary function is documented and primary hypothalamic failure is present. When no LH response to GnRH occurs, primary pituitary failure is the source of the problem.

It is important to realize that, just prior to birth, there is usually a surge of LH that may last a few weeks postnatally. Questionable serum testosterone levels within the first few weeks of life may be better clarified with a trial of hCG, as already noted. If no change in the baseline levels of testosterone occur after hCG treatment, the defect lies at the testicular level.

TREATMENT

Once the etiology of micropenis is determined, a more logically directed treatment plan can be devised. By employing the team approach to this problem, the family can be counseled appropriately. The mainstay of therapy is androgen replacement. Intramuscular injections of testosterone enanthate (25 mg) ideally should begin in the neonate and continue every 2 to 3 weeks for 3 months. Reassignment to female gender is considered only after failure to demonstrate adequate penile growth with androgen replacement, or if the phallus is so diminutive that any hope for further penile development is fruitless, or in cases in which certain congenital anomalies, such as cloacal exstrophy, preclude adequate male genital reconstruction and future sexual function.

A critical factor in the phallic response to androgen is not only the presence of functional androgen receptors but the volume of erectile tissue prior to treatment. The smaller the volume, the worse the response to androgens. If the penis responds satisfactorily to androgen therapy, brief repeated courses of testosterone should be administered up through puberty while monitoring bone age. This will allow for appropriate penile growth mimicking pubertal changes while minimizing the risks of accelerated skeletal maturation and potential short stature. Finally, any infants with undescended testes should undergo early orchidopexy to maximize any potential androgen production.

Suggested Readings

Burstein S, Grumbach MM, Daplan SL: Early determination of androgen responsiveness is important in the management of micropenis. Lancet 2:983–986, 1979

Feldman KW, Smith DW: Fetal phallic growth and penile standards for newborn male infants. J Pediatr 86:395–398, 1975

Lee PA, O'Dea LStL: Primary and secondary testicular insufficiency. Pediatr Clin North Am 37:1359–1387, 1990

Woodhouse CRJ (guest ed): Classification and management of micropenis. Dial Pediatr Urol 12(7):1–7, 1989

REDUCTION CLITOROPLASTY

Jacob Rajfer, M.D., F.A.C.S.

Torrance, California

The majority of cases in which reduction clitoroplasty is required occur in the female pseudohermaphrodite. The degree of phallus enlargement is a function of androgen effect. The anatomic defect may range from a mild clitoromegaly to a severe enlargement with labial fusion and a narrowing or absence of the vaginal introitus, a common urogenital sinus, or a completely masculinized phallus with or without hypospadias. Although the metabolic defect can be compensated with replacement corticosteroids, it is unlikely in most cases that genital shrinkage will occur with such treatment alone.

The two major principles of any surgical reconstruction of the external genitalia are normal appearance and normal sensation of the phallus or clitoris. In those patients with ambiguous external genitalia, normal appearance is achieved easily with any of a multitude of available techniques for reconstruction of the external genitalia. It is difficult to evaluate clinically whether the sensory function of the external genitalia has been left undisturbed after any operative procedure on the shaft of the phallus in an infant with ambiguous genitalia. Although there has been controversy in the literature as to whether normal sensory function of the clitoris is necessary for the attainment of sexual orgasm in women, there is a consensus that every attempt should be made to leave the normal sensory pathways of the clitoris undisturbed during reconstruction of the external genitalia.

A number of surgical procedures currently are available for repair of the hypertrophied clitoris, including total or partial amputation of the shaft of the clitoris, recession of the shaft of the clitoris under the pelvic bones, and concealment of the entire clitoris by the labia majora. The practice of simple phallectomy gives an acceptable cosmetic result but is not justifiable in light of its purported negative impact on later sexual functioning. Because the ideal end result of any such surgical procedure should be normal-appearing and functioning genitalia, the most appealing operative procedure to correct the hypertrophied clitoris would appear to be the concealment procedure, in which the clitoris itself is undisturbed. However, in the majority of patients with ambiguous external genitalia, the clitoris is much too large to perform a concealment procedure and patient discomfort can arise during clitoral tumescence. As a result, a one-stage, nerve-sparing partial amputation of the clitoris, which preserves the normal erectile and sensory function of the glans, would appear to be the procedure of choice.

Because the neurovascular bundle that provides sensation to the glans clitoris runs dorsally along the clitoral shaft, an alternate approach to the more commonly used dorsal approach for partial amputation of the hypertrophied clitoris was devised by Goodwin. In this procedure, the clitoris is approached ventrally on the inferior aspect of the shaft of the clitoris to minimize any potential damage to the dorsal neurovascular bundle. Kogan used a ventral incision to resect a segment of corporal spongy tissue beneath the tunica vaginalis. By remaining in the subtunical space, there is an added element of safety with a reduced risk of glans necrosis.

An alternative approach uses a circumcising incision that allows de-gloving of the entire clitoral shaft. A resection of a portion of corporal shaft can be performed after release of the neurovascular bundle adherent to the corpora. The clitoral shaft may be shortened to any desired length and the glans clitoris may be appropriately tailored, if necessary, to appear normal. Excess preputial skin can be divided in the midline and can aid in labia minora or vaginal reconstruction.

One-step clitoral reduction procedures are easy and quick to perform and do not interfere with other reconstructive procedures that may have to be performed simultaneously on the external genitalia, such as vaginoplasty. Therefore, the procedure may be performed in patients of any age, including the neonate. Early repair should be considered and undertaken before psychosexual identity has developed.

Suggested Readings

Goodwin WE: Partial (segmental amputation) of the clitoris for female pseudo-hermaphrodilism. Soc Pediatr Urol Newslett, January 21, 1981

Kogan SJ, Smey P, Bewitt SB: Subtunical total reduction clitoroplasty: a safe modification of existing techniques. J Urology 130:746–748, 1983

PRIAPISM

GERALD B. BROCK, M.D.

Montreal, Canada

Priapism, defined as a prolonged erection often characterized by pain and tenderness unaccompanied by sexual desire, ironically is a condition named after Priapus, the Greek god of fertility, luck, and gardens. Our knowledge of the normal physiologic steps and the possible pathophysiologic events during erection have expanded over the past 10 years. At present, failure of the erect penis to achieve detumescence is believed by most authorities to be the underlying pathogenic event leading to priapism.

Recently, a simplified physiology-based classification has gained general acceptance that helps to differentiate between the two major types of prolonged erections: high-flow arterial priapism and low-flow veno-occlusive priapism. The latter is the more common form; lacunar space drainage is obstructed persistently in these patients, thereby preventing detumescence. These men seek medical attention early in the course of their disease because of severe pain resulting from impaired arterial inflow consequent to high intracavernosal pressure; urgent treatment is required to reduce the risk of permanent impotence. Because of increasing use of pharmacologic erection programs, low-flow priapism is now familiar to most urologists. The other type of prolonged erection usually is caused by blunt perineal or penetrating trauma directly to the cavernosal artery, resulting in a high-flow, nonischemic type of prolonged erection. This form of priapism requires less urgent treatment because the risk of trabecular ischemic injury is small. Characteristically, these men often seek medical attention days after sustaining a perineal injury. The erection is not painful, but the penis can remain in a semirigid state without sexual stimulation, usually beginning within 24 to 48 hours after post-injury and lasting for several days to years. The underlying pathology is usually a laceration to the cavernosal artery, producing higher arterial inflow than is drained from the cavernosal bodies, thereby resulting in tumescence of a mild to moderate degree without evidence of tissue ischemia.

In cases of low-flow priapism, Spycher and Hauri showed clear histologic evidence of severe cellular and neural damage with sporadic necrosis within 24 hours. Cavernosal smooth muscle cells activated in the hypoxic low-flow environment were found to transform into more resistant fibroblasts that were capable of producing collagen. In cases of the high-flow type of priapism, the damage was limited to trabecular edema with preservation of potency.

ETIOLOGY

The underlying cause of priapism is highly dependent on demographics; the prevalence of sickle cell disease and the number of patients performing self-injection therapy with vasoactive agents for impotence are the two most important factors. In a review of the world literature in 1986, Pohl reported the etiologic factors of 230 cases: one third were idiopathic, 21 per cent were alcohol or drug related, 12 per cent were associated with perineal trauma, and 11 per cent occurred in men with sickle cell disease. In reviewing the literature since that publication, the number of iatrogenic-induced cases (with papaverine being the predominant culprit) has risen dramatically.

Within the past year, *intracavernous agents* that release nitric oxide have been tried in man, after experimental studies in which they were shown to relax cavernosal smooth muscle in vitro and to induce an erectile response in vivo. These agents have extremely short half-lives and may have a lower risk for priapism than currently is seen with papaverine or papaverine with phentolamine and prostaglandin E_1. However, at present, intracavernous injection of vasoactive substances remains the most likely cause of priapism confronting most urologists. In a worldwide review of the literature, Juenemann and Alkan reported that 5.3 per cent of patients had priapism at the initial diagnostic session and 0.4 per cent sustained a prolonged erection during self-administration. These cases of priapism are treated easily with intracorporeal aspiration alone or by aspiration and instillation of small doses of an alpha-adrenergic agent. There appears to be little risk of permanent impotence when detumescence is achieved within 4 to 6 hours, after which some ischemic injury has been reported to occur. In those rare cases that are refractory to alpha-adrenergic and aspiration therapy, or in situations in which the patient did not seek medical attention within 36 to 48 hours, surgical shunting procedures may be required (Table 1).

TABLE 1. Surgical Procedures for Reversal of Priapism

NAME	PROCEDURE TYPE	ADVANTAGES AND DISADVANTAGES
Winter	Corporoglanular	Minimally invasive, effective, permanent impotence risk low
Quackels	Corporospongiosal	Risk of urethrocorporeal fistula, urethral stricture, permanent impotence
Grayhack	Saphenous vein–cavernosum	Invasive, effective, long incision, risk of permanent impotence
Barry	Dorsal vein–cavernosum	Invasive, effective

Sickle cell disease, a condition resulting from inheritance of one or two genes coding for an abnormal S hemoglobin, affects 8 per cent of African-Americans. Vaso-occlusive events are a characteristic phenomenon of this disease and are caused by decreased erythrocyte pliability. Episodes of priapism are unusual in the sickle cell trait or one-gene population and much more common in the two-gene or homogenic S hemoglobin population (0.15 per cent of African-American men), in which prevalence rates of 40 per cent have been reported. These episodes usually occur at night when physiologic dehydration, metabolic acidosis, and nocturnal tumescence combine and prevent the less pliable erythrocytes of sickle cell disease from draining normally through the subtunical venules. Presentation with priapism is unusual before puberty (6 per cent of cases) but, once present, recurrent episodes are the rule. Treatment for these men is intravenous hydration, alkalinization, analgesia, and hypertransfusion to increase hemoglobin to more than 10 mg/dl and to reduce the hemoglobin S level to less than 30 per cent. Injection of alpha-adrenergic agents is appropriate if attempted early (less than 6 to 12 hours), before severe sludging has occurred.

Other causes of low-flow priapism are *drugs*, especially the antidepressant trazodone. Several antihypertensive agents (hydralazine, prazosin, and guanethidine) and antipsychotic drugs (chloropromazine) also have been associated with prolonged erections. Their alpha-adrenergic blocking effect is thought to induce vascular smooth muscle relaxation and subsequent erection. Several reports of priapism in men receiving 20 per cent *fat emulsion* have been documented. Fat emulsions accelerate thrombin production, leading to a shorter coagulation time; fat emboli and increased erythrocyte adhesiveness and aggregation can develop. This may account for the increased risk of priapism and has spurred the recommendation of reducing fat emulsions to 10 per cent. Idiopathic causes of low-flow priapism are prominent in most recent series; the cases usually follow sexual stimulation.

A less common presentation of priapism in which tumescence is seen in the absence of severe pain or ischemia usually is associated with *blunt perineal trauma or direct injury to the cavernous artery* (i.e., after intracavernous injection). In these situations, rapid differentiation from the ischemic low-flow form of priapism is important in choosing the most effective treatment. Aspiration of intracorporeal blood is an easy and reliable method for determining whether the prolonged erection is ischemic (low flow) or nonischemic (high flow). Duplex ultrasonography, if available, will provide objective evidence of high arterial inflow.

TREATMENT

Treatment options depend on several factors: (1) duration of erection; (2) rigidity (often this parallels the number of obstructed emissary veins); (3) presence or absence of ischemia; and (4) underlying cause. In all cases of low-flow priapism (except when contraindicated by the patient's medical history), an early attempt with alpha-adrenergic agents is indicated. In patients with a cardiac or cerebrovascular history, aspiration alone should be attempted. In the vast majority of patients, priapism secondary to vasoactive agents responds rapidly to pharmacologic therapy with little risk. Our agent of choice is phenylephrine. Using a 21-gauge scalp vein needle, 10 to 20 ml of blood is aspirated to permit phenylephrine, administered in increments of 250 to 500 μg intracavernosally at 5-minute intervals, to circulate. Systemic blood pressure often increases by 10 to 20 mm Hg, but the increase is of no clinical significance. The short half-life and high efficacy of phenylephrine make it a safe choice if aspiration alone fails.

In cases of marked hypoxia in which endothelial and/or smooth muscle destruction has been initiated, and in cases of long-standing erection (longer than 36 to 48 hours), more invasive therapy may be required. Venous drainage can be achieved surgically either by creation of a corporoglandular shunt (Winter procedure) using a trucut needle with multiple passes, or by direct visualization of the distal corpora and creation of a draining communication between the distal corpora and the glans as described by Metz. In cases of long-standing priapism, the distal corpora can be filled with old clotted blood, necrotic debris, and sloughed tissue that may prevent success of the corporoglanular shunt. Alternative procedures also have been described in which more proximal shunts are created. In the Quackels procedure reported in 1964, the proximal spongiosum is dissected and a shunt is created with a single corpus cavernosum. This technique provides substantial drainage, and unilateral or bilateral shunts can be fashioned. These procedures all facilitate detumescence through establishing a patent channel for venous outflow.

In cases of high-flow priapism refractory to conservative management (i.e., ice or compression alone), use of angiographic selective embolization has proved to be an effective treatment approach, often enabling return to normal sexual function within months. If embolization is not possible, open ligation of the traumatized artery, directed by ultrasound localization, is an alternative procedure. In our experience these cases can be treated effectively even after up to 3 years of priapism, but the degree of subsequent potency varies.

Suggested Readings

Levine FJ, Saenz de Tejada I, Payton TR, et al: Recurrent prolonged erections and priapism as a sequelae of priapism: Pathophysiology and management. J Urol 145: 764–767, 1991

Lue TF, Hellstrom WJG, McAninch JW, et al: Priapism: A refined approach to diagnosis and treatment. J Urol 136:104–108, 1986

Pohl J, Pott B, Kleinhans G: Priapism: A three phase concept of management according to etiology and prognosis. Br J Urol 58:113–118, 1986

Spycher MA, Hauri D: The ultrastructure of the erectile tissue in priapism. J Urol 135:142–147, 1986

Winter CC, Gladstone M: Experience with 105 patients with priapism: Update review of all aspects. J Urol 140: 980–983, 1988

SCROTAL TRAUMA, INCLUDING AVULSION AND LACERATIONS

JACK W. McANINCH, M.D.

San Francisco, California

SCROTAL LACERATION

Scrotal lacerations have a great variety of causes, ranging from shearing tears with relatively blunt objects to high-velocity gunshot wounds. Repair and management must take into consideration the cause of injury; for example, gunshot wounds need thorough débridement and delayed closure, whereas relatively uncontaminated wounds may be closed primarily.

Scrotal lacerations should be evaluated promptly and major bleeding controlled. The wound then should be packed with sterile gauze, and other significant injuries should be treated. The scrotal injury then requires careful exploration to ensure that no damage has occurred to the testicle, spermatic cord, or urethra. A urethrogram is necessary if urethral injury is suspected. The approach to management can be outlined as follows:

1. Hemostasis and cleansing.
2. Local anesthesia along wound edges with 1% lidocaine (Xylocaine).
3. Wound exploration to rule out associated injuries.
4. Débridement of wound edges back to viable tissue (noted by active bleeding).
5. Packing of wound with sterile gauze for delayed closure.

For primary closure:

1. A small Penrose drain may be utilized for drainage.
2. Deep tissues are approximated with interrupted 3-0 chromic catgut sutures.
3. Dartos fascia is closed with 3-0 chromic catgut sutures.
4. Skin is closed loosely with mattress sutures of 4-0 chromic catgut.

For delayed closure:

1. Daily dressing changes are done.
2. If the wound is free of infection after 5 days, delayed primary closure is performed using 3-0 and 4-0 chromic catgut sutures.
3. Drains are not required.

Pressure dressings should be utilized in

all scrotal lacerations to aid in preventing hematoma. The technique utilized is as follows:

1. Sterile fluffed gauze is applied to the wound area and entire scrotum.
2. Skin adhesive is applied to the perineum and suprapubic area.
3. Elastoplast tape is made to adhere firmly to the perineum and anteriorly to the anal orifice, extending up to the suprapubic area. Multiple layers may be required.
4. A large athletic supporter gives additional support.

Very little pain follows closure of scrotal lacerations, and generally minimal amounts of medications are required. Antibiotics usually are not indicated. Sitz baths twice daily once the skin edges are sealed promote healing.

Blunt, nonpenetrating trauma to the scrotum can cause severe contusion and development of hematocele from rupture of superficial veins in the scrotal wall or spermatic cord. Careful examination should ensure that testicle rupture is not present, and surgical exploration is indicated if the diagnosis is in question. Otherwise, the management is usually conservative: bed rest, scrotal elevation, and oral pain medication. If the hematocele is excessively large and evidence of continued bleeding is present, surgical drainage is indicated. A transverse incision over the hematoma with evacuation of clots and control of active bleeding is required. Penrose drains and pressure dressings should be utilized as described.

SCROTAL AVULSION

Skin avulsion represents the most massive scrotal injury. Commonly, these injuries are noted when the patient's clothing is caught in a revolving machine, tearing away the scrotal skin. Partial or total (uncommon) loss of scrotal skin may occur. The testicles and spermatic cord are frequently uninjured because of the multiple, distinct fascial layers surrounding the structures. The injury is seen more often in young men, for whom potency and spermatogenesis are of ultimate importance.

The approach to management is designed to cover the soft tissue defect and preserve testicular function. Reconstruction varies, depending on the extent of soft tissue loss and the viability of the testicle. In most cases, the testicle is found to be viable, and an attempt at preservation always is made, when possible.

Partial scrotal skin avulsions may denude one testicle and a portion of the other, leaving jagged skin edges. An excellent blood supply to the area exists, and minimal débridement should be done. The area should be irrigated liberally with Betadine solution for cleansing, and all foreign material and hair should be removed. Meticulous hemostasis is obtained. The remnant of scrotal skin then should be approximated over the testicle and soft tissue defect. Small Penrose drains may be used but should be removed within 48 hours. A supportive pressure dressing is applied, as previously described. Frequently, some tension on the suture line exists, but, because of the great elasticity and expansion ability of the tissues, a near-normal–appearing scrotum usually is seen when healing is complete.

A more massive but infrequent injury is total avulsion of the scrotal skin. The testicles and spermatic cords usually remain intact, and their blood supply is preserved. Penile skin often is lost in this type of injury, and its management is covered in another article.

The testicles and spermatic cords should be covered with moist, saline-soaked gauze while the patient is en route to the operating room. Under anesthesia, the area should be liberally irrigated and cleansed. Minimal débridement should be done and viability of each testicle should be established. Meticulous hemostasis is required.

Two techniques of repair are to be considered. If a cuff of scrotal skin is present and the testicles and cord maintain a good blood supply, a split-thickness skin graft is taken from the lateral thigh and utilized for soft tissue coverage. Drains are not necessary, and a supportive pressure dressing of fluffed gauze is used. Graft contracture will occur postoperatively, but the cuff of scrotal skin allows for a great deal of compliance and stretching. In time, the graft will soften, and an adequate scrotum will remain.

When no cuff of scrotum is present, or if the blood supply of the testicle and cord is in question, the testicle can be placed in a subcutaneous pouch on the lateral thigh. The pouch can be developed by gentle finger dissection and should be superficial to the thigh fascia to maintain lower temperatures for spermatogenesis. Should thigh skin be lost, then, alternatively, the testicle and cord can be placed subcutaneously on the lower abdomen. Owing to the higher temperature of the abdominal wall, spermatogenesis is more likely to be affected when the testicle is in this position. No tension should be present on the cord or testicle, to allow early ambulation without pain. Split-thickness skin grafts then may be applied to any existing soft tissue defects left uncovered. Some months later, reconstruction may be considered to form a more normal-appearing scrotum. Thigh flaps are raised on each side that include the attached cord and testicle and, when rotated together, form a scrotum that is sutured to the surrounding perineum and penile base. Skin grafts are used to cover the existing thigh flap defects.

Postoperative Care

Postoperative care is of great importance. The abundance of perspiration and tissue drainage makes moisture in the wound area continuously present, allowing bacteria to propagate and thus producing maceration of suture lines and delayed healing. The original dressing and drains should be removed within 48 hours. The area should be left open to air as long as possible, with continuous support of the scrotum and testicle. However, the patient should not walk without total scrotal support. Application of a drying agent (tincture of mercurochrome) to the skin edges is helpful and has antibacterial properties. Sitz baths, twice daily, followed by use of a heat lamp, should be started as soon as the patient can ambulate and will facilitate wound healing.

Careful daily inspection of the wound should be done to detect possible infection as early as possible. A wide variety of organisms are known to cause scrotal infections, including hemolytic streptococci, *Proteus*, staphylococci, and a large group of anaerobes. Infection is uncommon, but, when it occurs, rapid inflammation of the entire scrotum can develop in a matter of hours, resulting in a gangrenous loss of scrotal skin. Wound cultures followed by administration of appropriate antibiotics usually identify and control the problem.

SCROTAL BURNS

Thermal and electrical scrotal burns produce special problems in management because of the underlying vital organs and because massive edema can accumulate in the loose scrotal areolar tissues. A urethral catheter should be inserted in any major genital burn to prevent urinary retention and to monitor output.

Electrical burns are deceiving to the eye and initially appear less severe than they truly are. Marked tissue loss often is present, with associated loss of testicle and cord tissue from ischemia, necrosis, and thrombosis. Areas of demarcation should be débrided, and additional conservative débridement may be required on several occasions before all devitalized tissue is removed.

The extent of tissue in thermal burns is more obvious. First- and second-degree injuries usually heal primarily with local wound care and use of topical Silvadene after cleansing. When full-thickness skin is lost, split-thickness grafts are utilized for soft tissue coverage. The principles of management are as previously outlined.

Sepsis is the primary complication of major genital burns, and prevention by meticulous wound care is most successful.

Suggested Readings

Gomez RG, McAninch JW: Scrotal reconstruction using flaps and grafts. *In* Webster G, et al (eds): Reconstructive Urology. Boston, Blackwell Scientific Publications, 1993, pp 1059–1066

McAninch JW: Management of genital skin loss. Urol Clin North Am 16:387–398, 1989

Wolf JS Jr, Turzan CW, Cattolica EV, et al: Dog bites to male genitalia: Characteristics, management and comparison with human bites. J Urol 149:286–289, 1993

MALE GENITAL LYMPHEDEMA

SAKTI DAS, M.D.

Davis, California

Male genital lymphedema often manifests as gross swelling of the external genitalia secondary to impaired lymphatic drainage. Etiologies are classified into primary, or idiopathic, and secondary, or obstructive. Primary lymphedema is subdivided further either according to age of onset (i.e., lymphedema congenita, present at birth; lymphedema praecox, appearing before 35 years of age; and lymphedema tarda, appearing after 35 years of age) or anatomically based on lymphangiographic appearance of lymphatic aplasia, hypoplasia, or hyperplasia. The secondary group is subclassified according to the etiology of lymphatic obstruction:

1. Inflammatory (either parasitic, as in filariasis, or bacterial, as in lymphogranuloma, chancroid, erysipelas, tuberculosis, leprosy, syphilis).
2. Neoplastic (lymphatic permeation and blockage).
3. Iatrogenic (either surgical, following regional lymphadenectomy, or radiotherapy-induced blockage of draining lymphatics).

In the tropical and subtropical equatorial zone, filarial infestation accounts for a large population of patients, often with gigantic penoscrotal and lower extremity lymphedema. In other parts of the world, iatrogenic causes secondary to surgical or radiotherapeutic ablation of the regional lymphatic drainage are preponderant. Restricting the limits of lymphadenectomy or radiotherapy to the primary drainage areas and sparing the broader zones of neighboring lymphatic systems is a prudent step toward prophylaxis against distal lymphedema. Such therapeutic strategies have reduced the incidence of genital lymphedema in recent years.

NONSURGICAL MANAGEMENT

Conservative, nonsurgical therapy may be beneficial for milder degrees of genital lymphedema and often is reserved for elderly patients because the risk of surgery may be prohibitive. Elevation, scrotal support, and diuretics are of limited value in restricting progression of lymphedema. Benzopyrones are pharmacologic agents (not approved by the Food and Drug Administration) that stimulate circulatory macrophages to break down proteins of high molecular weight into substances of low molecular weight that can be handled by the hypoplastic lymphatic vessels. In general, results of conservative therapeutic measures are unsatisfactory, so that one must often resort to surgery.

Genital lymphedema in the pediatric population is usually primary or idiopathic. Surgical intervention is required at an early age to minimize physical and emotional strain on the child and the family.

SURGICAL REPAIR

A variety of surgical procedures have been available since the beginning of the century. These can be divided into two categories: (1) physiologic or nonexcisional procedures, and (2) excisional procedures. The physiologic procedures are designed to rectify or improve abnormal lymphatic drainage. They include the Gillies and Fraser procedure to bypass the abnormal region with a pedicle skin bridge from an area of presumed normal lymphatic flow; the Mielubowicz, Olszewski, Sokolowski lymphovenous shunting procedure, whereby a lymph node is transected and the capsule of the node is sutured to an open vein, allowing lymph drainage into the vein; and the Goldsmith and de los Santos procedure of omental transposition to bring unaffected omental lymphatic vessels into the diseased area. Such procedures have only occasional use in the management of genital lymphedema, especially when there is associated lymphedema of the lower limbs. In general, the bridging and shunting procedures are too complex to perform; moreover, the results for genital lymphedema with these procedures have been disappointing.

The excisional procedures include: (1) complete excision of the lymphedematous area followed by split-thickness skin grafting, and (2) excision of lymphedematous subcutaneous tissues followed by resurfacing with genital skin. With proper attention to technical details, these procedures often yield highly satisfactory functional and cosmetic results. Opinions differ as to which of the two types of excisional surgery is the more effective, complete excision with skin grafting or excision of lymphedematous tissue and reconstruction with penile skin without the use of skin grafts. More recently, the importance of completely excising the lymphedematous subcutaneous tissue from the penile flap has been emphasized to prevent recurrence of lymphedema. Recurrence and contracture, however, remain as rare possibilities in this procedure.

Complete excision of the skin and the subdermal lymphedema becomes mandatory in the presence of gross secondary cutaneous changes such as ulceration, chronic lymph leakage, dermal lymph varices, and vesiculation. In the absence of these overt cutaneous changes, relatively occult dermal involvement is often misjudged and can lead to recurrence of lymphedema if penile flap reconstruction is used instead of radical excision. In contrast, radical excision with split-thickness skin grafting offers a more consistent cosmetic result with comparatively less chance of recurrence. A few anatomic and technical details are of utmost importance in the surgical planning:

1. Complete excision of the involved area should be attempted to prevent recurrence.
2. Scrotal reconstruction should not require any skin grafting because the perineal area usually remains free from lymphedema. It is presumed that the perineal lymphatic drainage continues unimpaired through the superficial gluteal and deep anorectal lymph channels. Nonetheless, perineal skin can be pushed forward and closed transversely to cover the testes and cord even after extensive excision of scrotal lymphedema.
3. In an uncircumcised male, the inner lining of the prepuce is relatively uninvolved with lymphedema and can be unfurled to cover the distal penis.
4. Skin grafts wrapped around the denuded penis are joined ventrally in the midline. It is essential to make a few Z-plasty closures along this junction to prevent linear contracture with resultant ventral chordee. To prevent circumferential contracture, we also advocate several Z-plasties at the root of the penis where the graft meets the recipient area of the abdominal skin.

The grafted area often remains dry because of the lack of secretory dermal glands. Patients are instructed to use emollients such as cocoa butter or lanolin cream regularly. One of our patients had recurrent episodes of subcutaneous lymphangitis manifested by pain and redness in the area of reconstruction. He was treated successfully with oral penicillin followed by low-dose prophylaxis with penicillin for 1 year with no further recurrence. Although the reconstructed phallus is slightly different in color and texture after split-thickness skin grafting, the eventual cosmetic and functional results are quite acceptable and there is less chance of recurrence.

Suggested Readings

Das S, Tuerk D, Amar A, et al: Surgery of male genital lymphedema. J Urol 129:1240, 1983

Sauer PF, Bueschen AJ, Vasconez LU: Lymphedema of the penis and scrotum. Clin Plast Surg 15:507, 1988

FRACTURE OF THE PENIS

SAKTI DAS, M.D.

Davis, California

Fracture of the penis implies traumatic disruption of penile corporal bodies that is sustained while the penis is in a state of tumescence. Although only sporadically reported in the literature, such injuries are not uncommon. Minor fractures of the penis often pass undiagnosed or are diagnosed retrospectively from later manifestations of chordee or impotence.

A variety of direct blunt trauma or indirect bending injuries to the erect phallus can cause fracture of the penis. At least half of these injuries occurred from coital sexual athleticism, or the so-called *faux pas de coit*. The type or extent of injuries can be divided into three categories: (1) rupture of the corpora cavernosa only, (2) rupture of the corpora cavernosa and the urethra, and (3) isolated rupture of the urethra.

The diagnosis is often evident from the history of direct or indirect trauma to the erect phallus followed by acute pain, detumescence, swelling, and ecchymosis. Often these injuries are associated with a perceptible and at times audible crack at the rupture of the corpora. Urethral bleeding and voiding difficulty indicate urethral injury.

Corpus cavernosography helps delineate the site and extent of the tear in the tunica albuginea. Similarly, urethrography is indicated in the presence of urethral bleeding to establish the diagnosis and degree of urethral tear. These radiologic studies are of immense value in formulating treatment guidelines that are dependent on the type, extent, and severity of the injury.

Until around the middle of the century, conservative therapy in the form of compression bandage, local cold, urethral catheter drainage, antibiotics, and sedatives was advocated in treating fracture of the penis, and a reasonable degree of successful recuperation of sexual function was achieved by these means. However, complications such as delayed chordee, organized hematoma with or without infection, cavernous fibrositis, and impotence can result from such medical therapy. Conservative medical therapy therefore should be reserved for selected cases in which cavernosography and urethrography unequivocally delineate only a minor tear. Surgical exploration, evacuation of clots, and débridement, followed by necessary plastic repair of the tunica albuginea or urethra, have proved consistently successful and should be used promptly in patients with substantial rupture of the corpora and/or urethra.

SKIN LESIONS OF THE EXTERNAL GENITALIA

YOUNG C. KAUH, M.D.

Philadelphia, Pennsylvania

There are significant differences between circumcised and uncircumcised males in the incidence, severity, and clinical manifestations of dermatoses involving the glans penis and corona. Poor hygiene, moisture, and an overlapping prepuce make the uncircumcised penis more susceptible to infection, erosion, and carcinoma, particularly in weak, debilitated, and elderly people. The deeply rugose, thickened skin of the scrotum tends to be easily macerated and moisturized with tight clothing and heavy sweating, thus enhancing excellent absorption of topical contactants.

In the female external genitalia, the clitoris is equivalent to the penis and the labia majora to the scrotum. Loose connective tissue and abundant subcutaneous tissue of the labia majora become easily swollen by simple trauma. Inflammation may result in either minimal residual damage or scar tissue formation. As a result of moisture and proximity of body folds of the female external genitalia, the characteristics of common dermatoses often are not seen, consequently leading to misdiagnosis.

There are hundreds of conditions known to affect the external genitalia, male and female. However, this discussion is concentrated on describing primarily the dermatoses that we often are faced with in daily practice, in addition to a few interesting dermatologic conditions. Readers interested in learning about the rarer entities should refer to the references at the end of this article.

SCABIES

Scabies, caused by *Sarcoptes scabiei* is characterized clinically by the presence of burrows, which are produced by female mites. These are found mainly on the palms, finger webs, medial aspect of wrists, nipples, axillae, umbilicus, and external genitalia, particularly the glans penis and penile shaft. The burrows appear tortuous, and gray or skin colored, with fine ridges that are 5 to 15 mm long. A vesicle can be visible near the end of the burrow. They are directly associated with the presence of the mite. The main and most common complaint from patients is severe itching, particularly nocturnal itching that disturbs their sleep. The onset of itching is usually 2 weeks or longer after infestation.

Diagnosis. Finding the burrow, and a few erythematous small urticarial papules on the glans penis associated with nocturnal itching, is quite diagnostic. Scrapings from the burrows or papules confirms the presence of mites or ova by microscopic examination in 15 to 30 per cent of cases.

Treatment. Topical application of Elimite (Permethrin) 5% cream, Kwell (Lindane) 1% lotion, gamma benzene hexachloride or benzyl benzoate emulsion 10% to 25% is quite effective.

PEDICULOSIS PUBIS (CRAB LICE)

Increased sexual freedom has significantly and steadily contributed to the recent widespread increase of crab lice. Although pediculosis pubis is found primarily in pubic hair, it can be seen on the hair of the thighs, abdominal wall, axillae, and, rarely, even the eyebrows and eyelashes. Clinically, it is associated with severe itching, excoriations, and secondary bacterial infection. Maculae cerulae (blue-gray macules) are not infrequently found on the lower abdominal wall and thighs as a result of altered hemosiderin at the bite sites.

Four of the six legs of *Phthirus pubis* terminate in sturdy crab-like claws. The life span of the female is 3 to 4 weeks, and during that time she lays a maximum of 3 eggs a day to total 26 or more. The eggs are tightly cemented to the base of hair, where they hatch in 6 to 8 days.

Diagnosis. When crab lice and eggs are found on a patient with severe itching and a secondarily infected eczematoid eruption, the diagnosis is easily confirmed. However, it often can be overlooked.

Treatment. Kwell (Lindane) 1% lotion gamma benzene hexachloride application is quite successful.

PAPULOSQUAMOUS ERUPTIONS

Psoriasis

Silvery white, scaly and erythematous papules and plaques frequently are found on the scalp, elbows, knees, and lumbosacral areas, with characteristic fingernail involvement. Occasionally the glans penis is involved. Psoriasis, which may or may not be associated with itching, flares quite often in the winter, with improvement in the summer.

Treatment. Topical steroids, coal tar preparations, and systemic therapy consisting of cytotoxic antimetabolites are frequently successful. Retinoids and photochemotherapy also are available.

Lichen Planus

Lichen planus, a subacute and chronic dermatosis, is characterized by flat-topped, polygonal, small and violaceous papules. The predilection sites of lichen planus are the medial aspect of the wrists and ankles, buccal mucosa, and glans penis.

Treatment. Topical and systemic steroids can be beneficial, depending on the severity of the disease.

Lichen Nitidus

Lichen nitidus is an uncommon dermatosis of unknown etiology. It is characterized by asymptomatic, flat-topped, and shiny to flesh-colored papules, 2 to 3 mm in diameter, and commonly is seen in children. Its predilection sites are the penis, abdominal wall, and thighs.

Treatment. Mild topical steroids can be tried.

PEARLY PENILE PAPULE (HAIRY PENIS)

Pearly penile papules are seen mainly in men who are between 20 to 50 years old. No difference has been found in relation to race, circumcision, or sexual activity. Pearly penile papules are characterized clinically by small, pinhead-sized, smooth, dome-shaped, flesh-colored papules encircling the corona penis completely or partially. Occasionally, longer filiform lesions have been observed. Pearly penile papules are known to be a physiologic variant and are without any symptoms and functional significance. Treatment is not necessary, except reassurance given to the patient.

FIXED DRUG ERUPTION

Fixed drug eruption, which is one of the common drug eruptions, is characterized by recurrent episodes of pigmented skin lesions persistently at the same site with each administration of the allergenic drug. The skin lesions are usually well circumscribed and round. The initial fixed drug eruption consists of one or a few erythematous patches that may become bullous and, on healing, leave dusky, violaceous, brown or gray pigmented areas. Mild pruritus or burning sensations may be present. With reingestion of the same allergen, the eruption is manifested as a centrally erythematous to purple patch with or without blistering and marginal hyperpigmentation.

The involvement of external genitalia, penis, or vulva is common with or without other cutaneous involvement. Hyperpigmentation may last for weeks or months. The drugs most frequently involved are phenolphthalein, sulfonamides, tetracycline, barbiturates, phenylbutazone, and acetylsalicylic acid. Resolution of the fixed drug eruption on withdrawal of the drug can be incriminating evidence for the confirmation of the diagnosis.

ERYTHEMA MULTIFORME

Erythema multiforme, which is an acute self-limited dermatosis, is characterized by skin and mucous membrane lesions that may vary in severity and is prone to recurrence. Erythema multiforme usually occurs in the fall and spring, and affects men three to four times more often than women. The etiology of erythema multiforme may be idiopathic, but it often occurs as a reaction pattern to various stimuli, such as infections with herpes simplex virus, *Mycoplasma pneumoniae*, or *Yersinia enterocolitica*, radiation therapy, systemic lupus erythematosus, and reticulosis.

As the name implies, the eruptions are polymorphic. They include macules, papules, urticaria, and blistering with target or iris-like lesions. In one third of patients, prodromal symptoms of fever, malaise, headache, sore throat, and cough may precede skin eruptions by 5 to 10 days. The severe bullous form, Stevens-Johnson syndrome, is characterized by multiple organ involvement, including mouth, eyes, genitalia, skin, and lungs, with severe systemic illness. Involvement of the genitalia is common, with blistering, erosion, and ulceration of the glans penis, which may result in adhesion of the prepuce. In addition, genitourinary tract involvement may cause urinary retention, urethritis, vaginitis, proteinuria, hematuria, and vaginal stenosis.

Treatment. In the localized and mild form, systemic antihistamines can be very beneficial, and, for the severe form, systemic steroid therapy with prednisone 30 to 60 mg daily, tapering off over a period of 2 to 4 weeks, has been quite helpful in my experience. In the case of erythema multiforme secondary to herpes simplex virus infection, oral acyclovir is highly recommended for therapeutic and prophylactic purposes.

LICHEN SCLEROSUS ET ATROPHICUS (BALANITIS XEROTICA OBLITERANS, KRAUROSIS VULVAE)

Lichen sclerosus et atrophicus (LSA) also known as whitespot disease, is an uncommon disease with an unknown etiology. It is seen predominantly in women. The frequent onset of the disease with menopause and its spontaneous remission in girls after puberty suggest a possible hormonal etiology. Infection, trauma, and autoimmune reactions also may play a role in its pathogenesis.

LSA usually starts around the ages of 45 to 55, and the external genitalia are involved most frequently. They may be the only site of involvement. Cutaneous eruptions outside the genital area may be seen either in association with genital lesions or alone.

The ivory-white, sharply defined, atrophic papules and plaques with comedo-like follicular plugs often are found on the external genitalia. The lesion may become bullous and sometimes hemorrhagic, and may feel somewhat indurated. Patients may complain of soreness rather than itching. Balanitis xerotica obliterance of the glans penis and prepuce shows ivory-white, atrophic, sclerotic, and edematous changes that could result in phimosis, recurrent balanitis, and painful erection in uncircumcised patients.

Occasionally, LSA may coexist with morphea, and in 50 per cent of patients leukoplakia coexists with kraurosis vulvae. Squamous cell carcinoma also has been reported to occur with kraurosis vulvae.

Treatment. Topical corticosteroid preparations and testosterone propionate ointment 2.5% have been helpful for the condition. Oral vitamin E (1200 to 1600 units/day) also has been used. Vulvectomy is indicated if a squamous cell carcinoma develops. Otherwise, conservative therapy or limited excision is indicated because recurrences are common.

CONDYLOMA ACUMINATUM

Condyloma acuminatum, also known as anogenital wart, is sexually transmitted in most cases, and the incidence has been steadily increasing in recent years. Cloning for human papillomavirus (HPV) DNA has demonstrated that the majority of anogenital warts contain HPV DNA, consisting of HPV-6 and HPV-11 in addition to HPV-16 and HPV-18.

The incubation period of genital warts is between 2 and 3 months. In women with condyloma acuminatum of the vulva, gross vaginal involvement will be found in 20 per cent and cervical involvement in 6 per cent. Because HPV DNA has been detected in cervical anaplastic lesions, it is suspected that a significant number of patients with cervical anaplasia may have had subclinical condyloma acuminatum. Also, a recent study has shown that the majority of women with anogenital warts were infected by the same type of wart as their sexual consort and that one third of the group had cervical dysplasia.

Anogenital warts are clinically fairly soft, velvety, sessile verrucous papules that occasionally coalesce into cauliflower-like masses. In contrast, condyloma lata (secondary syphilis) is characterized by multiple, nonpainful, broad-topped, and wet papules. Giant condyloma accuminatum of Bushke-Lowenstein is characterized by relentless growth, infiltration, and invasion, with sinus and fistula formation and resistance to appropriate topical podophyllin therapy.

Because condyloma accuminatum is a sexually transmitted disease, both partners should be examined thoroughly by physical examination and other studies, including an application of 3% to 5% acetic acid solution (aceto whitening) and colposcopy.

Treatment. Application of podophyllin tincture 10% to 25% is the first choice of treatment except during pregnancy. About half of the patients treated with podophyllin may fail the first trial and may require a few more treatments. Because of potential carcinogenicity, cervical warts should not be treated with podophyllin. Other therapy, such as cryosurgery, electrosurgery, CO_2 laser, and interferons, may be required in severe and recalcitrant cases.

BOWENOID PAPULOSIS

Bowenoid papulosis, which was first described by Lloyd in 1970, is characterized clinically by multiple, verrucous or smooth-surfaced, small (2 to 10 mm in diameter, average 4 mm), asymptomatic, brown-red to violaceous or black papules. They commonly are found on the glans penis and shaft of the penis or the vulvar and perineal areas of young men and women. The histopathologic features may suggest carcinoma in situ (Bowen's disease), but the biologic course is most likely benign. However, one patient who was diagnosed as having bowenoid papulosis at the age of 42 developed true Bowen's disease on the scrotum 10 years later. Since then a few more cases have been reported. By molecular hybridization and immunostaining, HPV type 16 has been reported in most cases of Bowenoid papulosis. A significant and interesting finding is that HPV-16 also is found frequently in cervical carcinomas seen in female patients, and also in their sexual partners.

Diagnosis. Multiple brown-red to dark warty papules on the external genitalia of young patients may indicate bowenoid papulosis. Seborrheic keratosis, epithelial nevi, condyloma acuminatum, and verruca vulgaris should be differentiated.

Treatment. Because spontaneous regression has been well documented, bowenoid papulosis should be treated conservatively, and the patients may need long-term follow-up care.

ERYTHROPLASIA OF QUEYRAT (BOWEN'S DISEASE OF GLANS PENIS)

Erythroplasia of Queyrat is characterized clinically by a sharply defined, bright red, velvety, and slightly raised plaque on the glans penis and histologically by carcinoma in situ. This condition is seen almost exclusively in uncircumcised men. Bowen's disease of the vulva, which is an analogue of erythroplasia of Queyrat, is characterized by severe itching and multiple flat erythematous or pigmented, velvety or granular, and well-demarcated lesions. The existence of erythroplasia of female genitalia has been doubted by Graham and Helwig.

Treatment. Initial therapy can be a trial of topical 5-fluorouracil therapy, and, if not successful, cryosurgery and vulvectomy are next in order.

Suggested Readings

DeVillez RL, Stevens CS: Bowenoid papules of the genitalia. A case pregressing to Bowen's disease. J Am Acad Dermatol 3:149–152, 1980

Gissman L, Boshart M, Dierst M, et al: Presence of human papilloma virus in genital tumors. J Invest Dermatol (Suppl) 83:26–28, 1984

Ive FA: The umbilical, perianal and genital regions. *In* Champion RH, Burton JL, Ebling FJG (eds): Textbook of Dermatology, 5th ed. Oxford, England, Blackwell Scientific Publications, 1992, pp 2785–2858

Lever W, Schaumburg-Lever G: Diseases caused by viruses. *In* Histopathology of skin, 7th ed. Philadelphia, JB Lippincott, 1990, pp 411–418, 549–551

Silva PD, Micha JP, Silva DG: Management of condyloma acuminatum. J Am Acad Dermatol 13:457–463, 1985

HERPES GENITALIS

YOUNG C. KAUH, M.D.

Philadelphia, Pennsylvania

Herpes genitalis is one of the most common infections in humans throughout the world. It is caused by two viruses that do not show any cross-immunity: herpes simplex virus type 1 (orofacial, labial type, HSV-1) and herpes simplex type 2 (genital type, HSV-2).

ETIOLOGY AND PATHOGENESIS

Most herpes genitalis infections are caused by HSV-2; however, there has been a significant increase in the number of cases caused by HSV-1 infection over the last few decades. In recent studies, 20 to 40 per cent of cases of herpes genitalis have been found to be due to orogenital sexual contact. An interesting finding in one series is that herpes genitalis infections caused by HSV-1 are less likely to recur than those caused by HSV-2; the rate of recurrence was 60 per cent with HSV-2 versus 14 per cent with HSV-1. After primary infection, HSV-2 persists in the sensory nerve ganglia. It becomes dormant and recurs depending on the individual's humoral and cell-mediated immune mechanisms. Cell-mediated immunity seems to play a major role in the incidence and severity of genital herpes.

The incubation period of genital herpes is between 3 and 14 days, with 5 days being average. Primary infection with HSV-2 usually occurs on the genitalia, being contracted by sexual contact in early adult life. Occasionally, a newborn may be found to have contracted the disease by intrauterine infection or by direct exposure to the infected birth canal. Transmission of HSV to the infant occurs in 50 per cent of cases. Neonatal infection can be severe and fatal if maternal infection is primary and there is no maternal immune defense mechanism. Primary infection at the time of delivery or near the term of pregnancy is most risky for severe neonatal infection. However, if maternal infection is recurrent, genital herpes during pregnancy or at delivery very rarely results in serious morbidity, most likely as a result of protection by maternal antibodies. When there is a strong indication of primary herpes genitalis in woman around the time of delivery, a cesarian section is indicated.

PATHOLOGY

The characteristic lesion in herpes genitalis is an intraepidermal vesicle formed by ballooning degeneration and reticular degeneration, resulting in marked acantholysis. Specific changes are seen in the epidermal nuclei, with formation of intranuclear inclusions and multinucleated giant cells containing 2 to 15 nuclei. Viral particles can be identified by electronmicroscopy, and HSV-1 and HSV-2 can be differentiated.

SYMPTOMATOLOGY

Primary infection may be asymptomatic; however, it is usually more severe or widespread than recurrent infections. Often associated with primary infections are systemic symptoms of fever, restlessness, and general malaise.

The herpetic eruption often is preceded by the usual prodromal symptoms, such a local tingling, itching or burning sensation, fever, and general malaise. The eruption is characterized by a few grouped papules on erythematous bases, which develop into vesicles and pustules and rapidly break down to form grouped superficial erosions or painful and tender ulcers. In the male, the lesions are most frequent on the glans, prepuce, and frenulum, and the shaft of the penis often is not involved. In the female, similar eruptions are found on the external genitalia and mucous membrane of the vulva, vagina, and cervix. Generally speaking, if the herpetic eruptions occur on mucous membrane, the vesicles change quickly into erosions and ulcerations, whereas, on the skin, vesicles usually become pustular and then crusted. This disease process may last for 2 to 6 weeks. Dysuria, urinary retention, enlargement of regional lymph nodes, and cervicitis may occur. Neurologic symptoms and signs, such as meningeal involvement and radiculoneuropathy, have been reported rarely in both primary and recurrent herpes genitalis.

Recurrent herpes genitalis is often triggered by minor trauma, upper respiratory tract infection, menstruation, sunburn, and emotional stress. However, frequently no apparent reason for the recurrence is noted. Recurrent herpes genitalis differs most often from primary infection by the absence of systemic symptoms, shorter duration, and smaller, well-localized grouped eruptions. However, it can be quite distressingly painful and severe, or go unnoticed on occasion. Recurrences of herpes genitalis occur in about 50 per cent of infected patients, and asymptomatic attacks also occur in 50 per cent of cases.

It is very important to note that herpes genitalis can be contagious even during an asymptomatic attack, and that viral shedding has been identified in asymptomatic woman up to 6 months after a clinical attack of herpes genitalis. However, the amount of shedding from active lesions is 100 to 1000 times greater than that in a patient without lesions.

In immunocompromised patients, particularly in those with acquired immunodeficiency syndrome (AIDS), chronic ulcerative herpes simplex, generalized acute mucocutaneous herpes simplex, or acute systemic herpes simplex can be seen.

DIAGNOSIS

In the early stage of herpes genitalis, the grouped vesiculopustular lesions on erythematous bases are quite characteristic. However, in the later stage of the disease, the classic clinical manifestations may be lacking, inviting misdiagnosis. A Tzanck smear (cytologic examination of a smear taken from the floor of a new and freshly opened vesicle and stained with Giemsa stain or toluidine blue stain) reveals many acantholytic balloon cells and multinucleated giant cells.

Confirmation of the herpes virus can be obtained by electron microscopy, viral culture, or immunofluorescence studies for viral antigen. The complement fixation test and the neutralizing antibody test may provide evidence of rising antibodies or seroconversion in primary herpes infection. However, recurrent herpes infections seldom produce any significant change in antibody titer, and therefore these antibody tests are not helpful in the diagnosis or confirmation of recurrent herpes simplex infection.

TREATMENT

The most effective treatments for herpes simplex virus infections have been chemical compounds that specifically inhibit viral replication. Most of such medicines are nucleoside analogues, which inhibit viral DNA synthesis and thereby arrest viral replication. Idoxuridine (5′-iodo-2-deoxyuridine) was the first drug to be used. However, its effectiveness was limited because of poor tissue penetration, weak activity, and substantial toxicity.

Acyclovir (Zovirax) is by far the most effective antiviral chemical compound developed to date. It is the drug of choice for the majority of HSV infections and can be given topically, orally, and intravenously. Acyclovir is phosphorylated by the viral enzyme thymidine kinase and is activated once inside virus-infected cells. The phosphorylated form interferes with the viral DNA polymerase and blocks further synthesis of the viral DNA chain. These virus-specific steps of activation and chain termination are the reasons for acyclovir's specificity for HSV. Acyclovir is remarkably free of toxicity to humans because it is not a good substitute for cellular enzymes.

A single 200-mg oral dose of acyclovir reaches a peak serum level of approximately 1 μg/ml, which is 3 and 10 times the level required in vitro for a 50 per cent inhibition of HSV-1 and HSV-2, respectively. Serum levels with a dose of 5 mg/kg of body weight by intravenous administration are 5 to 10 times higher than those achieved with oral administration. Oral acyclovir, 200 mg taken five times a day for 10 days, is expected to result in a 70 to 80 per cent decrease in the duration of viral shedding, a 40 to 50 per cent decrease in the duration of symptoms, and a 30 to 40 per cent decrease in the time of healing. Oral therapy seems to be as effective as intravenous therapy and has the advantage of outpatient use, convenience, painlessness, and less expense. Topical acyclovir therapy should be given only for very mild primary herpes genitalis because oral therapy is far more effective. Initiation of therapy should be provided at the earliest stage in the course of recurrent herpes to achieve maximum benefit. Therefore, any patients with a history of recurrent disease should be instructed to start taking acyclovir at the onset of symptoms.

Continuous suppressive oral acyclovir, 400 mg taken twice a day, has been found to be effective and very well tolerated. Patients on up to 5 years of uninterrupted therapy for recurrent herpes genitalis have been followed, without any clinically significant changes in urinalyses, hematologic indices, or other laboratory values. The most frequently reported adverse reactions to acyclovir were nausea, vomiting, asthenia, headache, and skin rashes. During the 5 years of therapy, it was found that the frequency of false prodromes had decreased without any changes of lesion duration.

Viral Resistance to Acyclovir

HSV can develop resistance to acyclovir through mutations in the viral gene encoding thymidine kinase. Viral resistance to acyclovir was considered rare and the resistant virus was thought to be less pathogenic until many acyclovir-resistant HSV isolates from patients with AIDS were analyzed. These drug-resistant mutants, which are deficient in thymidine kinase, remain sensitive to vidarabine and foscarnet, because these drugs do not require viral thymidine kinase for activation.

Suggested Readings

Chang TW, Fiumara NJ, Weinstein L: Genital herpes. JAMA 229:544–545, 1974

Highet AS, Kurtz J: Viral infections. *In* Champion RH, Burton JL, Ebling FJG (eds). Textbook of Dermatology, 5th ed. Oxford, England, Blackwell Scientific Publications, 1992, pp 879–885

Kurtz T, et al: Safety and efficacy of long-term suppressive Zovirax treatment of frequently recurring genital herpes: Year 5 results. *In* Program and Abstracts of the 30th Interscience Conference on Antimicrobial Agents and Chemotherapy, Atlanta, October 21–24, 1990, p 270, abstract 1170 (1858570/2)

Lever W, Schaumburg-Lever G: Diseases caused by viruses. *In* Histopathology of Skin, 7th ed. Philadelphia, JB Lippincott, 1990, pp 400–404

Provost T, Farmer E: Herpes simplex. Curr Ther Dermatol 2:230–234, 1988

Whitley RJ, Gnann JW Jr: Acylovir: A decade later. N Engl J Med 327:782–789, 1992

CHANCROID

STEPHEN A. ZDERIC, M.D.

Philadelphia, Pennsylvania

Chancroid is an acute genital infection caused by the gram-negative organism *Haemophilus ducreyi.* It is a rare cause of the genital ulcer syndrome in the United States. Recently, its incidence has increased to 5000 cases reported in 1988 to the Centers for Disease Control. It is endemic in third-world nations, and thus a history of recent foreign travel is important when assessing any patient with a genital ulcer. The cases seen in the United States usually are in merchant marine or military personnel who have just returned from abroad, and tend to be clustered in seaport cities. The more likely causes of a genital ulcer in the United States are herpes or syphilis.

In contrast to syphilis, which presents as a painless ulcer with firm rolled edges, chancroid presents as a very painful ulcer with shaggy ragged edges. The trademark of herpes is the presence of painful vesicles on erythematous bases. The incubation period for chancroid is approximately 5 days, and the patient's initial complaint is the presence of one to three painful pustules on the penile shaft. These may coalesce together to form one giant ulcer. In a patient whose presentation is delayed, the inguinal lymph nodes already may have become fluctuant (buboes) and may ulcerate to create draining sinuses. If left untreated, the natural history of this disease is to produce chronic inflammation, scarring, and disfigurement of the genitalia.

A clinical diagnosis alone can lead to errors in diagnosis and therapy, and ancillary laboratory evaluation is needed when assessing any patient with a genital ulcer other than classic herpes. A VDRL or rapid plasma reagin test will allow the clinician to quickly (1 hour) rule out syphilis. Any patient with a genital ulcer should undergo human immunodeficiency virus (HIV) testing, because the spread of HIV is strongly associated with the genital ulcers. The diagnosis of chanchroid is established by culture of the ulcer or aspiration of a fluctuant lymph node. These should be plated on special media (chocolate agar with 1% isovitalex and vancomycin); the microbiology lab at each hospital should be consulted prior to specimen collection. A Gram stain may show a "school of fish" pattern of gram-negative rods, but these ulcers often become secondarily infected. There are no serologic tests for *H. ducreyi*, and the antigenic makeup of the organism is poorly understood. Identification by nucleic acid hybridization is currently in the research stages of development.

The treatment of chancroid is quite straightforward. Oral therapy with trimethoprim-sulfamethoxazole (160/180 mg, bid) or erythromycin (500 mg, qid) is carried out for 10 days or until all lesions have healed. Painful and fluctuant inguinal lymph nodes may require drainage or aspiration. Recent reports have described single-dose therapy with ceftriaxone, which offers the benefit of 100 per cent compliance. However, one must remember that *H. ducreyi* was at one time exquisitely sensitive to ampicillin, but most strains today have acquired the plasmid coding for penicillinase.

Suggested Readings

Boyd AS: Clinical efficacy of antimicrobial therapy in *Haemophilus ducreyi* infections. Arch Dermatol 125:1399, 1989

Jessamine PG, Ronald AR: Chancroid and the role of genital ulcer disease in the spread of human retroviruses. Med Clin North Am 74:1417, 1990

Ronald AR, Plummer F: Chancroid: A newly important sexually transmitted disease. Arch Dermatol 125:1413, 1989

GRANULOMA INGUINALE (DONOVANOSIS)

STEPHEN A. ZDERIC, M.D.

Philadelphia, Pennsylvania

Granuloma inguinale is a genital infection caused by the gram-negative rod *Calymmatobacterium granulomatis.* This bacterial species is unique in that it represents an intracellular pathogen that reproduces itself inside the lysosomes of the infected cells. This results in cells that contain a large phagosome filled with 20 to 30 of these gram-negative rods; this engorged vacuole is referred to as a Donovan body. Unfortunately, a large number of synonyms for this disease entity have evolved over the years, including donovanosis, granuloma donovani, granuloma pudenda tropicum, granuloma venereum, and, of course, granuloma inguinale. This often has led to its confusion with lymphogranuloma venereum, which is distinctly different and is caused by a chlamydial organism. For this reason, the term donovanosis or the etiologic agent *Calymmatobacterium* should be used primarily. Nevertheless these older terms persist, and one must remember to what they refer.

Fortunately, the incidence of donovanosis in the United States is low (10 to 20 cases reported in 1988), and it tends to be a disease that is acquired primarily in third-world nations. This diagnosis should be considered in any patient with a history of foreign travel and a genital ulcer or inguinal lymphadenopathy. It is important to remember that the incubation period is highly variable, ranging from 8 to 80 days, so the travel history may not be so apparent. The patients will present with a history of one or two painless beefy red lesions on the penile shaft that may coalesce to form a huge ulcer. If the disease has progressed, patients may present with massive inguinal adenopathy that ultimately may lead to ulceration with huge beefy red inguinal granulomas.

These granulomas are painless, and the primary concern is confusing the diagnosis with syphilis. The use of the VDRL or rapid plasma reagin serologic testing is of importance in making this distinction. Human immunodeficiency virus testing is important because of the association of heterosexual infection with open genital ulcerations. In some cases one might consider penile cancer in the differential diagnosis. No serologic tests exist for this organism, and microbiologic culture is impractical. The diagnosis is established by biopsy of the lesions and carrying out a "crush prep" between two glass slides and then applying Wright stain. The goal is to identify the Donovan bodies, which will clinch the diagnosis. At this point therapy is initiated with a 2- to 4-week course of tetracycline 500 mg PO, qid.

Suggested Reading

Schmid GP: Approach to the patient with genital ulcer disease. Med Clin North Am 74:1559, 1990

LYMPHOGRANULOMA VENEREUM

STEPHEN A. ZDERIC, M.D.

Philadelphia, Pennsylvania

Lymphogranuloma venereum (LGV) is due to a genital infection with a *Chlamydia trachomatis* organism. This chlamydial species has three major and distinct antigenic types (serotypes L1, L2, and L3) that can be tested for serologically to establish a diagnosis. These antigen structures are distinct from the more common *C. trachomatis* serotypes that are responsible for urethritis and epididymitis. All *Chlamydia* are mandatory intracellular organisms because they lack the ability to produce ATP, and simple techniques for culture are not feasible. This diagnosis should be suspected if there is a history of recent foreign travel to third-world nations. There are fewer than 500 cases of LGV annually in the United States.

The primary presenting complaint is impressive inguinal adenopathy that rapidly leads to suppuration and drainage. There is an initial painless and small ulcer that develops on the penile shaft from 3 to 12 days after the exposure. The patient often does not even recall the initial ulceration. About 1 week after this initial penile ulceration, the inguinal lymph nodes become painfully enlarged and fluctuant, and the patient seeks medical assistance. The characteristic physical finding on this evaluation is the "groove" sign, which is due to enlargement of nodes on both sides of the inguinal ligament (inguinal and femoral). If a diagnosis of LGV is suspected, serum should be sent for complement fixation tests to confirm the presence of the L serotypes.

This disease is primarily one that affects the lymphatics, and, if left untreated, there is a progression toward scarring and fibrosis of the nodes. This ultimately can result in genital elephantiasis. Other areas that may be infected include the rectal mucosa, which may result in strictures or fistulas. The therapy of LGV is based primarily on tetracycline 500 mg four times daily for 2 to 4 weeks. If tetracycline cannot be tolerated, erythromycin is an acceptable alternative. If the lymph nodes are large and fluctuant, aspiration is recommended so as to prevent ulceration and sinus formation. Surgical lymphadenectomy was recommended in the older literature, but is to be condemned because it probably was a major contributor to the resulting elephantiasis.

Suggested Readings

Burgoyne RA: Lymphogranuloma venereum. Primary Care 17:153, 1990

Schmid GP: Approach to the patient with genital ulcer disease. Med Clin North Am 74:1559, 1990

BALANITIS AND BALANOPOSTHITIS

GOPAL H. BADLANI, M.D.

New York, New York

Balanitis is an acute or chronic inflammation of the glans penis. "Posthitis" is the term denoting inflammation of the mucosal surface of the prepuce. When they coexist, the condition is called balanoposthitis.

PATHOGENESIS

Clinically, balanitis can be subdivided into infective and traumatic types, or can occur secondary to irritation. Factors predisposing to balanitis include long foreskin combined with poor hygiene, irritation by smegma, exposure to venereal and vaginal pathogens, friction and trauma, urine, and external irritants. When immune response is lowered, the normally saprophytic bacteria, yeast, and fusospiral organisms in the preputial sac may become pathogens. Other pathogenic organisms seen more commonly include *Chlamydia* and *Mycoplasma.* An indwelling Foley catheter and, especially, a Texas catheter can cause balanitis. Balanitis sometimes can be a presenting symptom of diabetes mellitus.

Infective Balanitis

Circinate erosive balanitis, acute infectious balanitis, trichomonal, mycoplasma, syphilitic, and chlamydial balanitis all have been described. The most common of the infective types is *Candida* balanitis. It may be primary or a complication of another dermatitis. *Candida* can be recovered from the vagina and, less commonly, from the coronal sulcus in the absence of clinical infection. Pathogenicity of the organism depends on the host factors, diabetes mellitus being the most important.

The characteristic appearance includes a glazed, nonpurulent surface, a scaling edge, and satellite pustules. Microscopy and culture confirm the diagnosis. Fissuring of the prepuce and fibrosis may result from recurrent candida balanitis.

PLASMA CELL BALANITIS (ZOON BALANITIS)

Seen in middle-aged or elderly men, the lesions are described as "cayene pepper" spots, circumcised plaques that are shiny, smooth, slightly moist, and stippled with minute red spots. Histologically, there is an intense plasma cell infiltrate.

BALANITIS XEROTICA OBLITERANS

A chronic sclerosing atrophic process of the glans penis, balanitis xerotica obliterans is considered by some to be akin to lichen sclerosis. Many patients with this condition present with urinary symptoms resulting from meatal stenosis. The lesions are whitish plaques on the surface of the glans and the prepuce. The foreskin is thickened, fibrous, and difficult to retract.

ERYTHROPLASIA OF QUEYRAT

These are usually asymptomatic, bright red, well-demarcated, shiny plaques in the glans penis. They represent carcinoma in situ of the glans penis and should be differentiated from balanitis.

MANAGEMENT

Patients often present with itching, pain, and drainage from the lesions. Advanced lesions may present with inability to retract the foreskin, voiding difficulty, fever, and inguinal adenopathy.

Initial management is medical, which focuses on local hygiene, keeping the area clean and dry. Patients are advised to retract the foreskin, wash the area, and then dry it before pulling the prepuce forward. Depending on the etiology, ointments such as Mycolog and Bacitracin may help. Oral antibiotics (e.g., tetracycline) are indicated when bacterial infection is present.

Predisposing factors such as diabetes mellitus, Foley catheter, and Texas catheter should be addressed. Patients should refrain from sexual activity. They should be advised to slightly retract the foreskin while voiding so that urine does not irritate the area. Circumcision should be considered strongly once the inflammation has subsided. A dorsal slit may be required on an urgent basis to treat severely inflamed cases in which the foreskin is difficult to retract. Underlying carcinoma of the penis can present as suppurative balanitis; hence, when the lesions fail to improve in a reasonable period of time, a biopsy should be performed.

Suggested Readings

Rook A, Wilkinson DS, Ebling FJG, et al (eds): Textbook of Dermatology, 4th ed, vol 3. Oxford, England, Blackwell Scientific Publications, 1986

Vohra S, Badlani GH: Balanitis and balanoposthitis. Urol Clin North Am 19:143–147, 1992

Wilson D: Dermatologic lesions of the penis. *In* Gillenwater J, Grayhack J, Howards S, et al (eds): Adult and Pediatric Urology, vol 2. Chicago Year Book Medical Publishers, 1987, pp 1484–1496

PHIMOSIS AND PARAPHIMOSIS

MICHEL A. PONTARI, M.D.

Philadelphia, Pennsylvania

Phimosis is the inability to retract the foreskin, or prepuce. This broad definition covers both the normal inability to retract the foreskin in infancy and early childhood and acquired phimosis, in which a narrowing of the distal prepuce prevents its retraction back of the glans penis.

Formation of the foreskin is completed by the fifth month of gestation. Once the glans penis is completely covered, the inner epithelium of the prepuce fuses with the epithelium on the glans itself. Both are stratified squamous epithelium. Later in gestation, the squamous cells keratinize and then degenerate, creating a space between the prepuce and glans. This separation process is usually incomplete at birth, and continues through childhood. At age 6 months, only 20 per cent of boys have a foreskin that can be fully retracted. This increases to 90 per cent at age 3, and nearly all 17-year-old boys can retract their foreskin fully. The foreskin should not be forcibly retracted at a young age, because this can lead to pain, bleeding, inflammation, and eventually to true phimosis as the injury leads to cicatrix formation and narrowing of the distal preputial opening.

Conditions leading to acquired phimosis include repetitive bouts of dermatitis induced by diaper rash, posthitis (preputial infection or inflammation), balanitis (infection or inflammation of the glans), local trauma, or a poorly performed circumcision. Clinically, phimosis is usually not painful. It does produce difficulty in maintaining adequate hygiene. Severe degrees of phimosis can lead to the accumulation of smegma and subsequent episodes of balanoposthitis. Very severe cases of phimosis have caused obstructive uropathy, including bladder decompensation and upper urinary tract deterioration. In these cases, voiding is difficult, the stream will be poor, the foreskin may balloon out with voiding and require manual decompression, and terminal dribbling may be apparent. Some evidence indicates that it is phimosis, and not just the presence of a foreskin, that predisposes to penile carcinoma. Prolonged phimosis may lead to balanitis xerotica obliterans, a chronic inflammatory process of the prepuce, glans, and urethral meatus.

The treatment for phimosis is a circumcision or dorsal slit. If superimposed balanoposthitis exists, the inflammation should be treated first and the circumcision delayed until this process has resolved. Circumcision in the neonatal period is carried out without anesthetic, although evidence shows that neonates do have physiologic responses from the pain of the procedure. In adults, circumcision can be performed under local anesthetic with a penile block proximally, supplemented by a circumferential block of the distal foreskin as needed. Young children (and their surgeons) are best served by a general anesthetic for this procedure.

PARAPHIMOSIS

Paraphimosis is the entrapment of the prepuce proximal to the coronal margin. This will not result from the retraction of a normal foreskin. If it occurs, one may assume that there is some underlying condition of the foreskin predisposing it to paraphimosis, such as phimosis, inflammation, or trauma. Paraphimosis is often iatrogenic and frequently occurs after failing to return the foreskin to its natural position after the insertion of a urethral catheter. Initially compression of the foreskin causes lymphatic congestion, but venous obstruction and arterial compromise may occur. Pain and swelling are common. Any superimposed infection will exacerbate the discomfort, and can lead to local cellulitis and inguinal adenopathy. Extension of the inflammation also has resulted in thrombophlebitis of the deep pelvic veins. If left untreated, penile ischemia and eventually gangrene may develop.

To reduce paraphimosis, gentle steady pressure must be applied to the foreskin to decrease swelling. This may be done manually or with an elastic wrap. When the swelling has decreased, the glans is pushed with the thumbs while the fingers pull on the foreskin. Because this tends to be a painful procedure, prolonged attempts at retraction of a paraphimotic foreskin should be accompanied by analgesia, such as intramuscular Demerol. In some cases, swelling of the glans occurs, which prevents reduction of the paraphimosis. This situation necessitates an emergency dorsal slit procedure, with an elective circumcision at a later date. Even if correctable in the emergency room, paraphimosis often recurs, so a circumcision is recommended in all cases.

Suggested Readings

Herzog LW, Alvarez SR: The frequency of foreskin problems in uncircumcised children. Am J Dis Child 140: 254, 1986
Poland RL: The question of routine neonatal circumcision. N Engl J Med 322:1312, 1990
Reddy CRRM, Devendranth V, Pratap S: Carcinoma of penis—role of phimosis. Urology 24:85, 1984
Schoen EJ: The status of circumcision of newborns. N Engl J Med 322:1308, 1990
Task Force on Circumcision: Report of the Task Force on Circumcision. Pediatrics 79:388, 1989

MANAGEMENT OF FOURNIER'S GANGRENE

MARK J. CHELSKY, M.D.

Philadelphia, Pennsylvania

Fournier's gangrene, defined as a synergistic necrotizing fascitis involving the perineum and genitalia, is a true urologic emergency. This entity was reported by A. J. Fournier in 1883. He described five patients with unexplained gangrene of the penis and scrotum all of whom had an abrupt onset, rapid progression, and the absence of a discernible cause. Today the term "Fournier's gangrene" is used to describe gangrene involving the genitalia with both abrupt and prolonged onset, and, in most cases, a precipitating cause is identifiable.

The rapidly progressive course of Fournier's gangrene makes it imperative that this entity be identified as early as possible and treated in an extremely urgent fashion. Possible sources of infection and immunologic compromise must be recognized, and the patient must be treated immediately with both broad-spectrum antibiotics and aggressive surgical débridement.

PRESENTATION

The onset of Fournier's gangrene in most recent series has been described as somewhat more insidious than that described by Fournier, often with symptoms existing for 3 to 4 days prior to presentation to a physician. Symptomatology usually includes pain or itching of the penis and scrotum out of proportion to the patient's clinical appearance. There is often an accompanying fever, chills, malaise, and elevated white blood cell count. Swelling and erythema of the genitalia usually are present and may progress to extreme proportions. If left untreated or treated inadequately, this process will progress to gangrene of the penile and scrotal skin with extension to the abdominal wall, and can lead quickly to septic shock.

ASSOCIATED CONDITIONS

The condition most commonly associated with Fournier's gangrene is diabetes. This is actually well-known as far back as Fournier's time. Underlying genitourinary and anorectal disease are also commonly associated etiologies. The most commonly associated genitourinary disorder is urethral stricture disease. Other genitourinary disorders include epididymo-orchitis, bladder carcinoma, balanitis, and venereal genital ulcers. The most common underlying gastrointestinal disorders are perirectal abscess along with perineal sinus, fissure in ano, anal fistulas, and sigmoid-vesical fistulas. Retroperitoneal diseases that have been associated with Fournier's gangrene include perforated colon carcinoma, perforated colonic diverticuli, pancreatis with retroperitoneal fat necrosis, ruptured retrocecal appendix, and perforated duodenal ulcer. A number of surgical procedures also have been noted to precipitate Fournier's gangrene, including vasectomy, prostate biopsy, internal urethrotomy, orchiectomy, circumcision, hydrocelectomy, and placement of a penile prosthesis.

PATHOPHYSIOLOGY OF INFECTION

Most cases of Fournier's gangrene are initiated by one of three mechanisms:

1. Trauma to the local area, providing direct access of the organism to the subcutaneous tissue.
2. Extension from a urinary tract infection, most commonly with infection of the periurethral glands and dissection along fascial planes to involve the penis and scrotum.
3. Extension of an infection from the perianal area of the retroperitoneal space along the fascial planes of the penis and scrotum.

This initial bacterial seeding usually includes both aerobic and anaerobic flora of the genitourinary or gastrointestinal tract. The organisms act in a synergistic fashion and pass through Buck's fascia to spread along the planes of dartos fascia of the scrotum and penetrate Colles' fascia of the perineum and Scarpa's fascia of the abdominal wall. An obliterative endarteritis occurs in the arteries of the involved region, resulting in exquisite pain along with inflammation and edema of the involved tissue. The oxygen tension in the involved tissue is reduced, inhibiting polymorphonuclear leukocyte activity and promoting growth of anaerobic and facultative aerobic organisms. This anaerobic metabolism is manifested by production of hydrogen and nitrogen, which are insoluble in tissue and may be detected as palpable crepitance.

BACTERIOLOGY

All recent series have reported mixed bacteria flora infections, including aerobic and anaerobic gram-positive cocci, gram-negative aerobic rods, and anaerobes including *Bacteroides fragilis* (most common), *Fusobacterium*, anaerobic streptococci, and clostridia. Flanigan noted the presence of *Pseudomonas* in all patients in a series with underlying colorectal etiology. Culture results in a series of 194 patients recently reported by Paty and Smith are shown in Table 1. In some cases, however, cultures will be unrevealing because of the inherent difficulties involved in anaerobic cultures and because virtually all patients will have received intravenous antibiotic therapy promptly at the time of diagnosis, prior to tissue débridement and culture collection. It is for this reason that careful preparation and analysis of intraoperative Gram stain is essential. Gram stain in some cases may reveal the large gram-positive "box car" bacilli of clostridia. However, anaerobic involvement can be assumed even in patients with negative cultures and an unrevealing Gram stain based on the pathognomonic feculent odor of the wound and the synergistic nature of the infection.

TABLE 1. Microbiologic Findings in 194 Cases of Fournier's Gangrene

ORGANISM	PREVALENCE (%)
Staphylococci	27
Streptococci	42
Escherichia coli	50
Klebsiella	16
Enterobacter	27
Proteus	23
Pseudomonas	26
Peptostreptococcus	34
Bacteroides	47
Clostridium	12

MANAGEMENT

Following the diagnosis of Fournier's gangrene, both blood and urine cultures should be obtained and a broad-spectrum triple antibiotic regimen should be initiated immediately. This should include a 1.5 mg/kg loading dose of an aminoglycoside with subsequent dosages of 3 to 5 mg/kg per 24 hours, with adjustments made for impaired renal function as necessary. In addition, peak and trough values should be followed closely. Clindamycin 600 mg IV q4–6h is used for anaerobic coverage, especially of *Bacteroides* organisms, and intravenous penicillin G (3 to 5 million units q6h) is used to provide coverage of clostridial organisms. Penicillin G is bacteriocidal and usually the best choice against anaerobes, with the exception of *B. fragilis.* Approximately 10 to 15 per cent of strains of clostridia and *Peptococcus* will be resistant to clindamycin. Because of resistant organisms such as these, the use of a multidrug regimen with overlapping sensitivities is justified for the initial treatment phase, and antibiotics can be adjusted based on subsequent culture results.

The importance of expedient surgical exploration and débridement cannot be overemphasized. Because many areas of tissue are necrotic and devascularized secondary to the synergistic infection, antibiotics will have no effect in these regions of tissue, and surgical débridement is the only effective treatment. If urethral pathology is suspected, the patient should have a retrograde urethrogram prior to exploration. In addition, careful rectal examination and possible endoscopy should be performed after induction of anesthesia if an anorectal source is suspected. The patient is then placed in the dorsal lithotomy position and a suprapubic cystotomy catheter is placed if necessary. All necrotic tissue is then débrided, and marginal tissue is either débrided or left for reinspection and possible repeat débridement depending on the surgeon's preference.

Postoperatively, wet-to-dry dressings with Dakin solution along with twice-daily whirlpool treatments hastens granulation. In addition, a number of groups have found hyperbaric oxygen therapy to be greatly beneficial in postoperative healing. The recommended treatment schedule is twice daily at 2.0 to 2.5 atm for 90 to 120 minutes until the patient's condition stabilizes. Treatments then are given once daily. Cohen reported a decrease in mortality rates from 66 to 25 per cent in diabetics and from 33 to 0 per cent in nondiabetics when hyperbaric treatment was utilized. In addition, duration of hospitalization is significantly decreased with hyperbaric treatment.

Despite today's universally aggressive approach to Fournier's gangrene, mortality rates are still quite significant, ranging from 7 to 60 per cent. This further underscores the necessity for prompt, aggressive antibiotic therapy and surgical débridement, along with meticulous attention to detail in postoperative care.

SUMMARY

There are a number of special urologic situations in which numerous secondary factors alter the immunologic milieu of the body and place the patient at significantly increased risk of developing infection or sepsis. With the careful selection of the proper antibiotic regimen, the risk of an infection and the possible development of sepsis in many of these patients can be reduced substantially if not eliminated. Although the regimens described in this article provide general guidelines, the importance of the patient's clinical condition and individual culture results cannot be overemphasized.

Suggested Readings

Baskin LS, Carroll PR, Cattolica EV, et al: Necrotizing soft tissue infections of the perineum and genitalia. Br J Urol 65:524–529, 1990

Kearney GP, Carling PG: Fournier's gangrene: An approach to its management. J Urol 130:695–699, 1983

Paty R, Smith AD: Gangrene and Fournier's gangrene. Urol Clin North Am 19:149–162, 1992

Spirnak JP: Fournier's gangrene: A true urologic emergency. Contemp Urol 4(1):46–52, 1992

Wolach MD, MacDermott JP, Stone AR, et al: Treatment and complications of Fournier's gangrene. Br J Urol 64: 310–314, 1989

CARCINOMA OF THE PENIS

PAUL F. SCHELLHAMMER, M.D.

Norfolk, Virginia

Penile carcinoma constitutes less than 1 per cent of all malignancies among the United States male population—an incidence of one to two cases per 100,000 persons per annum. Although penile carcinoma is an infrequently encountered tumor, its treatment has challenged and maintained the attention of the urologist because of the need to balance the morbidity and gain derived from surgical treatment of both the primary tumor and the first site of metastases, the inguinal nodes.

ETIOLOGY

The incidence of carcinoma of the penis varies markedly with the hygienic standards and the cultural and religious practices of different countries. Neonatal circumcision virtually eliminates the occurrence of penile carcinoma. However, among the uncircumcised African and Asian population, carcinoma of the penis accounts for 10 to 20 per cent of all malignancies in the male (carcinoma may arise in the scarred penile shaft skin after mutilating circumcision).

Publications have strongly criticized routine neonatal circumcision as a form of aesthetic and sexual mutilation. The 1971 edition of Standard and Recommendations of Hospital Care of Newborn Infants, by the Committee of the Fetus and Newborn of the American Academy of Pediatrics, stated that "there are no valid medical indications for circumcision in the neonatal period." However, data now suggest that the incidence of urinary tract infection in male infants may be reduced when circumcision is performed during the newborn period. Therefore, in 1988, the Task Force revised its assessment as follows: "Newborn circumcision has potential medical benefits and advantages as well as disadvantages and risks."

Of importance is the recent implication of a viral etiology of carcinoma. A three- to eightfold increase in the incidence of penile cervical carcinoma among the sexual partners of patients with penile carcinoma has been documented and may be related to infection with the herpes virus. Penile carcinoma also has been associated with the sexually transmitted human papillomavirus virus.

NATURAL HISTORY

Carcinoma of the penis usually begins with a small lesion that gradually extends to involve the entire glans, shaft, and corpora. Carcinoma in situ can precede and progress to invasive carcinoma. The terms "erythroplasia of Queyrat" and "Bowen's disease" have served to separate carcinoma in situ from the mainstream of thinking and reporting on penile carcinoma, but the epidemiology and natural history of this lesion parallel that of early carcinoma of the penis.

Among patients with invasive carcinoma, palpable adenopathy is found in 40 to 80 per cent at initial diagnosis. Approximately 50 per cent of adenopathy proves to be secondary to metastases, and the remainder to inflammatory reaction. Clinically detectable distant metastatic lesions to the lung, liver, bone, or brain are uncommon and are reported as occurring in 1 to 10 per cent of patients in large series. Carcinoma of the penis is characterized by a relentless progressive course, causing death for the vast majority of untreated patients within 2 years.

DIAGNOSIS

Identifying the malignant histology and depth of invasion of carcinoma of the penis by microscope study of a generous biopsy specimen is critical to planning therapy. Biopsy may be a separate procedure from amputation. However, biopsy with confirmation of tumor by frozen section followed by immediate surgical excision by partial or total amputation (with full prior informed consent from the patient) constitutes an efficient means of diagnosis and simultaneous treatment.

The vast majority of tumors of the penis are low-grade squamous cell carcinomas. A recent review emphasized that high-grade tumors frequently are associated with regional nodal metastases.

STAGING

The TNM staging system (Table 1, Fig. 1) most precisely describes depth of invasion. The Jackson system has been the most frequently employed staging system in the past but is deficient in defining depth of neoplastic infiltration.

The strongest prognostic indicator for survival is the presence and extent of nodal metastasis (Tables 2 and 3).

TREATMENT OF PRIMARY NEOPLASM

Stage TIS

Intraepithelial neoplasia is often termed Bowen's disease of the penis or erythroplasia of Queyrat. The two are similar on histologic examination and they are both characterized by the noninvasive epithelial cellular changes of carcinoma in situ. Confirmatory biopsies should be multiple and adequate to rule out invasion. When lesions are small and noninvasive, local excision that spares penile anatomic structure and function is adequate. If a lesion is preputial, circumcision will suffice. Mohs micrographic surgery (discussed later in this article) is another surgical option. Radiation therapy has been successful in eradicating the lesion, and appropriately delivered and planned radiation results in minimal morbidity. Topical 5-fluorouracil–base cream has been used with good therapeutic and cosmetic success. Isolated reports describe success with CO_2 and neodymium:yttrium-aluminum-garnet (Nd:YAG) laser therapy.

Stages T_a and T_1 through T_4

Amputation by partial or total penectomy has been the gold standard of therapy. However, the disfigurement that occurs with am-

TABLE 1. TNM Classification of Penile Carcinoma*

PRIMARY TUMOR (T)	
T_X	Primary tumor cannot be assessed
T_0	No evidence of primary tumor
TIS	Carcinoma in situ
T_a	Noninvasive verrucous carcinoma
T_1	Tumor invades subepithelial connective tissue
T_2	Tumor invades corpus spongiosum or cavernosum
T_3	Tumor invades urethra or prostate
T_4	Tumor invades other adjacent structures
REGIONAL LYMPH NODES (N)	
N_X	Regional lymph nodes cannot be assessed
N_0	No regional lymph node metastasis
N_1	Metastasis in a single superficial inguinal lymph node
N_2	Metastasis in multiple or bilateral superficial inguinal lymph nodes
N_3	Metastasis in deep inguinal or pelvic lymph nodes(s), unilateral or bilateral
DISTANT METASTASES (M)	
M_X	Presence of distant metastasis cannot be assessed
M_0	No distant metastases
M_1	Distant metastases

Adapted from Spiessel B, et al (eds): TNM Atlas: Illustrated Guide to the TNM/pTNM– Classification of Malignant Tumours, 3rd ed. New York, Springer-Verlag, 1989, pp 235–244; and American Joint Committee of Cancer: Manual Staging for Cancer, 3rd ed. Philadelphia, JB Lippincott, 1988, pp 189–191.

putation has directed efforts to organ-sparing techniques employing partial excision or Mohs surgery, or to nonsurgical techniques employing x-ray, laser, or cryodestruction. The necessary goal of any of these treatment modalities is complete destruction of the primary tumor.

Conventional Surgical Treatment

For lesions involving the glans and the distal shaft, even when apparently superficial, partial amputation with a 2-cm margin proximal to the tumor is necessary to minimize local recurrence. A recent series reported no local recurrences with total amputation and a 6 per cent local recurrence after partial amputation. In contrast, circumcision or local wedge excision has been associated with recurrence rates that approach 50 per cent.

If the proximal penile shaft is involved by malignancy, total penectomy is performed with perineal urethrostomy. In more advanced tumors with local extension to the scrotum or pubis, combination chemotherapy followed by surgery may be successful. Hemipelvectomy or hemicorporectomy merits consideration in certain well-selected individuals.

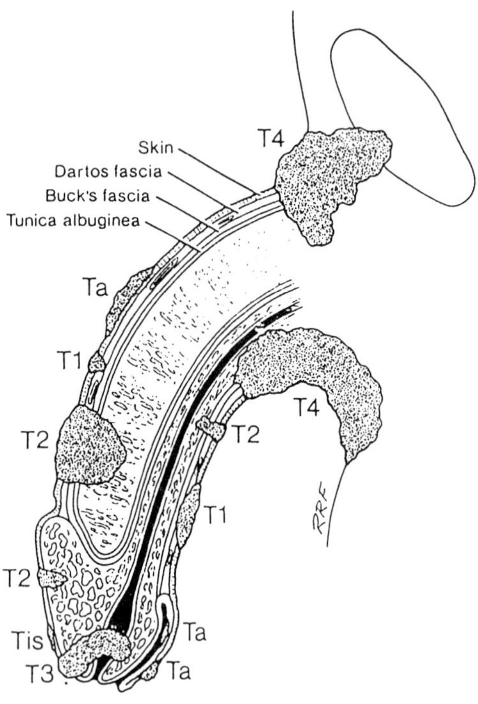

FIGURE 1. Staging of penile carcinoma by depth of invasion. (From Schellhammer et al: Tumors of the Pelvis. Campbell's Urology, 6th ed. Philadelphia, WB Saunders, 1992, p 1277, with permission.)

Mohs Micrographic Surgery

Mohs micrographic surgery (MMS) is a method of surgically removing skin cancer by the excision of tissue in thin layers. MMS includes color coding of excised specimens with tissue dyes, accurate orientation of excised tissue through construction of tissue maps, and microscopic examination of the horizontal frozen sections. The technique, first introduced in 1941 by Dr. Frederic Mohs, was described as microscopically controlled chemosurgery. The term "chemosurgery" has been replaced with the more up-to-date descriptive term "Mohs micrographic surgery."

MMS is a much more time-consuming modality than many of the traditional tissue-sparing techniques. The American College of Mohs Micrographic Surgery frowns on the use of additional personnel for the examination of these carefully prepared sections. They state that "the precise accuracy of MMS can be maintained only if the Mohs micrographic surgeon is responsible for all of the steps in the process. Variations from the technique or extra steps involving additional personnel may introduce errors which reduce the cure rate."

The capability of MMS to trace out silent tumorous "extensions," with a cure rate equivalent to the more radical surgical techniques, while allowing the maximum preservation of normal, uninvolved tissue makes it an attractive therapeutic modality for the treatment of select carcinomas of the penis. In Mohs' own series and other series, MMS seems to be ideally suited for small, distally located carcinomas. Mohs reported a 100 per cent cure rate in the lesions he treated that were less than 1 cm, but only a 50 per cent cure rate in lesions greater than 3 cm.

After MMS, healing is by secondary intention. Meatal stenosis can be a complication and an island flap or a Y-V advancement technique is required to relieve the stenosis.

Laser Surgery

Laser therapy has been used to treat Stages TIS, T_a, T_1, and some T_2 penile cancers. Potential advantages of laser therapy in penile cancer are destruction of the lesion with preservation of normal structures and function. The depth of laser destruction may be difficult to determine, and accurate histologic documentation of the depth of malignant penetration

TABLE 2. Clinical and Pathologic Characteristics of Inguinal Adenopathy

Series	Number of Patients	(Year)	Clinical False Negative: Impalpable Nodes with Positive Histology	5-Year Survival Rates: Inguinal Nodes Negative on Histology or Repeated Physical Examination	5-Year Survival Rates: Inguinal Nodes Resected and Positive
Beggs et al.	88	(1961)	20%	72.5%	45%
Kuruvilla et al.	153	(1971)	10%	69%	33%
Puras et al.	576	(1978)	38%[*]	89%	67%[†] 29%[‡]
Cabanas	80	(1977)	100%	90%	70%[§] 50%[‡] 20%[¶]
Fossa et al.	79	(1987)	13%	90%	80%[#] 20%[**]
Srinivas et al.	199	(1987)	18%	74%	82%[††] 54%[‡‡] 40%[§§] 12%[‖‖]
McDougal et al.	65	(1986)	66%	100%	83%[##] 66%[***] 38%[†††]

Modified from Campbell's Urology, 6th ed. Philadelphia, WB Saunders, 1992, p 1275.
[*]Histologic classification based on node biopsy, not node dissection.
[†]Positive findings in inguinofemoral nodes.
[‡]Positive findings in inguinofemoral and pelvic nodes.
[§]Single inguinal node with positive findings.
[‡]More than one inguinal node with positive findings.
[¶]Three-year survival with positive findings in inguinal and pelvic nodes.
[#]N_{1-2}.
[**]N_3.
[††]One node positive.
[‡‡]One to six nodes positive.
[§§]More than six nodes positive.
[‖‖]Bilateral nodes positive.
[##]Adjunctive adenectomy.
[***]Immediate therapeutic adenectomy.
[†††]Delayed therapeutic adenectomy.

may not be obtainable. Therefore, it is imperative to stage the tumor adequately with deep biopsies prior to applying laser therapy.

Treatment of TIS tumors (Bowen's disease, erythroplasia of Queyrat, bowenoid papulosis) can be achieved with any of the common surgical lasers. The Nd:YAG laser has been employed either as primary therapy or as an adjunct to excision of T_1 and T_2 tumors. Malloy reported successful ablation in six of

TABLE 3. Five-Year Survival Related to Extent of Nodal Metastasis

Series, Number of Patients (Year)	Number Positive Nodes: ≤2	Number Positive Nodes: >2	
Fraley et al., 31 (1989)	15/17 (88%)	1/14 (7%)	
Johnson et al., 22 (1984)	6/7* (85%)	2/15 (13%)	
Srinivas et al., 119 (1987)	5/6 (82%)	7/34 (20%)	9/16 (54%)[†]
Fossa et al., 18 (1987)	11/2 (88%)[‡]	2/6 (33%)[§]	

Modified from Campbell's Urology, 6th ed. Philadelphia, WB Saunders, 1992, p 1276.
*Approximate.
[†]A subset with one to six positive nodes.
[‡]Pathology: N_{1-2}.
[§]Pathology: N_3.

nine patients with Stage T_1 but failure in two patients with Stage T_2 tumors. Using knife excision or laser excision with the aid of a sapphire tip, followed by laser coagulation of the base of the tumor, Boon reported an 81 per cent success rate in the destruction of Stages T_1 and T_2 tumors. The largest series using Nd:YAG laser destruction for Stages TIS, T_1, T_2, and some T_3 tumors reported an actuarial survival at 5 years of 89 per cent for node-negative and 25 per cent for node-positive patients. Local recurrence was seen in only 2 of 28 patients with invasive tumor followed for 5 years.

Radiation Therapy

The sole advantage of initial radiation therapy over initial surgery relates to the preservation of penile anatomic structure and function—an end that also can be achieved with the advances in Mohs, laser, and reconstructive surgery already described.

Objections to radiation therapy are several. Squamous cell carcinoma is characteristically radioresistant, and the doses of radiation (6000 rads) necessary to sterilize deeply infiltrating penile tumors frequently result in complications that may require secondary penectomy. The lengthy treatment schedule of 3 to 6 weeks represents a formidable burden for the elderly. In contrast, partial penectomy represents a relatively simple and expeditious procedure. Long-term follow-up of the patient to detect recurrence is mandatory. In one series, 7 of 11 recurrences (63 per cent) were detected after 2 years and 2 of 11 (18 per cent) after 5 years.

TREATMENT OF INGUINAL NODES

The presence of inguinal metastases affects the prognosis more than tumor grade, gross appearance, or morphologic and microscopic patterns of the tumor, and presents a surgical challenge. Controversial issues center around the timing and extent of surgery.

Should lymphadenectomy be performed in the presence of clinically palpable inguinal nodes after appropriate treatment of the primary lesion and subsidence of inflammation? Yes! Twenty to 50 per cent of patients with clinically palpable adenopathy and histologically proven inguinal node metastases who are treated by inguinal lymphadenectomy achieve 5 years of disease-free survival. A series from Memorial Sloan-Kettering Cancer Center reported an 82 per cent 5-year survival after adenectomy for patients with a single positive node, and a series from the Norwegian Radium Hospital reported 88 per cent 5-year survival after adenectomy for patients with minimal nodal metastases (Table 3).

Should complete *inguinal lymphadenectomy* routinely *be performed in patients with clinically negative groin examination at the time of presentation of the primary lesion?* This question invites the greatest amount of controversy. Early complications of phlebitis, pulmonary embolism, wound infection, and flap necrosis and late complications of lymphedema can occur with disconcerting frequency after inguinal adenectomy. However, postoperative complications have been lessened in the last decade by: (1) improved pre- and postoperative care, (2) preservation of the dermis and Scarpa's fascia, and (3) preservation of the saphenous vein and modification of the extent of node dissection.

The incidence of metastases to the inguinal nodes has been reported as 2 to 25 per cent in patients presenting with penile carcinoma who have clinically negative inguinal examinations. Unfortunately, most series have not analyzed separately postlymphadenectomy survival of patients with clinically palpable nodes that are positive for neoplasm on histologic examination compared with survival of patients with clinically negative nodes that are positive for neoplasm on histologic examination. Three recent analyses did compare 5-year survival free of disease between patients who had either immediate adjunctive or delayed therapeutic lymphadenectomy. McDougal et al. (Table 2) reported a series of 23 patients with invasive primary lesions and nonpalpable nodes; 9 were treated with immediate adjunctive lymph node dissection (6 were node positive) and 14 by surveillance and delayed therapeutic lymph node dissection. The 5-year survival in the node-positive immediate adjunctive lymphadenectomy group was 88 per cent (five of six); in the surveillance group it was 38 per cent. A third subset in this series manifested adenopathy at presentation and had immediate therapeutic lymph node dissection, with 10 of 15 (66 per cent) surviving 5 years. The best results, therefore, were from *immediate* adjunctive lymph node dissection (88 per cent); the next best results were from immediate therapeutic lymph node dissection (66 per cent) and the worst results (38 per cent) were with surveillance and delayed lymph node dissection when nodes became palpable.

Fraley et al. reported that immediate adjunctive lymphadenectomy resulted in a survival free of disease at 5 years in 6 of 9 node-positive patients (66 per cent) compared to 1 of 12 patients (8 per cent) who had been followed and treated by delayed therapeutic lymphadenectomy. A series from the M.D. Anderson Hospital compared 5-year disease-free survival for 14 patients with early adjunctive lymphadenectomy for clinically impalpable but histologic node-positive disease with that for 8 patients who were followed and submitted to later lymphadenectomy when clinical nodal enlargement appeared. The primary tumors were of similar stage. The 5-year disease-free survival was 57 per cent with early adenectomy compared to 13 per cent with delayed adenectomy.

Should inguinal lymphadenectomy be bilateral rather than unilateral for patients presenting with unilateral adenopathy at initial presentation of the primary tumor? The answer to this question is yes. The anatomic crossover of lymphatics of the penis is well established. Clinical support for a bilateral procedure is based on the finding of subclinical contralateral metastases in greater than 50 per cent of patients so treated.

Should pelvic lymphadenectomy be performed in patients with positive inguinal metastases? Iliac nodes have been found to be positive for tumor metastases in 15 to 30 per cent of patients with positive inguinal nodes. Survival of patients with positive iliac nodes, although limited, has been documented (Table 2, Puras et al, Cabanas). The procedure is reasonable for the young male who is a good surgical risk.

Chemotherapy

The use of chemotherapy in the neoadjuvant and adjuvant setting was employed at the Milan National Tumor Institute. A protocol of 12 weekly courses of vincristine, bleomycin, and methotrexate was administered to 12 patients after adenectomy as adjuvant therapy and to 5 patients prior to node dissection as neoadjuvant therapy. The patients treated with adjuvant chemotherapy were at high risk (i.e., nine showed extranodal tumor growth, five had pelvic nodal involvement, and five had bilateral metastasis). At a follow-up ranging between 18 and 102 months, only one patient has recurred. The same regimen was used as neoadjuvant therapy for five patients with large nodal tumor metastasis (nodes ranged from 6 to 11 cm in size). Three achieved a partial response, were successfully resected, and continued without disease at 20 to 72 months.

Overview of Treatment Recommendations for Inguinal Nodes

Stages TIS, T_a, T_1, N_0M_0 (Jackson I and II)

This describes lesions that involve only the glans mucosa or shaft skin, are totally exophytic and superficial, and are very unlikely (<10 per cent) to have nodal metastases. Inguinal nodes should be followed by examination every 3 months for at least 2 years.

Stages T_2, T_3, N_0M_0 (Jackson I and II)

These lesions, while limited to the glans or shaft, demonstrate invasion of Buck's fascia, tunica albuginea, and corporal bodies. The incidence of nodal metastases increases significantly. Immediate adjunctive node dissection is indicated. Superficial node dissection may be employed initially. This involves removal of those nodes superficial to the fascia lata. Total lymphadenectomy (e.g., removal also of those nodes deep to the fascia lata contained within the femoral triangle) is performed if the superficial nodes are positive. Corporal lymphatics have been presumed occasionally to drain directly to the deep inguinal nodes. However, clinical experience and penile lymphatic studies show no evidence of direct pelvic node drainage. An alternative is to initially perform both a superficial and a deep node dissection, employing the limited boundary technique described by Catalona; the decision should be based on personal preference.

Stages TIS, T_a, T^-; M_0 (Jackson III)

Four to 6 weeks after treatment of the primary tumor, the nodes and control of infection are re-evaluated. If bilateral adenopathy persists, bilateral radical inguinal node dissections are recommended. If adenopathy is unilateral, ipsilateral superficial and deep node dissection is performed. Metastases are anticipated in approximately 50 per cent of the clinically normal contralateral groin. As noted above, a superficial node dissection only, if histology is negative, or a superficial and deep node dissection employing the limited boundary technique are options for the normal contralateral groin.

Stages Any T, Any N, M_1; T_4; Inoperable N (Jackson IV)

Treatment often is limited to palliative chemotherapy or radiotherapy. In selected patients with fixed nodes but no distant metastases, neoadjuvant chemotherapy is followed by inguinal and pelvic adenectomy.

Suggested Readings

Catalona WJ: Modified inguinal lymphadenectomy for carcinoma of the penis with preservation of saphenous veins: Technique and preliminary results. J Urol 140: 306, 1988

Fraley EE, Zhang G, Manivel C, et al: The role of ilioinguinal lymphadenectomy and significance of histological differentiation in treatment of carcinoma of the penis. J Urol 142:1478–1482, 1989

Johnson DE, Lo RK: Management of regional lymph nodes in penile carcinoma. Five-year results following therapeutic groin dissections. Urology 24:308–311, 1984

Kriegmair M, Rothenberger KH, Spitzenpfeil E, et al: Neodym-YAG-laser treatment for carcinoma of the penis (abstract #650) J Urol 143:351A, 1990

McDougal WS, Kirchner FK Jr, Edwards RH, et al: Treatment of carcinoma of the penis: The case of primary lymphadenectomy. J Urol 136:38, 1986

Mohs FE: Chemosurgery: A microscopically controlled method of cancer excision. Arch Surg 42:279, 1941

Pizzocaro G, Piva L: Adjuvant and neoadjuvant vincristine, bleomycin, and methotrexate for inguinal metastases from squamous cell carcinoma of the penis. Acta Oncolog 27:823–824, 1988

Srinivas V, Morse MJ, Herr HW, et al: Penile cancer: Relation of extent of nodal metastasis to survival. J Urol 137:880–882, 1987

TUMORS OF THE SCROTUM

GERALD L. ANDRIOLE, M.D.

St. Louis, Missouri

Tumors of the scrotum may run the gamut from benign to malignant. However, the large majority of scrotal wall tumors are benign. Nevi are the most frequent benign tumors of the scrotal wall; other common benign lesions that may arise at this site include sebaceous cysts, hemangiomas, leiomyomas, or manifestations of certain venereal diseases, especially condylomata acuminata. The most common malignant tumor of the scrotal wall is squamous cell carcinoma, followed by a variety of sarcomas such as leiomyosarcoma and Kaposi sarcoma. Melanoma, extramammary Paget disease, and basal cell carcinoma are even rarer malignant tumors of the scrotum.

Patients with scrotal wall lesions may complain of swelling, pain, or a nonhealing ulcer that is continuously moist. On physical examination, a subcutaneous tumefaction or a soft diffuse fullness of the scrotal wall may be palpated. Some scrotal wall lesions, especially vascular hemangiomas, may be difficult to distinguish from a varicocele on physical examination. This is especially true in prepubertal patients. For this reason, scrotal ultrasonography may be necessary to localize the lesion precisely to either the testicle or the scrotal wall. Physical examination of all patients with scrotal wall tumors should include palpation of the inguinal lymph nodes, because this site is the primary lymphatic drainage of the scrotum.

The histologic diagnosis and often the definitive treatment of scrotal wall tumors may be made by excisional biopsy. Ordinarily a partial scrotectomy may be accomplished with minimal cosmetic consequences and minimal morbidity. Such a procedure usually will be curative for benign lesions of the scrotum and also for some small malignant tumors. Squamous cell carcinoma, however, often is associated with lymph node metastases at the time of detection. This occurs because the time interval between the patient's initial suspicion of a problem to definitive therapy may exceed 3 years. For this reason, inguinal lymph node dissections generally are recommended for patients with squamous cell carcinoma of the scrotum. Ordinarily a modified superficial node dissection may be performed to determine if metastatic disease is present. If the modified groin dissection (one that removes lymph nodes medial and anterior to the femoral vein but not lateral to it) is negative, the patient may be followed. However, if microscopic disease is detected by the modified node dissection, a more complete radical inguinal lymph node dissection that includes the deep inguinal lymph nodes and the more proximal pelvic lymph nodes is warranted. As is true for patients with squamous cell carcinoma of the penis, those with scrotal squamous cell carcinoma who present with grossly palpable nodes are very infrequently cured by surgery. Adjuvant chemotherapy is recommended but also has generally not been very effective for these patients.

Sarcomas of the scrotum may arise from any layer of the scrotal wall. In the past, leiomyosarcoma was the most common sarcoma of the scrotum. The most important aspect of patient management is complete excision of the local lesion at the time of initial surgery. Locally recurrent sarcomas are often very difficult to manage and often are associated with distant disease. Regional lymphatic spread may occur with sarcomas of the scrotum and is often synchronous with hematogenous metastasis to the lung, liver, or bone. Because of this, surgery for advanced scrotal sarcoma is unlikely to be curative and chemotherapy is generally necessary.

Kaposi sarcoma may be a presenting sign of the acquired immunodeficiency syndrome. The scrotum is rarely the sole, initial area of involvement but may be one of several involved sites. Treatment of Kaposi sarcoma of the genital region is palliative and may include partial scrotectomy or neodymium:yttrium-aluminum-garnet laser obliteration of symptomatic lesions. Systemic medical therapy also is often given.

Melanoma and basal cell carcinoma of the scrotum are managed in a manner analogous to those that arise at other sites. Wide local excision with regional lymphadenectomy may be necessary for patients with large melanomas.

Suggested Readings

Dahl I, Angervall L: Cutaneous and subcutaneous leiomyosarcoma: A clinical pathological study of 47 patients. Pathol Eur 9:307, 1974

Kaufman DG, Kasznica J, Burbige KA, et al: Benign scrotal tumors masquerading as expanding varicoceles. Urology 29:612, 1987

McDonald MW: Carcinoma of the scrotum. Urology 19: 269–274, 1982

Ray B, Whitmore WF Jr: Experience with carcinoma of the scrotum. J Urol 117:741, 1977

Ritchie EL, Gonzales F, Zaontz M: Fibrous hamartoma of infancy masquerading as a rhabdomyosarcoma of the spermatic cord. J Urol 140:800, 1988

Siegal GP, Goffey TA: Solitary leiomyomas arising from the tunica dorcos scrotae. J Urol 116:69, 1976

WORK-UP OF THE IMPOTENT MALE AND SELECTION OF THERAPY

TOM F. LUE, M.D.

San Francisco, California

Recent advances in erectile physiology and pathophysiology have transformed our knowledge and approach to the impotent man. Elucidation of nitric oxide as the most likely neurotransmitter of erection and description of the venous compression mechanism, coupled with new treatment strategies, may lead to development of an optimal therapy for impotence in the next few years. However, there is still no "magic pill" available.

Many of the advances are directly attributable to the discovery and use of vasoactive agents capable of inducing corporeal smooth muscle relaxation. Currently, new diagnostic modalities, such as color duplex sonography, diagnostic use of intracavernous vasoactive agents, nocturnal penile tumescence testing, and cavernosometry, have given the clinician the ability to define rapidly and evaluate precisely the cause of erectile dysfunction. However, these advances have brought with them a dilemma for the impotent patient and treating urologist: Which tests are indicated, how reliable are the results, and in which patient should they be used?

Advances in technology also have provided the physician-urologist with a wealth of treatment choices. The simple penile prosthesis, the mainstay of treatment 10 to 15 years ago, now has evolved into a wide array of implantable, commandable, and near-physiologic devices. Self-injection programs using a myriad of agents are now commonplace. Improvements in vacuum devices and prototypes of other compression devices provide additional options to the patient and physician. Vascular reconstruction and venous ligation round out the list of treatment choices.

With this great availability of diagnostic and therapeutic choices, a simple approach to the impotent man is necessary. If impotence is thought of in the most basic of terms, it can be defined as (1) psychogenic, (2) neurogenic, (3) hormonal, (4) arterial, (5) cavernosal (as a consequence of dysfunction of the tunica albuginea, neurotransmitter-receptor coupling, trabecular smooth muscle, or endothelium), (6) drug induced, or (7) a combination of these etiologic elements. Currently, effective treatment approaches for all of these pathologies exist. The necessity to define the exact abnormality varies with each patient and should be based on his therapeutic goals and choice of preferred treatment; that is, the extent of the evaluation should be guided by the patient's goals and expectations. Use of an intracavernous vasoactive agent can be tried in the office setting during the initial visit and, if successful, may preclude further evaluation in some patients.

PATIENT WORK-UP

There exists a wide range of opinions on what is the most appropriate work-up for the impotent man. Recently, we have used a goal-directed approach for diagnosis and treatment that has proved satisfying for the patient. At the initial interview, the specific sexual defect that brought him to seek help is discussed and a therapeutic alliance with the patient is established. Important factors that determine the specific approach are the patient's physical and mental health, the underlying nature of the problem, and the patient's goals and degree of motivation. Education of the patient with details on what is expected with aging (i.e., loss of spontaneous, long-lasting psychogenic erections) and what is not expected (loss of reflexogenic erection during intercourse) is provided at the outset.

Many men confuse impotence with problems of ejaculation, libido, and orgasm. The nature and extent of sexual dysfunction that brought the patient into the office must be firmly established. The patient's motivation and expectations as well as the forms of therapy he will accept should be discussed during the initial encounter. We think this is of paramount importance in directing the work-up and treatment. We attempt to limit all invasive studies to those that can effect a change in management.

History, Physical Examination, and Laboratory Studies

A detailed history, physical examination, and several basic laboratory studies are essential features of the initial interview. The medical, surgical, and sexual history should be reviewed. Past problems of cardiac performance, diabetes, alcoholism, hypertension, hyperlipidemia, and psychologic or neurologic abnormalities must be addressed. Recent changes in bladder or bowel function may signal autonomic nervous system dysfunction. A history of smoking or recreational drug use should be determined. Common causes of sexual dysfunction, such as medication, past illness, and injury to the genitourinary system, also should be explored.

The physical examination can establish whether normal androgenic stimulation is present as assessed by development of secondary sexual characteristics. Sensation in sacral dermatomes combined with biothesiometry of the penis can test for the threshold of vibratory sensation, indicating an intact neurologic system or a gross neurologic deficit. The vascular status of the lower extremities can be evaluated by palpation initially. The penis, testes, and prostate should be examined. Evidence of trauma to the pelvis or genitalia and presence of a plaque (Peyronie's disease) are important clues to the cause of impotence in a small percentage of patients.

Essential laboratory studies at the initial interview are a complete blood count; measurement of serum urea, creatinine, and glucose; a lipid profile; and urinalysis. The cost effectiveness of endocrinologic screening in impotent men has been addressed recently, resulting in divergent screening practices. In cases in which both libido and testes size are normal, endocrine screening generally yields normal results and, as suggested by Johnson and Jarow, need not be performed. Others believe a higher incidence of endocrinopathy exists and continue to perform routine testosterone and prolactin tests in impotence screening.

Once the history, physical examination, and basic laboratory investigations are completed, the patient should be made aware of all available treatment options, success rates, relative advantages, disadvantages and cost. To those interested only in noninvasive forms of treatment, a choice of isoxsuprine, yohimbine, trazodone, or a vacuum constriction device (VCD) should be explained and offered. All patients need to be advised of any laboratory abnormality, and the appropriate therapy or referral should be suggested. Finally, the remaining patients comprise those who wish to undergo a more definitive evaluation.

Additional Diagnostic Tests

Patients whose impotence by history and physical examination is thought to be psychogenic are advised to undergo a Rigiscan (nocturnal penile tumescence test). If erections are of normal duration, frequency, and rigidity, referral for psychological or sexual counseling is arranged. Patients with high prolactin or abnormal testosterone levels should have repeat tests and measurement of follicle-stimulating hormone and luteinizing hormone.

An endocrinologist should evaluate all such patients for possible pituitary or hypothalamic dysfunction. For those patients with primary gonadal dysfunction, administration of testosterone enanthate (200 mg intramuscularly every 3 weeks) is suggested. In those patients at high risk for neurologic impairment, a neurologic consultation is recommended.

GOAL-DIRECTED EVALUATION AND TREATMENT

The majority of patients do not have either psychogenic- or endocrinologic-based impotence; instead, the cause is usually vascular or neurogenic. In those patients who seek active treatment of their impotence, a goal-directed approach is used (Fig. 1). Initially, we evaluate the arterial flow with what we have characterized as the CIS test (combined intracavernous injection and stimulation test). We currently inject 10 μg of prostaglandin E_1 intracavernously and assess tumescence after 10 to 15 minutes. In those patients who have a rapid rigid erection without manual stimulation, significant arterial or venous impairment can be ruled out and no further vascular evaluation is recommended. These patients comprise the group of men who are ideally suited for self-injection therapy. We give every patient a comprehensive instruction and consent form that includes the possible complications and specifically emphasizes the seriousness of priapism (see the article on Priapism for prevention and treatment). If, after intracavernous injection of a vasodilator, the erection is fully rigid at 1 hour, a preventative intracavernous injection of diluted phenylephrine hydrochloride (100 to 500 μg) is given to reverse the erection. All candidates for home therapy receive injections in the office at least twice with the same precautions until the lowest effective dose is determined. The patient is instructed to use this low dosage (usually titrated to provide an erection lasting 30 to 60 minutes) and not to increase it without consulting the physician.

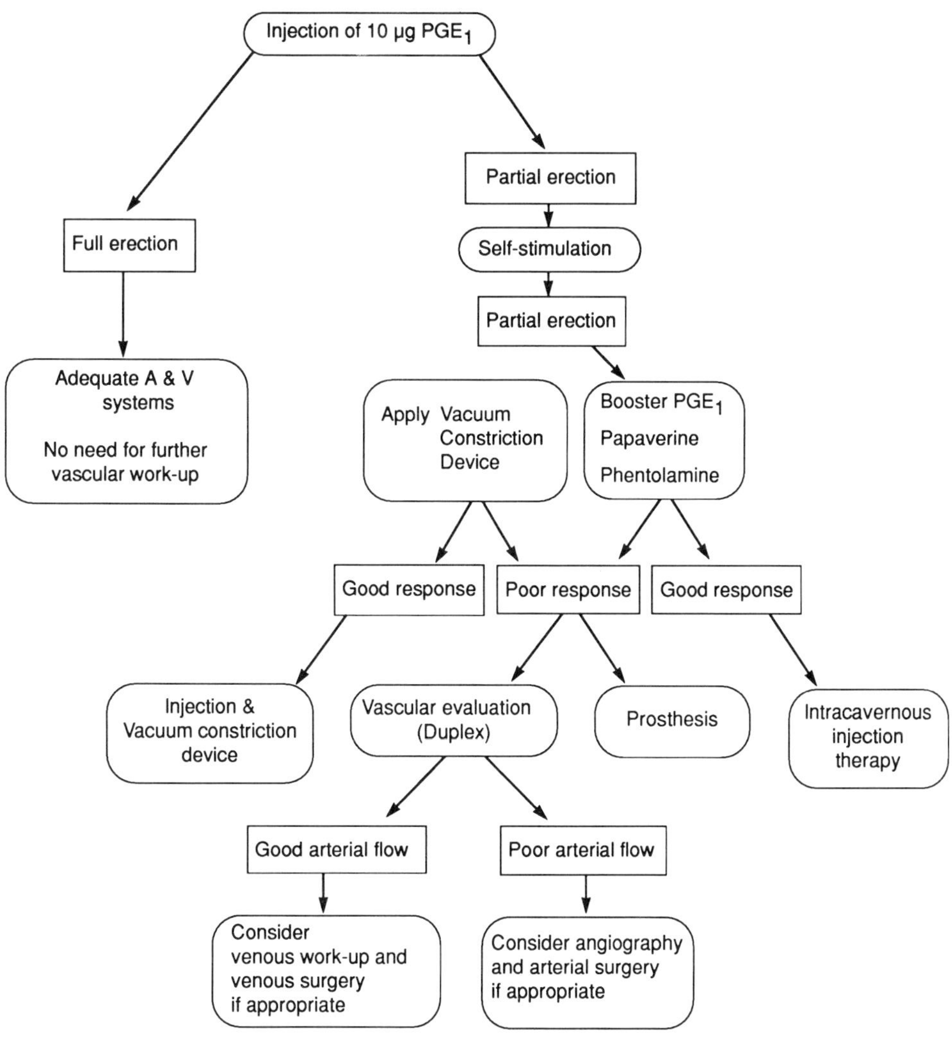

FIGURE 1. Algorithm for the diagnosis and treatment of impotence based on the patient's goals.

When a suboptimal erection is achieved with the initial injection and manual stimulation is required to attain a complete erection, two conclusions can be drawn: (1) the venous system is adequate and (2) the patient may have been inhibited initially, but the reflexogenic pathway is intact and the patient has overcome his centrally mediated inhibition. However, no statement about the arterial system can be made other than that it is not severely impaired. In this group of men, we again advise intracavernous therapy as first-line treatment.

In the patient who fails to achieve an adequate erection with stimulation, a booster dose of 0.5 ml of our "3P" solution (12 mg of papaverine, 9 μg of prostaglandin E_1, and 1 mg of phentolamine/ml) is injected and the patient is advised to repeat self-stimulation. If he is successful in achieving a complete erection, the patient is taught self-injection with the 3P combination. If the booster fails to work, a VCD is applied, providing a gross assessment of the significance of venous leak. If tumescence is maintained adequately for intercourse, a combination approach using intracavernous injection of a vasoactive agent with the VCD is suggested. In cases in which the VCD is unsuccessful, arterial and venous evaluation is recommended before contemplating vascular reconstructive surgery (arterial, venous or combination) or placement of a penile prosthesis. These remain as therapeutic options.

Among those patients who wish vascular reconstructive surgery or simply a more accurate assessment of the penile vascular supply, duplex ultrasonography is performed. This test uses a duplex scanner with 10-MHz ultrasound and 4.5-MHz pulsed Doppler to measure the diameter and flow of the cavernous arteries before and after intracavernous injection of a vasodilator. It allows assessment of the actual arterial flow, velocity, size, and dynamic characteristics of the vessels in the flaccid and erect states. The pulsatile nature of a normal vessel is readily apparent; when seen, this rapidly rules out significant arterial insufficiency as the cause of impotence. In our practice, pharmacologic cavernosometry (measurement of the flow required to maintain a full erection and the rate of drop in intracavernous pressure) and cavernosography (contrast-material study of the site of penile venous leakage) are used only among those patients who are candidates for venous surgery (i.e., those with poorly sustained erections with normal or near-normal arterial penile flow as documented by duplex ultrasonography). Recently, the efficacy of venous ablative procedures has been raised; most studies of large series show less than 50 per cent durable cures. The usefulness and ultimate indications for these procedures have yet to be defined fully.

Similarly, selective pudendal arteriography is indicated only for those patients without evidence of systemic vascular disease in whom duplex ultrasonography demonstrates impaired arterial flow to the penis. The angiogram is best used as a preoperative study to plan an arterial reconstructive procedure.

Among men with poor arterial flow or generalized atherosclerosis, or in cases in which the patient or partner are unable or unwilling to perform intracavernous injections, a penile prosthesis is a good choice. Although clearly invasive, this approach uniformly results in return of the patient's ability to engage in sexual activity. Penile prostheses have made great strides over the past 20 years. They have evolved into many different forms, including rigid, malleable, hinged, and inflatable devices. Improvements now result in excellent patient and partner satisfaction with an acceptably low complication rate. The semirigid and rigid prostheses are simpler and traditionally have had a lower failure rate than inflatable models. However, the more complex devices appear more natural in the flaccid state and allow the patient to control the timing of erection. Revision rates resulting from mechanical failure (fluid loss, pump migration, connector separation, or tubing kink) were high with earlier models, but these have declined.

CONCLUSION

Today's urologist is armed with a powerful armamentarium of diagnostic and therapeutic tools. Success (as defined as the ability to resume sexual activity) is possible for nearly every patient. Our goal as caregivers should be to achieve success in the least invasive and most natural way possible. This algorithm may facilitate that goal.

Suggested Readings

Lue TF: Erectile impotence: Diagnostic methods. Prob Urol 5:519–526, 1991

Melman A: Evaluation and management of erectile dysfunction. Surg Clin North Am 68:965–981, 1988

Sidi AA, Koleilat N, Fraley EE: Evaluation and treatment of organic impotence. Invest Radiol 23:778–789, 1988

MEDICAL AND SURGICAL TREATMENT OF PEYRONIE'S DISEASE

STEVEN M. SCHLOSSBERG, M.D.

Norfolk, Virginia

Peyronie's disease is a condition named for François de la Peyronie, who described the condition in 1743. A plaque or scar develops within the tunica albuginea that limits the elasticity of the penis. Typically, a deformity associated with constriction and curvature occurs with erection. In addition, men may notice a decrease in the quality of their erections that may result from organic and/or psychologic factors. Once a man develops Peyronie's disease, he should be told that the penis will never be exactly the way it was before the disease developed. Any therapy should be offered and accepted by the patient with this in mind.

DIAGNOSIS

Most men present in the fourth or fifth decade of life with a painful lump on the dorsum of the penis. Some will notice curvature as the presenting complaint. Most men have not heard of the condition and initially are concerned about malignancy or other unusual infiltrative conditions. A history should be obtained relative to trauma or any prior problems with sexual function. Risk factors for erectile dysfunction also should be reviewed. Some information about the relationship with the sexual partner is helpful in eventual counseling. At the initial visit, patients are encouraged to bring a photograph of the erect penis if a diagnosis has already been made.

A careful physical examination will help the patient understand the condition and demonstrate the extent of the disease. The glans is grasped by one hand to stretch the penis. At this point, the decrease in elasticity of the penis already may be apparent. The thumb and index finger are used to palpate the dorsal and ventral surfaces in a side-to-side fashion. The plaque may extend under the glans and/or to the penopubic angle dorsally. Lateral extension may be seen from a dorsal plaque. Although less common, many patients will have a concomitant ventral plaque under the urethra that balances the dorsal restriction. Many physicians and urologists may miss a ventral plaque if not specifically looking for one. Opposing plaques often lead to more complaints of a restrictive deformity and buckling with intercourse. In addition, an isolated ventral plaque may be seen in 10 per cent of patients. I often have the patients palpate the penis as well to try to show them the extent of the disease. During the explanation of therapy, their understanding of the location is quite helpful to them in planning management. All patients are checked for Dupuytren's contracture, which may be seen in 10 per cent of patients.

As part of the initial evaluation, a plain radiograph of the penis may be taken to look for calcification within the plaque. If calcification is present, it helps to determine which part of the disease will not change. In general, 25 per cent of plaques will calcify. Although other tests, including sonography, magnetic resonance imaging, and simple cavernosography, have been done, they add little to the careful physical exam and simple radiograph except in unusual cases.

ETIOLOGY AND NATURAL HISTORY

The etiology of Peyronie's disease is uncertain because no animal model exists to investigate it and patients are operated on at the end stage of their disease. However, a theory has been developed from both anatomic and investigational evidence. The tunica albuginea of the corpora cavernosa is made up of two layers: an inner circular and outer longitudinal layer. The corpora are separate structures proximally but fuse on the shaft of the penis. Their common wall results in a septum that fuses with the tunica in the dorsal and ventral midline. If the forces in the penis are compared to an I beam, the area of maximum stress occurs at the junction of the septum and the covering of the corpora cavernosa. This anatomic arrangement limits girth expansion and promotes lengthening during erection. With decrease in elasticity and possible decrease in rigidity, it may lead to microvascular injury as trauma occurs, associated with a decrease in elasticity and/or decrease in erectile function. A delamination occurs between the inner circular and outer longitudinal fibers, leading to a series of events that lead to plaque formation. From analysis of mature plaques, it is believed that fibrin deposition leads to fibroblast activation, blood vessel permeability, and accumulation of inflammatory cells. Pathologic examination reveals a perivascular infiltrate in the early stages of the disease. Later in the disease, the scar becomes more fibrous and may exhibit calcification and bone formation.

The natural history of the disease is variable, but some general observations are helpful in counseling patients. The disease process tends to run its course within 12 to 18 months. Although pain often may be an initial presenting complaint, it usually resolves within 6 months. In most men, when seen at the initial stages of the disease, stability or progression tends to be the rule in equal amounts. Although clearly seen, significant resolution and improvement are the exception rather than the rule. Men invariably develop a significant psychologic overlay to their condition that should be explored in the initial visit. They should be encouraged to develop a meaningful dialogue about the condition with their partner if not already present. Some men will be ashamed to discuss their frustration with the condition.

MEDICAL THERAPY

Initial therapy has been aimed at altering the inflammatory process. For the last 30 years, most patients have received either vitamin E or potassium para-aminobenzoate (Potaba) because reports appeared to suggest their usefulness in this condition. Although both have been used extensively, no randomized trial exists to substantiate their usefulness. I have preferred to use vitamin E (400 mg twice a day) because it is inexpensive and not associated with significant side effects. Medication typically is continued until the disease stabilizes. Potaba tends to be associated with poor compliance because of the dose (24 pills/day), cost, and gastric upset.

Other initial therapies have included intralesional steroids, steroids with ultrasound, and a variety of compounds introduced by iontophoresis. Because the plaque is so dense and I have seen exacerbation of the disease associated with steroid injection, I have advised patients against injection into the plaque. Radiation rarely is indicated and should be given only if severe pain exists. If pain is incapacitating after a significant period of time, a small dose may help (450 rad by the beta beam of a linear accelerator).

SURGICAL THERAPY

In the majority of patients, encouragement and medical therapy will suffice in the early stages of the disease. In some patients, this will be unsatisfactory because they can no longer function, and further therapy is warranted. After the disease has stabilized for at least 6 months and patients have had the disease for at least 12 months, surgical therapy can be considered.

Patients with Peyronie's disease who cannot function can be divided into three groups. In the first group, rigidity is normal but severe curvature prevents intercourse. In general, these are men with at least 45 degrees of dorsal or 30 degrees of ventral curvature. Many patients relate that their curvature is lateral rather than dorsal or ventral. Careful examination usually reveals that the penis rotates in a twisting fashion as it becomes erect. At the other end of the spectrum are patients with severe loss of rigidity that precludes intercourse. However, the majority of men present with a combination of the two complaints, exhibiting both a decrease in rigidity and curvature that makes intercourse awkward and difficult. During the initial visit, it is often helpful to get this information from both the patient and his partner.

In patients with poor rigidity and mild curvature, pharmacologic erection therapy may be helpful in getting patients through an initial difficult period. The safety of prostaglandin E_1 pharmacotherapy makes this a viable alternative in some patients for temporary or long-term treatment. Once the disease has stabilized, some patients may find a vacuum device suitable if the plaque is not too proximal.

Prior to offering surgical therapy, all patients should have an evaluation of vascular function to help plan therapy. A duplex ultrasound evaluation under pharmacologic stimulation will help determine if arterial or venous abnormalities are present. If veno-occlusive dysfunction is noted, dynamic infusion cavernosometry and cavernosography may be helpful in counseling patients as to the reliability of functional repair. If patients do not accumulate at least 40 mm Hg of intracorporal pressure, they will require some aid to help with rigidity after straightening. Typically, a prosthesis will be placed. With pressures above 40 mm Hg, functional repair still may be successful without placement of a prosthesis as long as arterial parameters are normal. Because falsely abnormal results may be seen with pharmacologic vascular function testing, sleep lab testing may be helpful in advising some patients.

Since almost all patients suffer some psychological problems from the disease, all patients are seen by a sex therapist prior to surgical therapy. This visit serves several purposes: it helps patients deal with their concerns about surgery, another independent evaluation occurs to determine if the patient understands the risks and benefits of surgery, and a discussion and plan for postoperative rehabilitation are developed.

Surgical therapy has been divided into three approaches. The plaque may be excised or incised and the defect grafted to lengthen the affected side. The opposite side may be shortened to straighten the penis. Some authors would advocate placement of a prosthesis with or without simultaneous straightening.

Although straightening by opposite shortening has been advocated by some authors, in my experience, most patients with Peyronie's disease complain of penile shortening and are not anxious to have any more done surgically. However, this approach should be considered in patients with adequate penile length or if vascular parameters are marginal and curvature is a problem. If a patient has marginal storage parameters, straightening the penis will maximize his axial rigidity and improve function while posing less risk of worsening erectile function after reconstructive surgery.

Excision and grafting have been the mainstay of functional reconstruction. Replacement grafts have come from dermis, tunica vaginalis, and temporalis fascia. If tunica vaginalis or temporalis fascia is the graft chosen, incision rather than excision of the plaque may be a better approach. With any approach, exposure of the plaque will be similar. A brief description follows.

For dorsal plaques, a circumcising incision is made and the penis is de-gloved in a plane between the dartos and Buck's fascia. Rather than elevating the dorsal neurovascular bundle from the side, we have chosen to go through the bed of the dorsal vein by excising it from the distal trifurcation to the suspensory ligament. The circumferential veins are ligated as well to prevent postoperative veno-occlusive dysfunction. Once the plaque is exposed, traction sutures are placed and the plaque is excised, preserving all erectile tissue. A dermal graft is harvested from the non–hair-bearing skin over the anterior superior iliac spine. The donor site is closed primarily. The graft is sutured in place to the free edge of the tunica albuginea and the septal fibers. Buck's fascia is reapproximated in the midline and the penile skin is closed after two suction drains have been placed. Patients are discharged in 3 to 4 days and are encouraged to begin having erections after 2 weeks. They may resume intercourse after 6 weeks, although graft and penile healing may not be complete for as long as 1 year. The results of this surgery in patients with good preoperative erectile function have been excellent.

In patients with poor preoperative erectile function, a penile prosthesis is an excellent method of management in this relatively young population. Recently, most patients have chosen an inflatable prosthesis that is placed through a penopubic incision. In a significant number, the prosthesis will straighten the penis. If correction of curvature is necessary, a circumcising incision is made and the plaque exposed. Typically, dorsal transverse incisions are made and the defect closed with either a dermal graft or a Gortex patch.

SUMMARY

The approach to patients with Peyronie's disease should be individualized. All patients should be tried with conservative therapy and only those who cannot function should be offered surgical therapy, with the understanding that the penis will never be the same as before the disease developed. The importance of psychological counseling by both the treating urologist and a sex therapist cannot be overemphasized.

Suggested Readings

Devine CD: Peyronie's disease. *In* Droller MJ (ed): Surgical Management of Urologic Disease: An Anatomic Approach. St. Louis, Mosby-Year Book, 1992, pp 901–915

Devine CD, Jordan GH, Schlossberg SM: Surgery of the urethra and penis. *In* Walsh PC, Retik AB, Stamey TA, et al (eds): Campbell's Urology, 6th ed. Philadelphia, WB Saunders, 1992, pp 2957–3032

Gelbard MK, Dorey F, James K: The natural history of Peyronie's disease. J Urol 144:1376, 1990

Jordan GH, Angermeier KW: Preoperative evaluation of erectile function with dynamic infusion cavernosometry/cavernosography (DICC) in patients undergoing surgery for Peyronie's disease: Correlation with postoperative results. J Urol 150:1138–1142, 1993

PENILE PROSTHESIS IN THE TREATMENT OF ERECTILE IMPOTENCE

TERRENCE R. MALLOY, M.D.

Philadelphia, Pennsylvania

In the past 20 years, outstanding advances have taken place in the diagnosis, testing, and evaluation of erectile dysfunction and impotence. Medical and surgical treatments have evolved to treat the various forms of sexual dysfunction. With better diagnosis and a more thorough understanding of the basic causes of erectile impotence, new and innovative forms of therapy have been developed.

Despite the outstanding improvement in the understanding and diagnosis of impotence, the various medical therapies have been successful in a limited number of patients. Despite the claims of success for intracavernosal pharmacotherapy, penile revascularization, venous ligation, and penile vacuum suction devices, penile prostheses remain the form of therapy with the highest rate of permanent success. The physician in the 1990s has a variety of types and manufacturers of prostheses for the impotent male.

PRESURGICAL EVALUATION

Prior to considering surgery, all patients should have a thorough evaluation to determine the etiology of their erectile impotence. It is essential that any alternative therapies that might benefit the patient have been discussed prior to surgery. A common claim in medical negligence cases involving prosthetic surgery has been the failure to pursue alternative conservative therapies before undertaking prosthetic surgery.

A complete history is essential in every patient, as well as a very thorough physical examination. On physical examination, a complete evaluation of the urologic, vascular, and neurologic aspects should be undertaken. Medical conditions that might influence surgery or the ability of the patient to use a prosthesis must be determined. A patient with impaired vision or decreased manual dexterity would have problems using an inflatable penile prosthesis. A urologic examination should determine that there are no urinary infections or urinary obstruction that should be corrected prior to the insertion of a penile prosthesis. Peyronie's disease often is undiagnosed until a careful physical examination of the penis has been performed. Corrective surgery to straighten the penis may be needed as well as to improve rigidity. Vascular assessment of the penile blood flow can be accomplished with a Doppler stethoscope. Determination of vasculogenic components can be assessed further with duplex ultrasonography or dynamic cavernosometry.

The patient should have a complete laboratory assessment, including a complete blood count, SMA-12, and measurement of serum testosterone and prolactin, and of prostate-specific antigen in patients over 50. These blood tests will help rule out medical conditions that might be affecting erectile function. Psychological testing, such as the Minnesota Multiphasic Personality Inventory, may be indicated, and nocturnal penile tumescence (NPT) studies are indicated when patients are considering prosthetic surgery. The NPT test is still the most commonly recognized test to establish the patient's legitimate claim with insurance companies. In any patients with erectile dysfunction secondary to trauma, the NPT test is essential to establish the organic etiology of the problem for any subsequent litigation.

In patients who are young and have suffered trauma, vascular reconstructive procedures may be beneficial. Penile arteriography may be indicated, and the pros and cons of this type of therapy should be discussed thoroughly with the patient before undertaking penile prosthesis surgery. In patients who are middle-aged or older or have diabetes mellitus, the results of revascularization procedures have been very poor, and testing probably would be nonproductive. Optional intracavernosal testing with papaverine or prostaglandin E_1 should be accomplished prior to doing prosthetic surgery so that the patient could have an experience of what intracavernosal drug therapy might do for his condition. The pros and cons of this therapy also should be discussed thoroughly with the patient.

DECISION TO PROCEED WITH PENILE PROSTHESIS SURGERY

With the conclusion of the diagnostic workup, the urologist and patient should discuss the findings. The tentative diagnosis of the type of erectile dysfunction should be obvious. If the patient is not satisfied with or is uncertain about his therapeutic options, more definitive tests may be contemplated. In certain patients, often elderly, the fact that the diagnosis has been made is sufficient. They may decide that they have no interest in surgery or further complicated tests and are willing to accept their condition or try alternate sexual behavior.

Other patients, including those with organic erectile impotence, also may benefit from sexual therapy either prior to surgery or concurrent with prosthetic implantation. In those patients who are hesitant to proceed with prosthetic surgery, a conservative course of sexual therapy often will alleviate their anxieties. At the same time, patients may benefit from conservative medical therapy with such drugs as yohimbine and isoxsuprine to improve their erectile function. If the serum testosterone is found to be low on two determinations, a conservative course of biweekly injections may be beneficial.

Intracavernosal drug therapy has received considerable attention in the recent urologic literature. Drugs such as papaverine and/or phentolamine, along with prostaglandin E_1, have been shown to have beneficial effects. The patient should be apprised of the availability of these drugs plus the chances of long-term success. Although these drugs are not approved by the Food and Drug Administration for use in impotence, there has been more than 5 years of experience in their use without significant problems. The patient may wish to start on a program of intracavernosal drugs prior to considering prosthetic surgery. This should be encouraged to be sure the patient has explored all alternative therapies before proceeding with the prosthetic device.

Vacuum "suction" devices that produce erection by limiting the outflow of venous blood have produced satisfactory results in certain patients. Long-term studies of success have been limited, however. The patient should be given literature about these devices, and should be made aware that there can be trauma to the base of the penis from the constrictive rings and that ejaculation may be retarded by the rubber binding at the base. Certainly, there is no harm if the patient wants to try the device prior to experiencing prosthetic surgery.

Revascularization surgery is available but, in general, has been successful only in younger patients who have experienced trauma.

PENILE PROSTHESIS SELECTION

The selection of the penile prosthesis that is ideal for the patient should be done after extensive consultation with the urologist. All the various types and forms of prosthetics should be explained to the patient. There are pamphlets and literature for each type prepared by the manufacturers that should be shown to the patient. Videotapes also are available that explain the types of prostheses. Long-term success rates should be discussed and the patient should be allowed to consider the various types of prostheses. It is essential that the patient receive the prosthesis that he is most comfortable in using and not that which is the easiest for the urologist to implant.

Rod Penile Prostheses

Rod penile prostheses have the advantages of simplicity of surgical insertion, long-term mechanical stability, and low malfunction rate. However, these devices all have the same major disadvantage in that there is no increase in girth or length with intercourse. Concealment in public places is difficult, and the device is easily palpated by the patient and partner alike, producing complaints of an artificial sensation. The devices can migrate proximally, producing an "SST"-type deformity in the penis that makes the glans droop like the nose of a supersonic transport plane. The rod also can produce constant pressure on the glans penis, which may lead to erosion in certain cases.

The earliest of these devices was the Small-Carrion device, which has a long history of success. In recent years, various rod prostheses have been produced by the Surgitek Corporation (Flexi-rod II), American Medical Systems (AMS 600), and the Bard Corporation (Jonas rod) that allow for better concealment. Many of these devices have an inner core consisting of stainless steel or silver alloy wires that allow for positioning of the rods.

In recent years, the Dacomed Corporation has produced the DuraPhase and OmniPhase prostheses, which have an inner core of ball-in-socket discs connected by a steel cable. Tension on these springs allows positioning of the device for intercourse and then concealment.

Fluid Malleable Prostheses

Fluid malleable prostheses have the advantage of better concealment than rod prostheses plus a more normal feel to palpation. However, the basic disadvantage still exists that there is no increase in length or girth with activation of the device; in addition, there is the chance of mechanical failure with loss of fluid. American Medical Systems produces the Dynaflex device, which has a fluid reservoir in the base of the prosthesis. Dual cylinders are placed into each corpora and are activated by pressure on a pump mechanism by squeezing the glans. This transfers the fluid to a central compartment, which allows for rigidity. At the completion of intercourse, deflation is accomplished by a release valve proximal to the pump. The principle disappointment with these devices has been the lack of increase of girth or length and some difficulty in learning how to use the pump and release mechanism.

Inflatable Penile Prostheses

The standard four-piece inflatable penile prosthesis (two cylinders, pump, and reservoir) still produces the most natural erection with the best rigidity and normal appearance. This device feels natural to palpation for both the patient and partner alike. When the device is deflated, the penis appears normal and causes no embarrassment in public places. There is no bulge in the pants that might indicate a prosthesis is present. The device presents no problems for endoscopic examination in patients requiring urologic procedures. When erect, the penis has increased circumference and, with certain devices, there is an increase in length. The American Medical Systems Model 700 Ultrex inflatable penile prosthesis allows for increase in circumference and length with a specially constructed three-ply cylinder. The cylinders are produced in various lengths and there is a rear tip extender that allows for exact fitting for the corporal cavernosal length in individual patients.

Mentor Corporation also has an inflatable penile prosthesis that has a record of satisfactory performance. The cylinders are a silicone-polyurethane blend that produces excellent durability. Early problems with the pump release mechanism in this device have been corrected. In the deflated state, the cylinders do not relax as naturally as silicone cylinders, but there is no major problem with concealment.

The principle criticism of the four-piece inflatable penile prosthesis in the past was related to its mechanical failure rate. In the early 1970s, there were considerable problems with mechanical stability. However, in the 1980s, with the introduction of the Mentor Corporation inflatable prosthesis and the American Medical Systems Model 700 Ultrex, stability has been excellent.

In recent years, three-piece inflatable penile prostheses (two cylinders and a combined pump-reservoir-scrotal mechanism) have been introduced. The Mentor Corporation and Surgitek have produced devices with a scrotal pump–reservoir combined mechanism. The advantage of both of these devices is the simplicity of surgery: There is no need to implant a separate abdominal reservoir. This is beneficial in patients with previous abdominal surgery during which the space of Retzius was obliterated, such as post–radical prostatectomy or cystectomy patients. The principle disadvantage of these devices is that the scrotal pump–reservoir does not hold sufficient fluid to allow maximum inflation of the cylinders. In patients with medium to large corporal length, there will not be sufficient fluid transfer to allow maximum expansion of the corpora cavernosa. Long-term success rates are not available for these types of devices, whereas there is more than a 15-year history of success with the four-piece inflatable penile prosthesis.

PROSTHETIC SURGERY

The patient should be given adequate time to select the prosthesis of his choice. The patient should be provided with literature to allow him to select the type of prosthesis that is most beneficial for his condition. If the surgeon is not experienced or comfortable implanting the patient's chosen type of prosthesis, he or she should refer the patient to a urologist with experience in that surgery.

Informed consent should be obtained prior to admission to the hospital. The consent form should be of the urologist's own design and not be a standard hospital consent form. The consent should include warnings of mechanical failure, possible infection, bleeding, and need for prosthesis removal. There should be a statement within the consent form indicating that no guarantee is made that the penis will be larger than in the premorbid condition. There should be no guarantee as to the performance of the device, because the manufacturers cannot guarantee the performance of the prosthesis. The patient should read and sign the consent form prior to admission so that no claim can be made that he did not have time to understand the proposed surgery prior to being hospitalized.

Preoperative preparation should consist of betadine scrubs to the surgical area the night prior to surgery. Infection in the urinary tract and on skin in the surgical area should be eliminated prior to surgery. Preoperative IV antibiotics are beneficial and should be administered beginning 12 hours prior to surgery. The surgical preparation should be done in the operating room just prior to surgery.

The surgical approach utilized should be one that is familiar so that the urologist may maximize results and minimize complications. Penile incisions should be avoided at all costs; potential damage to the neurovascular bundle may result. Infection or scarring also may cause problems with penile appearance. Excellent results have been obtained with the suprapubic incision or the scrotal approach, so there is no need for penile incisions for implantation of penile prostheses.

Prior to commencing surgery, an artificial erection should be performed to ascertain if there is an unsuspected angulation or Peyronie's plaque in the penis. Corrective corporaplasties may need to be performed after the prosthesis is inserted if the penis is not straight. The use of intraoperative antibiotic irrigation has produced beneficial results in preventing infection. Subcuticular closure of wounds has helped to obtain early healing of the wound without infection.

When implanting inflatable penile prostheses with scrotal pump mechanisms, Jackson-Pratt–type drains have proven very effective in preventing postoperative edema and hematoma. They generally are left in place for 18 hours and then removed.

Postoperatively, the patient is maintained on antibiotics to prevent infection. The Trendelenburg position plus ice to the scrotum helps prevent swelling and discomfort. The patient usually can be discharged on the first to third postoperative day depending on the type of prosthesis inserted.

On discharge, the patient should be maintained on antibiotics for 10 to 14 days. When swelling and pain have subsided, the patient will require careful instruction on the operation of the device. Literature should be provided to the patient to assure that he can properly utilize his prosthesis.

Suggested Readings

Bretan TN Jr: History of the prosthetic treatment of impotence. Urol Clin North Am 16:1–5, 1989

Furlow WL, Motley RC: The inflatable penile prosthesis: Clinical experience with a new controlled expansion cylinder. J Urol 139:945, 1988

Malloy TR, Malkowicz B: Pharmacologic treatment of impotence. Urol Clin North Am 14:297, 1987

Malloy TR, Wein AJ, Carpiniello VL: Comparison of inflatable penile prosthesis in the surgical treatment of erectile impotence. J Urol 123:678, 1980

Montague DK: Penile prosthesis: An overview. Urol Clin North Am 16:7, 1989

Scott FB, Byrd GJ, Karacan I, et al: Erectile impotence treated with an implantable penile prosthesis. J Urol 124:611, 1980

SALVAGE OF THE INFECTED INFLATABLE PENILE PROSTHESIS

J. KEITH LIGHT, M.D.

Syracuse, New York

The classical treatment for an infected inflatable penile prosthesis is removal of the whole device. However, this can be devastating for the patient, both financially and psychologically. The concept of the "salvage" or exchange operation for a known infected penile prosthesis arose because of the success in cardiac surgery in replacing infected artificial heart valves.

The reported incidence of device infection ranges from 0.5 to 3.1 per cent, with a higher incidence in paraplegics (6 per cent). Infection occurs in spite of perioperative coverage with both intravenous and oral antibiotics. The ability of bacterial contamination to survive the antibiotic regimen probably is related to the formation of a glycocalyx that surrounds the organism, preventing penetration by the antibiotics. This glycocalyx adheres to the device and coats the organisms, allowing them to survive the normal defense mechanisms of the body. The most common organism resulting in device infection is *Staphylococcus epidermidis*. This organism is usually of low pathogenicity but, in the presence of a foreign body, may result in a clinical infection. Infection—and its usual manifestation, erosion—commonly are delayed for more than 6 months following implantation or revision surgery in the majority of cases.

The clinical signs suggesting an infected prosthesis most often are confined to the pump and tubing. The systemic signs of fever, leukocytosis, and sepsis are rare, except in the diabetic patient. More commonly, one or more of the following signs will be present suggesting a low-grade infection:

1. Development of, or persistence of, pain with pump manipulation.
2. Thickened capsule around the pump and tubing.
3. Thinning of the skin over parts of the prosthesis, particularly over the pump and cylinder tips.
4. Persistent mild skin hyperemia over the pump.

5. Erosion of the pump without significant scrotal swelling.
6. Persistent attachment of the pump or tubing to the skin.
7. Absence of systemic signs of infection.

It should be remembered that the postoperative changes induced by the implantation surgery may take up to 3 months to resolve totally. Some of the above signs therefore may persist during the healing phase.

Oral antibiotics should be commenced if the clinical signs strongly suggest a low-grade device infection. However, the presence of systemic signs, especially in patients with diabetes mellitus, demands immediate and total removal of the device. If no response to the oral antibiotics occurs, strong consideration should be given to early surgery to establish the diagnosis. Procrastination in the presence of a persistent indolent device infection eventually will result in erosion of one or another of the components, usually the pump or cylinder tips.

Surgery is performed through the previous incision, usually a penoscrotal approach. The sheath surrounding the tubing and pump is opened with the aid of the Bovi. In the presence of significant tissue induration or frank pus, it is recommended that the entire device be removed with appropriate drainage. In the absence of the above two factors, device infection should be suspected if there is thickening of the sheath, which classically will be hyperemic or dull and opalescent. Intraoperative Gram stain from the exudate of the sheath frequently is performed. An exchange procedure is considered with absence of bacteria or the presence of gram-positive cocci on the stain. The presence of gram-negative rods, however, diminishes the chances of a successful salvage procedure.

The cylinders are removed through the penoscrotal incision and the corporeal bodies thoroughly irrigated with an antibiotic solution. The pump is removed through a separate scrotal incision and the soft tissue communications to the pump and reservoir areas are sutured closed before insertion of the new cylinders. The reservoir similarly is removed through a small incision directly over the reservoir site. A new pump and reservoir are placed on the contralateral side to the infected components and connected in the routine fashion. Drains are placed in the previous reservoir and pump spaces. The penoscrotal incision is closed primarily without drainage. Organism-specific antibiotics then are continued postoperatively, initially intravenously, for approximately 72 hours and then orally for up to 3 months.

Sixteen patients who underwent a salvage procedure for low-grade device infection were analyzed. *S. epidermidis* was cultured in 11 of the 16 patients (69 per cent), thus being the most common organism. Four patients had no growth on culture. Group D streptococcus and *Escherichia coli* were cultured from one patient. Cultures from 15 patients (94 per cent) therefore either grew *S. epidermidis* or were sterile. All the patients were treated with antibiotics prior to the salvage procedure. The clinical presentation of these patients was in accordance with a low-grade infection, with signs localized to the pump or cylinder tip. Furthermore, the time interval from the last operative procedure to the "salvage" operation ranged from 1 to 36 months, with a mean of 11.6 months. This relatively long duration is also in keeping with a low-grade infection. The follow-up period after the salvage procedure in these patients was 6 to 50 months, with a mean of 22.6 months. Eleven patients (69 per cent) had more than 1 year follow-up. Fifteen patients retained the inflatable prosthesis for this time period without clinical signs of device infection. One patient underwent insertion of a semirigid rod 1 month after the exchange procedure because of personal preference.

On the basis of these results, an exchange or "salvage" operation subsequently has been performed in all patients with a proven device infection with no intraoperative contraindications (i.e., presence of frank pus or significant tissue induration). Follow-up of these patients has confirmed the initial results. Overall, approximately 80 per cent of the patients managed in this fashion will retain their prosthesis for 18 months or longer. The remaining 20 per cent, however, will still lose the prosthesis, secondary to uncontrolled device infection.

Consideration should therefore be given to performing a salvage procedure in patients, especially the nondiabetic patient, who present with clinical signs of a device infection.

Suggested Readings

Carson CC: Infections in genitourinary prosthesis. Urol Clin N Amer 16:139, 1989

Furlow, WL, Goldwasser B: Salvage of the eroded inflatable penile prosthesis: a new concept. J Urol 138:312, 1987.

Montague, DK: Periprosthetic Infections. J Urol 138:68, 1987

SECTION 8

THE TESTIS AND EPIDIDYMIS

Congenital Disorders

CRYPTORCHIDISM

JACOB RAJFER, M.D., F.A.C.S.
Torrance, California

Although cryptorchidism remains one of the most common and frequently treated congenital disorders, great controversies exist regarding its etiology, natural history, and proper therapy. For the practicing physician, familiarity with the embryology and long-term sequelae of this disorder is mandatory in order to evaluate critically the evolving treatment strategies currently recommended and coming in the future.

EMBRYOLOGY

Normal testicular development begins at approximately 6 weeks of gestation with the migration of primordial germ cells to the genital ridge. A testis-determining factor produced by a testis-determining gene, now believed to be the SRY gene located on the short arm of the Y chromosome, is responsible for the differentiation of the indifferent gonad along the path to a testis. Meanwhile, the gubernaculum develops as a mesenchymatous column traversing from the gonad through an opening in the anterior abdominal wall to the scrotal swelling. Leydig cell differentiation along with testosterone production begins at approximately 8 weeks, while the cremaster muscle develops along the gubernaculum in the inguinal canal. Further sexual differentiation, including müllerian regression and formation of the vasa deferentia, epididymides, and external genitalia, begins at this time and is completed prior to the end of the first trimester. The testis then enters a dormant state, just inside the internal inguinal ring, until descent begins during the seventh month of gestation.

Testicular descent begins with marked swelling of the gubernaculum, especially the portion within the scrotum. The cremaster muscle and processus vaginalis also grow and extend distally. The testis rapidly descends through the open inguinal canal during the 28th week of gestation. Following descent, the gubernaculum differentiates into the internal and external cremasteric fasciae and the processus vaginalis obliterates.

The mechanism of normal descent remains unknown, as does the cause of its failure. Current theories suggest that descent is a complex and highly coordinated event requiring the action of hormonal factors (testosterone and dihydrotestosterone); biochemical changes (absorption of water by gubernacular hyaluronic acid, causing swelling and a marked change in consistency); mechanical factors (intra-abdominal pressure, gubernacular dilation by the growth of the epididymis); and possibly the influence of the genitofemoral nerve. Unfortunately, no single unifying theory presently can satisfy all experimental observations. Likewise, the cause of failure of descent is lacking a unifying theory. Hormonal disorders, mechanical obstruction, epididymal abnormalities, and an intrinsic testicular defect all have been proposed as etiologies.

INCIDENCE

At birth, approximately 30 per cent of premature and 3.4 per cent of term male newborns will have incomplete testicular descent. By 1 year of age, most cryptorchid testes will have completed descent, leaving a final incidence of 0.2 to 0.8 per cent. No racial or geographic difference in incidence has been reported. Retractile testes often are mistaken for cryptorchid testes and account for 50 to 80 per cent of testes referred for evaluation. Great care must be taken to exclude these testes because they do not pose any additional risk and do not require treatment.

The testis whose descent is arrested along the normal pathway without any evidence of obstruction accounts for 77 per cent of all cryptorchid testes. Of these, 64 per cent are located in the high scrotal region and 25 per cent in the inguinal canal, and 11 per cent are either intra-abdominal or absent. Testes that are obstructed in their normal descent account for 23 per cent of undescended testes, and ectopic testes occur in less than 1 per cent of patients.

DIAGNOSIS

An accurate diagnosis can be made most reliably during infancy, prior to age 2, while the scrotum is relatively large and the cremaster reflex poorly developed. Between ages 2 and 7, the cremasteric reflex is quite strong and definitive diagnosis can be very difficult. Following puberty, a majority of retractile testes will have descended permanently, thereby greatly simplifying diagnosis.

If the cryptorchid testes can be felt clearly and are not retractile, further diagnostic work-up is unnecessary and appropriate therapy should begin.

If both testes are impalpable, an evaluation to exclude anorchism is necessary. In boys less than 9 years of age, evaluation begins with measurement of basal serum levels of luteinizing hormone (LH) and follicle-stimulating hormone (FSH). Abnormally increased LH and FSH levels are diagnostic of bilateral anorchism and neither a human chorionic gonadotropin (hCG) stimulation test nor surgical exploration are necessary. After 9 years of age, elevated levels of serum gonadotropins are nondiagnostic. Normal gonadotropin levels at any age warrant surgical exploration. Unfortunately, there are no endocrine tests available that are able to differentiate a unilateral impalpable testis from an absent testis.

Following the diagnosis of an impalpable testis, an attempt often is made at localization. Ultrasound, computerized tomography, magnetic resonance imaging, venography, and laparoscopy all have been used, with laparoscopy appearing to be the most reliable. The need for preoperative localization remains controversial, with many authors questioning its necessity as opposed to a thorough exploration. Advantages of localization include diagnosis of testicular absence, altering of surgical approach for high intra-abdominal testis, and the laparoscopic placement of vascular clips on the testicular vessels in a two-staged Fowler-Stevens procedure.

RATIONALE FOR THERAPY

Critical to the understanding of any therapy is the rationale for intervention. In cryptorchidism, therapy is directed at preventing two well-described adverse consequences associated with cryptorchidism: subfertility and increased risk of testicular cancer. Unfortunately, therapy has not as yet been proven to be effective in preventing these sequelae.

The relative risk of developing testicular cancer is calculated to be from 10 to 40 times greater than in the normal population, depending on which incidence one chooses to accept (0.2 to 0.8 per cent), because cryptorchid patients account for 7.3 per cent of all testis cancer patients. Surgical therapy to date has failed to show a significant effect on reducing the risk.

The other important risk is that of infertility. Fertility rates of patients with cryptorchidism are controversial. Comparisons may vary depending on whether one is measuring sperm counts, tubular histology, or actual paternity. In bilateral untreated cryptorchid patients, 75 per cent have azoospermia, 25 per cent have oligospermia, and virtually none have reported fertility. Bilateral cryptorchid patients who have undergone therapy have been shown to have approximately 40 per cent azoospermia, 30 to 35 per cent oligospermia, and 30 to 35 per cent fertility.

In both treated and untreated unilateral cryptorchid patients, approximately 45 per cent will be oligospermic, although fertility rates differ significantly, with 35 per cent of untreated patients and 75 to 80 per cent of prepubertally treated patients being fertile. The cause for the wide discrepancy is unknown, although some believe that the untreated cryptorchid testicle exerts an adverse effect on the normal contralateral testis. Whether there will be improvement in cancer risk, sperm production, or fertility with earlier intervention, prior to age 2, as now advocated, remains to be seen.

MEDICAL THERAPY

The primary goal of therapy always has been to bring a viable testis into the scrotum, and thus the backbone of treatment has been surgical intervention. Attempts have been made to develop medical therapies in order to avoid the risks of surgery and anesthesia. The medical therapies typically have involved hormonal stimulation through the hypothalamic-pituitary-gonadal axis. The efficacy of these therapies remains very controversial. Treatment may consist of hCG injections (typically 10,000 to 12,000 U given in divided doses over 4 weeks), as used in the United States, or intranasal gonadotropin-releasing hormone (GnRH) (1.2 mg/day for 4 weeks), as used in Europe, or a combination of both. hCG is believed to act by imitating the effect of LH on Leydig cells, resulting in an increase in intratesticular testosterone production. GnRH acts to increase serum LH and FSH levels, thereby stimulating gonadal androgen production. Reported success rates for hCG range from 6 to 40 per cent, those for GnRH range from 9 to 59 per cent, and combination hCG/GnRH treatment has a success rate of 29 to 86 per cent. The wide discrepancy in results has not been explained, although some have attributed it to the possible inclusion of retractile testes in many of these studies.

Although the efficacy of hormonal therapy remains unproved, it continues to be a recommended first step in therapy because, even if the testis does not descend, such benefits as descent of retractile testes, growth of the testis and vasculature, and the possibility of making an impalpable testis palpable, thereby facilitating a difficult surgical repair, warrant its use.

SURGICAL THERAPY

As stated above, the primary goal of therapy is to bring a viable testis into the scrotum. Secondarily, the patent processus vaginalis is ligated. The timing of intervention is of critical importance because most cryptorchid testes will descend spontaneously during the first year of life, usually within the first few months. Therefore, treatment is safely delayed until after 1 year of age. Likewise, histologic signs of seminiferous tubular damage have been demonstrated as early as 2 years of age, prompting many to advocate early repair prior to age 2.

For those presenting later, orchiopexy should remain the treatment of choice up until puberty. For the postpubertal adolescent, orchiopexy has a very limited role because these testes generally will no longer have spermatogenic function and, despite surgery, still will pose a cancer risk. Thus, for the postpubertal adolescent and young adult, orchidectomy still could be considered the treatment of choice.

In the previously untreated adult, it is recommended that those under age 32 be treated in the same way as the postpubertal adolescent, with orchidectomy. In patients over 32 years of age, the risk of dying from the operation or anesthesia is greater than the risk of death from testicular cancer, and thus these patients should be followed without surgery. Of course, these are only general guidelines and treatment must always be individualized to the patient.

SPECIAL MANEUVERS

For the high-lying or difficult-to-bring-down testis, there are a variety of techniques available to overcome lack of adequate length, including the Prentiss and Fowler-Stevens procedures, two-stage repairs, and autotransplantation.

In the Prentiss technique, the floor of the inguinal canal is incised and the testis is brought into the scrotum in a straight line. This maneuver can gain an additional 2 to 3 cm of cord length.

In the Fowler-Stevens procedure, the testicular vessels are divided and the testis relies solely on collateral circulation from the vas. Prior to their division, the vessels are atraumatically clamped for 5 minutes and the tunica albuginea incised. Brisk bleeding from the tunica suggests adequate collateral perfusion. Great care must be taken during dissection because excessive trauma around the cord easily can damage the fragile collateral vessels and jeopardize the testicular blood supply. Preoperative localization of the impalpable testis can allow specific planning for this procedure and spare unnecessary dissection around the cord. Additionally, laparoscopically placed vascular clips also have been used in a two-stage Fowler-Stevens procedure, with the theoretical advantage of allowing time for the development of greater collateral flow. Success rates of the Fowler-Stevens procedure have been reported to range from 50 to 75 per cent.

Alternatively, a two-staged approach is possible in which the testis is anchored as far distally as possible and wrapped in Silastic to prevent adhesions during the first procedure. The second stage is performed 1 to 2 years later, when an attempt is made to place the testes into the scrotum. Success rates have been reported to be as high as 86 per cent.

Testicular autotransplantation involves microvascular anastomosis of the testicular vessels to the ipsilateral inferior epigastric vessels after placement of the testis into a dartos pouch. This technique can be used even in children as young as 2 to 3 years of age with acceptable results, although extensive experience with microvascular techniques is mandatory.

CONCLUSION

Cryptorchidism remains a common yet poorly understood congenital anomaly requiring careful diagnosis, timely intervention, and creative surgical management. It can be expected that, with further research, many of the controversies will be settled and current treatment strategies will continue to evolve.

Suggested Readings

Backhouse KM: Embryology of testicular descent and maldescent. Urol Clin North Am 9:315, 1988

Chilvers C, Dudley NE, Gough MH, et al: Undescended testis—the effect of treatment on subsequent risk of subfertility and malignancy. J Pediatr Surg 21:691, 1986

Farrer JJ, Walker AH, Rajfer J: Management of the postpubertal cryptorchid testis: A statistical review. J Urol 134:1071–1073, 1985

Lowe DH, Brock WA, Kaplan GW: Laparoscopy for localization of nonpalpable testes. J Urol 131:728–729, 1984

Scorer CG, Farrington GH: Congenital Deformities of the Testes and Epididymis. London, Butterworth & Co, 1971

A CLINICAL APPROACH TO TESTICULAR TORSION

HARRIS M. NAGLER, M.D.

New York, New York

Testicular torsion is an acute event requiring immediate diagnosis and treatment to prevent testicular loss. It is one of the few true urologic surgical emergencies. Although it occurs most commonly during adolescence, it can occur at any age. It has been demonstrated in experimental models that, unless detorsion is performed within 4 to 6 hours, irreversible testicular damage will occur. Unilateral testicular torsion has been reported to be associated with subfertility. The etiology of this diminished fertility is unclear. It has been hypothesized that there is an immunologic response that results in damage to the contralateral testis. Conversely, an underlying associated bilateral testicular abnormality has been reported in patients with testicular torsion.

CLINICAL PRESENTATION

The usual presentation of testicular torsion is acute scrotal pain. All prepubertal and young adults with a painful, swollen testis must be suspected of having testicular torsion. Often, erythema and scrotal edema follow the acute onset of scrotal pain. Although classic descriptions indicate that vigorous physical exercise is a frequent inciting event, our experience indicates that testicular torsion often occurs while the young adolescent is sleeping. The patient is awakened with acute onset of pain and presents at the emergency room at that time or early the next morning. The exact location of the pain may be unclear. The patient may complain of lower abdominal pain. It is important that the examination of any male patient with lower abdominal pain include a complete scrotal examination.

PHYSICAL EXAMINATION

The scrotum may be erythematous, edematous, and diffusely tender. The pain cannot be localized to the epididymal area; rather, the entire testicle is tender to the touch.

The location of the testicle within the scrotum should be noted. If the testicle can be identified clearly, its axis may be altered from the normal vertical position of the testicle. Additionally, the testicle may be elevated within the scrotum, occupying a more superior location. This is particularly helpful in diagnosis of left testicular torsion because the left testicle is often in a more dependent position in the normal condition. Patients may be aware of this alteration of testicular position.

When torsion is present, the examiner may not be able to differentiate the epididymis from the testes because of the associated congestion and edema, whereas, when the pain is secondary to epididymitis, the epididymis generally is differentiated clearly from the testicle and is the specific site of tenderness. A Prehn sign is unreliable in differentiating torsion from epididymitis. Unfortunately, physical examination will not always lead clearly to the appropriate diagnosis.

DIAGNOSTIC TESTS

The presence or absence of white blood cells within the urine does not allow for the differentiation of epididymitis from torsion. It has been demonstrated that rapid diagnosis of torsion is essential for testicular salvage. It must be emphasized that, if testicular torsion is suspected on the basis of clinical history and physical examination, the patient is best served by immediate scrotal exploration. Because the majority of acute scrotal pathology is treated nonoperatively, a less invasive, rapid, reliable technique is needed to diagnose testicular torsion.

Currently, the "gold standard" for the nonoperative diagnosis of testicular torsion remains radionuclide imaging studies. Radionuclide scanning with technetium-99m pertechnetate is an excellent diagnostic modality with a high degree of sensitivity and reliability. Gray-scale ultrasonography/Doppler flow studies of the scrotum previously have been demonstrated to be unreliable in the diagnosis of testicular torsion. More recently, color flow Doppler ultrasonography has been demonstrated to be as reliable as radionuclide scanning in the diagnosis of the acute scrotum. All of these modalities require the availability of expensive technology, a trained technician, and a radiologist. The color flow Doppler studies are less intensive in this regard, and, therefore, are becoming more widely utilized in the diagnosis of the acute scrotum. However, once again, it should be emphasized that, if testicular torsion is suspected, the appropriate management is acute surgical exploration.

Recently, our laboratory has explored the ability to diagnose testicular torsion on the basis of alterations in the intratesticular pH by the utilization of a percutaneous intratesticular pH probe. Although this technique has been studied only in animal models, it does appear to have the potential to be an inexpensive, reliable, and readily available diagnostic modality. Furthermore, no technical support is required. Further investigation must be carried out prior to the clinical application of this technology.

INITIAL THERAPY

At the time of presentation, an attempt at manual detorsion of the testicle may immediately restore blood flow to the compromised testicle. Because most testicular torsion occurs from outward to inward, the reduction process proceeds from inward to outward. However, torsion may occur to different degrees and in different directions. Therefore, manual detorsion is not generally successful. However, if this maneuver is successful, it may provide valuable time while awaiting an operating theater. The use of lidocaine infiltration of the cord for pain control, while attempting to detorse the testis, adds another risk of vascular compromise to an already compromised testis. We do not employ this therapy.

If detorsion is accomplished manually, the need for emergent surgery is obviated; however, bilateral orchiopexy is performed before discharging the patient. This surgery should be accomplished during the same hospitalization; otherwise, the patient may become complacent, develop a wait-and-see attitude, and not return until another event of testicular torsion occurs.

SURGERY

If testicular torsion is suspected and has not been ruled out, surgical exploration is undertaken as rapidly as possible. The surgical consent should include detorsion with orchiopexy, possible unilateral orchiectomy, and, importantly, orchiopexy of the contralateral testicle. Generally, when the diagnosis is clear, the surgical approach is through a transverse/transscrotal incision. If the scrotal pathology is unclear and the differential diagnosis includes an incarcerated hernia or a testicular tumor, an inguinal approach should be employed.

The more rapid the surgical exploration, the more likely that the testicle will survive. At the time of the procedure, the testicle is detorted. Generally, this is easily accomplished. If not, it may be because a prolonged period of torsion has resulted in a marked inflammatory response with associated vascular thrombosis and necrosis. If the testes is necrotic, the need for orchiectomy is obvious. Conversely, if detorsion results in "pinking up" of the testis with obvious reperfusion, the testis is salvaged and orchiopexy then is accomplished. The difficult clinical decision is what to do with the cyanotic but not frankly necrotic testis. Historically, the approach has been to detorse these testes and leave them in situ with the caveat that "it will either return to normal or at worst undergo secondary atrophy." Secondary atrophy has been reported to occur in 33 to 68 per cent of cases of "salvage." This indicates that a large number of testes that were left in situ had severe vascular compromise.

Although experimental evidence has demonstrated that testes that undergo secondary atrophy subsequently initiate an immunologic response that may affect the contralateral testes and lead to future infertility, this has not been demonstrated clearly to be the case in humans. It has been demonstrated that there may be pre-existing abnormalities in the contralateral testicle at the time of testicle torsion that may be associated with the pathology that allows testicular torsion to occur. Thus, the impact of a vascularly compromised testicle on future fertility remains controversial. Nevertheless, if a testicle is thought to be nonviable, it is best removed at the time of the initial operation to prevent secondary complications. The detorsed, nonviable testicle may simply undergo atrophy, but it also may develop into a necrotic phlegmon requiring secondary orchiectomy.

Although the duration of testicular torsion is significant in determining the subsequent outcome, it does not allow for the fact that the ischemia caused by a given degree of torsion may be accompanied by varying degrees of both arterial and venous obstruction. Therefore, no matter what the duration of the clinical history of torsion, patients should be treated in an emergent fashion. Thus, unless the patient presents with a fixed, nonmobile mass that is clearly the result of a necrotic testis, all patients must be treated emergently.

The classic intraoperative maneuvers (i.e., warming of the testis and checking for active bleeding on the cut surface) are, unfortunately, of limited value. When a testicle continues to be markedly cyanotic and edematous after detorsion, without signs of reperfusion, it is probably most reasonable to remove the testicle to avoid the secondary atrophy and phlegmon production that will be associated with a necrotic testis. Additionally, because the issue of contralateral alterations has yet to be resolved definitively, orchiectomy still may have some protective value.

ORCHIOPEXY

Once it has been determined that the testicle should be salvaged, orchiopexy should be performed. It is important that a nonabsorbable suture be utilized to carry out the "fixation." Testicular torsion after orchiopexy accomplished with absorbable sutures has been reported. For this reason, we use a nonabsorbable suture such as 4-0 silk.

The fixation is carried out by placing two sutures through the lateral aspect of the tunica albuginea and then passing them through the opposing dartos fascia. The tunica vaginalis may be traversed with the suture or removed to aid in this fixation process. One way of assuring an adequate "purchase" of the dartos fascia is to grasp the fascia with an Allis clamp. It is important that the dartos and not just the tunica vaginalis is grasped with this clamp to allow adequate fixation. Once the clamp has been appropriately positioned, 4-0 silk sutures with a "pop-off" needle can be passed into the dartos. One must be certain that the scrotal skin is not puckered or pierced by the suture. The positioning of these clamps is important to be certain that the testicle resides in a dependent location within the scrotum. After the initial sutures are placed, a third suture is placed on the medial aspect of the scrotal compartment. The sutures are then placed through the tunica albuginea of the testicle. Again, the position of the sutures will determine if the testicle will occupy a "comfortable" position within the scrotum. The tunica vaginalis and dartos fascia are then closed with running layers of absorbable suture. The skin is closed with absorbable vertical mattress sutures and Tegaderm is applied to the incision.

An identical procedure is carried out on the contralateral side to prevent contralateral testicular torsion. At times, bilateral orchiopexy can be accomplished through a single incision traversing the median raphe in a horizontal fashion. The dartos of each hemiscrotal compartment is entered directly, and the orchiopexy is carried out as described.

MISSED TESTICULAR TORSION

The patient with missed testicular torsion may present with a testicular mass or testicular atrophy. Although a scrotal abscess can be the result of testicular torsion, this is a rare presentation. Generally, the diagnosis of missed testicular torsion is made on the basis of history and physical examination. A diethylenetriaminepenta-acetic acid testicular scan reveals a "cold" testis surrounded by an area of increased perfusion. The cold area represents the area of absence of perfusion; the rim of increased perfusion results from the surrounding rim of inflammation. Although many of these testes will involute clinically and atrophy without morbidity, in general these are best removed surgically to hasten the recovery of the patient. Furthermore, the potential immunologic stimulus that may result from the atrophic testes is additional reason to remove these necrotic testes. Again, at the time of this exploration orchiectomy, the contralateral testicle must undergo orchiopexy. If the diagnosis of missed testicular torsion is unclear, an inguinal approach should be utilized.

TESTICULAR PROSTHESIS

In general, we do not advocate the placement of a testicular prosthesis at the time of orchiectomy for testicular torsion because of the intense inflammatory response that accompanies the necrotic testis.

SUMMARY

Testicular torsion is a true urologic emergency. An accurate and definitive diagnosis is mandatory. Generally, the history and physical examination will allow an appropriate diagnosis to be rendered, and surgical exploration can be based on these findings. However, when a low index of suspicion exists, adjunctive diagnostic tests can be utilized. Testicular radionuclide scanning remains a sensitive and specific test; however, it is cumbersome and costly. The advent and the ready availability of color flow Doppler ultrasonography have dramatically changed the approach to the low-suspicion acute scrotum. When surgery is performed, whether to remove or to fix the involved testis remains a difficult urologic decision that must be based on the clinical findings at the time of the procedure. The surgical approach of attempting to salvage all torsed testes at all costs, assuming the worst that can happen will be the occurrence of secondary atrophy, is no longer appropriate. However, the "wholesale" removal of testes is not advocated. Importantly, any patient who experiences testicular torsion must be treated surgically, and the appropriate surgical treatment must include orchiopexy of the contralateral testis.

Suggested Readings

Bartsch G, Frank S, Marberger H, et al: Testicular torsion: Late results with special regard to fertility and endocrine function. J Urol 124:375, 1980

Burks DD, Markey BJ, Burkhard TK, et al: Suspected testicular torsion and ischemia: Evaluation with color Doppler sonography. J Radiol 175:815–821, 1990

Hadziselimovic F, Snyder H, Duckett J, et al: Testicular histology in children with unilateral testicular torsion. J Urol 136(1 Pt 2):208–210, 1986

Krarup KS: The testis after torsion. Br J Urol 50:43, 1978

Nagler HM, Kogan S, Consentino MJ: Experimental aspects of testicular torsion. *In* R. Rabinowitz (ed): Dialogues in Pediatric Urology, vol. 8. Pearl River, WJ Miller Associates, 1985, pp 1–8

Nagler HM, White RV: The effect of testicular torsion in the contralateral testis. J Urol 128:1341, 1982

HYDROCELE AND SPERMATOCELE

STEPHEN A. ZDERIC, M.D.

Philadelphia, Pennsylvania

HYDROCELE

The fetal testes develops in the retroperitoneum and descends into its final scrotal position, bringing with it two investing layers of peritoneum. The tunica albuginea, which is intimately attached to the testes, is analogous to visceral peritoneum. The tunica vaginalis represents the parietal peritoneum, which forms a sack within the scrotal wall that contains the testes. Normally, within this sack a few drops of fluid are found that allow the visceral and parietal surfaces to slide over each other. The testes is prevented from twisting on its blood supply by an extension of visceral peritoneum that anchors the chord and part of the testes to the back of the scrotal wall and the tunica vaginalis. When this connection is missing, it is referred to as the bell clapper anomaly, which places a patient at risk for testicular torsion. Under normal conditions, only 1 to 3 ml of fluid are contained within this space, and a balance exists between fluid secretion and reabsorption. A hydrocele results when there is an imbalance between fluid production and reabsorption.

Diagnosis and Treatment in the Pediatric Patient

In the pediatric population, hydroceles commonly are diagnosed in the newborn nursery or in early infancy. Such hydroceles may be communicating and are characterized by a history of changes in size with position or crying. A communicating hydrocele must be assessed carefully to see if there is any evidence that abdominal visceral contents are passing into the scrotum, in which case a hernia is present. Communicating hydroceles result from a patent processus vaginalis that allows for entry of peritoneal fluid into the scrotum, where it becomes trapped. In some cases the fluid escapes intermittently, allowing for hydrocele resolution, and sometimes this occurs during the physical examination of the patient. Often one must rely on the history that is communicated by the family in arriving at the diagnosis. If the scrotal examination is normal, but there is a history of intermittent swelling, one should examine the spermatic cord by rolling the structures between the thumb and forefinger and feeling for a thickened sack (the "silk glove" sign). Noncommunicating hydroceles often are seen in infancy as well, and tend to resolve spontaneously.

The management of communicating and noncommunicating hydroceles in infancy is similar: with few exceptions most are followed conservatively and many resolve spontaneously by 12 months of age. The urologist always should remember that, in 20 per cent of asymptomatic adults at autopsy, a probe-patent processus vaginalis is found. It is rare that an infant hydrocele will require repair prior to 12 months of age. However, if the hydrocele is progressively enlarging, a sliding hernia develops that is not easily reduced, or a neurosurgical shunt must be placed, early inguinal exploration is permissible. Communicating hydroceles that have not resolved by 12 to 18 months of age are unlikely to do so, and may be surgically repaired.

The pediatric hydrocele is diagnosed clinically, and treatment should be based on clinical grounds. A cystic mass that transilluminates is the classic finding. If the testis cannot be palpated or feels abnormal, an ultrasound may be obtained, but this should not be performed routinely.

In a healthy child hydrocele repair is easily accomplished as a day surgery procedure. An inguinal approach is utilized; the external ring is identified and the fascia of the external oblique is opened to allow for exposure of the spermatic cord contents. The patent processus vaginalis lies on the upper outer aspect of the cord and may be teased away from the vessels and vas using blunt forceps. The dissection of the patent processus should proceed in a proximal fashion until the lip of the peritoneum is identified; at this point, a high ligation may be carried out with a vicryl suture. If the sack is very thin and difficult to handle, it is often better to open the sack and then carefully peel the layer off of the spermatic vessels and vas under direct vision. In infants and small children, loupes or other optical magnification are helpful with this dissection. If one cannot readily identify a patent processus vaginalis, the error to avoid is overdissection of the mid-cord structures. At this point the surgeon should focus attention on the internal ring and identify the peritoneum and its relationship to the gonadal vessels. In this manner one can identify the sack at its point of origin before it thins out.

In addition to ligation of the patent processus, it is worthwhile to bring the testes up into the incision, and open up the remaining investing layer of the tunica albuginea. It is my preference to fold the tunica back behind the testes and epididymis and tack it with one or two stitches so as to prevent a fluid accumulation in the scrotum postoperatively. If these basic principles are followed, repair of the pediatric hydrocele will give gratifying results.

Diagnosis and Treatment in the Adult Patient

Adult hydroceles are primarily of the noncommunicating variety. They may occur secondary to inflammatory (epididymitis), trauma, spermatic vein ligation, or, rarely, malignancy (primary testicular neoplasm or lymphoma). It generally is believed that most adult noncommunicating hydroceles have an inflammatory basis, and the process may often be subclinical. In third-world nations, the parasites *Wucheria bancrofti* and *Loa loa* may cause hydroceles. It is important to remember that 5 to 10 per cent of testicular neoplasms present with a hydrocele, and this makes careful palpation of the testes of paramount importance. If the testes cannot be palpated or if the exam is anything but normal, scrotal ultrasonography is indicated. Adult hydroceles of the communicating variety may present after the insertion of a peritoneal dialysis catheter, and these must be treated by surgical ligation of the patent processus vaginalis using the same techniques as outlined for the infant hydrocele.

The surgical management of the adult hydrocele differs from that in infancy in that a scrotal approach provides adequate exposure and an easier recovery. An inguinal incision is mandatory if there is any history of communication (variation in hydrocele size). The scrotum is prepped and draped, a transverse or median raphe incision is made, and dissection is carried down to the tunica vaginalis. The dartos muscle, fascia, and skin are peeled away from the tunica vaginalis as much as possible. This dissection is easiest when the sack is left intact, although, in the case of massive hydroceles, drainage of the fluid makes the case simpler. Once the hydrocele sack is entered, the testes, epididymis, and cord structures are identified, and this allows for the excess tunica vaginalis to be excised. It is my preference to do this with electrocautery to minimize any bleeding. At this point the excess sack may be wrapped around the testes and epididymis and the edges may be sutured to each other with two or three interrupted 3-0 vicryl sutures. An alternative method calls for running a chromic or vicryl stitch around the edges of the sack after the excision of the excess tunic.

Adult hydroceles may be managed "medically" with sclerotherapy if they are small enough or the patient presents a medical risk for anesthesia. This approach is absolutely contraindicated if there is any evidence to suggest a communicating hydrocele is present (after dialysis catheter placement). This technique evolved in England and is now favored over open surgery in Europe. The scrotum is scrubbed with betadine, and 1% lidocaine is used to numb the skin. The puncture into the scrotum should be made at the top of the scrotum so as to avoid the leakage of scleroscant. A 16-gauge angiocath is used to aspirate the hydrocele fluid, and the fluid is replaced with lidocaine or bupivicaine to allow for local anesthesia. The aspirated fluid must be perfectly clear; a bloody tap should raise the possibility of malignancy and the procedure should be abandoned in favor of open exploration. After 20 minutes to allow for numbing of the tunica vaginalis, the sclerosant should be injected into the hydrocele sack and the angiocath withdrawn. Anywhere from 4 to 10 ml of sclerosant may be used, and the higher the strength of the solution, the greater the need for instillation of local anesthesia. Lower strength solutions lessen the need for using lidocaine but increase the number of treatments required. Many choices for scleroscants are available, but the most popular choice is 5% tetracycline preceded by the instillation of 2 ml of 0.5% bupivicaine. Other alternatives include 5% ethanolamine, with which a success rate of 98 per cent was reported in a series of 158 patients. With scleroscant techniques success rates of 80 to 98 per cent may be attained depending on the series.

SPERMATOCELE

A spermatocele is a cystic dilation of the epididymis that is characterized by the inclusion of speramatozoa on examination of the fluid. These are usually painless swellings of the epididymis that are well circumscribed on physical examination, and may easily be diagnosed clinically. If there is any question as to the nature of any epididymal mass, an ultrasound is indicated. Most of these cysts may be followed conservatively and will need no further therapy. If the size is increasing or symptoms appear, open surgical excision is an option in management. However, the instillation of a scleroscant agent as outlined above will produce a 70 per cent success rate. The use of sclerotherapy in epididymal cysts should be limited to men for whom reproduction is no longer an issue because of a danger of epididymitis.

Suggested Readings

Epstein A, Novicki DE: Management of hydroceles. AUA Update Series, vol 7, lesson 19, 1988

Rodriguez WC, Rodriguez DD, Fortuno RF: The operative treatment of hydrocele: A comparison of 4 basic techniques. J Urol 125:804, 1981

Tammela T, Hellstrom PA, Mattila SP, et al: Ethanolamine oleate sclerotherapy for hydroceles and spermatoceles: A survey of 158 patients with ultrasound followup. J Urol 147:1551, 1992

Inflammations

EPIDIDYMITIS AND ORCHITIS

THOMAS P. BALL, Jr., M.D.

San Antonio, Texas

EPIDIDYMITIS

Acute epididymitis refers to inflammation or infection limited to the epididymis. It is the most common intrascrotal inflammation, now accounting for more than 600,000 yearly visits to health care providers in this country alone. Infection usually spreads to the epididymis in a retrograde fashion through the vas from the posterior urethra or prostate, although hematogenous dissemination doubtless occurs. In its mildest forms, it may involve only a portion of the epididymis, with localized tenderness, but most commonly it spreads to involve the entire epididymis and sometimes the vas deferens (deferentitis) or even the tissues of the spermatic cord (funiculitis), in which case the diagnosis even has been confused with appendicitis. In a small percentage of patients (usually in the older patient), the infection or inflammation may extend into the testis, making the diagnosis of epididymo-orchitis appropriate. Usually, however, epididymo-orchitis is a misnomer often applied to the patient who only has a severe epididymitis with an inflammatory hydrocele and edema of the overlying scrotal wall, making examination and differentiation of the scrotal contents quite difficult. In this situation, testicular torsion and tumor must be ruled out.

Types of Epididymitis

Epididymitis should be divided into three categories. In general terms, these categories are bacterial epididymitis, nonbacterial epididymitis (usually caused by *Chlamydia trachomatis* or mycoplasma organisms), and traumatic or chemical epididymitis. Infertility is a not infrequent result of epididymitis as a result of a sexually transmitted pathogen, but it can be seen with any form of this disease.

Bacterial Epididymitis

Acute bacterial epididymitis frequently is seen as a complication of prolonged catheter drainage, bacterial prostatitis, and gonococcal or nongonococcal bacterial urethritis. It occurs commonly in the presence of urethral pathology such as stricture disease and meatal stenosis and may follow self-instrumentation or instrumentation during urologic evaluation. Epididymitis is usually unilateral but may be seen bilaterally in rare cases. Aside from gonococcal infection, the most common bacterial etiologic agent is *Escherichia coli*, especially in homosexual men. However, virtually every known organism and type of infection has at one time been associated with epididymitis, including *Candida*, *Pseudomonas aeruginosa*, tuberculosis, brucellosis, coccidioidomycosis, blastomycosis, and even schistosomiasis. Cytomegalovirus epididymitis has been seen in immunocompromised patients following renal transplantation.

The patient usually presents with heaviness and dull, aching discomfort on the affected side of the scrotum. Fever, chills, and malaise may accompany the onset of epididymitis, and physical examination will reveal swelling, induration, and exquisite tenderness of part or all of the affected epididymis. The testis hangs low in the scrotum, and discomfort may be relieved somewhat by elevation and support (Prehn sign), as opposed to testicular torsion, in which the testis is usually high in the scrotum and pain is aggravated by further elevation. Pyuria and bacteriuria usually are present. In most cases, the infecting organism will be present in the urine or prostatic fluid and can be identified by culture of a freshly voided specimen, urethral smear, secretions obtained by gentle prostatic massage, or direct aspiration of the epididymis. In the presence of urethritis, the discharge should be cultured and sensitivities obtained to guide therapy. As always, tuberculosis must be considered in the differential diagnosis, particularly in protracted cases and when no bacterial organisms are identified. Appropriate cultures and skin tests should be performed.

Nonbacterial Epididymitis

Acute nonbacterial epididymitis is probably the most commonly encountered form of epididymitis. Most cases currently are thought to be secondary to infection by a sexually transmitted pathogen, usually *C. trachomatis*. It is occasionally found in the presence of a nonspecific urethritis, and, although the urine may show evidence of infection with mild pyuria, routine bacterial cultures are generally sterile. In laboratories capable of isolating the *Chlamydia* organism, a positive culture is confirmatory. *Ureaplasma urealyticum* likewise has been associated with nonspecific urethritis and epididymitis and also might serve an etiologic role. Antibiotic therapy is essential, as is treatment of the sexual partner.

Traumatic or Chemical Epididymitis

Traumatic or chemical epididymitis (recruit epididymitis) is common in the younger population and is one of the leading causes of disability and hospitalization in young males during basic military training. This condition is believed to be secondary to reflux of sterile urine down the vas with trauma or straining with a full bladder.

Reflux of urine from the prostatic fossa into the vas has long been known to occur and has been demonstrated repeatedly on voiding cystourethrograms, particularly in the presence of distal obstruction. Epididymitis has been shown to occur in infants with urethral valves through this mechanism, and, in all likelihood, the pressure and chemical irritation of urine within the delicate epididymis are all that is necessary to produce the typical clinical picture.

Symptoms here are generally secondary to an inflammation rather than an infection, although the presentation may be the same. The majority of patients are afebrile, but some present with a low-grade fever and scrotal findings that are identical to the bacterial form except that there is usually less involvement of the overlying skin. Urologic pathology is rare in the absence of preceding urologic symptoms. Not infrequently, the patient will give a clear-cut history of the onset of pain in the affected side of the scrotum while lifting, running, or straining with a full bladder.

Direct trauma also can produce epididymitis. This may occur as the result of a direct blow or even following a difficult vasectomy. In the latter instance, epididymitis most commonly is encountered about 3 to 4 weeks after vasectomy in patients in whom excessive epididymal trauma occurred during the procedure because of a short scrotum, tenseness of the patient, pre-existing pathology, or inexperience on the part of the operator. Repeated squeezing of the epididymis in attempts to both isolate and immobilize the vas seems to be a common factor, although entry of bacteria through the incision site could well be an additional source of infection in those with positive cultures. As in the case of chemical epididymitis, cultures in these patients are usually sterile, however.

Epididymitis in Children

The finding of acute epididymitis in children is rare, being noted in only 3 of 847 cases reviewed at our institution. Indeed, the differential diagnosis of acute testicular torsion must be entertained, because this is a far more common finding and one that requires immediate management. Also to be considered, even in the young child, are gonorrhea, testicular tumors, the fortunately rare rhabdomyosarcoma of the cord, and even child abuse.

The presence of epididymitis in children under the age of 10 should immediately suggest the possibility of obstructive disease involving the urethra, such as urethral valves, urethral stricture, meatal stenosis, or the presence of an acute urethritis. Urinary reflux into the vas deferens from the prostatic fossa already has been discussed as a possible etiology, and this has been particularly well demonstrated to occur in children, having been seen in over 10 per cent of voiding cystourethrograms of children with urethral valves.

Typically, epididymitis will be found in the child with one of the anatomic defects mentioned above and usually will be manifested by isolated tenderness and swelling of the epididymis, pyuria, and perhaps the presence of a mucoid or purulent urethral discharge. Often, the epididymitis will be of sufficient severity and duration to present with a tense, inflammatory hydrocele, which makes definitive examination of the scrotal contents impossible. Under these circumstances, surgical exploration is advisable unless pyuria is present and a typical history of gradual onset, urethral discharge, or instrumentation is obtained. Even in these latter instances it has been considered by many that the use of exploration and drainage of the tense, inflammatory hydrocele is the more conservative approach and may well hasten recovery.

Differential Diagnosis

Testicular scanning and the use of Doppler ultrasound have been recommended in children and adults as adjuncts in differential diagnosis of epididymitis and testicular torsion, and in some cases have been quite helpful. Scanning is performed by injecting 3 to 7 mCi of technetium-99m, followed by scanning 10 minutes later. In torsion, radioactive uptake will be decreased, whereas with epididymitis there will be increased uptake. With use of the Doppler ultrasound, it has been found that blood flow is decreased over the testis and epididymis in torsion but will be increased with the hyperemia and inflammation of epididymitis. If abscess is suspected, scrotal ultrasound may confirm the fluid loculation and lead to earlier exploration and a shorter period of disability.

Management

The management of epididymitis in general includes bed rest and scrotal elevation, both of which reduce the vascular engorgement and contribute to the relief of discomfort and resolution of the inflammatory response. Ice packs and cold compresses likewise are used to reduce hyperemia, inflammation, and discomfort. The pain is occasionally severe enough to require narcotics but most often can be managed with less potent analgesics such as oxycodone hydrochloride (Percodan) or hydrocodone bitartrate (Vicodin), one tablet every 4 to 6 hours, propoxyphene hydrochloride (Darvon) in combination with aspirin or acetominophen (Darvocet-N), or acetominophen compounds alone (especially in children). Codeine in doses of 0.5 grain either alone or in combination with aspirin-containing compounds is also effective, but one must be aware of the tendency for constipation with these medications, and it is advisable to avoid straining at stool if at all possible. Mild laxatives and stool softeners also have been of benefit in this regard.

Antibiotic therapy in all cases should be governed by the results of urine and semen cultures and sensitivities. This is certainly true in the case of those patients with indwelling catheters or pre-existing urinary tract infection. The fluoroquinolones are used most commonly in these cases unless the presence of sepsis dictates use of more potent IV antibiotic combinations.

In the absence of positive bacterial cultures, one should consider *C. trachomatis* as the likely etiologic organism, particularly in the presence of pyuria or irritative symptoms, and in this case one of the tetracyclines usually is employed. If the epididymitis follows gonococcal or nongonococcal (nonspecific) urethritis believed to be secondary to chlamydial infection, tetracycline usually is administered in doses of 1.5 gm stat, followed by 500 mg every 6 hours for 4 days. Suspected chlamydial epididymitis in the absence of urethritis may be managed with doxycycline 100 mg bid or 500 mg of tetracycline every 6 hours for the first 48 hours, reducing the dosage to 250 mg every 6 hours for the remainder of a 7- to 10-day course of therapy. In either event, sexual partners should be cultured or tested for serum antibodies to *C. trachomatis* and be treated simultaneously with tetracycline to eliminate the source of reinfection and to prevent possible complications in the female. In the absence of fever and pyuria, patients whose symptoms suggest "chemical epididymitis" usually are managed without antibiotics and respond well to nonspecific therapy. Tetracyclines also may be used in the older child who is past the age of dental development.

Ibuprofen (Motrin, Advil) and naproxen (Naprosyn) are frequently employed nonsteroidal anti-inflammatory agents, and their use is thought to hasten recovery. In view of the efficacy of steroids in mumps orchitis, one might suspect a similar effect with epididymitis, but this has not been the case. Intramuscular and oral enzyme preparations likewise have not proven effective in this condition.

Injection of the spermatic cord with 1% or 2% lidocaine is a very effective method of reducing pain in acute cases and often provides relief for many hours. Although it is not often employed, this modality is worthwhile in those with severe pain and as a prelude to examination when torsion is a reasonable consideration. Lidocaine may be combined in equal portions with bupivacaine (Marcaine) for longer lasting results, but the latter should not be used in children under the age of 12 years.

Extreme care must be taken with any patient who presents with the appearance of sepsis, as manifested by high fever and chills. Even healthy young adults have been known to die from sepsis secondary to epididymitis, and these patients should be treated as are those with sepsis resulting from any other cause, with (1) blood and other appropriate cultures; (2) intravenous fluids; (3) broad-spectrum antibiotics, such as the combination of gentamycin plus vancomycin or ampicillin; and (4) close monitoring of vital signs for early detection of hypotension or other evidence of sepsis.

In severe or recurrent cases of epididymitis, particularly in the elderly, one should consider prompt exploration with drainage and primary epididymectomy as definitive therapy. Removing the source of infection in this manner greatly hastens recovery and prevents further recurrence. Epididymectomy may be performed under local anesthesia if desired and involves simply delivering the testis through a midline raphe incision, then incising the tunica vaginalis at the attachment of the epididymis to the scrotal wall with a secondary parallel incision in the testiculo-epididymal groove. This delineates the epididymis and protects the testicular blood supply. The epididymis then can be bluntly and sharply dissected free of the testicular attachments. The vas is ligated, as are the vessels to the epididymis, and, after closing the fascia over the posterior aspect of the testicle, the scrotum is drained through a separate stab wound in its most dependent portion. Routine skin closure of the scrotum then is performed. By use of this method, hospitalization and absence from work have been reduced by half in several series.

Ambulation can be begun once the patient is free of pain and there is evidence of resolution of his inflammatory reaction. Snug diapers for children or jockey shorts should be advised once ambulation has begun. Because of the high incidence of infertility in those with a history of bilateral epididymitis (40 per cent in some series, and up to 25 per cent in those with unilateral epididymitis), urologic evaluation to determine the cause of the epididymitis and to rule out the presence of significant urologic pathology should be performed, and patients and their families should be warned of the advisability of immediate resumption of bed rest if pain should recur or develop on the opposite side.

Chronic Epididymitis

A small percentage of patients may have several recurrences of epididymitis and develop chronic induration and pain, especially if there is associated infection in the prostate or seminal vesicles. Although some will respond to long-term low-dose medication, such as trimethoprim-sulfamethoxazole, the majority benefit most from epididymectomy. If fertility is no longer a consideration, chronic epididymitis probably is best handled early by simple epididymectomy, although one must be aware that the incidence of persistent discomfort in this group may run as high as 25 per cent.

ORCHITIS

Orchitis refers to infection limited to the parenchyma of the testis itself. As mentioned in the introductory discussion of epididymitis, the testis can be involved with ascending infection from the epididymis through the ductuli efferentes to the seminiferous tubules. This is referred to as epididymo-orchitis. Primary orchitis is more rare, usually resulting from local involvement as a manifestation of a systemic disease.

The most frequent cause of orchitis is mumps. Most commonly the result of postpubertal infection, mumps orchitis can produce sufficient edema to result in bilateral atrophy and hypergonadotrophic hypogonadism with gynecomastia and infertility. Fortunately, the incidence of this condition is decreasing since the development of the mumps vaccine.

Other less common causes of orchitis include gonorrhea, syphilis, leprosy, tuberculosis, and filariasis. Hematogenous spread of *E. coli* has been reported to have occurred in a newborn.

Treatment is management of the basic disease, with supportive measures to include bed rest, ice packs, and elevation of the scrotum. Broad-spectrum antibiotics should be used pending results of specific cultures. Aspiration of the often-encountered tense hydrocele may result in significant symptomatic relief as well as provide fluid for culture.

Suggested Readings

Berger RE: Sexually transmitted diseases. Campbell's Urology, 6th ed, Philadelphia, WB Saunders, 1992, pp 830–832

Melekos MD, Asbach HW: Epididymitis: Aspects concerning etiology and treatment. J Urol 138:83, 1988

Mittemeyer BT, Lennox KW, Borski AA: Epididymitis: A review of 610 cases. J Urol 95:390, 1966

Tumors

SEMINOMA

E. JAMES SEIDMON, M.D.

Philadelphia, Pennsylvania

There are approximately 3000 to 4000 new cases of testicular carcinoma seen each year in the United States. Primary testicular tumors most commonly are found in patients ranging from 20 to 40 years of age, with a noted predominance in white males (3.7:100,000 versus 0.9:100,000 in black males), and account for 1 to 2 per cent of all neoplasms in males. Only two decades ago these tumors were the most common cause of solid tumor death, but, with the advancement of chemotherapy, radiotherapy, and improved diagnostic techniques as well as surgical skills, the survival rate now exceeds 90 per cent, making testis tumors the most curable cancer in all age groups. Treatment has progressed to the point at which radiotherapy alone or limited chemotherapy combined with a modified retroperitoneal lymph node dissection has led to decreased morbidity and improved quality of life for these patients.

The etiology of testicular tumors may relate to the essential development of the testes and may be affected by cryptorchidism (which accounts for 7 to 10 per cent of all testes tumors), environmental factors, age, gonadal dysgenesis, atrophy, heredity, and ethnic background. Hormonal excess by the mother in the form of diethylstilbestrol (DES) has been linked to the production of Leydig cell tumors. Less than 3 per cent of these tumors are bilateral and they are either synchronous or asynchronous. Histologically they may be the same, and they probably should be considered as new tumors.

CLASSIFICATION AND STAGING

Classification of testicular carcinoma has been limited to only the primary neoplasms. The vast majority of testicular tumors (90 to 95 per cent) arise from the germinal epithelium, and it is believed that a totipotential germ cell gives rise to both the seminoma and the nonseminomatous germ cell testis tumor. Nonseminomatous tumors undergo hematogenous spread more frequently and earlier than seminomas. There are three peak incidences for germ cell tumors: the most common is between the ages of 20 and 40, another peak occurs after the age of 60 (usually a lymphoma), and a third peak occurs at less than 2 years of age (usually a yolk sack tumor or occasionally a teratoma that acts in a benign manner).

For staging purposes, testicular germ cell tumors can be divided into pure seminoma and nonseminomatous categories (mixed tumors with seminoma fall into the latter category).

The staging of testicular carcinoma is presented in Table 1. Pathologic staging categories are Stage A: limited to the testis and cord; Stage B_1: microscopic metastases to six or fewer regional nodes or gross metastasis less than or equal to 2 cm in size; Stage B_2: microscopic metastases to more than six regional lymph nodes or gross metastases greater than 2 but less than 6 cm in diameter; Stage B_3: bulky retroperitoneal metastases greater than 6 cm; and Stage C: metastases above the diaphragm. Clinical staging uses corresponding Roman numerals (I, IIA, IIB, IIC, and III).

TABLE 1. Pathologic and Clinical Staging of Testicular Carcinoma

Stage A (I)	Tumor confined to the testis
Stage B_1 (IIa)	Few nodes in the retroperitoneum usually detected at time of node dissection
Stage B_2 (IIb)	Nodes greater than 2 to 6 cm
Stage B_3 (IIc)	Nodes greater than 6 cm
Stage C (III)	Spread above the diaphragm, especially to the lungs or involving abdominal solid organs

Computerized tomography (CT) remains the imaging method of choice for staging of patients with testicular germ cell tumor, with magnetic resonance imaging (MRI) reserved for selected problem cases.

TUMOR DISSEMINATION

The spread of testicular carcinomas occurs in a predictable fashion. Initially, dissemination is via the lymphatics. Testicular lymph drainage follows the gonadal veins: from the left testis to the para- and preaortic nodes just below the left renal vein (L1–L2), and from the right testis to the interaortic and paracaval nodes at the level of L2–L3 (right renal hilum, junction of right gonadal vein with the inferior vena cava). Crossover, particularly right to left, can occur via anomalous channels, but clinically some ipsilateral nodes almost always are present. Drainage into the ipsilateral upper external iliac nodes can occur but usually is seen only after adenopathy at the renal hilar level. Internal iliac and femoral nodes usually are not involved unless there has been trans-scrotal orchiectomy or other scrotal/inguinal surgery. If the primary tumor has spread beyond the capsule, atypical patterns of adenopathy can be seen.

From these sentinel nodes at the levels of the renal hila, which are rarely opacified by bipedal lymphangiography, spread occurs to the para-aortic/paracaval nodes and then the retrocrural nodes from T11 to L4. Dissemination then occurs to the posterior mediastinal, subcarinal, hilar, anterior mediastinal, and supraclavicular nodes or hematogenously to the lung, liver, bone, and brain. Chest metastases are usually to mediastinal nodes in patients with seminoma.

Unusual sites of testicular tumor metastasis include the kidney, adrenals, inferior vena cava, muscle, spleen, stomach, central pelvis, seminal vesicles, prostate, and pericardium. CT can depict these in previously untreated patients in the absence of retroperitoneal nodes, although unusual sites are far more likely to be seen in relapse after chemotherapy and/or retroperitoneal lymph node dissection.

CLINICAL PRESENTATION AND DIAGNOSIS

Clinically, the patient often will present with painless swelling or a heavy feeling in his scrotum. He may palpate the area and note a hardness or lump in the testicle. Pain and inflammation also may be the presenting factors and may cause the tumor to be confused with epididymitis, leading to delay in treatment. Clinical manifestations of advanced disease also may include a mass in the supraclavicular region, gynecomastia, or a palpable abdominal mass. Having ruled out epididymitis or orchitis, the differential diagnosis should include torsion or trauma.

Serum markers measured as a diagnostic aid include the β chain of serum human chorionic gonadotropin (hCG) and alpha-fetoprotein; the serum half-life for the former is approximately 45 minutes and that for the latter is 5 days. In pure seminoma, 5 to 10 per cent of patients will have elevated beta-hCG and histologic staining will demonstrate syncytiotrophoblast-like cells, whereas if there is an elevation of alpha-fetoprotein, one must look for a nonseminomatous element. A secondary serum marker, lactic dehydrogenase, also can be studied, especially in the treatment of advanced seminoma.

Ultrasound Diagnosis

Malignant testicular tumors produce a focal or diffuse alteration of the normal homogeneous testicular echo texture on ultrasound. Most frequently, the abnormality is a focal hypoechoic region without increased through transmission. With modern high-resolution, real-time equipment, 3- to 4-mm lesions can be detected. Necrosis and/or hemorrhage produces a complex mass with cystic and solid components. Occasionally there is total parenchymal replacement with a diffuse hypoechoic alteration in echo texture.

When a hypoechoic or complex intratesticular mass is seen, diagnostic considerations include abscess, orchitis, granulomatous disease, torsion, and infarct in addition to malignancy. Infarcts are generally indistinguishable from tumors, but sonographic clues to the other conditions exist. Findings of epididymal enlargement, indistinct and abnormal parenchyma surrounding a focal lesion, a large hydrocele, and scrotal skin thickening, separately or in combination, favor an inflammatory disease or torsion over neoplasm. Purely echogenic masses are often benign.

Differential diagnosis of a diffusely hypoechoic testis must include orchitis and global infarction (usually from torsion). Features favoring malignancy include heterogeneous testicular echo texture, lobular contour, and marked testicular enlargement. Features favoring benign disease include skin thickening, epididymal enlargement, smooth contour, homogeneous testicular texture, and no more than mild testicular enlargement.

Seminoma usually presents as a focal, homogeneous, poorly marginated, hypoechoic mass. Less common appearances are a well-marginated focal hypoechoic mass with an apparent capsule and an inhomogeneous focal mass with regions of increased echogenicity. A characteristic but uncommon sonographic appearance that suggests the specific diagnosis of seminoma is diffuse hypoechoic alteration of the echo texture of the entire testis accompanied by enlargement (acute lymphocytic leukemia will produce the same appearance).

It is unusual but not rare for germ cell tumors to present as mediastinal, retroperitoneal, or cervical masses with testes that are normal to palpation. The true incidence of this phenomenon is unknown because, prior to the advent of testicular sonography, many of these patients were presumed without proof to have extragonadal germ cell tumors. When testicular primaries are found by ultrasound in these patients, findings are reported to include: focal hypoechoic mass, diffusely hypoechoic testis, focal hypoechoic mass within a diffusely hypoechoic testis, and necrotic mass (anechoic center). Spontaneously regressed germ cell tumors are frequent findings in the testicle ipsilateral to adenopathy from purportedly extragonadal germ cell tumors. They manifest sonographically as small echogenic regions with or without shadowing. The pathologic correlate is a fibrotic scar. Calcification is generally present when there is shadowing.

Diagnosis with MRI

On MRI, seminomas are reported to be nearly isointense with testicular parenchyma on T_1-weighted images. T_2-weighted images depict seminomas as homogeneous or mildly inhomogeneous masses hypointense compared to residual parenchyma. The entire parenchyma can be replaced, and seminomas may be bilateral, making comparison with normal parenchyma impossible, so that knowledge of the expected parenchymal signal strength is important. Loss of the expected low-intensity rim of the tunica albuginea is a sign of invasion, and spread to the epididymis and spermatic cord may be seen as focal nodular enlargement of the same signal intensity as the primary tumor.

Metastatic lymph nodes usually are homogeneous on MRI; however, when necrosis, hemorrhage, or teratomatous change develops (CT correlate is cystic appearance), the MRI appearance will be altered. When the fluid in the mass is serous, it will appear more hypointense than usual on T_1-weighted images and more hyperintense than usual on T_2-weighted images. Subacute bleeding will result in hyperintensity on T_1-weighted images.

Currently, MRI is hampered relative to CT by less availability, greater cost, longer imaging time, inferiority for detecting small pulmonary parenchymal nodules, and lack of a suitable bowel contrast agent. Its advantages are lack of ionizing radiation, no need for intravenous contrast, good differentiation of lymph nodes from blood vessels, and little or no artifact from surgical clips.

TREATMENT

Initial treatment for testicular carcinoma includes measurement of serum markers followed by a radical orchiectomy via an inguinal approach. This approach is used because scrotal incision will lead to seeding of the superficial inguinal lymphatics. If the serum markers are elevated initially and return to normal following radical orchiectomy, and radiologic staging examinations of the retroperitoneum and chest are negative, the disease is probably confined to the testis and may have been eradicated by the orchiectomy. Elevation of serum markers may precede any other clinical detection method in the previously treated patient who is undergoing relapse.

Stage A (I) seminomatous tumors presently are treated with 2500 to 3000 rads to the periaortic and ipsilateral inguinopelvic lymph nodes, with a 5-year survival rate greater than 90 per cent. Surveillance of Stage A disease following radical orchiectomy is not recommended because limited radiotherapy offers excellent survival statistics with minimal side effects. Stage B_1 (IIa) tumors with limited nodal disease still are treated with radiotherapy up to 4500 rads. Concomitant mediastinal radiotherapy is withheld so that bleomycin may be utilized if the disease progresses or is recurrent. All of the more advanced stages of seminoma with bulky abdominal nodes and/or pulmonary nodules now are being treated essentially with the same chemotherapy as that used for nonseminomatous tumors, and survival is usually greater than 75 per cent.

It is important to stress that, to enter a surveillance regimen, a patient must have a negative chest radiography (preferably chest computerized tomography [CT]), lymphangiogram, abdominal CT scan, and serum markers. Patients should be excluded from a surveillance program if they have had a previous inguinal or scrotal operation or if the tumor invades the cord or inguinal lymphatics. These patients must be evaluated frequently in order to start therapy if recurrence is noted. Thus, they require measurement of serum markers and chest radiographs monthly for 1 year and then every 2 months for the second or third year. Abdominal CT scans should be obtained every 3 months for the first year and every 6 months for the second and third years. Appropriate follow-up after the third year is essential.

Chemotherapy for testes tumors was first reported in 1960 by Li et al., who reported the combination of actinomycin D, chlorambucil, and methotrexate. Single-agent therapy using vinblastine, mithramycin, or methotrexate was evaluated during that decade as well. Breakthrough chemotherapy began with the use of cis-platinum and combination therapy of vinblastine and bleomycin in the following decade. Finally, cytoreductive chemotherapy for minimal and moderate disease began using three courses of cisplatin, etoposide, and bleomycin, which showed excellent complete clinical remission; in advanced disease, four courses of the same regimen now are being used. Other treatment protocols include the use of cyclophosphamide and Adriamycin. Finally, in those patients who fail to have a complete response or have residual active tumor following retroperitoneal lymphadenectomy, salvage chemotherapy with cisplatin, etoposide, and ifosfamide appears to be effective.

Seminomas are extremely radiosensitive; therefore lymphadenectomy is rarely employed. Subclinical metastases in clinical Stage A diseases are controlled by elective radiotherapy to the para-aortic and ipsilateral iliac/inguinal nodes or chemotherapy. Chemotherapy rather than total abdominal irradiation is necessary for Stage B_2 or B_3 tumors because bulky adenopathy may lead to retrograde flow through the lymphatics, resulting in unusual sites of spread. Accurate CT localization of the sites and margins of tumor is important when reduced fields are used. Stage C disease is treated with chemotherapy or combined radiotherapy and chemotherapy. CT of the pelvis, abdomen, and chest should be used for initial staging. Mediastinal metastases (especially to subcarinal and posterior mediastinal nodes) are more prevalent than parenchymal metastases, and chest CT is superior to chest radiography in the depiction of both forms of metastatic disease. Knowledge that anterior mediastinal involvement is quite unusual for testicular germ cell tumors and posterior mediastinal involvement is not a feature of primary mediastinal germ cell tumors may abbreviate the search for a primary site in patients with anterior mediastinal seminoma.

After treatment, persistent but stable or slowly diminishing masses are common CT findings after chemotherapy for advanced seminoma. They usually represent fibrosis and/or necrosis in patients with normal serum markers and do not warrant excision or further chemotherapy. Benign teratomatous transformation does not occur in pure seminomas. Hilar and/or paratracheal lymphadenopathy appearing 1 to 8 years after successful radiotherapy for seminomatous tumors in patients who are otherwise disease free may be due to a sarcoid reaction. This lymph node reaction resolves spontaneously within 1 year. Biopsy for diagnosis is recommended. This phenomenon can occur with nonseminomatous tumors as well.

Suggested Readings

Blandy JP, Hope-Stone HF, Dayan AD: Tumors of the Testicle. New York, Grune & Stratton, 1970

Blei L, Sihelnik S, Bloom D, et al: Ultrasonographic analysis of chronic intratesticular pathology. J Ultrasound Med 2:17–23, 1983

Donohue JP: Selecting initial therapy: Seminoma and nonseminoma. Cancer 60:490–495, 1987

Einhorn LH, Donohue JP: Improved chemotherapy in disseminated testicular cancer. J Urol 117:65–69, 1977

Ellis JH, Bies JR, Kopecky KK, et al: Comparison of NMR and CT imaging in the evaluation of metastatic retroperitoneal lymphadenopathy from testicular carcinoma. J Comput Assist Tomogr 8:709–719, 1984

Higby DJ, Wallace HJ, Albert DJ, et al: Diaminodichloroplatinum: A Phase I study showing responses in testicular and other tumors. Cancer 33:1219–1225, 1974

Kirschling RJ, Kvols LK, Charboneau JW, et al: High-resolution ultrasonographic and pathologic abnormalities of germ cell tumors in patients with clinically normal testes. Mayo Clin Proc 58:648–653, 1983

Li MC, Whitmore WF, Golbey R, et al: Effects of combined drug therapy on metastatic cancer of the testis. JAMA 174:1291–1299, 1960

Oliver RT, Dhaliwal HS, Hope-Stone HF, et al: Short-course etoposide, bleomycin, and cisplatin in the treatment of metastatic germ cell tumours: Appraisal of its potential as adjuvant chemotherapy for stage 1 testis tumours. Br J Urol 61:53–58, 1988

Schmoll HJ: The role of ifosfamide in testicular cancer. Semin Oncol 16:82–95, 1989

NONSEMINOMATOUS TESTICULAR TUMORS

J. EDSON PONTES, M.D.

Detroit, Michigan

Significant progress has been made since the 1970s in the treatment of nonseminomatous testicular tumors (NSTTs) to the point that today these tumors are considered a model of curable neoplasms. A multidisciplinary approach combining solid principles of chemotherapy, appropriate timing of surgery, and pathologic understanding of the disease is responsible for this unparalleled success. In recent years, most of the trust has been placed on the outcome of surveillance protocols for patients with negative metastatic disease, on decreasing toxicity from chemotherapy in those patients with minimal disseminated disease, and on the identification of prognostic factors for patients with poor prognosis who may deserve more aggressive therapy.

DIAGNOSIS, STAGING, AND PATHOLOGY

Testicular tumors usually are diagnosed clinically. Patients generally feel a lump or detect progressive enlargement of the testis. Although a dull pain may be associated with the progressive enlargement of the testis, an acute episode of pain usually is associated with intratumor hemorrhage or infarct. Although testicular self-examination in the age-group population at risk of developing testicular tumors has been proposed, a recent study at our institution revealed that only a small percentage of the college students interviewed are aware of testicular self-examination. Some authors have proposed high-resolution ultrasonography as a highly sensitive method for the diagnosis of testicular tumors, but this technique is, in most cases, confirmatory of clinical findings. The most important facet of ultrasonography is the low false-positive results that preclude unnecessary removal of a testis. More recently, intraoperative biopsy with frozen sections has been demonstrated to be safe and accurate in the diagnosis of testicular malignancies.

Despite the advances in technology, radical inguinal orchiectomy is the initial step in the diagnosis of testicular tumors. Staging of testicular tumors should include both specific serum biologic markers, such as beta-human chorionic gonadotropin (β-hCG) and alpha$_1$-

fetoprotein (AFP), and nonspecific markers, such as lactic dehydrogenase (LDH) and Regan isoenzyme of alkaline phosphatase. These markers should be measured before orchiectomy and after, because they are good indicators of tumor activity. Up to 90 per cent of patients with NSTTs have elevated serum levels of β-hCG and AFP, depending on the stage of the disease. Clinical evaluation prior to retroperitoneal lymph node dissection demonstrates elevated markers in about 37 per cent of patients with N_1 disease, 57 per cent of those with N_2, and 88 per cent of those patients with N_3 retroperitoneal involvement. In patients with negative specific serum markers, elevation of LDH and Regan isoenzyme of alkaline phosphatase is useful in following response to therapy.

Additional staging procedures include intravenous urography, pulmonary tomography, bipedal lymphangiography, and computerized tomography (CT) of the abdomen and pelvis. Lymphangiography and CT will predict the absence of metastases in approximately 80 per cent of cases and will detect metastatic disease in 70 to 75 per cent of cases. CT is invaluable in assessing response to therapy in patients with bulky abdominal disease. Chest radiographs are an essential part of staging and follow-up of these patients. Bergman has shown that lung tomography may be more sensitive than chest radiography. Although CT scan of the chest detects smaller lesions than can be detected by chest radiographs, the possibility of differentiating metastatic lesions from benign conditions, including normal lymph nodes, makes the use of this technique less desirable.

Several classifications for clinical and pathologic staging of testicular tumors have been proposed. In general, they represent institutional variations reflecting individual preferences. In the past, most classifications were based on pathologic findings because all patients with NSTT underwent a retroperitoneal lymph node dissection. With the advent of surveillance protocols and the identification of prognostic factors associated with the primary tumor, the need to use the TNM system has increased. Table 1 shows the TNM system for testicular tumors.

It recently has become evident that there is a subgroup of patients who have disseminated disease with poor prognostic characteristics. Attempts to define this subgroup of patients have varied from the use of mathematical probabilities using marker levels, the number and site of metastatics used at Memorial Sloan-Kettering Cancer Center, and the evaluation of the extent of the disease in the chest, abdomen, and other visceral areas used by the National Cancer Institute, the European Organization for Research and Treatment of Cancer (EORTC), and Indiana University approaches. It is useful to define this group properly because responses to therapy in such patients differ significantly from those in patients with few metastatic nodules in the lungs, who also are classified as having metastatic disease. Pathologically, such tumors are thought to arise from totipotential germ cells, which give rise to a variety of histologic types. It has been proposed that a "histologic continuum" exists between classic seminoma and yolk sac tumor that is responsible for the variety of histologic types observed. In recent years, it has become evident that the primary chromosomal abnormality associated with germ cell tumors is an isochromosome of the short arm of chromosome 12. This abnormality is present in both seminomas and nonseminomas and offers strong evidence for the common origin of these tumors. Molecular studies that may provide prognostic characteristics are at an initial phase.

MANAGEMENT

Early-Stage Nonseminomatous Testicular Tumors

It has been recognized that, in patients with a negative metastatic work-up following radical orchiectomy for NSTT, only 20 to 30 per

TABLE 1. TNM Classification System for Testicular Tumors

PRIMARY TUMOR (T)	
T_X	Unknown
T_0	No evidence of primary tumors
T_2	Tumor confined to the testis
T_3	Tumor beyond the tunica albuginea
T_{4A}	Invasion of the cord
T_{4B}	Invasion of the scrotum
REGIONAL LYMPH NODES (N)	
N_1	Microscopic node involvement
N_2	Multiple node involvement
N_3	Extranodal extension (resectable)
N_4	Unresectable nodes of incomplete resection
DISTANT METASTASES (M)	
M_0	No evidence of metastasis
M_1	Metastatic disease

cent will have microscopic disease on the lymphadenectomy specimen. With the increased effectiveness of systemic chemotherapy, questions of submitting all patients with negative metastatic work-up to prophylactic lymphadenectomy are being evaluated. Surveillance protocols with well-defined criteria for entry have demonstrated the feasibility of this conservative approach to selected patients. Furthermore, evaluation of risk factors associated with primary tumors, such as invasion of the tunica albuginea or rete testis, and histologic subgroups, including the presence of embryonal cell elements and vascular and lymphatic involvement, has identified a subgroup with significant higher probability of lymph node metastasis. In this subgroup, retroperitoneal lymph node dissection is indicated. Surgical techniques that preserve ejaculatory function are now available, decreasing the morbidity associated with the procedure. The cornerstone of surveillance is a reliable, close monthly follow-up to detect early metastasis, which is likely to occur in about 20 per cent of such patients.

The management of patients with minimal metastatic disease, found during retroperitoneal lymphadenectomy (RPLND) or patients presenting initially with good prognostic metastatic disease has changed considerably in the last few years. After the initial success of systemic chemotherapy, attention has shifted toward obtaining similar results with less toxicity. Among patients found to have microscopic disease at the time of RPLND, the controversies are related to either a short course of adjuvant chemotherapy versus close follow-up with the treatment only of those patients who develop metastatic disease. Previous randomized prospective studies have shown relapse of approximately 40 per cent of patients following a positive RPLND as compared to 1 per cent of those patients receiving two courses of adjuvant chemotherapy. However, the overwhelming percentage of patients who relapse can be rescued with systemic chemotherapy. In patients with good prognosis metastatic NSTT, most of the present trends in treatment have been toward lower toxicity. In this regard, recent trials have shown that the combination of etoposide and cis-platinum (EP) or bleomycin, etoposide, and cis-platinum (BEP) is as effective as a combination containing vinblastine (VBP or VAB-6) with less toxicity. The overall response rate is over 90 per cent, with greater than 80 per cent of patients continuing to have no evidence of disease.

Advanced Nonseminomatous Testicular Tumors

Traditionally, patients with metastatic testicular tumors are treated initially with systemic chemotherapy, followed by surgical excision of residual masses. With modern chemotherapy, only approximately 20 per cent of the residual masses contain viable tumor. Most of the efforts of recent years have focused on the identification of prognostic factors that select a subgroup of patients not responsive to traditional chemotherapy. Chemotherapy regimens that include high doses of cis-platinum have demonstrated success in some centers. The use of ifosfamide as part of the initial regimen for the treatment of metastatic NSTT with poor prognostic characteristics has improved the outlook of some patients. In recent years, a tendency has developed to treat patients aggressively with high-dose chemotherapy and bone marrow autotransplant as the second line of therapy if the initial chemotherapy fails. Overall responses have been reported in approximately 44 per cent of patients. About 24 per cent of these are complete response. Although preliminary reports are encouraging, only time will allow for the ultimate evaluation of this approach.

TESTICULAR MALIGNANCY AFTER ORCHIOPEXY

KALISH R. KEDIA, M.D.

Cleveland, Ohio

The propensity of an undescended testis to develop a germ cell neoplasm has been long and widely recognized. Approximately 85 per cent of all testes are descended normally at birth, and the majority of the remaining testes usually descend in the first 12 months of life. Cryptorchidism affects about 1 in every 400 to 500 men. A review of well over 10,000 cases of testicular tumor has shown that approximately 10 per cent of all germinal cell tumors occurred in patients with undescended testes. These statistics suggest that the probability of a malignancy occurring in an undescended testis is 30 to 50 times greater than in a normally descended testis. The location of the undescended testis is also important with regard to the risk of tumorigenesis. Approximately 15 per cent of all undescended testes are located abdominally, and the risk factor for this group of patients is about six times greater than that for patients with palpable inguinal testes.

Two questions often are asked with reference to the management of patients with undescended testes:

1. Does orchiopexy decrease the increased incidence of testicular malignancy?
2. When should surgery be performed for undescended testes?

At present, the consensus in the literature is that the incidence does not decrease, but easy inspection of the gonad is permitted as a result of the orchiopexy. In 1978, Martin surveyed the literature and reviewed 220 cases of germinal cell tumors of the testes that had occurred after orchiopexy. Of these cases, 97 were accurately documented with details of age at orchiopexy and location of the testis at the time of tumor development. The age of the patients at the time of orchiopexy ranged from 5 to 48 years; it is significant that a large number of patients were subjected to orchiopexy between ages 10 and 15. Only six cases of tumor were reported after orchiopexy in children under age 10. The Memorial group recently reported 137 patients with history of cryptorchidism and testicular tumors. In the 93 cases in which cryptorchidism was corrected, the median age was 12 years, and only 10 cases of testicular tumors were reported in patients who had undergone orchiopexy before they were 10 years old. Kedia reported three patients who had undergone successful corrective surgery before their fifth year of life and subsequently developed germinal cell tumors. Two patients had undergone orchiopexy at age 3 and the remaining patient at age 4. An extensive review of the literature showed two additional cases of testicular tumors in patients who had undergone orchiopexy before age 6.

The paucity of tumors in patients with early orchiopexy suggests that an early operation may convey some protection against malignant degeneration. This observation as yet has little meaning, because the performance of orchiopexies before age 6 is a relatively recent phenomenon, and sufficient time has not yet elapsed to allow for the possible development of tumors. Most orchiopexies now are being done when the patient is at an early age (under 2 years); whether this will lower the incidence of malignant neoplasms remains to be seen. In a recent study from Switzerland, ultrastructural changes have been demonstrated in seminiferous tubules and Leydig cells in undescended testes beginning at age 6 months, and significant abnormalities by age 3 years. Recognition of histologic changes early in life suggests the question of whether earlier orchiopexy might reduce the chances of subsequent tumor development.

In another recent study from Copenhagen, 50 previously cryptorchid men were asked to undergo testicular biopsy. In three of these men, who had no clinical signs or symptoms of testicular tumor, biopsy specimens revealed carcinoma in situ, one with an adjacent invasive seminoma. A fourth man with an enlarged testis also had a carcinoma in situ pattern and an adjacent invasive embryonal carcinoma. It is also interesting to note that in approximately 6 to 10 per cent of patients with cryptorchid testis, tumors have developed in the opposite (normally descended) testis, suggesting that cryptorchidism may be a diffuse testicular abnormality and that there is a basic defect in gonadogenesis or primary dysgenesis of the germinal tissue in these patients. The age at diagnosis of testicular cancer does not differ appreciably among patients with cryptorchidism after orchiopexy versus patients with normally descended testes. The incidence of cell types of tumors occurring after orchiopexy is comparable to that of cell types among normally descended testes. The data reported in the literature also reveal that tumor stage and patient survival are similar for tumors developing after orchiopexy and those in normally descended testes.

The testis drains retroperitoneally to the area of its embryonic origin, whereas the scrotal skin, tunics, and epididymis drain into inguinal and pelvic lymph nodes. Scrotal and inguinal surgery may result in altered lymphatic drainage from the testis, and tumors that develop after orchiopexy may metastasize to the inguinal or iliac lymph nodes. In cases of seminoma after orchiopexy, the radiation should include the ipsilateral inguinal region, and, in cases of nonseminomatous tumor, the retroperitoneal lymphadenectomy also should include ipsilateral lymphadenectomy along the common and external iliac vessels. Although some surgeons have advocated ipsilateral inguinal lymphadenectomy in these cases, others believe that this is not necessary and that patients should be followed by careful clinical examination of the inguinal region and tumor markers.

In summary, the undescended testis is at increased risk for malignant degeneration, and orchiopexy does not protect the gonad from subsequent malignant changes. Unilateral cryptorchidism in teens should be treated by orchiectomy instead of orchiopexy, to prevent ipsilateral tumor development. After orchiopexy, patients must be examined regularly, perhaps for life, for early detection of cancer. It is hoped that prompt treatment of an undescended testis by age 2 will prevent the development of histologic changes that can lead to malignant degeneration.

BENIGN TESTICULAR MASSES

LEONARD G. GOMELLA, M.D.

Philadelphia, Pennsylvania

The majority of solid testicular masses in adults represent malignant tumors, predominantly of germ cell origin. Benign lesions are important because they may alter the management of a patient with a testicular mass. This is even more true in children, in whom most testicular tumors will prove to be benign.

Most intrascrotal masses are discovered incidentally by the patient or are due to unrelated trauma to the scrotal area. The patient's age, past medical history (undescended testicle, inguinal surgery, adrenal hyperplasia, inflammatory conditions such as epididymitis, etc.), the time of onset of puberty, and a family history of testicular tumors may give insight into the nature of the lesion. Patients with acute, painful scrotal swelling most often have acute inflammatory process such as orchitis or epididymitis.

During the patient's general physical examination, attention should be focused on the detection of any adenopathy or abdominal masses, the presence of gynecomastia, and any prior inguinal or scrotal incisions. The scrotum and its contents should be examined systematically with the patient standing. The testis should be palpated gently between the fingers from pole to pole, with the epididymis palpated with a distinct ridge separating it from the testicle. The size and consistency of each testicle should be compared to that of the opposite testicle and any masses diagrammed relative to the other scrotal contents. Next, the cord structures and the inguinal canal should be examined. Transillumination of testicular masses can be performed in a darkened room using a flashlight, and the results may support the diagnosis of a cystic structure such as an intrascrotal hydrocele or spermatocele. However, transcrotal ultrasound remains the initial imaging study of choice for all intrascrotal masses because it often can establish the diagnosis and guide further management decisions. In addition, the presence of a hydrocele makes the accurate evaluation of the testis by palpation virtually impossible, whereas ultrasound provides excellent resolution of the underlying testis. Scrotal scintigraphy has little value in the determination of the painless testicular mass and is used primarily with acute scrotal pain or swelling.

If the ultrasound examination confirms a solid lesion within the testis, further routine work-up should include measurement of tumor markers (alpha-fetoprotein and beta-human chorionic gonadotropin) and chest radiography in preparation for inguinal exploration with possible biopsy and/or radical orchiectomy.

The standard approach to the solid mass within the testis is the radical inguinal orchiectomy; in adults, 95 per cent of these masses will prove to be malignant. Through an inguinal incision, the canal is opened and the spermatic cord mobilized. The cord vessels are occluded with a Penrose drain or noncrushing vascular clamp before the testicle is mobilized into the wound. The operative field is redraped and the tunica vaginalis opened. At this point, a decision can be made as to management. In highly selected circumstances, if there is suspicion that the mass may be benign and the rest of the testicle is palpably and ultrasonographically normal, an excisional biopsy with frozen section histologic confirmation can be performed. This approach allows testicular preservation for a benign lesion. However, all patients should be counseled that a benign tumor may be discovered at the time of radical orchiectomy and that very often examination of the entire testicle is necessary to establish the definitive diagnosis. Testicular preservation is more likely to be attempted in children because the overwhelming majority of solid testicular masses in children are benign.

The following benign masses of the testicle have been described in the literature: adenomatoid tumor, teratoma of childhood, testicular cysts, Leydig cell tumor, Sertoli cell tumor, gonadoblastoma, granulosa cell tumor, nodular periorchitis (congenital adrenal hyperplasia), granulomatous orchitis, dilation of the rete testis, malakoplakia, lymphocytic orchitis, Brenner tumor, and various mesenchymal tumors.

ADENOMATOID TUMOR

These benign tumors are thought to be of mesothelial origin. Although more common in the epididymis, they can arise in the testicular tunics. There have been no reports of recurrence after local excision; therefore, conservative management based on inguinal exploration with histologic frozen section microscopic analysis is justified.

TERATOMA OF CHILDHOOD

Unlike the teratoma in the adult, which must be regarded as a malignancy, teratoma of childhood is a benign lesion. The majority of cases present between 20 and 30 months of age. Histologically, these lesions are usually encapsulated and have different germinal layers of endoderm, mesoderm, and ectoderm and often contain cystic structures. Any type of tissue, including cartilage, bone, mucus-secreting glandular epithelium, or neuronal tissue, may be found.

The lesion most often is treated by radical inguinal orchiectomy. There have been some reports of simple excision of the lesion with good results. If conservative testicular preservation is performed, the ipsilateral testicle should be biopsied to exclude any other abnormality, including carcinoma in situ. The teratoma of childhood has never been reported to metastasize; therefore, further therapy usually is not warranted. However, peripubertal and postpubertal adolescents should be treated as are adults with a malignant nonseminomatous germ cell tumor.

TESTICULAR CYSTS

Benign cysts of the testicle include epidermoid cysts, dermoid cysts, simple intratesticular cysts, hydatid cysts, and cysts of the tunica albuginea. Tunica albuginea cysts are discussed in the following article on "Paratesticular Masses and Tumors." Hydatid cysts are limited to the Middle East and will not be discussed.

The epidermoid cyst of the testicle is the most frequently occurring cyst. They occur most often in the third through fifth decade of life, but have been found in all age groups. Histologically, epidermoid cysts are composed entirely of keratin-producing stratified squamous epithelium and are distinct from the dermoid cyst. The dermoid cyst, the most common teratoma in females but rare in males, can consist of all elements of the integumentary system, including hair follicles, sweat glands, sebaceous glands, teeth, and appendages.

In order to be called a true epidermoid cyst, the following criteria must be met: (1) the cyst is within the testis itself, (2), the cyst contains keratinized material, and (3) the lining of the cyst wall is squamous epithelium and there are no teratomatous elements.

The epidermoid cyst tends to occur deep within the substance of the testicle and ranges from 0.5 to 10 cm, with an average size of 2 cm. Standard therapy has been radical orchiectomy. Although there have been reports of conservative management, this currently is not advocated. There have been several reports of concurrent malignant lesions and scars of presumed "burned out" germ cell tumors in the testicle. Although there have been no reports of metastasis of the epidermoid cyst, several cases of malignant testicular tumors in association with epidermoid cysts suggest that pathologic examination of the entire testicle is warranted.

Dermoid cysts are much more common in the ovary than in the testis. Dermoids can be differentiated from the more common epidermoid cyst using the histologic criteria noted above. Radical orchiectomy is recommended for definitive management.

Simple intratesticular cysts are an infrequent cause of a benign testicular mass. The etiology is uncertain, but trauma or a congenital origin has been postulated as a predisposing factor. Histologically, these thin-walled cysts are unilocular and lined by cuboidal cells and contain no cellular debris. They can be managed by simple excision, if appropriate, because there have been no reports of malignancy associated with these cysts.

LEYDIG CELL TUMORS

Leydig cell tumors, also known as interstitial cell tumors, are benign lesions in approximately 90 per cent of cases. This tumor can occur in all age groups, with the peak incidences being from 5 to 10 years and again from 30 to 35 years. In the prepubertal patient, the typical presentation relates to testosterone-induced precocious puberty and can include prominent external genitalia, pubic hair growth, and masculine voice. Older patients tend to present with a testicular mass. Because of the possibility of estrogen production by the tumor, between 20 and 40 per cent of older patients may present with gynecomastia, impotence, or infertility. Case reports have been published of occult, nonpalpable Leydig cell tumors discovered by ultrasound or selective venous sampling.

The Leydig cell tumor tends to be well defined, sometimes appearing encapsulated and being almost exclusively unilateral. The cells are typically polygonal and tightly packed, with abundant eosinophilic or vacuolated cytoplasm. The pathognomonic Reinke crystal, an eosinophilic structure with sharp borders, is seen in only 40 per cent of cases. Mitotic figures are typically absent. The differential diagnosis must include metastatic carcinoma (especially poorly differentiated prostate cancer), lymphoma, adrenal rests, or Leydig cell hyperplasia. The differentiation between benign and malignant forms is difficult and relies predominantly on the identification of metastasis. Malignant forms have been reported only in adults.

The treatment of Leydig cell tumor is radical orchiectomy. Although the endocrine effects tend to reverse in both adults and children, there may be persistent irreversible changes, such as residual gynecomastia. Further management is necessary only for malignant tumors.

SERTOLI CELL TUMOR

Sertoli cell tumors, also known as androblastomas, account for less than 1 per cent of testicular tumors, with 10 to 20 per cent being malignant. Approximately one third of Sertoli cell tumors are found during the first year of life, with an additional one third found in the 30 to 40 year age range. In distinction from Leydig cell tumors, malignant Sertoli cell tumors can be found in children. Up to 20 per cent of these tumors are associated with gynecomastia, a feature more likely associated with the malignant form of Sertoli cell tumor. Feminization, especially in children, is seen sometimes. Most patients, however, present with a scrotal mass.

Histologically, the tumor consists of a distinctive trabecular pattern, similar in morphology to an immature seminiferous tubule. Up to one third of Sertoli tumors can have Leydig cell elements, placing them in a category known as "mixed gonadal stromal tumor." Local invasion may suggest malignancy, which is confirmed by the identification of metastasis. Optimum management is radical orchiectomy.

GONADOBLASTOMA

This rare tumor is seen exclusively in intersex patients with dysgenetic gonads. The tumor has been reported in phenotypic males with scrotal testes, although this is more commonly associated with cryptorchidism. The gonadoblastoma is composed of both germ cells and gonadal stromal cells, such as Sertoli or Leydig cells. Malignancy is rare, and the lesion treated by radical orchiectomy.

GRANULOSA CELL TUMOR

The adult form of granulosa cell tumor often is associated with gynecomastia. The juvenile form of this tumor is the most common sex cord/gonadal tumor in infant males. These lesions tend to be benign, with only one case of an adult form metastasizing.

MALACOPLAKIA

This rare testicular lesion can be found after gram-negative urinary tract infections. This condition primarily affects males over the age of 40, and immunosuppression commonly is associated with malacoplakia. The clinical presentation is similar to that of chronic epididymo-orchitis. Pathologically, Michaelis-Gutman bodies are found.

GRANULOMATOUS ORCHITIS

Granulomatous orchitis can be secondarily caused by systemic illnesses such as tuberculosis or sarcoid. However, true granulomatous orchitis is a condition that is not associated with any identifiable pathogen. The patients with idiopathic granulomatous orchitis are usually in their 50s or 60s and typically present with epididymo-orchitis that is refractory to antibiotics. A persistent mass results in a radical orchiectomy. There have been no reports of this condition being diagnosed preoperatively. Granulomas in patients with systemic sarcoid can be managed by excisional biopsy and frozen section confirmation.

HYPERPLASTIC NODULES

Patients with congenital adrenal hyperplasia (CAH) can develop masses in the testes that are often bilateral. Most patients with the previous diagnosis of CAH present with palpable testicular masses and have an average age at diagnosis of 22 years. Although hyperplastic nodules often are diagnosed after radical orchiectomy, there have been case reports of dexamethasone treatment resolving these lesions. Histologically, the lesions consist of Leydig cell hyperplasia, and the differential diagnosis of these masses includes Leydig cell tumor.

DILATED RETE TESTIS

This lesion has a characteristic appearance on transcrotal ultrasound consisting of multiple small or spherical or tubular anechoic structures in the region of the mediastinum testis. They frequently are associated with epididymal cysts. Patients range in age from 31 to 76 years. The diagnosis frequently can be established with ultrasound, sparing the patient a surgical procedure.

MISCELLANEOUS BENIGN TUMORS

Tumors of the testicular supporting structures (hemangioma, fibromas, leiomyomas), nongranulomatous lymphocytic orchitis, and Brenner tumors all have been reported. Most are diagnosed after radical orchiectomy because their occurrence is infrequent.

CONCLUSIONS

Benign testis tumors are infrequent in adults and more commonly discovered in children. Although radical orchiectomy is considered standard therapy for many of these lesions, excisional biopsy with testicular preservation is appropriate in selected cases.

Suggested Readings

Feld R, Middleton WD: Recent advances in sonography of the testis and scrotum. Radiol Clin North Am 20: 1033–1051, 1992

Peterson RO: Urologic Pathology, 2nd ed. Philadelphia, JB Lippincott, 1992, pp 429–525

Rushton HG, Belman BA: Testis sparing surgery for benign lesions of the prepubertal testis. Urol Clin North Am 20:27–37, 1993

PARATESTICULAR TUMORS AND MASSES

LEONARD G. GOMELLA, M.D.

Philadelphia, Pennsylvania

Paratesticular masses and tumors can arise from the testicular tunics, epididymis, spermatic cord, or any of the surrounding connective tissues. Most are benign and consist of true solid tumors or fluid-filled cystic structures. Malignancy is rare in most paratesticular tissues, with the highest incidence of malignancy in the cord structures. Collectively, paratesticular neoplasms account for about 7 per cent of intrascrotal masses. Most testicular adnexal solid masses arise in the cord (50 to 60 per cent), with the remainder arising in the epididymis and testicular tunics.

Complete examination of the male external genitalia should include not only the testis but the paratesticular epididymal and cord structures, as outlined in the previous article on "Benign Testicular Masses."

Ultrasound is a useful adjunct to the physical examination of the scrotal contents, and often is the diagnostic test of choice, especially for "cystic" lesions such as hydrocele, spermatocele, and varicocele. Although ultrasound cannot distinguish reliably among solid paratesticular masses, it is useful in confirming the exact location of the lesion.

HYDROCELE

Hydrocele, the most common cause of scrotal swelling, results from a collection of serous fluid within the visceral and parietal tunica vaginalis. Hydrocele may be congenital or acquired. Congenital hydroceles are associated with a patent processus vaginalis in up to 6 per cent of newborn males, with many of these resolving by 1 year of age. Congenital hydrocele persisting beyond this time usually should be repaired through an inguinal incision that allows high ligation of the sac and repair of the associated hernia.

Adult hydrocele are usually "idiopathic" or can be associated with other conditions such as intrascrotal infection, systemic diseases (hypoalbuminemia, lymphedema caused by lymphatic obstruction), testicular neoplasm, or prior inguinal or scrotal surgery. The development of a hydrocele after a varicocele repair is a recognized complication of the procedure. Alterations in lymphatic drainage are thought to be the etiology of idiopathic hydrocele.

In adults, idiopathic hydrocele tend to be a painless, slowly growing mass associated with symptoms of "heaviness" or positional discomfort. The mass is cystic, nontender, and easy to transilluminate. Transcrotal ultrasound is diagnostic and usually demonstrates an anechoic fluid pattern. Septations are more likely to be associated with a reactive hydrocele. If the hydrocele precludes careful examination of the testicle, ultrasound usually can define testicular anatomy to rule out any lesion in the testicle that can cause a reactive hydrocele. Occasionally an asymptomatic hydrocele can bleed as a result of either trauma or underlying malignancy, resulting in a hematocele.

Idiopathic hydroceles do not require repair unless they are causing discomfort or are a cosmetic problem. Standard repair in adults involves a scrotal incision with complete excision of the walls of the hydrocele sac or opening the sac and reapproximating the everted edges of the sac behind the testis so that the fluid cannot collect again.

An alternative "nonoperative" approach is percutaneous aspiration with injection sclerotherapy. Agents used to sclerose the hydrocele sac can include tetracycline, sodium tetradecyl sulfate, and combinations of agents such as phenol, glycerine, and glucose. This approach often requires multiple treatments but can achieve an 80 to 90 per cent success rate. The treatments may cause pain and intrascrotal loculated adhesions that may make further attempts of sclerotherapy or formal surgical repair more difficult.

SPERMATOCELE

The spermatocele is technically a form of epididymal cyst and occurs most frequently in middle-aged men. The spermatocele typically presents as a painless mass above the testis and is palpably separate from the testis. Using high-resolution ultrasonography, these lesions may be discovered incidentally in 70 per cent of men. Spermatoceles have been postulated to be caused by infection, obstruction, or trauma. The lesion contains a clear or slightly milky fluid that contains spermatozoa. Ultrasound usually confirms the diagnosis, and these lesions usually require no further therapy unless the mass causes significant discomfort. A trans-scrotal approach with simple excision as an outpatient is usually sufficient.

VARICOCELE

Varicoceles are a dilation of the pampiniform plexus usually caused by incompetent valves of the spermatic veins. Approximately 15 per cent of the adult population has a varicocele, most frequently found on the left. The sudden onset of a varicocele should raise the suspicion of a retroperitoneal process, such as renal cell carcinoma or sarcoma, that is blocking the venous system.

These lesions are usually asymptomatic, although some patients have complaints of "fullness" in the area. In a small percentage of patients, the varicocele may cause oligospermia and fertility-related problems. The dilated veins become more distended with standing and the Valsalva maneuver. No treatment is usually necessary in patients with normal fertility unless there are severe symptoms related to the varicocele. Management of varicocele is discussed in Section 9.

POLYORCHIDISM

A supernumerary testis may be found at any point of descent of the normal gonad. The significance of this rare congenital anomaly is that it must be differentiated from other intrascrotal masses.

BENIGN EPIDIDYMAL LESIONS

The overwhelming majority of epididymal lesions are benign. Benign lesions of the epididymis that present as masses include adenomatoid tumor, cystadenomas, acute and chronic epididymitis, and a variety of benign mesenchymal lesions. Malignant lesions are rare but can include primary carcinoma of the epididymis, metastatic lesions, and malignant mesenchymal lesions such as rhabdomyosarcoma. Any patient who undergoes biopsy or excision of any or all of the epididymis should be counseled that the procedure may impact negatively on fertility.

The adenomatoid tumor accounts for over 50 per cent of solid epididymal neoplasms. The mass usually is discovered incidentally. Also called "benign nonpapillary mesothelioma," these lesions can be found at either pole of the epididymis; occasionally they have been described in the tunica vaginalis or cord. This neoplasm is of mesothelial cell origin and uniformly benign. The typical lesion is 2 cm, but lesions up to 6 cm have been reported. No treatment is necessary; however if the diagnosis is not clear, transinguinal exploration with histologic confirmation and simple excision is appropriate.

Papillary cystadenoma is a benign hamartoma of the epididymis most frequently found in the head of the epididymis. Up to one third of these lesions are associated with von Hippel–Lindau (VHL) disease, an autosomal dominant syndrome consisting of renal cell carcinoma, renal cysts, cerebellar hemangioblastoma, and other cystic lesions of the pancreas and lung. The cystadenoma can be bilateral, especially when associated with VHL disease. The lesion usually can be differentiated from a testicular neoplasm by ultrasound, and no specific treatment is needed unless the diagnosis is not clear. There have been no reports of recurrence after excision. However, patients in whom the diagnosis of cystadenoma is made should be monitored for other manifestations of VHL disease.

Inflammatory processes of the epididymis, such as acute epididymitis, typically are associated with pain and swelling that responds to antibiotics. Postinflammatory masses of the epididymis can be caused by resulting fibrosis. These masses are sometimes tender and are often clinically described as "chronic epididymitis."

Sperm granuloma are hard nodules that are usually less than 1 cm in size and often tender on palpation. Most patients are in their 30s and can give a specific history of trauma, epididymitis, or vasectomy. The histologic features are those of a typical granuloma, and the etiology is thought to be the release of sperm into the interstitium as a result of increased intraductal pressure. Simple excision can be performed if symptoms require removal.

Malakoplakia, often associated with testicular malakoplakia, can be found in the epididymis. Systemic sarcoid also can manifest as an epididymal lesion. Benign mesenchymal neoplasms can afflict the epididymis and are very rare. These can include leiomyoma, lymphangioma, and hemangioma.

MALIGNANT EPIDIDYMAL LESIONS

Primary malignancies of the epididymis are so infrequent that most appear in the literature as case reports. Collectively, they represent approximately 100 cases.

Primary epididymal carcinoma is an aggressive neoplasm, with most patients dying within 4 years of diagnosis. Patients have been reported to range from 22 to 78 years of age. The lesion can be up to 6 cm and often is associated with a hydrocele.

Leiomyosarcoma and rhabdomyosarcoma are similar in histology to their counterparts found elsewhere in the body. Aggressive multimodal therapy, including surgery, chemotherapy, and radiation, often results in long-term cure. Ten cases of extratesticular epididymal germ cell neoplasm have been reported and managed identically to their histologic testicular primary counterparts.

Approximately 59 cases of distant metastatic cancers have been described as epididymal masses. In approximately 30 per cent, the epididymal metastasis has been the first presentation of the disease. The most frequent primary sites include, in decreasing order, the prostate, kidney, stomach, and colon. Management is determined by the primary lesion.

BENIGN SPERMATIC CORD LESIONS

The spermatic cord elements include the vas deferens, blood vessels, nerves, and supporting stromal tissues. Spermatic cord lesions can account for 50 to 60 per cent of intrascrotal paratesticular masses. Intra-abdominal herniations around the spermatic cord should present no difficulty and can be distinguished readily by the physical exam; if there is concern, a transcrotal ultrasound should be diagnostic for intestinal herniation.

The benign cord lipoma is the most frequently encountered spermatic cord lesion. The etiology is usually simple herniation of preperitoneal fat into the cord. Histologically, these lesions consist of mature fat cells and no specific treatment is needed.

Ectopic tissues, such as adrenal rests, splenic tissues, and dermoid cysts, can present as masses of the cord. Benign mesenchymal lesions such as leiomyoma, neurofibroma, and myxoma have been reported rarely. Surgical inguinal exploration and excisional biopsy with frozen section confirmation is warranted because approximately 50 per cent of solid nodular masses in the stroma of the cord will be some form of malignant sarcoma.

Diabetics can manifest calcifications in the vas deferens that are of no clinical significance. Inflammatory lesions also can result in masses in the vas deferens. Tuberculous involvement of the vas can result in the characteristic "beaded" vas. Vasitis nodosa can present with discomfort and multiple nodules of the vas without previous history of tuberculous infection or vasectomy. The etiology is unclear in patients who have not undergone vasectomy, and the lesion is histologically characterized by sperm-containing ductules in the muscular coat of the vas, with or without sperm granuloma. Symptomatic, nonsurgical management is preferred for these conditions of the vas.

MALIGNANT NEOPLASMS OF THE SPERMATIC CORD

A high degree of suspicion should be used in the approach to the solid mass in the cord because up to 50 per cent can be malignant. Most of these lesions are painless and tend to arise from the intrascrotal portion of the cord. Most are sarcomas and can include rhabdomyosarcoma, liposarcoma, leiomyosarcoma, fibrosarcoma, angiosarcoma, malignant fibrous histiocytoma, neurofibrosarcoma, myxoid chondrosarcoma, and malignant rhabdoid tumor. The management of these tumors is virtually identical to the treatment of rhabdomyosarcoma.

Rhabdomyosarcoma is the most common type, and most commonly is found in children, with 80 per cent of cases described in patients less than 20 years of age. It tends to metastasize to regional nodes more readily than other cord sarcomas. The microscopic appearance is variable and typical for embryonal rhabdomyosarcoma, with strap cells, bizarre "tadpole" cells, and frequent mitotic figures being typical.

Management involves radical inguinal orchiectomy with high ligation of the cord. If the mass is adherent to the surrounding soft tissues, more aggressive resection may be required. Local radiation therapy may help prevent recurrence in the surgical field. Further multimodal therapy includes retroperitoneal lymphadenectomy, radiation therapy, and chemotherapy. Overall, survival with aggressive therapy approaches 75 per cent. Active combination chemotherapy agents include dactinomycin, doxorubicin, vincristine, and cyclophosphamide. Patients should be considered for treatment on current intergroup protocol standards.

There have been scattered case reports of metastasis to the cord from prostate, kidney, and gastrointestinal malignancies. Therapy is directed at excision of the cord mass and treatment of the primary malignancy.

MASSES OF THE TESTICULAR TUNICS

Fibrous pseudotumor, also called fibroma or nodular periorchitis, is a benign lesion of the tunica albuginea. It rarely is found in other paratesticular tissues. These lesions present as an asymptomatic, solid, smooth mass on the surface of the testicle. In 50 per cent of cases, they can be associated with a hydrocele. The etiology of the "scrotal pearl" discovered during the removal of a hydrocele is thought to be a fibrous pseudotumor that has broken off from the tunic. The etiology of fibrous pseudotumor may relate to previous trauma or infection. Histologically, these are simple fibromas.

Cysts of the tunica albuginea usually are palpable and nontender and lie outside of the testicular parenchyma. They are thought to arise from wolffian duct remnants and are uniformly benign.

The fibrous pseudotumor and tunica albuginea cyst are uniformly benign and can be managed by observation if the ultrasound is suggestive of the diagnosis. They require excision only if there is clinical difficulty differentiating them from testicular neoplasm.

Mesenchymal lesions of the tunics can include malignant mesothelioma, with 37 cases reported in the literature, and the occasional benign müllerian duct remnant and leiomyoma. There has been no uniformly successful approach to the malignant mesothelioma. Excision through a radical orchiectomy approach is required for diagnosis.

CONCLUSIONS

Solid lesions in the spermatic cord are at increased risk of representing a malignant sarcoma, whereas most other cystic and solid paratesticular lesions are benign. Ultrasound is helpful in establishing the diagnosis of many paratesticular lesions. If there is any doubt, exploration through inguinal incision is indicated.

Suggested Readings

Feld R, Middleton WD: Recent advances in sonography of the testis and scrotum. Radiol Clin North Am 20: 1033–1051, 1992

Orland SM, Schlecker BA, Wein AJ: Benign diseases of the testicle and paratesticular tissues. AUA Update, vol V, Lesson 24, 1986

Peterson RO: Urologic Pathology, 2nd ed. Philadelphia, JB Lippincott, 1992, pp 429–525

INTERSTITIAL CELL TUMORS OF THE TESTIS

S. BRUCE MALKOWICZ, M.D.

Philadelphia, Pennsylvania

Interstitial cell tumors of the testes are derived from gonadal mesenchyme cells and can develop into several lesions, including Sertoli cell tumors and their subtypes, Leydig cell tumors (which are discussed in a separate article), gonadoblastomas, and granulosa cell tumors. They are rare lesions that are generally benign and usually treated by inguinal orchiectomy. Malignant lesions are suggested by features such as vascular or lymphatic invasion, cellular anaplasia, and a high mitotic index, yet are only defined by the presence of metastases. The definition of malignancy is therefore tautological.

SERTOLI CELL TUMORS

These lesions are rare and make up approximately 1 per cent of testicular tumors in the adult or pediatric population. Interestingly, they are seen at a much greater frequency in dogs and other animals. These lesions are somewhat difficult to classify and range from Sertoli cell–only lesions to Sertoli-stromal cell variants. Sertoli cell–only tumors generally are associated with undescended testicles and also are found in cases of testicular feminization (25 per cent). They have a large range in size and are uniformly benign. Treatment consists of orchiectomy.

Sertoli cell tumors with stromal elements account for approximately 1 per cent of testicular neoplasms and almost 20 per cent of non–germ cell tumors of the testes. The majority of patients present under the age of 40, and there is a 10 to 20 per cent incidence of malignancy as defined by the presence of metastases. Malignancy has not been reported in patients under the age of 5, and most prepubertal patients present in infancy. The most common presentation is a painless testicular mass. Although the majority of these lesions are hormonally inactive, the most frequent endocrine manifestation is gynecomastia (up to one third of patients). Although rare, virilizing lesions have been reported. It is unclear if epithelial or stromal elements are responsible for hormone production.

Histologically, Charcot-Bottcher crystalloids are observed in pathologic and nonpathologic Sertoli cells. The arrangement of epithelial and stromal elements may vary from tubule-like structures to sheets of cells interspersed among stromal components. With respect to intermediate filaments, Sertoli cell tumors express cytokeratin and vimentin, whereas Leydig cell tumors express only vimentin.

In general, these lesions are cured by orchiectomy. Testis-sparing surgery in pediatric patients has not been advocated for these lesions. Tumors with malignant features may benefit from retroperitoneal lymph node dissection. Truly malignant lesions tend to be very aggressive and may benefit from multimodal therapy, including retroperitoneal lymphadenectomy, radiation therapy, and combination chemotherapy. Exact recommendations are difficult to make given the lack of significant aggregate clinical experience with the malignant form of these lesions.

One variation of these lesions includes the sclerosing Sertoli cell tumor. As the name implies, prominent sclerosis of cells is noted in these hard, usually small (0.4 to 1.5-cm) lesions. The median age of patients reported with this variant is 30 years (range of 18 to 80). None of the 10 described lesions were hormonally active, nor was any malignancy noted in the follow-up of five patients for a mean of 5.8 years, even in one patient whose primary tumor displayed malignant features.

Another variation includes large-cell calcifying Sertoli cell tumor. Nineteen cases have been reported. It has little malignant potential and usually occurs in the first two decades of life. The only patient with metastases was the oldest patient recorded (age 44). The lesions are usually tan to gray and exhibit amorphous or lamellar calcium throughout. Charcot-Bottcher crystalloids generally are noted. The tumor is bilateral and multifocal in more than one half of the cases. Of greater interest is the fact that this lesion has been associated with endocrine imbalances such as adrenal hyperplasia, hyperpigmentation of the skin, sexual precocity, and gynecomastia. Other lesions, such as tuberous sclerosis, Peutz-Jegher syndrome, and atrial myxomas, have been associated with this lesion. The treatment of choice is orchiectomy.

GONADOBLASTOMA

Gonadoblastoma is not a pure interstitial tumor of the testis, but is comprised of germ cell elements, interstitial tissue, and Sertoli cells. It comprises less than 0.5 per cent of testis tumors. These lesions are benign but have the capacity to degenerate into a dysgerminoma and should be removed. Eighty per cent of these patients are phenotypic females (testicular feminization or pure gonadal dysgenesis, XY type), who may present with primary amenorrhea and possibly an abdominal mass. The remainder are phenotypic males with cryptorchidism and hypospadias to a degree that suggests gender ambiguity. A Y chromosome cell line is present in these tumors. The lesion therefore may present as a streak gonad or indeterminate gonad. The tumor may be bilateral in one third to one half of cases; therefore, bilateral gonadectomy is recommended when gonadal dysgenesis is present.

GRANULOSA CELL TUMORS

Granulosa cell tumors are rare lesions that exhibit an internal architecture comprised of preovulatory granulosa cells and Sertoli cells. They generally present as a painless scrotal swelling in infants, with three quarters of them presenting in the first month of life. They appear cystic and often contain areas of solid cellular elements. Approximately 50 per cent of these lesions display Y chromosome abnormalities. No cases of metastases have been reported, and orchiectomy is curative.

Suggested Readings

Cortez JC, Kaplan GW: Gonadal stromal tumors, gonadoblastomas, epidermoid cysts, and secondary tumors of the testis in children. Urol Clin North Am 20:15–26, 1993

Sasano H, Hakashima N, Matsuzake O, et al: Testicular sex cord-stromal lesions: Immunohistochemical analysis of cytokeratin, vimentin and steroidogenic enzymes. Virchows Arch A Pathol Anat 421:163–169, 1992

Tetu B, Ro JY, Ayala AG: Large cell calcifying Sertoli cell tumor of the testis: A clinicopathological, immunohistochemical and ultrastructural study of two cases. Am J Clin Pathol 96:717–722, 1991

Zuckerberg LR, Young RH, Scully RE: Sclerosing Sertoli cell tumor of the testis: A report of 10 cases. Am J Surg Pathol 15:829–834, 1991

SERTOLI CELL TUMOR OF THE TESTIS

GABRIEL P. HAAS, M.D.

Detroit, Michigan

Interstitial stromal tumors of the testicle represent less than 5 per cent of testicular neoplasms. Sertoli cell tumors are the second most frequent interstitial tumors, following Leydig cell tumors, and constitute less than 1 per cent of all testicular tumors. The tumor may present at any age, with a number of pediatric cases reported. No particular predisposing factors have been identified, and most cases occur in the normally developed, intrascrotal testes.

The clinical presentation of Sertoli cell tumors is variable. Painless testicular enlargement or mass is the most common evidence of an abnormality, and this presentation is indistinguishable from the clinical presentation of the more frequent germ cell tumors. Evidence of endocrine abnormalities, particularly gynecomastia, has been reported in approximately one third of patients, and appears to be somewhat more common in prepubertal patients, in whom feminization or precocious puberty may be the first signs leading to the diagnosis in the course of a thorough physical examination. These endocrine manifestations are presumably the consequence of excessive estrogen and/or testosterone production, although, in many cases, the diagnosis was made following histologic evaluation of the radical orchiectomy specimen, and the results of preoperative endocrine work-up were not documented.

Work-up of these lesions should be the same as for any other testicular mass. History and physical examination should be complemented by testicular ultrasound examination and serum alpha-fetoprotein and beta-human chorionic gonadotropin levels. These serum studies should be negative in Sertoli cell tumor patients. Patients who present with endocrine manifestations should have their estrogen, testosterone, luteinizing hormone, and follicle-stimulating hormone levels evaluated. A number of cases of occult interstitial testicular tumors have been described in the literature. These tumors generally were suspected because of their endocrine activity; however, they were undetectable on physical examination. Testicular ultrasound often suggested an abnormality, which then led to the orchiectomy; however, occasionally even ultrasonography failed to demonstrate the lesion. These patients could be diagnosed by testicular vein sampling for excess hormonal production, and this technique could lateralize the location of the tumor. Several patients underwent inguinal exploration of a testicular mass with frozen section identification of the neoplasm.

Although most Sertoli cell tumors are 1 to 2 cm in diameter at the time of treatment, they may grow to significantly larger size with lengthy neglect. On cut surface, the tumor often has a pinkish or yellowish appearance and is well demarcated from the surrounding, compressed testicular parenchyma. Calcification and cystic degeneration in larger tumors have been described in some case reports. The histologic diagnosis is based on the presence of large, eosinophilic cells with abundant cytoplasm, resembling Sertoli cells. Individual cells are arranged in tubular or cord-like structures within a variable amount of myxoid connective tissue stroma. Mitotic activity is generally rare or absent, except in the malignant variety. Oval nuclei and prominent nucleoli are characteristic features. Infrequently, the presence of Reinke crystals or Call-Exner–like bodies also has been noted. Occasionally, Sertoli cell tumors may contain elements of other interstitial testicular tumors, such as Leydig cell tumors or gonadoblastomas.

Approximately 10 per cent of Sertoli cell tumors are malignant, or are likely to have a greater malignant potential. These lesions tend to be larger in size, are more infiltrative in appearance (invading surrounding tissues, blood vessels, and lymphatic channels), and have an increased prevalence of mitotic figures. However, as is the case with many other endocrine tumors, metastasis is the only certain indicator of a malignancy. Metastasis is sufficiently rare that the relative relationship of hematogenous or lymphatic routes of dissemination is yet to be elucidated.

Radical orchiectomy followed by close observation is the treatment of choice for clinically localized disease. Retroperitoneal lymph node dissection is not recommended in general, and particularly not in the pediatric age group, unless retroperitoneal lymphadenopathy can be demonstrated. The prognosis is good for the majority of tumors, which are localized; it is poor for advanced disease. Up to the present, the rarity of the condition precluded the development of effective therapy for metastatic tumors, although both radiation therapy and chemotherapy have been tried with limited results. Most cases of metastases occur within 6 months to 1 year from initial presentation, but presentation after several years has been reported. Possible sites of metastases are the retroperitoneal lymph nodes, liver, lung, and bone, so the metastatic work-up and consequent follow-up should include evaluation of these areas.

Suggested Readings

Buchino JJ, Buchino JJ, Uhlenhuth ER: Large-cell calcifying Sertoli cell tumor. J Urol 141:953–954, 1989

Gabrilove JL, Freiberg EK, Leiter E, et al: Feminizing and non-feminizing Sertoli cell tumors. J Urol 124:757–767, 1980

Haas GP, Pittaluga S, Gomella L, et al: Clinically occult Leydig cell tumor presenting with gynecomastia. J Urol 142:1325–1327, 1989

Haas GP, Shumaker BP, Cerny JC: High incidence of benign testicular tumors. J Urol 136:1219–1220, 1986

Perito PE, Ciancio G, Civantos F, et al: Sertoli-Leydig cell testicular tumor: Case report and review of sex cord/gonadal stromal tumor histogenesis. J Urol 148:883–885, 1992

Tokuc R, Sakr W, Pontes JE, et al: Accuracy of frozen section examination of testicular tumors. Urology 40: 512–516, 1992

LEYDIG CELL TUMORS OF THE TESTIS

S. BRUCE MALKOWICZ, M.D.

Philadelphia, Pennsylvania

Leydig cell tumors are relatively rare interstitial cell testicular lesions (1 to 3 per cent of all testicular tumors). These lesions are derived from the Leydig cells, which secrete testosterone in response to luteinizing hormone and are found in the connective tissue about the spermatogenic tubules. The cells are distributed in groups of 5 to 20 per tubule and account for 10 to 12 per cent of the testicular mass. The Leydig cells are derived from the mesenchymal cells about the seminiferous tubules. Many Leydig cell tumors will display pathognomic crystalloids of Reinke, yet it is not necessary to demonstrate them for a definitive diagnosis.

The majority of Leydig cell tumors present after puberty. Although 25 per cent may occur in childhood, Leydig cell tumors account for only 1 per cent of the lesions in the prepubertal testicular tumor registry. The peak age of presentation in this population is between ages 4 and 5 years. The majority of adult tumors present between 20 and 35 years of age, but the range can extend into old age (>80 years). There is no association between cryptorchidism and this disease. Distribution is equal for the right and left side. There is a 3 per cent frequency of bilaterality. Approximately 10 per cent of these tumors are malignant, and these occur exclusively in the adult population.

The etiology of this tumor is not well defined. Rodent models of this lesion have been developed by the exogenous administration of estrogen. In vivo data are rather sparse but do not suggest increased hormone levels as initiators or promoters of this tumor. Some immunohistochemical studies suggest that estrogen and progesterone receptor are expressed in Leydig cell tumor cells as opposed to normal Leydig cells, perhaps making them more sensitive to normal circulating levels of these hormones. Intermediate filaments are present in normal Leydig cells as well as tumor cells. Their expression in malignant Leydig cell tumors has not been well documented.

A Leydig cell tumor is usually solid, tan-red/brown, well circumscribed, and nonhemorrhagic/necrotic. These should be distinguished from hypertrophic nodules, which occur secondary to increased adrenal steroids, as in congenital adrenal hyperplasia. Not all cases of Leydig cell tumor will exhibit Reinke crystals, and a degree of seminiferous tubule atrophy is associated with these tumors.

The only true sign of malignancy in these lesions is metastases, making the definition of malignancy somewhat circular. It has been suggested that findings of a diameter greater than 5 cm, infiltrative margins, lymphatic/vascular invasion, necrosis, or high cellular grade/mitotic index are suggestive of but not diagnostic for malignancy. Metastases may develop as late as 8 years after the initial tumor diagnosis. The most common metastatic sites include the retroperitoneal or inguinal lymph nodes (68 per cent), lungs (45 per cent), liver (45 per cent), and bones (28 per cent). The tumor is essentially nonmalignant in the pediatric population.

In adults the most common clinical presentation is painless testicular swelling with or without an irregular mass. Gynecomastia may occur in 20 to 40 per cent of patients. Occasionally, the presenting symptom may be testicular pain. Other symptoms are associated with estrogen or progesterone imbalances, such as decreased libido and impotence. The mean time from recognition of symptoms to diagnosis is approximately 3 years. Other conditions in the differential diagnosis include Klinefelter syndrome and feminizing adrenogenital disorders.

In children, the most common presentation is isosexual precocious virilization. The diagnosis is made by the presence of a testicular mass, increased urinary 17-ketosteroids, and precocious puberty. Leydig cell tumors account for approximately 10 per cent of the cases of precocious puberty cases in male children. In addition to virilization, an overlay of feminization may occur (20 per cent gynecomastia).

The evaluation of such patients includes several biochemical studies to exclude congenital adrenal hyperplasia, adrenal carcinoma, and idiopathic precocious puberty. Biochemical evaluation entails serum testosterone, dehydroepiandrosterone, androstenediol, 17-hydroxyprogesterone, 11-desoxycortisol, and urine 17-ketosteroids. Boys with Leydig cell tumors will display increased testosterone, androstenediol, 17-hydroxyprogesterone, and 17-ketosteroids, with normal follicle-stimulating hormone and luteinizing hormone levels. A human chorionic gonadotropin stimulation test may distinguish Leydig cell hyperplasia from Leydig cell tumors. Additionally, adrenocortical hyperplasia can be corrected by replacement therapy, which suppresses adrenocorticotropic hormone secretion that, in turn, results in hyperplastic Leydig cell nodule regression.

In addition to laboratory findings, imaging studies may aid in the diagnosis of Leydig cell tumors. Leydig cell tumors usually appear as hypoechoic lesions on ultrasound, although this presentation is not pathognomonic. Resolution of such lesions can be quite good, with successful imaging of such lesions down to 3 mm. Testicular magnetic resonance imaging at 1.5 T also has been useful clinically if the suspicion of a Leydig cell tumor exists in the absence of other clinical signs.

Therapy for adult Leydig cell tumors usually consists of radical orchiectomy. Once a diagnosis is established, other imaging tests, such as a retroperitoneal computerized tomography scan and chest radiography, should be performed. Feminizing features may persist after surgery and are not an indication of metastatic or residual disease. In children, the standard therapy is simple orchiectomy, with testis-sparing surgery also available as an option. Retroperitoneal lymph node dissection is indicated in resectable malignant Leydig cell tumors. The poor response of these lesions to radiation therapy and chemotherapy supports the role of surgery in this disease, yet few sustained complete responses are documented after surgical excision. Uncertainty exists in the approach to those patients with worrisome pathologic features yet nonmetastatic disease. The development of template and nerve-sparing retroperitoneal lymph node dissection techniques has the potential to broaden the indications for performing surgery in patients with pathology suggestive for malignancy. Each case, however, must be individualized.

After the diagnosis of metastatic Leydig cell tumor, the survival is approximately 2 to 3 years. Long-term clinical follow-up is lacking in many reported cases. Approximately 20 per cent of well-documented cases were metastatic at initial presentation or on postoperative staging. The remaining patients with metastatic disease usually present in 16 to 28 months, with a range of 4 months to 8 years. Much of the follow-up on patients with benign histologic features is incomplete, but no patients with totally benign features and long-term follow-up are documented as undergoing malignant transformation. Few patients receive any benefit from external beam radiation therapy. No instances of tumor regression have been noted, and only some relief from bone pain has been documented. There are few data to support or disclaim secondary surgery in the face of tumor recurrence. If an isolated lesion is the only measurable disease, an attempt at surgery is not unreasonable. In more diffuse disease this is probably not effective.

Patients with malignant Leydig cell tumors have not benefited from classic platinum-based combination chemotherapy. Doxorubicin and cyclophosphamide have been equally ineffective. *o,p'*–DDD (mitotane) has displayed responses in three of eight patients. Only one complete response was obtained, yet this was durable (5 years), allowing the patient to live for 7 years after diagnosis of malignant disease.

Suggested Readings

Bertram KA, Bratloff B, Hodges GF, et al: Treatment of malignant Leydig cell tumor. Cancer 68:2324–2329, 1991

Buckspan MB, Klotz PG, Goldfinger M, et al: Intraoperative ultrasound in the conservative resection of testicular neoplasms. J Urol 141:326–327, 1989

Kay R: Prepubertal testicular tumor registry. Urol Clin North Am 20:1–5, 1993

Kim I, Young RH, Scully RE: Leydig cell tumors of the testis: A clinicopathological analysis of 40 cases and review of the literature. Am J Surg Pathol 9:177–192, 1985

van der Hem KG, Boven E, van Hennik MB, et al: Malignant Leydig cell tumor of the testis in complete remission on o,p'/dichlorodiphenyldichoroethane. J Urol 148:1256–1259, 1992

SECTION 9

INFERTILITY AND STERILITY

MALE SUBFERTILITY

JOEL L. MARMAR, M.D.

Camden, New Jersey

In the past, the treatment of male subfertility was often empirical. Men received hormone therapy for oligospermia despite normal serum levels of testosterone. Varicoceles were repaired without a clear understanding of the pathophysiology. Infections were treated without an understanding of sperm membrane physiology. Recently, information concerning molecular biology, genetics, and sperm function has been included in the male subfertility work-up. More specific treatment plans have been developed, including the use of assisted reproductive technologies to supplement conventional therapy.

This article reviews some of the assisted reproductive techniques that are used in clinical practice. Although the results may be variable, urologists must become familiar with these techniques. To illustrate the role of a comprehensive work-up, the molecular biology, genetics, and results of sperm function tests for some diagnoses of male subfertility are reviewed and the treatment plans that have been recommended for these cases are described.

ASSISTED REPRODUCTIVE TECHNOLOGIES FOR MALE SUBFERTILITY

Sperm Processing and Intrauterine Insemination

Sperm processing and intrauterine insemination (IUI) is a relatively simple technique that may be performed in an office setting. The whole semen is collected at the time of the procedure and the sperm are processed to remove seminal plasma. (Some of these techniques are described in the article on "Techniques of Andrology.") Ovulation must be predicted from either basal body temperature charts, ovulation predictor kits (documenting the luteinizing hormone [LH] surge), or ovarian ultrasound. IUIs may be performed with either unstimulated cycles or with combinations of ovulation inductions (oral clomiphene citrate or injections with Pergonal or Metrodin). These techniques require 5 to 10 million motile sperm in the final prepared specimen, and the fecundity rates (pregnancies per cycle) may range between 9 and 14 per cent.

The GIFT Procedure

Gamete intrafallopian transfer (GIFT) requires ovulation induction and egg retrieval by either laparoscopy or vaginal ultrasound. The oocytes and prepared sperm, separated by an air space, are drawn up into a small delivery canula (the techniques for sperm preparation are discussed in the article on "Techniques of Andrology"). The eggs and the sperm are introduced into the fallopian tube by laparoscopy. Fertilization occurs within the fallopian tube and implantation follows the wife's biologic responses. Approximately 200,000 to 400,000 motile sperm are utilized for this procedure, and the pregnancy rates have ranged between 20 and 35 per cent. This technique has been useful for male subfertility and in cases of unexplained infertility, but the female partner must have normal fallopian tube anatomy.

In Vitro Fertilization

Following ovulation induction, the oocytes are retrieved and incubated with prepared sperm in a test tube or Petri dish. These procedures require 25,000 to 50,000 motile sperm per oocyte. In cases of reduced sperm numbers, microinsemination techniques are utilized that employ microliter volumes of fluid, and in these cases as few as 10,000 to 15,000 motile sperm per oocyte have achieved fertilization.

Fertilization is determined by the presence of two pronuclei within the oocyte. The developing embryos are placed into the uterus as pronuclei or after cleavage occurs. In some cases, the embryos are placed into the fallopian tube as part of zygote intrafallopian transfer (ZYFT).

The fertilization rates may be related to the values of whole semen. If all semen parameters are normal, up to 80 per cent of the oocytes may be fertilized. If there is a one- or two-parameter defect of the semen values compared to the World Health Organization thresholds, the fertilization rate drops to between 45 and 50 per cent of the oocytes. In cases with three-parameter defects, the fertilization rates are reduced to less than 10 per cent. The overall pregnancy rates with in vitro fertilization (IVF) and male factor problems is approximately 12 to 18 per cent.

Micromanipulation

With failure of fertilization during IVF or in those cases with severely reduced sperm numbers, micromanipulation procedures may be utilized. Presently, three techniques are available. Partial zona dissection utilizes a finely ground glass canula to open one or two micro-holes in the zona pellucida for access of a limited number of sperm. Subzonal insertion places three to five sperm under the zona pellucida. The sperm must be preselected by processing techniques. Direct injection of a single sperm into the oocyte is yet another technique for micromanipulation, and this method requires only a single sperm for fertilization. New techniques now are being investigated that utilize predecondensed sperm as part of the direct injection process.

Micromanipulation offers options to some men with subfertility who have been foreclosed from treatment in the past, but the pregnancies have been limited. Men with three-parameter defects in whole semen may fertilize up to 20 to 25 per cent of the oocytes with micromanipulation, but the reported pregnancy rates have varied from 5 to 25 per cent per cycle from various centers. These techniques seem to require a long learning curve, but these methods will be the subject of much research in the future.

SPECIFIC DIAGNOSES OF MALE SUBFERTILITY

Hypogonadotropic Hypogonadism

This condition results from a genetic disorder that causes the neurons of the olfactory bulb to fail to migrate into their proper anatomic position. As a result, the mid-brain does not release the gonadotropin-releasing hormone (GnRH). These patients have delayed puberty, reduced testicular size, and azoospermia. The serum values for LH follicle-stimulating hormone (FSH), and testosterone are reduced. These patients often present with anosmia, which is part of Kallmann syndrome. Although this condition is rare, it represents a model that illustrates the importance of the complete work-up of the female partner.

These men respond to exogenous human chorionic gonadotropin and Pergonal (FSH) on alternate days. Over 3 months, the patients initiate spermatogenesis and motile sperm will appear in the ejaculate. Pregnancies have resulted with only 3 to 5 million sperm/ml in the whole semen. These cases illustrate that pregnancy may occur with relatively few sperm so long as there are no female factors. Furthermore, vigorous treatment of the female actually may overcome some minor problems with male subfertility. Therefore, it is important for the urologist to interact with the gynecologist and ensure that the female work-up and treatment is completed.

Androgen-Resistant Syndromes

The treatment of male subfertility with exogenous hormones has been disappointing for cases of idiopathic oligospermia. These patients usually have normal serum values for FSH, LH, and testosterone. An elevated FSH level usually suggests end-organ failure, and this condition is not responsive to therapy. Some patients with idiopathic oligospermia may go directly to assisted reproductive technologies. However, it seems as though there may be a subset of patients with mild forms of androgen-resistant syndrome who may be responsive to hormonal therapy.

The androgen receptor genes are located on the X chromosome and the genes for the enzyme 5-α-reductase are located on chromosomes 2 and 5. This enzyme converts testosterone to dihydrotestosterone, the most potent intracellular androgen. Defects among these genes may produce a faulty androgen receptor, leading to a spectrum of androgen-resistant disorders. For example, the extreme forms of androgen-resistant syndrome are manifested by testicular feminization and Reifenstein syndrome. In the former case, the patients are genetic males but phenotypic females. They are usually deficient in 5-α-reductase. They are raised as females and, after removal of the gonads, they receive a lifetime of estrogen replacement. Men with Reifenstein syndrome represent an intermediate stage of androgen resistance. These patients may present with severe oligospermia, azoospermia, and hypospadias. They usually have qualitative and quantitative defects of the androgen receptors and are poorly responsive to hormonal stimulation.

In contrast to these extreme forms, there are more common types of androgen-resistant syndromes that simply present with male infertility. Based on tests of androgen receptors in skin fibroblasts, it has been estimated that 40 per cent of men with oligospermia or nonobstructed azoospermia may have mild forms of androgen-resistant syndrome. More recently, Southern blot analysis and polymerase chain reactions have identified subfertile males with minor genetic deletions that seem to be responsible for mild forms of androgen-resistant syndromes. These patients have been treated with clomiphene citrate and/or tamoxifen and there has been improvement in the semen parameters. These cases may represent a subpopulation of patients who would benefit from hormonal stimulation therapy.

Some men with mild androgen-resistant syndrome demonstrate elevation of both LH and testosterone. Although this is a relatively easy test to obtain, it is not a consistent finding in all cases. In the future, it is hoped that less expensive genetic testing may be available to identify these patients. At the present time, the use of exogenous hormones is still empirical but may benefit some patients, especially those with mild forms of androgen-resistant syndrome.

Varicocele

The varicocele is one of the most common diagnoses among men with male infertility. Approximately 30 to 45 per cent of patients who present to infertility clinics have varicoceles. However, not all patients with varicoceles are infertile, and approximately 15 to 17 per cent of these men achieve fatherhood without therapeutic intervention. Therefore, it seems important to identify subfertile men with varicoceles before recommending surgery.

To help identify these men, the expanded semen analysis, sperm function test, and provocative tests of hormonal stimulation have been utilized. In some centers, the sperm penetration assay and hypo-osmotic swelling test have been helpful to select patients who may be candidates for varicocelectomy. Some men have received a GnRH stimulation test to identify Leydig dysfunction. Following surgery, approximately 30 to 45 per cent of these men may improve their function test results, leading to pregnancy rates of up to 40 per cent. In addition, the patients seem to be better candidates for assisted reproductive technologies following their varicocelectomies. For example, after varicocelectomy, the fecundity rate with IUI has been approximately 9 to 14 per cent per cycle, which is significantly higher than that for men who received medical therapy alone. Among patients who have been involved with the GIFT procedure, the postvaricocelectomy pregnancy rates have been reported to be between 30 and 35 per cent per cycle, which is also significantly greater than the rates for untreated men with varicoceles. After varicocelectomy, the pregnancy rate with IVF has been reported to be about 20 per cent among a group of men who had failed fertilization with IVF prior to surgery. Therefore, correction of varicoceles with outpatient procedures remains an important therapy for subfertile males, especially those who demonstrate abnormal sperm function on tests.

Congenital Absence of the Acrosome

The acrosome is derived from the Golgi apparatus during spermatogenesis. In some cases, the acrosome may be absent or there may be subtle forms of dysfunction. Men without acrosomes demonstrate round-headed sperm in the ejaculate, despite a normal sperm density and motility. These patients are unable to achieve pregnancy by coitus or with standard IVF techniques. These men may benefit by intra-oocyte injection in the future. Congenital absence of the acrosome is a relatively rare condition, but there seem to be more subtle forms that are more common and represent a spectrum of disorders related to the development and function of the acrosome.

When a group of infertile males were tested by acrosome stimulating protocols, some seemed to have a faulty response. Men with minor acrosomal defects may respond to sperm preparation techniques prior to IUI or other reproductive technologies. These subtle forms of acrosomal defects should be considered for the work-up of infertile men, especially those with unexplained infertility.

Immotile Sperm and Sperm Motility Defects

The development of the sperm tail is similar to that of other ciliated structures in nature, and the tails contain microtubules in a ratio of nine outer to two central tubules. In addition, there are dense fibers that surround the outer tubules in human sperm. Kartagener syndrome is a genetic defect of abnormal cilia development, including sperm tails. Although the sperm density may be normal and the acrosome may be well formed, electron microscopy of the sperm tail reveals a disordered configuration of the 9:2 relationship of the microtubules. These sperm are immotile and these men cannot fertilize by coitus. Although this specific condition is rare, there may be a spectrum of genetic defects that involve the sperm tail and affect sperm motility.

Other electron microscopy studies have indeed documented abnormalities of the microtubules and dense fibers in patients with subfertility and poor sperm motility. It is believed that these defects arise during spermatogenesis and may be related to the interaction of the late spermatocytes with Sertoli cells. Nevertheless, some of these sperm may respond to stimulation with compounds such as pentoxifylline, which leads to an increase of intracellular ATP. Patients with selective motility defects who prove to be responsive to stimulation may be candidates for sperm processing and either IUI or IVF.

CONCLUSION

This article has provided an overview of molecular biology and genetics as they relate to spermatogenesis. Although the cases illustrated here are limited, the principles should be considered in evaluating men with subfertility. Sperm function tests may help develop specific treatment programs for these men. In addition to the conventional therapies, the use of sperm processing and assisted reproductive technologies may prove beneficial for some men with subfertility and minor forms of genetic deletions. In the future, it seems important for urologists to have a working knowledge of the molecular biology and genetics for spermatogenesis. The use of sperm function testing also may be important for urologists to help select a treatment program for men with subfertility.

Suggested Readings

Acosta AA, Krager TF, Swanson RJ, et al: Human Spermatozoa in Assisted Reproduction. Baltimore, Williams & Wilkins, 1990

Akin JW: The use of clomiphene citrate in the treatment of azoospermia secondary to incomplete androgen resistance. Fertil Steril 59:223, 1993

Cohen J, Alikani M, Adler A, et al: Microsurgical fertilization procedures: The absence of stringent criteria for patient selection. J Assist Reprod Genet 9:197, 1992

Hennig W: Spermatogenesis Genetic Aspects. Berlin, Springer-Verlag, 1987

Marmar JL, Corson SL, Batzer FR, et al: Insemination data on men with varicoceles. Fertil Steril 57:1084, 1992

VARICOCELE

NELSON N. STONE, M.D.

New York, New York

Varicocele is a common finding, occurring in approximately 15 per cent of the male population. This condition results from a dilation of the internal spermatic vein. The majority of varicoceles occur on the left side. Bilateral varicoceles are present 15 to 20 per cent of the time, whereas a true right-sided varicocele is unusual (2 per cent of cases).

The abnormal dilation of the spermatic vein(s) is thought to result from any of a number of causes. Autopsy studies have demonstrated absent valves in the internal spermatic vein occurring much more commonly on the left side as compared to the right. It has been postulated that the right-angle takeoff of the left spermatic vein from the left renal vein may predispose to this condition. Another explanation theorizes the existence of a "nutcracker phenomenon" whereby the left renal vein is compressed between the superior mesenteric artery and aorta, resulting in increased venous pressure in the internal spermatic vein.

The recognition that the varicocele may be a factor in male infertility dates back to first-century Greece, where it was found that swollen scrotal veins were associated with an atrophic testicle. As early as 1929, fertility was successfully restored by performing a varicocelectomy. However, the presence of a varicocele does not always result in an impaired semen quality or impaired fertility. This is best illustrated by the fact that, even though

15 per cent of the male population have varicoceles, only about 5 per cent of men report a fertility problem.

Notwithstanding the above, the varicocele is a well-recognized cause of infertility. Various studies document, on average, that 34 per cent of men presenting with infertility have a varicocele. Perhaps the favored explanation as to how the dilated spermatic veins effect spermatogenesis was described by Zorgniotti and Mcleod. They found elevations of scrotal temperature of 0.6° to 0.8° C in infertile men with varicoceles and postulated an impairment in the countercurrent heat exchange mechanism. Although others also have documented the presence of this impairment in heat exchange mechanism associated with the varicocele, this explanation is not accepted by all. Other theories as to the causal relationship between the varicocele and impaired fertility include an alteration in the hypothalamic-pituitary-gonadal axis, stagnation of blood in the testicular circulatory system with hypoxia of the spermatogonia, and reflux of adrenal and renal metabolites down the spermatic vein.

In certain individuals with oligospermia and a varicocele there exists a significant suppression in testosterone production. Seminal luteinizing hormone levels were found to be decreased in patients with a varicocele compared to normal controls. Such individuals may respond to human chorionic gonadotropin or Clomid administration because both increase intratesticular testosterone.

The semen analysis associated with a varicocele and infertility often has been described as a "stress pattern." The typical findings are a decrease in the numbers of sperm, a decrease in the motility of the sperm, and an increase in the number of immature or abnormally formed sperm.

Although this description usually is encountered in the infertile patient with a varicocele, it is by no means pathognomonic of a varicocele. Several studies have demonstrated similar semen patterns in patients with infertility without evidence of a varicocele, as well as in normally fertile men who were evaluated during a viral illness.

PHYSICAL EXAMINATION

Patients with a varicocele usually present for evaluation of infertility rather than with a specific complaint. Alternately, a large varicocele may have been encountered during a routine physical exam, especially in an adolescent. If a varicocele is encountered in an adult who has not previously had a history of infertility, no specific further evaluation or treatment is necessary. The only exception is the sudden onset of a large left varicocele in an older male. In such cases a retroperitoneal or renal mass should be considered as a cause of the varicocele. Renal cell carcinoma has been known to result in obstruction of the spermatic vein, causing a varicocele. The presence of a large varicocele in an adolescent and the indications for treating it represent a controversial issue, and will be discussed later.

The physical exam begins with the patient standing. This position will increase the pressure in the spermatic vein and accentuate a varicocele if present. Large varicoceles can appear as distended veins in the upper scrotum, the so-called bag of worms. If a varicocele is not readily apparent, the cord structures should be palpated bilaterally. The thick, ropy feeling of dilated veins should be clearly palpable in the left upper scrotum. In questionable cases the Valsalva maneuver should further dilate the spermatic veins.

Varicoceles may be classified according to their size. Grade 1 varicoceles are small and difficult to palpate; Grade 2 are easy to feel and do not require the Valsalva maneuver to detect, and Grade 3 varicoceles are large and can be seen protruding in the scrotum.

Some conditions may be confused with a varicocele on physical exam. The dilated veins of the varicocele often will disappear when lying down. Thus, if a lipoma of the cord is mistakenly identified as a varicocele, when the patient becomes supine it will not disappear. An indirect inguinal hernia may sometimes mimic a varicocele. A hernia should be able to be pushed back inside the internal ring, leaving a normal-feeling cord when that has been accomplished.

The testes and adenexa always should be examined when evaluating the infertile male. The vas deferens and epididymis are palpated throughout their respective courses within the scrotum. The testicles should be felt for any abnormalities and the sizes of the left and right testicles compared. A difference of greater than 0.5 cm between the long axes of the two testes is considered abnormal.

RADIOGRAPHIC STUDIES

The majority of the time, no ancillary studies are needed to confirm the presence of a varicocele. Doppler ultrasound has been useful in questionable cases. The Doppler detects the venous reflux, which may be demonstrated as an audible signal or recorded on polygraph paper. Although Doppler flow studies are accurate for detecting clinically obvious varicoceles, their use in confirming a diagnosis of a subclinical varicocele is controversial. The controversy surrounds the decision to evaluate the patient in whom a varicocele is not clinically palpable and then to base the decision to treat the patient on the Doppler findings. Indeed, several investigators no longer use the Doppler flow studies in evaluating their infertile male patients.

Thermography occasionally has been used to help confirm the presence of a varicocele or to follow a case. Scrotal thermography measures the surface temperature of the scrotal skin and reflects the intratesticular temperature. This test is no longer used commonly because, as mentioned above, there is little indication to treat a subclinical varicocele not detected by physical exam.

Venography is used most commonly in conjunction with embolization of the spermatic vein and thus is discussed under Treatment of Varicoceles. This study may be useful in cases of recurrent varicocele to help localize the cause or location of the recurrence (Fig. 1).

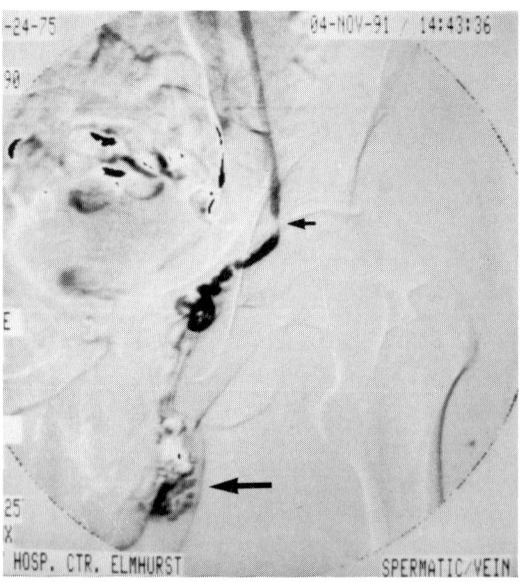

FIGURE 1. Recurrent varicocele. Venogram of spermatic vein demonstrates previously ligated area with persistence of smaller branch of spermatic vein (*small arrow*) and filling of veins in pampiniform plexus around testis (*large arrow*).

TREATMENT OF VARICOCELES

The ideal treatment of the varicocele requires interruption of the internal spermatic veins with preservation of the spermatic artery, the vas deferens with its blood supply, and the spermatic cord lymphatics. This may be accomplished by a number of surgical approaches or by radiographic embolization.

Surgical Techniques

Until recently there have been two surgical approaches to varix ligation, high inguinal and retroperitoneal. Within the last 2 years a third approach with the use of the laparoscope has been advocated by some.

The inguinal approach, as described by Ivanessevich and modified by Amelar and Dubin, requires an incision from the internal inguinal ring toward the external ring. The external oblique fascia is opened, exposing the spermatic cord, which is pulled up with a Penrose drain. The spermatic vein then is found, ligated, and divided. It is important to find all major branches of the spermatic veins with this approach. Because the spermatic artery is small (0.5 mm in diameter), it may be inadvertently ligated. In addition, lymphatic channels may be divided, leading to formation of a hydrocele in some patients.

Recently, Goldstein has advocated the lower inguinal approach with the use of the microscope to locate all the venous branches and preserve the spermatic artery. He performed 640 varicocelectomies on 429 men (211 bilateral) by making a short transverse incision at the level of the external ring. The distal spermatic cord and testis are delivered into the wound and, with the use of 8× magnification, all of the veins within the spermatic cord (with the exception of the deferential veins) are ligated and divided. The use of the microscope allows for identification and preservation of the testicular artery and lymphatics within the spermatic cord. The delivery of the testis into the wound allows for identification and division of any external spermatic and gubernacular veins. It is Goldstein's belief that division of these extra veins reduces the likelihood of any recurrence of the varicocele. With this technique he reported four recurrences (0.6 per cent) and no hydroceles.

The retroperitoneal approach was described originally by Palomo and required making a small transverse incision at the level of the internal ring to gain access to the spermatic cord. The cord, including the spermatic artery and vein, then was divided within the retroperitoneum proximal to the internal ring. The proximal division of the spermatic artery was thought not to compromise testicular blood supply because of adequate collaterals from the cremasteric and deferential arteries. A prior ipsilateral hernia repair or orchiopexy was a contraindication to this procedure.

Although the Palomo technique has been practiced successfully for many years, a modified approach that attempts to preserve the testicular artery and spermatic lymphatics still is preferred. The use of optical magnification or intraoperative Doppler probes has aided in the identification of the testicular artery. More recently, the laparoscope has been used to perform a type of modified Palomo procedure wherein retroperitoneal access is obtained by first moving intraperitoneally and incising the posterior parietal peritoneum over the spermatic vessels.

The laparoscopic technique requires general anesthesia and necessitates an intraabdominal approach. The Veress needle is inserted at the lower end of the umbilicus and the abdomen is insufflated with CO_2. A 10-mm trocar then is inserted into the distended abdomen with a laparoscopic lens and camera and the entire procedure is viewed on the monitor. Two or three ancillary trocars then are inserted under direct vision. The peritoneum just lateral to the varix is incised and the cord is identified. The large dilated spermatic vein is easily seen, grasped, and divided between clips (Fig. 2). After division of the main spermatic vein, smaller veins are identified and divided. The magnification from the laparoscopic lens and camera usually allows for identification and preservation of the spermatic artery (Fig. 3).

Information about the overall success of the laparoscopic technique has recently been published. Success rates appear to be similar to those for the open procedures. In a recent report, Mehan and Parra compared the open inguinal approach to the laparoscopic internal spermatic vein ligation. One hundred twenty-five consecutive open cases were compared to 70 laparoscopic ones. In all clinical parameters, including pregnancy rates (42 versus 28 per cent), hydrocele formation (1.5 versus 9 per cent), and shorter time to return to work, the laparoscopic approach was more successful.

Embolization

Embolization or sclerotherapy for varicoceles is relatively new, with the first reports published in 1978. The placement of a balloon or coil into the spermatic vein can be achieved through the femoral or internal jugular route. The complication rate is about 10 per cent, and the success rate for occlusion averages 73 per cent but varies from 50 to 100 per cent. Regardless of the technique used for varicocele repair, improvements in semen quality occur in 50 to 70 per cent of the patients undergoing correction of the varicocele, and pregnancy can be expected in 35 to 50 per cent of the couples. The differences in success

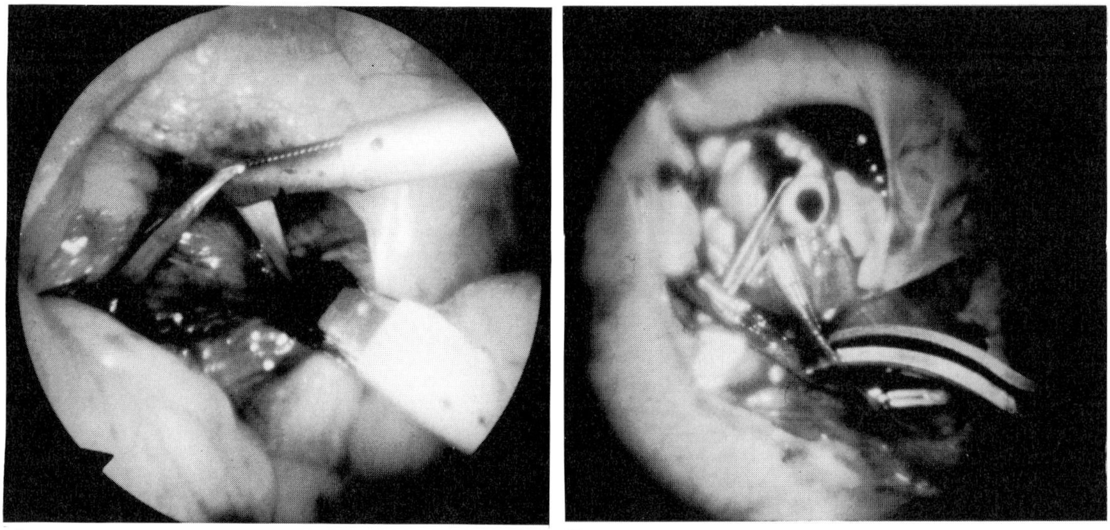

A B

FIGURE 2. Laparoscopic varicocelectomy. *A*, Endoscopic clip appliers ligate large internal spermatic vein. *B*, Vein has been clipped and divided.

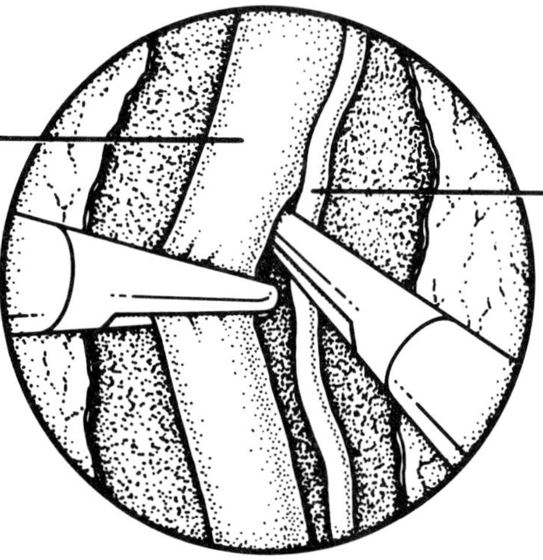

FIGURE 3. Laparoscopic varicocelectomy, schematic demonstrating how magnification from laparoscopic lens allows for identification and preservation of spermatic artery. (From Stone NN: Principles of laparoscopic surgery. *In* Droller MJ [ed]: Surgical Management of Urologic Disease: An Anatomic Approach. St. Louis, Mosby-Year Book, 1992, p 1269, with permission.)

rates are not related to the technique as much as to the preoperative sperm counts. In general, a patient with a sperm count of at least 10 million/ml has a 70 per cent chance of a successful outcome, compared to only 22 per cent in those patients with counts below 10 million/ml.

Varicocele in Adolescents

The treatment of a varicocele in an adolescent represents a special problem. These cases usually are discovered by the pediatrician during a school physical or identified by the child because of symptoms. The incidence of varicoceles in adolescents varies from 12.4 to 25.8 per cent, with an average of 16.3 per cent. The peak age of incidence is between 14 and 15 years of age. Although not all of these cases will need to be treated, repair might be indicated in any of the following circumstances:

1. Significant reduction in testicular volume.
2. Growth lag in the ipsilateral testis.
3. Symptoms (pain).
4. Bilateral varicoceles.

SUMMARY

Varicocele remains a common finding in the general population. Whereas 15 per cent of the male population have a varicocele, up to one-third of infertile men present with one. Surgical correction will result in improvement in semen quality in up to 70 per cent and pregnancy in 50 per cent of couples. Balloon embolization remains an alternative to surgical therapy and may be used preferentially in conjunction with venography in select cases of failed surgical therapy. A newer technique with the laparoscopic approach appears to be exciting but as of yet has not had a long enough track record to demonstrate superiority over the other methods.

Suggested Readings

Dubin L, Amelar R: Varicocele. Urol Clin North Am 5: 563, 1978

Goldstein M, Gilbert BR, Dicker AP, et al: Microsurgical inguinal varicocelectomy with delivery of the testis, an artery and lymphatic sparing technique. J Urol 148: 1808, 1992

Mehan DJ, Andrus C, Parra R: A comparative assessment of the open versus laparoscopic surgical treatment due to varicocele. J Urol 148:822a, 1993

Palomo A: Radical cure of varicocele by a new technique. Preliminary report. J Urol 61:604, 1949

Saypol DC, Lipschutz LH, Howards SS: Varicocele. *In* Lipschutz LH, Howards SS (eds): Infertility in the Male. New York, Churchill Livingstone, 1983, pp 299–313

Stone NN: Principles of laparoscopic surgery. *In* Droller MJ (ed): Surgical Management of Urologic Disease: An Anatomic Approach. St. Louis, Mosby-Year Book, 1992, p 1269

Zorgnitti A, McLeod J: Studies in temperature, human semen quality and varicocele. Fertil Steril 24:854, 1973

MICROSURGICAL VASOVASOSTOMY AND VASOEPIDIDYMOSTOMY

MARC GOLDSTEIN, M.D.

New York, New York

PREOPERATIVE EVALUATION

Physical Examination

Testis: Small or soft testes suggest impaired spermatogenesis and predict a poor outcome.

Epididymis: An indurated, irregular epididymis often predicts secondary epididymal obstruction, necessitating vasoepididymostomy.

Sperm Granuloma: A sperm granuloma at the testicular end of the vas means sperm has been leaking at the vasectomy site. This vents the high pressures away from the epididymis and improves the prognosis for restored fertility regardless of the time interval since vasectomy.

Vasal Gap: When a very destructive vasectomy has been performed, most of the scrotal straight vas may be absent, and the patient should be advised that inguinal extension of the scrotal incision will be necessary to enable a tension-free anastomosis.

Scars from Previous Surgery: Operative scars in the inguinal or scrotal region should alert one to the possibility of vasal obstruction at a site remote to the vasectomy. If two vasovasostomies are performed simultaneously in the same vas, devascularization of the intervening segments with subsequent fibrosis and failure could result.

Laboratory Tests

Semen analysis should be performed preoperatively to confirm the absence of sperm and document the diagnosis of azoospermia. Men with a low semen volume should have a transrectal ultrasound to alert one to the possibility of ejaculatory duct obstruction. The presence of serum or semen antisperm antibodies corroborates the diagnosis of obstruction.

Men with small, soft testes should have their serum follicle-stimulating hormone level measured. An elevated FHS level predicts impaired spermatogenesis and a poorer prognosis.

Anesthesia

General anesthesia is preferred. Slight movements are greatly magnified by the operating microscope and disturb performance of the anastomosis. If vasoepididymostomy is necessary, the operating time could exceed 4 or 5 hours. Muscle relaxation is necessary only when the incision is extended high into the inguinal region.

MICROSURGICAL VASOVASOSTOMY

Surgical Approaches

Scrotal

For vasectomy reversal, mark the external inguinal ring in case inguinal extension is necessary. Make 4-cm bilateral high vertical scrotal incisions beginning at the scrotal-inguinal junction and at least 1 cm lateral to the base of the penis. Deliver the testis to expose the entire scrotal vas.

INGUINAL INCISION

This is the preferred approach in men with suspected obstruction of the inguinal vas deferens from prior herniorrhaphy or orchiopexy. Incision through the previous scar usually leads directly to the site of obstruction.

Preparation of the Vasa

The vas is grasped with Babcock clamps. Penrose drains replace the Babcock clamps above and below the obstructed segment to facilitate dissection. The vas is mobilized for a distance of 3 to 4 cm on either side of the vasectomy site. Include the vasal vessels and periadventitial tissue. The vas should not be stripped of its sheath. The obstructed segment and, if present, the sperm granuloma at the vasectomy site should be removed.

When the vasal gap is large, dissect the entire convoluted vas free of its attachments to the epididymal tunic, allowing the testis to drop upside down (Fig. 1). These maneuvers can provide an additional 4 to 6 cm of length.

The testicular end of the vas is cut with an ultrasharp knife drawn through a slotted 2.5-mm diameter nerve clamp to yield a perfect 90 degree cut. The cut surface is inspected using $8 \times 15 \times$ magnification. A healthy white mucosal ring should be seen that springs back

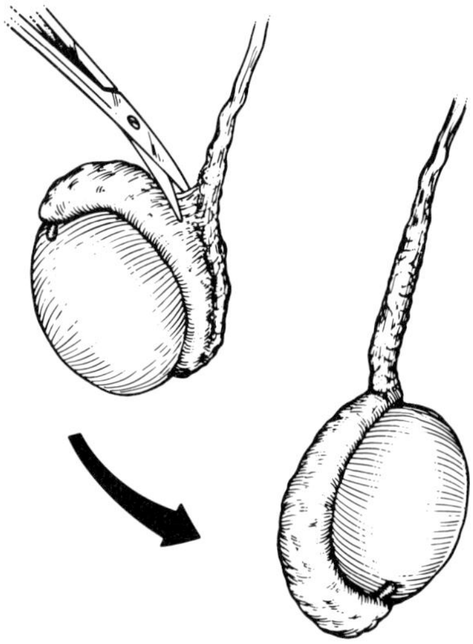

FIGURE 1. Dissection of the convoluted vas free of its attachments to the epididymal tunic allows the testis to drop down and provides 4 to 6 cm of additional length.

immediately after gentle dilation. If the blood supply is poor or the muscularis is gritty, the vas is recut until healthy tissue is found. The vasal artery and vein then are clamped and ligated with 6-0 nylon. Small bleeders are controlled with a micro-bipolar forcep. The vasal fluid is mixed immediately with a drop or two of saline and preserved under a cover slip for microscopic examination. The abdominal end of the vas deferens is cut in a similar manner and the lumen gently cannulated with a 24-gauge angiocath sheath. Injection of saline or Ringer lactate confirms its patency.

The ends of the vasa can be stabilized with a Goldstein Microspike approximating clamp. A sterile tongue blade covered with a Penrose drain is placed beneath the ends of the vasa to provide a platform on which to perform the anastomosis. Isolating the field through a slit in a rubber dam prevents micro-sutures from sticking to the surrounding tissue.

When To Perform Vasoepididymostomy

If microscopic examination of the vasal fluid reveals the presence of sperm with tails, vasovasostomy is performed. If no fluid is found, a 24-gauge angiocath sheath is inserted into the lumen and barbitage with 0.2 ml of saline performed while the convoluted vas is vigorously milked. *Men with large sperm granulomas often have virtually no dilation of the testicular end of the vas and little or no fluid may be noticed initially.* The barbitage fluid is expressed onto a slide and examined. *Invariably, when sperm granulomas are present, sperm are always found in this scant fluid.* If the vas is absolutely dry and spermless after multiple samples are examined, vasoepididymostomy should be performed. If the fluid expressed from the vas is found to be thick, white, water insoluble, and toothpaste-like in quality, examination rarely reveals sperm and vasoepididymostomy is performed. *When in doubt, and when the vasal fluid contains no sperm or sperm heads only, or if one is not very experienced with vasoepididymostomy, vasovasostomy should be performed.*

When copious, crystal clear, water-like fluid squirts out from the vas and no sperm are found in this fluid, a vasovasostomy is performed because the prognosis is good that sperm will return to the ejaculate.

Anastomotic Technique

All successful vasovasostomy techniques depend on adherence to surgical principles that are universally applicable to anastomoses of all tubular structures. These include:

1. Accurate mucosa-to-mucosa approximation.
2. Leakproof anastomosis.
3. Tension-free anastomosis.
4. Good blood supply.
5. Healthy mucosa and muscularis.
6. Good atraumatic anastomotic technique.

Microsurgical Multilayer Technique

Three 10-0 nylon sutures, double-armed with 70-μ taper-point needles with a fishhook configuration, are placed inside out in the mucosa under 20× to 32× magnification (Fig. 2). After these three mucosal sutures are tied, two 9-0 nylon deep muscularis sutures are placed exactly in between the previously placed mucosal sutures, just above but not through the mucosa (Fig. 3). These sutures seal the gaps between the mucosal sutures. A superficial adventitial 9-0 suture then is placed between these two muscularis sutures to provide additional strength. The vas is then rotated 180 degrees and three to five additional 10-0 sutures are placed to complete the mucosal portion of the anastomosis. Just prior to tying the last mucosal suture, the lumen is irrigated with heparinized Ringer solution to prevent the formation of clot in the lumen.

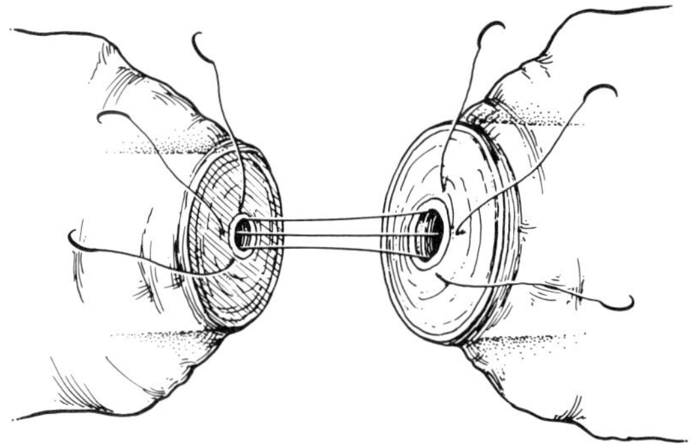

FIGURE 2. Three mucosal sutures are placed, inside out, and tied.

After completion of the 9-0 deep muscularis and superficial adventitial sutures, the anastomosis is finished by approximating the vasal sheath with six to eight sutures of 6-0 Proline. This layer completely covers the anastomosis and relieves it of all tension.

Anastomoses in the Convoluted Vas

Fear of cutting back into the convoluted vas in order to obtain healthy tissues may lead surgeons to complete an anastomosis in the straight portion when the testicular end of the vas has poor blood supply, unhealthy or friable mucosa, or gritty fibrotic muscularis. For anastomoses in the convoluted vas to succeed, a transverse cut yielding a round ring of mucosa and a lumen directed straight down is essential. A very oblique lumen with a thin flap of muscle and mucosa on one side is not acceptable. The vas should be recut at 0.5-mm intervals until a round lumen with good blood supply and healthy tissue is obtained. A slotted nerve clamp 3 to 4 mm in diameter and an ultrasharp knife facilitates this part of the procedure.

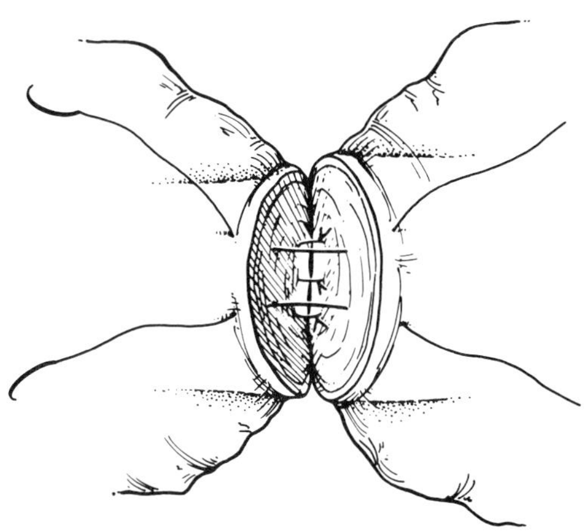

FIGURE 3. Deep submucosal sutures of 9-0 nylon, including all the muscularis and adventitia, are placed exactly in between each pair of mucosal sutures.

The convoluted vas should not be unraveled. This disturbs the blood supply at the anastomotic line.

The sheath of convoluted vas should be carefully dissected free of its attachments to the epididymal tunic (Fig. 1) to provide the necessary length to perform a tension-free anastomosis.

Crossed Vasovasostomy

Crossover is indicated in the following circumstances:

1. Unilateral inguinal obstruction of the vas deferens associated with an atrophic testis on the contralateral side.
2. Unilateral obstruction or aplasia of the inguinal vas or ejaculatory duct and contralateral obstruction of the epididymis.

Transect the vas attached to the atrophic testis at the junction of its straight and convoluted portion and confirm its patency with a saline vasogram. Dissect the contralateral vas toward the inguinal obstruction. Transect it and cross it through a capacious opening made in the scrotal septum and proceed with vasovasostomy as described above. This procedure is much easier than trying to find both ends of the vas within the dense scar of a previous inguinal operation.

It is preferable to perform one anastomosis with a high probability of success (vasovasostomy) than two operations with a much lower chance of success (i.e., unilateral vasovasoepididymostomy and contralateral transurethral resection of the ejaculatory ducts).

Long-Term Follow-Up Evaluation After Vasovasostomy

When sperm are found in the vasal fluid on at least one side at the time of surgery, carefully done microscopic anastomoses will result in appearance of sperm in the ejaculate in 90 to 98 per cent of men. Late obstruction, after initial patency, will occur in 5 to 10 per cent of men followed for at least 2 years. Pregnancy will occur in 50 to 60 per cent of couples followed for at least 2 years when female factors are excluded and sperm was found in the vas on at least one side at the time of vasovasostomy.

MICROSURGICAL VASOEPIDIDYMOSTOMY

End-to-End Anastomosis

End-to-end vasoepididymostomy is a most useful technique when the epididymal tubules are not markedly dilated or when vasal length is compromised, a situation commonly encountered during vasectomy reversal. The epididymis can be dissected off of the testis and flipped up to provide up to 5 cm of additional length.

The testis is delivered through a 3 to 4 cm high vertical scrotal incision. The vas deferens is isolated with a Babcock clamp and surrounded with a Penrose drain at the junction of the straight and convoluted portions of the vas deferens. Using 8× to 15× magnification, the vasal sheath is vertically incised with a microknife and a bare segment of vas, stripped of its carefully preserved vessels, is delivered. The vas is hemitransected with the ultrasharp knife until the lumen is entered. The vasal fluid is sampled. If microscopic examination of this fluid reveals the absence of sperm, the diagnosis of epididymal obstruction is confirmed. Saline vasography is performed as described earlier to confirm patency of the abdominal side of the vas deferens. The vas then is transected completely using a 2.5-mm slotted nerve clamp and the vas is prepared as described earlier for vasovasostomy. When end-to-end vasoepididymostomy is performed, as much sheath and periadventitial tissue should be left attached to the vas as possible.

The tunica vaginalis is opened and the testis delivered. The epididymis is encircled with a small Penrose drain and dissected proximally off of the testis to the vasoepididymal junction. The epididymis is encircled with a slotted nerve clamp of appropriate diameter (4 to 7 mm) and transversely sectioned using an ultrasharp knife. The distal epididymal stump is ligated and the proximal cut surface of the epididymis inspected under high-power magnification.

The epididymis is serially sectioned until a gush of cloudy fluid is seen effluxing from a single epididymal tubule. A touch prep of epididymal fluid is made. If many sperm are present, the single tubule continually effluxing fluid is identified by applying methylene blue to the cut surface of the epididymis. If no sperm are found or if the cut tubule is obliquely sectioned, the epididymis is recut until sperm-bearing fluid is found continually effluxing from a round, clearly visualized tubule.

The epididymis and vas deferens are stabilized with a Microspike approximating clamp so that the mucosa of the vas and single epididymal tubules are adjacent to each other. The anastomosis is begun under 32× magnification with the placement of two posterior mucosal sutures of 10-0 monofilament nylon double-armed with fishhook-shaped taper-point needles. Two to three additional anterior mucosal sutures are placed and all sutures are tied (Fig. 4).

After completion of the mucosal anastomosis, interrupted 9-0 nylon sutures are used to approximate the outer muscularis and adventitial layers of the vas deferens to the epididymal tunic. A Penrose drain is brought out in a dependent portion of the hemiscrotum.

End-to-Side Anastomosis

End-to-side vasoepididymostomy is most useful when vasal length is not compromised and marked dilation of the epididymal tubule is present.

Vasotomy, preparation of the vas, and opening of the tunica vaginalis is performed as described for end-to-end anastomosis. At a convenient point above the site of suspected obstruction, the epididymal tunic is incised with a microknife and trimmed with microscissors to create a round opening that

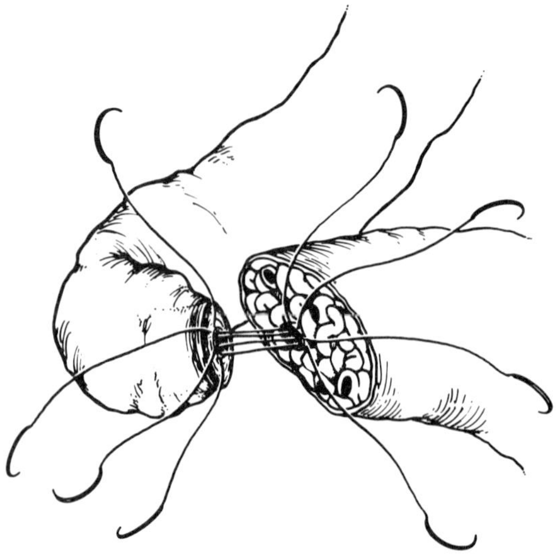

FIGURE 4. Placement of 10-0 mucosal sutures for end-to-end vasoepididymostomy.

matches the diameter of the previously prepared vas deferens. The tubules are dissected gently with a microscissors until a dilated loop of tubule is clearly exposed. The posterior edge of the epididymal tunic then is approximated to the posterior edge of muscularis and adventitia with three interrupted sutures of 9-0 nylon. This is done in such a way as to bring the vasal lumen into close approximation to the epididymal tubules selected for anastomosis. Under 25× to 32× magnification, using microscissors, the selected tubule is buttonholed and epididymal fluid is touched to a slide, diluted with saline, and inspected under the microscope for sperm. If no sperm are found, the opening in the tubule is closed and the procedure is repeated more proximally in the epididymis.

Once sperm are identified, methylene blue is dripped on the cut tubule to outline the mucosa. The posterior mucosal edge of the epididymal tubule is approximated to the posterior edge of the vasal mucosa with three sutures of 10-0 nylon double-armed with fishhook tapered needles. After these mucosal sutures are tied, the anterior mucosal anastomosis is completed with three additional 10-0 sutures. The outer muscularis and adventitia of the vas then are approximated to the cut edge of the epididymal tunic with 10 to 15 interrupted sutures of 9-0 nylon.

Long-Term Follow-Up Evaluation and Results

Microsurgical vasoepididymostomy in the hands of experienced and skilled microsurgeons will result in the appearance of sperm in the ejaculate in 50 to 80 per cent of men. Of men operated with long-term patency, about 43 per cent will impregnate their wives after a minimum follow-up of 2 years. Pregnancy rates are higher the more distal the anastomosis is performed. Additional pregnancies may be salvaged by redo operations in men who remain azoospermic, by in vitro fertilization (IVF) in men with very low counts but fairly good sperm quality, and by IVF combined with the micromanipulation techniques of partial zona dissection or subzonal insertion in men with poor sperm motility. In men who remain azoospermic despite repeated attempts at surgical reconstruction, microscopic epididymal sperm aspiration combined with IVF and oocyte micromanipulation offers hope.

Suggested Readings

Belker AM, Thomas AJ Jr, Fuch EF, et al: Results of 1,469 microsurgical vasectomy reversals by the Vasovasostomy Study Group. J Urol 145:505–511, 1991

Goldstein M: Surgery of male infertility and other scrotal disorders. *In* Walsh PC, Retik, AB, Stamey TA et al (eds): Campbell's Urology, 6th ed. Philadelphia, WB Saunders, 1992, pp 3114–3149

Schlegel PN, Goldstein M: Microsurgical vasoepididymostomy: Refinements and results. J Urol 150:1165–1168, 1993

Thomas AJ Jr: Vasoepididymostomy. Urol Clin North Am 14:527, 1987

TECHNIQUES OF ANDROLOGY

JOEL L. MARMAR, M.D.

Camden, New Jersey

The semen analysis has been the most widely used diagnostic test for the evaluation of male infertility for several decades, and the World Health Organization (WHO) has recommended fertility threshold levels of 20 million sperm/mL, 50 per cent motility, and 40 per cent normal morphologic forms. However, these threshold levels do not always distinguish fertile from infertile men. In recent years, the semen analysis has been expanded and sperm function tests have been utilized in clinical practice. These tests seem more predictive of fertility potential because they evaluate specific events of capacitation that occur after sperm leave the seminal plasma within the female reproductive tract. Subtle male factor problems may be identified with these tests, including changes related to hyperactivated motility, binding to the zona pellucida, completion of the acrosome reaction, and fusion of sperm to the oolemma membrane.

In addition to the diagnostic benefits, many of the methods used for sperm function tests have been adapted for assisted reproductive technologies, which have been used more often for the treatment of male subfertility. This article reviews some techniques of andrology, including the expanded semen analysis, sperm function tests, and sperm preparations. The intent is to point out the relevance of these techniques to the diagnosis and treatment of specific male factor problems.

LIQUEFACTION AND VISCOSITY

At the time of ejaculation, semen is normally thick because of coagulating proteins from the seminal vesicles. These specimens usually liquefy within 30 minutes because of the enzymatic action from the prostatic fluid. This process occurs more rapidly within a 37° C incubator. If a coagulum remains after incubation, this may be a cause of subfertility. These patients should be evaluated for prostatic inflammation and treated accordingly, and, if increased viscosity is noted on a postcoital test, a specific treatment plan is needed to deal with trapped sperm.

In the laboratory, the coagulum may be disrupted by transfer through a 21-gauge needle or by Percoll filtration and centrifugation. Small Percoll beads are available commercially and may be diluted into separate concentrations of 80, 60, and 40 per cent. An aliquot of 0.3 to 1.0 ml of the most dense concentration of Percoll (80 per cent) is placed at the bottom of a conical centrifuge tube and equal volumes of 60 and 40 per cent concentrations are layered on top in that order. The semen sample is placed above the Percoll and centrifuged at $300 \times g$ for 30 minutes. When the supernatant is removed, including the upper two thirds of the Percoll filter, the motile sperm remain at the bottom of the tube. After resuspension in 0.5 to 1.0 ml of Hams F-10 or other balanced salt solution, the sperm may be re-evaluated as part of an expanded semen analysis or this preparation may be used with assisted reproductive technologies.

ADVERSE EFFECTS OF POLYMORPHONUCLEAR LEUKOCYTES IN THE SEMEN

Polymorphonuclear leukocytes often are noted in the semen of subfertile men. Although these cells may be associated with infection, they may appear in semen without bacteria. It is now well known that the white blood cells produce oxygen free radicals that affect the sperm surface membrane. These radicals include hydrogen peroxide (H_2O_2), hydroxyl radicals (OH^-), and free oxygen ($O^{\cdot}$). These radicals may attack the phospholipid membrane of the sperm surface, and most laboratories now include sperm separation techniques as part of an expanded semen analysis to evaluate any negative effects of these cells or constituents of seminal plasma. Percoll filtration has been an effective method for eliminating white blood cells from the semen, and these preparations may be used in a variety of tests and procedures.

SPERM DENSITY

Sperm density may be determined with dedicated counting chambers. The Makler Chamber has been popular because it utilizes fresh semen and live sperm for evaluation of both sperm density and sperm motility. A drop of fresh whole semen is placed on the flat surface of the Makler Chamber. A special glass coverslip is positioned over the sample to create a depth of 10 μm. The coverslip contains a grid that is subdivided into 110 squares. The number of sperm counted in 10 separate squares is multiplied by 1×10^6 sperm/ml to give the sperm density. A hemocytometer may be used for the measurement of sperm density as well, but this method utilizes dead sperm. The semen is diluted 1:20 with water in a white cell pipette. A drop is placed on the slide of the chamber and the fluid spreads under the coverslip by capillary action. When the total sperm are counted within five red blood cell squares on the grid of the hemocytometer, this number is multiplied by 1×10^6 sperm/ml to give sperm density.

Despite careful laboratory technique, the value of sperm density may fluctuate on repeat analyses. For example, biweekly specimens from sperm donors usually demonstrate greater than 20 million sperm/ml. However, on some days, even donors will fall below this value. The results of longitudinal studies suggest that three specimens usually are needed to establish baseline values for 80 per cent of patients. If the discrepancies for sperm density are greater than 20 per cent after these three samples, additional specimens are needed to establish baseline values.

SPERM MOTILITY

Sperm motility may be assessed with a slide preparation. A drop of semen falling from the tip of a 21-gauge needle delivers approximately 10 to 15 μl of fluid. A 20×20-mm coverslip is placed over the fluid so that the depth is fixed at approximately 25 to 30 μm, which allows full expression of sperm motility. This preparation should settle for 1 minute and then be read at room temperature with 400× to 600× magnification or with a phase contrast microscope. The percentage of motile sperm is recorded from at least four to six fields and the number of motile sperm per 100 are recorded as the percent motility. The progressive motility of the sperm is scored in a semiquantitative manner: 1+ = immobile, 2+ = nonprogressive motility, 3+ = sluggish linear progression, and 4+ = rapid linear progression. Repeat motility studies should be carried out on prepared specimens after the seminal plasma has been removed. Observations at 2- and 6-hour intervals will document the preservation of sperm motility, which may be a problem for some subfertile men.

As the sperm undergo capacitation, a percentage of these cells will achieve "hyperactivation." They develop increased velocity, wide swings in lateral head displacement, and the lack of forward progression. Recently, computer-assisted semen analyzers have been utilized to provide objective measurements of sperm motility and hyperactivation, but these computerized systems are expensive ($30,000 to $40,000), and they are not cost-effective for most laboratories. As an alternative, the Makler Chamber may be useful for the evaluation of quantitative motility because the sperm movements between squares can be computed in microns per second. "Hyperactivation" may be estimated from these preparations without special equipment. This type of motility seems necessary for penetration into the zona pellucida, and unless 15 to 20 per cent of the sperm in a capacitated specimen achieve this motility, there may be a subtle male factor problem. When specimens fail to achieve a sufficient percentage of hyperactivated sperm, the specimen may be incubated with stimulants such as pentoxifylline as part of a diagnostic test or as a preparation for an assisted reproductive technology.

During evaluation of sperm motility, clumps of sperm may be observed on the slide preparation. In these cases, sperm antibody testing should be performed to document immunologic reactions. The immunobead test has been popular and utilizes small beads precoated with proteins specifically directed to the immunoglobulin IgA, IgG and IgM. If antibodies are present on the sperm surface, the beads will cling to the specific locations on the sperm head, midpiece, or tail. The immunobead test provides a semiquantitative assessment of the percentage of sperm involved with the antibody reaction as well as the location of the specific antibodies.

Not all cases of immunologic infertility present with clumping. The only finding in some cases may be reduced sperm motility. Patients with a selective motility defect on the semen analysis should be considered for sperm antibody testing. When the antibodies are detected, the laboratory may consider antibody elution. The semen is filtered through Percoll filtration and then incubated with immunobeads. Antibody-free sperm will "swim up" into the supernatant, and these sperm may be retrieved for assisted reproductive technologies. In the past, steroids have been used for the treatment of immunologic infertility, but this therapy has been used cautiously because of potential complications, including aseptic necrosis of the femoral head.

SPERM MORPHOLOGY

Recently, "strict criteria" have been used to evaluate normal sperm morphology. The sperm that meet these criteria seem capable of passage through cervical mucus, and of these sperm some will complete capacitation, a necessary step prior to fertilization. These strict criteria may be incorporated into an expanded semen analysis without additional special equipment.

The strict criteria require that normal sperm must have a smooth, oval head with a long axis of 5 to 6 μm and a short axis within 2.5 to 3.5 μm. The acrosome should cover 40 to 60 per cent of the sperm head. No neck, midpiece, or tail abnormality should be present. The midpiece is usually less than 1 μm in width and its entire length should be approximately 1.5 times the head length. No cytoplasmic droplets greater than one half the area of the sperm head should be present. The tail should be uniform and slightly thinner than the midpiece. The tail should appear uncoiled and measure approximately 45 μm in length. A variety of commercially available products may be used for staining, such as Papanicolaou stains, DIF-Quick, and Spermac.

The results with in vitro fertilization (IVF) have been uniformly poor without at least 14 per cent normal morphologic forms in whole semen as determined by strict criteria. The values for normal morphology by strict criteria also may be predictive of the outcome of other sperm function tests. The WHO has modified its standards for the semen analysis in its most recent publication to include strict criteria for sperm morphology.

TESTS OF SPERM FUNCTION

Acrosome Reaction

The acrosome reaction begins during capacitation, but it is completed on contact with the zona pellucida. Sperm washing techniques, exposure of the sperm to female steroids such as human follicular fluid or progesterone, or incubation with calcium iontophores may induce the acrosome reaction in the laboratory. The triple stain technique distinguishes live from dead sperm, and acrosome-reacted from unreacted sperm. This technique may be performed with standard laboratory equipment, including a light microscope. Special fluorescent stains such as the FITC-Lectin stain may be more specific and attach to the inner acrosomal membrane, which demonstrates completion of the acrosome reaction. However, a fluorescent microscope is required to read this preparation.

Standard protocols to induce the acrosome reaction have been utilized in many laboratories, and 15 to 20 per cent of the sperm are expected to complete the acrosome reaction in responses to these protocols. With this testing, some men may demonstrate subtle acrosome disorders, especially in cases of unexplained infertility.

Hemi Zona Assay

The zona pellucida from unfertilized eggs obtained at the time of IVF may be used for a sperm binding test. These zona are split with microdissection so that equal halves are retained. The patient's sperm is incubated with one half of the human zona and donor sperm is incubated with the other half. Fertile men have demonstrated a mean sperm binding of 34±8 sperm versus 5.9±2 for nonfertile men. Because the ZP3 protein within the zona pellucida completes the reaction, this test has been used as a functional assay. The results have been correlated with the outcome of IVF, but this method requires additional equipment and skill with microdissections.

Hypo-osmotic Swelling Test

The membrane surrounding the sperm head, midpiece, and tail is a living structure that contains phospholipids. After a 30-minute incubation with a hypo-osmotic solution (150 mOsm/liter), at least 60 per cent of the sperm tails should demonstrate swelling from a net transfer of water. This test documents the viability and function of the sperm membrane and may be utilized to evaluate damage from reactive oxygen species. Furthermore, it is inexpensive and the test may be predictive of the outcome of IVF. Some centers have utilized hypo-osmotic swelling as a functional test of infertile men with varicoceles. However, the results should be considered along with other aspects of the history and diagnostic work-up.

Sperm Penetration Assay

The sperm penetration assay (SPA) uses zona-free hamster eggs for incubation with human sperm after capacitation. Frozen zona-free eggs are commercially available or eggs may be obtained from young golden hamsters after superovulation. The cumulus is removed from the fallopian tube and the eggs are separated by hyaluronidase. The zona is digested with trypsin. After capacitation, human sperm may attach and penetrate through the membrane of the zona-free egg and decondense. A swollen sperm head may appear within the cytoplasm.

In its original form, this test had many false-negative results. Recently, the methodology has been modified to enhance capacitation. In some centers, sperm are treated with calcium iontophore to induce capacitation. Others utilize treatment with TEST-yolk buffer and thermal chill to 4° C. This enhancement seems to minimize the false-negative results.

Our own laboratory has utilized the combination of Percoll filtration, pentoxifylline stimulation, and incubation with human follicular fluid prior to exposure to the zona-free hamster eggs. These techniques are similar to the protocols that currently are used in our center for sperm preparations prior to IVF. Our data suggest fewer false-negative results with the enhanced SPA, and these results seem more predictive of the outcome of IVF. For example, if there is a positive score with the enhanced SPA, the patient may be expected to fertilize at least 80 per cent of his wife's eggs at the time of IVF. If there is a negative result with the enhanced SPA, 50 per cent of these patients will have no fertilization at all at the time of IVF. The remaining 50 per cent may fertilize only up to 40 per cent of their wives' eggs. Presently, the enhanced

SPA is performed before recommending costly assisted reproductive technologies.

CONCLUSIONS

An array of andrology techniques have been used in the laboratory to evaluate male fertility potential. No one test can assess all aspects of sperm function, and a panel of tests may be needed for treatment planning. An expanded semen analysis is used for observation of sperm in whole semen and after seminal plasma has been removed. As part of this test, morphology is evaluated by "strict criteria." Other more complex functional tests may be used to evaluate specific aspects of sperm function, especially when assisted reproductive technologies are contemplated. These tests and techniques now have become a basic part of the work-up for male subfertility.

Suggested Readings

Aitken RJ, Buckingham DW, Fang HG: Analysis of the responses of human spermatozoa to A23187 employing a novel technique for assessing the acrosome reaction. J Androl 14:132, 1993

Keel BA, Webster BW: Handbook of the Laboratory Diagnosis and Treatment of Infertility. Boca Raton, FL, CRC Press, 1990

Menkveld R, Swanson RJ, Oettle EE, et al: Atlas of Human Sperm Morphology. Baltimore, Williams & Wilkins, 1991

Siegel MS: The male fertility investigation and the role of the andrology laboratory. J Reprod Med 38:317, 1993

World Health Organization: WHO Laboratory Manual for the Examination of Human Semen and Semen-Cervical Mucous Interaction. Cambridge, England, Cambridge University Press, 1987

SECTION 10

MISCELLANEOUS

CIRCUMCISION

JOHN F. REDMAN, M.D.

Little Rock, Arkansas

Circumcision, the surgical removal of the prepuce, is the most frequently performed surgical procedure on males in the United States, with the vast majority of circumcisions being accomplished in the neonatal period. Because of the dissimilarity of neonatal circumcision from that of childhood and adult circumcision, the two groups will be considered separately.

NEONATAL CIRCUMCISION

With regard to neonatal circumcision, there are two primary controversial issues: the need for routine circumcision in newborn boys and analgesia for the procedure.

Indications and Contraindications

In 1975, an Ad Hoc Task Force on Circumcision of the American Academy of Pediatrics concluded that "there is no absolute medical indication for routine circumcision." However, since that report new evidence has suggested possible medical benefits from neonatal circumcision, prompting, in 1989, a revised statement from the Task Force on Circumcision: "Newborn circumcision has potential medical benefits and advantages as well as disadvantages and risks." It is agreed that phimosis, the diagnosis of the inability to retract the fully differentiated prepuce as a result of a stenosis of the preputial ring, cannot be made in neonates. The reasons for circumncision in the neonate, therefore, fall under the rubric of prophylaxis. The reasons given are to prevent the need for circumcision later in life, carcinoma of the penis, paraphimosis, infections of the foreskin (posthitis) or the glans (balanitis), urinary tract infections (particularly in the first year of life), and sexually transmitted diseases.

The contraindications to neonatal circumcision include hypospadias, megalourethra, penile curvature, penoscrotal webbing, a dorsal hood suggestive of penile deformity, or a small or short penis. An unstable or sick infant should not be circumcised, nor should a premature infant until the criteria for discharge are met. If it is obvious that the infant will require an operative procedure within the first year of life requiring a general anesthetic, consideration should be given to delaying the circumcision until that time. A history of a familial bleeding diathesis should prompt appropriate studies in the infant prior to circumcision.

Informed Consent

It has been stated that the circumcision decision in the United States is emerging as a cultural ritual rather than a medical misunderstanding among parents. Nonetheless, parents deserve a dispassionate presentation of the potential medical advantages of circumcision with an understanding that the procedure is still considered by most authorities to be cosmetic. Surgical risks, complications, and analgesia should be covered. As much as possible, the individual obtaining consent should refrain from trying to influence a decision.

Analgesia

Local anesthesia may be obtained by dorsal penile nerve block. The use of a nerve block in infants is controversial but is gaining increasing acceptance. The practitioner should be well familiar with the anatomy of the neurovascular bundle and understand that the vasculature of the glans is diminutive in the infant and closely entwined with the nerves. Not more than 1 ml of 0.25 per cent plain lidocaine is injected at the base of the penis as an annular subcutaneous or dorsal nerve block. The anesthetic is administered 30 minutes before the procedure.

Techniques

Generally, neonatal circumcision is performed with devices that produce simultaneous hemostasis and coaptation of the epithelial surfaces by crushing. The term "clamp" reflects the function of the instruments. For ritual circumcision, a Mogen (Bronstein) clamp generally is used. The prepuce is placed on stretch while the glans is depressed and shielded from the knife by the clamp itself, which is not wide enough for the glans to slip through. The two most common instruments utilized for routine neonatal circumcision are the Gomco clamp and the Plastibell. Both instruments require a dorsal slit of the prepuce to facilitate the placement of a bell-shaped shield over the glans. With a Gomco clamp, the prepuce is drawn through a template, following which a thumbscrew is tightened to crush the prepuce between the bell and the template. All adhesions of the glans to the inner leaf of the prepuce should be lysed prior to the placement of the bell. The prepuce then is excised with a knife along the template. With the Plastibell a suture, which remains in place, is secured in a groove in the base of the bell, which crushes the prepuce. The redundancy then is excised. The plastic bell, which remains in place, will fall off spontaneously after several days.

At times it is difficult to ascertain the correct amount of skin to excise. A helpful technique is to extend the dorsal slit to within 2 mm of the corona or mark with a skin pencil at the level of the corona and then use the apex of the slit or the mark to guide the placement of the template of the Gomco clamp, the groove of the Plastibell, or the clamp of the Mogen clamp. Likewise, attention should be paid to the ventrum of the penis to avoid excising or leaving too much prepuce. Under no circumstances should electrocautery be used to excise the prepuce in the presence of a metallic instrument.

Complications

The most common complication of neonatal circumcision is the incomplete removal of the foreskin. Although not pernicious, it may precipitate complaints from the parents, either because the child appears uncircumcised or there remains a rosette of redundant skin at the coronal level. A more distressing complication is the removal of too much skin, even to the point of denuding the shaft. This problem is best managed by doing nothing other than applying an antimicrobial ointment and waiting. With healing, the appearance is frequently surprisingly normal. An unusual complication is the concealed or buried penis, in which a cicatrix develops at the circumcision site with subsequent depression and engulfing of the glans. Skin bridges between the prepuce and the glans may occur if the prepuce is not completely freed from the glans prior to circumcision. Unique complications may occur with the Plastibell if the bell remains in place too long. Therefore, a retained Plastibell should be removed if it has not fallen off spontaneously after several days.

CHILDHOOD AND ADULT CIRCUMCISION

Indications and Contraindications

The medical indications for circumcision are better defined for boys and men, although, if strict conditions were applied, few circumcisions would be done. The indications are recurrent balanitis or balanoposthitis, phimosis, paraphimosis, condylomata acuminata, and precancerous or cancerous lesions. Frequently, patients or parents of boys will request circumcision for hygienic reasons or recircumcision for cosmetic reasons.

Contraindications are few, but do include conditions in which the prepuce may be required for subsequent reconstructive surgery. It should be emphasized that, for asymptomatic adults particularly, the motives leading to a request for circumcision should be scrutinized. Underlying psychiatric problems may be uncovered that would contraindicate surgery.

Analgesia

Circumcision in males over 6 weeks of age usually is done under general anesthesia, although in adults frequently regional or local anesthetic blocks are utilized. The dorsal penile nerve block with circumferential injection at the base of the penis can provide excellent analgesia for circumcision.

Techniques

Although circumcision clamps are available in sizes to accommodate older individuals, they are not truly suitable. The two primary techniques are the free-hand or dorsal slit technique and the sleeve technique. With the free-hand or dorsal slit technique, a straight hemostatic clamp is placed so that the lower jaw lies between the inner leaf of the prepuce and glans, being careful not to place the lower jaw of the clamp in the urethra. Following crushing of the prepuce with the clamp and incising in the area of the crush, all adhesions between the prepuce and the glans are lysed. Using scissors, both leaves of the prepuce then may be incised simultaneously along the coronal margin to the frenulum. The procedure also may be facilitated by adding a ventral slit prior to excising the lateral remaining halves of the prepuce. Hemostatis is secured with electrocautery, followed by approximation of the penile skin to the remaining inner leaf of the prepuce with interrupted or running absorbable suture. This technique is used most commonly if the prepuce cannot be retracted.

The preferred technique for circumcision is the sleeve technique. A traction suture is placed in the tip of the glans using a small atraumatic needle. The penis is extended to its full length with a moderate amount of stretching approximating erectile length, following which the skin is marked using a skin pencil at the level of the coronal sulcus. This maneuver will prevent the excision of an excess of skin, which may not be noted until the patient has an erection. The skin then is incised through the dartos tunic with a knife. The prepuce is retracted and the inner leaf of the prepuce is marked, leaving a 3.5-mm collar in a child and a 1- to 1.5-cm collar in the adult patient. Following the incision of the inner leaf, the two incisions are connected and the prepuce is dissected from the shaft circumferentially. Strict attention is paid to hemostasis, a process that is facilitated by retracting the shaft skin. Reapproximation of the penile skin is achieved with interrupted or running absorbable sutures. A light compressing dressing is optional if good hemostasis has been achieved.

Complications

The most common immediate postoperative complication is bleeding, which frequently requires a return to the operating room for identification of the site of bleeding and appropriate hemostasis. The evacuation of a hematoma may be required. The most common late complications, particularly in adolescents and adults, are the sequelae of the excision of too much skin. The result will be complaints of pain on erection, foreshortening of the erection, and penile curvature or deviation with erection. Impotence following circumcision has been reported, as has the precipitation of psychotic delusional behavior.

Suggested Readings

Brown MS, Brown CA: Circumcision decision: Prominence of social concerns. Pediatrics 80:215, 1987

Colen MS: Circumcision. *In* Fowler JE (ed): Mastery of Surgery: Urologic Surgery. Boston, Little, Brown, 1982, p 422

Kaplan GW: Complications of circumcision. Urol Clin North Am 10:542, 1983

Report of the Task Force on Circumcision. Pediatrics 84: 388, 1989

Wiswell TE, Hachey WE: Urinary tract infections and the uncircumcised state. Clin Pediatr 32:130, 1993

ENURESIS

GEORGE W. KAPLAN, M.D.

San Diego, California

Enuresis is a very common reason for urologic evaluation. At age 5 years, approximately 10 per cent of American children are still wetting their beds. At age 15 years, 1 per cent of children are still plagued with this problem. One occasionally will even encounter adults who admit to persistent nocturnal enuresis. The following discussion deals only with bed wetting and will not cover to any extent the problem of diurnal incontinence.

Enuresis can be defined as involuntary bed wetting beyond a certain age, at which time such behavior is considered inappropriate. Often enuresis is classified as primary or secondary. Primary enuresis refers to persistent bed wetting from the time of toilet training, whereas secondary enuresis refers to a prolonged dry interval between toilet training and the resumption of wetting. The implication is that secondary enuresis has a different etiology from primary enuresis. Actually, many patients who have primary enuresis will experience one or two dry intervals of as long as several months.

The age of toilet training seems to vary somewhat from society to society. For example, there has been reported an African tribe in which toilet training is accomplished by age 9 to 12 months. However, in the United States, most girls are toilet trained by age 2½ years and most boys by age 3. Certainly nocturnal enuresis is not a problem that is unique to our modern industrialized society, because there are references to it in antiquity and it is seen in some of the more primitive cultures of the world today.

Many possible etiologies have been proposed; a rational understanding of therapy is enhanced somewhat by reviewing some of them. One of the more constant observations has been that of a family history of enuresis. Roughly 65 per cent of the parents of enuretic patients acknowledged the familial nature of the problem when queried. The implication of this fact may be twofold: (1) enuresis may be developmental, and (2) enuretic parents may tolerate the problem more than those unfamiliar with the problem.

A frequent thought of both physicians and parents is that enuresis is caused by emotional conflict. It might be, however, that emotional symptoms are caused by enuresis rather than vice versa. In at least one study, the authors were unable to determine any psychiatric cause for bed wetting in their patients. Two other arguments against psychiatric conflict being the sole cause of enuresis are the observations that psychotherapy, in and of itself, is rarely beneficial, and that psychiatric disease, just like other disease, rarely has such a single-symptom presentation.

Parents often will say that enuresis occurs simply because the child is too lazy to arise and void in the toilet. A quotation from Samuel Adams in 1844, I believe, expresses most graphically my feelings in this regard:

> None of the brute creation will lie in their urine if they are not tied or penned; then why do we attribute this practice in the rational being to laziness? Simply because some are not able, by a careless and superficial examination, to find the cause, and well knowing that their reputations will be at stake if they do not account for the act, they too often condemn the helpless child to daily flogging.

There are many who feel that enuresis is more likely a developmental delay of sorts; I am somewhat inclined to agree. Certainly, if one compares the bladder capacity of the enuretic child with that of his nonenuretic sibling, the bladder capacity of the enuretic child is definitely smaller at a comparable age. Additionally, if one performs cystometry, the incidence of uninhibited contractions of the bladder (what some have termed "the immature pediatric bladder") is greater in the enuretic group than in an age- and sex-matched nonenuretic group. Campbell has studied a group of enuretic children with various forms of psychologic testing and found no evidence of emotional disease in enuretic patients as a group but did find evidence further supporting the hypothesis that enuresis indeed may be developmental.

Some Canadian workers have strongly suggested that enuresis is a manifestation of an allergic diathesis in many children. In their experience, the utilization of elimination diets has been quite beneficial. However, my own studies of immunoglobulin E (IgE) levels in enuretic patients demonstrated no difference between the levels obtained in enuretic children and those obtained in the general population. This suggests strongly that enuresis is not an IgE-mediated problem. Additionally, a study by Siegel et al. failed to confirm the Canadian results. It was their conclusion, as well as ours, that allergy is not a major factor in the etiology of enuresis.

Many workers think of enuresis as a sleep disorder, because many enuretic children are characterized as being very deep sleepers; such children tend not to awaken even when vigorous attempts are made to arouse them. Studies of rapid eye movement sleep in enuresis have proved to be conflicting. Additionally, there can be electroencephalographic abnormalities in some enuretic patients. It was on this latter basis that phenytoin once was suggested as a therapeutic modality for this disorder. Unfortunately, anticonvulsants have not proved efficacious in this regard.

It recently has been suggested that a significant percentage of cases of enuresis are secondary to a deficiency in the normal nocturnal increase in antidiuretic hormone levels. It is not clear whether this is a permanent difference from normal or a temporary part of a maturational delay. This does seem to be an isolated hormonal deficiency and is not related to any generalized pituitary defect.

Occasionally, children with urinary infection will present with nocturnal enuresis. When secondary enuresis is caused by urinary infection, the infection is documented easily by urinalysis and urine culture, and, more importantly, both the infection and the enuresis respond very promptly to medical management of the infection. More often, however, a child with primary enuresis may develop urinary infection. There is some suggestion in the literature that such infections and enuresis both are caused by a common factor, which is as yet unidentified. In any event, the enuresis in this instance usually does not abate with successful treatment of the infection. Another problem that occasionally has been seen in enuretic patients is bladder-sphincter dyssynergia. However, this is seen more often in children who have both day and night wetting than in those who have nocturnal enuresis alone.

A major concern of referring physicians and parents is that there may be some underlying obstructive or neurogenic lesion causing the enuresis. On this basis, intravenous urography, voiding cystourethrography, and cystoscopy have been utilized widely in the past to rule out such problems. It is my personal feeling that it is relatively rare for an "organic" lesion to cause pure nocturnal enuresis. A careful history and physical examination with urinalysis and urine culture should effectively detect most significant problems in this regard. Most of the lesions that have been detected by routine urography and cystoscopy when all other studies are normal are, in my opinion, usually coincidental rather than cause-and-effect problems.

Multiple agents have been utilized for the treatment of enuresis, because no single agent enjoys anything approaching consistent success. It is of interest that there is a great placebo effect in any therapeutic endeavor to treat enuresis; in one British study, almost 40 per cent of the children seen responded completely after merely talking to the physician. Imipramine (up to 2 mg/kg per day) has been shown to be of benefit in both double-blind and cross-over studies. Its major drawback is its toxicity, because there is relatively little margin of safety between the therapeutic effect and toxicity. The major toxicity is cardiac, but, fortunately, this can be reversed by the use of physostigmine. Desipramine is another agent that has demonstrated a similar but lesser efficacy in treating enuresis. Anticholinergics, by and large, have not been of great utility in the treatment of nocturnal enuresis. However, one newer anticholinergic, oxybutynin, has been shown, in double-blind studies, to be of some limited benefit. Alarm devices have been used by both the British and Canadians with a moderate amount of success. For some reason, this form of behavior modification has not been accorded great acceptance in this country; yet, in my own experience, it is often successful and deserves more emphasis. The success rate with behavior modification seems directly proportional to the motivation of both parent and child. Desmopressin acetate nasal spray (up to 40 mg nightly) has been used empirically with a great deal of success. It is safe in that there have been very few adverse reactions. Unfortunately, it is moderately expensive. Finally, manipulative urologic therapy (e.g., urethral dilation or meatotomy) has been utilized frequently with a great deal of anecdotal success. However, there is no rationale for such therapy, in my opinion, and I believe that it is best avoided.

Suggested Readings

Brock WA, Kaplan GW: Voiding dysfunction in children. Curr Prob Pediatr 10:1, 1980

Kolvin I, Keith RC, Meadow SR: Bladder Control and Enuresis. London, W Heineman Medical Books, 1973

Norgaard JP, Pedersen EB, Djurhuys JC: Diurnal antidiuretic hormone levels in enuretics. J Urol 134:1029, 1985

Rushton HG: Enuresis. *In* Kelalis PP, King LR, Belman AB (eds): Clinical Pediatric Urology, 3rd ed. Philadelphia, WB Saunders, 1992, pp 365–383

HYPERALIMENTATION IN UROLOGY

TERRY W. HENSLE, M.D.

New York, New York

The close relationship between nutritional status and surgical outcome has been acknowledged grudgingly for a number of years. It is now generally accepted that malnutrition significantly affects the hospital course of patients undergoing major surgery. Malnutrition also has direct bearing on the morbidity and mortality of badly traumatized and septic patients. Severe protein loss has been shown to impede tissue repair, reduce resistance to infections, and interfere with enzyme and plasma protein synthesis.

Malnutrition is a major risk factor for the development of infection in the general surgical population. Immune defects seen in malnutrition include low levels of complement, impaired opsonic and neutrophil function, impaired delayed hypersensitivity, decreased lymphoid mass and function, and a reprioritization of acute-phase proteins. Nutritional repletion reverses this immune dysfunction, resulting in a decrease in infectious morbidity and mortality.

Recent studies have demonstrated that up to 50 per cent of hospitalized general surgical or general medical patients are malnourished to some degree. This demonstration of the wide prevalence of in-hospital malnutrition has brought the problem into focus. If the clinician is to accept the responsibility for the delivery of optimal medical and surgical care, he or she must establish accurately the nature of the patients' nutritional status and the extent of his or her individual nutritional needs.

NUTRITIONAL ASSESSMENT

Nutritional assessment should be an integral part of the evaluation of all hospitalized patients who are scheduled for an extensive surgical procedure or for some form of antineoplastic therapy. It has been demonstrated clearly that such surveillance can minimize the risk of elective or semielective cardiac surgery or solid tumor surgery. A full nutritional assessment is not a time-consuming or expensive undertaking. In its simplest form, nutritional assessment includes the measurement of the body protein stores, fat stores, and energy expenditure. Nutritional assessment kits and explanatory material are readily available to the clinician from all the major manufacturers of parenteral products.

TYPES OF IN-HOSPITAL MALNUTRITION

Nutritional assessment makes it possible to identify and categorize patients with in-hospital malnutrition. Protein malnutrition (*kwashiorkor*) is a disease state associated with severe depletion of the visceral protein compartment, lowering of serum albumin and transferrin values, and a depression of cell-mediated immunity. There may be little or no associated change in anthropometric measurements or height-weight index in these patients. Protein-calorie malnutrition (*marasmus*) is the more common form of in-hospital malnutrition. There may be some depression of the visceral protein compartment; however, there is marked loss of skeletal muscle compartment and body fat stores, as demonstrated by reduction of all the anthropometric measurements. A combination of kwashiorkor and marasmus is a frequent accompaniment of chronic illness. This process leads to a depression of anthropometric measurements as well as measurements of the visceral protein compartment.

Once a nutritional defect has been identified, a period of at least 2 weeks is necessary for objective response to nutritional therapy. Only when there has been some measure of response (i.e., return of cellular immunity, increase in serum albumin levels, or weight gain) can a patient be considered an appropriate candidate for surgery. When one assesses the consequences of failing to treat malnutrition in terms of hospital cost and patient morbidity, it becomes essential to recognize malnutrition early, repair the deficit, and minimize complications.

THERAPY

Various forms of nutritional therapy are available to the clinician today. The best way to decide on the most appropriate form of therapy is to have a nutritional support plan. Several points must be considered in formulating a nutritional support plan: (1) category and extent of malnutrition (nutritional assessment), (2) extent of hypermetabolism (total urinary nitrogen), (3) individual protein and calorie requirements, (4) goal of nutritional therapy, (5) presence of functioning gastrointestinal (GI) tract, (6) appetite, (7) route of delivery of nutrients (central vein versus peripheral vein versus GI tract), and (8) presence of specific organ dysfunction.

Using this type of nutritional support plan, there are three forms of nutritional support available for consideration: enteral alimentation, hypertonic intravenous therapy, and isotonic intravenous therapy (protein sparing).

Enteral Alimentation

The enteral route remains the preferred method for nutritional support for patients who have a functioning GI tract. Enteral alimentation, if possible, appears to offer better gut preservation and immune stimulation than parenteral feeding. Glutamine is an amino acid nutrient that offers gut mucosal preservation during stress and sepsis. Enteral absorption of glutamine improves immune function by decreasing the incidence of bacterial translocation and preventing the decrease in secretory immunoglobulin A commonly seen with parenteral nutrition.

Many commercially prepared liquid diets and formulas for pediatric and adult use are available; these can provide 35 to 45 kcal/kg per day with a calorie-nitrogen ratio of about 300:1. High-nitrogen formulas have a calorie-nitrogen ratio of 150:1. The particular carbohydrate, fat, and protein content of these commercially prepared diets varies widely, and often it is necessary to have a number of preparations available to meet the particular pa-

TABLE 1. Enteral Nutrition Formulas

PRODUCT	CALORIE/ML	PROTEIN (AM/LITERS)	FAT (AM/LITERS)	CARBOHYDRATE (AM/LITER)	KCAL/N RATIO
Osmolite HN	1.06	44	37	141	150:1
Osmolite	1.06	37	39	145	178:1
Ensure	1.06	37	37	145	178:1
Vitaneed	1.0	40	40	128	156:1
Nutren Fiber	1.0	40	38	127	156:1
Peptamen	1.0	40	39	127	156:1
Vivonex TEN	1.0	38	3	206	175:1
Ensure Plus	1.5	55	53	200	170:1
Traumacal	1.5	83	68	142	116:1
Pulmocare	1.5	63	92	106	150:1
Isocal HCN	2.0	75	102	200	170:1
Suplena	2.0	30	96	255	427:1
Amin-aid	2.0	19.4	46	366	830:1
Pediasure	1.0	30	50	110	209:1

tient's needs (Table 1). Recent advances in the use of feeding modules, such as carbohydrate, fat, and protein, may allow more flexibility in the future to mix and match components without acquiring a large backlog of commercially prepared formulas.

The problems of nausea, vomiting, and diarrhea that have limited the use and acceptance of enteral preparations in the past now may be largely obviated by newer and more sophisticated methods of enteral feeding. Small Silastic feeding tubes have gained a high degree of patient acceptance as opposed to the usual plastic or rubber feeding tubes. These tubes, in conjunction with a careful stepwise increase in the infusion rate of the formula, have made the continuous administration of enteral preparations reasonable for most patients. Infusion rates begin at 10 ml/hr and may be increased to a maximum of 60 ml/hr. A minimum infusion rate of 20 ml/hr is needed for gut preservation and immune stimulation.

Great success has been achieved with enteral alimentation in support of the nondepleted, noncachetic patient. Unfortunately, delivery of adequate nutrition via the enteral route does not always prove to be rapid and efficient enough in the severely malnourished patient. Furthermore, malnutrition itself can cause anatomic changes in the GI tract that may lead to malabsorption. These changes are reversible with improvement in nutrition; however, this is a slow process. A more aggressive approach to nutritional restoration in the depleted patient often is warranted, because of either the time constraints or the degree of nutritional depletion.

Hypertonic Intravenous Nutrition

Once the patient has reached a state of nutritional depletion (Table 2), the only way to rebuild body cell mass and achieve anabolism rapidly is with total parenteral nutrition (TPN). The development of intravenous hyperalimentation by Dudrick et al. in 1968 was a significant advance in the care of critically ill and malnourished patients. At present, the delivery of hypertonic solutions of 25% dextrose and 4.25% amino acids with adequate amounts of vitamins, micronutrients, and cofactors has become a widely accepted form of therapy. Standard TPN solutions contain approximately 1000 calories/liter and 6 to 7 gm of nitrogen/liter, and exert 2000 mOsm of pressure at the point of delivery. A standard formulation for hyperalimentation solutions have been developed (Table 3). In addition to the listed ingredients, essential fatty acids are provided to the patient in the form of a continuous infusion of a 3% lipid (Intralipid) solution.

Because hyperalimentation solution is extremely hypertonic, it must be administered through a central venous line and its rate must be rigidly controlled. The central venous line must be placed with strict, sterile tech-

TABLE 2. Definition of Nutritional Depletion

A history of recent weight loss
A serum albumin level < 3.5 gm/100 ml
A total lymphocyte count < 1500/mm^3
Negative reactivity to a battery of recall skin test antigens

TABLE 3. Composition* of Standard Hyperalimentation Solution

Amino acids	100 g
Dextrose	200 g
Fat	100 g
Sodium	150 mEq
Potassium	82 mEq
Calcium	9 mEq
Magnesium	10 mEq
Chloride	150 mEq
Acetate	187 mEq
Zinc	3.5 mg
Copper	1.4 mg
Manganese	0.35 mg
Chromium	14 μg
Multivitamin 12	10 ml
Phosphorus	15 mM

*Composition per 2618 ml of solution.

nique in order to avoid infection. In patients with the need for a protracted course of TPN, a central venous catheter with a subcutaneous tunnel (i.e., Broviac, Groshong, or Hickman catheter) may be employed to minimize infection. The skin over the puncture site initially is defatted with ether and then cleansed with an iodine preparation. The line is placed into the superior vena cava by either the subclavian or the internal jugular route. Sterile dressings are applied, and antibiotic ointment is placed over the catheter entrance site. On alternate days, the dressing is changed, a new sterile dressing is applied, and an antibiotic ointment is reapplied to the puncture entrance in the skin. A Millipore filter is placed in the line, and the filter and IV tubing are changed every 24 hours. No medications, blood, or other fluids should be administered through the hyperalimentation line, nor should central venous pressure measurements be made utilizing the catheter through which the hyperalimentation solution is being administered.

Hyperalimentation solutions should be administered initially at low rates of infusion (50 ml/hr) until tolerance has been achieved, after which infusion may be increased gradually to the desired caloric need. Usually, between 2000 and 3000 ml of hyperalimentation solution, providing the patient with between 2000 and 3000 calories/24 hours, is the most desirable level for achieving anabolism.

Complete details regarding the insertion and care of the central venous line are easily available to the clinician from all the major manufacturers of hyperalimentation solutions. Visual aids directly related to catheter insertion also are available in the form of a movie and a slide series from other firms involved in the distribution of nutritional products.

Hypertonic Intravenous Nutrition in Acute Renal Failure

There is good evidence now available to suggest that both the clinical course and the overall outcome of the surgical patient with acute tubular necrosis can be altered nutritionally. Solutions of hypertonic glucose (70%) and essential amino acids delivered with a calorie-nitrogen ratio of 400:1 to 600:1 (versus the 150:1 ratio of the normal TPN solution) have proved effective in both the control of renal failure and the recovery of renal function in these patients.

Complications

Complications associated with TPN are not uncommon and can be divided into three groups: technical, septic, and metabolic.

Technical. Technical complications are associated mainly with placement of the central venous catheter and can include pneumothorax, hydrothorax, brachial plexus injury, arterial injury, venous thrombosis, and air embolism. The frequency of technical complications is related directly to the experience of the person inserting the catheter. Internal jugular line placement is technically less risky than the subclavian route; however, it is also less desirable in terms of patient comfort and ease of management.

Septic. Septic complications are related to either the catheter or the solution. Although septic rates of between 10 and 30 per cent have been reported in the past, most centers using hyperalimentation teams and a controlled approach to the manufacture and delivery of TPN solutions are reporting sepsis rates of between 2 and 3 per cent. Routine procedures have been established to evaluate and treat potential septic episodes in the patient on TPN.

Metabolic. There have been numerous metabolic complications associated with the use of TPN. The most common of these are related to alterations in glucose metabolism and result in degrees of either hyperglycemia or hypoglycemia, and the most dangerous of the metabolic complications is hyperosmolar, nonketotic coma. This condition results from unchecked hyperglycemia, glycosuria, and a massive osmotic diuresis. The resultant cerebral dehydration leads to coma and sometimes death. Although this problem was once prominent, it has become far less common with strict monitoring of TPN delivery and close supervision of the patient's metabolic parameters. Hyperglycemia and glycosuria alone are frequent sequelae of TPN. Control of glycosuria and hyperglycemia can be achieved easily and safely by adding small quantities of insulin (15 to 30 units) directly to the bottle of TPN solution. The use of a sliding scale and regular insulin coverage for glycosuria has little role in management of the patient on TPN.

Other metabolic complications, such as hypophosphatemia, hypercalcemia, hypocalcemia, and hypomagnesemia, tend to be simply problems in the amount of these substances delivered; these conditions are not life threatening and are easily reversible. Deficiencies in essential fatty acids and trace metals also have been associated with long-term use of intravenous hyperalimentation. Although these conditions can be worrisome and a diagnostic dilemma, they are easily remedied. In the case of essential fatty acid deficiency, the regular infusion of a commercial fat source remedies the problem in the most long-term TPN patients. Similarly, the routine daily or weekly addition of solutions containing the majority of trace metals to standard TPN preparations totally eliminates deficiencies.

Another metabolic abnormality linked to long-term administration of TPN is alteration in liver enzymes. This is based largely on the delivery of calories in excess of the optimal patient need. It is likely that the calories provided over and above those needed for anabolism stimulate an increased insulin response that leads to hepatic lipogenesis and hepatic enzyme derangement. Cyclic hyperalimentation has been proposed as one method of dealing with the problem of hyperalimentative liver.

Isotonic Parenteral Nutrition

Protein-sparing therapy is a form of nutrition in which isotonic amino acids are delivered via a peripheral vein in a 3% or 3.5% solution with appropriate vitamin, mineral, and electrolyte additives. The solution has an osmolarity of less than 600 mOsm and is well tolerated by peripheral veins. This form of therapy depends on the mobilization of endogenous fat stores for fuel and the provision of peripheral amino acids for obligate protein need. The ideal amount of protein needed to achieve nitrogen balance is probably between 1.5 and 2.0 gm/kg per day. Protein-sparing therapy is not a substitute for TPN. Amino acid infusions represent a satisfactory means of preserving the lean body mass of patients in the starved state and minimize catabolism as opposed to rebuilding body cell mass with TPN. In the well-nourished patient who faces a prolonged period of in-hospital starvation, amino acid infusions provide a more rational approach to the preservation of the body cell mass than do hypocaloric carbohydrate feedings (D_5W).

CONCLUSIONS

Nutritional support of the malnourished hospitalized patient must be viewed as a primary form of therapy today. Severe malnutrition is ominous for all hospitalized patients, especially those facing major surgery. If the clinician ignores the starving patient's nutritional needs, he or she cannot hope to have great success with other therapeutic modalities.

Suggested Readings

Buzby GP, et al: Perioperative total parenteral nutrition in surgical patients. N Engl J Med 325:525, 1991

Dudrick SJ, Latifi R: Total parenteral nutrition in surgery—current status. Contemp Surg 41:41, 1992

Hensle TW, Askanazi J: Nutritional support of the urological patient. *In* deVere White RW, Palmer JM (eds): New Techniques in Urology. Mount Kisco, NY, Futura Publishing Company, 1987

Kudsk KA, Zaloga GP (eds): Enteral Nutrition Support for the 1990s: Innovations in Nutrition, Technology, and Techniques. Report of the Twelfth Ross Roundtable on Medical Issues. Columbus, OH, Ross Laboratories, 1992

Nirgiotis JG, Andrassy RJ: Preserving the gut and enhancing the immune response: The role of enteral nutrition in decreasing sepsis. Contemp Surg 41:17, 1992

THE ACQUIRED IMMUNODEFICIENCY SYNDROME

ROBERT M. SWENSON, M.D.

Philadelphia, Pennsylvania

HUMAN IMMUNODEFICIENCY VIRUS EPIDEMIOLOGY OF INFECTION

The origins of the acquired immunodeficiency syndrome (AIDS) epidemic are unknown. However, it now seems clear that the oldest part of the epidemic is in central Africa, where human immunodeficiency virus (HIV) infection can be traced as far back as 1959. There, the predominant mode of transmission is as a heterosexually transmitted sexually transmitted disease (STD). Transmission of HIV clearly is facilitated by the presence of other STDs, particularly genital ulcer disease, in either or both partners. It is estimated that as many as 20 million Africans already may be infected.

With increasing worldwide travel, HIV infection, like other STDs, was spread widely throughout the world. In the United States, HIV infection was first introduced into the gay population in the late 1960s. Because the average time from initial infection to the development of AIDS is 10 years, the first AIDS cases in the United States began appearing in the late 1970s among homosexual men.

Unlike other highly communicable diseases (and like other STDs), the AIDS epidemic unfolded slowly and has had several distinct "epidemic curves." The second wave of the epidemic, beginning in approximately 1984, was among intravenous drug users. The third wave, beginning in approximately 1988, has been among sexual contacts of the first two groups infected. This is presently the fastest growing segment of the epidemic. The final wave of the epidemic will occur as AIDS cases begin appearing widely throughout the entire population.

An appropriate model for the AIDS epidemic is hepatitis B. Hepatitis B virus (HBV) is transmitted in similar ways and the hepatitis B epidemic is years ahead of the HIV epidemic. Screening of voluntary blood donors reveals that the endemic level of HBV infection throughout the United States ranges between 3 and 5 per cent. Eventually HIV infection also will become widely spread, at some lower level, throughout the United States. Estimates of what this level will be range from 0.2 to 0.5 per cent of the population.

WHO SHOULD BE TESTED FOR HIV INFECTION?

STDs such as HIV infection are distributed heterogeneously throughout populations. This makes it necessary to use "epidemiological clues" to identify those more likely to be infected. In the case of HIV infection these now include: (1) men who have sex with other men; (2) parenteral drug users; and (3) those who have sex with anyone who indulges in these activities. HIV infection is increasingly occurring along with other STDs. Thus, anyone who has a recently acquired STD or whose partner has an STD also should be tested. Because HIV infection is now widely spread throughout the heterosexual population, it now seems reasonable to test heterosexuals (as well as homosexual men) with more than one sexual partner. HIV testing also is indicated for any person exhibiting unusual manifestations or presentation of any infectious disease.

PATHOPHYSIOLOGY OF HIV INFECTION

HIV infects CD4 (helper/inducer) lymphocytes. These cells orchestrate the entirety of cellular immunity and have significant effects on the regulation of the humoral immune response. Over time, HIV infection slowly destroys CD4 cells, producing an increasingly severe cellular immune deficiency. As the immune deficiency increases, other infections occur more commonly and their clinical manifestations persist longer and eventually become less and less typical. As the CD4 count falls below 200/mm^3, opportunistic infections and malignancies occur. The latest Centers for Disease Control definition of AIDS now includes anyone with a CD4 count of less than 200/mm^3. The average time from initial infection with HIV to the development of AIDS is approximately 10 years.

THERAPY OF HIV INFECTION

Zidovudine (AZT, Retrovir) is effective in slowing the progression of HIV infection. The indication of zidovudine therapy is a CD4 cell count of less than 500/mm^3 even if the person is totally asymptomatic. The usual dose is 500 mg/day given every 4 hours while awake. Some recommend tid dosing (i.e., 200 mg tid) to improve compliance. Patients who begin AZT therapy should return for a follow-up evaluation with a complete blood count in 2 weeks, then monthly for 3 months and then every 3 months. Common side effects early in treatment include nausea, headache, insomnia, myalgias, flu-like symptoms, and fatigue. These usually resolve in 4 to 8 weeks if the drug is continued. The major side effect is bone marrow suppression, which occurs with a frequency that depends on the dose and duration of zidovudine therapy and the stage of HIV infection. The rate of dose-limiting marrow suppression increases from 3 per cent per year in asymptomatic patients to 40 per cent per year in patients with AIDS.

DDI (dideoxyinosine, Videx) has established merit in patients with advanced HIV infection (defined as a CD4 count of <200/mm^3 or symptomatic HIV infection with a CD4 count of <300/mm^3), those patients on prior treatment with zidovudine complicated by dose-limiting toxicity, or those who have developed clinical or immunologic deterioration despite appropriate zidovudine therapy. DDC (dideoxycytidine, Hivid) is of limited value for patients in advanced stages of HIV infection and should be used only in combination with zidovudine.

IMPACT OF HIV INFECTION ON THE DIAGNOSIS AND TREATMENT OF OTHER INFECTIONS

Early in HIV infection, before significant immune deficiency develops, the manifestations of other infections are unchanged and the treatment for most also is unchanged. As the immune deficiency progresses, complicating infections become increasingly difficult to treat. With profound immune deficiency, infections are more likely to become widely disseminated and are characterized by less and less of an inflammatory response. As a result, opportunistic infections increasingly may involve any part of the body, including the genitourinary tract. In addition, their clinical manifestations become increasingly different from the same infection in the normal host, and most become essentially impossible to eradicate. Because the treatment of active infections in a person with HIV infection and significant immune deficiency is extremely difficult, every effort should be made to prevent these complicating infections from developing.

PROPHYLAXIS FOR COMPLICATING INFECTIONS

Tuberculosis

After a continued decrease in tuberculosis in the United States every year since the turn of the century, there was a reversal of this trend in 1985 that is directly ascribed to the epidemic of HIV infection. Studies in New York City indicate that up to 40 per cent of patients with active tuberculosis have HIV infection. Observations regarding tuberculosis in patients with HIV infection indicate that this occurs relatively early in the sequential decline in immune competence, when the CD4 count averages approximately 200/mm^3, presumably reflecting the fact that this is a relatively virulent microbe compared to other opportunistic pathogens seen in this disease.

All patients with HIV infection should be screened by the Mantoux method (intradermal injection of five tuberculin units.) All patients also should be tested for cutaneous anergy with two of the three following antigens: *Candida albicans*, tetanus toxoid, and/or mumps. Induration of 5 mm or greater for the purified protein derivative (PPD) test is considered positive. Any induration is considered positive for the other antigens. Persons who should receive prophylaxis are: (1) those with HIV infection and a positive PPD or history of having a positive PPD; (2) those with HIV infection, anergy, and at high risk for tuberculosis (intravenous drug users, homeless persons, persons from areas with high rates of tuberculosis); and (3) any person with HIV infection and close personal contact with someone with tuberculosis. All candidates for prophylaxis should have a chest radiograph and an evaluation for extrapulmonary tuberculosis. Those with no evidence of active disease who fit the above criteria should receive isoniazid, 300 mg/day for 12 months.

Herpes Simplex Infections

Persons with HIV infection have a high prevalence of latent herpes simplex virus (HSV) infections. As their immune deficiency progresses, these latent infections may reactivate and result in progressive, locally invasive herpetic lesions (usually in the perianal region), which may be exceedingly difficult to control. For this reason, many advocate acyclovir prophylaxis to prevent the development of these lesions. Suggested doses are 400 mg PO bid or 200 mg PO three to five times/day.

TREATMENT OF GENITOURINARY TRACT INFECTIONS IN PERSONS WITH HIV INFECTION

Lower Urinary Tract Infection

Lower urinary tract infection results from infection of the bladder or urethra with *Escherichia coli*, other *Enterobacteriaceae, Staphylococcus saprophyticus*, or *Enterococcus* species. Because such infections occur most commonly in sexually active young women, they now are being seen with increasing frequency in women with concomitant HIV infection. At present, there is nothing to suggest that such patients require antimicrobial therapy different from someone without HIV infection. The results of a 3-day course of amoxicillin, trimethoprim, or doxycycline appear comparable to those achieved with longer courses of therapy. Sulfonamide-containing antimicrobials should be avoided in patients with HIV infection because such patients are far more likely to develop reactions to them.

Upper Urinary Tract Infections

Patients with acute pyelonephritis (APN) who do not have HIV infection can be divided into three groups: (1) those with complicated infection occurring in the setting of prior catheterization, hospitalization, urologic surgery, or known urologic abnormalities; (2) those with uncomplicated APN who are sufficiently ill to require hospitalization; and (3) those with mild APN that can be managed in the outpatient setting. Because bacterial infections tend to be more severe in persons with HIV infection, all those with APN should be hospitalized and treated with parenteral antibiotics unless they have very early immune deficiency and only the mildest disease. The bacteriology of APN does not seem to be different in those with HIV infection, so APN acquired outside the hospital may be treated with a variety of broad-spectrum antibiotics. The antibiotic chosen should be effective against potential infecting pathogens within the renal tissue as well as at sites beyond the urinary tract. In most instances, a third-generation cephalosporin, ampicillin-sulbactam, or ticarcillin–clavulinic acid is appropriate pending the results of cultures. The selection of which drug to use may depend on local sensitivity testing data. After 24 to 48 hours, therapy can be modified when susceptibility testing results are available. For patients with hospital-acquired or catheter-associated infections, it is advisable to broaden initial antibiotic coverage to include an antibiotic effective against *Pseudomonas aeruginosa*.

All patients with HIV infection and APN should be followed closely and managed aggressively. Follow-up urine cultures should be obtained after 72 or 96 hours to evaluate therapy because patients with HIV infection may remain febrile despite appropriate and ultimately effective antibiotic therapy. Therapy must be continued for a minimum of 14 days. Those with severe infection or a slow response to therapy should be treated longer, although there are few data to indicate a more precise duration of therapy.

Renal and Perirenal Abscess

Although persons with HIV infection have profound cellular immune deficiency, they also have some impairment of humoral antibody and phagocytic cell response. Thus, they have more difficulty controlling common bacterial infections. As a result, renal and perirenal abscess are probably more common in those with HIV infection. It is for this reason that all patients with apparent upper urinary tract infection who require hospitalization should be evaluated with ultrasonography and, if indicated, computerized tomography or an excretory urogram.

Most cases of renal cortical abscess (renal carbuncle) are due to *Staphylococcus aureus*. If this diagnosis is suspected from the history, physical examination, and ultrasonography and the microscopic urinalysis shows gram-positive cocci, antistaphylococcal therapy should be begun. A penicillinase-resistant penicillin (nafcillin) or first-generation cephalosporin (cefazolin) is appropriate. Drug users frequently are infected with methicillin-resistant *S. aureus* and should be begun on vancomycin. Third-generation cephalosporins should be avoided because of their lesser antistaphylococcal activity.

Renal corticomedullary abscess and perinephric abscess arise in the setting of underlying renal infection and are caused by a variety of gram-negative bacilli. When these are suspected, empirical antibiotic therapy should be directed against a broad range of urinary pathogens, including *P. aeruginosa*. Appropriate antimicrobial choices would include ceftazidime, ticarcillin–clavulinic acid, or an antipseudomonal penicillin (pipericillin) plus gentamicin or tobramycin. The indications for surgical drainage are similar to those in patients without HIV infection.

In patients with severe immune deficiency, a wide variety of other organisms such as mycobacteria or fungi may involve the kidney. This makes a presumptive microbiologic diagnosis (in the absence of positive blood cultures) very difficult. Every effort should be made to obtain material directly from the abscess by either percutaneous or open drainage. Any material obtained should be routinely examined and cultured for bacteria, mycobacteria, and fungi. Appropriate antimicrobial therapy would then be dictated by what micro-organism was identified.

TREATMENT OF STDs IN PERSONS WITH HIV INFECTION

Syphilis

Syphilis frequently occurs in persons with HIV infection. Early in HIV infection, the genital lesions, skin rash, and other clinical manifestations of syphilis are usually similar to those in persons without immune deficiency. As the CD4 count falls, the clinical and laboratory manifestations become increasingly variable from those in the normal host. For these reasons, all persons with HIV infection should be tested routinely for syphilis and those who are positive should be treated vigorously as soon as possible. At the present time, there is no clear consensus as to what is appropriate therapy. However, the following conclusions seem warranted:

1. Penicillin is the only effective therapy. Alternative regimens are completely unproven (tetracycline, erythromycin) or already have been shown to be ineffective (ceftriaxone).
2. All persons with HIV infection and a positive serologic test for syphilis should be evaluated further with cerebrospinal fluid examination.
3. All patients with later or neurologic syphilis of any stage should be treated with a regimen of high-dose daily penicillin. Thus, patients with primary, secondary, or latent syphilis of less than 1 year should be treated with the standard regimen of 2.4 million units IM of benzathine penicillin. All others should be treated with penicillin G, 12 to 24 million units IV/day in divided doses for 10 to 14 days. Patients allergic to penicillin should be desensitized and treated with penicillin rather than an alternative agent.

Herpes Simplex Infections

The initial treatment of mild mucocutaneous infections is acyclovir 200 mg PO five times per day for 10 days or until the lesions are crusted. More severe episodes may require intravenous acyclovir 15 mg/kg for at least 7 days. In each case, this should be followed by suppressive therapy as noted above.

Other STDs

Gonococcal infection occurs commonly in persons with HIV infection. Available evidence suggests that the clinical manifestations, laboratory diagnosis, and treatment are little different from those in the normal host. The standard treatment regimens (which also include treatment for chlamydial infection) are appropriate for persons with HIV infection.

Chancroid is a common disease in many developing countries. Since 1984, it has been occurring with increasing frequency in the United States and is now a common cause of genital ulcer disease. The diagnosis and treatment of chancroid is the same in those with and without HIV infection. Presently, erythromycin and ceftriaxone appear to offer effective therapy for most cases, although a few erythromycin-resistant strains now have appeared.

Suggested Readings

Barnes PF, et al: Tuberculosis in patients with human immunodeficiency virus infection. N Engl J Med 324:1644, 1991

Bartlett JG: Recommendations for the Medical Care of Persons with HIV infection, 2nd ed. Baltimore, Critical Care America, 1992

Hook EW III, Marra CM: Acquired syphilis in adults. N Engl J Med 326:1060, 1992

National Institute of Allergy and Infectious Diseases: State of the art conference on azidothymidine therapy for early HIV infection. Am J Med 89:335, 1990

Sande MA, Volberding PA (eds): Medical management of AIDS. Infect Dis Clin North Am 2:285–550, 1988

INDEX

Note: Page numbers in *italics* refer to illustrations; page numbers followed by t refer to tables.

ISBN 0-7216-5033-3